D1162782

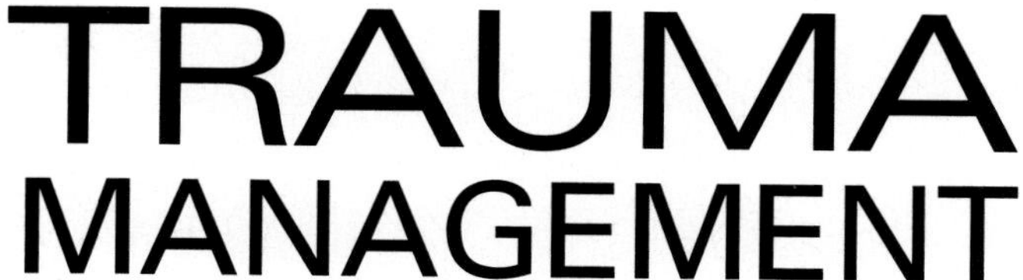
TRAUMA
MANAGEMENT
AN EMERGENCY MEDICINE APPROACH

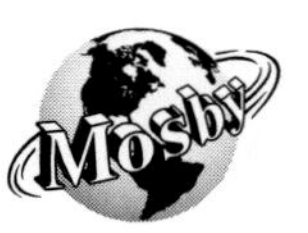

Visit our website at **www.mosby.com**

TRAUMA MANAGEMENT

AN EMERGENCY MEDICINE APPROACH

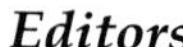

Editors

PETER C. FERRERA, M.D.
Staff Physician, Glens Falls Hospital, Glens Falls, New York
and Saratoga Hospital, Saratoga Springs, New York
Clinical Assistant Professor, Department of Emergency Medicine
Albany Medical Center, Albany, New York

STEPHEN A. COLUCCIELLO, M.D.
Assistant Chair and Director of Clinical Services and Trauma Coordinator
Department of Emergency Medicine, Carolinas Medical Center, Charlotte, North Carolina
Clinical Associate Professor of Emergency Medicine
University of North Carolina School of Medicine, Chapel Hill, North Carolina

JOHN A. MARX, M.D.
Chair, Department of Emergency Medicine, Carolinas Medical Center, Charlotte, North Carolina
Clinical Professor of Emergency Medicine, University of North Carolina School of Medicine
Chapel Hill, North Carolina

VINCENT P. VERDILE, M.D.
Associate Professor and Chair, Department of Emergency Medicine
Albany Medical College, Albany, New York

MICHAEL A. GIBBS, M.D.
Residency Program Director, Medical Director, MedCenter Air
Department of Emergency Medicine, Carolinas Medical Center, Charlotte, North Carolina
Associate Professor of Emergency Medicine, University of North Carolina at Chapel Hill
Chapel Hill, North Carolina

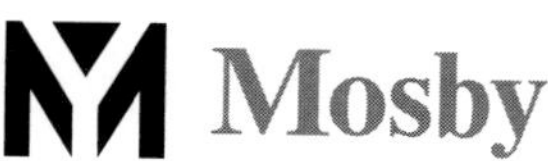

An Affiliate of Elsevier Science

St. Louis London Philadelphia Sydney Toronto

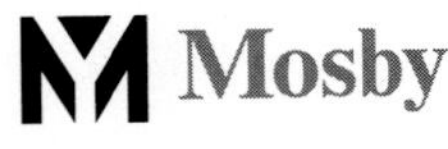

An Affiliate of Elsevier Science

Editor: Judith Fletcher
Senior Managing Editor: Kathy Falk
Project Manager: Patricia Tannian
Project Specialist: Melissa Lastarria
Book Design Manager: Gail Morey Hudson
Cover Design: Teresa Breckwoldt
Cover Art: Photographs by Eugene Richards, Inc., Brooklyn, New York

Mosby, Inc.
An Affiliate of Elsevier Science
11830 Westline Industrial Drive
St. Louis, Missouri 63146

Printed in the United States of America

International Standard Book Number 0-323-00210-2

02 03 04 GW/MVY 9 8 7 6 5 4 3 2

Contributors

Jean T. Abbott, M.D.
Attending Physician, Emergency Medicine
Associate Professor
University of Colorado School of Medicine
Denver, Colorado

James G. Adams, M.D.
Chief, Division of Emergency Medicine
Northwestern Memorial Hospital
Professor of Medicine
Division of Emergency Medicine
Northwestern University Medical School
Chicago, Illinois

Patric N. Anderson, M.D.
Attending Physician
Emergency Medicine Services Group, P.A.
Sparks Regional Medical Center
Fort Smith, Arkansas

Jon Apfelbaum, M.D.
McLeod Regional Medical Center
Florence, South Carolina

Andrew W. Asimos, M.D.
Director of Resource Utilization
Department of Emergency Medicine
Carolinas Medical Center
Charlotte, North Carolina
Clinical Assistant Professor of Emergency Medicine
University of North Carolina School of Medicine
Chapel Hill, North Carolina

Joel M. Bartfield, M.D.
Associate Professor and Residency Director
Department of Emergency Medicine
Albany Medical Center
Albany, New York

Jayne J. Batts, M.D.
Director, Clinical Forensic Medicine Program
Department of Emergency Medicine
Carolinas Medical Center
Charlotte, North Carolina

Robert Belfer, M.D.
Assistant Professor of Clinical Emergency Medicine and Pediatrics
Division of Pediatric Emergency Medicine
Robert Wood Johnson Medical School
University of Medicine and Dentistry New Jersey
Camden, New Jersey

Robert A. Bitterman, M.D., J.D.
Director of Risk Management and Managed Care
Department of Emergency Medicine
Carolinas Medical Center
Charlotte, North Carolina
Clinical Assistant Professor of Emergency Medicine
University of North Carolina School of Medicine
Chapel Hill, North Carolina

Eileen M.K. Bobek, M.D.
Clinical Instructor
Department of Emergency Medicine
University of Michigan Medical Center
Ann Arbor, Michigan

Michael J. Bosse, M.D.
Orthopaedic Trauma Surgeon
Department of Orthopaedic Surgery
Carolinas Medical Center
Charlotte, North Carolina

John D. Broderick, M.D.
Assistant Professor
Department of Emergency Medicine
Albany Medical Center
Albany, New York

Stephen A. Colucciello, M.D.
Assistant Chair and Director of Clinical Services and Trauma Coordinator
Department of Emergency Medicine
Carolinas Medical Center
Charlotte, North Carolina
Clinical Associate Professor of Emergency Medicine
University of North Carolina School of Medicine
Chapel Hill, North Carolina

William H. Cordell, M.D.
Clinical Professor of Emergency Medicine
Director, Section of Emergency Medicine Research
Department of Emergency Medicine
Indiana University School of Medicine
Indianapolis, Indiana

Carl C. D'Andrea, M.D.
Department of Emergency Medicine
New Milford Hospital
New Milford, Connecticut

Mohamud R. Daya, M.D.
Associate Professor
Department of Emergency Medicine
Orgeon Health Sciences University
Portland, Oregon

Theodore R. Delbridge, M.D., M.P.H.
Assistant Professor of Emergency Medicine
University of Pittsburgh
Medical Director, STAT MedEvac
Assistant Medical Director, Pittsburgh EMS
Pittsburgh, Pennsylvania

Edward Doolin, M.D.
Professor of Surgery and Pediatrics
Robert Wood Johnson School of Medicine
University of Medicine and Dentistry New Jersey
Camden, New Jersey

Robert M. Duchynski, M.D.
Kaiser Permanente Hospital Santa Rosa
Santa Rosa, California

Susan M. Dunmire, M.D.
Assistant Professor of Emergency Medicine
Department of Emergency Medicine
University of Pittsburgh School of Medicine
Pittsburgh, Pennsylvania

Jay L. Falk, M.D.
Director of Medical Education
Academic Chairman
Department of Emergency Medicine
Orlando Regional Healthcare
Clinical Professor of Medicine and Emergency Medicine
University of Florida College of Medicine
Orlando, Florida

Peter C. Ferrera, M.D.
Staff Physician, Glens Falls Hospital
Glens Falls, New York,
and Saratoga Hospital
Saratoga Springs, New York
Clinical Assistant Professor
Department of Emergency Medicine
Albany Medical Center
Albany, New York

Michael A. Gibbs, M.D.
Residency Program Director
Medical Director, MedCenter Air
Department of Emergency Medicine
Carolinas Medical Center
Charlotte, North Carolina
Associate Professor of Emergency Medicine
University of North Carolina at Chapel Hill
Chapel Hill, North Carolina

James E. Gruber, M.D.
Attending Staff Physician
Department of Emergency Medicine
Portercare Hospital
Denver, Colorado

E. Parker Hays, Jr., M.D.
Associate Residency Director
Department of Emergency Medicine
Carolinas Medical Center
Charlotte, North Carolina
Associate Professor of Emergency Medicine
University of North Carolina School of Medicine
Chapel Hill, North Carolina

Jennifer L. Isenhour, M.D.
Assistant Professor
Department of Emergency Medicine
Vanderbilt University Medical Center
Nashville, Tennessee

Stacy Weeks Jandreau, M.D.
Director
Department of Emergency Medicine
Aroostook Medical Center
Presque Isle, Maine

B. Tilman Jolly, M.D.
Associate Professor of Emergency Medicine
School of Medicine and Health Sciences
Associate Professor of Environmental and Occupational Health
School of Public Health and Health Services
The George Washington University Medical Center
Washington, DC

James B. Jones, M.D., PharmD
Associate Director
Emergency Medicine Research Program
Clinical Assistant Professor of Emergency Medicine
Department of Emergency Medicine
Indiana University School of Medicine
Indianapolis, Indiana

Lawrence E. Kass, M.D.
Associate Residency Director
Department of Emergency Medicine
State University of New York at Stony Brook
Stony Brook, New York

Jon R. Krohmer, M.D.
Medical Director
Kent County EMS
Associate Professor
Section of Emergency Medicine
College of Human Medicine
Michigan State University
Grand Rapids, Michigan

Patricia L. Lanter, M.D.
Clinical Assistant Professor
Department of Emergency Mediicne
Brown University
Providence, Rhode Island

Brian J. Levine, M.D.
Clinical Instructor in Emergency Medicine
Jefferson Medical College
Department of Surgery
Philadelphia, Pennsylvania
Attending Physician
Department of Emergency Medicine
Christiana Care Health System
Newark, Delaware

David B. Markowitz, M.D.
Clinical Instructor of Emergency Medicine
Albany Medical College
Albany, New York
Department of Emergency Medicine
A.O. Fox Hospital
Oneonta, New York

John A. Marx, M.D.
Chair
Department of Emergency Medicine
Carolinas Medical Center
Charlotte, North Carolina
Clinical Professor of Emergency Medicine
University of North Carolina School of Medicine
Chapel Hill, North Carolina

Thom A. Mayer, M.D.
Professor of Emergency Medicine
Georgetown University School of Medicine
George Washington University School of Medicine
Washington, DC
Chairman, Department of Emergency Medicine
Medical Director, Flight Services
Inova Fairfax Hospital
Falls Church, Virginia

Dennis P. McKenna, M.D.
Clinical Instructor
Department of Emergency Medicine
Albany Medical Center
Albany, New York

Joseph Messick, M.D. (deceased)
Department of General Surgery
Carolinas Medical Center
Charlotte, North Carolina

Kevin C. Meyer, M.D.
Department of Emergency Medicine
Orlando Regional Medical Center
Orlando, Florida

William S. Miles, M.D.
Director of Surgical Critical Care
Clinical Assistant Professor of Surgery
University of North Carolina School of Medicine
Chapel Hill, North Carolina
Clinical Instructor of Surgery, Trauma
Department of General Surgery
Carolinas Medical Center
Charlotte, North Carolina

Christine Milosis, M.D.
Department of Emergency Medicine
Medical Center of Delaware
Newark, Delaware

Vincent N. Mosesso, Jr., M.D.
Assistant Professor of Emergency Medicine
University of Pittsburgh
Medical Director, Prehospital Care
University of Pittsburgh Medical Center
Pittsburgh, Pennsylvania

Robert E. O'Connor, M.D., M.P.H.
Director of Education and Research
Emergency Medicine Residency Program Director
Department of Emergency Medicine
Christiana Care Health System
Newark, Delaware

Eric W. Ossmann, M.D.
Assistant Professor
Department of Emergency Medicine
Emory University School of Medicine;
Medical Director, Grady EMS
Atlanta, Georgia

Maria Pelucio, M.D.
Director of Medical Student Education
Department of Emergency Medicine
Carolinas Medical Center
Charlotte, North Carolina

Daniel M. Roberts, M.D.
Assistant Professor
Department of Emergency Medicine
Texas A&M University College of Medicine
EMS Medical Director
Scott and White Memorial Hospital
Temple, Texas

Carlo J. Rosen, M.D.
Program Director
Beth Israel Deaconess Medical Center
Harvard Affiliated Emergency Medicine Residency
Instructor of Medicine
Harvard Medical School
Boston, Massachusetts

Ronald N. Roth, M.D.
Associate Professor of Emergency Medicine
University of Pittsburgh School of Medicine
Pittsburgh, Pennsylvania

Thomas J. Russell, M.D.
Department of Emergency Medicine
Kaiser Permanente
Sacramento, California

Alfred D. Sacchetti, M.D.
Research Director
Department of Emergency Medicine
Our Lady of Lourdes Medical Center
Assistant Clinical Professor of Emergency Medicine
Thomas Jefferson University School of Medicine
Philadelphia, Pennsylvania

Robert Schneider, M.D.
Academic Faculty
Department of Emergency Medicine
Carolinas Medical Center
Charlotte, North Carolina

Suzanne M. Shepherd, M.D.
Associate Professor and Program Director
Department of Emergency Medicine
University of Pennsylvania Medical Center
Philadelphia, Pennsylvania

William H. Shoff, M.D., D.T.M.&H.
Assistant Professor
Director, Penn Travel Medicine
Department of Emergency Medicine
University of Pennsylvania Health System
Philadelphia, Pennsylvania

Susan A. Stern, M.D.
Assistant Professor
Department of Emergency Medicine
University of Michigan Medical Center
Ann Arbor, Michigan

Ronald L. Stram, M.D.
Assistant Professor and Associate Director
Department of Emergency Medicine
Albany Medical Center
Albany, New York

D. Matthew Sullivan, M.D.
Clinical Faculty
Department of Emergency Medicine
Carolinas Medical Center
Charlotte, North Carolina
Clinical Instructor of Emergency Medicine
University of North Carolina School of Medicine
Chapel Hill, North Carolina

Vivek Tayal, M.D.
Department of Emergency Medicine
Carolinas Medical Center
Charlotte, North Carolina

Michael H. Thomason, M.D.
Director, Trauma Service
Associate Chairman
Department of General Surgery
Carolinas Medical Center
Charlotte, North Carolina
Clinical Professor of Surgery
University of North Carolina School of Medicine
Chapel Hill, North Carolina

David P. Thomson, M.D.
Associate Professor
Department of Emergency Medicine
SUNY Upstate Medical University
Syracuse, New York

Vincent P. Verdile, M.D.
Associate Professor and Chair
Department of Emergency Medicine
Albany Medical College
Albany, New York

Richard E. Wolfe, M.D.
Assistant Professor
Harvard Medical School
Chief, Department of Emergency Medicine
Beth Israel Deaconess Medical Center
Boston, Massachusetts

Nestor R. Zenarosa, M.D.
Director of Emergency Services
Marshall Regional Medical Center
Marshall, Texas

Brian J. Zink, M.D.
Associate Professor
Department of Emergency Medicine
Assistant Dean for Medical Student Career Development
University of Michigan Medical School
Ann Arbor, Michigan

To my wife
Holly
and my daughter
Gabriella
the most meaningful parts of my life.
PCF

For my children
DJ, Nick, and **Vince**
(and of course grandbaby **Caylah**)
who taught me the important things.
And to my wife
Patti
who kept me on track, saying
"Just finish that book already!"
SAC

To the wit of my *colleagues*
the betterment of our *patients*
the spirit of my *children*
Connor and **Shelby**
and the soulful memory of my *mom*
Annie
JAM

To my wife
Lou-ann
For her constant love and support.
To all of my students and residents—
past, present, and future
And to the patients
who allow me the privilege of
caring for them.
VPV

To my wife and soul mate
Kimberly
who has been by my side at every
turn of this fascinating journey.
MAG

Preface

Over 34 million injured Americans receive care in emergency departments each year. The spectrum of the injuries encountered is enormous, ranging from benign to catastrophic. It is clear that the role of trauma management is a team effort between the emergency physicians and the various surgical subspecialty physicians. Since the emergency physician is the only member of this team who is assuredly present when the patient arrives, it is imperative that we become experts in the care of the trauma victim.

Although emergency physicians now conduct a significant portion of trauma research, most textbooks on trauma are written and edited by surgeons. This book is written by emergency physicians, for emergency physicians. We believe it will be useful in both the level I trauma center and the small community hospital. Practicing emergency physicians can refer to it for general reference and to assist in real-time decisions. Generous use of tables, graphics, and decision trees provides information at a glance.

Many chapters begin with a challenging clinical scenario and then discuss the selected topic in an evidence-based format. Each chapter answers the question, "What should the emergency physician do, and when?" Although pathophysiology and definitive operative principles are mentioned, each chapter emphasizes concerns central to emergency practice. The book highlights clinical pathways, evaluates cost-effective measures, and addresses controversies and cutting-edge technology. Tables emphasize common pitfalls and medicolegal issues.

Through the publication of this book we hope to increase the emergency physician's expertise in trauma management. We anticipate that you, our colleagues, will share the role of the traumatologist with confidence and pride.

The Editors

Contents

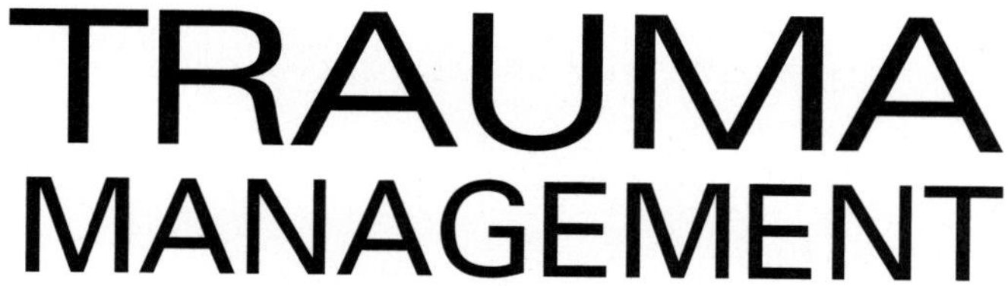

TRAUMA MANAGEMENT

AN EMERGENCY MEDICINE APPROACH

PART ONE
PREHOSPITAL CARE

Prehospital Care: Trauma Scoring Systems and Trauma Triage

1

RONALD N. ROTH

Trauma triage classifies patients based on the severity of their injuries and matches them to available resources. Several tools assist prehospital providers with these decisions, including triage algorithms, triage tags, and formal trauma triage scores. Accurate triage ensures that potentially salvageable patients with significant injuries receive the appropriate level of care.

TRAUMA TRIAGE

Military experience demonstrated that rapid triage and transport of injured soldiers to definitive care saved lives.[1] Despite these successes on the battlefield, in the mid 1960s the National Research Council noted that civilian trauma remained a neglected disease of modern society. Their publication identified the lack of suitable facilities and other problems associated with care of trauma victims.[2]

Optimal trauma care requires a systems-oriented approach that integrates field and hospital elements. A formal triage system requires two major components: trauma center designations and a means to direct victims to these centers.[3] Over the past two decades, these centers have improved survival for trauma patients.[1,4-6]

Unfortunately, there is no universally accepted mechanism for prehospital trauma triage. The ideal system would be very sensitive, identifying all patients who would benefit from treatment at a trauma center. Conversely, the ideal system would be specific enough to recognize trauma patients who can be managed at community hospitals.[7] The consequences of an inadequate system include over- and under-triage. In over-triage numerous patients with minor injuries go to a trauma center, creating the potential of overloading the system. In addition, costs for treating these less severely injured patients at a trauma center may be higher than at local facilities. Under-triage results in sending significantly injured patients to less prepared centers, which may increase morbidity and mortality.[3,7-9]

ON-SCENE TRAUMA TRIAGE OF MULTIPLE VICTIMS

The first responders often begin field triage. However, more experienced personnel should assume this responsibility on their arrival. Field triage is most efficient when victims are limited to a small geographic area. Large sites such as urban disasters and environmental emergencies (e.g., floods, earthquakes) may require multiple triage sites.

Field triage of multiple victims becomes necessary when the number of injured overwhelms the capabilities of the on-scene care providers or the resources of the closest receiving facility. At a multicasualty incident, if the number of patients and their injuries *do not* exceed the on-scene resources, all patients with life-threatening or potentially life-threatening injuries can be transported immediately. However, when the number of patients *does* exceed local resources, accurate and efficient triage defines the order of care. Potentially salvageable patients with life-threatening conditions require immediate treatment and transport, whereas more stable victims may be treated and transported later.

Although the disaster situation presents many challenges to prehospital care providers, the most difficult aspect to accept is the notion of an unsalvageable patient. In a single-victim incident, patients with a low probability of survival often receive tremendous attention. In the multicasualty incident, the philosophy of "the greatest good for the greatest number" must

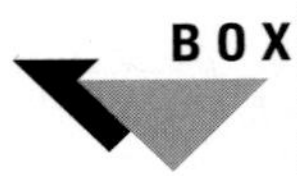

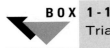

BOX 1-1
Triage Tag Categorization

RED
Most critically injured. Includes patients with major injuries to the head, thorax, and abdomen, and who require immediate surgical or specialty care.

YELLOW
Less critically injured. Includes patients who are less seriously injured who require surgical or specialty care within hours.

GREEN
Non–life or limb threatening. Such patients, the so-called *walking wounded,* do not require immediate stabilization or specialty care.

BLACK
Dead or unsalvageable. This category includes patients with nonsurvivable injuries, such as 90% burns in the elderly.

prevail. Medical resources wasted on the unsalvageable patient become unavailable to other patients who have a better chance of survival with immediate care. This notion of "allowing" a patient to die, although an anathema to many, is crucial in mass casualty triage.

Triage Tags

Triage tags are used by many prehospital systems during multicasualty events to identify the initial triage code of the patient. They are most effective in systems that use tags routinely for both large and small incidents. Triage tags work less well in systems that use them only for "the big one," since workers are unfamiliar with the tags. Problems with using triage tags include lack of familiarity by field and hospital providers, separation of the tag from the victim, contamination by blood or body fluids, and limited space for documentation and change in status.[10]

Color codes (Box 1-1) are commonly used to identify patient categorization by injury severity and need for transport.[10]

TRIAGE CRITERIA

No single triage criterion is definitive. Prehospital care providers must consider multiple factors, none of which are scientifically proven (Box 1-2). They must be familiar with anatomic and physiologic markers associated with significant trauma and understand the significance of mechanism of injury.[9,11-21]

The initial patient survey identifies most patients with immediate life-threats. Abnormal vital signs strongly suggest the need for transport to an appropriate facility. Although no formal scaling system accounts for premorbid conditions, many authorities suggest including them in triage decisions.[9]

Theoretically, analysis of injury mechanism at the scene may improve triage accuracy. The mechanism provides clues to both anatomic patterns of injury and the amount of kinetic energy transferred.[9,12] However, Henry et al[3,22] found that some mechanism criteria worsen triage specificity with little improvement in sensitivity, when used concurrently with physiologic and anatomic criteria.

The American College of Surgeons (ACS) Committee on Trauma and the American College of Emergency Physicians (ACEP) have published trauma triage guidelines to assist prehospital care providers with triage decisions.[11,12] The ACS committee acknowledges that their Triage Decision Scheme overtriages patients by approximately 30%. The ACEP guidelines include trauma triage algorithms to assist with the development of prehospital protocols, destination decisions, and trauma system design (Fig. 1-1). These algorithms emphasize the need to recognize unique requirements of an individual system and the importance of strong medical direction, continuous quality improvement, and support from all members of the trauma system.

TRAUMA SCORING

Over the past 20 years a number of groups have proposed a variety of trauma scoring techniques to determine the severity of injury both in-hospital and in the field. These scales categorize patients by severity using a variety of anatomic, physiologic, and mechanism of injury criteria.[9, 23]

Researchers often retrospectively use in-hospital scoring systems. However, many of these systems involve data points that encompass lesions found in surgery and cannot be employed in the emergency department (ED). However, some scoring systems can be used by the receiving ED to grade their trauma team response.[24-26] Over the past 25 years trauma scores using various physiologic, anatomic, and mechanistic criteria were developed to predict injury severity, need for trauma center care, and mortality.[9,27] Scoring systems tend to combine several variables, including cardiovascular system, respiratory system, central nervous system (CNS), type and location of injury, and abdominal examination.

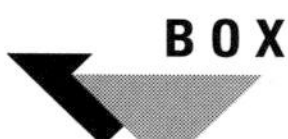

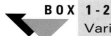

BOX 1-2
Variables Associated with a Higher Risk of Significant Injury

PATIENT ASSESSMENT
Pulse <60 or >100
Respiratory rate <10 or >29
Systolic blood pressure <90
Glasgow Coma Scale <13
Anatomic location of injuries may predict the need for emergent surgical or specialty care
- Penetration injuries to chest, abdomen, head, neck, or groin
- Flail chest
- Multiple proximal long bone fractures
- Burns with >50% body surface area; face or airway burns
- Pelvic fractures
- Paralysis
- Extremity amputation

MECHANISM OF INJURY
Ejection from automobile
Death of victim in the same passenger compartment
Extrication time >20 minutes
Fall >20 feet
Rollover accident
High-speed vehicle crash
Auto versus pedestrian >5 mph
Motorcycle crash >20 mph or separation of rider from bike

PREMORBID CONDITION
Age <5 or >55 years
Cardiac or respiratory disease
Psychosis
Diabetic taking insulin
Cirrhosis
Malignancy
Obesity
Coagulopathy

OTHER ISSUES
Potential for decline in patient condition
Availability of resources
Personnel and level of training
Equipment and supplies
Transport vehicles (ground versus air)
Turnaround time for vehicles
Local facilities and bed availability
Adult and pediatric trauma centers
- -Burn centers
- -Other specialized care centers

Presence of ongoing hazards or environmental dangers

An ideal scoring system should have predictive validity, correlate with outcome, be easily applicable in the field, and reliably applied amongst observers.[7,9,14,21,23] In practice, accurate prehospital trauma scores depend on the individual field provider's diagnostic skills. Environmental conditions, patient intoxication, and compensatory physiologic mechanisms that mask major injuries further limit these triage tools.

The Abbreviated Injury Scale (AIS) and the related Injury Severity Score (ISS) were developed as research tools to compare injuries suffered by trauma victims. Because both scoring systems require discharge data, these systems have no practical application in the ED or prehospital arena.[9]

Trauma Index

Developed in the early 1970s, the **Trauma Index (TI)** was one of the earliest scores used by prehospital providers to rate injury severity.[17] The TI was intended for prehospital use to determine the facility best suited for an individual trauma victim. The authors arbitrarily assigned numerical points to five variables: region of body injured, type of injury, cardiovascular status, CNS status, and respiratory status. In the original study they retrospectively applied the TI to inpatient trauma victims and then to patients evaluated in a single ED. Low scores correlated with minor injuries, whereas multiple-system trauma victims scored higher and suffered higher mortality.

Trauma Score/Revised Trauma Score

Two commonly used prehospital triage tools, the **Trauma Score (TS)** and the **Revised Trauma Score (RTS)** descended from the **Triage Index** proposed by Champion in 1980.[14] The Triage Index consisted of the Glasgow Coma Scale (GCS), capillary refill, and respiratory expansion. The original Triage Index was derived from data from over 1000 trauma patients. The authors identified variables with the greatest power to predict mortality, alone or in combination.[14]

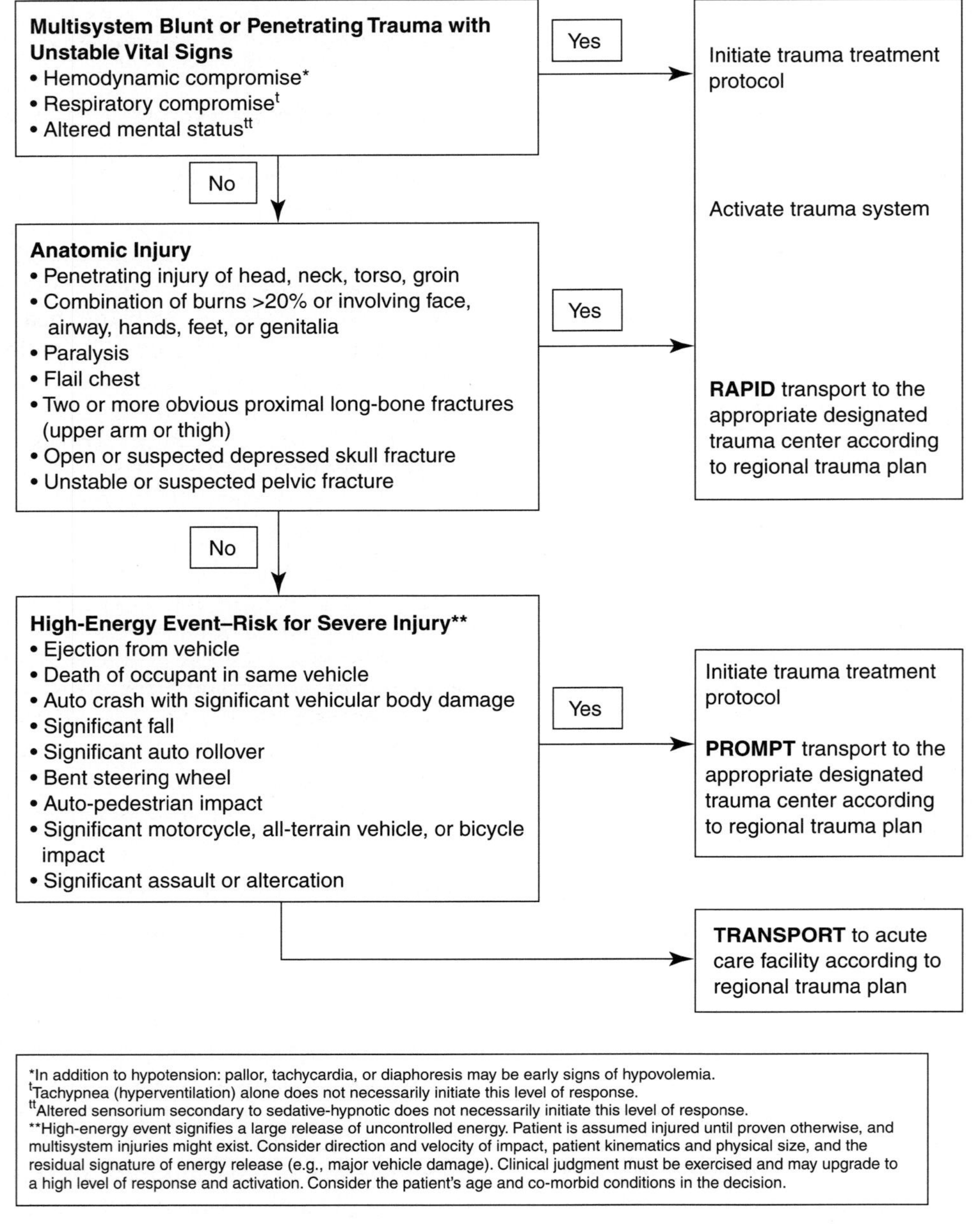

Multisystem Blunt or Penetrating Trauma with Unstable Vital Signs
• Hemodynamic compromise*
• Respiratory compromise†
• Altered mental status††
Yes
No
Initiate trauma treatment protocol
Activate trauma system
RAPID transport to the appropriate designated trauma center according to regional trauma plan
Anatomic Injury
• Penetrating injury of head, neck, torso, groin
• Combination of burns >20% or involving face, airway, hands, feet, or genitalia
• Paralysis
• Flail chest
• Two or more obvious proximal long-bone fractures (upper arm or thigh)
• Open or suspected depressed skull fracture
• Unstable or suspected pelvic fracture
Yes
No
High-Energy Event–Risk for Severe Injury**
• Ejection from vehicle
• Death of occupant in same vehicle
• Auto crash with significant vehicular body damage
• Significant fall
• Significant auto rollover
• Bent steering wheel
• Auto-pedestrian impact
• Significant motorcycle, all-terrain vehicle, or bicycle impact
• Significant assault or altercation
Yes
Initiate trauma treatment protocol
PROMPT transport to the appropriate designated trauma center according to regional trauma plan
TRANSPORT to acute care facility according to regional trauma plan
*In addition to hypotension: pallor, tachycardia, or diaphoresis may be early signs of hypovolemia.
†Tachypnea (hyperventilation) alone does not necessarily initiate this level of response.
††Altered sensorium secondary to sedative-hypnotic does not necessarily initiate this level of response.
**High-energy event signifies a large release of uncontrolled energy. Patient is assumed injured until proven otherwise, and multisystem injuries might exist. Consider direction and velocity of impact, patient kinematics and physical size, and the residual signature of energy release (e.g., major vehicle damage). Clinical judgment must be exercised and may upgrade to a high level of response and activation. Consider the patient's age and co-morbid conditions in the decision.

Fig. 1-1 Prehospital-model triage algorithm. (From ACEP: *Ann Emerg Med* 22:1088, 1993.)

The TS was developed in 1981 to increase the validity of the TI.[13] The TS evaluated respiratory rate, respiratory expansion, systolic blood pressure, capillary refill, and GCS.[15] Numbers were assigned to each parameter, with high numbers representing normal function. Total scores ranged from 1 to 16, and the authors suggested level I trauma care for trauma scores of 14 or less. When calculated from data recorded by paramedics and compared with the ISS, the TS showed a false-positive rate of 9.5% and a false-negative rate of 5.8%. Penetrating wounds were correctly classified in 73.2% of cases.[15] When data collected by field providers were compared with data collected by a nurse observer there was agreement in over 90% of assessments. Unfortunately, the field providers did not calculate the scores and during part of the study the nurse observer reminded personnel to gather missed variables.[28]

Concerns for the ability to assess capillary refill and respiratory effort along with the underestimation of the head injury severity lead to the revision of the score in 1989. The RTS consists of GCS, respiratory rate, and systolic blood pressure.[18] This score remains in common use today.

CRAMS

In 1982 Gormican[19] introduced a 10-point scale that measured five parameters: circulation, respiratory, abdomen, motor, and speech (**CRAMS**). These parameters were designed to simplify field trauma triage scoring. Each parameter was scored as normal (2), mildly abnormal (1), or severely abnormal (0). In an initial study of 500 trauma patients, the CRAMS score, as calculated by a mobile intensive care nurse or base station physician, correctly triaged 11 of 12 patients as major trauma victims (CRAMS ≤8).[19] Minor trauma victims were correctly categorized in nearly 90% of cases. Major trauma was defined as death in the ED or patients requiring immediate surgery, general surgery, or neurosurgery.

In a study performed in Salt Lake City, Kilberg et al[6] used field calculated CRAMS scores to direct patients with scores of <7 to a level I trauma center. They reported a significantly higher survival for severely injured patients (CRAMS <4) taken to a level I trauma center.

When applying the TS and the CRAMS scale via computer to over 5000 trauma patients, Ornato et al[29] found that both scales identified all major trauma patients who were dead on arrival or died in the ED. The TS was more sensitive to major trauma than CRAMS. Both systems failed to predict patients who were transferred directly from the ED to the operating suite.

Prehospital Index

The **Prehospital Index (PI)** is a scoring system developed through analysis of 313 trauma cases.[20] Systolic blood pressure, pulse, respiratory status, and level of consciousness were prehospital variables that correlated with the need for emergent surgery or mortality. Each variable received a score of 0 to 5, with normal variables scored 0. Scores range from 0 to 20, with patients scoring at least 4 having a higher incidence of surgery and mortality. In a validation study,[30] the PI incorporated a fifth variable of penetrating torso trauma, worth 4 points if present. In this prospective study of over 3000 patients, those with a PI of <4 had only a 0.6% incidence of surgery and no deaths. In the group of patients with scores >3, 47.3% required emergency surgery and 23% died. The authors recommend transport of patients with a PI above 3 to the highest level trauma center available.[30] In a retrospective Canadian study, a PI of >3 was very sensitive in identifying mortality (98%), but less sensitive in predicting patients who required surgery within 24 hours (59%).[31]

Trauma Triage Rule

The **Trauma Triage Rule (TTR)**, proposed by Baxt et al,[21] was derived retrospectively from a cohort of 1004 adult trauma patients. The TTR defined a major trauma victim with the following variables: systolic blood pressure <85 mmHg, a GCS motor score of <5, or penetrating injuries of the trunk, head, or neck. The authors noted a sensitivity of 92% (patients who died or required a surgical procedure) and a specificity of 92% when applied to the 1004 patient cohort.

The TTR is simple to apply and does not require mathematical calculations. The prehospital care provider need only consider three variables (two in blunt trauma), and blood pressure and GCS are routinely measured by most systems. The authors recommend that patients identified by the TTR as major trauma victims be taken to higher level trauma centers.[21]

Emerman et al[7] retrospectively compared the TTR, the RTS, the PI, and the CRAMS scale. They found that all four scales identified adult trauma patients who died or required emergent operation with sensitivities of at least 85%. The specificity of the TTR (90%) exceeded that of the CRAMS scale (83%).

Paramedic Judgment

The literature is generally positive regarding the ability of prehospital providers to predict serious injury and need for a trauma center. Ornato et al[29] described paramedic judgment to be almost as good (more than 90% sensitive and specific) as CRAMS and the TS. Fries et al[23] found that field provider judgment, without the use of formal trauma scoring techniques, was more sensitive but less specific than the TTR in identifying life-threatening injuries. Emerman et al[8] showed provider judgment to be as accurate as the RTS, the PI, and the CRAMS scale. A different study showed that a paramedic's perception of injury severity enhanced trauma triage.[32]

Despite these testimonials to paramedic judgment, conflicting data exist. One study suggests that paramedic judgment alone was insensitive in identifying major trauma.[33] Patients who were also incorrectly categorized by the formal triage instruments tended to be hemodynamically stable.

CONCLUSIONS

In general, prehospital trauma triage scoring systems accurately identify trauma victims who will die en route or in the ED. However, because most of these patients have profoundly abnormal vital signs, they do not present triage dilemmas. Scoring systems may identify only a subset of patients who will benefit from trauma center care. However, systems based solely on physiologic criteria tend to miss hemodynamically stable victims with major injuries.

Unfortunately, the definition of a "major trauma victim" varies between studies, making comparisons of scoring systems difficult. Also, many of the scoring systems were derived and examined retrospectively and lack validation by large prospective studies. Because most studies calculated scores "after the fact" through a chart review, their direct application as field triage tools is severely limited.

Prehospital provider level of training, response times, distance to trauma centers, and the availability of rotorcraft may influence the accuracy of a scoring system in a specific locale. In addition, a scoring system validated in an urban system may not be as accurate in a rural area. Interobserver variability is another concern. Scoring systems vary in the number of parameters measured and calculated by the field crews (Table 1-1). Accuracy and reproducibility of a scoring system may decrease as the number of calculations and data points increases.

TABLE 1-1
Comparison of Variables Among Scoring Systems

SCORING SYSTEM	VARIABLES
Trauma Index	Region of body injured, type of injury, cardiovascular status, CNS status, and respiratory status
Trauma Score	Respiratory rate, respiratory expansion, SBP, CR, and GCS
Revised Trauma Score	GCS, respiratory rate, and SBP
CRAMS	Circulation, respiratory, abdomen, motor, and speech
Prehospital Index	SBP, pulse, respiratory status, level of consciousness, penetrating torso trauma
Trauma Triage Rule	SBP, GCS, or penetrating injuries of the trunk, head, or neck

CNS, Central nervous system; *SBP,* systolic blood pressure; *GCS,* Glasgow Coma Scale; *CR,* capillary refill.

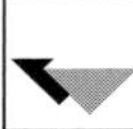

PEARLS & PITFALLS

- The goal of any triage scheme is to separate major trauma victims from the overall population of trauma victims.
- Ideally a trauma triage system would avoid both under- and over-triage.
- Paramedic judgment independent of formal trauma scoring systems is relatively sensitive in identifying patients who benefit from trauma center care.
- All of the scoring systems require initial prehospital provider training and continuing education.
- Each trauma system must determine acceptable rates of under- and over-triage and the best method of achieving local success.

REFERENCES

1. Arroyo JS, Crosby LA: Basic rescue and resuscitation: trauma system concept in the United States, *Clin Orthop Rel Res* 318:11-16, 1995.
2. Division of Medical Sciences, National Academy of Sciences: *Accidental death and disability: the neglected disease of modern society,* Washington, 1966, National Research Council.
3. Henry MC, et al: Evaluation of American College of Surgeons trauma criteria in a suburban and rural setting, *Am J Emerg Med* 14:124-129, 1996.
4. West JG, Trunkey DD, Lim RC: Systems of trauma care: a study of two counties, *Arch Surg* 114:455-460, 1979.
5. West JG, Cales RH, Gazzaniga A: Impact of regionalization: the Orange County experience, *Arch Surg* 118:740-744, 1983.
6. Kilberg L, et al: Effectiveness of implementing a trauma triage system on outcome: a prospective evaluation, *J Trauma* 28:1493-1498, 1988.
7. Emerman CL, Shade B, Kubincanek J: Comparative performance of the Baxt Trauma Triage Rule, *Am J Emerg Med* 10:294-297, 1992.
8. Emerman CL, Shade B, Kubincanek J: A comparison of EMT judgement and prehospital trauma triage instruments, *J Trauma* 31:1369-1375, 1991.
9. Maslanka AM: Scoring systems and triage from the field, *Emerg Med Clin North Am* 11:15-27, 1993.
10. Vayer JS, Eyck RP, Cowan ML: New concepts in triage, *Ann Emerg Med* 15:927-930, 1986.
11. American College of Surgeons Committee on Trauma: *Prehospital resources for optimal care of the injured patient,* Chicago, 1993, American College of Surgeons.
12. American College for Emergency Physicians: Guidelines for trauma care systems, *Ann Emerg Med* 22:1079-1100, 1993.
13. Champion HR, et al: Trauma Score, *Crit Care Med* 9:672-676, 1981.
14. Champion HR, et al: An anatomic index of injury severity, *J Trauma* 20:197-202, 1980.
15. Morris JA, et al: The Trauma Score as a triage tool in the prehospital setting, *JAMA* 256:1319-1325, 1986.
16. West JG, et al: A method for evaluating field triage criteria, *J Trauma* 26:655-659, 1986.

17. Kirkpatrick JR, Youmans RL: Trauma Index: an aide in the evaluation of injury victims, *J Trauma* 14:711-714, 1971.
18. Champion HR, et al: A revision of the Trauma Score, *J Trauma* 20:188, 1989.
19. Gormican SP: CRAM scale: field triage of trauma victims, *Ann Emerg Med* 11:132-135, 1982.
20. Koehler JJ, et al: Prehospital Index: a scoring system for field triage of trauma victims, *Ann Emerg Med* 15:178-182, 1986.
21. Baxt WG, Jones G, Fortlage D: The Trauma Triage Rule: a new, resource-based approach to the prehospital identification of major trauma victims, *Ann Emerg Med* 19:1401-1406,1990.
22. Henry MC, et al: Incremental benefit of individual American College of Surgeons Trauma Triage Criteria, *Acad Emerg Med* 3:992-100, 1996.
23. Fries GR, et al: A prospective comparison of paramedic judgement and the trauma triage in the prehospital setting, *Ann Emerg Med* 24:885-889, 1994.
24. Tinkoff GH, O'Conner RE, Fulda GJ: Impact of a two tier trauma response in the emergency department: promoting efficient resource utilization, *J Trauma* 41:735-740, 1996.
25. Philips JA, Buchman TG: Optimizing prehospital triage criteria for trauma team alerts, *J Trauma* 34:127-132, 1993.
26. Simon BJ, et al: Vehicular trauma triage by mechanism: avoidance of the unproductive evaluation, *J Trauma* 37:645-649, 1994.
27. Baxt WG, Berry CC, Epperson MD: The failure of prehospital trauma prediction rules to classify trauma patients accurately, *Ann Emerg Med* 18:1-8, 1989.
28. Moreau M, et al: Application of the trauma score in the prehospital setting, *Ann Emerg Med* 14:1049-1054, 1985.
29. Ornato, et al: Ineffectiveness of the Trauma Score and the CRAMS Scale for accurately triaging patients to trauma centers, *Ann Emerg Med* 14:1061-1064, 1985.
30. Koehler JJ, et al: A multi-center validation of the prehospital index, *Ann Emerg Med* 16:380-385, 1987.
31. Plant JR, MacLeod DB, Kortbeek J: Limitation of the prehospital index in identifying patients in need of a major trauma center, *Ann Emerg Med* 26:133-137, 1995.
32. Simmons E, et al: Paramedic injury severity perception can aid trauma triage, *Ann Emerg Med* 26:461-468, 1995.
33. Hedges JR, et al: Comparison of prehospital triage instruments in a semi-rural population, *J Emerg Med* 5:197-208, 1987.

On-Line Medical Command

2

JON R. KROHMER

Teaching Case

The emergency medical service (EMS) radio in your emergency department (ED) crackles: a 32-year-old male victim of a motor vehicle collision. The paramedics indicate that this unrestrained driver of a car lost control and collided with a tree. There is significant damage to the car, and there will be a prolonged extrication. The victim is unresponsive with severe head, chest, and lower extremity injuries. Current vital signs include BP 110/60, pulse 125, and respirations are 32 and shallow. They have applied a cervical collar and immobilized the spine. They estimate a 15- to 20-minute extrication and 15-minute transport.

How should you manage on-line command? ■

Although EMS personnel deliver medical care, they do not practice autonomously. Instead they function under the direct and indirect supervision of physicians. Medical oversight is "the ultimate responsibility and authority for the medical actions taken by a prehospital provider or an EMS system," and includes the "physician or medical groups with such authority."[1] This medical oversight is an integral component of all EMS systems. Regardless of whether EMS personnel are licensed or certified in their particular state, all states require that EMS personnel account to a medical director. In some states, the regulations stipulate that EMS personnel function directly under a physician's license.

The concept of medical oversight has jointly evolved with EMS. Several terms refer to this function, including *medical control, medical direction,* and *medical oversight*. Although some see significant distinctions among these terms, they are generally used interchangeably. Additionally, *medical command* frequently includes providing specific direction to EMS personnel either via radio or telephone in *real time*—concurrent with the prehospital care of an individual.

MEDICAL OVERSIGHT

Historically, medical oversight consists of two major functions: on-line (direct) and off-line (indirect) supervision. On-line functions originally referred to direct supervision of the EMS personnel via either radio or telephone. Off-line activities referred to all of the other medical oversight functions (Box 2-1). More recently, authorities categorize medical oversight functions as *prospective, concurrent* (or *contemporaneous*), and *retrospective* depending on the timing relative to the actual patient encounter (Box 2-1).

OFF-LINE MEDICAL DIRECTION

As noted in Box 2-1, many medical oversight activities occur before (prospective) and after (retrospective) the actual patient encounter. Patient care protocols and other policies and procedures are crucial elements of oversight.

Patient care protocols define the level of care provided. For trauma patients the EMS medical director should develop the protocols with input from other system participants, including emergency physicians (EPs) and trauma surgeons. Protocols promote uniformity of care and educate field personnel in the expected standards. They also serve as an objective basis for the quality improvement (QI) program. Specific protocol issues should address the appropriate assessment of injuries, airway management, and other prehospital procedures. These protocols outline the scope

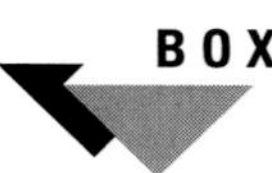

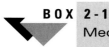

BOX 2-1
Medical Oversight Activities

PROSPECTIVE ACTIVITIES (OFF-LINE)
Initial education
Prehospital personnel
Hospital personnel
Protocol, policy, and procedure development
Personnel selection and retention
Total Quality Management Program development
Political/legislative process
Disaster planning

CONCURRENT ACTIVITIES (ON-LINE OR DIRECT)
Radio/telephone
On-scene

RETROSPECTIVE ACTIVITIES (OFF-LINE OR INDIRECT)
Total Quality Improvement program
Routine review (e.g., major trauma, cardiac arrest)
Special review
Random audit
Continuing education
Remedial education
Counseling/disciplinary process

of prehospital care and identify situations that require on-line medical direction.

Standing orders are a central component of protocols. These preauthorized directives empower EMS personnel to intervene before establishing on-line medical direction. Standing orders typically instruct personnel regarding routine procedures (e.g., spinal immobilization) or critical, time-dependent interventions (e.g., intubation in an apneic patient) before contacting an on-line physician. Standing orders mandate a vigorous QI program to audit both compliance and patient outcomes.

The *procedures* aspect of Policy and Procedures defines how activities are to be performed. For example, specific techniques for immobilization, airway management (e.g., ventilation, intubation, and surgical techniques, if available), and fluid administration must be defined for system personnel.

Policies typically define administrative activities that occur in the EMS system. Policies that outline hospital destinations for prehospital triage categories (e.g., critical trauma, pediatric trauma, hyperbaric oxygen therapy, and burn treatment) must be prospectively established. If local trauma centers are not available, transport via helicopter air ambulance may be required. In this case, a policy should indicate which patients require air-medical service and define the process for activating the helicopter.

Other prospective activities specific to the trauma patient include the education of personnel in trauma management (such as basic and advance trauma life support) and instruction regarding established protocols, policies, and procedures.

The medical director or his or her designate must establish and maintain the QI process. Continuing education should address educational needs identified by the QI process.

Retrospective activities include review of paramedic run sheets and performance audits. These QI activities should involve other team members in the trauma system such as other prehospital agencies, emergency departments, and trauma facilities.

ON-LINE MEDICAL DIRECTION

On-line (concurrent) medical direction provides direct communication between field providers and supervisory personnel. Typically, on-line direction occurs over radio or telephone between the field and ED. All EMS personnel, including basic life support (BLS) personnel, should have access to on-line resources. For the trauma patient, on-line direction may clarify the appropriate destination. There are several potential models for these activities. On-scene oversight by the medical director or other personnel, such as other physicians or field supervisors, can be an important aspect of concurrent medical direction.

During the early days of EMS, on-line medical direction was required before field personnel performed any advanced life-support intervention. With increasing education and experience of EMS personnel, many procedures are now accomplished under standing orders. There are complex situations, however, that benefit from on-line control and consultation with a physician. This direct contact also reinforces the team nature of EMS. The on-line interaction between physician and medic does not reflect inadequate training, but rather elevates the quality of prehospital care.

On-line direction is also very helpful when EMS personnel deviate from protocols. High-risk legal issues are best managed by on-line direction. These issues include the treatment and transport of minors, use of restraints on combative patients, field pronouncement of death, and EMS-initiated refusal of transport. Paramedics should consult with the on-line physician for other medicolegal hazards such as patient refusal of treatment or when a bystander physician attempts to control the scene.

Finally, the information provided to ED personnel via direct communication enables the ED to adequately prepare for the patient's arrival. This communication is particularly important when special resources are needed. Such situations include patients who require trauma team activation or specialty team response (as in the case a of a seriously injured trauma victim who is more than 20 weeks pregnant).

Models for On-Line Command

In some systems, each receiving hospital speaks directly with EMS personnel via radio or telephone. This model promotes close communication and continuity of care. Direct interaction reduces the risk of miscommunication that may arise if information is relayed from another facility. However, this system involves more on-line participants (multiple personnel from multiple hospitals) and requires more effort to educate and monitor. The content and style of medical direction varies proportionately to the size of the pool of physicians providing the on-line command.

Another model of on-line direction involves centralized control of on-line activities. This control can occur either through one hospital (resource hospital) or through one centralized facility (medical command center). Under the resource hospital model, all on-line direction originates from one hospital facility. The designated resource hospital is responsible for medical direction of a particular geographic area or for a specific group of EMS agencies. With a centralized facility (which does not necessarily have to be a hospital), on-line personnel are available specifically for EMS consultation. Personnel may be physically present at that facility or available by radio. For example, at some centers, resident and attending physicians are available via portable radio and are contacted by the communications center for on-line direction. Information about the patient is then relayed by the communications center to the receiving hospital in preparation for the patient's arrival. This centralized system may be more consistent, because it originates from a smaller number of personnel. Continuing experience yields a better understanding of the protocols, ease of education, and QI follow-up.

Concern has been raised that a resource hospital might inappropriately divert patients to its hospital rather than to other hospitals in the system for financial gain. In studies from Oregon,[2,3] implementation of a resource hospital system did not increase the percentage of patients transported to the resource hospital. Quite the opposite, critical cases were more frequently diverted to outlying community hospitals, away from the urban resource hospital.

ON-SCENE MEDICAL OVERSIGHT

Another important aspect of concurrent medical oversight is on-scene supervision, usually by the medical director or similar personnel. The medical director must spend time in the field, both to ensure quality care and to build *esprit de corps*. The medical director must be familiar with the system, its personnel, and have first-hand knowledge of the daily challenges of prehospital care. Continuing field experience also increases the medical director's credibility with EMS personnel. Additional benefits of on-scene control include QI, education, and patient care.

Directly observing the care provided by personnel is one of the most valuable QI tools available to a medical director. Although directors can glean information by reviewing run forms and audits, the best way to identify problems is to physically observe care. Run form review can identify that the patient was intubated, but only on-scene observation confirms technique, time to intubation, number of attempts, and other issues that may not be evident on the run form.

The field is an ideal setting to educate EMS personnel. If the oversight personnel on-scene identify a problem (e.g., a field provider having difficulty intubating patients), the supervisor can instruct the field provider in real time.

Occasionally, on-scene care by medical supervisors may expand care options. In some systems, field supervisors receive special training in advanced field techniques or carry medications beyond those available on the ambulance. Some systems have physicians respond to the scene.

MEDICAL OVERSIGHT PERSONNEL

Traditionally, physicians have provided medical oversight. Certainly, each EMS system must identify a physician to serve as the medical director for the system.[4-6] Although the medical director leads the EMS system, they cannot function independently. The director must interact and cooperate with numerous members of the system: administrators, educators, QI personnel, field personnel, specialty physicians in the community, and others involved in trauma care.

Although the medical director is ultimately responsible for EMS oversight, a number of other personnel perform supervisory functions. Frequently, physicians provide on-line direction via radio or telephone, whether they are in the ED or in a centralized communications facility. However, in some systems specially trained nurses or paramedics perform those on-line activities. Generally they have additional training and experience above that of most field providers. Radio control can encourage or calm anxious field personnel and on-line supervisors can refer to written protocols when necessary.[7] A designated physician should be immediately available as needed.

On-line supervisors require special training. Some locations provide courses and real-time experience (e.g., regular on-line audit review, annual field ride-alongs).[8] This training applies to physicians and nonphysicians alike. Training is also provided in Emergency Medicine residency programs.[9] Some states require completion of a one-day base station course.[7]

EFFECTIVENESS OF ON-LINE MEDICAL DIRECTION

The value of on-line medical direction remains unknown. Does it improve outcomes or is it a waste of time? If it needlessly prolongs scene time with no apparent outcome benefit, on-line command should be strictly limited. Several studies have investigated on-line direction for medical patients, particularly those with cardiac and respiratory problems.[10-12] Unfortunately, there is little research on the impact in trauma patients.

In a retrospective review of ALS run sheets, Holliman et al[13] identified on-line errors by physicians in 4.4% of the runs reviewed and identified six types of errors, which accounted for 80% of the total errors. They used this information to reshape education for medical command physicians. Looking at the same system several years later, Wuerz et al[14] conducted a blinded, prospective study of direction provided by EPs in a university hospital. They found that physician orders were given in 19% of the study cases. However, many of these orders were for care preauthorized by standing orders, which the paramedics had not followed. On-line direction time averaged 4 minutes and comprised one third of the total field treatment time. The authors felt that on-line medical direction improved quality control by reducing omissions in prehospital care.

Another trial demonstrated that on-line direction is more common in cardiac (78% of cardiac cases) than in trauma (35% of cases) patients.[15] In this study, physician-direction rarely deviated from standing orders (3.7% of all on-line calls). On-line direction prolonged in-field scene time by an average of 8 minutes. However, the authors felt that on-line direction may have improved outcomes.

Other researchers argue that on-line direction needlessly prolongs field scene time. In a retrospective review, Pointer et al[16] showed that on-line direction lengthened the scene time by almost 4.5 minutes compared to patients managed by standing orders. Protocol compliance was found to be similar among the groups. However, this study did not investigate types of patients, nor did it indicate change in patient conditions or outcomes. Hunt et al[10] found no difference in on-scene times for cardiac arrest patients with or without on-line direction.

Standing orders have nearly replaced on-line control in many locals. However, standing orders do not always shorten prehospital time intervals. Gratton et al[17] reviewed cases of major trauma patients transported to a level I trauma center before and after implementation of standing orders for invasive procedures. They found that standing orders did not decrease scene time in unstable trauma patients and had no impact on the number of procedures performed.

RISK MANAGEMENT ISSUES

There is very little information available about the legal threats of on-line medical direction. One article examined eight cases of EMS litigation that included references to on-line activities. It suggested several risk management considerations regarding on-line direction (Box 2-2).[18] Interestingly, none of those cases included "the contention that the prehospital provider functions as an agent or extension of a physician or that a patient-physician relationship is established by virtue of the EMS contact."[18]

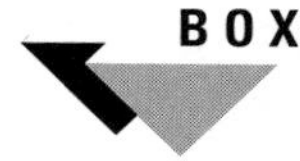

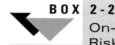

BOX 2-2
On-line Medical Direction Risk Management Recommendations

- Only physicians or other persons knowledgeable in the emergency medical service (EMS) protocols should provide on-line medical direction.
- EMS Medical Directors should be involved in the development and implementation of nontransport, diversion, and bypass protocols.
- Base station orders, particularly bypass and diversion events should be reviewed by EMS and emergency department (ED) medical directors. Recordings of base station communication should be required for quality assurance.
- EMS Medical Directors should educate prehospital providers on the importance of timely and accurate communication to the base station physician.
- Destination policies must be motivated by the medical needs of the patient in conjunction with the receiving facility capabilities.

From Shanaberger CJ: *Prehosp Disast Med* 10(2):75-81, 1995.

The physician who takes on the responsibility of on-line medical command also is at potential risk for liability in cases of maloccurrence. EMS provider malpractice may incur medicolegal risk for the on-line physician who has not even seen the patient. However, the on-line physician is named as a codefendant less than 10% of the time.[19,20]

Potential problems the on-line physician may encounter include the following:

1. Competent patient who withdraws initial consent to treatment
2. Treatment of minors without parental consent resulting from nonavailability of the parent
3. Impaired patients (caused by trauma, drugs, hypoxia) who cannot refuse treatment
4. Bystander physician who assumes medical command at the scene

Documentation of a patient's competence at the scene is necessary in cases when the patient refuses treatment. A common situation EPs encounter is the hypoglycemic patient who initially was lethargic or obtunded and resumes a normal mental status after infusion of intravenous glucose. These patients are instructed that they are welcome to be evaluated in the ED and that they may seek medical assistance anytime after refusal.

In the treatment of minors, it is always in the patient's best interest to take him or her to the ED for medical assistance even when a parent or guardian cannot be contacted. Commission is always medicolegally safer than omission.

Impaired patients cannot make informed decisions with regard to their well-being. Once again, commission (in this case, transporting to the hospital against the patient's will) is medicolegally safer than omission (leaving the patient at the scene).

If a bystander physician tries to assume medical command at the scene, the EMS personnel should contact the medical control physician. Since the EMS personnel must follow predetermined orders with regard to patient care, they should not deviate if the bystander physician gives different orders. It is not wise for the on-line physician to relinquish control to the bystander physician, since the bystander physician is covered by Good Samaritan laws and the on-line physician is not.

CONCLUSION

The paramedics now radio the ED with an update. The patient has been extricated, immobilized, and they are en route to the hospital, with an ETA of 10 minutes. The patient remains unresponsive but without external hemorrhage. They were able to intubate him and are ventilating with a bag-valve device with 100% O_2. An intravenous line has been placed. Secondary survey reveals probable bilateral flail chests, and the abdomen is firm. Multiple lower extremity fractures have been splinted with the pneumatic antishock garment. Current vital signs: BP 80/36, P 130, and assisted ventilations 24. The paramedic indicates that he is experiencing increasing resistance to ventilations. You suggest bilateral needle decompression of the chest. After decompression, medics report that the ventilations are easier and the blood pressure is normalizing. You notify the trauma team of the patient's impending arrival and prepare the trauma suite.

PEARLS & PITFALLS

- ◆ EMS personnel are accountable to a medical director.
- ◆ Medical command frequently involves providing specific direction to EMS personnel via radio or telephone concurrent with the prehospital care of the patient.
- ◆ Standing orders typically instruct EMS personnel regarding routine procedures or critical time-dependent interventions before contacting an on-line physician.
- ◆ Retrospective review of EMS run sheets aid in identifying problems and help to educate prehospital providers, but direct field observation is an even better method of quality improvement.

REFERENCES

1. Kuehl AE (editor): *Prehospital systems and medical oversight,* ed 2, St Louis, 1994, Mosby.
2. Neely KW, et al: The effect of base station contact on ambulance destination, *Ann Emerg Med* 19:906-909, 1990.
3. Waddington N, et al: The effect of on-line medical control centralization on ambulance destination, *J Emerg Med* 5:299-303, 1987.
4. *Emergency medical services base station function and design: on-line medical control,* Position Statement, Lenexa, KS, 1989, National Association of EMS Physicians.
5. *Medical direction of emergency medical services,* ACEP Policy Statement, Dallas, TX, 1997, American College of Emergency Physicians.
6. *Medical direction of prehospital emergency medical services,* Policy Resource and Education Paper, Dallas, TX, 1997, American College of Emergency Physicians.
7. Delbridge TR, et al: Contemporaneous medical direction. In Paris PM, Roth RN, Verdile VP (editors): *Prehospital medicine: the art of on-line medical command,* St Louis, 1996, Mosby.
8. Pointer JE: The emergency physician and medical control in advanced life support, *J Emerg Med* 3:31-35, 1985.

9. Swor RA, Chisolm C, Krohmer J: Model curriculum in emergency medical services for emergency medicine residencies, *Ann Emerg Med* 18:418-421, 1989.
10. Hunt RC, et al: Standing orders versus voice command, *JEMS* 7(11):26-31, 1982.
11. Peacock JB, Blackwell VH, Wainscott M: Medical reliability of advanced prehospital cardiac life support, *Ann Emerg Med* 14: 407-409, 1985.
12. Rottman SJ, et al: On-line medical control versus protocol-based prehospital care, *Ann Emerg Med* 30:62-68, 1997.
13. Holliman CJ, Wuerz RC, Meador SA: Medical command errors in an urban advanced life support system, *Ann Emerg Med* 21: 347-350, 1992.
14. Wuerz RC, et al: On-line medical direction: a prospective study, *Prehosp Disast Med* 10(3):174-177, 1995.
15. Erder MH, Davidson SJ, Cheney RA: On-line medical command in theory and practice, *Ann Emerg Med* 18:261-268, 1989.
16. Pointer JE, Osur MA: Effect of standing orders on field times, *Ann Emerg Med* 18:1119-1121, 1989.
17. Gratton MC, el al: Effect of standing orders on paramedic scene time for trauma patients, *Ann Emerg Med* 20:1306-1309, 1991.
18. Shanaberger CJ: Case law involving base-station contact, *Prehosp Disast Med* 10(2):75-81, 1995.
19. Soler JM, et al: The ten year malpractice experience of a large urban EMS system, *Ann Emerg Med* 14:982-985, 1985.
20. Goldberg RJ, et al: A review of prehospital care litigation in a large metropolitan EMS system, *Ann Emerg Med* 19:557-561, 1990.

Controversies in Prehospital Trauma Care

3

DAVID P. THOMSON

Medicine has been called "The Youngest Science," and nowhere is this designation more evident than in the prehospital care of the trauma victim.[1] Although ambulances have responded to trauma for over 150 years, only in the past quarter century has science been applied to prehospital medicine. Much of the care rendered is based on the medical "art" of preceding generations.

The scientific era of prehospital trauma care began with the 1966 paper, "Death and Disability in America," which outlined the plight of victims of motor vehicle crashes.[1] Before this time, ambulance drivers, often funeral home employees with little medical training, provided prehospital trauma care. Their goal was to get to the hospital in the shortest amount of time. Interventions, if any, consisted of splinting long bone fractures and, rarely, giving oxygen. Spinal immobilization was unknown, and intravenous (IV) cannulation was restricted to hospitals.

The other major force impacting prehospital care was the Vietnam War. Physicians who had served in Vietnam realized that the same techniques used to stabilize wounded soldiers might benefit civilian trauma victims. They argued that providers other than physicians and nurses could render care in the streets, just as corpsmen and medics had done on the battlefield.

These pioneers borrowed techniques from a variety of disciplines. If an intervention worked in one setting, it was assumed applicable to the streets. Because the Pneumatic Anti-Shock Garment (PASG), also known as Military Anti-Shock Trousers (MAST), appeared useful in Vietnam, it was introduced to civilian prehospital care. Intravenous fluid resuscitation, used in stabilizing hypotensive patients in the hospital, was now performed in the ambulance. Immobilization, which had previously consisted of applying boards to deformed extremities, was adapted to the spine. All of these interventions took time, leading to growing prehospital delays. Before anyone thought to evaluate these interventions, many had been codified into law, making randomized prospective trials legally risky, if not impossible.

In this chapter, we consider the scope of prehospital interventions, and how prolonging field time affects survival. Next, we examine the literature surrounding prehospital treatment of the hypotensive trauma patient, both with the PASG and IV fluids. We discuss what is known about spinal immobilization. Although we try to present a balanced perspective, none of these problems has been definitively studied.

"STAY AND PLAY" VERSUS "SCOOP AND RUN"

The debate over whether to stabilize the patient at the scene or to rush to the hospital is not new. Techniques such as starting IV lines and administering medications were first applied to trauma patients during the early 1970s. At the same time, the concept of the trauma "golden hour" gained acceptance. This notion suggested that severely injured trauma patients need definitive surgical care within 1 hour of injury to optimize survival. The tension between prehospital interventions and rapid transport continues to divide the medical community.[3]

To determine the priorities for a specific patient, the paramedics must answer several questions: What is the mechanism of injury? How stable is the patient, and how far is the hospital? What resources are available in the community?

Patient-specific factors are extremely important in deciding how much time to spend in the field. On the one hand, operative delays may be detrimental to certain patients. On the other, some patients require field intubation, chest decompression, and other advanced prehospital techniques. Patients suffering blunt trauma have different needs than those with stab wounds to the chest. While field intubation is an important maneuver in the hypercarbic head-injured patient, the most important intervention in penetrating cardiac trauma is emergent thoracotomy.

Resources differ dramatically for urban victims with nearby trauma centers and rural patients located hours from the nearest facility.[4] Paramedics and the medical directors must ensure expedient transport to the emergency department (ED) and limit time-consuming interventions to the immediately lifesaving.

TREATMENT OF THE HYPOTENSIVE TRAUMA PATIENT

Generally accepted medical practice affirms that normotension is good. Pressures above or below this poorly defined range are considered "bad." The traditional medical response to hypotension is to normalize the blood pressure. In 1903 Crile[5] used compression garments to increase the blood pressure of surgical patients. Since that time, conventional practice has mandated that hypotensive trauma patients receive lots of blood and fluid. For years, controversies raged over using colloids or crystalloids, but crystalloids and blood won the day. Currently, the most pressing question is how much fluid, if any, is needed before surgical control of bleeding.

Previous hemorrhagic shock models from the 1950s to 1980s relied on a controlled hemorrhage model. Animals were bled down to a certain pressure or volume, at which point the hemorrhage was stopped. However, this model may not apply to patients with trauma, where victims often suffer uncontrolled hemorrhage. In the uncontrolled hemorrhage studies using an aortotomy, Bickell et al,[6] Kowalenko et al,[7] and Stern et al[8] discovered that outcomes were worse if swine were subsequently resuscitated to a normal pressure. To the surprise of many, at least some fluid restriction improved survival. Both the rate and volume of infusion affect the dynamics of bleeding. Although explanations for this phenomenon abound, a definitive answer remains unknown. One theory suggests that when pressures fall, the wound thromboses, allowing recovery. Raising the pressure without fixing the lesion disrupts the clot and increases hemorrhage. Others dispute this explanation.[9,10]

The group in Houston took the research to the streets, and randomized hypotensive EMS patients to IV or no IV fluids in the field.[11] The researchers found that in hypotensive patients with penetrating torso injuries, delay of aggressive fluid resuscitation until operative intervention improved outcome. Another retrospective study was unable to demonstrate any survival advantage conferred by prehospital fluids.[12]

Overall, it appears that in the urban setting of penetrating trauma, aggressive fluid resuscitation at best does no harm, and at worst may result in increased bleeding. Further research is needed to define which patients, if any, may benefit from fluid resuscitation, as well as what rate and volume of fluid will maximize survival.

INTRAVENOUS ACCESS—THE IV START

If one accepts that the prehospital trauma patient should receive blood pressure support, there are two major alternatives: IV fluids and the PASG. Each of these interventions is contentious. Although the most apparent benefit for IV access in the trauma patient is administration of fluids or blood, it may serve other uses. The IV start may be used to obtain blood samples such as a type and crossmatch and hemoglobin, and the IV may be used to administer medications.

Time

Many prehospital debates center on time spent in the field. Does the benefit justify the time required to perform a procedure? The argument boils down to the familiar "stay and play," versus the "scoop and run" philosophies. All procedures consume time, a precious commodity in the field. Intravenous access in the trauma patient is no exception. The first question is *when* the IV should be started. In the medical patient, paramedics became accustomed to starting the IV at the scene, before transport. In the cardiac patient, this "stay and play" approach is appropriate, since many medical resuscitations can occur outside the hospital. But in the trauma patient, any delay in definitive care (i.e., operation) may increase morbidity. One trauma center concluded that the lag caused by starting an IV significantly delayed the patient's arrival at the hospital.[13] Since the amount of fluid infused in the ambulance is small, they argued that most patients benefit more from early transport than from an IV. This argument is countered by the concept of a "zero-time IV," in which the IV is started en route to the hospital.[14] This approach has been championed in studies from Denver, Los Angeles, and Atlanta.[15-17]

Complications

Like all procedures, IV access has associated complications. The question is whether the complication rate for EMS IV lines is significantly greater than lines begun in the ED. Lawrence and Lauro[18] examined this question during the late 1980s. In their study, they found that IV lines started by EMS providers had a complication rate nearly six times higher than those started in the ED. Of note, glove use was rare at the time of their study. In another trial from the late 1980s, researchers showed that they could start high-flow central lines in the ED more quickly and as safely as basilic vein lines.[19]

The "Bottom Line"

From these studies, it appears that the fluid administered in the field may not harm the patient, so long as the infection rate remains low. However, no study has ever shown an advantage to prehospital fluids in the trauma victim. Until more research is available, we should not abandon prehospital IV lines in trauma patients. Instead EMS medical directors must monitor this procedure to ensure safety and timeliness of transport.

PNEUMATIC ANTI-SHOCK GARMENT

Once the mainstay of prehospital blood pressure support, the PASG has fallen into disfavor. Although primitive devices were used at the turn of this century, the PASG only became popular after the Vietnam War. After enjoying apparent success in Vietnam, the device was introduced to the United States in Miami, Florida. A case series described the use of the PASG in both medical and trauma patients in the field.[20] Although the authors found that the garment improved blood pressure, they expressed two concerns: (1) the device is a temporary solution, not intended to replace rapid transport to definitive care, and (2) the increased blood pressure might increase bleeding from wounds not covered by the trousers. The authors also recommended a controlled study. Unfortunately, before a well-designed, randomized clinical trial was undertaken, the garment became a "standard of care." Nearly a decade passed before anyone had the courage to rigorously study the PASG.

Beginning in 1983, Bickell et al[21,22] at Baylor University and the City of Houston EMS conducted prospective studies of the PASG in hypotensive trauma patients. In the first of these trials they were unable to find any improvement in the trauma score when the PASG was used. In the later study, they looked at penetrating abdominal injuries, a subset many supposed would benefit from the garment. Even in this population, there was no survival advantage. A retrospective study from San Francisco mirrored these results.[23]

In contrast with the Houston studies, Cayten et al[24] looked at this problem in New York City. Their conclusions, based on several years of data, indicated an increase in survival in severe hypotension, defined as an initial blood pressure of less than or equal to 50 mmHg. Since there were no survivors of abdominal trauma in the non-PASG group, they concluded that use of the PASG should be continued. However, its findings remain suspect as this study was neither randomized nor prospective.

O'Connor and Domeier[25] recently reviewed the literature on the PASG in both trauma and medical patients. They concluded that the PASG may support severely hypotensive patients with abdominal injuries, but other indications remain unproven. The garment may be contraindicated in thoracic trauma. These data was synthesized by the National Association of EMS Physicians.[26] The position paper classified each indication for the PASG using a familiar system.[27] Most of the indications for PASG were class II, suggesting an acceptable but unproven modality. The only class I indication was for hypotension resulting from a ruptured abdominal aortic aneurysm.

Although many centers use the PASG to stabilize pelvic fractures, the only evidence supporting its use comes from small case series.[28-30] Although it appears reasonable that the PASG would assist hemorrhage control in unstable pelvic fractures, no large randomized controlled trials have been conducted to evaluate this indication.

Certain traumatic conditions were considered *inappropriate* for use of the PASG (class III): diaphragmatic rupture, penetrating thoracic injury, lower extremity fractures, extremity trauma, abdominal evisceration, and cardiac tamponade.

SPINAL IMMOBILIZATION

Spinal immobilization, like the PASG, became the standard of care without scientific evidence. That is not to say that it is a bad standard; in the 1970s, patients frequently arrived in EDs with complete spinal cord lesions. By the 1980s, most spinal cord injury victims arrived with incomplete lesions, leading Green et al[31] to suggest that spinal immobilization was responsible for the improvement. One group retrospectively examined the relationship between spinal immobilization and neurologic injury.[32] Their study paired trauma victims from the University of New Mexico and the University of Malaya. In New Mexico, spinal immobilization was standard, while in Malaya none of the patients were immobilized. Surprisingly, their results suggest that spinal immobilization has little or no effect on the outcome of blunt spinal injury. Some data suggest that immobilization may increase spinal hypoxia, while others propose the opposite.

At present, there are no data to conclusively support or refute the use of spinal immobilization. However, until there are definitive studies showing harm, it will likely remain a standard of care. Perhaps it is more relevant to ask who might benefit from this procedure and who is most at risk if immobilization is abandoned?

Domeier et al[33] looked retrospectively at patients who suffered spinal fractures or spinal cord injuries to define important risk factors. Their data show that patients with altered mental status, intoxication, spinal pain, and extremity fracture are in danger of spinal injury. They also reported that patients with isolated spinal tenderness are not at risk, a finding that conflicts with most other research. These data suggest ways to decrease the use of immobilization, thus dramatically reducing prehospital costs.

Studies conflict regarding the amount of agreement between prehospital providers and emergency physicians regarding the need for spinal immobilization in individual patients. A study performed by Sahni et al[34] showed that paramedics can safely determine the need for spinal precautions. Using standardized patients, emergency physicians and paramedics usually agreed on immobilization decisions. While another study demonstrated similar findings,[35] a third study showed that prehospital personnel and emergency physicians *disagreed* nearly one quarter of the time on the need for cervical immobilization.[36] These data indicate that any system, that permits prehospital discretion in immobilization, must audit the program.

CONCLUSIONS

Care of the prehospital trauma patient continues to evolve. New techniques are introduced and old techniques are discarded or transformed. In the end, the medical director must not only study the current literature, but must be familiar with the daily realities of prehospital care. Reliable, state-of-the-art prehospital care requires constant evaluation of performance.

REFERENCES

1. Thomas L: *The youngest science,* New York, 1983, Viking Press.
2. National Academy of Sciences—National Research Council: *Accidental death and disability: the neglected disease of modern society,* Washington, DC, 1966, National Academy Press.
3. Border JR, et al: Panel: prehospital trauma care–stabilize or scoop and run, *J Trauma* 23:708-711, 1983.
4. Demetriades D, et al: Paramedic vs. private transportation of trauma patients: effects on outcome, *Arch Surg* 131:133-138, 1996.
5. Crile GW: *Blood pressure in surgery: experimental and clinical research,* Philadelphia, 1903, Lippincott.
6. Bickell WH, et al: The detrimental effects of intravenous crystalloid after aortotomy in swine, *Surgery* 110:529-536, 1991.
7. Kowalenko T, et al: Improved outcome with hypotensive resuscitation of uncontrolled hemorrhagic shock in a swine model, *J Trauma* 33:349-353, 1992.
8. Stern SA, et al: Effect of blood pressure on hemorrhage volume and survival in a near-fatal hemorrhage model incorporating a vascular injury, *Ann Emerg Med* 22:155-163, 1993.
9. Silbergleit R, et al: A new model of uncontrolled hemorrhage that allows correlation of blood pressure and hemorrhage, *Acad Emerg Med* 3:917-921, 1996.
10. Silbergleit R, et al: Effect of permissive hypotension in continuous uncontrolled intra-abdominal hemorrhage, *Acad Emerg Med* 3:922-926, 1996.
11. Martin RR, et al: Prospective evaluation of preoperative fluid resuscitation in hypotensive patients with penetrating truncal injury: a preliminary report, *J Trauma* 33:354-362, 1992.
12. Kaweski SM, Sise MJ, Virgilio RW: The effect of prehospital fluids on survival in trauma patients, *J Trauma* 30:1215-1219, 1990.
13. Smith JP, et al: Prehospital stabilization of critically injured patients: a failed concept, *J Trauma* 25:65-70, 1985.
14. O'Gorman M, Trabulsy P, Pilcher DB: Zero-time prehospital IV, *J Trauma* 29:84-86, 1989.
15. Pons PT, et al: Prehospital venous access in an urban paramedic system: a prospective on-scene analysis, *J Trauma* 28:1460-1463, 1988.
16. Jones SE, Nesper TP, Alcouloumre E: Prehospital intravenous line placement: a prospective study, *Ann Emerg Med* 18:244-246, 1989.
17. Slovis CM, et al: Success rates for initiation of intravenous therapy en route by prehospital care providers, *Am J Emerg Med* 8:305-307, 1990.
18. Lawrence DW, Lauro AJ: Complications from IV therapy: results from field-started and emergency department-started IVs compared, *Ann Emerg Med* 17:314-317, 1988.
19. Arrighi DA, et al: Prospective, randomized trial of rapid venous access for patients in hypovolemic shock, *Ann Emerg Med* 18: 927-930, 1989.
20. Civetta JM, et al: Prehospital use of the military anti-shock trouser (MAST), *J Am Coll Emerg Phys* 5:581-587, 1976.
21. Bickell WH, et al: Effect of antishock trousers on the trauma score: a prospective analysis in the urban setting, *Ann Emerg Med* 14:218-222, 1985.
22. Bickell WH, et al: Randomized trial of pneumatic antishock garments in the prehospital management of penetrating abdominal injuries, *Ann Emerg Med* 16:653-658, 1987.
23. Mackersie RC, Christensen JM, Lewis FR: The prehospital use of external counterpressure: does MAST make a difference? *J Trauma* 24:882-888, 1984.
24. Cayten CG, et al: A study of pneumatic antishock garments in severely hypotensive trauma patients, *J Trauma* 34:728-735, 1993.
25. O'Connor RE, Domeier RM: An evaluation of the pneumatic anti-shock garment (PASG) in various clinical settings, *Prehosp Emerg Care* 1:36-44, 1997.
26. Domeier RM, et al: Use of the pneumatic anti-shock garment (Position paper), *Prehosp Emerg Care* 1:32-35, 1997.
27. Emergency Cardiac Care Committee and Subcommittee, American Heart Association: Guidelines for cardiopulmonary resuscitation and emergency cardiac care. 1: Introduction, *JAMA* 268: 2172-2188, 1992.
28. Bruining HA, et al: Clinical experience with the medical antishock trousers (MAST) treatment of hemorrhage, especially from compound pelvic fracture, *Neth J Surg* 32:102-107, 1980.

29. Moreno C, et al: Hemorrhage associated with major pelvic fracture: a multispecialty challenge, *J Trauma* 26:987-994, 1986.
30. Brunette DD, Fifield G, Ruiz E: Use of pneumatic antishock trousers in the management of pediatric pelvic hemorrhage, *Pediatr Emerg Care* 3:86-90, 1987.
31. Green BA, Eismont FJ, O'Heir JT: Prehospital management of spinal cord injuries, *Paraplegia* 25:229-238, 1987.
32. Hauswald M, et al: Out-of-hospital spinal immobilization: its effect on neurologic injury, *Acad Emerg Med* 5:214-219, 1998.
33. Domeier RM, et al: Prehospital clinical findings associated with spinal injury, *Prehosp Emerg Care* 1:11-15, 1997.
34. Sahni R, Menegazzi JJ, Mosesso VN Jr: Paramedic evaluation of clinical indicators of cervical spine injury, *Prehosp Emerg Care* 1:16-18, 1997.
35. Brown LH, Gough JE, Simonds WB: Can EMS providers adequately assess trauma patients for cervical spine injury? *Prehosp Emerg Care* 2:33-36, 1998.
36. Meldon SW, et al: Out-of-hospital cervical spine clearance: agreement between emergency medical technicians and emergency physicians, *J Trauma* 45:1058-1061, 1998.

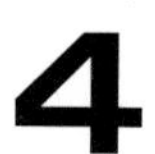

4 Air-Medical Transport

THEODORE R. DELBRIDGE

Teaching Case

A 75-year-old man traveling on the interstate was struck on his driver-side door by a truck. On arrival at the scene, the paramedics find he has no pulse or respirations. They intubate him and begin CPR. The monitor shows a slow, wide-complex rhythm that is unresponsive to fluid, epinephrine, and atropine. The scene is 20 miles north of the trauma center, surrounded by rush-hour traffic. The paramedics have called on the medic radio and are requesting a helicopter.

What should you do?

HISTORICAL PERSPECTIVE

The 1966 paper, *Accidental Death and Disability: The Neglected Disease of Modern Society,*[1] included 29 recommendations for improving the American healthcare system's response to trauma. The paper suggested pilot programs to evaluate automotive and helicopter ambulance services in sparsely populated areas and in regions that lacked hospital facilities adequate for seriously injured persons. Currently, approximately 200 air-medical services now deploy helicopters throughout the United States. Approximately 45% of their flights are for trauma patients, and 30% of the flights go directly to the scene.[2]

The first air-medical transport occurred during the retreat of the Serbian Army from Albania in 1915. A French pilot transported an injured Serbian officer in an unmodified fighter aircraft.[3] In subsequent decades the military increasingly used aircraft to transport wounded soldiers. During the Korean conflict the mortality rate among wounded U.S. soldiers was less than during World War II; at least some of this benefit was a result of the use of helicopters. The helicopters used during the Vietnam War, unlike their predecessors, allowed the wounded to be carried and treated inside the aircraft. The mortality rate during the Vietnam War decreased to less than 1 per 100 casualties. Air evacuation of wounded soldiers certainly contributed to improved survival. More than 370,000 soldiers were transported by helicopter in Vietnam. The average time for them to reach definitive care was 35 minutes, compared with 2 to 4 hours during the Korean conflict, and 6 to 12 hours during World War II.[4-6]

Because of its success with air evacuation in Vietnam, the Army initiated programs to respond to civilian emergencies in the United States. During 1966 and 1967, Army helicopters from Ft. Rucker, Alabama, and Ft. Sam Houston, Texas, evacuated 40 patients to medical facilities.[7] From 1967 to 1970, the government funded several civilian projects that verified the utility of helicopters for air-medical missions. Collectively, these projects revealed that helicopters could evacuate rural patients, make safe landings in metropolitan areas, and save valuable time.[7] In some metropolitan areas, such as Los Angeles and Chicago, police and fire department helicopters were occasionally pressed into service for medical missions.[4]

In July 1970 the federal government initiated the Military Assistance to Safety and Traffic (MAST) project. Eventually this project came to serve 23 communities.[7] Under this program, personnel and air-medical resources on stand-by for military units could respond to civilian needs. The early experience was positive; helicopters saved an average of 53 minutes compared with ground ambulances.

Also in 1970 the Maryland State Police initiated formal operations of its Med-Evac program as a component of a statewide emergency medical services program.[8] Dispersion of air-medical resources throughout the state resulted in shorter response times. During its first 5 years of operation, the

Med-Evac program transported more than 3000 patients, nearly half directly from the scenes.[9]

The first civilian hospital-based medical helicopter program commenced operations in October 1972 at St. Anthony Hospital Systems in Denver, Colorado.[10] Some of the initial issues faced by the program remain critical to air-medical programs today. These issues include maintaining complex communications systems, providing adequate preparation and monitoring of the medical flight crew, integrating the air-medical program into the trauma system, and addressing concerns regarding appropriate utilization.

Air-medical programs have evolved substantially over the past three decades. Early programs used single-engine helicopters, provided service primarily to their own hospitals, and had inappropriately low transport service charges. The current generation of air-medical programs more often deploys twin-engine aircraft, are focused on safety standards, seek appropriate utilization, and are attempting to balance financial realities with the desire to provide a community service.[4] Throughout the United States several models exist for air-medical services. These models include programs that are based within single hospitals, within hospital consortiums, within public safety agencies, and as independent entities. No matter what the model, air-medical services should integrate with the emergency medical services (EMS) and regional trauma care systems.[11]

ADVANTAGES

Air-medical services potentially offer two main advantages over ground EMS ambulances. These advantages are speed and the ability to overcome geographic obstacles.[12] When utilized appropriately, the aircraft's speed, combined with the ability to overcome geographic barriers, can accelerate transport to a trauma center. At least one study suggests that the earlier a trauma patient arrives at a trauma center, the lower the morbidity and mortality.[13]

Many different events comprise the prehospital phase of care. These events include prehospital dispatch, response to the scene, accessing and extricating the victim, providing on-scene treatment (often simultaneous with extrication activities), and transport to the trauma center. When an air-medical service is used, additional factors arise. Aircraft liftoff may take several minutes, depending on the organization of the service and the type of aircraft being used. Once in the vicinity of the landing zone, landing may take 3 to 5 minutes, since the aircraft's crew surveys the area to identify hazards. Sometimes the landing zone may be closer to the trauma scene than ground EMS vehicles were able to get, saving significant time. Alternatively, the landing zone may be at a site further from the trauma scene, requiring the patient to be moved to the landing zone. Finally, in general, loading and securing a patient into an aircraft is a more hazardous and complicated process than placing a patient in an ambulance.

Speed of Transport

It is possible to dispatch a medical helicopter at various points in the preshospital timeline: at the same time that ground EMS units are dispatched, immediately after EMS personnel assess the situation, or after victim extrication is complete.[7,14-19] The most timesaving course is to summon the air-medical service as soon as there is adequate information to indicate its need.

The potential for an air-medical service to expedite transport depends on many factors. When considering deployment, weigh the total in-transit time of the medical helicopter from the time of dispatch to delivery of the patient at the destination hospital. It is this cycle time that must be compared with ground transport intervals.[15,18]

Helicopters are generally not useful for short transports or in urban areas. In general, when the helicopter is responding from the same trauma center to which it will transport the patient, significant time can be saved when the scene is more than 26 to 41 miles away, and the patient is "ready" to be transported at the time the helicopter is dispatched.[18,20] The effective radius for helicopter transport shrinks to as little as 20 miles, if only 5 minutes of extrication remain at the time of helicopter dispatch.[20] Many air-medical transports occur within 25 miles of the helicopter base and trauma center and are felt to be justified from a time perspective.[10] Because air-medical responses may not begin at the same point to where the patient will be delivered, the response distance may be shorter or longer than the transport distance. When air-medical resources are geographically dispersed, additional timesavings are realized.[8,9]

Fixed-wing aircraft also speed transport to trauma centers. Compared to helicopters, fixed-wing aircraft offer the advantages of faster air speed, longer range, ability to fly in adverse weather conditions, and lower operating costs. Their major disadvantage is the need to land at an appropriate-sized airport, thus necessitating ground transport at each end of the patient transfer. When the response and transport distances are more than 100 nautical (air) miles, fixed-wing transport costs significantly less than helicopter transport.[21] Furthermore, when the fixed-wing aircraft can lift off in a timely manner, the total time required for the patient to reach the trauma center may be the same compared with a helicopter.[21] For this reason, fixed-wing aircraft may be preferred in remote areas. In parts of the Pacific Northwest, after initial stabilization at a level III trauma center, patient transport by fixed-wing aircraft may be only one half to one tenth the duration of ground transport.[22]

In metropolitan areas, aircraft offer few advantages in trauma transport. Except in rare circumstances, urban scene flights do not accelerate trauma center arrival.[23] In some cases air-medical services actually prolong prehospital time, especially when an efficient ground EMS system meets no unusual impediments.[7,15,17,18,23] Although helicopter use promotes delivery of the patient to a trauma center,[15,17] it is often the severity of a patient's injury that prompts helicopter activation.

Whether or not an air-medical service is directly affiliated with a trauma center, it should function as an integral part of the EMS and trauma care systems, especially for rural areas.[24] Air-medical service programs should function as extensions of trauma centers, and can profoundly affect the operation of the center.[25]

Effects on Mortality

Although transport time is crucial, it is not the only advantage of air-medical services.[26] Several studies suggest air transport may improve survival even in cases of prolonged prehospital time. However, in evaluating the literature comparing ground transport with air transport, it is important to realize that none of these studies are blinded or randomized. No trial has randomized trauma patients to helicopter or ground transport; differences in patient selection may have profoundly affected the outcome of published studies.

Baxt and Moody[14] compared the mortality of matched patients who sustained severe brain injuries and were transported to a trauma center by either a community advanced life support EMS system or a hospital-based medical helicopter. The mortality of the EMS-transported patients was 40%, whereas that of the helicopter-transported patients was 31%. Among survivors, morbidity was also less in the helicopter-transported group. These differences were found even though the EMS-transported patients arrived at the trauma center an average of 33 minutes *earlier* than the air-medical patients. However, the level of care available during transport was higher in the air-medical group. A physician and nurse staffed the helicopter, whereas paramedics staffed the EMS ambulances. Patients in the air-medical group had the advantage of airway control by endotracheal intubation, instead of esophageal obturator airway (EOA) as in the EMS group. Additional medications, such as mannitol, were also available in the helicopter. Thus the sophistication of the transport teams and their abilities to provide certain interventions may have influenced patient outcomes.

These same authors noted similar results in another evaluation of trauma patients transported from the scene by either ground EMS or medical helicopter. Baxt and Moody[12] compared the outcomes of 150 trauma patients in each group with a standard derived from the Trauma Score and Injury Severity Score (TRISS). For the ground EMS patient group, the mortality rate was actually higher than predicted. For the air-medical patient group, the mortality rate was 52% less than predicted. Ground EMS patients were injured predominantly in urban areas, whereas the air-medical patients were injured mostly in rural areas. Paramedics treated and transported the EMS group, whose average time from injury to arrival at the trauma center was 35 minutes. The air-medical group was initially treated by diverse first responders, followed by the physician/nurse helicopter staff, and arrived at the trauma center 58 minutes after their injuries occurred. However, because a physician was on the helicopter, the time to initial physician contact was similar for the two groups. If these results are valid, the air-medical service provided some advantage to its patients despite a prolonged prehospital time. This advantage applied mostly to the subset of severely injured patients.

In another large study, seven hospital-based air-medical programs compared their trauma patient mortality with a predicted standard. They used the TRISS methodology to compare the actual outcomes with predicted outcomes of 1273 adult trauma patients transported by helicopter directly from the scene.[27-29] Overall, the air-medical programs had a 21% lower mortality rate than expected.[30] Patients whose predicted probability of survival was less than 75% benefited the most. However, the precise factors that reduced mortality remained unclear.

Additional evaluations of the effectiveness of air-medical services have found similar results. In North Carolina, patients with Trauma Scores between 5 and 10 had an 82.8% survival when transported by helicopter directly from the scene, compared with a 53.5% survival for those patients transported by ground EMS.[31] The time intervals from injury to arrival at the trauma center were similar in the two groups, but the air-medical group was more likely to receive endotracheal intubation, larger volumes of resuscitation fluid, and blood transfusions.

In many areas of the country, EMS helicopters respond directly to the scene. In rural areas a helicopter can transport a patient to a trauma center in the same time it takes a ground ambulance to arrive at a community hospital. Although air-medical services provide a survival advantage for many trauma patients, the greatest benefit occurs when a patient is brought directly from the scene to a trauma center.[32]

Contrary to the studies discussed earlier, several studies show little advantage of helicopter transport over ground transport of trauma patients. Brathwaite et al[33] compared 15,938 helicopter-transported patients with 6473 ground-transported patients and found that the estimated odds of survival were not affected by helicopter transport. Cunningham et al[34] reviewed 1346 helicopter-transported patients with 17,144 ground-transported patients; all patients were taken directly from the scene to the trauma center. Although there was a tendency towards increased survival among helicopter-transported patients with higher injury severity scores, the great majority of patients transported by both ground and air had low injury severity measures. These studies suggest that a more defined and limited subset of patients be identified as appropriate candidates for air-medical transport.

The Flight Team

The sophistication of the air-medical flight crew improves care of trauma victims during transport. In general, air-medical personnel have more experience in caring for critical patients, whereas severely injured victims comprise only a small percentage of EMS transports. Furthermore, several states allow for medications and procedures by nurses and paramedics unavailable to ground EMS personnel.[35]

The most appropriate composition of air-medical crews is the subject of continuing controversy. In some cases experienced physicians add value to the air-medical flight crew. At their initiation, several hospital-based air-medical programs provided physicians as part of the regular flight team.[36-38] Baxt and Moody[36] noted that when a physician and nurse team staffed a medical helicopter, the mortality rate from blunt trauma was 35% less than predicted, whereas nurse/nurse teams achieved predicted mortality for their patients. However, as air-medical services have matured, these findings have not been reproduced.[39-41]

Flight physicians are more likely to make independent judgments,[38,42] which may lead to additional interventions for the patient.[41] However, physicians' technical skills alone rarely augment the proficiency of air-medical crews.[38,42] Furthermore, as flight nurses and paramedics gain experience, the proportion of missions to which a physician adds significant value decreases.[43] An analysis of procedures performed by flight nurses and physicians revealed few differences. Flight nurses who are routinely accompanied by qualified physicians may be less skilled in cricothyrotomy, endotracheal intubation, and pericardiocentesis than their counterparts who are not. However, when flight nurses work without an accompanying physician, they are able to perform most of the procedures a flight physician might perform, except central venous cannulation and saphenous vein cutdown.[44]

Evaluations of STAT MedEvac systems show that physician judgment made an important contribution in 22% to 25% of cases, including situations other than trauma.[38,42] When a physician is not part of the flight team, a communications system can connect the flight crew with a medical control physician. Currently only 11% of air-medical services routinely deploy flight physicians at least part of the time. The most common air-medical crew configuration is flight nurse/flight paramedic followed by flight nurse/flight nurse.

For a select group of seriously injured patients, air-medical transport rapidly expands the capabilities of the EMS and trauma systems.[32] It can quickly deliver expertise and equipment to the patient's side and expedite evacuation to a trauma center. Its benefits, however, come with limitations.

DISADVANTAGES OF AIR-MEDICAL TRANSPORT

There are three principal disadvantages associated with utilizing air-medical services to transport trauma victims. These disadvantages relate to logistical considerations, safety, and cost.

Logistics

The task of summoning an EMS helicopter to the scene of a trauma victim can be complex. The ability to communicate among EMS and public safety officials at the scene, their communications center(s), the air-medical service communications center, and the responding helicopter is paramount. The first step is notification of the air-medical service. At the communication center, calls for service arrive by telephone or radio. The communications personnel must determine the location to which a helicopter is to respond, assess the resources closest to the scene, and dispatch the appropriate aircraft. In some regions more than one air-medical service is available. It is the obligation of the air-medical service to determine the fastest way to deliver assistance, even if that entails coordination with another service. Scene location must be translated into information the pilot can use to navigate efficiently. Longitude and latitude can be obtained from charts or computer programs.

As the aircraft is being dispatched, it is important that its pilot remain unaware of particular details of the medical situation that might influence the decision to attempt the mission. From a pilot's perspective, such flight decisions should be made based on current and predicted weather conditions in the area and the known capabilities of the aircraft. The pilot must not choose to fly based on patient factors, such as an injured child or other tragic circumstance. Changing weather conditions or mechanical failure may cause a mission to be suspended, and a contingency plan should exist for getting the patient to the trauma center or other appropriate hospital. Pilots must not attempt to complete a transport in unsafe conditions.

The **visual flight rules (VFR)** under which most medical helicopters operate require the daytime visibility and cloud ceiling to be at or better than 1 mile and 500 feet, respectively. At nighttime, the visibility and ceiling must be at or better than 2 miles and 500 feet, respectively. Depending on local conditions, these parameters may be more restrictive. As helicopter and navigational technologies have improved, some medical helicopters operate under **instrument flight rules (IFR).** With the necessary equipment and training, the pilot can navigate under inclement conditions to fixed locations. These locations are usually airports, although **global positioning systems (GPS)** technology allows for other locations, including hospital helipads. Nevertheless, some weather restrictions remain, and helicopters cannot operate in all conditions.

Once an EMS helicopter is airborne, the need for coordination intensifies. The ability to provide the air-medical crew with updates regarding patient(s) condition is important. These updates allow them to make timesaving preparations while en route to the scene or referring hospital. When the response is to a scene, the helicopter must be able to communicate with the ground team to identify hazards and prepare the landing zone. At the landing zone, safety concerns take priority. Designated personnel must maintain a safe perimeter and control all approaches to the helicopter. These logistical considerations are also important when a helicopter lands at a hospital helipad.

Merely requesting a helicopter significantly increases the work for on-scene EMS, public safety workers, and the associated communications centers. Resources at the scene must be sufficient to coordinate the helicopter's arrival. This endeavor must not distract medical personnel from providing optimal patient care.

Safety

Weather is the greatest single factor in medical helicopter crashes. Unfortunately, the safety record of air-medical services within the United States is far from perfect. Helicopter EMS is inherently more dangerous than other routine helicopter operations. For the period 1982 to 1987, the overall accident rate for EMS helicopters in the United States was 11.7 per 100,000 hours of flight operations, compared with 6.7 per 100,000 hours for helicopter taxi services.[45] Accidents were defined as occurrences involving serious or fatal injury or extensive helicopter hull damage. A 1986 survey of 100 air-medical programs in the United States revealed that 14 had experienced a fatal crash during their existence, accounting for 42 deaths of crew members and patients.[46] From 1986 to 1988 there were 17 accidents among 173 air-medical services that transported approximately 308,000 patients.[47] Factors that lowered accident rates were high flight volume and pilots' abilities to change flight plans from VFR to IFR in deteriorating weather conditions.[47] Although 1989 to 1991 was a safer period, 10 deaths resulted from helicopter crashes during 1991 and 1992.[48] At least 10 more deaths occurred in 1997 and 1998.

Each tragic event reminds us that every request for an EMS helicopter places lives at risk. Strict adherence to safety standards is mandatory, both for people in the helicopter and people on the ground. During its first 16 years of operation the Maryland State Police Aviation Division experienced four helicopter crashes resulting in six fatalities. Subsequently, a training/safety section was developed within the division, and there were no crashes during the subsequent 13 years.[9]

One of the factors that undoubtedly contributes to the danger of air-medical transport is the necessity to land in unfamiliar, makeshift landing zones. Medical helicopters commonly land at fully certified, illuminated helipads, other predesignated landing zones, or make-shift landing zones at trauma scenes.[5] Illuminated helipads familiar to the pilot offer the safest option, and predesignated landing zones are the preferred alternative. Air-medical services designate these sites in conjunction with local EMS and public safety officials. Makeshift landing zones at the trauma scene present the greatest danger, and comprise 30% of medical helicopter responses.[2] Nearby hazards such as tall structures and high-tension wires menace the flight. At night, these structures are hidden and increase the risk during the most hazardous phases of flight: landing and takeoff. It is imperative that the personnel responsible for establishing the helicopter landing zone be familiar with its requirements, diligent about identifying all hazards, and reliable in communicating important information to the aircraft crew. Many air-medical services provide training for public safety personnel to help them perform these duties.

Cost

The cost of providing air-medical services is considerable. Maintaining an EMS helicopter base requires a significant investment. Depending on the specific type of helicopter, the qualifications of the air-medical crew (i.e., physician, nurse, paramedic), and the ability to achieve economies of scale, the fixed cost per year for operating an EMS helicopter can range from approximately 1.5 to 2 million dollars. Completing one additional transport adds relatively little to the overall costs. The incremental costs associated with each mission (i.e., fuel and aircraft maintenance expense) is approximately $800 and depends on the specific aircraft and distance traveled. Most of the expense associated with providing air-medical services is attributed simply to making them available.

APPROPRIATE UTILIZATION

Since the initial deployment of EMS helicopters for civilian use in the United States, there has been concern regarding their overuse. An evaluation of a U.S. Army air-medical unit revealed that helicopter use saved approximately 48 minutes compared with ground ambulance. However, only 33% of patients directly benefited from air transport.[49] Most patients flown had neither a true medical nor surgical emergency. Among transports to a trauma center, use of a helicopter was essential or helpful for 23%, and not a factor for 57%.[50,51] Patients likely to benefit from air-medical transport had lower trauma scores and Glasgow Coma Scale scores.

One approach to determining appropriate EMS helicopter use is the number and type of interventions required during transport. The Therapeutic Intervention Scoring System serves this purpose.[52] Among all medical helicopter flights, approximately 42% (range 29% to 53%[53,54]) are appropriate by virtue of the intensity of care required during transport, trauma score, or physiologic scores. An additional one third of flights have 50% probability of being appropriate. In one evaluation involving six air-medical service programs, 54% of all trauma patients, including 49% of scene response patients, were critical and appropriate for medical helicopter use.[54]

Both the Association of Air-Medical Services and the National Association of EMS Physicians have developed criteria for appropriately using air-medical services, including for cases of trauma.[55,56] They indicate that a helicopter scene response may be justified if there is evidence of critical injuries by virtue of an objective score, certain anatomic injuries, or physiologic derangement. Other considerations include a serious mechanism of injury; difficulty in accessing the patient by ground; and a significant decrease in transport time.[55,56] Presence of abnormal vital signs increases the specificity and is 98% sensitive in identifying patients appropriate for triage to a trauma center. When the helicopter saves more than 20 minutes or the scene is otherwise inaccessible, then its use is also justified.[57] A scoring system in the field might add unnecessary complexity to the task of identifying patients who need to be transported to a trauma center, whether by helicopter or not.[57]

Certain patients, despite the obvious severity of their injuries, are not appropriate for air-medical transport. When a patient is nonsalvageable, helicopter evacuation serves no purpose, and exposes people to the risk of flying and working around the operating aircraft. For example, patients who suffer blunt cardiac arrest at the scene will not survive, regardless of means of transport.[58,59] In these cases, helicopter use cannot be justified.

Interfacility Transport

Interfacility air-medical transport is often indicated when trauma patients are initially stabilized at a community hospital and require transfer to a trauma center. Criteria similar to those for appropriate scene responses apply to interfacility transports as well. The use of a helicopter or fixed-wing aircraft is justified when there is an urgent need for a trauma center, and air-medical transport results in significant timesaving. Their use is also reasonable when the level of care required by the patient is available from the air-medical service, but not from ground transport systems.

When hospitals are more than 25 miles apart, helicopters save significant time. Using the TRISS methodology to predict survival, one study found a 25% reduction in expected mortality when trauma patients were transported between distant hospitals by helicopter instead of by ground.[60] This effect predominated among patients with a probability of survival less than 0.9%. Additionally, trauma patients transported up to 800 miles by helicopter or fixed-wing aircraft, after stabilization at a level III trauma center, experience outcomes similar to trauma patients within a metropolitan area.[61]

The effects of transporting trauma patients first to a community hospital, followed by transfer to a trauma center, remains unclear. Some data suggests that trauma patients transported by helicopter directly to the trauma center may experience slightly better outcomes.[62] However, initial transfer of a trauma patient from the scene to a community hospital is appropriate in many cases. Transfer to a community hospital is indicated when stabilization is urgently required and the local hospital has adequate resources to intervene.

Local stabilization is also indicated if the ground transport time to the community hospital is significantly shorter than the time a helicopter requires to transport the patient directly to the trauma center. Additionally, the need for transfer to a trauma center might not be evident until an emergency physician at a local hospital evaluates the patient.

Unfortunately, evaluation of trauma patients in an ED is associated with significant delays in transfer. One study indicated that an average of 70 minutes elapsed between arrival at a community hospital and the initial request for a helicopter. It was only 34 minutes for children less than 16 years old.[63]

Emergency physicians and others involved in preparing trauma patients for interhospital transfer should prepare the patient for flight. As many as one third of air-medical interfacility transfer patients require interventions by the flight crew before they can be safely evacuated. The need to perform these tasks, such as endotracheal intubation, central venous cannulation, and thoracostomy, increases the medical helicopter's ground time by as much as 84%.[64] In general, the priorities in preparing patients for air-medical transport are airway control, treatment of known pneumothoraces, and intravenous access if possible. Therefore plans for air-medical service utilization to evacuate trauma patients should include a standardized approach for assessing their suitability and preparing them for transport.

Despite objective measures of injury severity, it is not always clear who will benefit from air-medical transport. Analyses of appropriateness have evaluated data available retrospectively. The challenge is to prospectively identify those factors that improve survival.[4] If the patient does not require the immediate services of a trauma center or the specialized interventions of the flight team, then a medical helicopter may be unnecessary.

CLINICAL CONSIDERATIONS

Air transport personnel face several major challenges when caring for a seriously injured patient aboard an aircraft. Some challenges are best managed if the flight crew prepares both the helicopter and the patient before flight.

Organization and Aircraft Design

Organization within the helicopter is essential. The majority of medical helicopters in the United States furnish close quarters. Space is at a premium, and the medical interior is carefully designed. With the patient and necessary equipment on board, there is little room for maneuvering. Furthermore, if the flight crew is appropriately restrained, necessary equipment must be within easy reach. The flight team must arrange intravenous lines, blood pressure cuffs, pulse oximetry probes, and airway equipment for ready use. Aircraft design may pose obstacles to care during transport. For example, the ability to perform effective CPR varies by aircraft.[65] Except for obtaining intravenous access and administering emergency treatment, the helicopter should be the location of last resort for initiating new therapy or performing important procedures.

Flight Physiology

Routinely, medical helicopter missions are completed within 2500 feet above ground level. Thus the spectrum of issues related to flight physiology does not usually come into play. For example, with an altitude change of 2000 feet, a patient's oxygen requirement increases by only approximately 8%. Air-filled spaces will also increase their volumes by approximately 8%. Nevertheless, all trauma patients should receive supplemental oxygen while being transported. If adequate oxygenation cannot be achieved at ground level, the situation will only worsen at altitude. When pneumothorax is present, the crew or transferring physician should place a chest tube before transport. Without a chest tube, the potential for expansion resulting from the primary injury and difficulty in continually assessing breath sounds create a dangerous situation.

Flight physiology concerns become greater during fixed-wing transport and in helicopters flying in IFR conditions. The ability to maintain a specific cabin pressure is a function of a particular aircraft's design. Depending on the distance of the flight and the type of aircraft being used, a pressurized medical fixed-wing aircraft will be able to maintain a cabin altitude of 1000 to 5000 feet. Helicopters flying in IFR conditions are typically at altitudes in the range of 5000 feet. At such altitudes the atmospheric pressure can significantly expand air-filled spaces (e.g., pneumothorax, gastric distention, pneumatic antishock garments [PASG], IV fluid bags, endotracheal tube cuffs). Pneumatic antishock garments may expand and increase muscle compartment pressures. Patients who have suffered SCUBA diving accidents (dysbarism) may also decompensate. Altitude will also increase oxygen requirements and decrease ambient temperature.

Airway

As in every other aspect of trauma care, airway control is paramount for patients transported by helicopter. The threshold for securing an adequate airway via endotracheal intubation must be lowered for such patients. Engine noise hampers the ability to perform ongoing physical assessments. Breath sounds are drowned out, even with the aid of an amplified stethoscope.[66] Blood pressures are hard to auscultate, and vibrations render pulses difficult to palpate.[67] Thus the flight crew must rely on visual cues, including the patient's appearance, cardiac monitor, noninvasive blood pressure monitor, and pulse oximeter. Whenever there is doubt regarding the security of a patient's airway, the prudent course is to perform endotracheal intubation under the most controlled circumstances. The helicopter is not such a place. Once loaded in the aircraft, the adult patient is usually not easily repositioned. In many medical helicopters, the patient's head rests on the stretcher between a caregiver's legs. Although intubation has certainly been accomplished under these conditions, they are far from ideal. Patients with borderline airways should be intubated *before* boarding the helicopter.

The Combative Patient

The combative patient presents another dilemma. Agitation is multifactorial, but always presents a safety risk. Unlike a ground ambulance, which can stop and pull off the road if a situation gets out of control, a helicopter cannot "pull over." The potential for a patient to injure himself or herself or a crewmember, damage the aircraft, or distract the pilot is real and catastrophic. Sedating agents can be useful, but time and care are required for titration. Furthermore, over-sedation may depress respirations—a dangerous situation during transport. Thus some patients are best managed by sedation, chemical paralysis, and intubation.

CONCLUSION

In the opening scenario regarding the blunt trauma arrest, helicopter transport is unnecessary; the patient will not survive. Medics should be instructed to either pronounce the patient in the field if permitted by local regulations or transport the patient by ground to the trauma center.

Air-medical services rapidly transport severely injured patients, and increase access to trauma centers. The utility of an air-medical service depends both on the urgent need for a trauma center and the expertise of the flight team. These considerations vary with locality. Although criteria for air-medical service utilization have been proposed, each EMS system and community hospital should adjust them to accommodate their particular situation. Plans should standardize ways to request air-medical response, coordinate a helicopter's or fixed-wing aircraft's arrival, and prepare a patient for transport.

Emergency physicians must become familiar with air-medical services and their appropriate utilization. To continuously improve care, medical directors must audit flight team performance. Only under these circumstances can air-medical transport become an effective tool to reduce trauma-related morbidity and mortality.

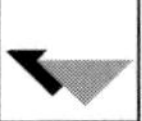

PEARLS & PITFALLS

- Advantages of air-medical transport include speed and the ability to overcome geographic obstacles.
- Flight crews may have more experience, medications, and procedural skills available than EMS ground units. Air transport is more effective when the incident occurs 20 or more miles from a trauma center. Do not transport the dead or victims of blunt trauma arrest by aircraft.
- The transferring hospital should:
  —Request the air-medical unit as soon as need for transfer recognized
  —Intubate patients with borderline airways (i.e., patients with a high probability of losing the ability to maintain their airways)
  —Place chest tubes in patients with known pneumothoraces
  —Obtain intravenous access
  —Immobilize the spine (if indicated)
  —Comply with federal transfer regulations (EMTALA)
  —Contact the trauma center, fill out paperwork, send medical records and radiographs
  —Provide blood for transport
  —Compress pelvic fractures (pneumatic anti-shock garment, "bean-bag" splint, towel wrap)
  —Sedate or intubate combative patients

REFERENCES

1. National Academy of Sciences, National Research Council: *Accidental death and disability: the neglected disease of modern society,* Washington, DC, 1966, National Academy Press.
2. Rau W, Lathrop G: 1998 Transport statistics and fees survey, *Air Med* 4:19-22, 1998.
3. Macnab AJ: Air-medical transport: "Hot Air" and a French lesson, *J Air Med Transport* 11:15-18, 1992.

4. Gabram SG, Jacobs LM: The impact of emergency medical helicopters on prehospital care, *Emerg Med Clin North Am* 8:85-102, 1990.
5. Jacobs LM, Bennett B: A critical care helicopter system in trauma, *J Natl Med Assoc* 81:1157-1167, 1989.
6. Neel S: Army aeromedical evacuation procedures in Vietnam:implications for rural America, *JAMA* 204:309-313, 1968.
7. Felix WR Jr: Metropolitan aeromedical service: state of the art, *J Trauma* 16:873-881, 1976.
8. Cowley RA, et al: An economical and proved helicopter program for transporting the emergency critically ill and injured patient in Maryland, *J Trauma* 13:1029-1038, 1973.
9. Cowley RA, Gretes AJ: Providing safe med-evac helicopter transport: Maryland's 18-year experience, *Md Med J* 37:521-524, 1988.
10. Cleveland HC, et al: A civilian air emergency service: a report of its development, technical aspects, and experience, *J Trauma* 16: 452-463, 1976.
11. Moylan JA: Impact of helicopters on trauma care and clinical results, *Ann Surg* 208:673-678, 1988.
12. Baxt WG, Moody P: The impact of a rotorcraft aeromedical emergency care service on trauma mortality, *JAMA* 249:3047-3051, 1983.
13. Cales RH, Trunkey DD: Preventable trauma deaths: a review of trauma care systems development, *JAMA* 254:1059-1063, 1985.
14. Baxt WG, Moody P: The impact of advanced prehospital emergency care on the mortality of severely brain-injured patients, *J Trauma* 27:365-369, 1987.
15. Burney RE, Fischer RP: Ground versus air transport of trauma victims: medical and logistical considerations, *Ann Emerg Med* 15:1491-1495, 1986.
16. Freilich DA, Spiegel AD: Aeromedical emergency trauma services and mortality reduction in rural areas, *NY State J Med* 90:358-365, 1990.
17. Schiller WR, et al: Effect of helicopter transport of trauma victims on survival in an urban trauma center, *J Trauma* 28:1127-1134, 1988.
18. Smith JS, et al: When is air-medical service faster than ground transportation? *Air Med J* 258-261, August 1993.
19. Spaite DW, et al: A new model for evaluating the impact of major system changes on emergency air-medical scene responses in a regional EMS system, *Prehosp Disast Med* 7:19-23, 1992.
20. Peckler S, Rogers R: Air versus ground transport from the trauma scene: optimal distance for helicopter utilization, *J Air Med Transport* 8:44, 1989.
21. Thomas F, et al: Outcome, transport times, and costs of patients evacuated by helicopter versus fixed-wing aircraft, *West J Med* 153:40-43, 1990.
22. Sharar SR, et al: Air transport following surgical stabilization: an extension of regionalized trauma care, *J Trauma* 28:794-798, 1988.
23. Fischer RP, et al: Urban helicopter response to the scene of injury, *J Trauma* 24:946-951, 1984.
24. Law DK, et al: Trauma operating room in conjunction with an air ambulance system: indications, interventions, and outcomes, *J Trauma* 22:759-765, 1982.
25. Schwab CW, et al: The impact of an air ambulance system on an established trauma center, *J Trauma* 25:580-586, 1985.
26. Rhee KJ, et al: Trauma Score change during transport: is it predictive of mortality? *Am J Emerg Med* 5:353-356, 1987.
27. Champion HR, et al: The major trauma outcome study: establishing national norms for trauma care, *J Trauma* 30:1356-1365, 1990.
28. Champion HR, et al: Trauma score, *Crit Care Med* 9:672-676, 1981.
29. Copes WS, et al: The injury severity score revisited, *J Trauma* 28:69-77, 1988.
30. Baxt WG, et al: Hospital-based rotorcraft aeromedical emergency care services and trauma mortality: a multicenter study, *Ann Emerg Med* 14:859-864, 1985.
31. Moylan JA, et al: Factors improving survival in multisystem trauma patients, *Ann Surg* 207:679-685, 1988.
32. Champion HR: Helicopters in emergency trauma care, *JAMA* 249:3074-3075, 1983.
33. Brathwaite CE, et al: A critical analysis of on-scene helicopter transport on survival in a statewide trauma system, *J Trauma* 45:140-144, 1998.
34. Cunningham P, et al: A comparison of the association of helicopter and ground ambulance transport with the outcome of injury in trauma patients transported from the scene, *J Trauma* 43:940-946, 1997.
35. Delbridge TR, Verdile VP, Platt TE: Variability of state-approved emergency medical services drug formularies, *Prehosp Disast Med* 9:S55, 1994.
36. Baxt WG, Moody P: The impact of a physician as part of the aeromedical prehospital team in patients with blunt trauma, *JAMA* 257:3246-3250, 1987.
37. Duke JH Jr, Clarke WP: A university-staffed, private hospital-based air transport service: the initial two-year experience, *Arch Surg* 116:703-708, 1981.
38. Rhee KJ, et al: Is the flight physician needed for helicopter emergency medical services? *Ann Emerg Med* 15:174-177, 1986.
39. Burney RE, et al: Variation in air-medical outcomes by crew composition: a two-year follow-up, *Ann Emerg Med* 25:187-192, 1995.
40. Burney RE, et al: Comparison of aeromedical crew performance by patient severity and outcome, *Ann Emerg Med* 21:375-378, 1992.
41. Hamman BL, et al: Helicopter transport of trauma victims: does a physician make a difference? *J Trauma* 31:490-494, 1991.
42. Snow N, Hull C, Severns J: Physician presence on a helicopter emergency medical service: necessary or desirable? *Aviat Space Environ Med* 57:1176-1178, 1986.
43. Schwartz RJ, Jacobs LM, Lee M: The role of the physician in a helicopter EMS system, *Prehosp Disast Med* 5:31-37, 1990.
44. Thomas F, Clemmer TP, Orme JF: A survey of advanced trauma life support procedures being performed by physicians and nurses used on hospital aeromedical evacuation services, *Aviat Space Environ Med* 56:1213-1215, 1985.
45. Rhee KJ, et al: A comparison of emergency medical helicopter accident rates in the United States and the Federal Republic of Germany, *Aviat Space Environ Med* 61:750-752, 1990.
46. Carter GL, et al: Safety and helicopter-based programs, *Ann Emerg Med* 15:1117-1118,1986.
47. Low RB, et al: Factors associated with the safety of EMS helicopters, *Am J Emerg Med* 9:103-106, 1991.
48. Mikat A: Air-medical safety: paying the price, *J Air Med Transport* 11:26-30, 1992.
49. Reddick EJ: Evaluation of the helicopter in aeromedical transfers, *Aviat Space Environ Med* 50:168-170, 1979.
50. Urdaneta LF, et al: Role of an emergency helicopter transport service in rural trauma, *Arch Surg* 122:992-996, 1987.
51. Urdaneta LF, et al: Evaluation of an emergency air transport service as a component of a rural EMS system, *Am Surg* 50:183-188, 1984.
52. Savitsky E, Rodenberg H: Prediction of the intensity of patient care in prehospital helicopter transport: use of the revised trauma score, *Aviat Space Environ Med* 66:11-14, 1995.

53. Burney RE, et al: Evaluation of hospital-based aeromedical transport programs using therapeutic intervention scoring, *Aviat Space Environ Med* 59:563-566, 1988.
54. Rhee KJ, et al: Differences in air ambulance patient mix demonstrated by physiologic scoring, *Ann Emerg Med* 19:552-556, 1990.
55. Air-medical Services Committee of the National Association of Emergency Medical Services Physicians: Air-medical dispatch: guidelines for scene response, *Prehosp Disast Med* 7:75-78, 1992.
56. Association of Air-medical Services: Position paper on the appropriate use of emergency air-medical services, *J Air Med Transport* 9:29-33, 1990.
57. Rhodes M, et al: Field triage for on-scene helicopter transport, *J Trauma* 26:963-969,1986.
58. Lindbeck GH, Groopman DS, Powers RD: Aeromedical evacuation of rural victims of nontraumatic cardiac arrest, *Ann Emerg Med* 22:1258-1262, 1993.
59. Wright SW, et al: Aeromedical transport of patients with post-traumatic cardiac arrest, *Ann Emerg Med* 18:721-726, 1989.
60. Boyd CR, Corse KM, Campbell RC: Emergency interhospital transport of the major trauma patient: air versus ground, *J Trauma* 29:789-793, 1989.
61. Valenzuela TD, et al: Critical care air transportation of the severely injured: does long distance transport adversely affect survival? *Ann Emerg Med* 19:169-172, 1990.
62. Jacobs LM, et al: A three-year report of the medical helicopter transportation system of Connecticut, *Conn Med* 53:703-710, 1989.
63. Garrison HG, Benson NH, Whitley TW: Helicopter use by rural emergency departments to transfer trauma victims: a study of time-to-request intervals, *Am J Emerg Med* 7:384-386, 1989.
64. Leicht MJ, et al: Rural interhospital helicopter transport of motor vehicle trauma victims: causes for delays and recommendations, *Ann Emerg Med* 15:450-453, 1986.
65. Thomas SH, Stone CK, Bryan-Berge D: The ability to perform closed-chest compressions in helicopters, *Am J Emerg Med* 12: 296-298, 1994.
66. Hunt RC, et al: Inability to assess breath sounds during air-medical transport by helicopter, *JAMA* 265:1982-1984, 1991.
67. Low RB, Martin D: Accuracy of blood pressure measurements made aboard helicopters, *Ann Emerg Med* 17:604-612, 1988.

Prehospital Approach to Common Difficult Scenarios

5

JON APFELBAUM

Prehospital providers must often deal with situations in which they are potentially open for liability. One such instance occurs when the decision is made to bypass nearby community hospitals to take injured patients directly to a more distant trauma center. Another circumstance arises when a patient refuses medical care after prehospital personnel arrive at the scene. In the latter instance, documentation of the patient's level of competence, factoring in common confounding variables such as head injury or alcohol intoxication, is crucial in protecting the prehospital personnel from potential litigation. In either case, the prehospital personnel should always act in the patient's best interest, using clinical judgment and weighing in the resources of the surrounding hospitals.

TRAUMA TRIAGE PROTOCOLS AND PITFALLS

Teaching Case

At 2:57 AM on a Sunday morning, your local emergency medical service (EMS) squad is called to a scene where a 27-year-old male struck a tree with his motorcycle. He was traveling at a high rate of speed and was not wearing a helmet. His obvious injuries include massive facial trauma, chest contusions, and an angulated left leg. His vital signs are a systolic blood pressure of 80 by palpation, a pulse of 128 beats per minute (bpm), and a respiratory rate of 28 with poor air movement. Physical findings include an open mandibular fracture; decreased breath sounds on his right side; a tense and tender abdomen; and an apparently fractured left femur. He also smells strongly of alcohol. After properly immobilizing him with a cervical collar and a long spinal board, he is loaded into the ambulance. En route to the regional level I trauma center airway support is maintained, two large-bore intravenous lines are established, a fluid bolus is initiated, and his leg is splinted using Hare traction. The transport time is 17 minutes. Two other hospitals are bypassed on the way to the level I center. The patient subsequently requires operative intervention, has a prolonged hospital course, and is discharged to a rehabilitation facility with extensive neurologic deficits. The patient's family brings a lawsuit against your agency, claiming that care was delayed because of bypassing other facilities, which therefore contributed to his poor outcome.

What Are the Components of Prehospital Trauma Triage?

The decision that a patient requires a trauma center is based on physiologic abnormalities, anatomic criteria, mechanism of injury, and the medical provider's clinical suspicion.[1] The patient's associated medical conditions may also play a factor. The ideal trauma triage system identifies patients who require rapid transport to a dedicated trauma center. It is estimated that the incidence of major trauma requiring a trauma center is approximately 1000 patients per 1 million people per year (~250,000 patients/year), or about 5% to 7% of the 3.6 million patients hospitalized annually for trauma.[2]

Over-triage is defined as sending low-risk patients to a trauma center. **Under-triage** means transporting seriously injured patients to a hospital that is not dedicated to trauma. Over-triaging increases the trauma center volume and may dilute the resources available to other victims, whereas under-triaging leaves critical trauma patients without the resources of a dedicated center.

What Are the Scoring Systems for Field Triage?

Anatomic criteria, physiologic abnormalities, mechanism of injury, and the medical provider's clinical suspicion form the basis for a variety of scoring systems.

Scoring Systems

ANATOMIC

The **Abbreviated Injury Scale (AIS)** and the **Injury Severity Scale (ISS)** are based on anatomic criteria. Both of these scales were developed to evaluate outcomes and are not practical for prehospital use. Most applicable anatomic criteria are based on clinically apparent injuries, such as:[1,3,4]

- Penetrating trauma to head, neck, trunk, or proximal extremities
- Flail chest
- Amputation proximal to wrist or ankle
- Two or more proximal long bone fractures
- Pelvic fracture
- Paralysis or neurologic deficit
- Burn >10% of total body surface area or with inhalation injury

PHYSIOLOGIC

Physiologic scoring systems incorporate the patient's vital signs and clinical condition. Various scoring systems have been developed that include components of the following:[1,3-5]

- Blood pressure
- Heart rate
- Capillary refill time
- Respiratory rate
- Glasgow Coma Scale (GCS)
- Abdominal examination

MECHANISM OF INJURY AND SITUATIONAL

Mechanism of injury implies that an event with a significant energy transfer confers a greater risk of injury. Such situations may include:[1,3,4]

- Death of same car occupant
- Fall of >15 feet
- Pedestrian struck at greater than 5 to 10 miles per hour (mph) or run over
- Ejection from vehicle
- Prolonged extrication
- Vehicle rollover
- Motorcycle or bicycle crash at >20 mph or with ejection
- Automobile deformity with >12 to 20 inches of intrusion
- Age <12 or >60
- Environmental extremes
- Co-morbid serious medical problems
- Intoxication
- Pregnancy

COMBINED

Research has determined that the combination of certain aspects of these scoring systems might provide a more useful tool for prehospital trauma triage. Champion et al[6] devised the **triage index** through retrospective analysis of trauma patients and subsequently developed the **trauma score (TS)**.[7] The TS consists of the GCS, capillary refill, systolic blood pressure, respiratory rate, and respiratory expansion. In 1989 the TS became the **revised trauma score (RTS)**, incorporating the GCS, respiratory rate, and systolic blood pressure.[8] In 1982 the **CRAMS** scale was introduced[9]; it is composed of circulation, respiration, abdominal examination, motor, and speech. Both the CRAMS and the RTS are no more effective as triage tools as compared with the paramedic's clinical judgment.[1] To further differentiate the degree of severity in the field setting, the **prehospital index** was established in 1986.[10] This scoring system includes systolic blood pressure, heart rate, respiratory rate, and level of consciousness. Once again, it performs no better than clinical judgment.

Researchers hoped that incorporation of mechanism of injury would improve triage. Studies showed that the combination of CRAMS or TS with mechanism of injury aided recognition of serious trauma.[4,11] The 1990 American College of Surgeons Committee on Trauma field triage criteria initially assessed physiologic derangement, anatomic injury, mechanism of injury, and co-morbid factors.[12] This assessment was revised in 1993 to exclude mechanism of injury alone as a criteria for transport to a trauma center. At that time, they recommended on-line medical control to assist in trauma triage.

A combination of anatomic, physiologic, and mechanism factors, in conjunction with the prehospital provider's clinical judgement, is the best trauma triage tool currently available.

How Good Are These Systems?

All the current triage methods have about an 85% sensitivity and specificity for the need for trauma center care.[1,3] Medical systems try to minimize over- and under-triage. However, on balance, triage systems should protect patients and, when necessary, err on the side of over-triage. Although over-triaging patients stresses the resources of the trauma center, under-triaging risks inadequate care.

How Valid Is the Prehospital Medical Care Provider's Assessment of the Severity of Injury?

At this time, the EMS provider's "injury severity perception" remains as good as, if not better than, formal triage scoring systems.[1,3,5] However, this statement does not imply that formal triage criteria should not be used. The various scores may aid prehospital providers in making clinical decisions, as well as developing a method to review triage decisions. In addition, certain healthcare systems may have specialty centers for treating patients with specific injuries or conditions.

Is Bypassing Hospitals to Transport Seriously Injured Patients to Trauma Centers Associated with Worse Outcomes?

This question has not been fully answered. Multiple studies have shown the benefits of regional trauma centers.[13-18] However, few studies have analyzed the time from an injury to the arrival at the trauma center as it compares with survival. One study showed that bypassing other hospitals in favor of a trauma center adds an average of 3 minutes to the transport time in an *urban* setting.[19] Patient outcomes were not adversely affected by this short delay. However, the issue of extended transport times, such as bypassing rural hospitals to go directly to an urban trauma center, has not been studied. The benefits of trauma center transport appear to outweigh the risks of bypassing the nearest hospital. However, there may be benefits in going to the nearest hospital initially if the patient requires immediate lifesaving interventions, such as endotracheal intubation, chest tube insertion, or replacement of blood products.

How Does Involving a Physician Change the Triage Process?

Involving an on-line physician in the triage process improves the system. Physician input can decrease over- or under-triage.[2,5,11] The 1993 American College of Surgeons' Committee on Trauma criteria advocates on-line medical control to assist with the trauma triage decision.[11] A detailed discussion of on-line medical command occurs in Chapter 2.

What Are Some Other Factors Involved in the Triage Decision-Making Process?

Local politics, economic impact, and hospital resources can all factor, indirectly or directly, into the destination choice. Triage decisions may place the prehospital personnel in a hostile environment and under significant pressure.[1]

Bypassed community hospitals may feel medically affronted and financially slighted. The prehospital personnel should not have to contend with political issues when faced with a hypotensive patient; a triage policy developed in conjunction with regional hospitals may avoid such pitfalls. Patient care is improved by adoption and compliance with physician-directed prehospital trauma triage.

Economic factors have a profound impact on trauma systems. Los Angeles County + University of Southern California (LAC+USC) Medical Center was on the verge of closing in 1995. This situation was in part caused by their financial losses maintaining one of the busiest trauma centers in the United States.[20] A high volume of patients sustaining penetrating trauma and a population that tends to be uninsured or under-insured may be the main reason for the financial difficulties. To maintain a viable trauma system, planners (not the individual medic caring for a gunshot victim) must weigh community resources to balance excellent care with prudent distribution of patients.[21]

REFUSAL OF PREHOSPITAL CARE

Teaching Case

Paramedics are called to the scene of a motor vehicle crash at 10 PM on a Friday night. A 35-year-old male drove his car into a telephone pole at approximately 40 mph. He was apparently unrestrained; medics note a starred windshield and bent steering wheel. He is bleeding from a cut on his forehead, walking around his vehicle inspecting the damage, and cursing. He is markedly ataxic and smells strongly of alcohol. He refuses their offer of medical attention and transport. After consulting with medical control by radio and the on-scene police, the medics take the patient against his will to the hospital for further evaluation in full spinal immobilization. En route the patient is verbally abusive and threatens to sue "everyone."

■

Can Patients Refuse Medical Care, Even If It Is Not in Their Best Interest?

Lucid patients have the right to refuse medical care. The law states that a person has the right to choose what is, or is not, done to his or her body, even if refusing treatment entails grievous harm or death. The essential component is that the person must be of sound mind and able to understand the nature of the treatment offered, the alternatives, and the potential consequences of his or her refusal.[22,23]

The word "capable" is a medical term that describes a patient's ability to understand such considerations. Although most healthcare providers use the word "competent," it is best reserved for situations where a judge or magistrate renders a legal decision regarding a person's mental state.

A capable patient may exercise his or her right to autonomy and refuse even lifesaving therapy. In such a case, the prehospital personnel must document the patient's mental status and competency. They should discuss the treatment options, treatment alternatives, and risks of refusing care with the patient. An incapable patient cannot refuse medical care or observation. Clinically intoxicated or head-injured persons are unable to make informed decisions, and prehospital providers need to act in the patient's best interest.[24]

Can a Medical Provider be Held Liable for Transporting a Patient Against His or Her Will?

Yes, but a prehospital provider is more likely to be held responsible for allowing an incompetent patient to refuse care. Should the above patient die or suffer permanent disability, the bereaved family could claim gross negligence by the prehospital personnel. It is a "catch-22," where the medical providers can be accused of wrongdoing no matter which choice they make. The three central principles that guide situations regarding refusal of care are:

1. Act in the patient's best interest
2. Act within the protocols and policies defined by the parent EMS agency
3. Appropriately document the encounter

When the individual described in the above scenario brought a lawsuit against the EMS providers, appropriate documentation provided the best defense. Because the patient was not capable because of intoxication and head injury, the prehospital providers appropriately transported him against his will, and documented their reasons. Principles of acceptable legal medical care typically follow good medical care and concern for the patient's health and rights.[24] As such, acting in the patient's best interest is the optimal "rule-of-thumb" policy.

What Should the Prehospital Provider Do When Faced with a Patient Who Refuses Care?

When faced with this dilemma, the EMS provider must perform a mental status examination to determine the patient's competence. The examination should involve several factors:

1. Is the patient oriented to person, place, and time?
2. Does the patient appear to understand the care offered?
3. Does the patient understand the alternatives and the potential consequences of refusal?

If the patient is oriented, not clinically intoxicated, and appears to understand the above issues, he or she is presumed to be competent to refuse care. However, patients who have just attempted suicide cannot refuse transport. Also, patients who appear clinically intoxicated, despite being oriented to person, place, or time, should still be transported for evaluation if potential for serious injury exists.

Certainly, allowing a competent patient to refuse transport may pose medical risks to the patient (and if a bad outcome occurs, legal risk to the medical personnel). Among those who refuse care, at least 30% do not recall the potential risks of refusing care.[25]

Several alternatives exist to minimize the risk involved with refusal of care. Prehospital providers should involve the on-line medical control physician. Having a physician discuss the need for EMS transport with the patient via radio or cellular phone increases the likelihood that a patient will agree to treatment.[26,27] Current recommendations suggest that prehospital providers use all available methods to convince patients who appear seriously injured to consent to transport.[23] Police presence on-scene may also aid the prehospital providers in dealing with difficult patients.

What Are the Risks of Lawsuits Against Prehospital Providers?

The single largest legal risk faced by EMS providers is the failure to treat or transport a patient requesting care. Nontransport, or delayed transport, accounts for 34% to 90% of litigation directed at EMS providers.[25,28,29] In systems where paramedics can initiate refusal of care, errors in triage may occur in up to 20% of cases. In the same study, 90% of patients who expressed dissatisfaction with EMS providers had previously been refused care. Perceived indifference or hostility by the medical provider is associated with litigation.[25] Failure to provide appropriate spinal immobilization is another cause of frequent lawsuits.

Other frequent sources of litigation include ambulance vehicle collisions, especially during emergency operations, and the failure of emergency equipment. Liability caused by equipment failure is difficult to defend if the malfunction is due to inadequate or incomplete maintenance. Recently, claims have been associated with increased demands for services in the presence of decreasing funding and resources. Overburdened, understaffed, and poorly equipped EMS systems are a "legal disaster."[22]

REFERENCES

1. Maslanka AM: Scoring systems and triage from the field, *Emerg Med Clin North Am* 11:15-27, 1993.
2. Champion HR, et al: The effect of medical direction on trauma triage, *J Trauma* 28:235-239, 1988.
3. Simmons E, et al: Paramedic injury severity perception can aid trauma triage, *Ann Emerg Med* 26:461-468, 1995.
4. Bond RJ, Kortbeek JB, Preshaw RM: Field trauma triage: combining mechanism of injury with the prehospital index for an improved trauma triage tool, *J Trauma* 43:283-287, 1997.
5. Blackwell TH: Prehospital care, *Emerg Med Clin North Am* 11:1-14, 1993.
6. Champion HR, et al: An anatomic index of injury severity, *J Trauma* 20:197-202, 1980.
7. Champion HR, et al: Trauma score, *Crit Care Med* 9:672-676, 1981.
8. Champion HR, et al: A revision of the Trauma Score, *J Trauma* 29:623-629, 1989.
9. Gormican SP: CRAMS scale: field triage of trauma victims, *Ann Emerg Med* 11:132-135, 1982.
10. Koehler JJ, et al: Prehospital index: a scoring system for field triage trauma victims, *Ann Emerg Med* 15:178-182, 1986.
11. Knudson P, Frecceri CA, DeLateur SA: Improving the field triage of major trauma victims, *J Trauma* 28:602-606, 1988.
12. Norcross ED, et al: Application of American College of Surgeons' field triage guidelines by prehospital personnel, *J Am Coll Surg* 181:539-544, 1995.
13. Shackford SR, et al: The effect of regionalization upon the quality of trauma care as assessed by concurrent audit before and after institution of a trauma system: a preliminary report, *J Trauma* 26:812-820, 1986.
14. Shackford, SR, et al: Impact of a trauma system on outcome of severely injured patients, *Arch Surg* 122:523-527, 1987.
15. West JG, Trunkey DD, Lim RC: Systems of trauma care: a study of two counties, *Arch Surg* 114:455-460, 1979.
16. Cales RH: Trauma mortality in Orange County: the effect of implementation of a regional trauma system, *Ann Emerg Med* 13:1-10, 1984.
17. West JG, Cales RH, Gazzaniga AB: Impact of regionalization: the Orange County experience, *Arch Surg* 118:740-744, 1983.
18. Teufel WL, Trunkey DD: Trauma centers: a pragmatic approach to need, cost, and staffing patterns, *J Am Coll Emerg Phys* 6:546-551, 1977.
19. Sloan EP, et al: The effect of urban trauma system hospital bypass on prehospital transport times and level 1 trauma patient survival, *Ann Emerg Med* 18:1146-1150, 1989.
20. Cornwell EE III, et al: Health care crisis from a trauma center perspective: the LA story, *JAMA* 276:940-944, 1996
21. Boyd DR: Trauma: a controllable disease in the 1980's (Fourth Annual Stone Lecture, American Trauma Society), *J Trauma* 20:14-24, 1980.
22. Ayres RJ Jr: Legal considerations in prehospital care, *Emerg Med Clin North Am* 11:853-867, 1993.
23. Burstein JL, et al: Outcome of patients who refused out-of-hospital medical assistance, *Am J Emerg Med* 14:23-26, 1996.
24. Siegel DM: Consent and refusal of treatment, *Emerg Med Clin North Am* 11:833-840, 1993.
25. Zachariah BS, et al: Follow-up and outcome of patients who declined or are denied transport by EMS, *Prehosp Disast Med* 7:359-364, 1992.
26. Alicandro J, et al: Impact of interventions for patients refusing emergency medical services transport, *Acad Emerg Med* 2:480-485, 1995.
27. Burstein JL, et al: Refusal of out-of-hospital medical care: effect of medical-control physician assertiveness on transport rate, *Acad Emerg Med* 5:4-8, 1998.
28. Shanaberger CJ: The sharing of responsibilities, *JEMS* 11:58-59, 1986.
29. Morgan DL, Wainscott MP, Knowles HC: Emergency medical services liability litigation in the United States: 1987-1992, *Prehosp Disast Med* 9:214-221, 1994.

PART TWO

RESUSCITATION

Priorities and Pitfalls in Trauma Management

6

STEPHEN A. COLUCCIELLO AND PETER C. FERRERA

Teaching Case

A 27-year-old third-trimester pregnant female on subcutaneous heparin is involved in a high-speed motor vehicle crash. She is obtunded and makes only slight respiratory effort. Her teeth are clenched, and she has markedly decreased breath sounds on the left. The initial blood pressure is 70/40 mmHg with a pulse of 130 beats per minute (bpm).

Without a word from you, the team leader, the nurses obtain intravenous (IV) access, apply supplemental oxygen, and cut off her clothes. In minutes, you have continuous data from pulse oximetry, automatic blood pressure, and cardiac monitors. While the nurses are busy, you perform a left-sided needle thoracentesis. With a rush of air, her blood pressure rises to 100/50 mmHg. You direct the nurses to elevate the backboard on the right, tilting her uterus to the left. The unit clerk places stat calls to the trauma surgeon, obstetrician, and neonatologist.

Neurologic examination reveals a Glasgow Coma Scale (GCS) score of 8, equal pupils at 4 mm, and no obvious hemiparesis. You intubate her orally after ascertaining she has a withdrawal response to pain in all four extremities. The nurse has already drawn up IV lidocaine, etomidate, and succinylcholine, and gives it on your command. You intubate her, apply an end-tidal CO_2 detector, and ascertain breath sounds. A thoracostomy tube placed in the left chest returns 400 cc of blood.

A secondary survey shows a left hemotympanum and large ecchymoses across her chest and abdomen. Her uterus is gravid and her pelvis unstable. Her left leg is shortened, and externally rotated. The nurses have run point-of-care (POC) labs and coagulation studies, placed an orogastric tube and Foley catheter, and have ordered type-specific blood at your direction. Fresh frozen plasma is also ordered to reverse the patient's coagulopathy. While the radiology technician is completing the chest, pelvis, and cervical spine films, the respiratory therapist places the patient on the ventilator, targeting her pCO_2 for eucapnia.

A chest radiograph shows the endotracheal and chest tubes in excellent position but demonstrates a left pulmonary contusion and a wide mediastinum. A pelvic radiograph shows an open-book fracture and a fetal skull fracture. Your bedside ultrasound shows free fluid in Morison's pouch and a fetal heart rate of 170 bpm. The nurses obtain a second IV line and report a BP of 80 systolic. They tell you that the urine is grossly bloody and report the initial values from the POC labs: hematocrit 28%, lactate 4.

You place additional calls to neurosurgery, orthopedics, and cardiothoracic services while you wrap the pelvis and place the left femur in a Hare traction splint, quickly rechecking the distal pulse. Tetanus toxoid is given.

The trauma surgeon arrives and you report your findings. You suggest immediate laparotomy, and advise the neurosurgeon to place an intraventricular pressure monitor during surgery. You also suggest an intraoperative transesophageal echocardiogram (TEE) to evaluate the aorta, while monitoring the baby with cardiotocography.

The trauma surgeon agrees. The nurses have already placed the patient on a transport monitor and O-negative blood is running under pressure. The patient and her escorts slip into the waiting elevator, and they are gone. ■

Although no single chapter can "sum up" trauma management in the emergency department (ED), a discussion of central principles is useful. This chap-

TABLE 6-1
Common Errors in Trauma Resuscitation: Blunt Trauma

CONDITION	ERROR
General	Failure to appreciate occult shock Failure to recognize high-risk patients (elderly, children, pregnant women) Failure to log-roll the patient Failure to examine the perineum
Hypotension	Failure to prioritize injuries Failure to quickly involve surgeon or initiate transfer Sending the hypotensive patient to CT scanner Delaying therapy or transfer for low-priority tests or interventions Failure to transfuse or delayed transfusion
Altered mental status	Failure to evaluate abdomen with CT, US, or DPL Failure to measure bedside glucose Failure to obtain CT scan of head Assuming alcohol is cause of altered mental status
Cervical injury	Failure to immobilize neck Failure to obtain adequate radiographs "Clearing" the neck of a comatose patient
Spinal injury	Failure to initiate high-dose steroid protocol for cord injury Assuming shock is due to cord injury rather than blood loss
Chest trauma	Failure to appreciate radiographic signs of aortic injury Failure to empirically treat tension pneumothorax Failure to appreciate radiographic signs of diaphragmatic rupture
Abdominal trauma	Relying on physical examination alone to evaluate the abdomen in a patient with altered mental status, multiple injuries, or who has been intubated Relying on physical examination alone to evaluate the abdomen during the second half of pregnancy, or in the patient with spinal cord injury
Pelvic trauma	Failure to compress pelvis with PASG or tight sheet in trauma room Failure to evaluate the abdomen for hemoperitoneum Failure to transfuse Delay in transfer to trauma center
Extremity trauma	Failure to immediately reduce fractures or dislocations that compromise distal circulation Failure to recognize compartment syndrome Failure to splint fractures
Pain	Failure to provide timely analgesia Failure to provide adequate analgesia

CT, Computed tomography; *US,* ultrasound; *DPL,* diagnostic peritoneal lavage; *PASG,* pneumatic anti-shock garment.

ter critically examines those precepts and addresses some common errors in ED resuscitations (Tables 6-1 and 6-2).

The successful management of the trauma patient depends on an organized approach to resuscitation. The familiar hierarchy of Airway, Breathing, and Circulation (ABCs) remains a useful starting point. However, the priorities in trauma management extend far beyond these fundamental precepts.

During the evaluation, the emergency physician (EP) must quickly determine the severity of injury and decide if transport to a trauma center is in the patient's best interest. The physician can often determine the need for trauma center transport based on the primary and secondary survey alone, without the need for extensive diagnostic testing. In many cases, an immediate "gestalt" regarding severity of illness is more important than an exhaustive enumeration of injuries.

Disposition often takes precedence over diagnosis. From the emergency medicine perspective, whether the patient has something as common as a ruptured spleen or as unusual as a gallbladder avulsion is immaterial. The key issue is recognition of a surgical emergency. Once the EP deals with life-threats such as airway compromise or tension pneumothorax, a

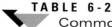

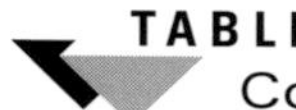
TABLE 6-2
Common Errors in Trauma Resuscitation: Penetrating Trauma

CONDITION	ERROR
General	Failure to examine the back Failure to look for injury in axilla or perineum Assuming bullets take a straight trajectory within the body Failure to appreciate that bullets that enter extremities may violate torso Failure to appreciate the occult injuries that may occur with the multiple pellets from a shotgun
Hypotension	Failure to quickly involve surgeon or initiate transfer Using CT to evaluate the hypotensive victim of penetrating trauma Delaying therapy or transfer for low-priority tests or interventions Failure to clinically detect and empirically treat tension pneumothorax
Head trauma	Failure to manage airway Failure to appreciate cranial violation in the conscious patient with a head wound
Cervical injury	Failure to appreciate violation of platysma Failure to involve surgeon when platysma is violated Failure to manage airway early and definitively if expanding hematoma
Chest trauma	Failure to empirically treat tension pneumothorax Failure to appreciate signs of pericardial tamponade Failure to appreciate diaphragm violation
Abdominal trauma	Relying on physical examination alone to evaluate the abdomen in a patient with altered mental status, multiple injuries, or who has been intubated. Use of CT to evaluate visceral injury (can be used in some experienced centers to evaluate isolated RUQ injuries and determine peritoneal violation)
Extremity trauma	Failure to measure arterial-brachial index Failure to give antibiotics for open joints or fractures

CT, Computed tomography; *RUQ,* right upper quadrant.

crucial question must be answered: "Does this patient need an operation (and if so, how quickly)?"

TRAUMA TEAM

Successful management of the injured patient depends on a well-organized team of physicians, nurses, and other personnel. The trauma response team should not be a peculiarity of a trauma center, but common to all EDs that treat injuries. The team composition and size depend on the institution. The number of personnel should also vary with patient acuity. A radio report from the prehospital providers allows EDs to determine the necessary initial response.

Larger teams are not necessarily more efficient than smaller teams.[1] However, several aspects remain consistent.

Team Captain

An experienced team captain is crucial to a well-run resuscitation.[2] Identify the captain before the patient arrives. In larger teams, the captain may refrain from performing resuscitative procedures that may distract from his or her supervisory role.

Horizontal Versus Vertical Resuscitation

Another important aspect of trauma care involves "horizontal" as opposed to "vertical" resuscitation. The horizontal approach involves multiple tasks performed *simultaneously* as opposed to sequentially. Trauma team performance is optimized when each team member completes his or her allocated task while other team members are performing theirs.[3]

Standard protocols empower nurses to start IVs, apply cardiac monitors, oxygen masks, noninvasive blood pressure cuffs, and draw blood all without specific direction by the trauma captain. The radiology technician would prepare to obtain a chest radiograph during this same period, while the examining physician is calling out the physical findings of the primary survey. Waiting to perform each task in sequence is less efficient.

Precautions

One important aspect of the trauma protocols is the use of barrier precautions for team members. However, compliance with these safety measures is spotty. The so-called "universal precautions" of gown, gloves, facial protection, and shoe covers are now termed *standard precautions*, perhaps because it is standard to ignore them. They are disregarded during at least one third of invasive trauma procedures.[4] The team captain should ensure compliance.

PRIMARY SURVEY AND RESUSCITATION

During the initial evaluation of the trauma patient, the trauma team must quickly address life-threats. Evaluation and resuscitation are simultaneous. The Advanced Trauma Life Support (ATLS) course sponsored by the American College of Surgeons emphasizes the hierarchy of Airway, Breathing, Circulation, Disability, and Exposure/Environment. Although the validity of this sequence has not been subject to scientific scrutiny, most authorities support this approach. During the primary survey, the physician should address life-threats to each of these systems before moving forward in the evaluation.

Airway

The primacy of airway is well justified in trauma management. Simple interventions such as the jaw-thrust or suctioning may be life-saving. However, the EP must also be an expert at advanced techniques.

Orotracheal intubation is a skill essential for the EP. Rapid sequence intubation (RSI) has reduced the complications of emergency airway management.[5] This sequence of interventions is designed to facilitate intubation while minimizing the risk of increasing intracranial pressure and aspiration. Pharmacologic agents may include a neuroprotective drug (e.g., lidocaine), an induction agent (e.g., etomidate), and a neuromuscular blocker (succinylcholine) to produce paralysis. In the trauma patient with overt or occult shock, the physician should avoid drugs that can produce hypotension (e.g., barbiturates).

Regardless of the skill of the intubator, a "back-up" plan is essential in case of failed intubation. Although cricothyroidotomy remains the common final pathway to failed intubation, other interventions, such as the laryngeal mask, are useful in the trauma patient. Chapter 7 discusses alternative airway maneuvers.

After every intubation, endotracheal tube placement must be confirmed with either measurement of end-tidal CO_2 or with an esophageal detector device. Any other methods, such as auscultation or chest radiography, are inadequate.

Breathing

The distinction between an airway problem and a breathing problem is crucial. Not all patients in respiratory distress require intubation. Hypotensive patients with absent or markedly diminished breath sounds on one side need emergent decompression of their chest. Remember that a chest radiograph is a poor substitute for a plastic tube between the ribs. Unstable patients cannot tolerate the time necessary for radiographic corroboration of tension pneumothorax.

Circulation

Until ***proven*** (not assumed) otherwise, hypotension in the trauma patient is due to blood loss. Although tension pneumothorax, pericardial tamponade, myocardial contusion, and neurogenic shock may all produce hypotension in the trauma patient, hemorrhage is statistically the prime offender (Figs. 6-1 and 6-2).

CONTROL BLEEDING

The EP should control external bleeding by direct pressure. Splinting can decrease internal bleeding from skeletal injuries. Femur fractures should be splinted with Sager or Hare traction. Unstable pelvic fractures can produce life-threatening hemorrhage and may ultimately require angiographic embolization, external fixation, or both. However, in the trauma room pelvic compression can quickly reduce pelvic volume and decrease retroperitoneal bleeding. Interventions can be as simple as a bed sheet wrapped tightly around the pelvis or involve the use of the pneumatic antishock garment (PASG, formally known as the MAST suit).

When it comes to organ rupture, only surgery provides definitive control of massive intraabdominal hemorrhage.

RESTORE VOLUME

Although current research is focusing on hypotensive resuscitation, its clinical use is restricted to a few centers in patients with penetrating truncal injuries. In penetrating trauma, rapid transport to the operating suite is more important than aggressive fluid administration.

In nearly all patients hypotensive after blunt trauma, volume resuscitation is indicated. Infuse crystalloids concurrent with evaluation and treatment of tension pneumothorax or suspected pericardial tamponade.

Venous access can be achieved in a variety of ways. Antecubital cannulation is the most obvious approach but some patients may require venous cutdowns or central lines. The interosseous route is useful in small children with no other access. At least two large-bore

Primary Survey and Resuscitation
Intubate as needed
Establish intravenous access

Clinical evidence of tension pneumothorax?

Yes → Decompress chest

No

Obtain CXR and complete primary and secondary survey
Give fluids and blood as needed

Does the patient need transfer or emergent surgical consult?

Yes → Place initial call to surgeon trauma center

No, or unclear at this time

Unstable pelvic fracture?

Yes → Decrease pelvic volume (PASG, blanket wrapped around pelvis, beanbag device)

No

Complete examination and diagnostic studies as indicated

Persistent hypotension despite resuscitation?

No → Complete examination and diagnostic studies as indicated

Yes → Scenario I: Trauma center or tertiary care hospital

Yes → Scenario II: Smaller hospital See Fig.6-2

Perform DPL or bedside ultrasound

Hemoperitoneum?

Yes → Emergent laparotomy

No

Search for and manage other causes of blood loss:
Pelvic, femur, or long bone fractures
Retroperitoneal bleed
Occult penetrating trauma
Cardiogenic shock
Distributive shock
Neurogenic shock
Reevaluate for hemoperitoneum (e.g., repeat ultrasound)

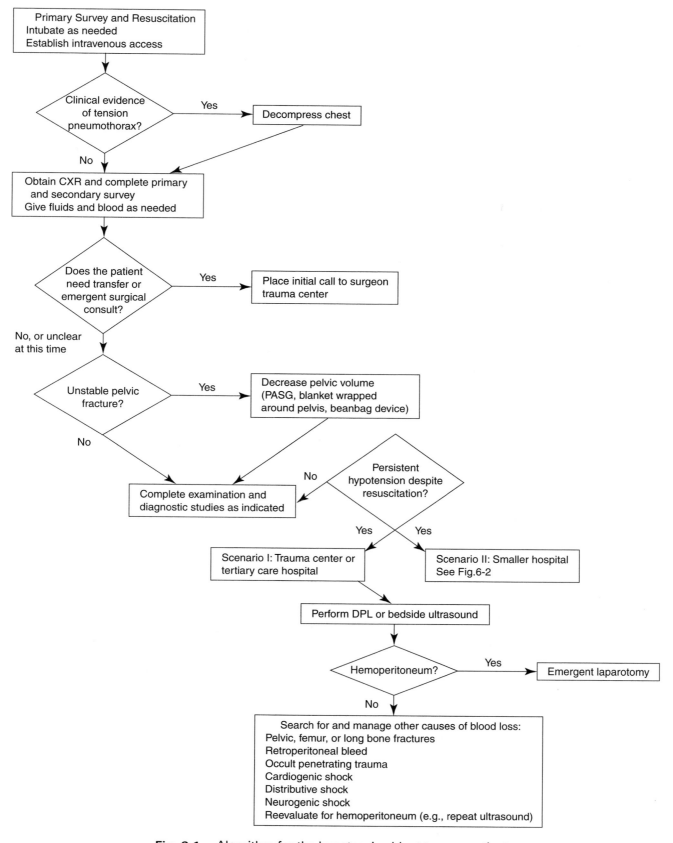

Fig. 6-1 Algorithm for the hypotensive blunt trauma patient.

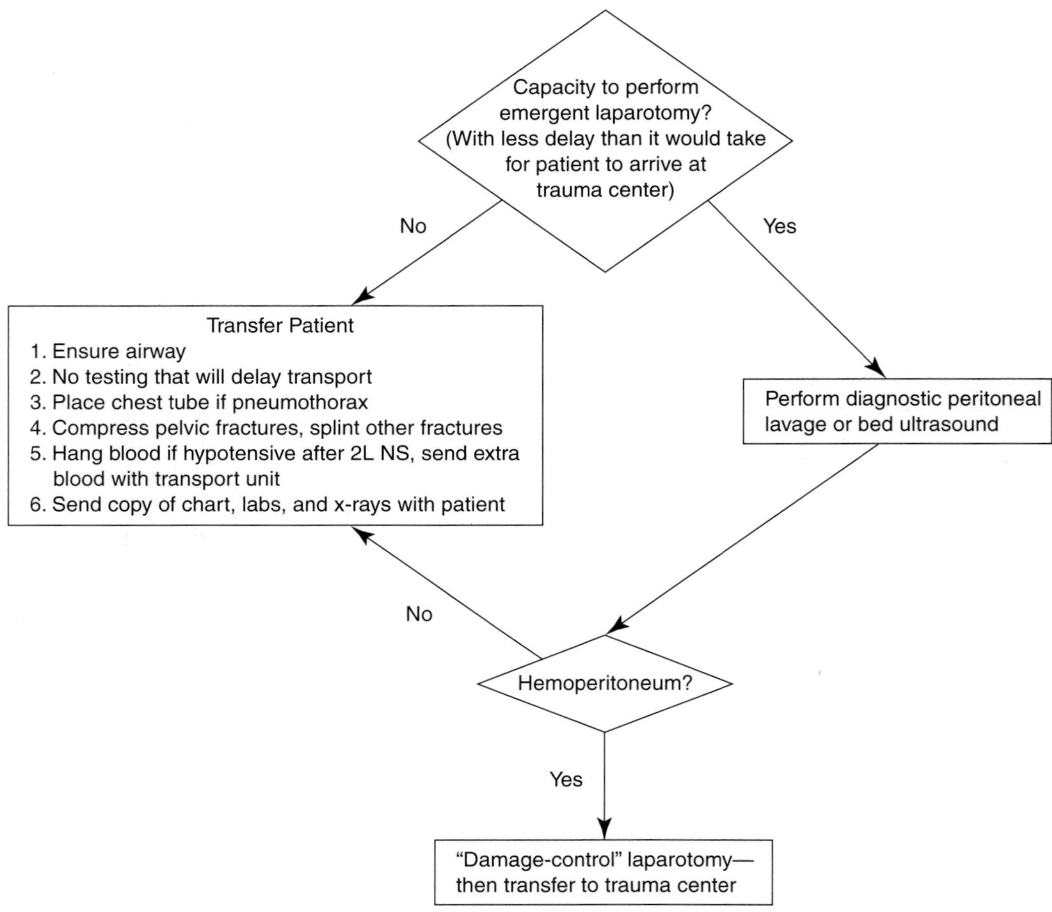

Fig. 6-2 Algorithm for persistent hypertension in the blunt trauma patient at a smaller hospital.

IVs of crystalloid solution given "wide-open" is standard in the hypotensive blunt trauma patient. High-volume resuscitation requires large tubing and large short catheters. The use of a cordis port (size 8 French or higher) permits dramatic flow rates.[6]

The end points of volume resuscitation remain unclear. Return to normal parameters of blood pressure, heart rate, and urine output may be inadequate. As many as 50% to 85% of patients remain in a dangerous state of "compensated" shock, despite relatively normal vital signs.[7] For this reason, normalization of lactate and base deficit are receiving greater scrutiny as markers for appropriate resuscitation.

GIVE BLOOD

The criteria for blood transfusion have not been strictly defined. It is generally accepted that emergency transfusion is necessary in the presence of persistent hypotension despite fluid resuscitation. Certain patients may require early transfusion in anticipation of ongoing hemorrhage. Early transfusion is especially helpful in cases of severe pelvic fractures, particularly those that involve the disruption of the posterior elements. Once hospitalized, trauma patients may be given blood to optimize oxygen transport. Some centers use a hematocrit of 30% as a trigger for transfusion in the seriously injured patient.

When blood is transfused, the IV line cannot be attached to any other fluid apart from normal saline (the calcium in Ringer's lactate can produce clotting in the tubing). When massive transfusions are required, blood can be given through a high-volume warmer (infuser). Alternatively, 250 cc of warmed saline added to the unit in conjunction with a pressure bag will dramatically increase flow.[8,9] Red cells tolerate saline heated to 70° C. A 250 cc aliquot of 70° C saline will warm a unit of blood to 44° C.[8]

Disability

The *D* for "disability" in the ATLS algorithm refers to a rapid neurologic evaluation. Note the level of consciousness (the Glasgow Coma Scale), pupillary size and reactivity, and the symmetry of the motor and sensory examinations.

Cerebral resuscitation is an important concern in the head-injured patient and should begin early during care. Early cerebral resuscitation must avoid the two most dangerous insults to the traumatized brain: hypotension and hypoxia. Other interventions can include the administration of mannitol, moderate hyperventilation (to a pCO_2 between 30 and 35 mmHg), and elevation of the head of the bed to 30 degrees. Adjuncts such as mannitol and moderate hyperventilation are best restricted to patients with lateralizing signs or neurologic deterioration.[10] However, ensuring adequate cerebral blood flow and oxygenation is more important during the initial resuscitation than any adjunctive measures.

Exposure

Removing the clothes facilitates the physical examination of the severely injured patient. At the same time, it predisposes them to hypothermia. Hypothermia is deadly in the multiply-injured patient. Hypothermia in the trauma patient is associated with dysrhythmias, coma, coagulopathy, decreased cardiac output, and increased mortality.[11,12] The chance of survival falls with every degree drop in core temperature. Mortality rates are 40% with a core temperature of <34° C, 69% at temperatures <33° C, and 100% at <32° C.[13]

In the trauma room, cover the patient with warmed blankets and use warmed IV fluids and blood. Attention to a patient's temperature may easily be overlooked and nursing protocols should include measurement of a rectal or core temperature. Some trauma centers use thermistors built into the Foley catheter to monitor core temperature.

SECONDARY SURVEY

History

The history obtained from the patient, paramedics, or witnesses allows the EP to anticipate injuries. Patients who jump from heights are prone to fractures of the calcaneus, tibial plateaus, lumbar spine, and pelvis, and often suffer retroperitoneal bleeds.[14] Pedestrians, bicyclists, and motorcyclists struck by cars or trains are likely to have intraabdominal and skeletal injuries.

The history of loss of consciousness (LOC) is especially important in victims of blunt trauma. In one study, transient LOC in the field was associated with both neurosurgical and nonneurosurgical injuries. Nearly 20% of these patients required surgery for life-threatening injuries, the vast majority being extracranial.[15]

Although a list of the patient's medications can be helpful from a variety of perspectives, obtaining information regarding one particular drug—warfarin (Coumadin)—is essential. Patients on warfarin are at high risk for life-threatening hemorrhage even after relatively minor trauma.[16]

Physical Examination

The physical examination propels much of the further evaluation of the trauma patient. It often determines the direction and scope of diagnostic testing. An experienced clinician can ascertain the need for admission, operation, or transfer within minutes of examining the patient.

However, this section focuses on the *limitations* of the physical examination. The physical examination may mislead the physician. As many as 25% of seriously injured trauma patients have at least one injury that is overlooked at the time of initial evaluation.[17,18] The most commonly missed injuries are musculoskeletal and typically involve the thoracolumbar spine, pelvis, hip, and knee.[19-21]

Fortunately, there are patterns to this deception. Missed injuries are particularly likely in patients who have altered mental status, those who are intubated, and those requiring immediate operation.[22,23] The experienced EP can recall countless cases where alcohol has muddied the diagnostic waters. Alcohol use is especially problematic in cases of apparently mild head trauma, where alterations of mental status may be incorrectly attributed to intoxication.

The most frequently overlooked life-threats to the trauma patient occur within the mysterious confines of the abdomen. Missed intraabdominal injury is the most common preventable cause of death.[24]

Abdominal tenderness is neither sensitive nor specific for significant intraabdominal injury. Decreased levels of consciousness, alcohol intoxication, spinal cord injury, and distracting injuries all impair the accuracy of the abdominal examination. Overall, the physical examination of the abdomen is only 65% accurate in detecting intraabdominal trauma.[25,26] Most authorities assume that serial examinations provide more reliable data.

RECOGNITION OF SHOCK

The recognition of shock is one of the most important challenges in trauma care. There are numerous and occasionally subtle physical signs of shock, including diaphoresis, clammy skin, cyanotic nail beds, and altered mental status. However, many physicians mistakenly rely on profound tachycardia or frank hypotension to make the diagnosis, findings that may represent *irreversible* shock.

Vital signs are ***insensitive*** indicators of blood loss.[27,28] Hypotension is often a late finding, and as many as 30% of patients in shock may have normal heart rates.[29] Certain subgroups of trauma patients are more likely to have relatively normal vital signs until they decompensate precipitously. These high-risk groups include children, the elderly, and pregnant females.

INJURIES THAT DISTRACT THE PHYSICIAN

The most spectacular injuries are not necessarily the most life-threatening. Facial injuries, although dramatic, do not pose an immediate life-threat unless they jeopardize the airway. These wounds should not distract the physician from concomitant injuries to intracranial, thoracic, or abdominal structures. Similarly, an open tibial fracture, although "eye-catching," is ultimately less significant than a grade 4 laceration of the spleen.

INJURIES THAT DISTRACT THE PATIENT

The gating theory of pain explains why one injury may divert attention from another. This phenomenon may be most dangerous in patients who suffer a painful extraabdominal injury that distracts them (and the physician) from coexisting intraabdominal trauma. Patients with distracting injuries may have little or no abdominal tenderness despite significant intraabdominal pathology. In one prospective study, 7% of alert trauma patients had intraabdominal injury despite the lack of abdominal pain or tenderness. All of these patients suffered distracting injuries.[30]

Clinically occult intraabdominal injury should be considered in the presence of multiple extremity, pelvic, and rib fractures, as well as those with pulmonary injuries. Patients sustaining injuries to the chest wall who complain of isolated chest pain may also have intraabdominal injury, especially in the presence of rib fractures and pneumothoraces.[30]

Diagnostic Studies

Although diagnostic studies can provide crucial information in the trauma patient, there is tension between the need to know and the need to treat. A moribund patient with a rigid belly may die during the performance of diagnostic tests. Here, fleeting moments are better spent transporting the patient to the operating suite. The EP must always consider the benefits versus risks of tests, especially when the investigations require transport out of the ED. Nowhere is this more apparent than in the use of computed tomography (CT) in trauma.

RADIOGRAPHIC STUDIES

Computed Tomography Scanning. Although CT scanning provides unquestioned benefit in trauma management, its inappropriate use can be deadly. Hypotensive patients may die on the scanner table. In some trauma centers, it is wryly called "the circle of death." For many critically injured patients, head CT may be safely delayed until other life-threats are managed. One study of 462 consecutive patients with blunt trauma showed that although head trauma was the most common reason for admission, few patients (5%) required neurosurgical intervention. The study emphasized that management of the airway, and laparotomy to control hemorrhage, were more important to outcome than "routine" head CT scans.[31]

Another common pitfall involves the limitations of testing. The EP must recognize that many studies are falsely normal despite significant pathologic conditions. For example, CT of the abdomen may overlook injury to the diaphragm, intestine, or bladder.

Plain Films. Although there is no uniform radiographic series applicable to all trauma victims, certain films are *almost* routine. Chest radiography should be universal in victims of significant blunt trauma and in those with penetrating torso injuries. However, the film should be delayed to treat a clinically apparent tension pneumothorax. A potentially lethal pitfall involves overlooking the abnormal mediastinum and the associated aortic disruption.[32] Although cervical and pelvic films are frequently ordered in the multiply-injured patient, they may be obtained on a selective basis.

LABORATORY TESTING

Few laboratory tests change the initial management of the trauma patient. However, the following tests may be valuable in the severely injured.

Glucose. Patients with altered mental status require bedside testing of glucose. Although it is easy to assume that altered mental status is secondary to head injury, hypoglycemia may have precipitated the trauma. The patient who presents with confusion, seizures, coma, or focal neurologic deficit may require dextrose, as opposed to CT scanning.[33]

Blood Typing. What is the single most important blood test in the trauma patient? Could it be the crossmatch? Emergency blood transfusion can be lifesaving for the severely injured trauma patient. Although uncrossmatched blood is indicated in extreme circumstances, crossmatched or type-specific blood will suffice in most case of hemorrhage.[34] In the severely traumatized patient, obtain a specimen for blood bank analysis.

Stat Hemoglobin/Hematocrit. A bedside test for hemoglobin is standard in most trauma resuscitations. The EP must recognize the limitations of this test. Although a low hemoglobin level after injury usually indicates serious hemorrhage, it is insensitive to acute blood loss.[35] However, serial levels provide evidence of persistent or significant hemorrhage.

Other factors besides hemorrhage may be responsible for a low hemoglobin. One liter of intravenous fluids alone (without blood loss) may decrease hemoglobin by a point or more.[36] In addition, certain patients, such as those with AIDS, sickle cell disease, or chronic renal failure, may also present with an initially low value.

Lactate and Base Deficit. Measures of acidosis, such as lactate or base deficit (BD), rise with shock. Such parameters may be more sensitive to early blood loss than invasive monitoring. In one large study, admission BD (especially more negative than –6) identified patients likely to require early transfusion. It also predicted increased ICU and hospital stays, as well as those at risk for shock-related complications.[37] Because of the likelihood of subsequent transfusion, the authors suggested that patients with BD <–6 should undergo type and crossmatch rather than type and screen. An elevated BD is especially ominous in the elderly.[38] Although not well studied for this indication, acidosis may become an important criteria for transfer to a trauma center.

EVALUATING FOR HEMOPERITONEUM—BLUNT TRAUMA

Of all (preventable or potentially preventable) trauma patient deaths, the most common single error across all phases of care was failure to appropriately evaluate the abdomen.[24]

Recognizing intracavitary hemorrhage is a primary goal for EPs. Massive hemothorax is readily apparent on chest radiograph, although life-threatening retroperitoneal bleeding occurs primarily in patients with unstable pelvic fractures. It is the rapid assessment of intraperitoneal blood that remains problematic in multitrauma. The three primary modalities to detect hemoperitoneum include diagnostic peritoneal lavage (DPL), ultrasound (US), and CT scans. The choice of these studies depends on a variety of factors including hemodynamic stability of the patient, concurrent injuries, and hospital resources (including the time required to obtain a final interpretation of the study).

Diagnostic Peritoneal Lavage

Diagnostic peritoneal lavage is especially useful for the hemodynamically unstable patient. Within minutes of ED arrival, a positive aspirate can determine the need for laparotomy in the hypotensive patient. In the absence of unequivocal clinical indicators for laparotomy, the more unstable the patient, the greater the utility of DPL.[39]

DPL is useful in both penetrating and blunt abdominal trauma. A reduced red cell threshold (5000 cells/mm) makes it sensitive to abdominal violation in patients with penetrating injuries to the low chest.[40]

Computed Tomography Scanning

The latest generation of helical scanners provides rapid and accurate diagnostic information regarding most body compartments. CT scanning is the imaging modality of choice in the ***hemodynamically stable*** trauma victim who needs further evaluation of the head or torso. Because of this diagnostic prowess, the real and important limitations of CT scans are not appreciated by many physicians.

In a study involving 1331 abdominal CT scans for trauma, the authors found a complication rate of 3.4%, including 25 false-negative scans, 3 false-positive scans, and 18 delays to the operating suite.[41] The authors remarked that in their institutions DPL was associated with fewer complications than CT scanning. In another review of 2047 CT scans in trauma patients, less than 30% of the scans contributed to management. In this series, 6% of CT scans were falsely positive, 2 patients died in the CT suite, 6 more died shortly after completion of the scan, and 12 were transported emergently from CT to the operating suite.[42]

Although CT scanning is accurate for intraabdominal injury in blunt trauma, it has limited utility in cases of penetrating abdominal trauma. It should not be used to determine hollow viscus injury in patients with penetrating abdominal trauma (although it can provide information regarding trajectory in those with tangential wounds that do not clearly endanger the abdomen). Triple-contrast CT scanning (rectal, oral, and intravenous) is useful in managing patients with penetrating trauma to the back and flanks.

Ultrasound: The Fast Examination (Focused Abdominal Sonography in Trauma)

In much of the world, ultrasound has long been the primary means of evaluating the traumatized abdomen. Only in the past several years has it become an important diagnostic tool in U.S. trauma centers. The

FAST examination differs from traditional US techniques in that it does not attempt to identify specific organ injury. Instead, the EP uses trauma US to search for hemoperitoneum.

Like DPL, trauma US is best used to determine the need for urgent laparotomy in the hypotensive victim of blunt trauma.[43] Although US is less sensitive than DPL, it is very accurate in the hypotensive patient and can determine the presence of hemoperitoneum within minutes. It provides some advantages over DPL, since it is noninvasive and does not require a special approach in the patient with previous laparotomies.

In a growing number of trauma centers, US is used as the initial screen for hemoperitoneum. Hypotensive patients with free fluid in the abdomen proceed directly to laparotomy. Hemodynamically stable patients with negative US either undergo CT scanning or serial examinations as indicated. This algorithm using abdominal US can safely decrease the number of nontherapeutic laparotomies, without delaying diagnosis of hemoperitoneum.[44]

EVALUATING FOR AORTIC INJURY

Exclusion of aortic injuries is an important concern in multiple trauma. Although it is easy to miss subtle findings of aortic injury, the EP can detect at least 95% of all aortic injuries by scrupulously examining the initial chest film.

A chest film showing a wide mediastinum, blunted aortic knob, or deviation of the trachea or nasogastric tube suggests aortic injury. An upright or reverse Trendelenburg inspiratory film is helpful, since a significant number of patients *without* aortic injury demonstrate a wide mediastinum on the supine view.[45]

Although aortography has been the traditional standard for evaluating aortic injury, helical CT scanning is emerging as an important diagnostic modality in stable patients. Recent studies show that helical CT scanning is very sensitive for aortic injury when compared with aortography.[46,47]

The use of transesophageal echocardiogram (TEE) for suspected aortic injury depends on operator and institutional factors. It is especially useful in unstable patients.[48-51] It can be performed in the ED or in the operating suite on patients undergoing emergent abdominal or neurosurgical procedures.

PENETRATING ABDOMINAL TRAUMA

Victims of penetrating abdominal trauma often pose less of a diagnostic challenge than their blunt trauma cohorts. Most gunshot wound victims with abdominal wounds undergo immediate laparotomy because of the high incidence of visceral injury. Tangential wounds that do not obviously endanger the abdomen can be evaluated using DPL or diagnostic laparoscopy. Conservative management is also appropriate for stab wound victims without peritonitis or evisceration, using local wound exploration, DPL, diagnostic laparoscopy, or serial physical examinations. For wounds with the potential for diaphragmatic perforation, diagnostic laparoscopy can accurately detect serious injuries, and curtail unnecessary laparotomies.[52-54]

PRIORITIES IN THE MULTIPLY-INJURED PATIENT

The multiply-injured blunt trauma victim presents unique challenges. In this population, competing life-threats vie for attention. Which surgical emergency is most important to address, a wide mediastinum or decorticate posturing? Should a hypotensive patient with a pelvic fracture go to the operating suite for a laparotomy or to the angiography suite for embolization of the pelvic vasculature? The most frequently encountered life-threats include neurosurgical emergencies (coma with or without lateralizing signs), intraabdominal hemorrhage, major pelvic fractures, and aortic injury. What does the EP do when faced with a patient who is posturing, hypotensive, and has an open-book pelvic fracture and a wide mediastinum?

Role of Bedside Test for Hemoperitoneum

Although the management of the multiply-injured patient depends on the severity and type of specific injuries, certain broad principles apply. In general, apart from respiratory failure or tension pneumothorax, the immediate life-threat in the victim of multiple trauma is uncontrolled intraabdominal hemorrhage. Thus early detection of hemoperitoneum with diagnostic peritoneal aspiration or bedside US is essential in the hypotensive patient. In most cases, hemoperitoneum plus shock equals laparotomy.

Combined Head and Abdominal Trauma

Consultants pull the comatose patient with hemoperitoneum in opposite directions: the surgeon towards the OR, the neurosurgeon towards CT. The literature provides equivocal answers for this conundrum.

It is rare that a patient will have both an operable intracranial lesion *and* a surgically correctable intraabdominal injury.[55,56] Patients with suspected brain injuries who are hemodynamically stable are appropriate candidates for CT scanning of both the brain and torso. It is in the unstable patient where the priorities of the trauma surgeon and neurosurgeon collide.

A bedside test for hemoperitoneum can determine the order of subsequent interventions. If the patient has hemoperitoneum but can be stabilized with fluid and or blood administration, a head CT may be indicated. Head CT scanning is most important in the patient with lateralizing findings (asymmetry between right and left side neurologic examination or unilateral "blown" pupil).

Patients with hemoperitoneum and lateralizing signs are candidates for emergent head CT *if* their blood pressure stabilizes with fluids or blood.[57] However, in the patient who remains hemodynamically unstable, immediate laparotomy is necessary.[55] In the persistently hypotensive patient, defer the CT for laparotomy. In this case, the neurosurgeon may perform empiric burr holes or place an intraventricular pressure monitor in the operating suite concurrent with the laparotomy. In addition, mannitol and initiating moderate hyperventilation are indicated for declining neurologic status or lateralizing signs.

Combined Abdominal and Pelvic Trauma

Patients with major pelvic fractures, especially those with disruption of the posterior elements, may die of uncontrolled retroperitoneal hemorrhage. On the other hand, many patients with pelvic fractures have massive intraabdominal injury. Here again, a bedside test for hemoperitoneum is a crucial deciding factor.

Because a positive DPL can lead to a nontherapeutic laparotomy in a patient with a pelvic fracture, a diagnostic peritoneal ***aspirate*** is a better choice in the hypotensive patient. A positive aspirate should direct the patient to the operating suite, a negative aspirate to the angiography suite.[58] Alternatively, a large hemoperitoneum on bedside US should prompt laparotomy in the hypotensive patient.

Wide Mediastinum in Multiple Trauma

The vast majority of patients with aortic injuries die before ever reaching the hospital. Those who arrive alive to the ED are likely to survive their aortic injury for several hours. Pericardial tamponade from a traumatic retrograde aortic dissection is almost unknown.[59,60] Therefore hypotensive patients with a wide mediastinum without hemothorax are likely to have abdominal or retroperitoneal hemorrhage.

Ninety-five percent of patients with aortic disruption have associated injuries requiring operative intervention.[61] Although at least one author suggests that identification and repair of aortic injuries is paramount,[62] most authorities recognize the primacy of hemoperitoneum in the "pecking order" of life-threats.[61,63,64]

Antihypertensive therapy with IV β-blockers alone (esmolol) or in combination with nitroprusside may decrease the incidence of rupture in patients with aortic injuries.[46]

RECOGNIZING FUTILITY

It is important for the EP to recognize the limits of futility in trauma resuscitation. Although CPR occasionally results in dramatic "saves" in the medical arrest, it is no understatement to say traumatic arrest is a bad prognostic sign. The one exception is the victim of penetrating mediastinal trauma who arrests in the ED or while en route to the hospital. In this group, prompt ED thoracotomy may be lifesaving. However, the combination of blunt trauma and cardiac arrest is almost uniformly fatal. With one exception,[65] essentially all reviews on ED thoracotomy for blunt trauma arrest suggest it is ultimately futile.

Attempting to resuscitate patients with essentially no chance of survival wastes valuable resources. Resources are best applied to patients who might live with aggressive interventions. Pronouncing the patient with blunt trauma arrest can have a significant financial impact without decreasing the number of ultimate survivors.[66]

The principle of the greatest good for the greatest number becomes most evident in a disaster where multiple victims compete for care. Those with ultimately fatal injuries must be allowed to die to save those who could benefit from interventions.[67] Such moribund patients, if conscious, need adequate analgesia including perhaps a morphine drip, as in the case of an 80-year-old patient with 90% burns.

SUMMARY

During the trauma resuscitation, the EP must ask several questions. These self-queries must be insistent and recurrent. They should be asked and answered repeatedly during each phase of resuscitation.

1. Does this patient need an ED procedure such as intubation, chest tube, fluid challenge, transfusion, or pelvic compression? If so, how soon?
2. Should I call a surgeon or initiate transfer **now**?
3. Is this patient in shock? If so, where is the bleeding?

And the final most frustrating question in regard to the unstable patient is:

4. Why are they still here? Why is the patient not in the operating suite or in transit to the trauma center?

Trauma resuscitations can vary from the maniacal to nearly serene, from chaotic entropy to focused energy. Although difficult to prove in a randomized controlled trial, the quality of leadership and teamwork has a more profound impact on the tenor of the event than does the patient's injuries. By fostering teamwork and focusing on these core questions, the EP can redirect the frenzied "Brownian motion" of trauma resuscitation.

REFERENCES

1. Deo SD, Knottenbelt JD, Peden MM: Evaluation of a small trauma team for major resuscitation, *Injury* 28:633-637, 1997.
2. Hoff WS, et al: The importance of the command-physician in trauma resuscitation, *J Trauma* 43:772-777, 1997.
3. Driscoll PA, Vincent CA: Variation in trauma resuscitation and its effect on patient outcome, *Injury* 23:111-115, 1992.
4. Evanoff B, et al: Compliance with universal precautions among emergency department personnel caring for trauma patients, *Ann Emerg Med* 33:160-165, 1999.
5. Li J, et al: Complications of emergency intubation with and without paralysis, *Am J Emerg Med* 17:141-143, 1999.
6. Scalea TM, et al: Percutaneous central venous access for resuscitation in trauma, *Acad Emerg Med* 1:525-531, 1994.
7. Porter JM, Ivatury RR: In search of the optimal end points of resuscitation in trauma patients: a review, *J Trauma* 44:908-914, 1998.
8. Iserson KV, Knauf MA, Anhalt D: Rapid admixture blood warming: technical advances, *Crit Care Med* 18:1138-1141, 1990.
9. Zorko MF, Polsky SS: Rapid warming and infusion of packed red blood cells, *Ann Emerg Med* 15:907-910, 1986.
10. Bullock R, et al: *Guidelines for the management of severe head injury*, New York, 1995, Brain Trauma Foundation.
11. Jurkovich GJ, et al: Hypothermia in trauma victims: an ominous predictor of survival, *J Trauma* 27:1019-1024, 1987.
12. Gentilello LM, et al: Is hypothermia in the victim of major trauma protective or harmful? A randomized, prospective study, *Ann Surg* 226:439-447, 1997.
13. Luna GK, et al: Incidence and effect of hypothermia in seriously injured patients, *J Trauma* 27:1014-1018, 1987.
14. Scalea T, et al: An analysis of 161 falls from a height: the "jumper syndrome," *J Trauma* 26:706-712, 1986.
15. Owings JT, et al: Isolated transient loss of consciousness is an indicator of significant injury, *Arch Surg* 133:941-946, 1998.
16. Ferrera PC, Bartfield JM: Outcomes of anticoagulated trauma patients, *Am J Emerg Med* 17:154-156, 1999.
17. Chan RN, Ainscow D, Sikorski JM: Diagnostic failures in the multiple injured, *J Trauma* 20:684-687, 1980.
18. Dove DB, Stahl WM, DelGuercio LR: A five-year review of deaths following urban trauma, *J Trauma* 20:760-766, 1980.
19. Enderson BL, Maull KI: Missed injuries: the trauma surgeon's nemesis, *Surg Clin North Am* 71:399-418, 1991.
20. Hirshberg A, et al: Causes and patterns of missed injuries in trauma, *Am J Surg* 168:299-303, 1994.
21. Laasonen EM, Kivioja A: Delayed diagnosis of extremity injuries in patients with multiple injuries, *J Trauma* 31:257-260, 1991.
22. Aaland MO, Smith K: Delayed diagnosis in a rural trauma center, *Surgery* 120:774-778, 1996.
23. Rizoli SB, et al: Injuries missed during initial assessment of blunt trauma patients, *Accid Anal Prev* 26:681-686, 1994.
24. Davis JW, et al: An analysis of errors causing morbidity and mortality in a trauma system: a guide for quality improvement, *J Trauma* 32:660-665, 1992.
25. Olsen WF, Hildreth DH: Abdominal paracentesis and peritoneal lavage, *J Trauma* 11:824-829, 1971.
26. Powell DC, Bivins BA, Bell RM: Diagnostic peritoneal lavage, *Surg Gynecol Obstet* 155:257-264, 1982.
27. Abou-Khalil B, et al: Hemodynamic responses to shock in young trauma patients: need for invasive monitoring, *Crit Care Med* 22:633-639, 1994.
28. Scalea TM, et al: Central venous blood oxygen saturation: an early, accurate measurement of volume during hemorrhage, *J Trauma* 28:725-732, 1988.
29. Demetriades D, et al: Relative bradycardia in patients with traumatic hypotension, *J Trauma* 45:534-539, 1998.
30. Ferrera PC, et al: Injuries distracting from intraabdominal injuries after blunt trauma, *Am J Emerg Med* 16:145-149, 1998.
31. Fulton RL, et al: Ritual head computed tomography may unnecessarily delay lifesaving trauma care, *Surg Gynecol Obstet* 176: 327-332, 1993.
32. McLellan BA, et al: Role of the trauma-room chest x-ray film in assessing the patient with severe blunt traumatic injury, *Can J Surg* 39:36-41, 1996.
33. Luber SD, et al: Acute hypoglycemia masquerading as head trauma: a report of four cases, *Am J Emerg Med* 14:543-547, 1996.
34. Gervin AS, Fischer RP: Resuscitation of trauma patients with type-specific uncrossmatched blood, *J Trauma* 24:327-331, 1984.
35. Knottenbelt JD: Low initial hemoglobin levels in trauma patients: an important indicator of ongoing hemorrhage, *J Trauma* 31:1396-1399, 1991.
36. Kass LE, et al: Prospective crossover study of the effect of phlebotomy and intravenous crystalloid on hematocrit, *Acad Emerg Med* 4:198-201, 1997.
37. Davis JW, et al: Admission base deficit predicts transfusion requirements and risk of complications, *J Trauma* 41:769-774, 1996.
38. Davis JW, Kaups KL: Base deficit in the elderly: a marker of severe injury and death, *J Trauma* 45:873-877, 1998.
39. Blow O, et al: Speed and efficiency in the resuscitation of blunt trauma patients with multiple injuries: the advantage of diagnostic peritoneal lavage over abdominal computerized tomography, *J Trauma* 44:287-290, 1998.
40. Merlotti GJ: Peritoneal lavage in penetrating thoraco-abdominal trauma, *J Trauma* 28:17-23, 1988.
41. Davis JW, et al: Complications in evaluating abdominal trauma: diagnostic peritoneal lavage versus computerized axial tomography, *J Trauma* 30:1506-1509, 1990.
42. Rizzo AG, Steinberg SM, Flint LM: Prospective assessment of the value of computed tomography for trauma, *J Trauma* 38:338-342, 1995.
43. Wherrett LJ, et al: Hypotension after blunt abdominal trauma: the role of emergent abdominal sonography in surgical triage, *J Trauma* 41:815-820, 1996.
44. Shih HC, et al: Noninvasive evaluation of blunt abdominal trauma: prospective study using diagnostic algorithms to minimize nontherapeutic laparotomy, *World J Surg* 23:265-269, 1999.
45. Schwab CW, et al: Aortic injury: comparison of supine and upright portable chest films to evaluate the widened mediastinum, *Ann Emerg Med* 13: 896-899, 1984.
46. Fabian TC, et al: Prospective study of blunt aortic injury: helical CT is diagnostic and antihypertensive therapy reduces rupture, *Ann Surg* 227:666-677, 1998.

47. Gavant ML, et al: Blunt traumatic aortic rupture: detection with helical CT of the chest, *Radiology* 197:125-133, 1995.
48. Kearney PA, et al: Use of transesophageal echocardiography in the evaluation of traumatic aortic injury, *J Trauma* 34:696-701, 1993.
49. Cohn SM, et al: Exclusion of aortic tear in the unstable trauma patient: the utility of transesophageal echocardiography, *J Trauma* 39:1087-1090, 1995.
50. Chirillo F, et al: Usefulness of transthoracic and transesophageal echocardiography in recognition and management of cardiovascular injuries after blunt chest trauma, *Heart* 75:301-306, 1996.
51. Vignon P, et al: Role of transesophageal echocardiography in the diagnosis and management of traumatic aortic disruption, *Circulation* 92:2959-2968, 1995.
52. Ivatury RR, Simon RJ, Stahl WM: A critical evaluation of laparoscopy in penetrating abdominal trauma, *J Trauma* 34:822-827, 1993.
53. Zantut LF, et al: Diagnostic and therapeutic laparoscopy for penetrating abdominal trauma: a multicenter experience, *J Trauma* 42:825-829, 1997.
54. Fernando HC, et al: Triage by laparoscopy in patients with penetrating abdominal trauma, *Br J Surg* 81:384-385, 1994.
55. Wisner DH, Victor NS, Holcroft JW: Priorities in the management of multiple trauma: intracranial versus intra-abdominal injury, *J Trauma* 35:271-276, 1993.
56. Thomason M, et al: Head CT scanning versus urgent exploration in the hypotensive blunt trauma patient, *J Trauma* 34:40-44, 1993.
57. Winchell RJ, Hoyt DB, Simons RK: Use of computed tomography of the head in the hypotensive blunt-trauma patient, *Ann Emerg Med* 25:737-742, 1995.
58. Evers BM, Cryer HM, Miller FB: Pelvic fracture hemorrhage: priorities in management, *Arch Surg* 124:422-424, 1989.
59. Goverde P, et al: Traumatic type B aortic dissection, *Acta Chir Belg* 96:233-236, 1996.
60. Gammie JS, et al: Acute aortic dissection after blunt chest trauma, *J Trauma* 40:126-127, 1996.
61. Lee RB, Stahlman GC, Sharp KW: Treatment priorities in patients with traumatic rupture of the thoracic aorta, *Am Surg* 58:37-43, 1992.
62. Kirsh MM, et al: The treatment of acute traumatic rupture of the aorta: a 10-year experience, *Ann Surg* 184:308-316, 1976.
63. Richardson JD, Wilson ME, Miller FB: The widened mediastinum: diagnostic and therapeutic priorities, *Ann Surg* 211:731-736, 1990.
64. Borman KR, Aurbakken CM, Weigelt JA: Treatment priorities in combined blunt abdominal and aortic trauma, *Am J Surg* 144:728-731, 1982.
65. Branney SW, et al: Critical analysis of two decades of experience with postinjury emergency department thoracotomy in a regional trauma center, *J Trauma* 45:87-94, 1998.
66. Pasquale MD, et al: Defining "dead on arrival": impact on a level I trauma center, *J Trauma* 41:726-730, 1996.
67. Kennedy K, et al: Triage: techniques and applications in decision making, *Ann Emerg Med* 28:136-144, 1996.

Airway Management in the Trauma Setting

7

ROBERT E. O'CONNOR AND BRIAN J. LEVINE

Teaching Case

A 20-year-old man was shot in the left mandible, with the bullet exiting his right cheek. He traveled by foot to the nearest hospital and collapsed in the doorway. He was breathing on his own, but his airway was filled with blood. He was given 10 mg of vecuronium but could not be intubated. Cricothyroidotomy was ultimately performed, but the patient sustained at least 30 minutes of cerebral anoxia. On arrival at the trauma center 2 hours later, he was brain dead.

In this situation it is clear that the patient's airway status was precarious. However, since he still was making respiratory efforts, an attempt at an awake oral intubation could have been made using a sedative and spraying the oropharynx with a local anesthetic. If a paralytic is necessary, a short-acting agent such as succinylcholine should be used; if the airway still cannot be secured, at least the paralytic effect will wear off in 5 minutes. ■

Failure to properly manage the airway is a major cause of early preventable deaths in trauma patients. Although most patients require intubation for airway compromise, head trauma, profound shock, or respiratory failure, some seriously injured and combative patients require paralysis to protect them from harm.

Problems unique to trauma airway management include cervical spine instability, thermal inhalation, penetrating neck trauma, and severe closed-head injury. Delays in definitive airway management can result in rapid and often irreversible deterioration. The solution is the right therapy, in the right amount, at the right time. Often, the simple administration of supplemental oxygen is all that is required. However, in other patients the airway may need to be urgently secured. Because of their unpredictability, these airway procedures are the primary responsibility of the emergency physician (EP) and cannot be delegated to others.[1,2]

RECOGNIZING AIRWAY DIFFICULTY

Airway compromise takes many forms, ranging from gradual to sudden, partial to complete, and intermittent to recurrent. Not only assess, but continually reassess, the severely injured patient. A common error in airway management involves the failure to recognize marginal airway function. Key issues include the following:

1. Deliver adequate oxygen to vital organs
2. Maintain a patent airway
3. Ensure adequate ventilation
4. Protect the cervical spine
5. Recognize the need for endotracheal intubation
6. Know when and how to utilize rapid sequence intubation (RSI)
7. Be proficient in surgical airway techniques[3]

Assessment of airway patency is the first priority in trauma management. Trauma patients may have a partial or complete airway obstruction as a result of facial injury.[4] The upper airway may be partially or completely obstructed by the tongue, dislodged dentures, or teeth. Blood, vomitus, foreign body, or swollen tissues may also occlude the airway. If the obstruction is due to tissue laxity or posterior displacement of the tongue, simple maneuvers may quickly alleviate the problem. However, if the blockage is due to a for-

The authors would like to acknowledge Teresa Thuet for her assistance in the preparation of this manuscript.

eign body, distorted tissues, or vomitus, clearing the airway becomes problematic. In the case where swollen tissues obstruct the airway, establish an airway before worsening edema limits therapeutic options.

CERVICAL SPINE

In terms of cervical spine motion, bag-valve-mask (BVM) ventilation appears to produce the most neck movement. Oral endotracheal and nasotracheal intubation are roughly equivalent and produce less cervical motion.[5] Regardless of which technique is used, it is clear that maintaining in-line stabilization is essential to protect the cervical spine and facilitates laryngoscopy.[6] Both techniques are safe, provided that inline cervical spine immobilization can be maintained. When confronted with a combative patient or one in whom in-line stabilization is not possible using an awake technique, sedation and neuromuscular blockade may reduce cervical injury.

AIRWAY MANEUVERS

Three common maneuvers used to open the airway are the combination neck-lift/head-tilt, chin-lift, and jaw-thrust techniques. Because of the potential for spinal injury, the combination neck-lift/head-tilt is contraindicated in the victim of blunt trauma. In the trauma patient, either the jaw-thrust or chin-lift maneuver should be employed to open the airway, particularly if BVM ventilation becomes necessary. It is imperative that in-line stabilization of the head and neck is maintained throughout all maneuvers.

Chin Lift

Of the three techniques, the chin-lift is the easiest to perform.[7] This technique avoids unnecessary neck displacement and, according to one study, produces the greatest airway patency. To perform the chin-lift maneuver, the rescuer places his or her fingertips, palm side up, beneath the patient's chin to gently lift the chin forward. This passively opens the patient's mouth. Because the tongue and other soft tissues are attached to the mandible, the simple maneuver of lifting the mandible moves contiguous soft tissues away from the posterior pharynx.

Jaw Thrust

In the jaw-thrust maneuver, the rescuer places his or her thumbs on the mandibular rami and pulls the jaw forward. This moves the tongue and other soft tissues out of the hypopharynx. Both of these methods open an airway occluded by the tongue or tissue laxity. The jaw-thrust and chin-lift maneuvers can be performed in a totally immobilized patient without moving the neck.[3,8,9]

At times, patient positioning and airway opening are ineffective. Airway obstruction caused by vomitus, copious secretions, foreign material, or ongoing hemorrhage requires suctioning. Either a dental or tonsil tip (Yankauer) suction device should be used.[10,11] Although the widely available catheter tip device can suction an endotracheal tube after the patient has been intubated, it is virtually useless in clearing copious secretions, blood, or other material from the pharynx. Ideally, all three catheter tips should be readily available at the head of the patient's bed. When suction is needed, there is no time for a frantic search.[3,8,9]

ARTIFICIAL AIRWAY DEVICES

After the airway has been opened and suctioned, the patient may still require an artificial airway. If the chin-lift or jaw-thrust maneuver merely opens the airway temporarily, either a nasopharyngeal (NP) or oropharyngeal (OP) device can maintain patency if immediate intubation is not anticipated. These devices facilitate BVM ventilation and provide an artificial lumen through the pharynx, which displaces the tongue and soft tissues.

Insert the OP airway by placing the device in an inverted position on the patient's hard palate and then rotating it 180° to its final position behind the patient's tongue. An alternate procedure is to use a tongue blade. The blade pulls the tongue off the posterior pharynx so the airway may slide behind the tongue. This latter technique does not require rotation of the device. Shoving an oral airway in place without using these techniques is not only traumatic, but forces the tongue against the posterior pharynx, resulting in complete airway obstruction. Once inserted, the oral airway may be taped into position to prevent expulsion. Do not cover the lumen of the airway with tape. The oral airway should not be used in the conscious patient; such patients are likely to vomit with insertion.

The NP airway can be used in patients with trismus or teeth clenching. Unlike the oral airway, conscious or semiconscious patients are usually able to tolerate this device. An NP airway is placed directly into the nostril after lubrication and advanced along the nasal floor towards the nasopharynx. When in position, the flared external end should rest at the nasal entrance.

Either of these artificial airways provides airway patency equivalent to the chin-lift or jaw-thrust techniques and frees the operator's hands for BVM ventilation. Both devices are temporary measures and cannot substitute for definitive interventions. Once an artificial airway is in place, reassess the patient.

MASK VENTILATION

The most common and effective means of supporting ventilation is the BVM device. BVM ventilation is extremely effective, but requires careful attention to maintain a tight mask seal, airway patency, and delivery of adequate ventilation. This seemingly simple skill must be mastered by anyone involved in airway management. If at all possible, two rescuers should perform BVM ventilation, preferably with an artificial airway already in place.[12] In patients with heavy beards and midface crush injuries, a mask seal may be difficult to obtain. If adequate ventilation is unsuccessful with the BVM device, the critical patient may require an immediate surgical airway.

The BVM device should be attached to high-flow supplemental oxygen with delivery of at least 15 liters per minute to avoid hypoxia. A common pitfall is an inadvertent disconnection from the oxygen wall supply.

Even in skilled hands, BVM ventilation requires continuous monitoring of mask seal, airway patency, tidal volumes, and foreign material in the airway. If vomitus, blood, or other debris is not cleared, it may be forced down the trachea during ventilation. Another hazard of BVM ventilation is insufflation of the stomach, with subsequent passive regurgitation and aspiration of gastric contents. The likelihood of gastric insufflation is much higher if airway patency is not secured.

A few important caveats apply to BVM ventilation regardless of whether there are one or two rescuers performing the technique. Leave dentures in place to help ensure a better mask seal—they can be removed just before intubation. In addition, strict attention should be paid to adequate compression of the bag and to the ventilatory rate so that high-flow oxygen is delivered. Many BVM devices are equipped with a pressure-regulated pop-off valve. This valve should be disabled, since airway pressures higher than the valve limit may be required.

To reduce the chance of gastric distention secondary to air insufflation, apply firm posterior pressure on the cricoid ring to compress the esophagus in unconscious patients. This technique, known as Sellick's maneuver, reduces gastric air insufflation and the subsequent risk of vomiting and aspiration.[13,14] The amount of pressure required should be equal to that which would cause discomfort if one were to compress the bridge of the nose.

The procedure is contraindicated in the conscious patient who is likely to gag. A common pitfall of Sellick's maneuver is compression of the thyroid rather than cricoid cartilage. Pressure on the thyroid cartilage cannot occlude the esophagus because of its open posterior structure. If a patient vomits during Sellick's maneuver, release pressure and roll the patient to the side to avoid gastroesophageal injury. Maintain spinal precautions during the log roll.

ENDOTRACHEAL INTUBATION

There are several major reasons for endotracheal intubation (ETI). Failure to maintain adequate oxygenation and ventilation, despite opening or clearing the airway secretions, is a primary indication. Patients who are not spontaneously breathing also require ETI.

The second most common reason for ETI includes patients unable to protect their airway as a result of loss of airway patency or protective reflexes. Patients who have lost these reflexes risk aspiration of gastric contents.[9,15-17] It is commonly taught that patients who have lost their gag reflex require ETI. Although it is important to determine the patients' ability to handle secretions, "testing the gag reflex" is generally not recommended, since this maneuver may precipitate vomiting and worsen intracranial hypertension. In addition, up to 40% of the general population may not have a gag reflex.[18] Instead, observe the patient's ability to swallow. Intact swallowing generally confirms retained airway protection. Although there is no single, clear-cut test that the clinician can use to assess the need for intubation, any patient who needs continuous suctioning or an artificial airway, or who is unable to swallow usually requires intubation. Other indications for ETI include the following:

1. Impending airway obstruction
2. Severe head injury (Glasgow Coma Scale ≤8)
3. Need to perform diagnostic studies in uncooperative patients

Equipment

Preparation is essential for success. The primary cause of chaos during intubation is lack of readiness. The rare patient requires immediate intubation or cricothyroidotomy on arrival. During the initial minutes, most critically ill trauma patients may be managed with simple maneuvers, including mask ventilation.

To avoid pandemonium, use a mental or physical checklist to verify that all elements are ready *before* attempting the procedure. The essential steps include the following:

1. Verify that the required intubation equipment is available and functioning
2. Establish intravenous access

3. Prepare for administration of pharmacologic aids
4. Attach a pulse oximeter and cardiac monitor and ensure that they are functioning
5. Assess the patient for presence of a difficult airway
6. Proper patient positioning
7. A backup plan

It is essential that the physician follow these steps at every intubation. Failure to include all of the essential steps in the preintubation checklist invites disaster. Seemingly minor omissions such as the failure to draw up the proper dosage of medications, or failure to prepare adequate suctioning equipment, can have serious consequences. In addition, the operator should minimize exposure to potentially infectious materials by employing universal precautions. Operators should wear gloves and an impervious gown and use a mask with protective eyewear.

Many trauma centers find that an airway cart ensures that all necessary equipment is within reach. These carts must be routinely checked before each shift and restocked after each use. The ideal cart is open, organized, and labeled so that essential equipment can be identified. Airway carts should contain, at a minimum, the following:[19,20]

- A variety of adult and pediatric endotracheal tubes (cuffed and uncuffed)
- Adult and pediatric laryngoscope handles
- A variety of adult and pediatric straight and curved blades
- Endotracheal tube stylettes
- Syringes
- Topical anesthetics
- Magill forceps
- End-tidal CO_2 detectors or esophageal detector devices
- Oropharyngeal and nasopharyngeal airway devices
- Various sized bag-valve masks
- A selection of suction catheters
- Pharmacologic adjuncts necessary for intubation
- Extra laryngoscope batteries and bulbs
- A separate locked "airway drug box" for controlled medications

A separate cart or drawer may be used for the patient with a difficult airway. Equipment may include the following:

- Cricothyroidotomy tray
- Equipment for percutaneous transtracheal ventilation
- Laryngeal mask airway (LMA) or intubating LMA
- Bullard laryngoscope blade
- Intubating fiberoptic bronchoscope
- Lighted stylet
- Combitube or other esophageal-tracheal combination airway
- Equipment for retrograde intubation

Laryngoscope Blades

Selection of either a straight or curved blade is largely a matter of personal preference, but there are some properties unique to each. The following differences are mostly anecdotal, and no well-designed study has proven the purported advantages of one blade over another.

A curved blade (MacIntosh) is inserted into the vallecula, where indirect pressure lifts the epiglottis free of the hyoepiglottic ligament to expose the vocal cords and larynx. The curved blade reduces the risk of dental trauma and, according to some, requires less forearm strength to visualize the vocal cords. The curved blade is also useful in pushing the tongue out of the way to permit visualization of the vocal cords.

In contrast, the straight blade (Miller) is used to directly lift the epiglottis. The straight blade may be a better choice in pediatric patients, in whom the epiglottis is floppy, or in patients requiring spinal immobilization. Disadvantages include increased dental trauma and increased risk of laryngospasm. The clinician should become adept at using each blade and select the blade that is most appropriate for the clinical circumstance. There are a variety of other specialized laryngoscope blades, but they are not widely available and merely represent a variation on the basic theme of straight versus curved.[21]

Endotracheal Tubes

Endotracheal tubes are made of plastic and labeled according to internal diameter. Linear markings are usually imprinted on the exterior of the tube for determining the distance from the tip. These markings help determine the proper depth of tube insertion. Selection of the proper tube size is important in ensuring the success of ETI especially in infants and children. In infants and children the following formula[22] is usually used to determine tube size:

$$\text{Endotracheal Tube Size (internal diameter in mm)} = 4 + (\text{age in years}/4)$$

An alternative to this method is to use the width of the nail on the patient's little finger to gauge the approximate endotracheal tube size. Selection of proper tube size in the pediatric patient is of paramount importance because of the fact that children younger than 8 years of age are often intubated with an uncuffed tube. If an inappropriately small size is used, there will be an inadequate seal within the trachea, resulting in an air leak. An excessively large tube will not pass beyond the cricoid ring, the narrowest portion of the pediatric airway. If a caregiver is able to pass the endotracheal tube through the cords, but then encounters resistance as the tube abuts the cricoid ring, the tube should be removed and the next smallest size tube (0.5 mm internal diameter smaller) inserted following reoxygenation.

The proper depth of insertion for any endotracheal tube can be estimated by multiplying the internal diameter by three and aligning this mark at the lip. For example, a 4-year-old patient who requires an endotracheal tube with an internal diameter of 5 mm should have a 15 cm depth of insertion.[23-26] Alternatively, the black line that is embedded near the end of the tube should pass through the cords.

A cuffed endotracheal tube may be used in patients over the age of 8, although some centers safely use cuffed tubes in younger children. Adult women will generally accept a 7 to 8 mm tube, whereas adult men will generally accept a 7.5 to 9 mm endotracheal tube, although 7.5 and 8 mm tubes are most commonly employed. In general, the largest acceptable tube should be used so that resistance to airflow within the tube is minimized. This is especially important when intubating patients with chronic obstructive pulmonary disease, since the effort of breathing increases exponentially with decreasing internal diameters. A small tube can subsequently be replaced with a larger tube in most cases, most easily with a tube-changing guide threaded through the original tube.

It is essential to check the cuff of the endotracheal tube for air leaks before intubation. Once the patient is intubated, determine appropriate cuff inflation by slowly injecting air into the cuff while the patient is being ventilated until no air leak is audible. In general, approximately 5 to 8 ml of air will suffice. The caregiver may also compress the pilot balloon to test for adequate inflation pressures. For long-term use, measure cuff pressure and maintain between 20 and 25 mmHg; cuff pressure exceeding 30 mmHg compromises capillary blood flow to the trachea.

Preparation of the endotracheal tube deserves special mention. A flexible stylette may be lubricated and passed down the tube to increase its stiffness and ability to direct the tube anteriorly if necessary. Do not permit the stylette to extend beyond the tip of the endotracheal tube, since it may lacerate the trachea. The stylette should have the proximal end bent to prohibit distal migration of the stylette. The tip of the endotracheal tube, as well as the cuff, may be lubricated with a water-soluble lubricant. On occasion however, the excessive lubricant accidentally transferred to the physician's hands makes equipment slippery.

Monitoring

ELECTROCARDIOGRAPHY

The use of an electrocardiograph (ECG) monitor and pulse oximetry should be standard in emergency department intubations. These devices will alert the physician to untoward events more quickly than changes in the vital signs. The ECG will detect bradycardia or asystole that is occasionally seen with rapid sequence intubation, particularly in the elderly.

PULSE OXIMETRY

The old saw regarding holding one's breath to determine the length of an intubation attempt is outdated. Pulse oximetry is an objective means to reduce the frequency and duration of hypoxemia associated with emergency intubation.[27]

END-TIDAL CO_2

Once the patient is intubated, confirm placement with an objective test such as the end-tidal CO_2 detector or the esophageal detector device (see the following discussion). The use of continuous end-tidal CO_2 monitoring in intubated patients is becoming widespread in trauma centers.

Factors Contributing to Difficult Airway Management

The optimal position for ETI is one in which the patient is placed in the "sniffing position" with the occiput raised 7 to 10 cm above the stretcher. The head should be extended and the neck slightly flexed to align the oropharyngeal and laryngeal axes. In the acutely injured trauma patient who has not had clearance of the cervical spine, this position endangers a potentially unstable cervical spine. Therefore the "sniffing position" should not be used in a trauma patient unless the cervical spine has been cleared. Continuous immobilization by an assistant is required throughout the procedure. Immobilized trauma patients, by definition, have a potentially difficult airway, since in-line stabilization prevents optimal head and neck positioning.

Trauma patients have other characteristics that contribute to the difficult airway (Box 7-1).[28-35] An early determination of the difficult airway allows the EP to plan ahead and consider airway alternatives, including involvement of an anesthesiologist (Fig. 7-1).

Several steps can help predict the difficult airway. The conscious patient should be asked to open his or her mouth as wide as possible. It may be difficult to

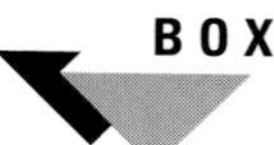

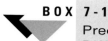

BOX 7-1
Predictors of the Difficult Airway

Narrow submental angle
Submental swelling
Submandibular swelling
Suprahyoid notch to chin distance <6
Deviated trachea
Neck swelling
Neck scars
Limited mouth opening
Narrow mouth width
Small intraoral cavity
Poor view of fauces
Large tongue
Cleft lip/palate
Long teeth

Adapted from McIntyre: *Can J Anaesth* 34:204-13, 1987.

perform laryngoscopy in patients with limited jaw openings. Look for signs of maxillofacial or laryngeal trauma, which complicate airway management. A receding mandible, prominent upper incisors, and a short neck reduce the angles necessary to visualize the vocal cords and render intubation difficult.[34,36-40]

The degree of difficulty, represented by the patient's ability to open his or her mouth, can be assessed using the Mallampati score (Fig. 7-2).[36] Although facial fractures themselves do not always make intubation more difficult, bleeding may be profuse, and the clinician must have adequate suction available to keep the airway clear. Bleeding may be compounded by a diminished ability of the patient to protect his or her airway, as shown by the pooling of blood or secretions in the hypopharynx.

Severe perioral fractures, both mandibular and maxillary, pose additional problems. If the patient's face is unstable, a proper mask seal may be impossible. Such a patient cannot be ventilated by BVM if the patient is paralyzed and intubation unsuccessful. In such cases, prep the patient's neck and open a cricothyroidotomy tray in case surgical access becomes necessary.

Upper airway trauma may involve expanding hematomas, burns, penetrating neck injuries, and blunt contusions, thus making intubation extremely difficult because of the disruption of normal anatomy and landmarks.[37] Airway trauma can be classified as either open or closed. In open injuries, there is a direct communication between the airway and the outside. The open trachea may be intubated directly through the skin if needed.

Closed injuries represent a challenge since airway landmarks may be obscured or the trachea disrupted. One such presentation is the "clothesline injury" that a snowmobile rider suffers when speeding under a low-slung wire. Tracheal disruption is suspected based on the mechanism of injury, massive subcutaneous air, and a persistent pneumothorax despite a functioning chest tube under suction. In a patient with a clothesline injury and suspected tracheal disruption, avoid neuromuscular blockade. The patient's airway and neck muscles hold the severed airway in apposition and paralysis may make intubation impossible. If such a patient is encountered, immediately prepare for a surgical airway. Awake intubation using a laryngoscope or a fiberoptic device is an alternative to cricothyroidotomy, as long as the physician is prepared to surgically intervene.

Regardless of the particular problem encountered, it is best to identify the difficult airway before attempting intubation. This allows the EP to anticipate and compensate for anatomic or traumatic hurdles. Preparation and forethought help avoid disaster.

Intubation Process

The ability to manage the airway of a trauma patient requires a thorough understanding of airway anatomy (Fig. 7-3, *A*). After making the necessary preparations, the physician managing the airway should stand at the head of the bed with the patient raised to the level of the physician's lower sternum. The laryngoscope should be grasped with the left hand, and the patient's lower lip is drawn down with the right thumb. The jaw is pulled forward, and the tip of the laryngoscope is introduced into the right side of the mouth. The blade is then advanced along the right side of the mouth, gradually displacing the tongue to the left as the blade is moved to the center. Failure to place the blade in the middle of the mouth or move the tongue to the left are common errors that may result in an inability to visualize the vocal cords. If the blade tip is off center, the cords will not be seen and intubation will be rendered impossible.

The operator exerts a force along the axis of the laryngoscope handle, lifting it upward and forward at a 45° angle. With this motion, the pharyngeal tissues are displaced anteriorly to enhance visualization of the cords. Immediately upon performance of this maneuver, the epiglottis should come into view. If the epiglottis is not visible, an assistant should exert downward pressure on the thyroid cartilage.

Once the epiglottis is seen, the next step is cord visualization, accomplished by inserting the curved blade into the vallecula, or if the straight blade is

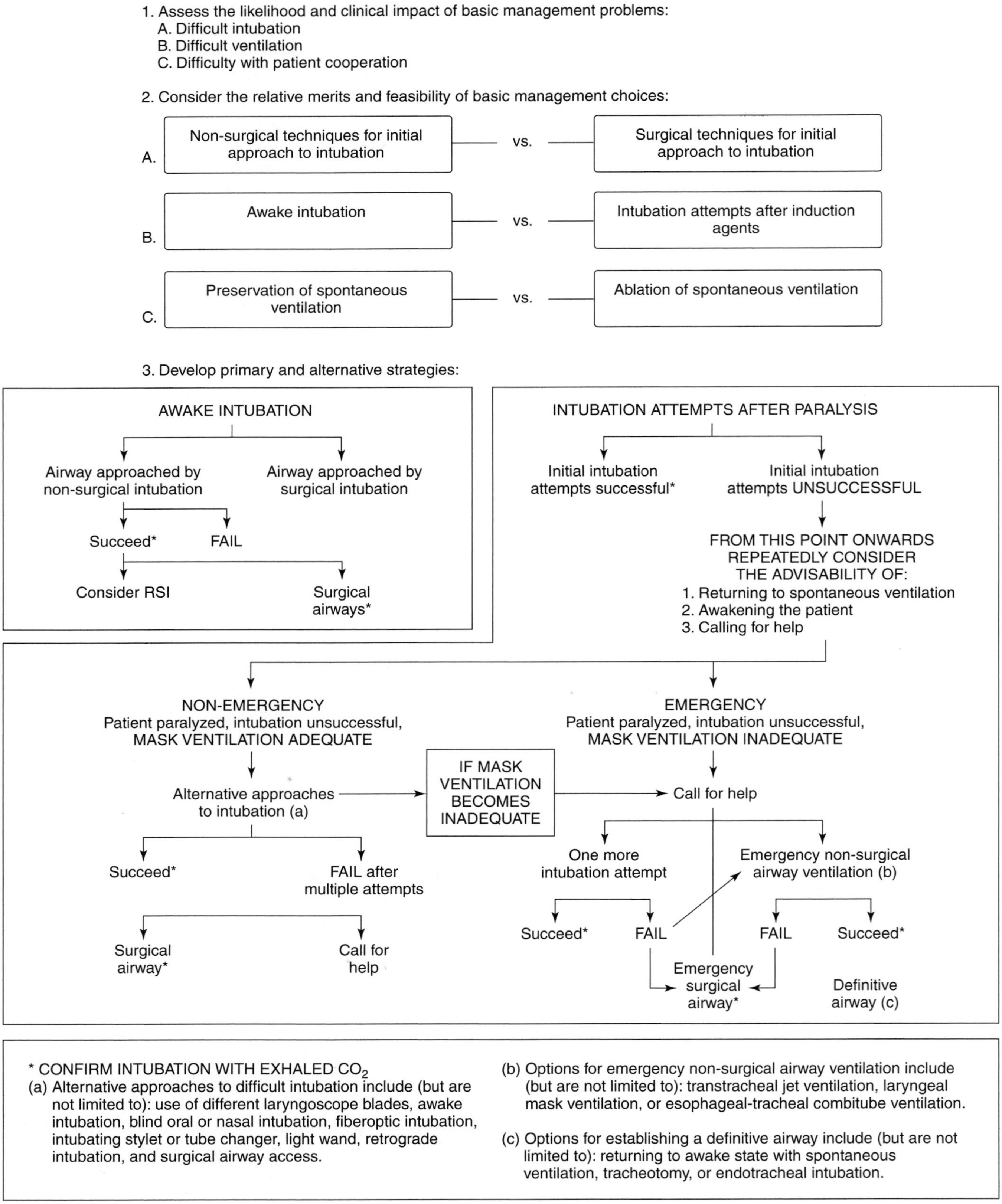

1. Assess the likelihood and clinical impact of basic management problems:
A. Difficult intubation
B. Difficult ventilation
C. Difficulty with patient cooperation
2. Consider the relative merits and feasibility of basic management choices:
A.
Non-surgical techniques for initial approach to intubation
vs.
Surgical techniques for initial approach to intubation
B.
Awake intubation
vs.
Intubation attempts after induction agents
C.
Preservation of spontaneous ventilation
vs.
Ablation of spontaneous ventilation
3. Develop primary and alternative strategies:
AWAKE INTUBATION
Airway approached by non-surgical intubation
Airway approached by surgical intubation
Succeed*
FAIL
Consider RSI
Surgical airways*
INTUBATION ATTEMPTS AFTER PARALYSIS
Initial intubation attempts successful*
Initial intubation attempts UNSUCCESSFUL
FROM THIS POINT ONWARDS REPEATEDLY CONSIDER THE ADVISABILITY OF:
1. Returning to spontaneous ventilation
2. Awakening the patient
3. Calling for help
NON-EMERGENCY
Patient paralyzed, intubation unsuccessful, MASK VENTILATION ADEQUATE
Alternative approaches to intubation (a)
Succeed*
FAIL after multiple attempts
Surgical airway*
Call for help
IF MASK VENTILATION BECOMES INADEQUATE
EMERGENCY
Patient paralyzed, intubation unsuccessful, MASK VENTILATION INADEQUATE
Call for help
One more intubation attempt
Emergency non-surgical airway ventilation (b)
Succeed*
FAIL
FAIL
Succeed*
Emergency surgical airway*
Definitive airway (c)
* CONFIRM INTUBATION WITH EXHALED CO2
(a) Alternative approaches to difficult intubation include (but are not limited to): use of different laryngoscope blades, awake intubation, blind oral or nasal intubation, fiberoptic intubation, intubating stylet or tube changer, light wand, retrograde intubation, and surgical airway access.
(b) Options for emergency non-surgical airway ventilation include (but are not limited to): transtracheal jet ventilation, laryngeal mask ventilation, or esophageal-tracheal combitube ventilation.
(c) Options for establishing a definitive airway include (but are not limited to): returning to awake state with spontaneous ventilation, tracheotomy, or endotracheal intubation.

Fig. 7-1 Difficult airway algorithm. (Adapted from Caplan R, et al: *Anesthesiology* 78:597-602, 1993.)

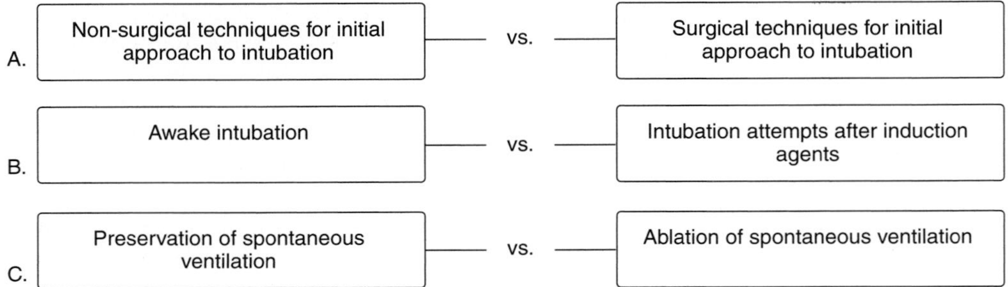

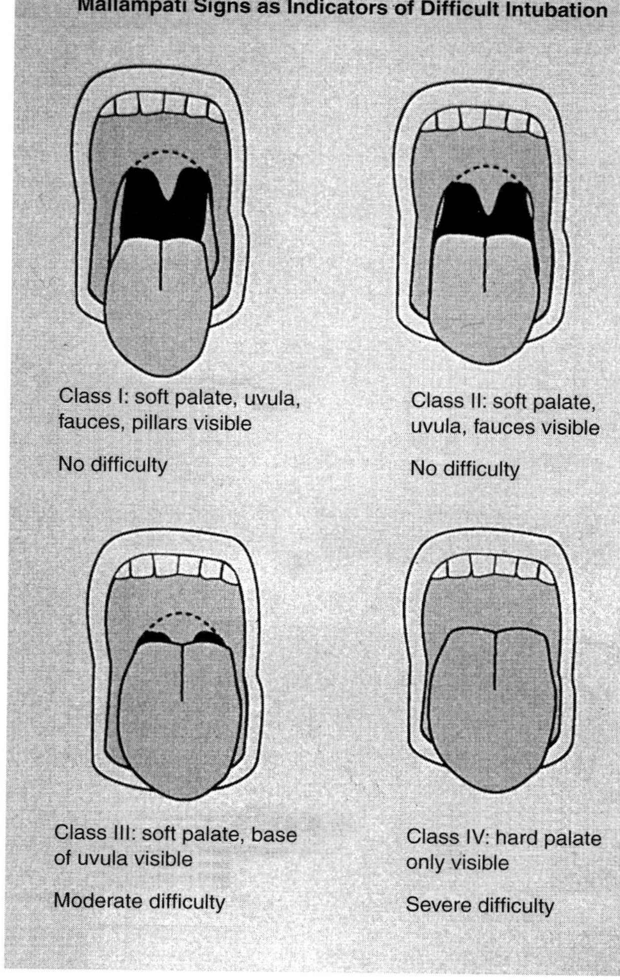

Fig. 7-2 The Mallampati Score for prediction of difficulty on intubation. (Courtesy KW Publications. In Walls RM: Airway management. In Rosen P, et al [editors]: *Emergency medicine: concepts and clinical practice,* ed 4, St Louis, 1998, Mosby.)

used, by directly lifting the epiglottis. Copious secretions may require suctioning of the airway.

If the cords are not visible, have the assistant perform a BURP (Backwards, Upwards, and Rightward Pressure) maneuver.[41,42] Each step should be executed separately while the intubator looks for the cords. First, exert downward pressure on the thyroid cartilage to displace the airway posteriorly into the operator's line of sight, then upwards and finally rightward. In some cases, visualization is improved if the assistant hooks a finger inside the right cheek of the patient and pulls it laterally.

Once the vocal cords have been visualized (Fig. 7-3, *B*), the tube may be passed. The operator holds the tube with his or her right hand and inserts it into the right side of the patient's mouth carefully so the tip of the tube does not obscure the line of sight. If thyroid cartilage pressure had been required to visualize the cords, it should be maintained. The tube is then advanced towards the patient's vocal cords. Once the tube is in the vicinity of the cords, the operator should pass it through the cords under direct visualization until the cuff goes through the glottis. Passage should require little effort, and if resistance is encountered, the tube should be repositioned, or a smaller tube should be used. Excessive force during tube passage may result in damage to the vocal cords. Once the tube has been passed through the cords, the laryngoscope is removed and the endotracheal tube cuff is inflated. The operator should hold on to the tube securely until it can be taped or tied into place. At this point, verification of tube placement is the next important step.

Verification of Endotracheal Intubation

Always use an objective test of endotracheal tube placement such as the end-tidal CO_2 detector or an esophageal detector device. Other means are inadequate.

The importance of verifying endotracheal placement cannot be overemphasized, since unrecognized esophageal placement is rapidly fatal. Verification of tube placement in the trauma patient is made more difficult because the intubation process is performed under adverse conditions. It is important to note that although esophageal intubation is undesirable, it is not harmful if *quickly* recognized. Although there are many ways to verify endotracheal tube placement, none is completely reliable in all circumstances.

Although direct visualization of tube passage is comforting, it is not sufficient. By visualizing the tube as it passes through the cords, the operator can be reasonably assured that the tube has been placed in the trachea. However, problems arise if the cords are not visible or if the tube becomes dislodged before it has been secured. It is essential that the operator maintain the proper depth of insertion while the tube is being taped in place. Although neck flexion should not apply to the immobilized trauma patient, cervical motion can propel the endotracheal tube as much as 3 to 5 cm, which may result in tube dislodgment.[43]

Another method for verifying tube placement involves a combination of clinical assessment and direct measurements. Chest rise with ventilation is inadequate,[44-47] and auscultation of breath sounds in the axilla and epigastrium are fallible.[48-50] Changes in exhaled tidal volumes, reservoir bag compliance, endotracheal tube cuff stiffness, tube fogging, and the

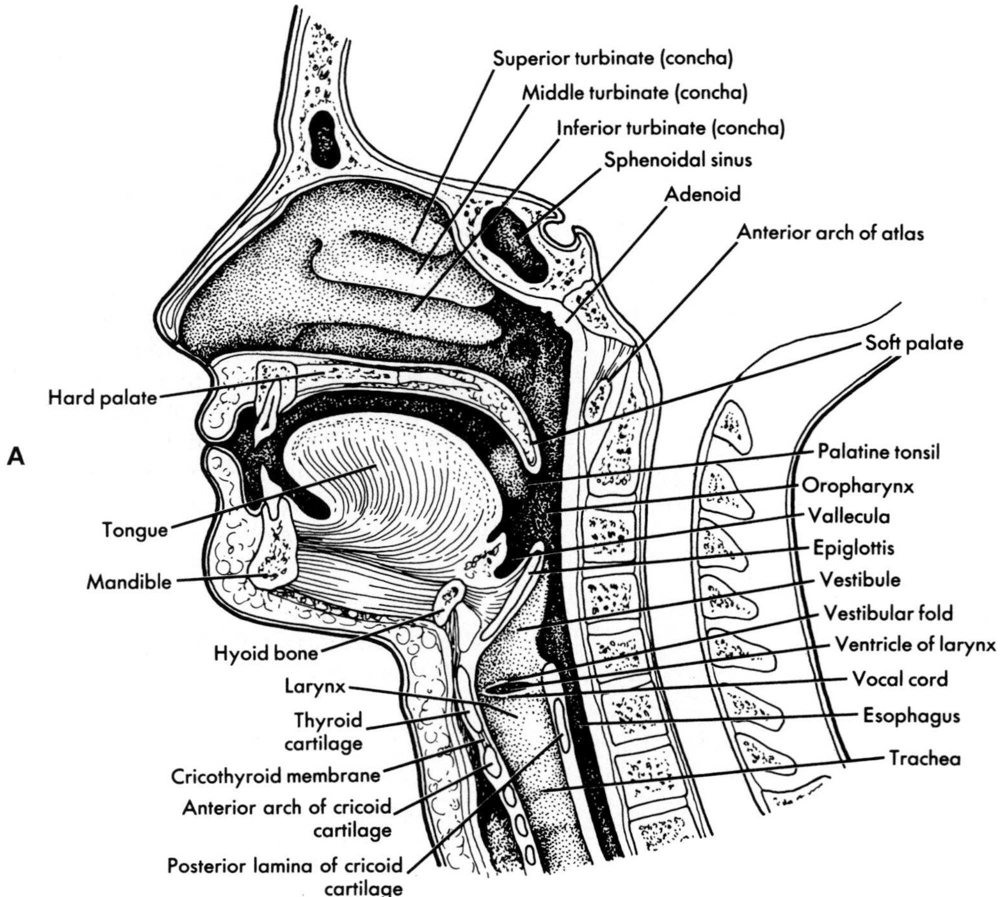

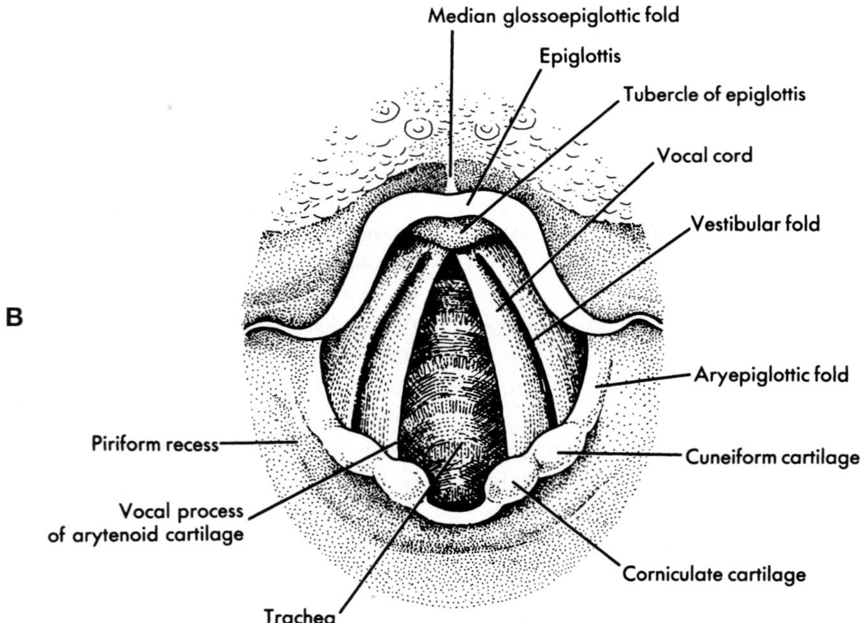

Fig. 7-3 **A,** Sagittal view of the airway. **B,** Laryngoscopic view of the airway. (From Morris I: Airway management. In Rosen P, et al [editors]: *Emergency medicine: concepts and clinical practice,* ed 3, St Louis, 1992, Mosby.)

presence of gastric contents cannot distinguish tracheal versus esophageal placement.[44,45,48,51-53]

Chest radiography squanders valuable time if a patient has an esophageal intubation. An anterior-posterior view alone may falsely conclude that a midline tube is in the trachea. Pulse oximetry takes too long to detect esophageal intubation. With esophageal intubation, adequate oxygen saturation may be seen for up to 5 minutes despite the absence of lung ventilation.[44,48,54] In addition, pulse oximetry readings lag a minute or two behind actual oxygen saturation as measured by arterial blood gas.

The esophageal detector device is "low-tech," inexpensive, and reliable.[55,56] The operator can connect either a self-inflating bulb or syringe to the ET tube.[57] Free aspiration of air occurs with tracheal intubation, whereas difficult aspiration is due to esophageal intubation. Although very accurate, there are some cases where the device can mislead the operator.[58] The esophageal detector device tends to be less precise in patients who are morbidly obese, and the performance is highly dependent on the experience of the observer.[59] Its accuracy in the prehospital arena is poor.[60]

The most reliable method for verifying tube placement is end-tidal carbon dioxide ($ETCO_2$) detection.[61] This measurement is highly sensitive and specific in verifying tube placement in patients with a perfusing rhythm. The technique is less sensitive but still highly specific in low perfusion states. During cardiac arrest, endotracheal tube placement may result in a low $ETCO_2$ reading resulting from the minimal blood flow back to the lungs; but if a high $ETCO_2$ reading is seen, endotracheal placement is assured.[62] The basic methods of $ETCO_2$ detection include qualitative colorimetric and quantitative digital measurements. The digital quantitative method yields much more information than the basic colorimetric device in terms of physiologic status and arterial carbon dioxide saturation. However, the colorimetric device appears to be adequate in verifying tube placement (Fig. 7-4).

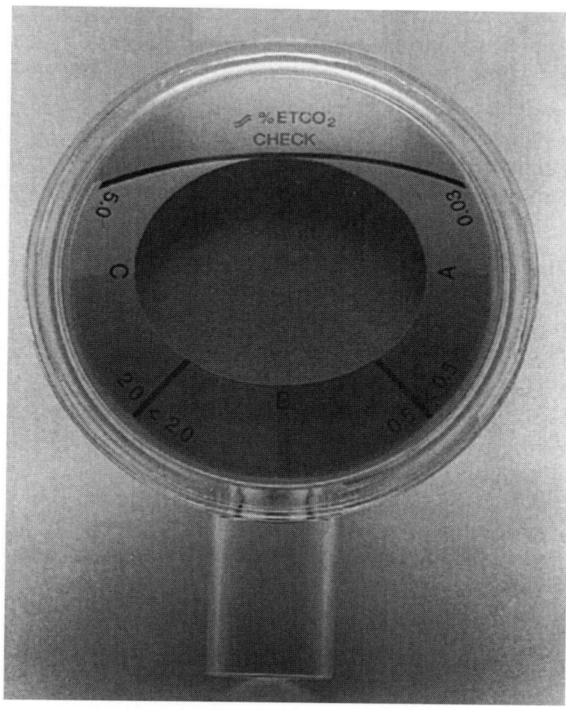

Fig. 7-4 Colorimetric end-tidal CO_2 detector. The central disk changes color to match a color scale with indicated concentrations of CO_2. (From Walls RM: Airway management. In Rosen P, et al [editors]: *Emergency medicine: concepts and clinical practice,* ed 4, St Louis, 1998, Mosby.)

RAPID SEQUENCE INTUBATION

Rapid sequence intubation (RSI) is the preferred method of intubation in the trauma patient who requires emergent airway management. The technique is termed *rapid sequence* because it involves the simultaneous induction of general anesthesia and a neuromuscular blockade, usually with succinylcholine (Fig. 7-5). This technique is preferred in trauma patients because they are frequently combative, may have recently eaten, and may have unstable cervical spine or increased intracranial pressure.[4,6] The purpose of RSI is to induce a state of unconsciousness and neuromuscular paralysis, to reduce the risk of aspiration, prevent secondary brain injury, and facilitate successful intubation.[63] As with all airway procedures, RSI requires careful preparation and training to maximize the chance of success.

No randomized controlled trial has yet tested the utility of neuromuscular blockade in the emergency department. However, one study did compare complications during intubation before and after the introduction of neuromuscular blockers in the ED. Complications were greater in both number and severity in the nonparalyzed group and included aspiration (15%), airway trauma (28%), and death (3%). None of these complications occurred in the rapid sequence group who received neuromuscular blockade.[64]

Preparation

While preparing for RSI, look for signs of a difficult intubation. Determine a backup plan, as well as the likelihood of using it. In addition, all pharmacologic adjuncts should be drawn into syringes for quick use, and the laryngoscope and proper-sized endotracheal tube selected. Place the patient on a pulse oximeter

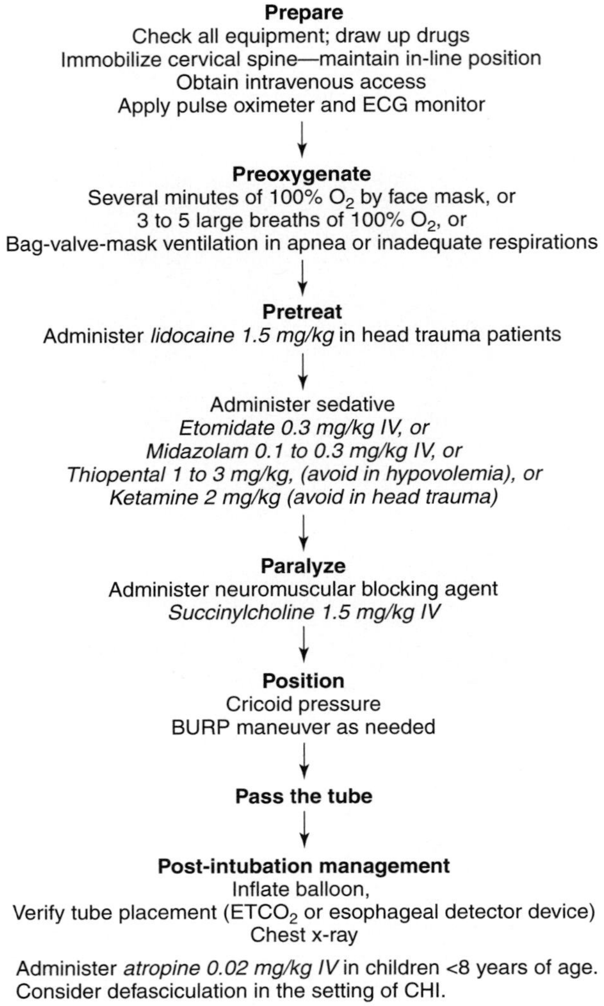

Prepare
Check all equipment; draw up drugs
Immobilize cervical spine—maintain in-line position
Obtain intravenous access
Apply pulse oximeter and ECG monitor

↓

Preoxygenate
Several minutes of 100% O_2 by face mask, or
3 to 5 large breaths of 100% O_2, or
Bag-valve-mask ventilation in apnea or inadequate respirations

↓

Pretreat
Administer *lidocaine 1.5 mg/kg* in head trauma patients

↓

Administer sedative
Etomidate 0.3 mg/kg IV, or
Midazolam 0.1 to 0.3 mg/kg IV, or
Thiopental 1 to 3 mg/kg, (avoid in hypovolemia), or
Ketamine 2 mg/kg (avoid in head trauma)

↓

Paralyze
Administer neuromuscular blocking agent
Succinylcholine 1.5 mg/kg IV

↓

Position
Cricoid pressure
BURP maneuver as needed

↓

Pass the tube

↓

Post-intubation management
Inflate balloon,
Verify tube placement ($ETCO_2$ or esophageal detector device)
Chest x-ray

Administer *atropine 0.02 mg/kg IV* in children <8 years of age.
Consider defasciculation in the setting of CHI.

Fig. 7-5 Proposed sequence of RSI. (Adapted from Walls RM, et al: *Manual of emergency airway management,* ed 3, Philadelphia, 2000, Lippincott, Williams & Wilkins.)

and a cardiac monitor. Decide whether ventilation can be performed if intubation fails. The inability to adequately provide ventilation in the setting of failed intubation mandates preparation for a surgical airway.[28-35] If time permits, a second intravenous line should be started. Prepare the end-tidal CO_2 detector for use.

Preoxygenation

The purpose of preoxygenation is to wash out the nitrogen reserve present in the pulmonary dead space, using oxygen. Preoxygenation creates an oxygen reservoir, which should allow at least 3 minutes of apnea in the normal adult before desaturation occurs. Administering 100% oxygen for 5 minutes, using a nonrebreather oxygen mask if the patient is spontaneously ventilating, accomplishes this goal. If there is insufficient time for the full 5 minute preoxygenation phase, approximately two thirds to three fourths of the effect can be achieved if the patient takes four vital capacity breaths with 100% oxygen.[65] If the patient is not spontaneously ventilating and requires BVM ventilation, it is imperative that an assistant apply cricoid pressure (Sellick's maneuver) to reduce the risk of gastric insufflation. Avoid BVM ventilation in patients with adequate respirations, since gastric distention increases the risk of aspiration during RSI. Many overeager respiratory therapists begin bagging the patient as soon as succinylcholine is administered. Help them resist this temptation.

Pressure (Intracranial)

While the patient is being preoxygenated, address a number of considerations, the first of which is suspected increased intracranial pressure (ICP).[66] Lidocaine 1.5 to 2.0 mg/kg given 5 minutes before intubation will blunt the pressor response that occurs with manipulation of airway structures.[67] Some authorities also suggest an opioid such as fentanyl, in a dose of 3 to 5 μg (micrograms)/kg, or a defasciculating dose of a nondepolarizing neuromuscular blocking agent. These agents may also reduce ICP spikes in response to depolarizing blockers. In general, the defasciculating dose is approximately 10% of the dose needed to induce paralysis. *Although this step is sometimes recommended for patients with increased ICP, there is no objective evidence that pretreatment with a defasciculating dose has any clinical benefit.* In addition, the clinician should be forewarned that 3 to 4 minutes should elapse between the administration of the defasciculating dose and succinylcholine. To achieve the desired effect, this delay must be weighed against the theoretical bene fit of reducing the pressor response and rise in ICP in response to airway manipulation. "Mini-dose" succinylcholine (one tenth of the paralyzing dose) given several minutes before the paralyzing dose, can also decrease fasciculations.[68] Again, the clinical significance of this in trauma resuscitation is unknown.

Paralysis And Sedation

The next step involves the rapid administration of two drugs: a sedative and neuromuscular blocking agent. This renders the patient unconscious and provides ideal intubating conditions. As the patient loses con-

TABLE 7-1
Neuromuscular Blockers

DRUG	COMMENTS	DOSAGE
Succinylcholine—depolarizing	Drug of choice for trauma intubation; fast onset, reliable	1-1.5 mg/kg (peds 2 mg/kg with atropine)
Atracurium—nondepolarizing	Useful in renal failure	0.4-0.5 mg/kg IV
Cis-atracurium—nondepolarizing		0.1-0.2 mg/kg IV
Pancuronium—nondepolarizing	Older drug, cardiac side effects	0.1 mg/kg IV
Rocuronium—nondepolarizing	Useful in children if muscular dystrophy known or suspected; fast onset	0.6-1.2 mg/kg IV
Vecuronium—nondepolarizing	Useful for prolonged paralysis	0.1 mg/kg IV

sciousness with sedation, an assistant should apply cricoid pressure to reduce the risk of aspiration.[13]

The choice of neuromuscular blocking agents is restricted to two general categories, depolarizing and nondepolarizing agents (Table 7-1). The only widely available depolarizing agent at this time is succinylcholine. A variety of nondepolarizing agents are available, such as pancuronium, vecuronium, rocuronium, and other agents such as atracurium and cis-atracurium.

DEPOLARIZING NEUROMUSCULAR BLOCKING AGENTS

Succinylcholine is the preferred neuromuscular blocking agent in most EDs. The recommended dose of succinylcholine is 1 to 1.5 mg/kg given by rapid intravenous push. It has a rapid onset (30 to 60 seconds) and short duration of action (10 to 15 minutes). Avoid using inadequate doses, since appropriate dosing guarantees complete relaxation and avoids repeat dosing. Once succinylcholine is given, the operator should expect about 45 seconds before complete relaxation. If a defasciculating dose of a competitive neuromuscular blocker had not been given previously, generalized muscle fasciculations occur in approximately 10 to 15 seconds. A defasciculating dose prevents these fasciculations.

A number of adverse effects may be seen with succinylcholine. The most clinically apparent are muscle fasciculations. Some authorities consider these fasciculations problematic in the setting of suspected elevated ICP, globe ruptures, and skeletal fractures or dislocations. However, these theoretical concerns may not outweigh the proven benefits of succinylcholine. Other adverse effects include myalgias, hyperkalemia, stimulation of autonomic ganglia (negative inotropy), malignant hyperthermia, prolonged apnea, and histamine release.

With succinylcholine administration, the plasma potassium may rise up to 0.5 mEq/L. In otherwise healthy patients, this rise may be of little consequence. However, in patients with late severe burns, renal failure, major muscle trauma (crush injury), or upper motor neuron disease, hyperkalemia may induce a lethal arrhythmia. *For patients with burns or crush injuries, it takes several days after the trauma for the muscles to become vulnerable to the potassium-releasing effects of succinylcholine. For this reason, these are not important concerns in most ED patients.*

Malignant hyperthermia, a syndrome of excessive muscular contractions, may occur in approximately 1 in 50,000 adults. This autosomally dominant clinical syndrome consists of cardiac arrhythmias, hyperpyrexia, coagulation defects, hypoxia, acidosis, and myoglobinuria. Treatment of malignant hyperthermia is largely supportive. The administration of benzodiazepines and dantrolene is also recommended.

NONDEPOLARIZING (COMPETITIVE) NEUROMUSCULAR BLOCKING AGENTS

Nondepolarizing neuromuscular blocking agents are classified as either steroids (pancuronium, rocuronium, and dacuronium) or benzylisoquinolines (d-tubocurare, mivacurium, doxacurium, metocurine, atracurium, cis-atracurium). Problems with the neuromuscular blocking agents include promotion of histamine release, which is especially pronounced with d-tubocurare, an agent rarely used today.[69] In general, nondepolarizing neuromuscular blocking agents have a slower onset of action and a longer half-life than succinylcholine. Both the onset of action, as well as duration of action, can be shortened by using a technique known as priming. Priming involves the preadministration of a small dose (5% to 10% of the dose required for neuromuscular blockade) approximately 3 to 4 minutes before administering the paralyzing dose.[70] Priming promotes an onset of action within 60 to 90 seconds, which is comparable to succinylcholine.

Although the duration of action using the priming method is shortened compared with just a single paralyzing dose of the nondepolarizing agent, it is still much longer than succinylcholine. Unfortunately, priming may cause problems in emergency airway management. If the priming dose is too large, it may cause premature respiratory failure and hypoxia.

Induction Agents

A large array of pharmacologic adjuncts is available to the EP to sedate the patient for intubation. These agents include barbiturates, benzodiazepines, opiates, and specific agents such as ketamine, propofol, and etomidate. The choice should depend mostly on the clinical situation and to a lesser extent on clinician preference or institutional protocol. The physician must consider the effects of the agents on the individual patient and, in particular, anticipate the possibility of occult blood loss (Table 7-2).

BENZODIAZEPINES

Of all the benzodiazepines, midazolam (Versed) is the best suited as an induction agent.[71,72] It shares with the other benzodiazepines the following effects: anxiolytic, hypnotic, sedative, anticonvulsive, skeletal muscle relaxant, and amnestic properties. Benzodiazepines have no analgesic effects and only induce sedation and amnesia.

Midazolam has often been compared with diazepam (Valium). Midazolam offers a number of advantages over diazepam, including increased potency, more rapid onset of action, shorter half-life, less cardiopulmonary depression, and decreased tissue irritation. Although the recommended dose for conscious sedation is 0.05 to 0.1 mg/kg, the induction dose ranges from 0.1 to 0.3 mg/kg intravenously. Following this higher dose, loss of consciousness occurs in about 30 to 45 seconds with the duration of action of 10 to 20 minutes and elimination half-life of 1 to 4 hours.[73]

Midazolam has achieved widespread clinical use and is safe and effective. However, in the trauma setting, administration of midazolam may cause a moderate to marked systolic hypotension as a result of decreased vascular tone.[74,75] Cardiac output and coronary artery blood flow are not affected. Respiratory depression is another common side effect of benzodiazepines and appears to be more pronounced if doses are given very rapidly, in large quantities, or if the patient has an underlying co-morbidity or pulmonary compromise.[76] Overall complication rates are low, making midazolam an acceptable choice as an induction agent.

BARBITURATES

The two agents in this class that have been primarily used to induce anesthesia in the ED are thiopental and methohexital (Brevital). Although these agents have been widely used for elective procedures in the operating suite, they have been used less frequently in the ED setting. Although these agents are excellent sedatives, they may be dangerous in the setting of multisystem trauma.[77-79] The barbiturates depress the vasomotor centers and myocardial contractility, and may cause severe hypotension. Patients with ongoing hem-

TABLE 7-2
Induction Agents and Pharmacologic Airway Adjuncts

DRUG	COMMENTS	DOSAGE
Etomidate	A drug of choice in trauma intubations. Minimal chance of hypotension.	0.3 mg/kg IV over 30-60 sec
Fentanyl	Good for painful conditions. Avoid rapid infusion.	3-5 μg/kg IV
Ketamine	Avoid in head trauma. Useful in the hypotensive patient as it can increase blood pressure.	1-2 mg/kg IV over 1 min
Lidocaine	Useful in head trauma. Give at least 5 minutes before intubation if time allows.	1.0-1.5 mg/kg IV
Methohexital	Avoid in hypovolemia. Good in isolated head trauma without hypotension.	1-3 mg/kg IV
Midazolam	Avoid in hypovolemia. Good in isolated head trauma without hypotension.	5 mg or 0.2-0.3 mg/kg IV
Propofol	Avoid in hypotension. Rapid onset, short acting.	40 mg IV q 10 sec until induction (2-2.5 mg/kg)
Thiopental	Avoid in hypovolemia. Good in isolated head trauma without hypotension.	3-5 mg/kg IV

orrhage or left ventricular dysfunction are especially vulnerable. Nonetheless, the EP should be familiar with their use as they offer some advantages in *isolated* head trauma.

The recommended dose of thiopental is 3 to 5 mg/kg IV administered over 60 seconds. The normal dose of methohexital is 1 to 3 mg/kg IV over 30 to 60 seconds. Following intravenous injection, thiopental and methohexital quickly accumulate in the brain, with peak levels attained within less than 1 minute.[80,81] In this manner, first-pass deep sedation is achieved. The duration of action for methohexital is 4 to 6 minutes compared with 5 to 10 minutes for thiopental. Both agents exert their effect by acting on the gamma-aminobutyric acid (GABA) receptors to produce profound depression of central nervous system activity. Barbiturates are capable of producing a wide range of dose-dependent levels of sedation ranging from mild sedation to deep coma. Although the patient loses consciousness, barbiturates do not block afferent impulses. If a painful procedure is contemplated, the coadministration of opioid analgesia is warranted.

Barbiturates have been widely advocated to induce anesthesia in patients with head injury. It is argued that the administration of barbiturates is somehow neuroprotective and therefore the drug of choice in this setting. The reader should note that the neuroprotective effects of barbiturates during intubation have never been proven. In addition, many head-injured patients have multiorgan system trauma with ongoing blood loss, a situation in which the administration of barbiturates could be disastrous.

Thiopental can promote the release of histamine, leading to bronchoconstriction; therefore it should be avoided in patients with asthma, chronic obstructive pulmonary disease, reactive airway disease, or chronic bronchitis. In addition to exacerbating bronchospasm, barbiturates may also produce laryngospasm.

OPIOIDS

Of the numerous opiates available, fentanyl is best suited for RSI. The drug has a high potency, minimal histamine release, rapid serum clearance, and rapid onset of action, with analgesia produced in as little as 90 seconds. The duration of effect is approximately 30 to 40 minutes, and longer analgesic effect requires repeat dosing.[82-86]

Doses of 3 to 5 μg/kg are adequate to produce effective analgesia. When fentanyl is used as a primary anesthetic agent in the OR, much higher doses are used (50 to 100 μg/kg). Even these high doses produce minimal side effects. Fentanyl is unique among the opiates in that it produces minimal, if any, histamine release, and therefore is seldom associated with vomiting or hypotension. The drug is ideally suited for administration in patients with head injury, as well as in patients with hypotension or reactive airway disease.

One commonly cited, but rarely seen, side effect is skeletal muscle and chest wall rigidity.[87] This phenomenon has only been observed when doses in excess of 10 μg/kg are given, but usually the dose is much higher (50 to 100 μg/kg). Skeletal muscle rigidity can be completely overcome with succinylcholine or naloxone.[88]

PROPOFOL

Propofol is an ultra–short-acting, nonbarbiturate sedative-hypnotic agent derived from the alkylthenols. The onset of action following intravenous administration is extremely rapid, since the agent is highly lipid soluble. The level of sedation produced by propofol is dose-dependent, and ranges from light sedation to general anesthesia. The drug has an onset of action within 30 to 60 seconds, a 10-minute duration, and an elimination half-life of 1 to 3 hours. In general, the dose is 2 to 2.5 mg/kg. It has the additional benefit of reducing the risk of emesis and lowering ICP. Patients who are hypovolemic may become hypotensive, especially if the drug is given rapidly. Propofol is also water insoluble and causes burning at the site of injection. The drug has been reported to cause respiratory depression and apnea if given by rapid bolus.

ETOMIDATE

Some authorities consider etomidate the sedative drug of choice for RSI. This imidazole derivative is a short-acting nonbarbiturate sedative-hypnotic. It has a number of beneficial properties, such as rapid onset of action, rapid peak activity, and brief duration of action. It differs from thiopental in that it has no cardiodepressant effects, making it ideally suited for administration to patients in shock.

Like propofol, etomidate produces anesthesia during first-pass circulation so that peak sedation is attained within 1 minute of IV infusion. The duration of action is approximately 10 minutes, while its elimination half-life is 2 to 4 hours.

The induction dose is 0.3 mg/kg intravenously, which may be repeated as needed since there is virtually no accumulation of the drug. Beneficial effects of etomidate include reduced intracranial pressure, reduced cerebral blood flow, and reduced cerebral metabolic rate. The systemic mean arterial pressure is maintained constant, thus maintaining cerebral perfusion pressure. This agent is suitable for patients with head injury where elevated ICP is suspected.[89-92]

The most common adverse effects of etomidate are nausea and vomiting. In addition, up to two thirds of patients complain of pain at the site of injection, which can be attenuated by simultaneous saline infusion or premedication with an opiate. The use of etomidate in the operating suite has been associated with suppression of endogenous cortisol production; however, these reports have generally followed repeated dosing or continuous infusion of the agent. It is unlikely that clinically significant effects occur following a single dose.

KETAMINE

Ketamine, a derivative of phencyclidine (PCP), possesses the unique property of producing a dissociative anesthesia. This is characterized by an inability of the subject to react to visual, auditory, or painful stimuli while appearing awake. It does not affect the reticular activating system, but rather interrupts the association pathways between the thalamocortical and limbic system. The drug induces a trancelike state without affecting skeletal muscle tone, respiratory effect, or airway reflexes. One advantage of ketamine is its ability to produce bronchial smooth muscle relaxation, thereby making the drug extremely useful in the treatment of status asthmaticus, bronchospasm, or reactive airway disease.[93-95] Some effects that can theoretically benefit a hypovolemic trauma patient are increased blood pressure, heart rate, and cardiac output following ketamine administration. These effects are most likely mediated by the central nervous system rather than direct cardiovascular effects.[96,97] Ketamine should not be used in patients with myocardial ischemia or head trauma, since it will increase blood pressure, myocardial oxygen consumption, and ICP.[98,99]

The recommended dosage of ketamine is 1 to 2 mg/kg given intravenously over 1 minute. The clinical duration of action is approximately 5 to 15 minutes. The elimination half-life is approximately 2 to 3 hours, and complete recovery usually requires 1 to 2 hours.

Ketamine can produce post-anesthesia emergence reactions. These reactions are attenuated by the coadministration of benzodiazepine.[100] Emergence reactions have been reported in from 5% to 30% of patients given the drug, although they are more common in adults, women, and patients receiving higher doses. Because this agent does not induce skeletal muscle relaxation, it should be used with a paralytic agent to facilitate ETI.[101,102] Ketamine is associated with increased salivary and respiratory secretions, which may be attenuated by simultaneous administration of atropine or glycopyrrolate.

Passing the Endotracheal Tube

Once the patient is fully relaxed, the endotracheal tube should be inserted under direct visualization into the trachea. If intubation is unsuccessful or the cords are not visualized, the patient may be ventilated briefly with a BVM between attempts. It is imperative that cricoid pressure is maintained during BVM ventilation while the patient is paralyzed to prevent passive regurgitation. As soon as the endotracheal tube has been placed, the cuff should be inflated and tube position verified by measurement of end-tidal CO_2 or with an esophageal detector device. Cricoid pressure should not be discontinued until proper tube placement is assured. Once proper tube placement has been confirmed, begin mechanical ventilation and obtain a chest x-ray to determine ET tube depth.

Paralysis After Intubation

Once the patient has been successfully intubated, long-term paralysis may be desirable to prevent the patient from "fighting the ventilator," to prevent self-extubation, and to facilitate radiographic studies. In general, the nondepolarizing neuromuscular blocking agents are used to achieve prolonged paralysis primarily because of their longer duration of action. *It should be administered in conjunction with ongoing sedation.* The terror a patient experiences if paralyzed but awake must be avoided. Vecuronium is an excellent choice because of its limited side effects.

PEDIATRIC CONSIDERATIONS

The pediatric patient who requires airway management differs from the adult in several ways. Some differences are anatomic, whereas others include altered responses to the pharmacologic adjuncts. Relative to the torso, the child's head is much larger, making the vocal cords difficult to visualize during laryngoscopy. Adding to this difficulty is a short neck and a high larynx. The epiglottis is high and very soft, which may obscure visualization of the vocal cords (Fig. 7-6). The trachea in the child is relatively short, thereby making inadvertent right main stem bronchus intubation more likely.

In a young child, a towel placed under the shoulders can compensate for the large occiput and facilitate intubation. However, this is potentially dangerous in the child with potential C-spine injury. Because of a floppy epiglottis, a straight laryngoscope blade is preferable, especially in very young children.

Considerable controversy surrounds the choice of neuromuscular blocking agent to be used and facilitated in the ETI of children. Cautions against the use

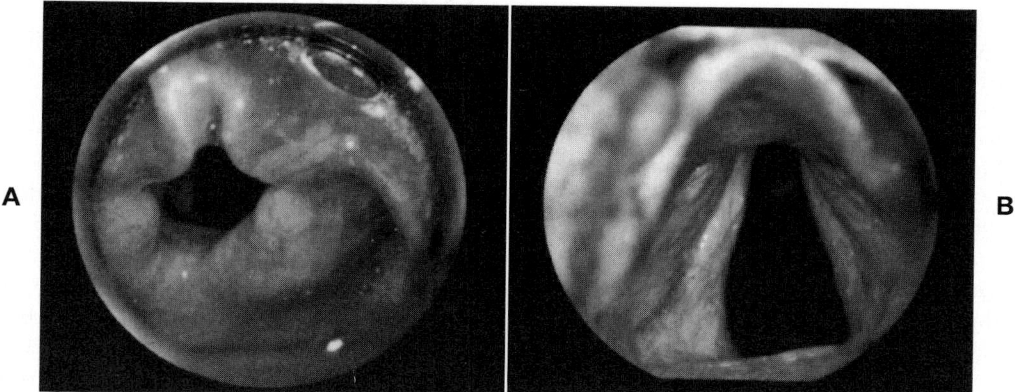

Fig. 7-6 **A,** Infant glottis; **B,** adult glottis. Note the soft, edematous appearance of infant tissue and folded, omega (Ω) or U shape of the infant glottis. (Courtesy Dr. Hollinger, Chicago. In Motoyama EK, Davis PL: *Smith's anesthesia for infants and children,* ed 6, St Louis, 1996, Mosby.)

of succinylcholine stem from its propensity to cause excessive bradycardia and even asystole in children, as well as untoward reactions in children with unrecognized muscular dystropy.[103,104] This sensitivity to the vagal effects of succinylcholine decline with age, and after age 6 it is unlikely to be a problem. Premedication with atropine (0.01 to 0.02 mg/kg, minimum dose 0.1 mg) should ameliorate the problem of bradycardia in the younger child. The dose of succinylcholine in infants needs to be increased to 2 mg/kg to achieve complete paralysis. Although the package insert for succinylcholine cautions against its use in children, succinylcholine is used both widely and safely to achieve neuromuscular blockade in children. Some authors recommend nondepolarizing neuromuscular blockers such as rocuronium to facilitate ETI, but prolonged paralysis occurs with these agents.

Induction agents may be used in children with the same caveats as adults. At least theoretically, etomidate would appear to be an excellent choice for RSI in children.

COMPLICATIONS OF ENDOTRACHEAL INTUBATION AND THE TRAUMA PATIENT

The Cardiac Patient

The pressor response is not a major concern in most trauma patients. This reflex is of minor consequence in the normal patient, but can have some effect in the setting of elevated ICP or cardiovascular dysfunction. Special attention is warranted in patients with ischemic heart disease, myocardial infarction, cardiogenic shock, aortic dissection, cerebral vascular insufficiency, congestive heart failure, and coronary artery disease.

The pressor response to airway stimulation occurs with both laryngoscopy and intubation. Stimulation of the hypopharynx, as well as manipulation of the upper airway, elicits a potent sympathetic discharge.[105] The magnitude of the pressor response increases with the duration of the stimulus, which generally peaks within 45 seconds and persists for as long as 5 minutes.[106,107] In general, the mean arterial pressure increases by approximately 30 mmHg while the heart rate tends to increase by an average of 30 beats per minute (the "30-30" rule).

Since the pressor response is based on the reflex release of catecholamines, it may be blunted by the administration of ß-blocking agents such as esmolol, or opiates such as fentanyl.[108,109] There is evidence that high-dose fentanyl (50 μg/kg) effectively suppresses the pressor response.[110] Other studies have shown effective but incomplete suppression of the pressor response at much smaller doses in the range of 3 to 5 μg/kg, especially when the drug is coadministered with etomidate. Lidocaine has been extensively evaluated for its ability to blunt the pressor response during ETI, but results have been inconclusive. It is known that lidocaine, when given in a dose range of 1.5 to 2.0 mg/kg, will attenuate the response; however, it is unclear whether the reported reduction has any clinical significance.[111-115]

The Head-Injured Patient

A rise in ICP is also triggered with ETI, separate from the blood pressure response. Although the mechanism of this rise is unknown, it is most likely associated with catecholamine release. In a head-injured patient, the baseline ICP is elevated, and further increases in ICP are undesirable. Lidocaine has been commonly promoted to blunt the rise in ICP associated with intubation.[116,117] Although results are somewhat conflicting, most studies indicate that when administered at a dose of 1.5 mg/kg IV, lidocaine ameliorates elevations in ICP resulting from manipulation of the airway. As with the pressor response, fentanyl at a dose of 3 to 5 µg/kg is also effective in preventing further elevations in ICP associated with laryngoscopy and intubation.[118]

Blunting of the intracranial hypertensive reflex is perhaps best achieved with deep sedation and neuromuscular blockade. Ironically, succinylcholine may increase ICP by causing fasciculations. The nondepolarizing neuromuscular blockers do not appear to cause this phenomenon. Giving a defasciculating dose of a nondepolarizing neuromuscular blocker will blunt the elevated ICP seen with succinylcholine. There are no good studies demonstrating the clinical significance of either the ICP spike or the pressor response to intubation in the trauma patient. However, there are numerous and strongly held opinions.

Hence, in the setting of head injury the clinician has a number of options. In the first option, succinylcholine can be used without the addition of a nondepolarizing agent. Under these circumstances, the patient should be premedicated with lidocaine and perhaps fentanyl, to blunt the ICP and pressor responses to intubation. Such patients also require a sedating agent such as etomidate. If there is sufficient time, a second option is to administer a competitive (nondepolarizing) agent in place of the succinylcholine. The third option is to give a defasciculating dose of the nondepolarizing agent, followed by succinylcholine along with lidocaine and an induction agent.

ALTERNATIVE AIRWAY MANAGEMENT TECHNIQUES

Blind Nasotracheal Intubation

The technique of blind nasotracheal intubation (BNTI) should be avoided in the setting of head injury for two reasons. Patients with head injury may have undiagnosed midface fractures, in which case the technique of BNTI is risky. Although there are several reports regarding safety of nasotracheal intubation in facial injury, this cannot be recommended.[119,120] Secondly, BNTI produces dramatic increases in ICP and has a lower success rate than ETI with sedation and neuromuscular blockade (RSI). In the past, BNTI was advocated as the method of choice in patients with potential C-spine injury, but this recommendation has not withstood scientific scrutiny.[121,122] Despite these concerns, BNTI still has its advocates. In experienced hands, intubation success rates may be high.

Cricothyrotomy

Most ED intubation attempts are successful. However, regardless of the experience of the EP, ETI is at times difficult, contraindicated, or impossible. If intubation is unsuccessful, ventilation must be preserved, usually by mask ventilation. When both intubation and ventilation have failed, cricothyrotomy is necessary. There are other indications for cricothyrotomy besides failed ETI, including traumatic injuries that make oral and nasal ETI difficult or hazardous, maxillofacial hemorrhage in which BVM ventilation risks introducing blood into the airway, or complete obstruction of the pharynx and hypopharynx.[123,124] Relative and absolute contraindications include tracheal transection, disruption of the cricoid cartilage or larynx, age less than 8 years of age (transtracheal jet ventilation is the method of choice), and patients with bleeding disorders.

Because of the "crash" nature of this procedure, equipment to perform a cricothyrotomy should be readily available and, in the case of predictable difficulties, open before RSI. Recommended equipment for the procedure is listed in Box 7-2.

Initially expose the patient's neck and identify landmarks. Right-handed operators should stand on the patient's right side, allowing the left hand to immobilize the larynx and locate landmarks while the right hand operates. The physician identifies the cricothyroid membrane by palpating the laryngeal prominence and running a finger down until the indentation of the cricothyroid membrane is palpated. If time permits, use local anesthesia (using lidocaine with epinephrine) and aseptic skin preparation. A midline vertical skin incision approximately 3 to 4 cm long is made over the cricoid membrane. Care must be taken to avoid injury of the thyroid gland because massive bleeding may result.

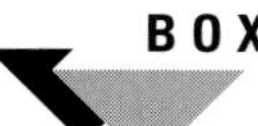

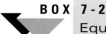

BOX 7-2
Equipment for a Standard Cricothyrotomy Tray

10 ml syringe	Scalpel
#11 blade	Scissors
4×4 gauze pads	Small curved hemostats
Lidocaine + epinephrine	Syringe with 25-gauge needle
Trousseau dilator	Tracheal hook
Needle holder	Tracheal suction catheter
Prep solution	Cuffed tracheostomy tubes—size 4, 5, 6 for adults

Once the skin incision has been completed, stabilize the larynx by holding it between the nondominant thumb and middle finger. Once the cricothyroid membrane is identified, make a horizontal (transverse stabbing) incision about 1 cm in length in the lower cricothyroid membrane near the cricoid cartilage, avoiding the arterial supply to the thyroid cartilage. Ensure that only the tip of the scalpel blade enters the trachea. Curved Mayo scissors are then inserted beside the scalpel blade and spread horizontally to widen the space. Curved hemostats or preferably a Trousseau dilator is then inserted into the incision site of the cricothyroid membrane and the tracheostomy tube is inserted between the opened blades. Some authorities recommend insertion of the dilators immediately after the cricothyroid membrane is incised. The purpose of the dilator is to hold the larynx anteriorly and to widen the vertical incision so the tracheostomy tube may be passed.

Percutaneous Cricothyrotomy Using the Seldinger Technique

This technique has been widely advertised but has not been well tested in the setting of acute trauma. Until experience using this device has been published, it should be avoided in favor of the surgical cricothyrotomy or transtracheal jet ventilation.

Transtracheal Jet Ventilation

Percutaneous transtracheal jet ventilation (PCTV) is the surgical rescue of choice in patients under 10 years of age.[125,126] It can be utilized effectively in the adult or child with a difficult airway. The properly placed catheter can be used to allow definitive cricothyroidotomy in the adult, particularly when identification of landmarks is difficult. Although complete airway obstruction is cited as the only contraindication to this procedure, it may be lifesaving even in this event, if no other technique is available.

Percutaneous transtracheal jet ventilation involves percutaneous puncture of the cricothyroid membrane with a large needle, preferably 10 to 12 gauge. Once inserted, this needle is used to ventilate the patient with a 50 pound per square inch (psi) standard unregulated wall oxygen source. It is essential that the regulator use oxygen in a 50 psi source to achieve optimal ventilation. This entails removing the "Christmas-tree" adaptor from the wall O_2 outlet and using a wall plate to directly access the oxygen supply. Other methods of ventilation, such as attaching a BVM with an adaptor, are inadequate. Perform this technique by identifying the landmarks as noted for the surgical cricothyrotomy, preparing the skin, and if time permits, injecting local anesthesia. A large (10- or 12-gauge) needle is then inserted through the skin with syringe aspiration while directing the needle caudally. Once the trachea is encountered, air will be aspirated through the syringe. At this point, advance the catheter and withdraw the needle. The catheter is then secured into place while attached to high-pressured ventilation tubing connected to the standard wall oxygen outlet at 55 psi. Although the PCTV is available commercially, it may be assembled using commonly stocked ED equipment. The physician controls airflow into the device using a trigger or by occluding an open port in the circuit. The inspiratory-to-expiratory ratio should be at least 1 to 3, allowing air to escape from the lungs and minimize the risk of barotrauma.

Complications of this procedure include minor bleeding at the puncture site, tracheal trauma secondary to high airway pressures, vocal cord damage, pneumothorax, and hypercarbia. Improper tube placement may result in the percutaneous insufflation of air with resulting subcutaneous emphysema. If this complication is encountered, the needle should be removed and reinserted to ensure that it is the trachea. Above all, once the needle is in proper position, it should be secured to the neck. It is important to note that transtracheal jet ventilation is only a temporary measure until a more definitive airway can be obtained. The device does not protect the patient from gastric aspiration, and after approximately 40 minutes significant hypercarbia may develop.

Esophageal Tracheal Combitube

Personnel not trained in ETI use the Combitube most commonly. It should be considered a temporary measure whose use is restricted to rescue placement after failed oral intubation. This device is a double lumen tube with one lumen functioning as the esophageal airway and the other functioning as a tracheal airway. The tube is placed blindly, preferably into the esophagus (but occasionally into the trachea) and a large proximal balloon is inflated to prevent escape of air into the pharynx, the mouth, or nose. A second balloon is located distally and occludes the esophagus (following esophageal placement) or acts as a tracheal cuff (following tracheal placement). The esophageal lumen is ventilated first. If this lumen appears to be ventilating the esophagus, then the tracheal lumen is ventilated. Standard methods for confirming tube placement such as end-tidal CO_2 can then be used to determine the site of placement. In the setting of a trauma patient with possible cervical spine injury, the Combitube is unproven and in general should not be used by personnel who are trained in the techniques of ETI, RSI, and performing a surgical airway.[127-130]

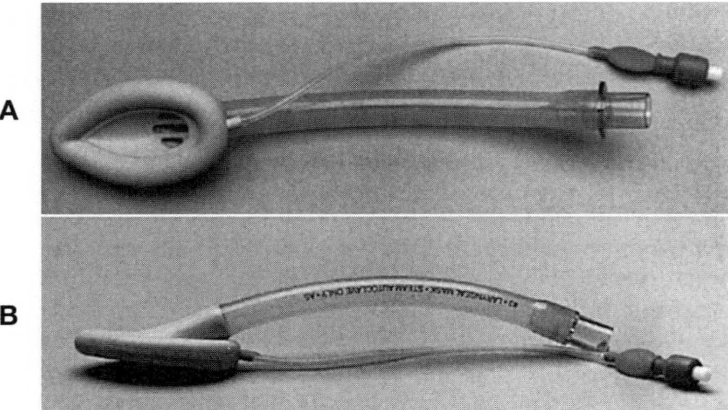

Fig. 7-7 The laryngeal mask airway (LMA). **A,** Front view; **B,** side view. (From Walls RM: Airway management. In Rosen P, et al [editors]: *Emergency medicine: concepts and clinical practice,* ed 4, St Louis, 1998, Mosby.)

Laryngeal Mask Airway

The laryngeal mask airway (LMA) consists of an irregular silicone mask with an inflatable rim connected to a tube that permits ventilation (Fig. 7-7). The tube is blindly inserted into the pharynx and then inflated, providing a seal over the larynx that permits ventilation of the trachea with minimal gastric insufflation. Its use has been widespread, with millions of patients being ventilated in the operating suite using this device. Although the LMA has a theoretical benefit in the emergency setting, studies to date have focused on its use during cardiopulmonary arrest. In the trauma setting, an experienced operator might use the LMA as a temporizing measure following a failed intubation. The device in no way protects the airway from aspiration, should vomiting occur during airway manipulation. Until further studies are available, its use cannot be promoted by personnel who are well versed in other forms of securing the airway.[131,132]

A recent advance in the LMA is the development of an "intubating" LMA. This device allows the EP to establish an airway using a variation of the laryngeal mask airway. Once the airway is in place, the physician then inserts a specially adapted endotracheal tube through this device and removes the laryngeal mask.

Bullard Laryngoscope

The Bullard laryngoscope is a fiberoptic rigid laryngoscope advocated for endotracheal intubation in the setting of a difficult airway. The scope is a long smooth curved blade with a fiberoptic channel and suction port (Fig. 7-8).[133] Its use has been proposed in situations where ETI has failed or in cases of awake intubations where cervical spine movement is to be avoided.[134] Studies to date have indicated that use of the Bullard laryngoscope causes less cervical spine movement when compared with a standard-straight or curved-blade laryngoscope. The disadvantage of this device is that it requires significant practice to master.[135]

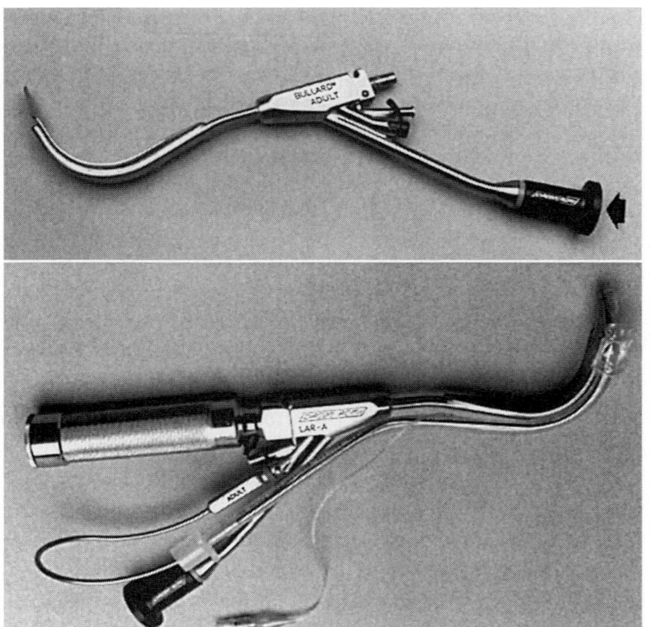

Fig. 7-8 The Bullard laryngoscope. **A,** The laryngoscope blade with fiberoptic viewing port *(arrow).* **B,** The laryngoscope blade with stylet attached and endotracheal tube loaded. (From Walls RM: Airway management. In Rosen P, et al [editors]: *Emergency medicine: concepts and clinical practice,* ed 4, St Louis, 1998, Mosby.)

CONCLUSION

Managing the trauma airway is an essential emergency medicine skill. Keys to success involve preparation and the anticipation of difficulties. A mental or physical checklist helps to prevent disaster. The trauma patient may require four practitioners to accomplish intubation: the nurse to administer medications, someone to immobilize the patient's head, another to provide Sellick's maneuver, and the intubator. Drugs for intubation may range from none in the moribund patient who requires an immediate airway to a complex scheme of five agents or more in the hemodynamically stable trauma victim. Although theoretical concern for the ICP spike associated with intubation is appropriate, no well-designed prospective study provides answers regarding optimal drug selection for RSI. Before administering any drugs, determine any impediments to either RSI or mask ventilation. The greater the impediments, the more important the backup plan. Alternative airway plans should include cricothyroidotomy. Checking the equipment before each shift, formulating an airway strategy early in patient management, and anticipating the difficult airway provides the greatest chance of success.

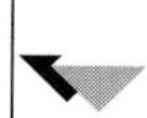

PEARLS & PITFALLS

- Be prepared.
  - Check laryngoscope bulbs, suction equipment, BVM before each shift.
  - Immediately restock after each intubation.
- Look for trouble.
  - Anticipate the difficult airway *before* paralyzing the patient (see Box 7-1).
  - Have a backup plan, particularly for patients with an anticipated difficult airway.
- Use monitors.
  - End-tidal CO_2—Clinical signs of esophageal intubation are unreliable.
  - Pulse oximetry—Pulse oximetry during intubation can prevent desaturation.
- Drugs.
  - Nothing paralyzes faster than succinylcholine.
  - Suspect occult shock; etomidate is a safe and effective in hypovolemia.
- Trauma patients have "full bellies and tight heads."
  - Avoid aspiration by:
    - No BVM ventilation in the spontaneously breathing patient
    - No BVM between the time the patient is given succinylcholine and intubation; preoxygenate instead
    - Apply Sellick's maneuver during intubation
  - Avoid increases in ICP by:
    - Lidocaine 1.5 mg/kg before intubation (5 minutes best)
    - Induction agent (Barbiturates dangerous if hypovolemia)
- Sedate. Paralyzed patients may be awake and suffering. Always sedate patients who are given paralytics.

- Don't lose the hole! When performing a cricothyroidotomy, always keep something (either a finger, instrument, or tracheal tube) in the incised membrane.

REFERENCES

1. Ma OJ, Bently B II, DeBehnke DJ: Airway management practices in emergency medicine residencies, *Am J Emerg Med* 13: 501-504, 1995.
2. Koenig KL: Survey of airway management in emergency medicine residencies, *Acad Emerg Med* 1:200, 1994.
3. Emergency Cardiac Care Committee and Subcommittees A-H: Guidelines for cardiopulmonary resuscitation and emergency cardiac care. III. Adult advanced cardiac life support, *JAMA* 268:2199-2241, 1992.
4. Walls RM: Management of the difficult airway in the trauma patient, *Emerg Med Clin North Am* 16:45-61, 1998.
5. Holley J, Jorden R: Airway management in patients with unstable cervical spine fractures, *Ann Emerg Med* 18:1237-1239, 1989.
6. Walls RM: Airway management in the blunt trauma patient: how important is the cervical spine? *Can J Surg* 35:27-30, 1992.
7. Guildner CW: Resuscitation—opening the airway: a comparative study of techniques for opening an airway obstructed by the tongue, *J Am Coll Emerg Phys* 5:588-590, 1976.
8. Alexander RH, Proctor HJ: *Advanced trauma life support course for physicians,* ed 5, Chicago, 1993, American College of Surgeons.
9. *Textbook of advanced cardiac life support,* Dallas, 1994, American Heart Association.
10. Naigow D, Powasner MM: The effect of different endotracheal suction procedures on arterial blood gases in a controlled experimental model, *Heart Lung* 6:808-816, 1977.
11. Ruben H, Hansen E, MacNaughton FI: High capacity suction technique: a method of reducing the aspiration hazard during induction, *Anaesthesia* 34:349-351, 1979.
12. Jesudian MC, et al: Bag-valve-mask ventilation: two rescuers are better than one—preliminary report, *Crit Care Med* 13:121-123, 1985.
13. Sellick BA: Cricoid pressure to control regurgitation of stomach contents during induction of anaesthesia, *Lancet* 2:404-406, 1961.
14. Petito SP, Russell WJ: The prevention of gastric inflation—a neglected benefit of cricoid pressure, *Anaesth Intens Care* 16: 139-143, 1988.
15. Mendlson CL: The aspiration of stomach contents into the lungs during obstetric anesthesia, *Am J Obstet Gynecol* 52:191-205, 1946.
16. Roberts RB, Shirley MA: Reducing the risk of acid aspiration during cesarean section, *Anesth Analg* 53:859-868, 1974.
17. Gutsche BB: *Pulmonary aspiration of gastric contents in the obstetric patient,* Baltimore, 1979, Williams & Wilkins.
18. Davies AE, et al: Pharyngeal sensation and gag reflex in health subjects, *Lancet* 345:487-488, 1995.
19. Greenberg M, Hedges J: The trauma room, *J Trauma* 18:261-262, 1978.
20. Yaron M, Ruiz E, Baretich MF: Equipment organization in the emergency department adult resuscitation area, *J Emerg Med* 12:845-848, 1994.
21. Applebaum EL, Bruce DL: *Tracheal intubation,* Philadelphia, 1976, Saunders.

22. King BR, et al: Endotracheal tube selection in children: a comparison of four methods, *Ann Emerg Med* 22:530-534, 1993.
23. Cole F: Pediatric formulas for the anesthesiologist, *Am J Dis Child* 94:672-673, 1957.
24. Morgan GA, Steward DJ: Linear airway dimensions in children: including those from cleft palate, *Can Anaesth Soc J* 29: 1-8, 1982.
25. Owen RL, Cheney FW: Endobronchial intubation: a preventable complication, *Anesthesiology* 67:255-257, 1987.
26. Roberts JR, Spadafora M, Cone DC. Proper depth placement of oral endotracheal tubes in adults prior to radiographic confirmation, *Acad Emerg Med* 2:20-24, 1995.
27. Mateer JR, et al: Continuous pulse oximetry during emergency endotracheal intubation, *Ann Emerg Med* 22:675-679, 1993.
28. American Society of Anesthesiology: Practice guidelines for management of the difficult airway: a report by the American Society of Anesthesiologists Task Force on Management of the Difficult Airway, *Anesthesiology* 78:597-602, 1993.
29. Bellhouse CP, Dore C: Criteria for estimating likelihood of difficulty of endotracheal intubation with the MacIntosh laryngoscope, *Anaesth Intens Care* 16:329-337, 1988.
30. Benumof JL: Management of the difficult adult airway: with special emphasis on awake tracheal intubation, *Anesthesiology* 75:1087-1110, 1991.
31. McIntyre JW: The difficult tracheal intubation, *Can J Anaesth* 34:204-213, 1987.
32. Norton ML, Brown AC: Evaluating the patient with a difficult airway for anesthesia, *Otolaryngol Clin North Am* 23:771-785, 1990.
33. Schwartz DE, Wiener-Kronish JP: Management of the difficult airway, *Clin Chest Med* 12:483-495, 1991.
34. White A, Kander PL: Anatomical factors in difficult direct laryngoscopy, *Br J Anaesth* 47:468-474, 1975.
35. Wilson ME, et al: Predicting difficult intubation, *Br J Anaesth* 61:211-216, 1988.
36. Mallampati SR, et al: A clinical sign to predict difficult tracheal intubation: a prospective study, *Can Anaesth Soc J* 32:429-434, 1985.
37. Walls RM, Wolfe R, Rosen P: Fools rush in? Airway management in penetrating neck trauma (editorial), *J Emerg Med* 11: 479-480, 1993.
38. Cormack RS, Lehane J: Difficult tracheal intubation in obstetrics, *Anaesthesia* 39:1105-1111, 1984.
39. Mathew M, Hanna LS, Aldrete JA: Pre-operative indices to anticipate difficult tracheal intubation, *Anesth Analg* 68:S187, 1989.
40. Cass NM, James NR, Lines V: Difficult direct laryngoscopy complicating intubation for anaesthesia, *Br Med J* 1:488-489, 1956.
41. Takahata O, Kubota M, Mamiya K, et al: The efficacy of the "BURP" maneuver during a difficult laryngoscopy, *Anesthesia Analg* 84:419-21, 1997.
42. Knill RL: Difficult laryngoscopy made easy with a "BURP," *Can J Anaesth* 40:279-282, 1993.
43. Conrardy PA, et al: Alteration of endotracheal tube position: flexion and extension of the neck, *Crit Care Med* 4:7-12, 1976.
44. Pollard BJ, Junius F: Accidental intubation of the oesophagus, *Anaesth Intens Care* 8:183-186, 1980.
45. Howells TH, Riethmuller RJ: Signs of endotracheal intubation, *Anaesthesia* 35:984-986, 1980.
46. Ogden PN: Endotracheal tube misplacement [letter], *Anaesth Intens Care* 11:273-274, 1983.
47. Cundy J: Accidental intubation of oesophagus, *Anaesth Intens Care* 9:76, 1981.
48. Linko K, Paloheimo M, Tammisto T: Capnography for detection of accidental oesophageal intubation, *Acta Anaesthesiol Scand* 27:199-202, 1983.
49. Peterson AW, Jacker LM: Death following inadvertent esophageal intubation: a case report, *Anesth Analg* 52:398-401, 1973.
50. Howells TH: Oesophageal misplacement of a tracheal tube [letter], *Anaesthesia* 40:387, 1985.
51. Robinson JS: Respiratory recording from the oesophagus, *Br Med J* 4:225, 1974.
52. Stirt JA: Endotracheal tube misplacement, *Anaesth Intens Care* 10:274-276, 1982.
53. Birmingham PK, Cheney FW, Ward RJ: Esophageal intubation: a review of detection techniques, *Anesth Analg* 65:886-891, 1986.
54. Batra AK, Cohn MA: Uneventful prolonged misdiagnosis of esophageal intubation, *Crit Care Med* 11:763-764, 1983.
55. Williams KN, Nunn JF: The oesophageal detector device: a prospective trial on 100 patients, *Anaesthesia* 44:412-414, 1989.
56. Wee MY, Walker AK: The oesophageal detector device: an assessment with uncuffed tubes in children, *Anaesthesia* 46:869-871, 1991.
57. Wee MY: The oesophageal detector device: assessment of a new method to distinguish oesophageal from tracheal intubation, *Anaesthesia* 43:27-29, 1988.
58. Jenkins WA, Verdile VP, Paris PM: The syringe aspiration technique to verify endotracheal tube position, *Am J Emerg Med* 12:413-416, 1994.
59. Marley CD Jr, et al: Evaluation of a prototype esophageal detection device, *Acad Emerg Med* 2:503-507, 1995.
60. Pelucio M, Halligan L, Dhindsa H: Out-of-hospital experience with the syringe esophageal detector device, *Acad Emerg Med* 4:563-568, 1977.
61. Ornato JP, et al: Multicenter study of a portable, hand-size, colorimetric end-tidal carbon dioxide detection device, *Ann Emerg Med* 21:518-523, 1992.
62. Garnett AR, et al: End-tidal carbon dioxide monitoring during cardiopulmonary resuscitation, *JAMA* 257:512-515, 1987.
63. Stept WJ, Safar P: Rapid induction-intubation for prevention of gastric-content aspiration, *Anesth Analg* 49:633-636, 1970.
64. Li J, et al: Complications of emergency intubation with and without paralysis, *Am J Emerg Med* 17:141-143, 1999.
65. Gambee AM, Hertzka RE, Fischer DM: Preoxygenation techniques: comparison of three minutes and four breaths, *Anesth Analg* 66:468-470, 1987.
66. Walls RM: Rapid sequence intubation in head trauma, *Ann Emerg Med* 22:1008-1013, 1993.
67. Bedford RF, et al: Lidocaine or thiopental for rapid control of intracranial hypertension? *Anesth Analg* 59:435-437, 1980.
68. Koenig KL: Rapid-sequence intubation of head trauma patients: prevention of fasciculations with pancuronium versus minidose succinylcholine, *Ann Emerg Med* 21:929-932, 1992.
69. Sohn YJ, et al: Comparative pharmacokinetics and dynamics of vecuronium and pancuronium in anesthetized patients, *Anesth Analg* 65:233-239, 1986.
70. Baumgarten RK, et al: Priming with nondepolarizing relaxants for rapid tracheal intubation: a double-blind evaluation, *Can J Anaesth* 35:5-11, 1988.
71. Whitwam JG, Al-Khudhairi D, McCloy RF: Comparison of midazolam and diazepam in doses of comparable potency during gastroscopy, *Br J Anaesth* 55:773-777, 1983.
72. Baker TJ, Gordon HL: Midazolam (Versed) in ambulatory surgery, *Plast Reconstr Surg* 82:244-246, 1987.
73. Samuelson PN, et al: Hemodynamic responses to anesthetic induction with midazolam or diazepam in patients with ischemic heart disease, *Anesth Analg* 60:802-809, 1981.

74. Kawar P, et al: Haemodynamic changes during induction of anaesthesia with midazolam and diazepam (Valium) in patients undergoing coronary artery bypass surgery, *Anaesthesia* 40:767-771, 1985.
75. Adams P, et al: Midazolam pharmacodynamics and pharmacokinetics during acute hypovolemia, *Anesthesiology* 63:140-146, 1985.
76. *Physician's Desk Reference,* Montvale, NJ, 1995, Medical Economics Data.
77. Bischoff KB, Dedrick RL: Thiopental pharmacokinetics, *J Pharm Sci* 57:1346-1351, 1968.
78. Eckstein JW, Hamilton WK, McCammond JM: The effect of thiopental on peripheral venous tone, *Anesthesiology* 22:525-528, 1961.
79. Frankl WS, Poole-Wilson PA: Effects of thiopental on tension development, action potential, and exchange of calcium and potassium in rabbit ventricular myocardium, *J Cardiovasc Pharmacol* 3:554-565, 1981.
80. Olsen RW: Barbiturates, *Int Anesthesiol Clin* 26:254-261, 1988.
81. Price HL, et al: The uptake of thiopental by body tissues and its relation to the duration of narcosis, *Clin Pharmacol Ther* 1:16-22, 1960.
82. Mostert JW, et al: Clinical comparison of fentanyl with meperidine, *J Clin Pharmacol* 8:382-391, 1968.
83. Rosow CE, et al: Histamine release during morphine and fentanyl anesthesia, *Anesthesiology* 56:93-96, 1982.
84. Rosow CE, et al: Hemodynamics and histamine release during induction with sufentanil or fentanyl, *Anesthesiology* 60:489-491, 1984.
85. Flacke JW, et al: Histamine release by four narcotics: a double-blind study in humans, *Anesth Analg* 66:723-730, 1987.
86. Martin DE, et al: Low-dose fentanyl blunts circulatory responses to tracheal intubation, *Anesth Analg* 61:680-684, 1982.
87. Comstock MK, et al: Rigidity and hypercarbia associated with high dose fentanyl induction of anesthesia [letter], *Anesth Analg* 60:362-363, 1981.
88. Hill AB, et al: Prevention of rigidity during fentanyl-oxygen induction of anesthesia, *Anesthesiology* 55:452-454, 1981.
89. Langley MS, Heel RC: Propofol: a review of its pharmacodynamic and pharmacokinetic properties and use as an intravenous anaesthetic, *Drugs* 35:334-372, 1988.
90. Sebel PS, Lowdon JD: Propofol: a new intravenous anesthetic, *Anesthesiology* 71:260-277, 1989.
91. White PF: Propofol: pharmacokinetics and pharmacodynamics, *Semin Anesth* 7 [Suppl 1]:4, 1988.
92. Mackenzie N, Grant IS: Propofol for intravenous sedation, *Anaesthesia* 42:3-6, 1987.
93. Lundy PM, Gowdey CW, Colhoun EH: Tracheal smooth muscle relaxant effect of ketamine, *Br J Anaesth* 46:333-336, 1974.
94. Fisher MM: Ketamine hydrochloride in severe bronchospasm, *Anaesthesia* 32:771-772, 1977.
95. Betts EK, Parkin CE: Use of ketamine in an asthmatic child: a case report, *Anesth Analg* 50:420-421, 1971.
96. Wong DH, Jenkins LC: An experimental study of the mechanism of action of ketamine on the central nervous system, *Can Anaesth Soc* J 21:57-67, 1974.
97. Schwartz DA, Horwitz LD: Effects of ketamine on left ventricular performance, *J Pharmacol Exp Ther* 194:410-414, 1975.
98. Gardner AE, Dannemiller FJ, Dean D: Intracranial cerebrospinal fluid pressure in man during ketamine anesthesia, *Anesth Analg* 51:741-745, 1972.
99. Shapiro HM, Wyte SR, Harris AB: Ketamine anaesthesia in patients with intracranial pathology, *Br J Anaesth* 44:1200-1204, 1972.
100. White PF, Way WL, Trevor AJ: Ketamine—its pharmacology and therapeutic uses, *Anesthesiology* 56:119-136, 1982.
101. Dundee JW, Lilburn JK: Ketamine-lorazepam: attenuation of the psychic sequelae of ketamine by lorazepam, *Anaesthesia* 32:312-314, 1977.
102. Chasapakis G, et al: Use of ketamine and pancuronium for anesthesia for patients in hemorrhagic shock, *Anesth Analg* 52: 282-287, 1973.
103. Leigh MD, et al: Bradycardia following intravenous administration of succinylcholine chloride to infants and children, *Anesthesiology* 18:698-702, 1957.
104. Nugent SK, Laravuso R, Rogers MC: Pharmacology and use of muscle relaxants in infants and children, *J Pediatr* 94:481-487, 1979.
105. Bond AC, Davies CK: Ketamine and pancuronium for the shocked patient, *Anaesthesia* 29:59-62, 1974.
106. Wycoff CC: Endotracheal intubation: effects on blood pressure and pulse rate, *Anesthesiology* 21:153-158, 1960.
107. Takeshima K, Noda K, Higaki M: Cardiovascular response to rapid anesthesia induction and endotracheal intubation, *Anesth Analg* 43:201-208, 1964.
108. Hartigan ML, et al: A comparison of pre-treatment regimens for minimizing the haemodynamic response to blind nasotracheal intubation, *Can Anaesth Soc J* 31:497-502, 1984.
109. Derbyshire DR, et al: Plasma catecholamine responses to tracheal intubation, *Br J Anaesth* 55:855-860, 1983.
110. Russell WJ, et al: Changes in plasma catecholamine concentrations during endotracheal intubation, *Br J Anaesth* 53:837-839, 1981.
111. Dahlgren N, Messeter K: Treatment of stress response to laryngoscopy and intubation with fentanyl, *Anaesthesia* 36:1022-1026, 1981.
112. Denlinger JK, Ellison N, Omnisky AJ: Effects on intratracheal lidocaine on circulatory responses to tracheal intubation, *Anesthesiology* 41:409-412, 1974.
113. Derbyshire DR, Smith G, Achola KJ: Effect of topical lignocaine on the sympathoadrenal responses to tracheal intubation, *Br J Anaesth* 59:300-304, 1987.
114. Youngberg JA, Graybar G, Hutchings D: Comparison of intravenous and topical lidocaine in attenuating the cardiovascular responses to endotracheal intubation, *South Med J* 76:1122-1124, 1983.
115. Helfman SM, et al: Which drug prevents tachycardia and hypertension associated with tracheal intubation: lidocaine, fentanyl, or esmolol? *Anesth Analg* 72:482-486, 1991.
116. Poulton TJ, James FM: Cough suppression by lidocaine, *Anesthesiology* 50:470-472, 1979.
117. Yukioka H, et al: Intravenous lidocaine as a suppressant of coughing during tracheal intubation, *Anesth Analg* 64:1189-1192, 1985.
118. Martin DE, et al: Low-dose fentanyl blunts circulatory responses to tracheal intubation, *Anesth Analg* 61:680-684, 1982.
119. Rosen CL, et al: Blind nasotracheal intubation in the presence of facial trauma, *J Emerg Med* 15:141-145, 1997.
120. Why KS: A technique of nasotracheal intubation in patients with recent facio-maxillary injury, *Anaesth Intensive Care* 3:152-153, 1975.
121. Horellou MF, Mathe D, Feiss P: A hazard of naso-tracheal intubation, *Anaesthesia* 33:73-74, 1978.
122. Zwillich C, Pierson DJ: Nasal necrosis: a common complication of nasotracheal intubation, *Chest* 64:376-377, 1973.
123. Jacobson S: Upper airway obstruction, *Emerg Med Clin North Am* 7:205-217, 1989.
124. Yealy DM: Surgical methods of airway control, *Emerg Care Q* 3:11, 1987.

125. Stewart RD: Manual translaryngeal jet ventilation, *Emerg Med Clin North Am* 7:155-164, 1989.
126. Neff CC, Pfister RC, Van Sonnenberg E: Percutaneous transtracheal ventilation: experimental and practical aspects, *J Trauma* 23:84-90, 1983.
127. Frass M, et al: Ventilation with the esophageal tracheal Combitube in cardiopulmonary resuscitation: promptness and effectiveness, *Chest* 93:781-784, 1988.
128. Frass M, et al: The esophageal tracheal Combitube: preliminary results with a new airway for CPR, *Ann Emerg Med* 16: 768-772, 1987.
129. Frass M, et al: Esophageal tracheal Combitube (ETC) for emergency intubation: anatomical evaluation for ETC placement by radiography, *Resuscitation* 18:95-102, 1989.
130. Frass M, et al: Esophageal tracheal Combitube, endotracheal airway and mask: comparison of ventilatory pressure curves, *J Trauma* 29:1476-1479, 1989.
131. Pennant JH, White PF: The laryngeal mask airway: its uses in anesthesiology, *Anesthesiology* 79:144-163, 1993.
132. Brimacombe J, Berry A: Insertion of the laryngeal mask airway—a prospective study of four techniques, *Anaesth Intensive Care* 21:89-92, 1993.
133. Cooper SD, Benumof JL, Ozaki GT: Evaluation of the Bullard laryngoscope using the new intubating stylet: comparison with conventional laryngoscopy, (published erratum appears in Anesth Analg 80:434, 1995) *Anesth Analg* 79:965-970, 1994.
134. Cohn AI, Zornow MH: Awake endotracheal intubation in patients with cervical spine disease: a comparison of the Bullard laryngoscope and the fiberoptic bronchoscope, *Anesth Analg* 81:1283-1286, 1995.
135. Hikawa Y, et al: Use of Bullard intubating laryngoscope in emergency room, *Masui J* 43:1761-1765, 1994.

Resuscitation: Management of Shock

8

SUSAN A. STERN AND EILEEN M. K. BOBEK

Teaching Case

A 37-year-old man was thrown off his motorcycle into a tree. He arrives at the emergency department (ED) with a blood pressure of 80/50 mmHg and a pulse of 100 beats/min. Physical examination is remarkable for no sensory or motor function below T4. His abdomen is soft, nontender, and nondistended. Chest and pelvic radiography are normal except for a T3 fracture. Abdominal ultrasound shows a large amount of free fluid in his peritoneal cavity. After 2 liters of normal saline his blood pressure remains at 80/50 mmHg. He is given 2 units of uncrossmatched O-positive blood via a blood warmer. Methylprednisolone is started, and the patient is taken rapidly to the operating suite for laparotomy. His devitalized grade IV splenic laceration prompts a splenectomy. Postoperatively his blood pressure is 100/50 mmHg. After 3 days his neurologic status remains unchanged.

This case highlights that shock in trauma is hemorrhagic in nature until other causes are excluded, even in the face of spinal cord injury. A chest radiograph will exclude obvious tension pneumothorax or hemothorax, and a pelvic radiograph will determine the presence of any major pelvic fractures. This patient's abdominal examination is limited by his inability to detect pain below the level of his spinal cord injury; therefore hemoperitoneum must be rapidly excluded by either ultrasound or diagnostic peritoneal lavage.

■

The clinical syndrome of shock has both fascinated and perplexed scientists and physicians for centuries. Researchers have devoted vast amounts of time and resources to studying the manifestations and pathophysiology of this condition.

The definition of shock is in continuous evolution. In 1743 Henri Francois LeDran coined the term *choc* to describe the progressive collapse of vital organ function that occurred after injury or surgery. He observed that some soldiers injured in battle survived their initial trauma, only to succumb hours or days later. Various theories were offered to explain this phenomenon, the most popular of which invoked a circulating toxin.[1] In 1872 Samuel D. Gross[2] described shock as a "rude unhinging of the machinery of life." Although this industrial metaphor lacks scientific rigor, it portrays the core disruption of normal homeostasis.

By 1917 clinicians believed that hypotension was a consistent manifestation of shock.[3] In 1940 Blalock[4,5] provided a more refined description, and defined shock as "peripheral circulatory failure, resulting from a discrepancy in the size of the vascular bed and the volume of the intravascular fluid." Gross physiologic indices of heart rate and blood pressure became essential to the diagnosis. Because hypovolemia was a central concept, aggressive fluid resuscitation became the standard treatment. This approach has remained constant for decades.

More recently, shock research has focused on defining the alterations in cellular physiology. In addition, investigators have developed laboratory models to better define and emphasize the pathophysiologic processes specific to the various stages of trauma. This has resulted in the realization that the pathophysiologic processes that predominate immediately following a traumatic event are different from those that dominate the later stages. Hence, clinicians are beginning to recognize that the patient encountered soon after the traumatic event by the emergency physician is likely to have ongoing uncontrolled hemorrhage and therefore may respond differently to aggressive volume replacement than the patient encountered in the intensive care unit after bleeding has been controlled. This enhanced understanding of the hemodynamic, cellular, and biochemical processes characteristic of shock have led clinicians to question the appropriateness of currently accepted diagnostic and treatment modalities. Even the once universally accepted therapy of aggressive volume resuscitation is now considered controversial. The timing and amount of volume resuscitation has become a critical issue.

The shock syndrome is now more accurately defined as a state in which tissue perfusion is inadequate to meet metabolic demands. Even this definition is somewhat vague, reflecting our continued ignorance of fundamental processes in shock. Future advances will depend on uncovering the biochemical and cellular complexities of this condition.

EPIDEMIOLOGY

Researchers have identified three major patterns of death from trauma. **Immediate deaths** occur shortly after injury and are usually the result of devastating wounds such as lacerations of the brainstem, heart, or major blood vessels. **Early deaths** occur within several hours and most commonly result from acute hemorrhage and traumatic brain injury. Finally, **late deaths** occur days to weeks after injury and result from infection or multiple organ failure.[6] Epidemiologic data show that immediate and early deaths account for approximately 80% of trauma-related fatalities, and the majority are secondary to rapid exsanguination.[6-9] Most importantly, a significant portion of early deaths are preventable by aggressive trauma care.

Several investigators have studied the preventable death rate (PDR) from injury and its association with inappropriate care.[10-14] These studies demonstrate an overall PDR of approximately 13%. In addition, for patients dying after transport to a hospital, the PDR is as high as 27%. The most common cause of preventable death was acute hemorrhage followed by central nervous system (CNS) injury, and the most frequent type of inappropriate care *was failure to recognize and adequately treat acute hemorrhage*. These data suggest that the development and implementation of improved treatment strategies could greatly reduce injury-related fatalities.

PATHOPHYSIOLOGY

Shock occurs when there is disruption of the physiologic processes that govern cellular perfusion and oxidative metabolism. Under normal circumstances, delivery of metabolic substrate to the cell and removal of waste products are finely balanced by neuroendocrine control. The body regulates cardiac contractility, circulating blood volume, and vasomotor tone to ensure adequate cellular perfusion. This intricate system of control is vulnerable at many points. When trauma disrupts one or more of these variables, the body activates a complex cascade of compensatory mechanisms. If the imbalance between oxygen delivery and oxygen supply is not rapidly corrected, the ability to compensate is overwhelmed and cellular energy metabolism becomes anaerobic.

Historically, shock has been described as occurring in three stages according to the degree of compensation. These stages are compensated, decompensated, and irreversible shock. However, it is more accurate to describe shock as a continuum of progressive deterioration in cellular perfusion, which if not interrupted, culminates in death. Early in this continuum, compensatory mechanisms can maintain vital organ perfusion at normal or near-normal levels. However, if the primary defect responsible for the "shock state" is not corrected, the body's compensatory mechanisms can no longer maintain adequate tissue perfusion. Irreversible shock results when cellular damage is so extensive that the organism dies despite appropriate therapy. Regardless of shock's origin, the final common pathway is decreased oxygen delivery to the capillary exchange beds, resulting in critically impaired oxidative metabolism.

Therapy is usually directed at correcting the underlying pathophysiologic process. For this reason, it is convenient to categorize the shock states as follows: **hypovolemic**, **distributive**, **cardiogenic**, and **obstructive**. The most common cause of shock in the trauma victim is hypovolemia, specifically acute hemorrhage, and much of the following discussion emphasizes this etiology. However, many of the pathophysiologic processes observed in hypovolemic shock are also common to other forms of shock. Those pathophysiologic features unique to distributive, cardiogenic, and obstructive shock are discussed separately.

Hypovolemic (Hemorrhagic) Shock

In the trauma patient, hypovolemic shock usually means hemorrhagic shock. The primary pathophysiologic event is an interruption in the vascular circuit. The patient bleeds either internally or externally, and circulating blood volume drops. Blood loss reduces preload and stroke volume, and ultimately decreases cardiac output. Several compensatory mechanisms initially sustain blood pressure and tissue perfusion. These mechanisms fall into two general categories: vasoconstriction and increase in intravascular volume.

VASOCONSTRICTION

The initial fall in blood pressure inhibits the afferent discharge of baroreceptors in the aortic arch and carotid sinus, while the decrease in blood volume inhibits the discharge of stretch receptors in the right atrium. The reduction in baroreceptor discharge triggers the midbrain to increase sympathetic nervous system output. The decrease in effective blood volume also stimulates afferent discharge from chemoreceptors in the aortic arch and carotid bodies, further activating the sympathetic nervous system. This increased sympathetic tone releases epinephrine and norepinephrine, intensifying venomotor tone, heart rate, and myocardial contractility, and, subsequently, cardiac output.[15-17]

Arteriolar constriction caused by catecholamines is not homogeneous. The body preserves blood flow to the heart and brain at the expense of skeletal muscle, skin, and the gastrointestinal tract. Blood flow to the liver is also reduced, but to a lesser extent than in the peripheral tissues. Although renal blood flow is preserved with small to moderate hemorrhage, renal vessels constrict with larger hemorrhage.[15,17,18]

Although volume depletion seems to be the most likely stimulus for increased epinephrine release, acidosis may also trigger this phenomenon. Laboratory studies demonstrate that elevations in plasma epinephrine during hemorrhage parallel the onset of acidosis. Intravenous administration of sodium bicarbonate blunts the epinephrine release.[19]

PLASMA VOLUME

Vasoconstriction shifts fluid between the vascular compartment and the interstitium. Normally, little or no net movement of fluid occurs between these two compartments. However, during early or compensated hemorrhagic shock a decrease in effective circulating volume and diminished precapillary arteriolar vasoconstriction reduce capillary hydrostatic pressure. This reduction ultimately moves protein-free fluid from the interstitium to the vascular space, thus increasing intravascular volume and decreasing interstitial volume. This extracellular fluid mobilization occurs over a 6- to 12-hour period and does not account for large-volume changes during the early phases of hemorrhagic shock.[15,17,20-23]

The hypothalamic-pituitary-adrenocortical axis mediates other significant hormonal responses. Decreased renal blood flow activates the renin-angiotensin system and stimulates production of angiotensin I. Angiotensin I is subsequently converted to angiotensin II, a potent vasoconstrictor that stimulates aldosterone release from the adrenal cortex. In addition, angiotensin II potentiates the action of adrenocorticotropic hormone (ACTH) on the adrenal cortex and epinephrine release from the adrenal medulla.[15,17,24,25] Aldosterone is the most potent mineralocorticoid released from the adrenal cortex. Aldosterone increases renal sodium and water retention, and renal potassium excretion, which augments the intravascular volume.[15,17,26,27] Accelerated release of ACTH from the anterior pituitary enhances cortisol production during shock. In addition, the posterior pituitary releases additional antidiuretic hormone (ADH) or vasopressin, which promotes reabsorption of solute-free water in the distal tubules and collecting ducts of the kidneys. ADH also further stimulates peripheral vasoconstriction.[15,17,26,27]

CATABOLISM

The increased catecholamine output and glucocorticoid production characteristic of shock results in a catabolic state, with increases in the plasma concentration of glucagon. Glucagon and catecholamines promote liver gluconeogenesis, glycogenolysis, and lipolysis. As shock progresses, it impairs fatty acid oxidation and increases dependence on glycolysis. Consequently, during shock caregivers observe hyperglycemia, as well as elevated lactate and fatty acid levels.[28,29]

IMPAIRED CELLULAR PUMPS AND CELL DISRUPTION

The intense and complex neuroendocrine response allows the victim to tolerate a significant volume loss before exhibiting signs of shock. However, if the effective circulating blood volume is not eventually corrected, compensatory mechanisms begin to fail and tissues become ischemic, compromising cellular respiration. As cells shift from aerobic to anaerobic metabolism, cellular adenosine triphosphate (ATP) levels fall, and energy-dependent cell functions begin to deteriorate. One of the most important ATP-dependent functions maintains ion gradients across cell membranes. Normally, there is a high ratio of intracellular to extracellular potassium and a low ratio of intracellular to extracellular sodium. These concentration gradients are sustained by the sodium-potassium-ATPase pump (Na^+-K^+ ATPase), which extrudes three sodium ions from the cell for every two potassium ions it allows to enter. As shock progresses, ATP levels dwindle, and the Na^+-K^+ ATPase pump fails. Sodium leaks down its concentration gradient into the cell, and potassium moves out of the cell. Since water enters the cell passively with sodium, this energy deficit ultimately results in cellular swelling and ultrastructural changes in cellular organelles such as mitochondria and lysosomes.[15,17,30]

The decrease in cellular ATP levels also affects calcium homeostasis. Normally, intracellular calcium concentration $[Ca]_{IC}$ is 0.1 μmol/L as compared to an extracellular calcium concentration $[Ca]_{EC}$ of 1 mmol/L. Because calcium acts as a second messenger for stimulus-response coupling in many biologic processes, calcium homeostasis is essential to normal physiology. In addition, elevation of intracellular and intramitochondrial calcium concentration may disrupt cellular physiology and morphology during shock. Sarcolemmal calcium ATPase (Ca^{+2}-ATPase) and Na^+-K^+ ATPase pumps maintain the large calcium concentration gradient. The Ca^{+2}-ATPase pump extrudes one calcium ion in exchange for two hydrogen ions. The high extracellular sodium ion concentration created by the Na^+-K^+ ATPase pump produces enough energy to transport one calcium ion outside of the cell for every three sodium ions that move into the cell. The decreased cellular ATP during shock disrupts calcium homeostasis and elevates intracellular calcium.[31-34] This increased $[Ca]_{IC}$ is directly cytotoxic, separating cell junctions and altering cytoskeleton structures, thus changing cell shape and organelle orientation. As $[Ca]_{IC}$ increases, the rate of mitochondrial calcium uptake is enhanced, so that these organelles accumulate calcium, which initially protects the cell against calcium overload. However, the high calcium concentration in the mitochondrial cytosol eventually interferes with ATP synthesis and uncouples oxidative phosphorylation, further exacerbating the cellular energy deficit of shock. In addition, the elevated $[Ca]_{IC}$ leads to activation of membrane phospholipases and release of acid hydrolases from cellular organelles, further decaying membranes and damaging energy production.[31-37]

ACID-BASE DISTURBANCES

Shock is also characterized by the development of acid-base disturbances. In mild-to-moderate or compensated shock, the most frequently observed acid-base abnormality is respiratory alkalosis. Alkalosis results from a combination of factors, including hypoxic or hypotensive stimulation of aortic and carotid chemoreceptors, the presence of a metabolic acidosis, and painful stimuli. All of these mechanisms activate the respiratory center and produce hyperventilation. As shock progresses, however, anaerobic metabolism predominates, stimulating lactate production and subsequent metabolic acidosis. This metabolic acidosis may further exacerbate the shock state, causing decreased myocardial contractility, decreased sensitivity to catecholamines and other stress hormones, and predisposing to cardiac dysrhythmias.

A TOXIC CASCADE

As bleeding continues, ischemia worsens and cellular damage becomes widespread. Shock leads to failure of cellular respiration, decreased energy production, and disruption of energy-dependent cellular functions. The result is widespread abnormalities in cellular morphology and physiology, and activation of membrane phospholipases. The activated membrane phospholipases promote release of fatty acids and the formation of prostaglandins, yielding further tissue injury and inflammation. Damage to organelles such as lysosomes releases acid hydrolases into the cytoplasm, further injuring cells. Large quantities of waste products spew into the circulation. In addition, injured cells release potent vasoactive mediators such as arachidonic acid metabolites, kinins, histamines, serotonin, and vasoactive peptides. These mediators produce numerous deleterious effects: alteration of vascular tone, increased capillary permeability, decreased myocardial contractility, and redistribution of blood from vital organs.[15,17]

Injured tissues release mediators, which exacerbate the shock state through both local and systemic effects. Endothelial disruption at sites of injury and ischemia exposes subendothelial collagen and basement membrane, which ultimately initiates both the coagulation and complement cascades. Activation of complement promotes an aggressive inflammatory response. Tissue injury also triggers arachidonic acid metabolism, accelerating production of prostaglandin and leukotrienes, which mediate vascular tone and inflammation. Platelet activating factor (PAF) is another byproduct of arachidonic acid release from the cell membrane and is a potent stimulator of platelet and neutrophil activation. PAF production results in microvascular thrombosis at injury sites and further contributes to tissue injury and inflammation.[38-41]

HEART OF THE MATTER

During the initial phase of shock, sympathetic nervous system outflow increases, resulting in increased heart rate, myocardial contractility, stroke volume, and subsequently enhanced cardiac output. Hence during this early phase, blood pressure and tissue perfusion are maintained via augmentation of myocardial pump function. However, if shock persists or progresses, myocardial function becomes impaired. In 1942 Carl Wiggers[42] first suggested that myocardial depression occurs during shock. He observed that during protracted hemorrhagic hypotension, elevations of venous pressure fail to increase cardiac output or arterial blood pressure. Since the 1940s, the accumulated experimental and clinical evidence supports the concept of progressive cardiac deterioration in hemorrhagic shock. Several theories attempt to explain this phenomenon, and hypotheses include global ischemia, acidemia, myocardial depressant factors, and diastolic dysfunction.[42-47]

Diastolic dysfunction is one of the first cardiac manifestations of shock. Ventricular filling depends on myocardial compliance and active ventricular relaxation (in addition to venous return). The ventricular relaxation relies on ATP-dependent sarcoplasmic reticular calcium re-uptake. Because calcium re-uptake is disrupted during shock, stiff ventricles and impaired ventricular filling occurs.[48,49]

The concept of a **toxic humoral substance** generated during circulatory shock is an engaging and widely studied theory. This theory explains much of the pathophysiology of the shock state and accounts for the observation that myocardial depression does not occur until the later phases of shock. Several circulating cardiotoxic substances with a wide variety of chemical characteristics have been reported.[43-45] Additional support for this theory is provided from studies in which plasma ultrafiltrate from animals subjected to prolonged hypotension was used to perfuse hearts excised from normal animals; the isolated hearts demonstrated myocardial depression.[46,50]

Distributive (Neurogenic) Shock

Distributive shock occurs when abnormalities in vascular resistance cause maldistribution of blood flow. Specifically, low vascular resistance increases intravascular capacity; the expanded vascular capacity in the setting of a normal or low intravascular volume results in a functional hypovolemia and inadequate tissue perfusion. Common causes of distributive shock include sepsis, anaphylaxis, drug ingestions, and spinal cord injury (neurogenic shock). **Neurogenic ("spinal") shock** is the most common etiology of distributive shock in the setting of trauma. Central neurogenic shock was first described approximately 150 years ago and occurs only with physiologic or anatomic transection or near-transection of the spinal cord.

Outflow from the sympathetic nervous system originates in the hypothalamus and the nucleus tractus solitarius of the medulla, and descends to the preganglionic cell bodies located in the intermediolateral columns of the spinal cord from segments T1-L2/3. These preganglionic fibers then exit via ventral roots T1-L2/3 and terminate in paravertebral ganglia of the sympathetic trunk. This trunk extends from the base of the skull to the coccyx along the anterolateral surfaces of the vertebral column. These ganglia then give rise to the postganglionic sympathetic fibers that innervate the target organs. The heart and blood vessels lying above the diaphragm are supplied primarily by preganglionic cell bodies in thoracic spinal cord segments T1-T7, whereas vasculature below the diaphragm is supplied by thoracic cord segments T5 and below. Hence, all sympathetic outflow occurs below the cervical segments. In contrast, the parasympathetic outflow originates in the nucleus ambiguus of the medulla, exits the skull via the vagus nerve (cranial nerve X), and descends in the carotid sheath; these fibers do not pass through the spinal cord.

Spinal cord injury occurring above T1 results in loss of excitatory and inhibitory input to all preganglionic sympathetic neurons and therefore largely unopposed parasympathetic tone. Unopposed vagal tone explains the lack of tachycardia seen in patients with neurogenic shock. The loss of sympathetic tone also explains why neurogenic shock is known as "warm" shock. Patients do not vasoconstrict and may lack the cool and clammy skin of those in hemorrhagic shock. Transection of the cervical spinal cord often impairs cardiovascular control. Thoracic lesions produce less cardiovascular derangement because they result in only partial loss of sympathetic control, depending on the level of cord injury.[51,52] Lesions below T6 rarely produce spinal shock.

Loss of sympathetic innervation to the heart and blood vessels from a T1-T4 cord level injury results in unopposed cardiac vagal tone and subsequent bradycardia, as well as loss of arterial tone and hypotension. Bradycardia in the presence of a spinal cord injury occurs most frequently in patients with a complete cervical cord injury. It is significant that these patients are exceptionally prone to hypotension, particularly when the circulatory volume is further compromised by acute hemorrhage from injury. Temperature control can also be affected by the loss of sympathetic tone. These patients lose their ability to sweat in hot environments and to vasoconstrict in cooler settings. Therefore these patients must be kept warm in the often-frigid trauma room.[53-58]

Shock in a patient with a spinal cord injury is fraught with hazard for the physician and especially the patient. All-to-often hypotension is assumed to be caused by the spinal injury, although in fact the patient may have hemorrhagic shock, or a combination of hemorrhagic or distributive shock. Paralyzed trauma victims with massive hemoperitoneum may have warm extremities, bradycardia, and because of their spinal injury, a nontender abdomen. Always assume that shock in a spinal cord–injured patient is due to hypovolemic and not neurogenic shock. Only after blood loss is objectively ruled out (e.g., chest radiograph, abdominal ultrasound) should the physician entertain the diagnosis of neurogenic shock.

Obstructive Shock (Tamponade, Pneumothorax)

In obstructive shock the heart cannot generate adequate cardiac output because of a mechanical obstruction. Intrinsic cardiac pump function and intravascular volume may be normal. The most common causes of obstructive shock are pericardial tamponade, tension pneumothorax, and pulmonary embolus, the former two being more likely in trauma.

In **pericardial tamponade**, fluid accumulates in the pericardial space, elevating intrapericardial pressure. This fluid impairs ventricular filling and subsequently reduces stroke volume and cardiac output. When intrapericardial pressure approximates atrial and ventricular end-diastolic pressures, the aortic pressure falls, choking coronary blood flow. Because this decrease in coronary blood flow occurs when there is increased myocardial oxygen demand, rapid myocardial failure, shock, and ultimately cardiac arrest may ensue.[59]

In **tension pneumothorax** the air accumulates in the intrathoracic cavity and compresses the vena cava and the cavoatrial junction. This compression decreases venous return to the heart, which limits cardiac output.

TABLE 8-1
Differential Diagnosis of Shock in Trauma

CLASSIFICATION	ETIOLOGY
Hypovolemia	Hemorrhage* Burns Plasma losses (peritonitis, sepsis)
Obstructive	Pericardial tamponade* Tension pneumothorax* Pulmonary embolism
Cardiogenic	Myocardial infarction* Myocardial contusion* Dysrhythmia* Drug intoxication*
Distributive	Spinal cord injury* Sepsis

*Indicates acute cause.

Cardiogenic Shock

Cardiogenic shock is defined as the inability of the heart to maintain adequate tissue perfusion because of impaired pump function. As with other forms of circulatory failure, activation of the autonomic nervous system occurs as a compensatory mechanism. However, unlike any other forms of shock, these compensatory responses are rarely effective and even harmful. For example, in cardiogenic shock the heart typically cannot increase stroke volume in response to catecholamines. The arteriolar constriction secondary to the increased sympathetic outflow elevates afterload and therefore increases left ventricular workload. The compensatory increase in heart rate may also be harmful because it increases myocardial oxygen demand when myocardial oxygen supply is limited.[60]

Cardiogenic shock in the setting of trauma most commonly occurs secondary to an acute myocardial infarction (AMI) that either precipitated or resulted from the traumatic event, or from direct myocardial injury. Causes of direct myocardial injury following blunt trauma include myocardial contusion, or rarely, valvular disruption. After penetrating trauma, cardiogenic shock may result from chamber rupture or transection of a coronary artery.

DIFFERENTIAL DIAGNOSIS

The most common cause of shock in the trauma victim is acute hemorrhage. When evaluating and treating trauma victims, however, the emergency physician (EP) must also consider several other potential etiologies (Table 8-1). Failure to consider these diagnoses causes missed opportunities to correct potentially reversible pathologic processes, such as tension pneumothorax.

Hypotensive patients who sustain a high spinal cord injury present the greatest diagnostic challenge. Consider the possibility of distributive shock in any patient whose findings are consistent with spinal cord injury—once occult blood loss is excluded.

Obstructive shock resulting from pericardial tamponade or tension pneumothorax is most likely in patients who sustain penetrating or blunt trauma to the thorax or upper abdomen. Decreased unilateral breath sounds in the presence of hypotension mandates immediate chest decompression. In less obvious cases, a chest radiograph will demonstrate impending tension pneumothorax. Patients with pericardial tamponade may have distended neck veins and muffled heart tones, although these findings are often absent or equivocal.

Finally, although less common in the trauma setting, cardiogenic shock remains a potential cause of circulatory failure. Patients with cardiac causes of shock usually have a distinctly abnormal ECG. Ischemic-type chest pain, pulmonary edema, or loud systolic murmurs may also suggest the diagnosis. Immediate bedside echocardiography can elucidate a cardiac etiology of shock. If the patient is conscious, a history of antecedent chest pain or syncope may identify patients who sustain trauma secondary to a cardiac event.

Diagnosis is complicated when more than one cause of circulatory failure is present in the same patient. For example, the victim of blunt trauma who suffers a cardiac contusion may have both pump failure and hypovolemic shock.

PREHOSPITAL INTERVENTION

Widely accepted goals of prehospital treatment include timely extrication, establishment of a patent airway, provision of adequate ventilation and oxygenation, control of obvious hemorrhage, and rapid transport to an appropriate hospital. Two other prehospital interventions once widely accepted have recently engendered controversy: the application of the pneumatic antishock garment (PASG) and the infusion of intravenous fluids.

Pneumatic Antishock Garment

The PASG was originally developed in 1903 by Crile to prevent postural hypotension in neurosurgical patients.[61] It was not until the Vietnam War that this device was extensively used to treat hemorrhagic shock. It was subsequently popularized as an integral part of civilian prehospital care.[62-64] When first introduced, it was believed that the PASG elevated blood pressure through autotransfusion; specifically, inflation of the PASG was thought to translocate blood from the lower extremities to the central circulation. More recent investigations, however, demonstrate that the blood pressure elevation results from an increase in total peripheral resistance.[65,66] Despite a wealth of experimental data, few reports document its efficacy in hemorrhagic shock. In fact, data from controlled trials of the PASG in the trauma setting fail to demonstrate any benefit.[67-70] In addition, harmful effects, including higher mortality, occur when the PASG is used on patients with penetrating chest trauma.[71]

PASG is an effective splint for immobilization of lower extremity fractures. In addition, several case reports document its utility in limiting retroperitoneal hemorrhage resulting from pelvic fractures.[72,73] One retrospective study suggests a possible benefit for severely hypotensive patients (systolic blood pressure of less than 50 mmHg). In this prehospital study, PASG may have provided a slightly better outcome than anticipated in profoundly hypotensive patients who had no contraindications to its use.[74]

Absolute contraindications to the use of the PASG include pulmonary edema, penetrating thoracic trauma, and known or suspected ruptured diaphragm. Relative contraindications include pregnancy, evisceration, impaled foreign body, lower extremity compartmental syndrome, and lumbar spine instability.[72]

If using the PASG for hypotension, reconsider this decision. If it is used, inflate the leg compartments simultaneously, before inflating the abdominal compartments. Inflation of the PASG is targeted to achieve a systolic blood pressure exceeding 100 mmHg with the lowest possible inflation pressure. Deflate the PASG only when there has been adequate fluid resuscitation and stabilization of vital signs. Deflation must be gradual, while closely monitoring the patient's blood pressure. Deflate the abdominal compartment first; if systolic blood pressure falls more than 5 mmHg, discontinue deflation until fluid resuscitation restores blood pressure.[72]

Intravenous Fluids

The second controversial topic concerning the prehospital care of the hypotensive trauma victim regards intravenous (IV) fluid resuscitation. Since the Vietnam era, prehospital care of the civilian trauma victim has included aggressive administration of IV fluids. Now, many clinicians and investigators question this strategy.

Advocates of prehospital administration of IV fluids argue that paramedics can initiate IV lines with minimal or no delay in transport. They postulate that the prehospital infusion of large volumes of crystalloid may improve blood pressure and vital organ perfusion.

Opponents cite the fact that no controlled clinical trials demonstrate benefit to early aggressive crystalloid resuscitation. Animal data suggest that aggressive fluid resuscitation may actually increase bleeding in an uncontrolled hemorrhage model, worsening outcome. In addition, initiation of prehospital IV fluid therapy may delay transport to definitive care. Even if the line is started in the moving ambulance, the volume of fluid that paramedics can infuse during transport is inadequate to keep pace with severe bleeding. However, it is still useful to have two large-bore IVs in place to permit expedient administration of blood products when the patient reaches the ED.

This fluid controversy was studied in Houston in a series of nearly 600 hypotensive patients with *penetrating* torso injuries.[75] In half the patients fluids were delayed until operation, whereas the control group was managed with immediate fluid resuscitation. Strictly limiting prehospital fluids improved outcomes; patients in this group demonstrated both lower mortality and fewer complications. Sampalis et al[76] also looked at mortality in trauma (both blunt and penetrating) patients receiving prehospital on-site IV fluid replacement. Compared with patients who did not receive on-site IV fluids, mortality was higher in those patients receiving IV fluids. This higher mortality was also significant even after controlling for injury severity, mechanism of injury, prehospital time, age, and gender.

Currently, the fluid controversy remains unresolved. It seems likely, however, that prehospital IV fluid therapy is beneficial only in very specific settings, and that transport time and hemorrhage severity must be considered. A reasonable recommendation is to place IV lines only while en route to the hospital or during patient extrication to avoid potentially lethal delays in transport and maximize the potential benefit of IV fluid therapy. Rapid transport to definitive care always takes precedence over attempts at fluid resuscitation.[77-80]

EMERGENCY DEPARTMENT EVALUATION

Few clinical entities are as challenging to the EP as that of a trauma victim in shock. These patients often have multiple injuries affecting several organ systems. Because timely diagnosis and treatment are essential for a good outcome, quickly begin resuscitation while simultaneously performing the history and physical examination to ascertain the etiology of shock.

Historical Assessment

Historical features and mechanism of injury are important in determining the etiology of shock. For example, a patient may present to the ED with evidence of uncompensated shock after a motor vehicle crash in which there was little damage to the vehicle. In this case, the EP must consider both hemorrhagic and nonhemorrhagic causes of shock. The differential diagnosis in this patient is quite broad and should include cardiogenic shock from acute myocardial infarction (AMI), distributive shock secondary to spinal cord injury or a drug reaction, or even obstructive shock from a pulmonary embolism. Obviously, hemorrhagic shock remains high in the differential of *all* trauma patients.

The clinical course immediately after injury is also important. Question the paramedics regarding the lowest blood pressure, the fastest heart rate, and the volume of prehospital fluids. Knowledge of prehospital vital signs, as well as interventions, may influence the patient's initial presentation in the ED. For example, a trauma victim who was hypotensive at the scene but is normotensive after prehospital fluids may have occult hemorrhage.

Similarly, information regarding the patient's past medical history is helpful. Compensatory responses may be less effective in the elderly and patients with comorbidities such as hypertension, cardiovascular, or pulmonary disease. In addition, the patient's ED presentation may be significantly affected by underlying illness and prescribed medications. An example is the patient who cannot develop a tachycardic response because of concomitant presence of β-blocker medication for control of hypertension.[81,82]

Initial Clinical Assessment

VITAL SIGNS

Normal vital signs do not rule out the diagnosis of shock. This statement is especially true in children, in pregnant patients, and in the elderly, who are often on medications that impair normal physiologic responses. Some trauma victims demonstrate overt circulatory shock characterized by pale, cool, and diaphoretic skin; tachycardia; hypotension; and a decreased level of consciousness. In such cases, the diagnosis is obvious at a glance. However, the majority of injured patients do not present in such dramatic fashion. More common is the patient in compensated shock with only minimal abnormalities in vital signs. This patient represents the greatest diagnostic challenge. Although these patients may appear stable, the patient may deteriorate unless the underlying lesion is identified and corrected.

Alterations in vital signs and other physical findings observed during the early or compensated phase of shock reflect the stress response and associated increase in sympathetic tone. With relatively small hemorrhage (<15% of the total blood volume), tachycardia may be present but the patient's blood pressure and respiratory status generally are within normal limits. As hemorrhage volume increases, so does sympathetic outflow, dramatizing the clinical picture. At blood loss of approximately 25% to 30%, blood pressure falls, pulse pressure narrows, and the patient may become agitated secondary to compromised cerebral perfusion. If this shock state persists or if blood loss progresses, tachypnea, confusion, and lethargy result. At blood volume losses of 40% or greater, the patient is often in a moribund state (Table 8-2).[83]

Not all patients exhibit tachycardia with shock. Age, cardiac disease, and medications may all prevent compensatory tachycardia. However, relative bradycardia is also a frequent response to traumatic blood loss in the otherwise healthy adult. "**Relative bradycardia**" describes a heart rate that is normal despite significant blood loss. As many as 30% of hypotensive patients may have a normal heart rate.[84]

Changes in the respiratory pattern are also common in circulatory shock. However tachypnea is nonspecific and may have multiple etiologies, including pain, fear, anxiety, acidosis, and hypoxia. Patients with mild-to-moderate shock generally exhibit a respiratory alkalosis as a result of direct stimulation of the respiratory center. If the shock state persists and metabolic acidosis progresses, tachypnea may become more pronounced. Hypoventilation is an ominous

TABLE 8-2
Clinical Manifestations of Hemorrhagic Shock and Initial Therapy

PERCENT BLOOD LOSS	PHYSICAL SIGNS	INITIAL TREATMENT
10%-15% Up to 750 ml*	Tachycardia	2 L crystalloid; then reevaluate
20%-25% (1000 to 1250 ml)*	Tachycardia Delayed capillary refill Narrow pulse pressure ± hypotension	2 L crystalloid Blood transfusion if still hypotensive after 2 L crystalloid (type and crossmatched)
30%-35% (1500 to 1750 ml)*	Tachycardia Tachypnea Marked hypotension Agitation and confusion Acidemia	Immediate infusion of crystalloid and uncrossmatched blood
40%-45% (2000 to 2500 ml)*	Moribund	Immediate infusion of crystalloid and uncrossmatched blood

*Estimated blood loss in a 70 kg adult.

sign seen in decompensated shock, but also may indicate chest or pulmonary injury, CNS depression as a result of traumatic brain injury or intoxication, respiratory muscle fatigue, or diaphragmatic or spinal cord injury. Labored respirations accompany direct chest or pulmonary injury, or airway obstruction.[17]

Temperature is a frequently omitted vital sign, but its importance cannot be overestimated. As many as two thirds of severely injured patients are hypothermic, and protection from thermal stress is often overlooked during the evaluation and resuscitation of the trauma victim. Hypothermia is associated with increased mortality, the development of coagulopathies, and if severe, ventricular dysrhythmias and depressed cardiac function.[85,86] Because resuscitation often causes hypothermia, some trauma centers use continuous temperature monitoring in these patients. A Foley catheter equipped with a special thermistor is a convenient means of monitoring core temperature.

Pulse oximetry is often considered the fifth vital sign. Pulse oximetry may be unobtainable in patients with profound shock. Values below 91% represent significant hypoxia and may be secondary to airway compromise, respiratory insufficiency, pulmonary complications, and other traumatic sequelae.

OTHER PARAMETERS

Capillary refill is an easily obtained, noninvasive measure of circulatory status. In 1947 Beecher et al[87] first advocated capillary refill as a parameter for grading the severity of shock. They correlated "normal," "definite slowing," and "very sluggish" capillary refill with "no," "slight to moderate," and "severe shock," respectively. They provided no time values as standards for these categories. Currently a capillary refill time of less than 2 seconds is considered normal, although no controlled studies support this standard.[88,89] In healthy volunteers, several factors influenced capillary refill other than volume status, including age, skin temperature, and gender. Hence the usefulness of capillary refill as an estimate of circulatory impairment is questionable; it is potentially insensitive, as well as nonspecific.[88]

In addition to assessing heart rate, evaluate peripheral pulses for volume and symmetry. The classic "weak and thready" pulse characterizes uncompensated hemorrhagic shock. In contrast, a bounding pulse may indicate a distributive etiology for circulatory failure such as neurogenic shock.

Occult hemorrhage generally occurs in one or more of five main anatomic regions: the chest, abdomen, retroperitoneum, pelvis, and femur. Pain, swelling, ecchymosis, or deformity in any of these areas should suggest the possibility of internal hemorrhage. Physical examination findings may also be helpful in identifying other etiologies of circulatory compromise. For example, the presence of distended neck veins and muffled heart sounds suggests pericardial tamponade, whereas tracheal deviation and decreased breath sounds may herald a tension pneumothorax. Similarly, signs of spinal cord injury such as paralysis and loss of sphincter tone may portend neurogenic shock in a hypotensive patient.

Laboratory and Radiographic Data

Appropriate use of ancillary laboratory tests and radiography can provide valuable diagnostic information.

A chest radiograph identifies signs of thoracoaortic injury, or hemothoraces and pneumothoraces otherwise missed on physical examination. A pelvis film may identify fractures associated with significant hemorrhage. However, in most cases, the need for a pelvis film is based on clinical criteria (see Chapters 22 and 46). The computed tomography (CT) scan has become the most widely used imaging technique in the United States to determine hemoperitoneum and retroperitoneal bleeding. However, *unstable patients should not be sent to CT.* Bedside ultrasound, diagnostic peritoneal lavage (DPL), and exploratory laparotomy remain the procedures of choice for the unstable trauma patient (see Chapter 19). For the trauma victim who requires immediate operation, some studies may need to be obtained in the operating suite or postoperatively as indicated. Radiographic studies should not delay resuscitation or other immediate interventions.

Initial laboratory evaluation of the trauma victim in shock is of limited use. The most important initial blood test in the trauma victim with suspected hemorrhagic shock is the type and crossmatch. Hemoglobin and hematocrit determinations, although universally obtained, may be misleading in early hemorrhagic shock. In acute hemorrhage, the initial hematocrit does not accurately reflect the degree of blood loss, and a normal value does not rule out the possibility of significant or ongoing hemorrhage. The trauma hematocrit may also reflect a combination of premorbid value, hemodilution from fluid administration, and endogenous plasma refill. Nonetheless, a hematocrit of less than 35% even in the early stage of shock may be significant, possibly indicating hemorrhage or a preexisting anemia. Serial hematocrits over several hours are more useful in detecting ongoing hemorrhage and guiding transfusion.[90]

MEASURES OF ANAEROBIC METABOLISM

Measures of anaerobic metabolism provide an important clue to occult shock. Measures of anaerobic metabolism include serum bicarbonate, pH, base excess, and lactate. Of these, lactate is the most sensitive indicator of occult shock (see Chapter 9). Although these parameters are superfluous in obvious circulatory collapse, they may be useful in patients with a significant mechanism of injury and near-normal vital signs. Elevations suggest an advanced stage of shock and the need for immediate resuscitation and aggressive search for blood loss.

Circulatory shock represents a state of inadequate tissue perfusion that ultimately results in a shift from aerobic to anaerobic metabolism and increased lactate production. **Serum lactate** levels provide an indirect measure of the imbalance between tissue oxygen supply and oxygen demand, an important surrogate for tissue perfusion. In fact, serum lactate level estimates both the severity of shock and adequacy of resuscitation. A high lactate suggests inadequate tissue perfusion. A correlation between increasing serum lactate level and increasing mortality in critically ill patients was first demonstrated over 30 years ago.[91-93] Since that time, several laboratory and clinical studies have confirmed those initial observations.[94-97] In a study of patients with circulatory shock from varying etiologies, Vincent and colleagues[94] evaluated the usefulness of serial lactate measurements in predicting outcome of patients with circulatory shock. In this study, lactate concentrations that decreased within the first 60 minutes of treatment predicted survival. In addition, the *change* in lactate concentration over time in response to resuscitation better predicted outcome than the initial value. Several studies of trauma victims have confirmed these data. The trials demonstrate that both initial lactate and change in serum lactate level with resuscitation correlate with death or development of organ failure.[98-102] If serum lactate concentration remains elevated, initiate enhanced resuscitative efforts. In the past, lactate level determinations were not immediately available, so their usefulness in the ED was limited. However, the recent bedside lactate analyzers provide accurate serum lactate determinations within minutes.[103]

Base deficit is defined as the amount of base, in millimoles, required to titrate 1 liter of whole arterial blood to a pH of 7.40, when the sample is completely saturated with oxygen at 37° C and has a pCO_2 of 40 mmHg. Several investigators suggest using base deficit as a measure of global tissue acidosis. It serves both as an index of the severity of shock and the adequacy of resuscitation. Several studies correlate elevations in base deficit (more negative numbers) with subsequent mortality after trauma, as well as the amount of crystalloid and blood replacement required for resuscitation in the initial 24 hours.[96,104-108] In contrast, a recent study by Mikulaschek and colleagues[109] showed that base deficit measurements did not predict outcome and did not correlate with serum lactate concentrations. However, all of these studies have been retrospective; to date, no prospective clinical trial has demonstrated that changes in base deficit during resuscitation correlate with survival. Although base deficit may be a reliable indicator of tissue hypoperfusion, measurements should be interpreted in conjunction with other indicators of tissue perfusion during trauma resuscitation. In addition, the recent availability of bedside lactate analyzers may make this parameter a less optimal assessment variable.

Arterial blood gases will assess the patient's acid-base, ventilatory, and oxygenation status. Measurement of arterial pCO_2 provides information about the patient's ventilation and may guide the decision to intubate.[110] Knowledge of the patient's oxygenation status, obtained from the blood gas or pulse oximetry is essential in patients suspected of circulatory shock. Hypoxemia exacerbates the tissue oxygen deficit that accompanies hemorrhage.

Monitoring During Shock and Resuscitation

Trauma victims who initially come to the ED in compensated shock may quickly decompensate. Frequent reassessments and continuous monitoring is essential to facilitate early detection and correction of ongoing hemorrhage or other causes of circulatory compromise.

Initiate continuous cardiac monitoring as soon as possible in all trauma victims with presumed or potential circulatory shock, since changes in heart rate may guide resuscitation. Tachycardia secondary to hemorrhage usually resolves with adequate resuscitation; persistent tachycardia despite aggressive resuscitation suggests ongoing hemorrhage or other physiologic stress. Dysrhythmias may cause or contribute to the shock state.

Urine output is a well-established method of assessing circulatory status. It reflects renal perfusion and therefore overall central perfusion, provided the patient does not have preexisting renal disease. Perform urinary catheterization on any patient with suspected or ongoing circulatory shock. A urine output of 1 to 2 ml/kg/hr is normal, although in patients without underlying renal disease, output of less than 1 ml/kg/hr denotes inadequate resuscitation and poor perfusion.[110]

CENTRAL VENOUS PRESSURE

Most patients who come to the ED with acute shock can be adequately resuscitated and monitored using peripheral venous access, continuous heart rate and blood pressure monitoring, and measurement of urine output. Central venous monitoring, however, may be useful in a selected patient population. **Central venous pressure (CVP)** reflects the relationship between the blood volume, venous capacitance, and cardiac function, and estimates volume status and the adequacy of resuscitation in the critically ill. It is most accurate in patients without preexisting cardiac and pulmonary disease. With hemorrhagic shock the initial CVP is low, but increases as intravascular volume is replaced. Persistently low CVP measurements despite volume replacement suggest ongoing bleeding. CVP measurements may also help diagnose the cause of shock. For example, an initially elevated CVP with hypotension, or an increased CVP after fluid resuscitation not accompanied by increased blood pressure suggests certain etiologies for shock, including poor pump function (e.g., as seen with myocardial ischemia or a myocardial contusion) or an obstructive etiology (e.g., pericardial tamponade, tension pneumothorax, or pulmonary embolus).[110,111]

There are several limitations to CVP monitoring during acute shock. First, it is an invasive technique. Second, CVP reveals right heart function and reflects left heart performance only in an otherwise healthy patient. In a patient with cardiac or valvular disease, CVP may not follow volume status. Changes in intrathoracic pressure (e.g., as noted with positive pressure ventilation or pneumothorax) also affect measurements. Finally, data from several studies comparing CVP and blood volume measurements during fluid resuscitation indicate that a 20% to 30% blood volume deficit may exist, despite a normal CVP and blood pressure.[110,111] As with other physiologic parameters, it is most useful to follow trends and changes in CVP rather than placing undue emphasis on an isolated measurement. Indications for emergent placement of a central venous catheter in a patient with traumatic shock include the following:

1. The inability to establish adequate peripheral IV access
2. Prolonged and extensive resuscitation, including multiple blood transfusions
3. To aid in the diagnosis of undefined shock
4. Close monitoring of volume status in patients with co-morbidities such as congestive heart failure or renal insufficiency (see Table 8-2)

If placement of a central venous catheter is deemed appropriate, place a large central line (Cordis sheath) via the Seldinger technique.[110,111]

LIMITATIONS OF CLINICAL PARAMETERS OF SHOCK

Current teachings define shock as "an abnormality of the circulatory system that results in inadequate organ perfusion and tissue oxygenation." However, the conventional parameters of heart rate, blood pressure, and CVP are not measures of tissue perfusion. These indices are nonspecific and are affected by multiple factors, including age, anxiety, temperature, and various medications. The parameters are imprecise and insensitive in patients with compensated shock. Vital signs are particularly misleading. In several studies, patients resuscitated from shock continued to suffer from inadequate tissue perfusion (defined as decreased mixed venous oxygen saturation and elevated serum lactate levels), despite normal vital signs. If resuscitation is discontinued based on the traditional end-points of normal blood pressure and heart rate, a significant portion of patients remain in compensated shock, placing them at risk of morbidity and mortality.[112-117] Based on these shortcomings, investigators have recently suggested several alternative parameters for assessment of shock and the adequacy of resuscitation.

PULMONARY ARTERY CATHETERS

Pulmonary artery catheters provide extensive hemodynamic and metabolic information. These devices permit direct measurement of cardiac output, as well as the opportunity to obtain mixed venous oxygen blood samples. Therefore this procedure monitors the balance of tissue oxygen supply and demand.[110,111] The primary indication for pulmonary artery catheterization (PAC) in the critically ill ED trauma patient is undifferentiated shock, when additional hemodynamic and metabolic data would be helpful in diagnosis. In addition, PAC may be helpful in patients with co-morbidities such as congestive heart failure and renal insufficiency. Volume replacement in these patients is problematic and not easily managed through less invasive techniques such as CVP (Table 8-3). A major limitation of PAC, however, is that it is invasive and time-consuming.

Another potentially useful measure of tissue perfusion is **mixed venous oxygen saturation**. Mixed venous oxygen saturation reflects the degree of oxygen extraction by the tissues and thereby estimates the balance of oxygen supply and demand. It is not commonly used in the ED setting, and it is further discussed in Chapter 9. Other shock parameters such as end-tidal CO_2 ($ETCO_2$) monitoring and the shock index are also addressed in that chapter.

TABLE 8-3
Indications for Invasive Monitoring in the Shock Patient

ACCESS	INDICATIONS
Central venous catheter	Inability to establish adequate peripheral intravenous access Large-volume and prolonged fluid resuscitation Diagnosis of undifferentiated shock Continuous SVO_2 measurements Close volume status monitoring
Pulmonary artery catheter	Necessity for continuous SVO_2 and cardiac output measurement Atypical response to fluid resuscitation Diagnosis of undifferentiated shock Patients in whom volume status monitoring is critical but may be difficult to assess (e.g., preexisting cardiovascular disease and the elderly)

EMERGENCY DEPARTMENT MANAGEMENT

Hemorrhagic Shock

The primary goals in the management of shock of any etiology are to restore adequate tissue perfusion and correct the primary pathophysiologic process. If adequate oxygenation is not assured, cellular function deteriorates even with appropriate circulatory support. Respiratory support is a primary goal of resuscitation. Although respiratory failure is uncommon during the early phase of shock, if circulatory compromise is not corrected, respiratory muscle fatigue leads to hypoventilation and hypoxemia. Use of accessory muscles increases oxygen consumption and therefore total body oxygen requirements, exacerbating the shock state. Restoration of an effective circulating blood volume is crucial. However, the *timing* of fluid resuscitation is now being challenged. Recent research may force us to abandon traditional approaches to fluid resuscitation.

TRADITIONAL MODEL OF FLUID RESUSCITATION

For decades, the mainstays of therapy for hemorrhagic shock remained unchanged. These four principles included rapid volume expansion, restoration of normal blood pressure, control of ongoing external hemorrhage, and rapid operative control of internal bleeding.[110] In the "push the fluids" paradigm, adults are initially resuscitated with 2 to 3 liters of isotonic crystalloid infused as rapidly as possible to restore blood pressure and circulating volume. This practice is based on laboratory studies that used modified Wiggers preparations of protracted hemorrhagic hypotension to evaluate the effects of various fluids on survival rate. These studies demonstrated the presence of an interstitial fluid deficit and the phenomenon of transcapillary refill after several hours of hemorrhagic shock. Investigators observed that this extracellular fluid deficit was corrected only with the administration of sodium-containing electrolyte solutions in a volume equal to approximately three times the estimated blood loss. They noted that survival was greatest in animals that received the electrolyte solutions. Early researchers concluded that correction of the extracellular fluid deficit was essential for optimal resuscitation.[118-121] These results led to the practice of aggressive administration of isotonic crystalloids and blood products for patients in hemorrhagic shock (Table 8-4), infused in a ratio of approximately 3 ml of

TABLE 8-4
Resuscitation Fluids

FLUID	CONTENT	DOSING	INDICATIONS	ADVANTAGES	DISADVANTAGES
Crystalloids: Normal saline (NS) Lactated Ringer's (LR)	154 mEq/L Na 154 mEq/L Cl 130 mEq/L Na 109 mEq/L Cl 28 mEq/L lactate 4 mEq/L K	*Initial bolus* Adults 2 L PEDS 20 cc/kg 3 ml crystalloid/ml blood loss as a general guideline for replacement	Volume expansion	May obviate need for blood No risk of disease transmission Inexpensive	Lacks O_2 carrying capacity Hemodilution Non–anion-gap hyperchloremic metabolic acidosis with NS Metabolic alkalosis with LR
Whole blood	450-500ml/unit (includes RBC's, WBCs, plasma constituents, platelets) Hct 35%-40%	10-20 cc/kg or as needed based on clinical assessment	Acute blood loss ≥30% Hct 30%	Increase 0_2 carrying capacity Volume expansion	Storage and cost limitation Infectious disease transmission Transfusion reaction Citrate toxicity Platelets and coagulation factors not functional
Packed RBCs	300-350 ml RBCs Hct 70%-80%	10-20 cc/kg or as needed based on clinical assessment	Acute blood loss ≥30% Hct 30%	Greatest increase in 0_2 carrying capacity	Storage and cost limitation Infectious disease transmission Transfusion reaction Citrate toxicity No platelets or coagulation factors
Fresh frozen plasma	180-300 ml Contains plasma proteins, labile and nonlabile coagulation factors	1 u FFP/5-6 u PRBCs or whole blood transfused if coag. studies are not available If coag. studies available, use PT/PTT as guide	PT/PTT 1.5 × nl DIC Anticoagulation with Coumadin	Volume expansion Provides clotting factors	Allergic reaction
Platelets	1 unit = 5.5×10^{10} platelets in 40-70 ml of plasma	1 unit/10 kg (6-10 units)	Known platelet dysfunction ptl. count <100,000 in presence of active hemorrhage	May decrease FFP requirement	Allergic reaction

crystalloid per 1 ml of blood.[122] These classic laboratory studies, the escalating cost of blood products, along with the infectious risks of blood transfusion, made asanguineous fluids the agent of choice for the initial resuscitation of hemorrhagic shock.

COLLOIDS VERSUS CRYSTALLOIDS

Although it is generally accepted that initial resuscitation with asanguineous fluid is appropriate in the trauma victim with mild-to-moderate hemorrhage, the choice of asanguineous fluid remains somewhat controversial. Options include isotonic crystalloid, hypertonic crystalloid, and colloid. The crystalloid versus colloid debate is largely centered on the effect of these fluid types on the lung. Colloid supporters argue that maintenance of the plasma colloid oncotic pressure (PCOP) is necessary to minimize interstitial edema, especially in the lungs. They argue that hemodilution of serum proteins and the subsequent decrease in PCOP resulting from large-volume crystalloid resuscitation create an oncotic pressure gradient favoring movement of fluid out of the intravascular space into the pulmonary interstitium. Careful analysis of the Starling microvascular forces, however, indicates that this assumption is incorrect. The pulmonary capillary endothelia are normally more "leaky" than the systemic capillary endothelia and permit considerable flow of fluid, including plasma proteins, between the capillaries and the pulmonary interstitium. Consequently, the interstitial oncotic pressure of the lung is relatively high, approximately 70% of intravascular values. Therefore, as PCOP decreases, the interstitial oncotic pressure decreases proportionally and the difference between the two changes minimally.[118,119,123-130]

Proponents of colloid resuscitation also argue that because colloids remain primarily in the intravascular space, they are more effective volume expanders and yield less peripheral edema as compared with crystalloids. Systemic capillary endothelia are less leaky than pulmonary capillary endothelia, so the systemic interstitial oncotic pressure is only 20% to 30% of intravascular values. Because of this larger transcapillary oncotic gradient, peripheral tissues are affected more by protein hemodilution; therefore marked peripheral edema occurs 2 to 3 days after large-volume crystalloid resuscitation.* In contrast, proponents of crystalloid resuscitation argue that this peripheral edema does not appear to have any harmful effects and there is no correlation between peripheral edema and pulmonary edema. Crystalloid supporters also point out that balanced salt solutions effectively correct the interstitial fluid deficit associated with hypovolemic shock, whereas colloids do not.[123-125,129-131]

Extensive review of the literature comparing crystalloid and colloid resuscitation in hemorrhagic shock fails to support a superior efficacy of one asanguineous solution over the other. Although studies have demonstrated that smaller volumes of colloid are required as compared with crystalloid for restoration of vital signs, they fail to demonstrate any reduction in mortality.[131-133] Crystalloids, however, are more readily available and significantly less expensive than colloids, and therefore are recommended as the agent of choice for initial shock resuscitation.

HYPERTONIC SALINE

Over the past several decades, numerous laboratory and clinical studies have investigated another class of resuscitation agents—hypertonic solutions, most commonly hypertonic saline (HTS, 7.5% sodium chloride). This research stemmed from the pursuit of a more effective prehospital and battlefield resuscitation solution. Although IV fluid administration has been the mainstay of the prehospital and preoperative management of hypotensive trauma victims for several decades, the development of more rapid and efficient prehospital transport systems has brought this practice into question.[77-80] Two factors propelled development of a new resuscitation fluid: recognizing that the volume of isotonic fluid given in the prehospital setting is often insufficient to compensate for blood loss sustained from trauma, and the need to limit the volume and weight of supplies in the military setting. This ideal fluid could be administered in small volumes, yet still yield significant intravascular expansion.

Numerous laboratory studies demonstrate that small-volume infusions of HTS more effectively increase blood pressure, raising cardiac output and providing volume expansion, than conventional isotonic crystalloids.[134-141] The hemodynamic response to HTS infusion is well documented; it results in rapid increases in mean arterial pressure and cardiac output, a decrease in systemic vascular resistance, and improved renal and splanchnic blood flow.[136,142,143] At the cellular level HTS infusions improve resting membrane potential and decrease intracellular water content.[144] The observed effects on cardiovascular function are attributed to several factors. First, laboratory studies demonstrate that HTS infusion expands intravascular volume by shifting fluid from the intracellular to the extracellular space.[140,145,146] In addition, hypertonic solutions promote precapillary dilatation and an overall decrease in systemic vascular resistance, further inducing fluid shifts into the vascular compartment.[145,147,148] HTS solutions also reduce edema

*References 118, 119, 123, 124, 126, 128.

of endothelial cells in the microvasculature, therefore enhancing microcirculatory flow and peripheral perfusion.[145,149,150] Some investigators suggest that HTS directly improves cardiac contractility.[140,142,151-153] The latter issue remains controversial, however, since other studies suggest that the improved cardiac output associated with infusion of hypertonic solutions is secondary to augmented preload and decreased afterload rather than increased cardiac contractility.[138,154-157] More recently, hypertonic solutions have been combined with dextran. Typically, these solutions consist of 7.5% sodium chloride and a 6% solution of dextran 70. The dextran transiently partitions the recruited fluid in the plasma space and prolongs the beneficial hemodynamic effects of the hypertonic solution.[146,158-161]

Early laboratory studies that demonstrate the efficacy of small-volume infusions of HTS were conducted in controlled hemorrhage models, in which bleeding occurs atraumatically via an intraarterial catheter. More recently, a few studies have used uncontrolled or vascular injury hemorrhage models to study the efficacy of HTS. In these latter investigations, the administration of HTS resulted in increased hemorrhage from sites of vessel injury and subsequent increased short-term mortality as compared with either withholding resuscitation or the use of conventional isotonic crystalloids. The authors of these investigations caution against the use of HTS in uncontrolled hemorrhage from trauma.[162-165]

Hypertonic solutions may prove most beneficial in the multiple trauma victim in hemorrhagic shock who has sustained traumatic brain injury. Clinical studies demonstrate that morbidity and mortality from traumatic brain injury (TBI) is significantly increased when associated with hemorrhagic hypotension. The poorer outcome is thought to result from a secondary brain injury attributable to impaired cerebral oxygen delivery;[166-171] therefore it is reasonable to use a resuscitation regimen that restores cerebral oxygen delivery as soon as possible. A major concern with conventional resuscitation is that infusion of large volumes of isotonic crystalloids increases cerebral edema and intracranial pressure in TBI and may further compromise cerebral oxygen delivery.[172-175] In contrast, laboratory studies of small-volume infusions of hypertonic solutions produce rapid volume expansion while improving cerebral hemodynamics after hemorrhagic shock. In addition, several studies demonstrate that hypertonic resuscitation after hemorrhagic shock either with or without concomitant TBI results in smaller increases in ICP and improves cerebral hemodynamics, including cerebral blood flow and cerebral oxygen delivery, compared with standard isotonic regimens. Hypertonic solutions may be a better resuscitative agent for the patient with combined TBI and hemorrhagic shock.[176-181]

Over the past decade, several human trials have evaluated the safety and efficacy of hypertonic solutions for trauma victims. In all of these trials, the IV infusion of 250 ml of 7.5% sodium chloride increased blood pressure more effectively than the infusion of isotonic crystalloids. There were no differences, however, in the overall survival rates. Unfortunately, all of these trials have been small and lack statistical power to adequately assess mortality as an outcome.[160,182-185]

There are potential risks associated with the use of HTS-dextran solutions. If hypernatremia or rapid elevations in serum osmolality occur, neurologic complications, including confusion, seizures, and central pontine myelinolysis, could theoretically develop. In addition, there are hypothetical concerns of metabolic acidemia resulting from rapid increase in the plasma chloride concentration.[186-188] Another potential complication is anaphylaxis from the administration of dextran solutions. However, the incidence of dextran-induced anaphylactic reactions is very low, estimated to be 0.025% per unit administered.[189] Dextran solutions may induce coagulopathies thought to be related to the inhibition of platelet aggregation. However, the prolonged bleeding time associated with dextran occurs with large doses or during prolonged infusion, far exceeding the small single dose administered in combination with hypertonic saline solution in trauma.[190,191] Although these potential risks appear numerous, none have been observed or reported in any of the animal or human trials to date.[161]

BLOOD TRANSFUSION

In general, hemorrhage of up to approximately 20% of the total blood volume can be safely replaced solely with crystalloids administered in a volume equal to 3 ml of crystalloid per milliliter of estimated blood loss. Patients who have sustained hemorrhage of approximately 20% to 40% of their blood volume, or those demonstrating continued shock despite aggressive resuscitation with 2 to 3 liters of crystalloid, require blood transfusion (see Table 8-2).[110] Although it is often possible to wait for fully typed and crossmatched blood, the decision to transfuse must be based on multiple factors, including the assessment of ongoing blood loss, the patient's ability to compensate, and the efficiency of the local blood bank in performing crossmatches.

Traditionally, in the hospitalized medical or surgical patient, transfusion is indicated if the hemoglobin is below 10 g/dl or the hematocrit is less than 30%. These guidelines may be inappropriate in acute hemorrhage because the initial hematocrit often does not reflect the degree of blood loss. In fact, the initial hematocrit may be normal even with 30% volume loss. In a patient not receiving intravenous fluids, it may be hours before fluid shifts reduce hematocrit. Therefore the clinical picture should guide transfusion decisions, possibly aided by a serum lactate. The decision to transfuse must also consider the patient's age and co-morbidities. Young otherwise healthy trauma victims tolerate a greater degree of reduction in their oxygen-carrying capacity than elderly patients with cardiac or pulmonary disease.

Blood Types. Use type-specific or type O blood if significant ongoing hemorrhage is expected, the patient's ability to compensate is in question, or there are anticipated delays in acquiring crossmatched blood. Usually the patient's ABO group and Rh factor can be determined within 5 to 10 minutes; however, if a longer delay is expected, do not hesitate to transfuse type O packed red blood cells (PRBCs).

More aggressive therapy is indicated for patients with persistent hypotension who have likely sustained hemorrhage of 40% to 50% of their blood volume or greater. Transfuse these patients immediately with type O blood. Infusion of large volumes of crystalloids in this setting may result in profound hemodilution and critical decreases in oxygen-carrying capacity beyond which the patient can compensate. Before giving type O blood, draw a specimen for type and crossmatch.[83,192,193]

Although clinicians have raised the concern about the safety of transfusion with uncrossmatched blood, several large studies demonstrate that transfusion of type-specific and type O blood is safe. Failure to provide timely replacement of PRBCs and oxygen-carrying capacity poses a much greater risk to the patient than does the transfusion of type-specific and type O blood.[193-197]

Rh Issues. Rh-negative group O PRBCs has long been considered the blood of choice for emergency situations. However Rh-negative blood is often in short supply and stocks may be inadequate in many hospitals at various times. It is safe to use the more abundant Rh-positive group O PRBCs in all men and in women older than 45. Since naturally occurring anti-Rh antibodies do not exist, there is no advantage in the use of Rh-negative blood. There is a theoretical concern that Rh-negative patients may have been sensitized from pregnancy or previous transfusions and may develop a delayed hemolytic transfusion reaction if Rh-positive blood is used. However, this situation is rare and several studies have demonstrated that type O-positive blood can be transfused with little risk.[194,197] Therefore use group O-Rh-positive PRBCs as the first choice for emergency transfusions, and reserve type O-Rh-negative PRBCs for females with childbearing potential.

High-Volume Transfusions. Recent animal studies on uncontrolled hemorrhage question the wisdom of large-volume fluid and blood resuscitation before operation. Rapid infusion systems, now common in many trauma centers, quickly infuse dramatic amounts of warmed blood and fluids compared with conventional IV techniques. A recent clinical study showed that trauma patients who received large amounts of warmed blood and fluids had a higher mortality than matched controls who were managed without the use of a rapid infusion device.[198] The clinical questions of "who needs large-volume resuscitation?, when do they need it?, and how much do they need?" remains unanswered. However, EPs are often faced with situations that they believe necessitate massive transfusions. How is this best accomplished?

Blood flow through a catheter increases in proportion to the square of the radius of the smallest aspect of the IV circuit, which is usually the IV catheter itself (Poiseuille's law). The use of large-bore catheters such as an 8-French line, combined with high-volume IV tubing, provides the fastest blood administration. Pressure bags applied to the blood increase flow rates considerably.

Addition of 200 to 250 cc of warmed saline to the PRBCs guards against iatrogenic hypothermia and doubles the flow rate of blood through the IV circuit.[199] The temperature of the warmed saline can be quite high. Saline at 70° C (nearly 160° F) raises the temperature of refrigerated blood to about body temperature without significant hemolysis, or change in RBC survival.[200,201] However, most physicians may be reluctant to employ such high temperatures for added saline. Regardless of the temperature of fluid added to the blood, normal saline is the *only fluid* that can be used in conjunction with blood transfusions. Ringers lactate will cause precipitation of blood within the tubing.

Component Therapy. Component therapy is the current standard for blood transfusion. The separation of blood into its components has significantly increased the efficiency of transfusion. Blood component therapy generally includes PRBCs, fresh frozen plasma (FFP), platelets, and cryoprecipitate. A unit of whole blood contains 200 ml of red blood cells (RBCs) and 250 ml of plasma, and the latter provides coagulation factors. Theoretically, whole blood is a better resuscitative agent because it can correct volume deficit, increase oxygen-carrying capacity, and provide coagulation factors. Several factors, however, suggest that whole blood offers little or no advantage to component therapy. First, because of cost and storage issues whole blood is often not readily available. Second, evidence suggests that PRBCs and component therapy are as effective as whole blood. For example, the assumption that whole blood may avoid a dilutional coagulopathy may not be valid. Platelets are not well preserved in whole blood, and become essentially functionless within 24 to 36 hours at blood storage temperatures (1° to 6° C). In addition, there is a significant decrease in clotting factors with increasing storage time. By 14 days, factor VIII activity decreases to approximately 25%, whereas factor V activity drops to approximately 60%.[90,197,202] Third, volume expansion can be achieved as readily with crystalloids combined with PRBCs as with the plasma component of whole blood. An advantage of component therapy is that infusions can be specified according to the needs of the individual patient. In trauma this need is often confined to increasing oxygen-carrying capacity and therefore to transfusion of PRBCs. In fact, PRBC infusions increase oxygen-carrying capacity more efficiently than whole blood.[90,203] Unfortunately, to date no well-controlled studies compare whole blood with component therapy. Therefore, based on the economic, storage, and supply and demand issues, PRBC infusion and component therapy are considered the method of choice for increasing RBC mass and oxygen-carrying capacity in hemorrhagic shock.

Complications of Transfusions. Most complications of transfusions occur with massive transfusions, often considered 10 units or more. Because such patients are unstable and need to move out of the ED for continuing care, most of these complications occur in the operating suite or intensive care unit.

Platelets and Coagulation Factors. Transfusion of large volumes of blood products, as well as crystalloids, carries a number of physiologic consequences. Coagulation factors and platelet number and function are significantly diminished during RBC storage. Massive blood and fluid administration dilute the number of circulating platelets (**dilutional thrombocytopenia**) causing clotting abnormalities (**hemorrhagic diathesis**). Timely administration of platelets and FFP may prevent this complication. In the past, recommendations for the infusion of platelets and FFP were based on the number of units of RBCs transfused. However, recent clinical and laboratory studies demonstrate no correlation between the volume of transfusions and abnormal laboratory coagulation studies and clinical evidence of a bleeding diathesis. More commonly, bleeding disorders correlate with injury type and severity and the occurrence of disseminated intravascular coagulation.[204-206] Therefore transfuse platelets and FFP according to clinical evidence of impaired hemostasis and documented abnormalities of the prothrombin time (PT), partial thromboplastin time (PTT), and platelet count.[90,207] The most common recommendation is to administer FFP if the measured PT and PTT exceed 1.5 times the normal value if there is continued hemorrhage. Prolongation of the PT and PTT by themselves does not necessarily correlate with actual hemorrhage, and correction of these laboratory abnormalities does not necessarily restore normal clotting. FFP is generally stored in volumes of 200 to 250 ml, and coagulation factor levels are approximately the same as in fresh whole blood, except factors V and VIII. Although the levels of the latter two coagulation factors are lower than in fresh whole blood, they are generally adequate for hemostasis. Cryoprecipitate contains concentrated factor VIII, von Willebrand factor, and fibrinogen and is rarely required in acute trauma except for patients with von Willebrand disease or documented hypofibrinogenemia. As with FFP, prophylactic platelet transfusion is no longer appropriate. Generally, initiate platelet transfusion if counts fall below 100,000/mm^3 in trauma with continued hemorrhage.[90,202] In an average-sized adult, transfusion of six pooled platelet concentrates immediately raises the platelet count by 40,000 to 60,0000/mm^3. Because response is affected by many factors, measure the platelet count after transfusion to see if further infusions are needed. In addition, each 5 to 6 units of platelets contains 250 to 350 ml of plasma and may decrease the FFP requirement.

Electrolyte Disorders. Massive transfusion can produce significant electrolyte and acid-base disorders. One possible complication is **hypocalcemia**. Each unit of PRBCs contains approximately 20 ml of citrate solution, which binds to ionized calcium in vivo. The liver rapidly metabolizes citrate, and in healthy, well-perfused patients with normal hepatic function, this amount of citrate is well-tolerated. However, larger citrate doses associated with massive transfusion may be toxic and precipitate hypocalcemia. In addition, citrate metabolism may be impaired in patients with underlying liver dysfunction, a poorly perfused liver resulting from circulatory shock, or cardiac failure. Clinical signs of hypocalcemia include prolongation of the QT segment on the electrocardiogram, skeletal muscle tremors, and perioral tingling. Empiric calcium is not recommended; rather, monitor serum calcium levels closely during blood transfusions since hypocalcemia may aggravate the shock state.[90,197,208] Treatment of citrate toxicity and hypocalcemia includes the intravenous administration of 10% solution of calcium chloride. Citrate also has the potential to precipitate hypomagnesemia. Given the association between hypocalcemia and hypomagnesemia, some authors suggest the administration of magnesium chloride concomitantly with calcium chloride in massive transfusion. Magnesium chloride is preferred, since the sulfate form may bind calcium and further aggravate the hypocalcemia.[90]

Hyperkalemia is a theoretic concern during massive transfusion. Potassium levels are significantly elevated in banked blood secondary to leakage from intact cells and cell lysis that occurs during collection and storage of blood. In clinical practice, hyperkalemia is rarely observed during massive transfusion because the RBCs quickly reestablish their ionic pumping mechanism and the potassium is rapidly absorbed. In fact, **hypokalemia** is a more common finding because the metabolic alkalosis associated with massive transfusion moves potassium into the cells. Because of these potential imbalances, monitor serum potassium levels in patients with massive transfusions.[90,208]

Acid-Base Disorders. Banked blood is relatively acidic due to its citrate content, as well as lactate accumulation during storage. There is a theoretic concern that large-volume transfusion results in acidemia. However, if liver perfusion is adequate, most of the lactate is converted to bicarbonate in a single pass through the liver, producing a post-transfusion alkalosis rather than an acidosis.[90,208] Do not consider a metabolic acidosis a consequence of transfusion.

If the patient is acidotic, correct the underlying cause of the acidosis by improving tissue perfusion and oxygenation. Search for occult hemorrhage that requires surgery to control internal bleeding. Do not treat acidosis with bicarbonate. Controlled studies have failed to demonstrate a beneficial effect of bicarbonate administration, and it may even be detrimental in hemorrhagic shock.[209] In laboratory studies, sodium bicarbonate administration resulted in higher serum lactate levels and lower measured tissue pO_2. Potential consequences of bicarbonate infusion include the development of hypernatremia, hypokalemia, hyperosmolarity, volume overload, and a leftward shift of the oxyhemoglobin dissociation curve and subsequent decrease in tissue oxygen delivery.[210,211]

In rare cases, a trauma victim may demonstrate a significant metabolic acidosis from a cause other than circulatory shock. Examples include the patient with diabetic ketoacidosis, a toxic ingestion, or carbon monoxide poisoning.

Hypothermia. Hypothermia is another frequently observed and serious consequence of massive blood transfusion. Hypothermia causes the oxyhemoglobin dissociation curve to shift to the left, impairing oxygen delivery and exacerbating the shock state. In addition, hypothermia slows liver metabolism and, specifically, breakdown of citrate and lactate. Lower body temperatures interfere with platelet function and the clotting cascade, which exacerbates coagulopathy. Hypothermia also increases the potential for cardiac dysrhythmias. Hypothermia is easily preventable through the use of a high-volume fluid warmer whenever massive fluid resuscitation is indicated.[90,208]

Transfusion Reactions. Hemolytic transfusion-mediated reactions represent another potential consequence of massive blood transfusion. At least 70% to 80% of transfusion reactions result from ABO incompatibility, which is also the most common cause of acute fatalities from blood transfusion. ABO incompatibility is almost always a result of a patient identification error, not because of a problem with blood typing itself. The initial blood sample is either mislabeled when sent from the ED, or the nurse does not properly match the number on the blood unit with the number on the patient's ID band. These errors can be avoided by scrupulously matching all samples and blood units with the patient's ID band.

Morbidity and mortality from hemolytic transfusion reactions are directly related to the amount of incompatible blood infused. The incidence of hemolytic transfusion reactions is one event per every 6000 blood units transfused, with a mortality of 1/100,000 units transfused.[202] Clinical manifestations of acute hemolysis include fever, chills, tachycardia, hypotension, abdominal pain, and back pain. In addition, it may precipitate hemoglobinuria and disseminated intravascular coagulation. Many of these clinical signs are also attributable to shock, so a hemolytic transfusion reaction may go unrecognized unless the EP remains vigilant.

Transfusion-Transmitted Disease. Improved screening has significantly decreased the incidence of **transfusion-transmitted disease** (TTD). However, TTD remains an important concern and is the most common cause of late death from transfusion. The four major blood-borne viruses are **hepatitis C virus** (HCV), **hepatitis B virus** (HBV), human **immunodeficiency virus** (HIV), and **human T-cell lymphotropic virus** (HTLV). Data from 1992 estimate the incidence of transfusion-related HCV to be 1 case for every 3300 units of blood transfused; the risk of HIV is 1 per 225,000 units of blood; and the risk of HBV is 1 per 200,000 units transfused. Although the risk of transmission of HIV, HTLV, HBV, and HCV is relatively small, the often fatal outcome from these illnesses remains of considerable concern.[90,212-214]

Approximately 50% of patients who contract hepatitis C develop chronic hepatitis, and about 20% of this group develop cirrhosis. Hepatitis C also predisposes to hepatocellular carcinoma. Previously, HCV (formerly known as non-A, non-B hepatitis [NANB]) was the most common infectious complication associated with blood transfusion. However, the development of screening methods has decreased the incidence of

HCV transfusion transmission considerably. An estimated 50% of patients with post-transfusion HBV infection become symptomatic, with a mortality of 1% to 2%.

Autotransfusion. The demand for blood products often exceeds the supply. Patients who undergo surgery for blunt or penetrating trauma require an average of 5 units of blood, with an occasional patient requiring more than 50 units.[215] An alternative to the transfusion of banked blood is **autotransfusion**, that is, the "collection and reinfusion of the patient's own blood for volume replacement."[216] The advantages of autotransfusion in trauma patients with hemorrhagic shock include the following:

1. The blood is readily available in the ED.
2. Autotransfused blood is normothermic and does not predispose to hypothermia.
3. There is no risk of incompatibility.
4. No risk of patient-to-patient transmission of infectious disease.
5. Higher levels of 2,3-diphosphoglycerate in autotransfused as compared with stored blood.
6. Acceptable to patients with religious convictions that prohibit transfusion with homologous blood.
7. Preserve limited stores of banked blood.[217-219]

The authors have proposed a range of indications for autotransfusion of the ED trauma patient, including (1) exsanguination from trauma, (2) moderate blood loss when banked blood is not available (i.e., because of a blood shortage or a difficult crossmatch), (3) massive blood loss in which autotransfusion is used as a supplement to banked blood, and (4) religious beliefs against banked blood.[220-223] Contraindications to the use of autotransfusion include the presence of malignant lesions or infection in the area of traumatic blood accumulation, gross contamination of the blood as with trauma to the gastrointestinal tract, wounds older than 4 to 6 hours, and known renal and hepatic insufficiency.

Because of the risk of enteric contamination of blood collected from the intraperitoneal cavity after trauma, ED autotransfusion is generally limited to acute hemothorax and the collection of shed blood from the intrathoracic cavity.[221] Potential complications from autotransfusion include the development of transient disseminated intravascular coagulation characterized by hypofibrinogenemia, the presence of fibrin split products, thrombocytopenia, and prolongation of the PTT, PT, and thrombin time.[217,223] Increased RBC hemolysis with concomitant increase in free plasma hemoglobin and serum potassium levels has also been observed.[222-224] These complications are generally of little clinical significance and can be avoided through the use of proper technique and limiting the volume of autotransfused blood to less than 3 liters. Another potential complication is air embolism. Although rare, this complication is potentially fatal and almost always occurs as a result of error in technique.[215,225,226]

There are two general methods currently available for autotransfusion of trauma patients. In the simplest, the blood is collected from thoracostomy tubes into a reservoir with an anticoagulant and then reinfused as whole blood through a filter. In the alternative technique, the collected blood is washed with isotonic saline solution, particulate matter is separated, and the RBCs are washed, resuspended, and reinfused. Although the unwashed method is simpler and faster, there is a theoretical concern that particulate matter may be infused into the patient.[227] Plaisier and colleagues[228] compared these two techniques of autotransfusion in trauma patients with blood collected at the time of laparotomy and observed the two methods to be equally effective. The simple device that reinfuses unwashed blood is appropriate for major trauma in the ED.

Potential benefits of autotransfusion in trauma outweigh the risks. Symbas and colleagues[229] reviewed their experience with autotransfusing 200 patients with traumatic hemothorax and found no significant morbidity related to the procedure. Mattox et al[215] reported on 69 patients who underwent autotransfusion; these authors reported that the one death attributable to the autotransfusion procedure was from air embolism. O'Riordan[223] described the use of autotransfusion in a smaller series (8 trauma cases) and observed no morbidity or mortality related to the procedure except evidence for mild disseminated intravascular coagulation that completely resolved by 72 hours. In a larger review of over 1000 cases, Klebanoff et al[230] reported no morbidity or mortality related to the procedure of autotransfusion. The Council on Scientific Affairs of the American Medical Association has endorsed autotransfusion as an "effective, safe, and cost-effective" treatment for trauma patients.[227]

Neurogenic Shock

The cardiovascular abnormalities that arise from acute spinal cord injuries reflect an imbalance in the autonomic nervous system. The injury decreases sympathetic tone without affecting parasympathetic output. Bradycardia and hypotension are the primary cardiovascular manifestations of this form of circulatory shock.[56-58] In a study of patients with acute spinal cord injury, bradyarrhythmias were the most frequently observed complications and were universally present with severe cervical cord injury.[55] In this series, 29% of patients with cervical injuries resulting in complete loss of motor function required either atropine or pacemaker therapy for symptomatic bradycardia. Sixty-eight percent of patients in that same group experienced hypotension, while 35% required vasopressor therapy.

Treat bradycardic episodes with atropine. Occasionally, atropine may be ineffective since the underlying pathophysiology is inadequate sympathetic tone rather than excessive parasympathetic tone. If symptomatic bradycardia does not respond to medical measures, initiate temporary cardiac pacing.[54,55] Typically, bradycardia resolves spontaneously 3 to 5 weeks after injury and does not require permanent pacemaker therapy. Treat hypotension associated with spinal cord injury initially with volume infusion. If hypotension persists and acute hemorrhage has been ruled out by objective tests such as CT, give vasopressors such as dopamine or norepinephrine. The use of a pulmonary artery catheter may be necessary to guide volume replacement.[54,55]

PEDIATRIC TRAUMA RESUSCITATION

Although the general principles of evaluation and resuscitation of the pediatric trauma patient do not differ from those for adults, there are physiologic, as well as psychologic, differences to consider. The initial evaluation of a pediatric patient offers unique challenges that reflect the patient's age and ability to communicate and comprehend the situation. Since a child may not be able to verbalize specific complaints, it may be more difficult to detect specific injuries (see Chapter 33). This diagnostic challenge is further exacerbated by the child's ability to compensate during periods of hypoperfusion. The latter reflects the sensitivity to catecholamine release and the subsequent marked increases in venomotor tone. Children can compensate for as much as 20% of circulating volume blood loss with little or no change in vital signs. Frequent serial evaluations are essential despite initially normal vital signs.

The cardiovascular response to circulatory shock differs within the pediatric population based on age. As in the adult, the primary determinants of cardiac output are heart rate and stroke volume; their relative contributions differ by age. The myocardium of the young infant has relatively less contractile tissue per unit mass, exhibits a disorganized pattern of muscle fiber arrangement, and is less responsive to inotropic stimulation than older children and adults. Also, resting and stress level heart rates of young children are generally greater than in adults. The infant depends on preload to increase stroke volume and on heart rate to augment cardiac output more than does the older child.[231,232]

Another issue complicating the assessment of the pediatric trauma victim is that normal heart rate and blood pressure in children vary widely by age. The normal vital signs are easily memorized or calculated. The upper limits of normal for heart rates are as follows: less than 140/min for infants; less than 120/min for preschool children; and less than 100/min for school-age children. An estimate of the normal systolic blood pressure can be obtained by adding 70 to twice the child's age in years. For example a normal 2-year-old child's pressure should be 74 (i.e., 70 + [2 × 2]). The normal diastolic blood pressure is two thirds of the normal systolic pressure.[233,234]

Standard blood pressure measurement techniques can be unreliable in small children. Accurate blood pressure measurements require the use of an appropriately sized blood pressure cuff. Because there is a wide range of extremity size in the pediatric age group, blood pressure cuffs are often too large or too small relative to the extremity circumference, and the measured pressures are then falsely depressed or elevated, respectively. The proper-size cuff will cover two thirds of the distance between the child's shoulder and the olecranon process.[234,235]

The general principles of treatment of circulatory shock are the same in the pediatric population as in the adult population. In general, a pediatric patient with blood loss of approximately 25% to 30% can tolerate replacement solely with crystalloid. Infuse an initial bolus of 20 ml/kg of crystalloid, then give a second bolus if hypoperfusion persists. If the patient continues to demonstrate signs of circulatory shock or has experienced a known blood volume loss of 40% or greater, transfuse PRBCs as a bolus of 10 ml/kg. Although these are helpful guidelines, the amount of blood and crystalloid administered must be determined by frequent assessment of the patient's clinical status, with the end-point being objective evidence of adequate tissue perfusion.[233,236]

One of the most difficult problems in pediatric resuscitation is that of establishing IV access. If peripheral venous access is not readily achievable, place a central venous catheter. The femoral vein is usually accessible, and the subclavian vein is an alternative. Consider intraosseous lines in children under 5 years of age, when vascular access is difficult; fluid can be rapidly infused if the IV bag is pressurized, or fluid may be pumped by hand using a large bore syringe. A final option is to perform a venous cutdown using the same technique as in the adult.

GERIATRIC TRAUMA RESUSCITATION

The geriatric trauma population also poses a unique challenge to the EP. Although the incidence of trauma is lower in the elderly population than in any other age group, geriatric patients are more likely to die or require prolonged hospitalization. The elderly in-hospital case fatality rate is 15% to 30%, compared with a 4% to 8% case fatality rate for younger trauma patients. An understanding of the physiologic changes characteristic of the normal aging process facilitates diagnosis, treatment, and optimal outcome in the geriatric trauma victim (see Chapter 34).[237-240]

Changes of the cardiovascular system are among the most notable in this age group. Advancing age reduces the number of α-adrenergic receptors, and diminishes sensitivity to catecholamines, which impairs the ability to increase heart rate and force of myocardial contraction in response to stress. In addition, age-related changes in left ventricular function occur even in the absence of cardiac disease. Maximum stroke volume and heart rate decrease, the pericardium and myocardium stiffen, and diastolic dysfunction develops. These changes increase myocardial oxygen demand.

Atherosclerotic heart disease is common in the elderly, affecting up to 60% of the population, and these patients are predisposed to cardiac ischemia during even mild circulatory shock. If myocardial ischemia develops, ventricular diastolic compliance is impaired, which in turn increases myocardial oxygen demand and further reduces cardiac output.

All of these physiologic alterations limit the geriatric patient's physiologic reserve and ability to compensate for the circulatory shock. In addition, many of these patients are taking prescription medications (such as β-blockers) that may further impair their compensatory mechanisms.

Aggressively identify and treat hypotension and hemorrhage in the geriatric trauma population. Based on their limited ability to tolerate and compensate for a decrease in oxygen carrying capacity, and the possibility for cardiac ischemia, consider transfusion of PRBCs early in the resuscitation.[241-244]

These physiologic changes with aging also make diagnosis of shock more difficult. Characteristic changes in vital signs are often blunted. However, invasive monitoring may be necessary to guide fluid resuscitation because volume status may be difficult to assess, and these patients are at high risk for volume overload. Elevated lactate is an important clue in occult shock in the elderly.

In a study of elderly patients undergoing elective surgery, 80% of patients initially considered stable for surgery (after undergoing invasive monitoring) had significant physiologic deficits that increased their perioperative risk.[245] Several of these patients had advanced functional defects and these individuals all died in the immediate postoperative period. Significantly, *vital signs did not predict the presence or absence of physiologic impairment or outcome*. Similarly, Scalea and colleagues[246] described a series of geriatric trauma victims with an overall mortality of 44%. One third of these deaths were unexpected based on injury severity. When they instituted invasive monitoring in apparently stable patients, more than 60% had significant physiologic abnormalities, including depressed cardiac output, depressed mixed venous oxygen saturations, or both. Based on their findings, these authors recommend early invasive monitoring with pulmonary artery catheterization and attempts to optimize perfusion with volume, transfusion, and inotropic support. The appropriate timing and necessity of invasive monitoring and the efficacy of the latter treatment strategy has yet to be studied in a prospective controlled trial.

CONCLUSIONS

Until recently, recommendations for the preoperative management of hemorrhagic shock include early aggressive fluid resuscitation with the goal of restoring normotension. These standards were universally accepted for several decades. Recently, however, this treatment strategy has come under considerable attack. The debate primarily centers on the timing and amount of resuscitation. One camp of investigators advocates delayed or at least limited resuscitation until operative control of hemorrhage. They note that the current standards were implemented despite a complete lack of controlled clinical trials evaluating their safety and efficacy. In addition, they argue that the *current recommendations are based on data from laboratory studies using hemorrhage models that do not adequately replicate the pathophysiologic events that occur in traumatic hemorrhage*. Specifically, these studies used controlled hemorrhage models in which animals were bled via a surgically implanted catheter. In the clinical setting, hemorrhage occurs from a disruption in the vascular circuit. Although some degree of clotting may occur immediately after injury, further hemorrhage is possible until operation. Controlled or catheter bleed models do not account for these physiologic processes, undermining their clinical relevance. A growing number of studies use uncontrolled hemorrhage models, wherein blood loss occurs as a direct result of vascular injury. Theoretically, this model better mimics clinical reality. In these studies, aggressive crystalloid resuscitation before operative control of hemorrhage resulted in increased hemorrhage volume and short-term mortality as compared with limited or no resuscitation.[165,247,248]

Debate still rages as to which hemorrhage model, uncontrolled or controlled hemorrhage, best approximates the human experience. Only one prospective clinical trial has compared immediate with delayed resuscitation of traumatic hypotension.[75] This study looked only at patients hypotensive (defined as a systolic blood pressure ≤90 mmHg) from penetrating torso trauma. Survival to hospital discharge was significantly greater in the delayed resuscitation group (70%) as compared with the immediately resuscitated patients (62%). Patients in the delayed resuscitation group also demonstrated a trend toward fewer postoperative complications. Although this study had several limitations, it is significant that the majority of patients in whom resuscitation was withheld until operative intervention survived to hospital discharge without major complications.

In contrast, arguments supporting the current early aggressive resuscitation protocols are based on the assumption that hypotension from acute hemorrhage, if left untreated, will rapidly progress to irreversible shock. Advocates of the current "aggressive fluids" approach argue that the need for increasing cardiac output and oxygen delivery exceeds any risk of accentuating hemorrhage. This assumption is unsupported by clinical or laboratory data. As described in this chapter, untreated hemorrhagic hypotension leads to a cascade that results in diffuse tissue injury and ultimately death of the organism. The time interval, however, over which this process becomes irreversible remains undefined. Clinical data from World War II[249,250] and the recent clinical trial by Bickell et al,[75] as well as laboratory data, suggest that moderate hypotension (i.e., MAP = 50 to 60 mmHg) can be tolerated for several hours before resuscitation and rarely results in irreversible shock. These data illustrate the principle that simple hemorrhagic hypotension and hemorrhagic shock are distinct entities and should be treated differently.

Although the recent data supports limiting or withholding resuscitation until operative control of hemorrhage is obtained, it is insufficient to revolutionize practice guidelines. Before making drastic changes in the current treatment recommendations, we must address several issues. We require a better understanding of the physiology of injury and acute hemorrhage, as well as the limits of physiologic compensation. It is essential to define the severity and duration of hemorrhage that provoke multisystem organ failure (MSOF) or death. These parameters probably differ for the pediatric patient, the healthy adult, and the geriatric patient. In addition, the risk of MSOF or death may also vary depending on whether the patient has sustained blunt versus penetrating trauma, and the presence of a concomitant traumatic brain injury. Future studies of novel resuscitation regimens must use appropriate models that mirror the physiology of hemorrhagic shock in human victims of trauma. These models will allow the investigator to evaluate the impact of new treatment strategies on intrinsic hemostasis and the normal physiologic response to injury. Finally, additional human trials are needed in both blunt and penetrating trauma victims to determine optimal fluid strategies. Only through an improved understanding of these principles will we be able to determine the appropriate timing and end-points of resuscitation, as well as the most efficacious resuscitation regimen(s).

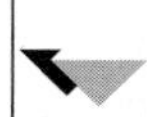

PEARLS & PITFALLS

Shock Research

- Controlled hemorrhage models do not adequately replicate the pathophysiologic events that occur in traumatic hemorrhage.
- Regardless of shock's origin, the final common pathway is decreased oxygen delivery to the capillary exchange beds, resulting in critically impaired oxidative metabolism.
- The most common cause of shock in the trauma victim is acute hemorrhage

Recognition of Shock

- The most frequent cause of preventable trauma deaths *is failure to recognize and adequately treat acute hemorrhage.*
- *Normal vital signs do not rule out the diagnosis of shock,* especially in children, during pregnancy and in the elderly.
- Do an initial assessment rapidly to evaluate end-organ perfusion, as well as to detect any acute life-threatening but treatable injury. Include an evaluation of the airway and respiratory status, heart rate, blood pressure, skin color and temperature, and level of consciousness.
- Assume that shock in a spinal cord–injured patient is due to hypovolemia, not neurogenic shock. Only after blood loss is objectively ruled out (e.g., by chest radiograph, abdominal ultrasound) should the physician entertain the diagnosis of neurogenic shock.

- The most promising and well-studied noninvasive modality for assessing the presence of shock and the adequacy of resuscitation appears to be serum lactate level.

Treatment of Shock

- It is safe to use the more abundant Rh-positive group O PRBCs in all men and in women older than 45. Reserve type O-Rh-negative PRBCs for use in females with childbearing potential.
- Potential benefits of autotransfusion in trauma outweigh the risks.
- The proper timing and amount of resuscitative fluids (blood and crystalloid) for hemorrhagic shock remains unanswered. Using resuscitative fluids to achieve normotension in patients with penetrating torso injuries may worsen outcomes. Hypotensive patients with such injuries need immediate operation once tension pneumothorax is ruled out.

REFERENCES

1. Simeone FA: Shock, trauma and the surgeon, *Ann Surg* 158: 759-774, 1963.
2. Gross SG: *A system of surgery: pathological, diagnostic, therapeutic, and operative,* Philadelphia, 1872, Lea & Febiger.
3. Archibald EW, McLean WS: Observations upon shock with particular reference to the condition as seen in war surgery, *Ann Surg* 66:280, 1917.
4. Blalock A: Shock: further studies with particular reference to the effects of hemorrhage, *Arch Surg* 29:837-857, 1934.
5. Blalock A: Experimental shock: the cause of the low blood pressure produced by muscle injury, *Arch Surg* 20:959-996, 1930.
6. Trunkey DD: Trauma, *Sci Am* 249:28-35, 1983.
7. Bellamy RF: The causes of death in conventional land warfare: implications for combat casualty research, *Mil Med* 149:55-62, 1984.
8. McKoy C, Bell MJ: Preventable traumatic deaths in children, *J Pediatr Surg* 18:505-508, 1983.
9. Acosta JA, et al: Lethal injuries and time to death in a level I trauma center, *J Am Coll Surg* 186:528-533, 1998.
10. Maio RF, et al: A study of preventable trauma mortality in rural Michigan, *J Trauma* 41:83-90, 1996.
11. Esposito TJ, et al: Analysis of preventable trauma deaths and inappropriate trauma care in a rural state, *J Trauma* 39:955-962, 1995.
12. Certo TF, Rogers FB, Pilcher DB: Review of care of fatally injured patients in a rural state: 5-year followup, *J Trauma* 23:559-565, 1983.
13. Dykes EH, et al: Preventable pediatric trauma deaths in a metropolitan region, *J Pediatr Surg* 24:107-111, 1989.
14. Root GT, Christensen BH: Early surgical treatment of abdominal injuries in the traffic victim, *Surg Gynecol Obstet* 105:264-267, 1957.
15. Gann DS, Amaral JF: Pathophysiology of trauma and shock. In Zuidema GD, et al (editors): *The management of trauma,* Philadelphia, 1985, Saunders.
16. Guyton AC: Arterial pressure regulations: rapid pressure control by nervous reflexes and other mechanisms. In Guyton AC (editor): *Textbook of medical physiology,* Philadelphia, 1986, Saunders.
17. Baue AE: Physiology of shock and injuries. In Geller ER (editor): *Shock and resuscitation,* New York, 1993, McGraw-Hill.
18. Slater GI: Sequential changes in distribution of cardiac output in hemorrhagic shock, *Surgery* 73:714-722, 1973.
19. Darby TD, Watts DT: Acidosis and blood epinephrine levels in hemorrhagic hypotension, *Am J Physiol* 206:1281-1284, 1964.
20. Moss GS, Saletta JD: Traumatic shock in man, *N Engl J Med* 290:724-726, 1974.
21. Drucker WR, Chadwick CDJ, Gann DS: Transcapillary refill in hemorrhage and shock, *Arch Surg* 116:1344-1353, 1981.
22. Cloutier CT, Lowery BD, Carey LC: The effect of hemodilutional resuscitation on serum protein levels in humans in hemorrhagic shock, *J Trauma* 9:514-521, 1969.
23. Moore FD: The effects of hemorrhage on body composition, *N Engl J Med* 273:567-577, 1965.
24. Lefer AM, Hock CE: Vascular mediators in circulatory shock. In Hardaway RM (editor): *Shock: the reversible stage of dying,* Littleton, CO, 1988, PSG Publishing.
25. Carey LC, Cloutier CT, Lowery BD: Growth hormone and adrenal cortical response to shock trauma in the human, *Ann Surg* 174:451-460, 1971.
26. Campbell ITG, Newbegin HE: Endocrine aspects of shock. In Hardaway RM (editor): *Shock: the reversible stage of dying,* Littleton, CO, 1988, PSG Publishing.
27. Trachte GJ: Endocrinology of shock. In Altura BM, Lefer AM, Schumer W: *Handbook of shock and trauma: basic science,* vol 1, New York, 1983, Raven Press.
28. Stoner HB: Metabolism after trauma and in sepsis, *Circ Shock* 19:75-87, 1986.
29. Wood CD, et al: Carbohydrate metabolism and the hemodynamic response to shock, *J Surg Res* 38:1-6, 1985.
30. Illner H, Shires GT: The effect of hemorrhagic shock on potassium transport in skeletal muscle, *Surg Gynecol Obstet* 150:17-25, 1980.
31. Kihara Y, Grossman W, Morgan JP: Direct measurement of changes in intracellular calcium transients during hypoxia, ischemia, and reperfusion of the intact mammalian heart, *Circ Res* 65:1029-1044, 1989.
32. Rasmussen H: The calcium messenger system (first of two parts), *N Engl J Med* 314:1094-1101, 1986.
33. Rasmussen H: The calcium messenger system (second of two parts), *N Engl J Med* 314:1164-1170, 1986.
34. Carpenter MA, Trunkey DD, Holcroft J: Ionized calcium and magnesium in the baboon: hemorrhagic shock and resuscitation, *Circ Shock* 5:163-172, 1978.
35. Carafoli E: Membrane transport and the regulation of the cell calcium levels. In Trump BF, Cowley RA (editors): *Pathophysiology of shock, anoxia, and ischemia,* Baltimore, 1982, Williams & Wilkins.
36. Borle AB: Control, modulation and regulation of cell calcium, *Rev Physiol Biochem Pharmacol* 90:13-153, 1981.
37. Blaustein MP: The interrelationship between sodium and calcium fluxes across cell membranes, *Rev Biochem Pharmacol* 70: 33-82, 1974.
38. McEver RP: Role of the endothelium on the inflammatory response. In *Critical care: state of the art,* vol 12, Fullerton CA, 1991, Society of Critical Care Medicine.
39. Fosse E, et al: Complement activation following multiple injuries, *Acta Chir Scand* 153:325-330, 1987.

40. Zimmermann T, et al: The role of the complement system in the pathogenesis of multiple organ failure in shock, *Prog Clin Biol Res* 308:291-297, 1989.
41. Feuerstein G, Siren AL: Platelet-activating factor and shock, *Prog Biochem Pharm* 22:181-190, 1988.
42. Wiggers CJ: The present status of the shock problem, *Physiol Rev* 22:74-123, 1942.
43. Goldfarb RD: Characteristics of shock-induced circulating cardiodepressant substances: a brief review, *Circ Shock* 1(suppl): 23-33, 1979.
44. Greene, LJ, et al: Isolation of myocardial depressant factor from plasma of dogs in hemorrhagic shock, *Biochim Biophys Acta* 491:275-285, 1977.
45. Lundgren O, et al: Effects of myocardial contractility of blood-borne material released from the feline small intestine in simulated shock, *Circ Res* 38:207-315, 1976.
46. Hallstrom S, et al: Negative inotropic and cardiovascular effects of a low molecular plasma fraction in prolonged canine hypovolemic traumatic shock—papillary muscle and isolated heart preparation, *Prog Clin Biol Res* 308:231-235, 1989.
47. Barry WH, et al: Changes in diastolic stiffness and tone of the left ventricle during angina pectoris, *Circulation* 49:255-263, 1974.
48. Marban E, Koretsune Y, Kusuoka H: Disruption of intracellular Ca^{2+} homeostasis in hearts reperfused after prolonged episodes of ischemia, *Ann NY Acad Sci* 723:38-50, 1994.
49. Kusuoka H, Marban E: Cellular mechanisms of myocardial stunning, *Annu Rev Physiol* 54:243-256, 1992.
50. Parker JL, Adams HR: Myocardial effects of endotoxin shock: characterization of an isolated heart muscle model, *Adv Shock Res* 2:163-175, 1979.
51. Arrowood JA, Mohanty PK, Thames MD: Cardiovascular problems in the spinal cord injured patient, *Phys Med Rehab* 1:443-456, 1987.
52. Atkinson PP, Atkinson JL: Spinal shock, *Mayo Clin Proc* 71:384-389, 1996.
53. Zipnick RI, et al: Hemodynamic responses to penetrating spinal cord injuries, *J Trauma* 35:578-582, 1993.
54. Levi L, Wolf A, Belzberg H: Hemodynamic parameters in patients with acute cervical cord trauma: description, intervention, and prediction of outcome, *Neurosurg*ery 33:1007-1016, 1993.
55. Lehmann KG, et al: Cardiovascular abnormalities accompanying acute spinal cord injury in humans: incidence, time course and severity, *J Am Coll Cardiol* 10:46-52, 1987.
56. Meyer GA, et al: Hemodynamic responses to acute quadriplegia with or without chest trauma, *J Neurosurg* 34:168-77, 1971.
57. Eidelberg EE: Cardiovascular response to experimental spinal cord compression, *J Neurosurg* 38:326-331, 1973.
58. Alexander S, Kerr FW: Blood pressure responses in acute compression of the spinal cord, *J Neurosurg* 21:485-491, 1964.
59. Shoemaker WC: Pericardial tamponade. In Grenvik A, Holbrook PR, Shoemaker WC (editors): *Textbook of critical care,* Philadelphia, 1995, Saunders.
60. Rodgers KG: Cardiovascular shock, *Emerg Med Clin North Am* 13:793-810, 1995.
61. Crile GW: *Blood pressure in surgery: experimental and clinical research,* Philadelphia, 1903, Lippincott.
62. Gardner WJ, Storer J: The use of the G-suit in control of intraabdominal bleeding, *Surg Gynecol Obstet* 123:792-798, 1966.
63. Cutler BS, Daggett WM: Application of the G-suit to the control of hemorrhage in massive trauma, *Ann Surg* 173:511-514, 1971.
64. Kaplan BC, et al: The military anti-shock trouser in civilian pre-hospital emergency care, *J Trauma* 13:843-848, 1973.
65. McSwain NE: Pneumatic trousers and the management of shock, *J Trauma* 17:719-724, 1977.
66. Gaffney FA, et.al: Hemodynamic effects of medical anti-shock trousers (MAST garment), *J Trauma* 21:931-937, 1981.
67. Mattox KL, et al: Prospective randomized evaluation of anti-shock MAST in post-traumatic hypotension, *J Trauma* 26:779-786, 1986.
68. Mattox KL, et al: Prospective MAST study in 911 patients, *J Trauma* 29:1104-1111, 1989.
69. Chang FC, et al: PASG: does it help in the management of traumatic shock? *J Trauma* 39:453-456, 1995.
70. Bickell WH, et al: Randomized trial of pneumatic antishock garments in the prehospital management of penetrating abdominal injuries, *Ann Emerg Med* 16:653-658, 1987.
71. Honigman B, et al: The role of the pneumatic antishock garment in penetrating cardiac wounds, *JAMA* 266:2398-2401, 1991.
72. Norton R: Pneumatic antishock garment. In Roberts JR and Hedges JR (editors): *Clinical procedures in emergency medicine,* ed 3, Philadelphia, 1998, Saunders.
73. Brunette DD, Fifield G, Ruiz E: Use of pneumatic antishock trousers in the management of pediatric pelvic hemorrhage, *Pediatr Emerg Care* 3:86-90, 1987.
74. Cayten CG, et al: A study of pneumatic antishock garments in severely hypotensive trauma patients, *J Trauma* 34:728-733, 1993.
75. Bickell WH, et al: Immediate versus delayed fluid resuscitation for hypotensive patients with penetrating torso injuries, *N Engl J Med* 331:1105-1109, 1994.
76. Sampalis JS, et al: Ineffectiveness of on-site intravenous lines: is prehospital time the culprit? *J Trauma* 43:608-615, 1997.
77. Kaweski SM, Sise MJ, Virgilio RW: The effect of prehospital fluids on survival in trauma patients, *J Trauma* 30:1215-1218, 1990.
78. Smith JP, et al: Prehospital stabilization of critically injured patients: a failed concept, *J Trauma* 25:65-70, 1985.
79. Trunkey DD: Is ALS necessary for pre-hospital trauma care? *J Trauma* 24:86-87, 1984.
80. Border JR, et al: Panel: Prehospital trauma care: stabilization or scoop and run, *J Trauma* 23:708-711, 1983.
81. Herndon JG, et al: Chronic medical conditions and risk of fall injury events at home in older adults, *J Am Geriatr Soc* 45:739-743, 1997.
82. Sacco WJ, et al: Effect of pre-injury illness on trauma patient survival outcome, *J Trauma* 35:538-543, 1993.
83. Saxe JM, Ledgerwood AM, Lucas CE: Principles of resuscitation. In Geller ER (editor): *Shock and resuscitation,* New York, 1993, McGraw Hill.
84. Demetriades D, et al: Relative bradycardia in patients with traumatic hypotension, *J Trauma* 45:534-539, 1998.
85. Luna GK, et al: Incidence and effect of hypothermia in seriously injured patients, *J Trauma* 27:1014-1018, 1987.
86. Jurkovich GJ, et al: Hypothermia in trauma victims: an ominous predictor of survival, *J Trauma* 27:1019-1024, 1987.
87. Beecher HK, et al: The internal state of the severely wounded man on entry to the most forward hospital, *Surgery* 22:672-711, 1947.
88. Schriger DL, Baraff L: Defining normal capillary refill: variation with age, sex, and temperature, *Ann Emerg Med* 17:932-935, 1988.
89. Schriger DL, Baraff LJ: Capillary refill: is it a useful predictor of hypovolemic states? Ann Emerg Med 20:601-605, 1991.
90. Nacht A: The use of blood products in shock, *Crit Care Clin* 8:255-291, 1992.

91. Huckabee WE: Abnormal resting blood lactate. I. The significance of hyperlactatemia in hospitalized patients, *Am J Med* 30:833-839, 1961.
92. Huckabee WE: Abnormal resting blood lactate. II. Lactic acidosis, *Am J Med* 30:840-848, 1961.
93. Broder G, Weil MH: Excess lactate: an index of reversibility of shock in human patients, *Science* 143:1457-1459, 1964.
94. Vincent JL, et al: Serial lactate determinations during circulatory shock, *Crit Care Med* 11:449-451, 1983.
95. Weil MH, Afifi AA: Experimental and clinical studies on lactate and pyruvate as indicators of the severity of acute circulatory failure (shock), *Circulation* 41:989-1001, 1970.
96. Dunham CM, et al: Oxygen debt and metabolic acidemia as quantitative predictors of mortality and the severity of the ischemic insult in hemorrhagic shock, *Crit Care Med* 19:231-243, 1991.
97. Stacpoole PW, et al: Natural history and course of acquired lactic acidosis in adults, *Am J Med* 97:47-54, 1994.
98. Manikis P, et al: Correlation of serial blood lactate levels to organ failure and mortality after trauma, *Am J Emerg Med* 13: 619-622, 1995.
99. Siegel JH, et al: Early physiologic predictors of injury severity and death in blunt multiple trauma, *Arch Surg* 125:498-508, 1990.
100. Milzman D, et al: Admission lactate predicts injury severity and outcome in trauma patients, *Crit Care Med* 20 (suppl):S94, 1992 (abstract).
101. Abramson D, et al: Lactate clearance and survival following injury, *J Trauma* 35:584-589, 1993.
102. Mizock BA, Falk JL: Lactic acidosis in critical illness, *Crit Care Med* 20:80-93, 1992.
103. Aduen J, et al: The use and clinical importance of a substrate-specific electrode for rapid determination of blood lactate concentration, *JAMA* 272:1678-1685, 1994.
104. Davis JW, et al: Base deficit as a guide to volume resuscitation, *J Trauma* 28:1464-1467, 1988.
105. Davis JW, et al: Admission base deficit predicts transfusion requirements and risk of complications, *J Trauma* 41:769-774, 1996.
106. Davis JW: The relationship of base deficit to lactate in porcine hemorrhagic shock and resuscitation, *J Trauma* 36:168-172, 1994.
107. Davis JW, Shackford SR, Holbrook TL: Base deficit as a sensitive indicator of compensated shock and tissue oxygen utilization, *Surg Gynecol Obstet* 173:473-476, 1991.
108. Rutherford EJ, et al: Base deficit stratifies mortality and determines therapy, *J Trauma* 33:417-423, 1992.
109. Mikulaschek AS, et al: Serum lactate is not predicted by anion gap or base excess after trauma resuscitation, *J Trauma* 40:218-222, 1996.
110. Wilson RF: Techniques of resuscitation. In Geller ER (editor): *Shock and resuscitation,* New York, 1993, McGraw-Hill.
111. Shoemaker WC, Parsa MH: Invasive and noninvasive physiologic monitoring. In Ayres SM, et al (editors): *Textbook of critical care,* ed 3, Philadelphia, 1995, Saunders.
112. McNamara JJ, et al: Resuscitation from hemorrhagic shock, *J Trauma* 23:552-558, 1983.
113. Abou-Khalil B, et al: Hemodynamic responses to shock in your trauma patients: need for invasive monitoring, *Crit Care Med* 22:633-639, 1994.
114. Bland RD, et al: Hemodynamic and oxygen transport patterns in surviving and nonsurviving postoperative patients, *Crit Care Med* 13:85-90, 1985.
115. Rady MY, et al: Continuous central venous oximetry and shock index in the emergency department: use in the evaluation of clinical shock, *Am J Emerg Med* 10:538-541, 1992.
116. Wo CC, et al: Unreliability of blood pressure and heart rate to evaluate cardiac output in emergency resuscitation and critical illness, *Crit Care Med* 21:218-223, 1993.
117. Rady MY: The role of central venous oximetry, lactic acid concentration and shock index in the evaluation of clinical shock: a review, *Resuscitation* 24:55-60, 1992.
118. Carrico CT, et al: Fluid resuscitation following injury: rationale for the use of balanced salt solutions, *Crit Care Med* 4:46-56, 1976.
119. Shires GT: Pathophysiology and fluid replacement in hypovolemic shock, *Ann Clin Res* 9:144-150, 1977.
120. Dillon J, et al: A bioassay of treatment of hemorrhagic shock, *Arch Surg* 93:537-555, 1966.
121. Lowery BD, Cloutier CT, Carey LC: Electrolyte solutions in resuscitation in human hemorrhagic shock, *Surg Gynecol Obstet* 133:273-284, 1971.
122. Committee on Trauma. American College of Surgeons: *Advanced trauma life support manual,* Chicago, 1997, American College of Surgeons.
123. Tranbaugh RF, Lewis FR: Crystalloid versus colloid for fluid resuscitation of hypovolemic patients, *Adv Shock Res* 9:203-216, 1983.
124. Peters RM, Hargens AR: Protein vs. electrolytes and all of the Starling forces, *Arch Surg* 116:1293-1298, 1981.
125. Guyton AC, Lindsey AW: Effect of elevated left atrial pressure and decreased plasma protein concentration on the development of pulmonary edema, *Circ Res* 7:649-657, 1959.
126. Virgilio RW, Smith DE, Zarins CK: Balanced electrolyte solutions: experimental and clinical studies, *Crit Care Med* 7:98-106, 1979.
127. Mackersie RC, Durelle J: Differential clearance of colloid and crystalloid solutions from the lung, *J Trauma* 35:448-453, 1993.
128. Holcroft JW, Trunkey DD: Extravascular lung water following hemorrhagic shock in the baboon: comparison between resuscitation with Ringer's lactate and Plasmanate, *Ann Surg* 180: 408-417, 1974.
129. Tranbaugh RF, et al: Determinants of pulmonary interstitial fluid accumulation after trauma, *J Trauma* 22:820-826, 1982.
130. Moss GS, et al: Effects of saline and colloid solutions on pulmonary function in hemorrhagic shock, *Surg Gynecol Obstet* 133:53-58, 1971.
131. Moss GS, et al: Colloid or crystalloid in the resuscitation of hemorrhagic shock: a controlled clinical trial, *Surgery* 89:434-438, 1981.
132. Hauser CJ, et al: Oxygen transport responses to colloids and crystalloids in critically ill surgical patients, *Surg Gynecol Obstet* 150:811-816, 1980.
133. Velanovich V: Crystalloid versus colloid fluid resuscitation: a meta-analysis of mortality, *Surgery* 105:65-71, 1989.
134. Kramer GC, et al: Small-volume resuscitation with hypertonic saline dextran solution, *Surgery* 100:239-247, 1986.
135. Lopes OU, et al: Hemodynamic affects of hypertonic NaCl infusions during hemorrhagic shock in dogs, *Proc Physiol Soc* (Dec):64-65, 1979.
136. Maningas PA: Resuscitation with 7.5% NaCl in 6% dextran 70 during hemorrhagic shock in swine: effects on organ blood flow, *Crit Care Med* 15:1121-1126, 1987.
137. Maningas PA, et al: Small-volume infusion of 7.5% NaCl in 6% dextran 70 for the treatment of severe hemorrhagic shock in swine, *Ann Emerg Med* 15:1131-1137, 1986.
138. Nakayama S, et al: Small-volume resuscitation with hypertonic saline (2,400 mOsm/L) during hemorrhagic shock, *Circ Shock* 13:149-159, 1984.
139. Traverso LW, et al: Hypertonic sodium chloride solutions: effect on hemodynamics and survival after hemorrhage in swine, *J Trauma* 27:32-39, 1987.

140. Velasco IT, et al: Hyperosmotic NaCl and severe hemorrhagic shock, *Am J Physiol* 239:H664-H673, 1980.
141. Wade CE, et al. Cardiovascular, hormonal and metabolic responses to resuscitation with small volumes of hypertonic solutions following hemorrhage, *Fed Proc* 46:805, 1987 (abstract).
142. Rowe GG, et al: Hemodynamic effects of hypertonic sodium chloride, *J Appl Physiol* 32:182-184, 1972.
143. Rocha-e-Silva M, et al: Hypertonic resuscitation from severe hemorrhagic shock: patterns of regional blood flow, *Circ Shock* 19:165-175, 1986.
144. Nakayama S, et al: Infusion of very hypertonic saline to bled rats: membrane potentials and fluid shifts, *J Surg Res* 38:180-186, 1985.
145. Mazzoni MC, et al: Dynamic fluid redistribution in hyperosmotic resuscitation of hypovolemic hemorrhage, *Am J Physiol* 255:H629-H637, 1988.
146. Smith GJ, et al: A comparison of several hypertonic solutions for resuscitation of bled sheep, *J Surg Res* 39:517-528, 1985.
147. Nerlich M, Gunther R, Demling RH: Resuscitation from hemorrhagic shock with hypertonic saline or lactated Ringer's (effect on the pulmonary and systemic microcirculations), *Circ Shock* 10:179-188, 1983.
148. Gazitua S, et al: Resistance responses to local changes in plasma osmolality in three vascular beds, *Am J Physiol* 220:384-391, 1971.
149. Mazzoni MC, et al: Capillary narrowing in hemorrhagic shock is rectified by hyperosmotic saline-dextran reinfusion, *Circ Shock* 31:407-418, 1990.
150. Behrman SW, et al: Microcirculatory flow changes after initial resuscitation of hemorrhagic shock with 7.5% hypertonic saline/6% dextran 70, *J Trauma* 31:589-600, 1991.
151. Wildenthal K, Mierzwiak DS, Mitchell JH: Acute effects of increased serum osmolality on left ventricular performance, *Am J Physiol* 216:898-904, 1969.
152. Kien ND, et al: Cardiac contractility and blood flow distribution following resuscitation with 7.5% hypertonic saline in anesthetized dogs, *Circ Shock* 35:109-116, 1991.
153. Koch-Weser J: Influence of osmolarity of perfusate on contractility of mammalian myocardium, *Am J Physiol* 204:957-962, 1963.
154. Ogino R, et al: Effects of hypertonic saline and dextran 70 on cardiac contractility after hemorrhagic shock, *J Trauma* 44:59-69, 1998.
155. Suzuki K, et al: Effects of hypertonic saline and dextran 70 on cardiac function after burns, *Am J Physiol* 268:H856-H864, 1995.
156. Goertz AW, et al: Effect of 7.2% hypertonic saline/6% hetastarch on left ventricular contractility in anesthetized humans, *Anesthesiology* 82:1389-1395, 1995.
157. Welte M, et al: Hypertonic saline dextran does not increase cardiac contractile function during small volume resuscitation from hemorrhagic shock in anesthetized pigs, *Anesth Analg* 80:1099-1107, 1995.
158. Velasco IT, et al: Hypertonic and hyperoncotic resuscitation from severe hemorrhagic shock in dogs: a comparative study, *Crit Care Med* 17:261-264, 1989.
159. Wade CE, et al: Resuscitation of conscious pigs following hemorrhage: comparative efficacy of small-volume resuscitation, *Circ Shock* 29:193-204, 1989.
160. Vassar MJ, Perry CA, Holcroft JW: Prehospital resuscitation of hypotensive trauma patients with 7.5% NaCl versus 7.5% NaCl with added dextran: a controlled trial, *J Trauma* 34:622-633, 1993.
161. Dubick MA, Wade CE: A review of the efficacy and safety of 7.5% NaCl/6% dextran 70 in experimental animals and in humans, *J Trauma* 36:323-330, 1994.
162. Gross D, et al: Treatment of uncontrolled hemorrhagic shock with hypertonic saline solution, *Surg Gynecol Obstet* 170:106-112, 1990
163. Gross D, et al: Quantitative measurement of bleeding following hypertonic saline therapy in 'uncontrolled' hemorrhagic shock, *J Trauma* 29:79-83, 1989.
164. Gross D, et al: Is hypertonic saline resuscitation safe in 'uncontrolled' hemorrhagic shock? *J Trauma* 28:751-756, 1988.
165. Bickell WH, et al: Use of hypertonic saline/dextran versus lactated Ringer's solution as a resuscitation fluid after uncontrolled aortic hemorrhage in anesthetized swine, *Ann Emerg Med* 21:1077-1085, 1992.
166. Shackford SR, et al: The epidemiology of traumatic death: a population-based analysis, *Arch Surg* 128:571-575, 1993.
167. Adams JH, Graham DI, Scott G: Brain damage in fatal non-missile head injury, *J Clin Pathol* 33:1132-1145, 1980.
168. Miller JD, et al: Early insults to the injured brain, *JAMA* 240: 439-442, 1978.
169. Chesnut RM, et al: The role of secondary brain injury in determining outcome from severe head injury, *J Trauma* 34:216-222, 1993.
170. Wald SL, Shackford SR, Fenwick J: The effect of secondary insults on mortality and long-term disability after severe head injury in a rural region without a trauma system, *J Trauma* 34:377-382, 1993.
171. Miller JD, Becker DP: Secondary insults to the injured brain, *J R Coll Surg Edinb* 27:292-298, 1982.
172. Poole GV Jr, et al: Effects of resuscitation from hemorrhagic shock on cerebral hemodynamics in the presence of an intracranial mass, *J Trauma* 27:18-23, 1987.
173. Gunnar W, et al: Head injury and hemorrhagic shock: studies of the blood brain barrier and intracranial pressure after resuscitation with normal saline solution, 3% saline solution, and dextran-40, *Surgery* 103:398-407, 1988.
174. Prough DS, et al: Effects of hypertonic saline versus lactated Ringer's solution on cerebral oxygen transport during resuscitation from hemorrhagic shock, *J Neurosurg* 64:627-632, 1986.
175. Prough DS, et al: Effects on intracranial pressure of resuscitation from hemorrhagic shock with hypertonic saline versus lactated Ringer's solution, *Crit Care Med* 13:407-411, 1985.
176. Prough DS, et al: Regional cerebral blood flow following resuscitation from hemorrhagic shock with hypertonic saline: influence of a subdural mass, *Anesthesiology* 75:319-327, 1991.
177. Ducey JP, et al: A comparison of the cerebral and cardiovascular effects of complete resuscitation with isotonic and hypertonic saline, hetastarch and whole blood following hemorrhage, *J Trauma* 29:1510-1518, 1989.
178. Shackford SR, Norton CH, Todd MM: Renal, cerebral, and pulmonary effects of hypertonic resuscitation in a porcine model of hemorrhagic shock, *Surgery* 104:553-560, 1988.
179. Walsh JC, Zhuang J, Shackford SR: Fluid resuscitation of focal brain injury and shock, *Surg Forum* 41:56-59, 1990.
180. Walsh JC, Zhuang J, Shackford SR: A comparison of hypertonic to isotonic fluid in the resuscitation of brain injury and hemorrhagic shock, *J Surg Res* 50:284-292, 1991.
181. Zornow MH, Scheller MS, Shackford SR: Effect of a hypertonic lactated Ringer's solution on intracranial pressure and cerebral water content in a model of traumatic brain injury, *J Trauma* 29:484-488, 1989.
182. Holcroft JW, et al: 3% NaCl and 7.5% NaCl/dextran 70 in the resuscitation of severely injured patients, *Ann Surg* 206:279-288, 1987.
183. Mattox KL, et al: Prehospital hypertonic saline/dextran infusion for post-traumatic hypotension, *Ann Surg* 213:482-491, 1991.

184. Younes RN, et al: Hypertonic solutions in the treatment of hypovolemic shock: a prospective, randomized study in patients admitted to the emergency room, *Surgery* 111:380-385, 1992.
185. Vassar MJ, et al: A multicenter trial for resuscitation of injured patients with 7.5% sodium chloride: the effect of added dextran 70, *Arch Surg* 128:1003-1013, 1993.
186. Norenberg MD, Leslie KO, Robertson AS: Association between rise in serum sodium and central pontine myelinolysis, *Ann Neurol* 11:128-135, 1982.
187. Laureno R: Central pontine myelinolysis following rapid correction of hyponatremia, *Ann Neurol* 13:232-242, 1983.
188. Sterns RH, Riggs JE, Schochet SS Jr: Osmotic demyelination syndrome following correction of hyponatremia, *N Engl J Med* 314:1535-1542, 1986.
189. Ljungstrom KG, et al: Adverse reactions to dextran in Sweden 1970-1979, *Acta Chir Scand* 149:253-262, 1983.
190. Ross AD, Angaran DM: Colloids vs crystalloids: a continuing controversy, *Drug Intell Clin Pharm* 18:202-212, 1984.
191. Berliner AD, Lackner H: Hemorrhagic diathesis after prolonged infusion of low molecular weight dextran, *Am J Med Sci* 263:397-403, 1972.
192. Schwab CW, Civil I, Shayne JP: Saline-expanded group O uncrossmatched packed red blood cells as an initial resuscitation fluid in severe shock, *Ann Emerg Med* 15:1282-1287, 1986.
193. Schmidt PJ, Leparc GF, Samia CT: Use of Rh positive blood in emergency situations, *Surg Gynecol Obstet* 167:229-233, 1988.
194. Blumberg N, Bove JR: Un-cross-matched blood for emergency transfusion: one year's experience in a civilian setting, *JAMA* 240:2057-2059, 1978.
195. Sohmer PR, Dawson RB: Transfusion therapy in trauma: a review of the principles and techniques used in the MIEMS program, *Am Surg* 45:109-125, 1979.
196. Lefebre J, McLellan BA, Coovadia AS: Seven years experience with group O unmatched packed red blood cells in a regional trauma unit, *Ann Emerg Med* 16:1344-1349, 1987.
197. Kruskall MS, et al: Transfusion therapy in emergency medicine, *Ann Emerg Med* 17:327-335, 1988.
198. Hambly PR, Dutton RP: Excess mortality associated with the use of a rapid infusion system at a level I trauma center, *Resuscitation* 31:127-133, 1996.
199. Zorko MF, Polsky SS: Rapid warming and infusion of packed red blood cells, *Ann Emerg Med* 15:907-910, 1986.
200. Iserson KV, Knauf MA, Anhalt D: Rapid admixture blood warming: technical advances, *Crit Care Med* 18:1138-1141, 1990.
201. Wilson EB, et al: Red blood cell survival following admixture with heated saline: evaluation of a new blood warming method for rapid transfusion, *J Trauma* 28:1274-1277, 1988.
202. Propp DA: Transfusion therapy: blood and blood products. In Roberts JR, Hedges JR (editors): *Clinical procedures in emergency medicine*, Philadelphia, 1998, Saunders.
203. Shackford SR, Virgilio RW, Peters RM: Whole blood versus packed-cell transfusions: a physiologic comparison, *Ann Surg* 193:337-340, 1981.
204. Hewson JR, et al: Coagulopathy related to dilution and hypotension during massive transfusion, *Crit Care Med* 13:387-391, 1985.
205. Harke H, Rahman S: Haemostatic disorders in massive transfusion, *Bibl Haematol* 46:179-188, 1980.
206. Harrigan C, et al: Primary hemostasis after massive transfusion for injury, *Am Surg* 48:393-396, 1982.
207. Labadie LL: Transfusion therapy in the emergency department, *Emerg Med Clin North Am* 11:379-406, 1993.
208. Schiffer CS: Transfusion therapy in the critical care setting. In Shoemaker WC, et al (editors): *Textbook of critical care*, Philadelphia, 1989, Saunders.
209. Cooper DJ, et al: Bicarbonate does not improve hemodynamics in critically ill patients who have lactic acidosis: a prospective, controlled, clinical study, *Ann Intern Med* 112:492-498, 1990.
210. Makisalo HJ, et al: Effects of bicarbonate therapy on tissue oxygenation during resuscitation of hemorrhagic shock, *Crit Care Med* 17:1170-1174, 1989.
211. Iberti TJ, et al: Effects of sodium bicarbonate in canine hemorrhagic shock, Crit Care Med 16:779-782, 1988.
212. Schreiber GB, et al: The risk of transfusion-transmitted viral infections, *N Engl J Med* 334:1685-1690, 1996.
213. Donahue JG, et al: The declining risk of post-transfusion hepatitis C virus infection, *N Engl J Med* 327:369-373, 1992.
214. Dodd RY: The risk of transfusion-transmitted infection, *N Engl J Med* 327:419-421, 1992.
215. Mattox KL, et al: Blood availability for the trauma patient—autotransfusion, *J Trauma* 15:663-669, 1975.
216. Young FP, Purcell TB: Emergency autotransfusion, *Ann Emerg Med* 12:180-186, 1983.
217. Silva R, et al: The risk:benefit of autotransfusion: comparison to banked blood in a canine model, *J Trauma* 24:557-564, 1984.
218. Orr M: Autotransfusion: the use of washed red cells as an adjunct to component therapy, *Surgery* 84:728-732, 1978.
219. Dixon JL, Smalley MG: Jehovah's Witnesses: the surgical/ethical challenge, *JAMA* 246:2471-2472, 1981.
220. Reul GJ, et al: Experience with autotransfusion in the surgical management of trauma, *Surgery* 76:546-555, 1974.
221. Rakower SR, Worth MH Jr, Lackner H: Massive intraoperative autotransfusion of blood, *Surg Gynecol Obstet* 137:633-636, 1973.
222. Weekes LR: A second look at autotransfusion, *J Natl Med Assoc* 66:367-371, 1974.
223. O'Riordan WD: Autotransfusion in the emergency department of a community hospital, *JACEP* 6:233-237, 1977.
224. Brener BJ: Autotransfusion: safe at any speed? *Arch Surg* 108: 761, 1974.
225. Duncan SE, Klebanoff G, Rogers W: A clinical experience with intraoperative autotransfusion, *Ann Surg* 180:296-304, 1974.
226. Bretton P, Reines HD, Sade RM: Air embolization during autotransfusion for abdominal trauma, *J Trauma* 25:165-166, 1985.
227. Council on Scientific Affairs, American Medical Association: Autologous blood transfusions, *JAMA* 256:2378, 1986.
228. Plaisier BR, et al: Autotransfusion in trauma: a comparison of two systems, *Am Surg* 58:562-566, 1991.
229. Symbas PN: Extraoperative autotransfusion from hemothorax, *Surgery* 84:722-727, 1978.
230. Klebanoff G, Phillips J, Evans W: Use of a disposable autotransfusion unit under varying conditions of contamination: preliminary report, *Am J Surg* 120:351-354, 1970.
231. Wetzel RC: Shock in neonates and children. In Hardaway RM (editor): *Shock: the reversible stage of dying*, Littleton, CO, 1988, PSG Publishing.
232. Friedman WF: The intrinsic physiologic properties of the developing heart, *Prog Cardiovasc Dis* 15:87-111, 1972.
233. Mayer T: Management of hypovolemic shock. In Mayer TA (editor): *Emergency management of pediatric trauma*, Philadelphia, 1985, Saunders.
234. American Heart Association: *Recognition of respiratory failure and shock: anticipating cardiopulmonary arrest: pediatric advanced life support*, Philadelphia, 1988, American Heart Association.
235. Kirkendall WM, et al: Recommendations for human blood pressure determination by sphygmomanometers, *Circulation* 36:980-988, 1967.
236. American Heart Association: *Fluid therapy and medications: pediatric advanced life support*, Philadelphia, 1988, American Heart Association.

237. Champion HR, et al: Major trauma in geriatric patients, *Am J Public Health* 79:1278-1282, 1989.
238. *Statistical Abstract of the United States,* ed 114, Washington, DC, 1994, U.S. Department of Commerce.
239. Schwab CW, Kauder DR: Trauma in the geriatric patient, *Arch Surg* 127:701-706, 1992.
240. Osler T, et al: Trauma in the elderly, *Am J Surg* 156:537-543, 1988.
241. Kostis JB, et al: The effects of age on heart rate in subjects free of heart disease: studies by ambulatory electrocardiography and maximal exercise stress test, *Circulation* 65:141-145, 1982.
242. Weisfeldt ML, Lakarra EG, Gerstenblith G: Aging and cardiac disease. In Braunwald E (editor): *Heart disease: a textbook of cardiovascular medicine,* Philadelphia, 1988, Saunders.
243. Elveback L, Lie JT: Continued high incidence of coronary artery disease at autopsy in Olmstead County, Minnesota, 1950-1979, *Circulation* 70:345-349, 1984.
244. Walsh RA: Cardiovascular effects of the aging process, *Am J Med* 82(suppl 1B):34-40, 1987.
245. Del Guercio LR, Cohn JD: Monitoring operative risk in the elderly, *JAMA* 243:1350-1355, 1980.
246. Scalea TM, et al: Geriatric blunt multiple trauma: improved survival with early invasive monitoring, *J Trauma* 30:129-136, 1990.
247. Bickell WH, et al: The detrimental effects of intravenous crystalloid after aortotomy in swine, *Surgery* 110:529-536, 1991.
248. Stern SA, et al: Effect of blood pressure on hemorrhage volume and survival in a near-fatal hemorrhage model incorporating a vascular injury, *Ann Emerg Med* 22:155-163, 1993.
249. Beecher HK: Treatment of wounded men. In *Resuscitation and anesthesia for wounded men,* Springfield, IL, 1949, Charles C. Thomas.
250. Wiggers CJ: Experimental hemorrhagic shock. In *Physiology of shock,* New York, 1950, Commonwealth Fund.

Emergency Department Monitoring of Trauma Patients

9

JAY L. FALK, PATRIC N. ANDERSON, AND KEVIN C. MEYER

Many patients sustaining serious traumatic injury present with obvious signs of shock. Tachycardia and hypotension trigger aggressive resuscitation. However, other patients with substantial blood loss, but who have normal or near-normal vital signs, may not be recognized as being seriously ill. Recent data indicate that traditional vital signs and clinical assessments are insensitive at identifying patients with inadequate tissue perfusion (shock),[1] especially when patients have received prehospital fluid resuscitation.

More sensitive markers of tissue hypoperfusion than traditional vital signs include the shock index,[2] arterial lactate levels,[3] base deficit (BD),[4] mixed venous oxygen saturation (SvO_2),[5] expired carbon dioxide (CO_2) levels,[6] and most recently, tissue CO_2 levels.[7] These markers identify compromised patients in the trauma room who may have relatively normal heart rate and blood pressure. High-risk patients include those with altered mental status (secondary to head trauma or intoxication), the elderly, the pregnant trauma victim, and those with altered sensation resulting from spinal cord injury. Although it is not entirely clear which patients benefit from such monitoring, these newer modalities, when coupled with astute clinical assessment, may improve outcome for trauma patients.

PHYSIOLOGY OF HYPOPERFUSION

Under ordinary circumstances, the human organism exists in a state of oxygen (O_2) excess. Each minute, tissues extract only 25% of the O_2 delivered by the blood, resulting in a mixed venous oxygen saturation (SvO_2) of 75%. Systemic oxygen delivery (DO_2) is the product of arterial oxygen content (CaO_2) and cardiac output (CO). CaO_2 is primarily determined by the amount of hemoglobin (Hb) and the level to which it is saturated with O_2. In the trauma patient DO_2 may be compromised by decreases in Hb level (i.e., bleeding), hemoglobin saturation (e.g., hypoxemia), or by falling CO. Hypovolemia and cardiac factors such as contusion, ischemia, infarction, or tamponade can reduce CO.

Oxygen consumption (VO_2) is the rate of oxygen usage by the various tissue beds. Initially, reductions in DO_2 do not result in corresponding decreases in VO_2 because of O_2 reserves. When DO_2 is further reduced, systemic O_2 extraction increases from 25% to a maximum of 75%, which initially maintains total body VO_2.[8] This increased O_2 extraction in the face of decreased DO_2 forms the basis of SvO_2 monitoring in shock patients.[9] An SvO_2 below normal (75%) suggests that tissue O_2 demands have exceeded supply, activating compensatory mechanisms. When DO_2 falls below a "critical" level, this compensatory mechanism is overwhelmed and VO_2 decreases in parallel with systemic DO_2 (Fig. 9-1).

Tissue hypoxia is associated with lactic acidosis because of cellular anaerobic metabolism.[3] Lactate is a measure of O_2 debt. Lactate rises when O_2 supply is inadequate to meet O_2 demand. In a canine model of hemorrhagic shock, increases in O_2 debt (and lactate) correlated with mortality.[10] In the early 1970s Weil and Afifi[11] demonstrated that in patients in an intensive care unit (ICU), arterial blood lactate levels less than 2 mmol/L were associated with a 90% survival rate, whereas increases in lactate to a level of 8 mmol/L or more were associated with survival rates of $<10\%$. Some patients with decreased O_2 demands (e.g., in the setting of hypothermia or sedative drug overdose) may tolerate substantial reductions in DO_2 without producing lactate. Conversely, some patients have supranormal O_2 needs (e.g., those with high work of breathing, fever, seizures, and stimulant drug

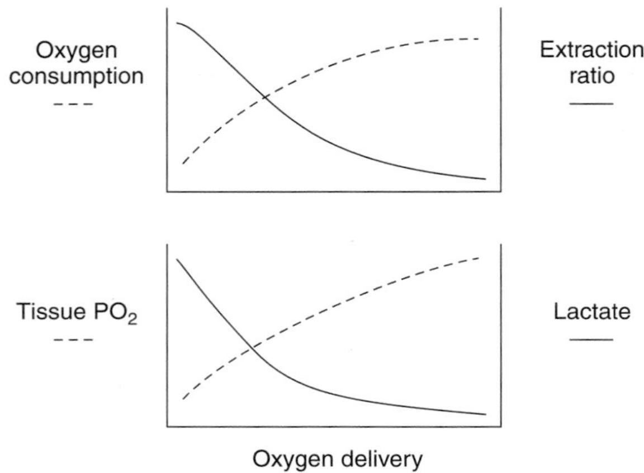

Fig. 9-1 Physiology of hypoperfusion. In circulatory shock, compensatory mechanisms are evoked when decreases in oxygen delivery to tissues reach critical levels. Oxygen extraction ratio increases, and oxygen consumption and tissue oxygen tension are thereby maintained. When delivery falls further, oxygen consumption decreases, indicating a state of delivery-dependent oxygen consumption representative of tissue hypoxia. Under these conditions, tissue oxygen tension is reduced and systemic lactate level rises. Such changes may precede obvious hemodynamic instability. (From Falk JL, et al: *J Cardiothorac Vasc Anesth* 2[suppl 6]:33-38, 1988.)

intoxication) and develop lactic acidosis despite "normal" DO_2. Therapies directed at reducing O_2 demands (e.g., ventilatory support, cooling measures) might improve tissue perfusion in these instances by better matching of O_2 demand with available O_2 supply.

TRAUMA PATIENT MONITORING

Traditional Vital Signs

The extent of hemorrhage can be estimated by using a combination of heart rate, respiratory rate, and blood pressure (Table 9-1).[12] Sympathetic response to blood loss defends against hypotension via vasoconstriction and tachycardia.[13] More subtle clinical signs such as agitation, piloerection, narrowed pulse pressure, and delayed capillary refill may be present in compromised patients who are successfully compensating for substantial blood volume losses.[8]

HEART RATE

The absence of tachycardia should not lull the clinician into a false sense of security. *Many patients in shock have normal or even slow heart rates.*[14] **Relative bradycardia** is defined as a systolic pressure ≤90 mmHg and a pulse rate ≤90 beats per minute (bpm). As many as 30% of hypotensive patients may have relative bradycardia.[15] In patients with abdominal trauma and shock, vagal mechanisms may blunt the tachycardic response. Patients with exsanguinating hemorrhage may suffer from coronary hypoperfusion with resultant bradycardia **(central hemodynamic collapse).**[14]

Other causes of relative bradycardia include preexisting cardiac disease **(chronotropic incompetence).** β-blockers can similarly prevent tachycardia. Head-injured patients with increased intracranial pressure **(Cushing's reflex)** and patients with spinal cord injury may be bradycardic despite concomitant hemorrhagic shock.[14]

RESPIRATORY RATE

The respiratory rate is an unreliable indicator of shock. One would expect that the patient in shock would be tachypneic, as a compensatory measure in the face of developing metabolic acidemia. Tachypnea has multiple etiologies, including (1) compensation for metabolic acidosis, (2) hypoxia from lung injury or airway compromise, (3) pneumohemothorax, (4) pain, (5) anxiety, or (6) anemia resulting from hemorrhage. Sedative drugs or severe head injury may depress respiratory drive even in the face of shock.

BLOOD PRESSURE

Blood pressure is universally accepted as an important parameter in trauma management. However, accurate measurement may be difficult during resuscitation. Accordingly, it has been recommended that clinicians obtain a rough estimation of blood pressure by palpation of major arterial pulses during initial resuscitation.[13] The presence of the following pulses suggest minimum systolic pressures: radial, 80 mmHg; femoral, 70 mmHg; and carotid, 60 mmHg.[13] However, these parameters are not substantiated by an authoritative database.

Noninvasive assessment of blood pressure relies on the detection of oscillatory waves generated by blood flow reexpanding vessels occluded by a pressurized cuff **(Korotkoff sounds).** Vasoconstriction resulting from low CO (e.g., hypovolemia or cardiogenic causes) severely impairs the generation of these waves. Vasoconstricted shock patients may have true intraarterial pressures substantially higher than simultaneously obtained noninvasive readings.[14,16,17] All noninvasive techniques, including auscultation, palpation, Doppler, and oscillometric techniques may give erroneous data compared with directly-measured intraarterial pressures.[16]

Intraarterial line placement during trauma resuscitation can provide accurate data with a continuous digital display. Arterial lines are used routinely in the operating suite and in the ICU. In addition, a portable transport monitor can track intraarterial pressures in

TABLE 9-1
Estimated Fluid and Blood Requirements* (Based on Patient's Initial Presentation)

	CLASS I	CLASS II	CLASS III	CLASS IV
Blood Loss (ml)	up to 750	750-1500	1500-2000	≥2000
Blood loss (% blood volume)	up to 15%	15%-30%	30%-40%	≥40%
Pulse rate	<100	>100	>120	≥140
Blood pressure	Normal	Normal	Decreased	Decreased
Pulse pressure (mmHg)	Normal or increased	Decreased	Decreased	Decreased
Capillary refill test	Normal	Positive	Positive	Positive
Respiratory rate	14-20	20-30	30-40	>35
Urine output (ml/hr)	≥30	20-30	5-15	Negligible
Central nervous system–mental status	Slightly anxious	Mildly anxious	Anxious and confused	Confused, lethargic
Fluid replacement (3:1 rule)	Crystalloid	Crystalloid	Crystalloid + blood	Crystalloid + blood

From Falk JL, O'Brien JF, Kerr R: *Crit Care Clin* 8(2):323-340, 1992.
*For a 70-kg male patient.

patients who spend considerable time in a computed tomography (CT) scanner, radiography suite, hallway, or transport vehicle. Intraarterial lines allow serial blood sampling for arterial blood gases (ABGs) or lactate levels. Despite the advantages, it is unclear which patients should receive an intraarterial line in the trauma room. Patients in shock may benefit if definitive therapy is not delayed by line placement. Geriatric patients may also profit from such invasive monitoring.[18]

Shock Index

In an effort to increase the sensitivity of vital signs for detecting shock, Allgower and Burri[19] first described the shock index (SI) in 1967. They defined the SI as the ratio of heart rate over systolic blood pressure, which normally ranges from 0.5 to 0.7. The higher the SI, the greater the mortality. In their study, mortality was 40% among blunt abdominal trauma patients with SI values >1. Elevation of the SI indicates a deterioration in the left ventricular stroke work index and heralds acute circulatory failure. An SI of 0.9 or higher reportedly has a better sensitivity than the individual measurements of heart rate or systolic blood pressure to identify critically ill patients in the ED.[2] However, other investigators found that the SI (based on the initial vital signs taken within 5 minutes after the patient's arrival in the ED) is not superior to the heart rate or systolic blood pressure alone, and all three variables have low sensitivities (typically near or below 50%) for significant injuries or hypoperfusion.[20] Although insensitive, an elevated SI (on arrival to the ED) is frequently associated with the need to triage to a high level of care and possibly ICU admission.[21] Overall, the SI appears to have limited value in the ED compared with traditional vital signs that do not require calculation in this frenetic circumstance. Further prospective study comparing SI with other markers of tissue hypoperfusion such as lactate are needed.

Serum Lactate

Virchow poetically stated that shock is "a rude unhinging of the machinery of life." More prosaically, shock is an imbalance between tissue O_2 demands and tissue O_2 supply.[8] Impaired DO_2 is the primary problem in all shock states, regardless of etiology. Increased tissue O_2 demands from concomitant acute respiratory failure (and increased work of breathing), shivering, seizures, or hypercatabolic states may contribute to the imbalance.

When tissue hypoxia occurs, pyruvate oxidation in the Krebs cycle decreases. Lactate production rises, and adenosine triphosphate (ATP) formation continues via glycolysis.[3] This anaerobic metabolism is much less efficient and results in only 2 moles of ATP produced per mole of glucose compared with 38 mol ATP per mole under aerobic conditions.[3] The amount of lactate correlates with the total O_2 debt, the magnitude of the hypoperfusion, and the severity of shock. Blood lactate concentration in states of normal perfusion and physiologic demand is 1.0 ± 0.5 mml/L.

Blood lactate concentrations may have prognostic value.[3,6,11,22-26] Broder and Weil[25] documented that only 11% of patients with excess lactate concentrations

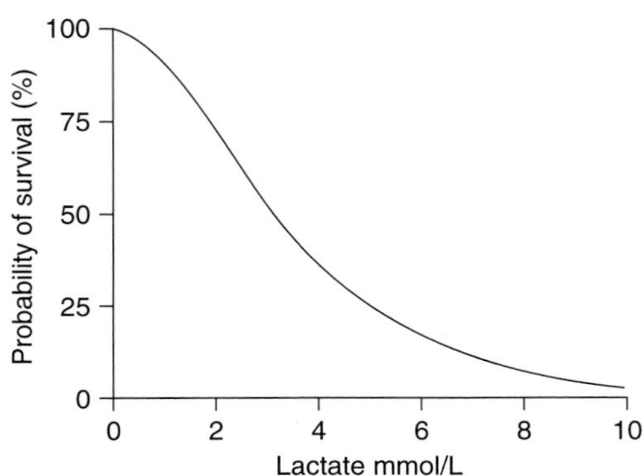

Fig. 9-2 Probability of survival based on initial arterial blood lactate level (mmol/L) in intensive care unit patients. Severity of perfusion failure and probability of survival are identified by the magnitude of lactate acidosis. (From Falk JL, et al: *J Cardiothorac Vasc Anesth* 2[suppl 6]:33-38, 1988.)

(>4 mmol/L) survived circulatory shock. In a study of patients with circulatory shock, Weil and Afifi[11] subsequently demonstrated that as lactate concentration increased from 2 to 8 mmol/L, the estimated probability of survival decreased from 90% to 10% (Fig. 9-2). Vitek and Cowley[26] confirmed these observations and demonstrated that the etiology of shock influenced survival. Patients in hemorrhagic shock tolerate higher levels of lactic acidosis than those in cardiogenic shock. Although hemorrhagic shock can be corrected with aggressive transfusion and surgical intervention, cardiogenic shock remains largely untreatable. Likewise, several studies show that patients in septic shock have lower blood lactate than those in hemorrhagic shock.[27-29] This discrepancy may be secondary to greater hepatic blood flow in the septic patients, leading to improved lactate clearance.

Peretz and colleagues[30] noted that the mortality rate increased from 18% to 73% in critically ill patients who presented with lactate levels >4.4 mmol/L. In critically ill patients there is a striking increase in mortality as lactate concentrations rise above 2.5 mmol/L.[23] Likewise, a persistent metabolic acidosis is strongly associated with high mortality in patients with the adult respiratory distress syndrome.[31]

The presence of underlying liver disease affects the relationship between elevated serum lactate level and tissue hypoperfusion.[28,29,32-35] Cirrhotic patients have normal baseline blood lactate concentrations, but demonstrate a decreased ability to clear lactate during periods of increased production. This decreased hepatic reserve and the significance of a single lactate level may vary considerably among cirrhotic patients. Nevertheless, in a study of patients with chronic liver disease, Kruse et al[35] confirmed the utility of lactate as a metabolic marker of shock. Despite the variability in lactate clearance, the degree of increase in lactate levels correlated with mortality.

Difficulties in the interpretation of peak lactate concentration as a prognostic indicator have led investigators to examine the utility of sequential determinations of lactate during resuscitation. Falk et al[36] monitored sequential lactate concentrations in 24 patients with circulatory shock. All patients received a fluid challenge to optimize hemodynamics, and data was collected for 24 hours after resuscitation. Survivors progressively cleared their lactate at a rate of approximately 2.5% per hour, and 18 hours into the resuscitation, lactate levels declined to half their peak values. In contradistinction, patients who expired during the study period failed to clear the lactic acidosis despite similar volumes of fluid and hemodynamic response. In studies of patients with septic shock, initial blood lactate concentrations did not differ between survivors and nonsurvivors, although a greater reduction of lactate in the survivors relative to nonsurvivors was demonstrated.[37,38] Patients in circulatory shock who experience a reduction in lactate of more than 5% during the first hour of treatment have a better prognosis than those who do not.[39]

We believe these data have relevance to the clinician at the bedside. When patients are resuscitated to the clinician's satisfaction, serial lactate concentrations are followed over time. If the lactate fails to clear or levels increase, then interventions directed at increasing DO_2 and VO_2 are indicated.

Serial lactate determinations may also be helpful in the trauma room when assessing patients with altered mental status or other factors that preclude adequate history taking. Many patients present with obtundation following seizures that may have been precipitated by head trauma or intoxication. These patients may have severe metabolic acidosis, which is often accompanied by lack of respiratory compensation. On initial assessment, differentiation of patients who are simply post-ictal from patients who may have other serious conditions (e.g., septic shock or severe poisonings) may be difficult. Since the lactate clearance in the former group of patients is rapid (half-life 60 min)[40] compared with the latter group (half-life 18 hr),[36] repeat lactate determination can substantially assist the clinician in differentiating between these two patient groups.

The use of lactate as an index of tissue perfusion has several limitations. Foremost, for significant increases in blood lactate to occur, lactate must not only accumulate in tissues and spill into the systemic circulation, but its rate of production must exceed hepatic, renal, and skeletal muscle uptake.[39] Therefore regional hypoperfusion may be present despite normal blood lactate concentrations. Recent work[41-43] has focused on the splanchnic circulation. The results of these studies suggest that the presence of normal blood lactate concentration in critically ill patients does not ensure that splanchnic perfusion is adequate. Metabolic monitoring of regional circulations may improve detection of organ hypoperfusion. Although some techniques currently remain experimental, such as tissue O_2 monitoring, innovative approaches may soon be common, such as gastric mucosal pH monitoring as a reflection of splanchnic perfusion, or monitoring of sublingual tissue CO_2 levels.[7,43,44]

Base Deficit

Base deficits (BDs) are easily and rapidly obtained in the trauma room and have been used as a substitute for lactate. Variables that disturb the relationship between lactate and BD during resuscitation, such as the administration of bicarbonate, make lactate more reliable. Base deficit measurements may guide fluid resuscitation and are also predictive of mortality.[10,45-48] A significant BD is an ominous sign in patients with serious head injury and in the pregnant trauma victim.[46,49]

Davis et al[45] evaluated the usefulness of BDs as indicators of hypovolemia in trauma patients. They reviewed 209 trauma patients with serial ABGs drawn during their resuscitation. The volume of fluid required for resuscitation was greater in the group with more negative BDs. They found that the initial BD is a reliable early indicator of volume loss. Additionally, ongoing hemorrhage was suggested by a progressively worsening serial BD despite fluid resuscitation. Sixty-five percent of the patients with persistent occult bleeding were identified with an increasing (i.e., becoming more negative) BD. Accordingly, in the trauma centers participating in these studies, any trauma patient with a BD more negative than –5 receives aggressive resuscitation.[45] The ABG is repeated after infusion of 2 to 3 liters of crystalloid or after any decrease in blood pressure to assess changes in the BD. A BD that worsens or does not improve necessitates a diligent search for hemorrhage, even in the face of stable vital signs.[45]

Base deficit measurements may be as accurate in the detection of shock as invasive parameters. Researchers have compared it with measurements of mean arterial pressure, central venous pressure, CO, arterial-venous oxygen difference, SvO_2, DO_2, VO_2, and the ratio of DO_2 to VO_2. In a swine hemorrhage model, BD closely paralleled invasive hemodynamic variables and accurately reflected the changes in DO_2 and VO_2.[47] Although BD worsened with hemorrhage and improved with resuscitation, it did not return to baseline. Not only did BD indicate shock, but also normalization of the BD tracked improvement when invasive monitoring was impractical. A canine model also demonstrated that BDs more negative than –16 mmol/L correlated with increased mortality.

Human studies also demonstrate an association between BD and mortality. In a retrospective study of 3791 trauma patients, ABGs were drawn within 24 hours of admission. Both an injury score and BD predicted mortality, along with injury mechanism, age, and the presence of a head injury. Patients with BDs more negative than –15 mmol/L were most likely to die.[48] Such patients may benefit from aggressive monitoring and resuscitation.

LIMITATIONS OF BASE DEFICIT IN TRAUMA

Although the most common cause of a large BD is hemorrhagic shock and associated lactic acidosis, metabolic acidosis may be a result of other factors. The use of cocaine, recent seizures, uremia, hypoxia, diabetic ketoacidosis, and a variety of toxins will result in a significant BD. The use of bicarbonate may obscure the deficit but does not correct the underlying problem.

The clinical role of BD and lactate in the trauma room is not fully defined. Who deserves measurement of these parameters, and when are serial studies indicated? Some trauma centers use lactate or BD as a routine point-of-care test, and serial levels are obtained in those with abnormal results or potential for ongoing blood loss. They can be used in smaller hospitals, along with other indicators, to assess the need for trauma center transfer. Suggestions for selective use of BD or lactate are outlined in Box 9-1.

MIXED VENOUS OXYGEN SATURATION

Mixed venous oxygen saturation (SvO_2) measurements are used extensively in ICUs to assess the balance between VO_2 and DO_2. Mixed venous blood drawn from the pulmonary artery (PA) port of a PA catheter represents an average or mixing of the blood returning from all perfused tissue, including the heart. Fiberoptic catheters provide continuous venous oximetry and correlate well with intermittent measurements of SvO_2.[5] A low (<65%) or rapidly falling SvO_2 indicates inadequate DO_2. This imbalance may be caused by on-going hemorrhage, decreased CaO_2, low CO, or an increase in tissue O_2 demands. A low or falling SvO_2 provides an "early warning" for impending decompensation.[5]

The hazards and time constraints of PA catheterization complicate the use of these measurements in the ED. On the other hand, central lines placed in the su-

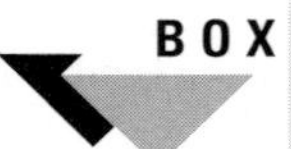

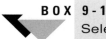

BOX 9-1
Selective Use of Lactate and Base Deficit in Trauma

THE POOR HISTORIAN
Intoxication
Significant head trauma

COMPROMISED PHYSICAL EXAMINATION
Altered mental status
Spinal cord injury

COMPROMISED PATIENT
Elderly victims
Pregnant females

LIKELY ONGOING BLOOD LOSS
History of prehospital hypotension
Patient with posterior pelvic fractures
Low or dropping hemoglobin
Blunt abdominal trauma

LIMITED RESOURCES
Small hospital with limited surgical backup
(Abnormal values may prompt trauma center transfer)

perior vena cava are common. Central SvO_2 obtained from these lines could substitute for true mixed venous measurements. The central SvO_2 is usually higher than PA SvO_2 because of desaturation of myocardial venous blood, which drains into the heart via the coronary sinus. A canine model showed a 96% to 97% correlation between central venous and mixed venous O_2 saturations.[9]

In an effort to identify the earliest and most reliable indicator of occult blood loss, Scalea et al[50] studied a canine shock model. They progressively bled 16 dogs and monitored vital signs, hemodynamic parameters, and mixed and central venous O_2 saturations. Tachycardia, hypotension, and narrowed pulse pressure correlated poorly with blood loss. SvO_2 was the most sensitive indicator of shock and progressively decreased in all the dogs. There was a very high correlation for the mean SvO_2 versus percent hemorrhage ($r = 0.98\%$). Changes in SvO_2 are apparent with as little as 3% blood loss. Although central SvO_2 and cardiac index demonstrated a 92% correlation with blood loss, the correlation of mixed SvO_2 was 98%.

In a clinical study examining the use of central SvO_2 monitoring in trauma patients, 26 stable trauma patients with suspected blood loss were evaluated. Despite stable vital signs, 10 patients (39%) had central SvO_2 less than 65%. These patients had more serious injuries, larger estimated blood losses, and greater transfusion requirements than those with higher central SvO_2. Accordingly, the researchers suggest that central SvO_2 monitoring is a useful tool to assess blood loss and the efficacy of resuscitation.[51]

END-TIDAL CO_2

End-tidal CO_2 ($ETCO_2$) is determined by the body's CO_2 production, minute ventilation (V_E) and pulmonary perfusion (Q). When the circulatory status and Q are normal, $ETCO_2$ is determined primarily by V_E. Under normal circumstances, $ETCO_2$ approximates arterial pCO_2.[52] This situation changes when Q is low, usually as a result of decreased CO during shock states or cardiac arrest.[14,53-58] In these settings, the $ETCO_2$ varies according to pulmonary blood flow (CO) rather than V_E. Under conditions of very low pulmonary blood flow, delivery of CO_2 to the lungs is markedly reduced and minimal CO_2 is exhaled.

Numerous investigators have demonstrated the linear correlation between $ETCO_2$ and CO at low flow states.[56-58] At low flows, $ETCO_2$ varies with CO, whereas at normal or high flows it does not.

Techniques for monitoring expired CO_2 in the operating suite, recovery suite, and ICU include the use of mass spectrometry and infrared absorption systems.[52] Portable infrared CO_2 monitors can be used successfully in the ED. Current versions of these portable devices provide simultaneous pulse oximetry data. Warm-up time is minimal, calibration is simple, and the devices are durable enough to be utilized in the field.

Clinical Use of $ETCO_2$ in Trauma

Endotracheal intubation should always be confirmed by an objective test, since clinical assessment may be inaccurate. $ETCO_2$ monitors or the esophageal detection device have been successfully utilized in this context. The quantitative $ETCO_2$ detector with capnographic waveform is an excellent means to ensure proper intubation. However, in patients with spontaneous circulation, a qualitative end-tidal detector, which changes color in the presence of CO_2, is an inexpensive alternative. The advantages of alphanumeric display, waveform, and trending data capabilities of the quantitative detector often outweigh the utility of the colorimetric devices. The electronic quantitative detector allows the physician to achieve desired eucapnia in head trauma victims, without the need for frequent ABGs.

$ETCO_2$ and Shock

Circulatory shock consists not only of failure of DO_2, but also of failure of carbon dioxide excretion.[59] The venoarterial CO_2 gradient reported during circulatory arrest and resuscitation[60,61] is simply a dramatic example of this phenomenon.[62-65] Patients with normal circulation have normal venoarterial CO_2 gradients (<6.0 mmHg), whereas those in shock have venoarterial CO_2 gradients of 24 mmHg or more.[64] Patients in circulatory arrest have venoarterial gradients of 49 mmHg. Others have made similar observations in patients with sepsis and septic shock.[65]

Venous hypercarbia during cardiac arrest results from decreased Q and CO_2 excretion by the lungs, yielding very low levels of $ETCO_2$.[53,57,66] Similar pathophysiology is likely in the hypoperfusion states seen during circulatory shock.[10,11]

Currently, $ETCO_2$ monitoring is not widely used to monitor patients in circulatory shock. It is likely that severe circulatory compromise and obvious hemodynamic instability would occur before any aberration in $ETCO_2$. However, $ETCO_2$ monitoring has potential utility during resuscitation of severely compromised trauma victims. These patients are usually intubated, and in the early minutes of resuscitation traditional methods of assessing circulatory status are difficult to use. Auscultated blood pressures are unreliable in patients with low-output, vasoconstricted states.[17] Placement of intraarterial lines takes time and personnel, both of which may be limited in the ED. Many of these victims receive massive fluid resuscitation and are at risk of fluid overload. Administration of fluids is especially relevant in patients with concomitant shock and closed head injury or pulmonary contusion. Currently, there are only very limited parameters to guide fluid therapy in this setting.

We reported a case in which $ETCO_2$ monitoring was used in a patient with head trauma, severe hemorrhagic shock, and central circulatory collapse (Fig. 9-3).[14] $ETCO_2$ increased from 10 mmHg to 25 mmHg during the first several minutes of fluid resuscitation. This increase occurred while V_E was held as constant as possible with bagged ventilation. Hemodynamic parameters improved along with the rise in $ETCO_2$. Additional studies to determine the correlation of $ETCO_2$ with other hemodynamic and cardiorespiratory parameters are in progress.

Intubated patients often are transported from the trauma room to the CT scanner or other diagnostic areas in the hospital. Patients who appear stable may suddenly decompensate in these areas where monitoring is less than ideal. $ETCO_2$ may drop before traditional vital signs deteriorate. Certainly a precipitous fall in $ETCO_2$ would alert the physician to possible accidental extubation.

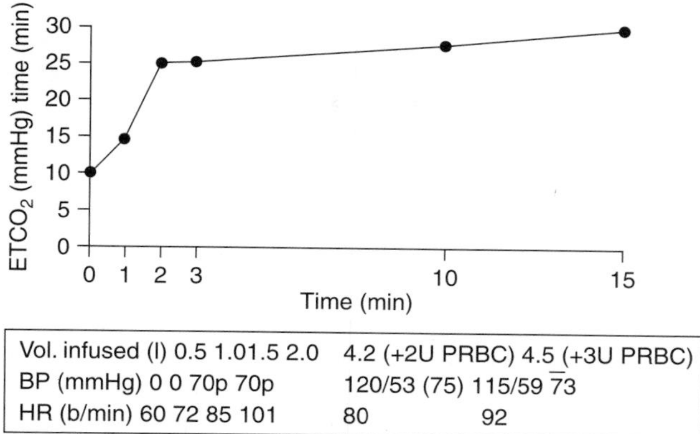

Fig. 9-3 The response of end tidal CO_2 ($ETCO_2$) to fluid resuscitation in a patient with central hemodynamic collapse following traumatic hemorrhagic shock. The $ETCO_2$ increased from very low levels on presentation in response to aggressive fluid resuscitation in this severely traumatized patient. This response appears to correspond to increases in total systemic flow and the hemodynamic parameters delineated in the figure. (From Falk JL, O'Brien JF, Kerr R: *Crit Care Clin* 8[2]:323-340, 1992.)

TISSUE CO_2 MONITORING

Although shock has traditionally been conceptualized as an impairment in DO_2, more recently it has also been viewed as an alteration of CO_2 excretion.[59,67] Tissue hypoperfusion resulting in ischemia causes lactic acidosis, which is buffered by tissue bicarbonate, which generates more CO_2.[68] Tissue CO_2 levels increase to extraordinary levels in the heart during cardiopulmonary resuscitation. During all forms of circulatory shock, the splanchnic bed has been shown to receive even less blood flow than other tissue beds.[69] Accordingly, CO_2 accumulation in gut mucosal tissue has been advocated as an early harbinger of shock.[70] Unfortunately, the technique of gastric tonometry is cumbersome, requires long equilibration times and H_2 blockade of gastric acid secretion, rendering it virtually useless in the trauma room.

Recently, a tissue CO_2 probe utilizing a fluorescent optode technology has been developed that is capable of measuring sublingual mucosal tissue CO_2 quickly and reliably. Preliminary studies in animal models[7] and patients (unpublished data) suggest that this technique may be very useful in identifying patients with compensated shock following trauma. Tissue CO_2 seems to increase more rapidly than lactate as hypoperfusion develops, and it returns to normal far more quickly than lactate following resuscitation,[7] making it a more "real-time" monitor than other metabolic markers of shock.

PULSE OXIMETRY

Pulse oximetry is useful as a monitor of oxygenation in the trauma room but is not particularly useful as a monitor of tissue perfusion. Accurate pulse oximetry requires the presence of good pulsatile blood flow in the tissues. Oximetry is a plethysmographic technique that requires detectable pulsations to distinguish between light absorption of arterial blood and the background absorption that is associated with venous blood and tissues.[71] In vasoconstricted and low-flow states such as hemorrhagic shock, pulse oximetry may be unable to give a reading or may potentially give an inaccurate reading.[72] Trauma patients who have been in or around fires may have high carboxyhemoglobin levels that will be erroneously read as oxyhemoglobin by the pulse oximeter, giving a false sense of security. Accordingly, all burn victims should have ABGs and co-oximetry to assess their state of oxygenation and level of carboxyhemoglobin. Similarly, methemoglobinemia will confound pulse oximetry readings.

The pulse oximeter can be an invaluable tool during rapid sequence intubation in the trauma victim. After adequate preoxygenation in patients with good pulsatile signal, the pulse oximeter allows for deliberate control of the airway without concern for hypoxemia. Desaturation in this setting alerts the clinician to the immediate need to stop intubation attempts and proceed with bag-mask ventilation with high-flow O_2 until O_2 saturation returns to acceptable levels.

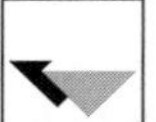

PEARLS & PITFALLS

- Vital signs may be insensitive indicators of systemic hypoperfusion (shock)
- Hypotension is a late finding in shock, and both auscultated and automated cuff pressures are frequently inaccurate in this setting; direct measurement of intraarterial pressures provides a more accurate assessment
- Biochemical markers of O_2 debt, such as BD and lactate, provide the best early warning of occult tissue hypoxia
- Worsening BD or lactate should prompt increased resuscitative efforts and a search for occult hemorrhage
- In patients with a central line, measurement of central SVO_2 also helps diagnose compensated shock and allows the physician to adjust fluid and blood product administration

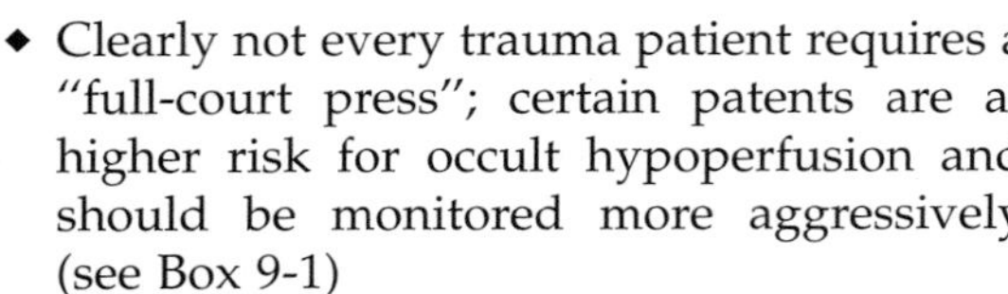

- Clearly not every trauma patient requires a "full-court press"; certain patents are at higher risk for occult hypoperfusion and should be monitored more aggressively (see Box 9-1)

REFERENCES

1. Shippy CR, Appel Pl, Shoemaker WC: Reliability of clinical monitoring to assess blood volume in critically ill patients, *Crit Care Med* 12:107-112, 1984.
2. Rady MY, et al: Shock index: a re-evaluation in acute circulatory failure, *Resuscitation* 23:227-234, 1992.
3. Mizock BA, Falk JL: Lactic acidosis in critical illness, *Crit Care Med* 20:80-93, 1992.
4. Rutherford EJ, et al: Base deficit stratifies mortality and determines therapy, *J Trauma* 33:417-423, 1992.
5. Nelson LD: Continuous venous oximetry in surgical patients, *Ann Surg* 203:329-333, 1986.
6. Falk JL, et al: Fluid resuscitation in shock, *J Cardiopulm Resusc* 10:275-288, 1993.
7. Nakagawa Y, et al: Sublingual capnometry for diagnosis and quantitation of circulatory shock, *Am J Respir Crit Care Med* 157: 1838-1843, 1998.
8. Falk JL, et al: Fluid resuscitation in shock, *J Cardiothorac Anesth* 6:33-38, 1988.
9. Reinhart K, et al: Comparison of central-venous oxygen saturation during changes in oxygen supply/demand, *Chest* 95:1216-1221, 1989.
10. Dunham CM, et al: Oxygen debt and metabolic acidemia as quantitative predictors of mortality and the severity of the ischemic insult in hemorrhagic shock, *Crit Care Med* 19:231-243, 1991.
11. Weil MH, Afifi AA: Experimental and clinical studies on lactate and pyruvate as indicators of the severity of acute circulatory failure (shock), *Circulation* 41:989-1001, 1970.
12. Cornwell EE III, Kennedy F, Rodriguez J: The critical care of the severely injured patient. I. Assessing and improving oxygen delivery, *Surg Clin North Am* 76:959-969, 1996.
13. *Advanced trauma life support,* Chicago, 1998, American College of Surgeons.
14. Falk JL, O'Brien JF, Kerr R: Fluid resuscitation in traumatic hemorrhagic shock, *Crit Care Clin* 8:323-340, 1992.
15. Demetriades D, et al: Relative bradycardia in patients with traumatic hypotension, *J Trauma* 45:534-539, 1998.
16. Carroll GC: Blood pressure monitoring, *Crit Care Clin* 4:411-434, 1988.
17. Cohn JN: Blood pressure measurement in shock: mechanisms of inaccuracy in auscultatory and palpatory methods, *JAMA* 199: 118-122, 1967.
18. Scalea TM, et al: Geriatric blunt multiple trauma: improved survival with early invasive monitor, *J Trauma* 30:129-136, 1990.
19. Allgower M, Burri C: Shock index, *Dtsch Med Wochenschr* 92: 1947-1950, 1967.
20. King RW, et al: Shock index as a marker for significant injury in trauma patients, *Acad Emerg Med* 3:1041-1045, 1996.
21. Rady M, et al: A comparison of the shock index and conventional vital signs to identify acute critical illness in the emergency department, *Ann Emerg Med* 24:685-690, 1994.
22. Mizock BA: Controversies in lactic acidosis: implication in critically ill patients, *JAMA* 258:497-501, 1987.
23. Kruse JA, Mehta KC, Carson RW: Definition of clinically significant lactic acidosis, (abstr) *Chest* 92(suppl):100, 1987.

24. Cryan L, Ledinham I: The significance of lactate in intensive care, *Intensive Crit Care Diag* 5:15-17, 1986.
25. Broder G, Weil MH: Excess lactate: an index of reversibility of shock in human patients, *Science* 143:1457-1459, 1964.
26. Vitek V, Cowley RA: Blood lactate in the prognosis of various forms of shock, *Ann Surg* 173:308-313, 1971.
27. Rosenberg JC, Rush BF: Blood lactic acid levels in irreversible hemorrhagic and lethal endotoxic shock, *Surg Gynecol Obstet* 126:1247-1250, 1968.
28. Perret C, Enrico J: Lactic acid in shock and liver failure. In Moret P, Weber J (editors): *Lactate: physiologic, methodologic and pathologic approach,* New York, 1980, Springer-Verlag.
29. Cowan BN, et al: The relative prognostic value of lactate and haemodynamic measurements in early shock, *Anaesthesia* 39: 750-755, 1984.
30. Peretz DI, et al: The significance of lacticacidemia in the shock syndrome, *Ann NY Acad Sci* 119:1133-1141, 1965.
31. Fowler AA, et al: Adult respiratory distress syndrome: prognosis after onset, *Am Rev Respir Dis* 132:472-478, 1985.
32. Perret C, Enrico J: Lactate in acute circulatory failure. In Bossart H, Perret C (editors): *Lactate in acute conditions,* New York, 1979, S Karger.
33. Woll PJ, Record CO: Lactate elimination in man: effects of lactate concentration and hepatic dysfunction, *Eur J Clin Invest* 9:397-404, 1979.
34. Owen OE, et al: Hepatic, gut and renal substrate flux rates in patients with hepatic cirrhosis, *J Clin Invest* 68:240-252, 1981.
35. Kruse JA, Zaidi SA, Carlson RW: Significance of blood lactate levels in critically ill patients with liver disease, *Am J Med* 83:77-82, 1987.
36. Falk JL, et al: Delayed lactate clearance in patients surviving circulatory shock, *Acute Care* 11:212-215, 1985.
37. Parker MM, et al: Serial cardiovascular variables in survivors and nonsurvivors of human septic shock: heart rate as an early predictor of prognosis, *Crit Care Med* 15:923-929, 1987.
38. Vincent JL, et al: Serial lactate determinations during circulatory shock, *Crit Care Med* 11:449-451, 1983.
39. Kruse JA, Carlson RW: Lactate metabolism, *Crit Care Clin* 3:725-746, 1987.
40. Orringer CE, et al: Natural history of lactic acidosis after grand-mal seizures: a model for the study of an anion-gap acidosis not associated with hyperkalemia, *N Engl J Med* 297:796-799, 1977.
41. Bihari D: Multiple organ failure: role of tissue hypoxia. In Bihari D, Cerra F (editors): *Multiple organ failure,* Fullerton, CA, 1989, Society of Critical Care Medicine.
42. Haglund U, Fiddian-Green RS: Assessment of adequate tissue oxygenation in shock and critical illness: oxygen transport in sepsis, *Intensive Care Med* 15:475-477, 1989.
43. Fiddian-Green RS, Baker S: Predictive value of the stomach wall pH for complications after cardiac operations: comparison with other monitoring, *Crit Care Med* 15:153-156, 1987.
44. Fiddian-Green RS: Should measurements of tissue pH and PO_2 be included in the routine monitoring of intensive care unit patients? *Crit Care Med* 19:141-143, 1991.
45. Davis JW, et al: Base deficit as a guide to volume resuscitation, *J Trauma* 28:1464-1467, 1988.
46. Siegel JH, et al: Early physiologic predictors of injury severity and death in blunt multiple trauma, *Arch Surg* 125:498-508, 1990.
47. Davis JW, Shackford SR, Holbrook TL: Base deficit as a sensitive indicator of compensated shock and tissue oxygen utilization, *Surg Gynecol Obstet* 173:473-476, 1991.
48. Rutherford EJ, et al: Base deficit stratifies mortality and determines therapy, *J Trauma* 33: 417-423, 1992.
49. Scorpio RJ, et al: Blunt trauma during pregnancy: factors effecting fetal outcome, *J Trauma* 32:213-216, 1992.
50. Scalea TM, et al: Central venous blood oxygen saturation: an early, accurate measurement of volume during hemorrhage, *J Trauma* 28:725-732, 1988.
51. Rady MY, et al: Continuous central venous oximetry index in the emergency department: use in the evaluation of clinical shock, *Am J Emerg Med* 10:538-541, 1992.
52. Moon R, Camporesi E: Respiratory monitoring. In Miller R (editor): *Anesthesia*, ed 3, New York, 1990, Churchill Livingstone.
53. Falk JL, Rackow EC, Weil MH: End-tidal carbon dioxide concentration during cardiopulmonary resuscitation, *N Engl J Med* 318:607-611, 1988.
54. Tang W, et al: $ETCO_2$ as a hemodynamic determinant of hemorrhagic shock in the rat, (abstr) *Chest* 100(suppl):134, 1991.
55. Sun S, et al: End-tidal PCO_2 and arterial PCO_2 indicate severity of perfusion failure during anaphylactic shock, *Clin Res* 39: 422-A, 1991.
56. Ornato JP, Garnett AR, Glauser FL: Relationship between cardiac output and the end-tidal carbon dioxide tension, *Ann Emerg Med* 19:1104-1106, 1990.
57. Gudipati CV, et al: Expired carbon dioxide: a noninvasive monitor of cardiopulmonary resuscitation, *Circulation* 77:234-239, 1988.
58. Weil MH, et al: Cardiac output and end-tidal carbon dioxide, *Crit Care Med* 13:907-909, 1985.
59. Johnson BA, Weil MH: Redefining ischemia due to circulatory failure as dual defects of oxygen deficits and of carbon dioxide excesses, *Crit Care Med* 19:1432-1438, 1991.
60. Duggal C, et al: Effect of duration of cardiac arrest on coronary perfusion pressure and end-tidal CO_2 as predictors of resuscitability, *Crit Care Med* 18(suppl):222, 1990.
61. Weil M, et al: Difference in acid-base state between venous and arterial blood during cardiopulmonary resuscitation, *N Engl J Med* 315:153-156, 1986.
62. Halmagyi DF, Kennedy M, Varga D: Hidden hypercapnia in hemorrhagic hypotension, *Anesthesiology* 33:594-601, 1970.
63. Benjamin E, et al: Venous hypercarbia in canine hemorrhagic shock, *Crit Care Med* 15:516-518, 1987.
64. Adrogue HJ, et al: Assessing acid-base status in circulatory failure: differences between arterial and central venous blood, *N Engl J Med* 320:1312-1316, 1989.
65. Mecher CE, et al: Venous hypercarbia associated with severe sepsis and systemic hypoperfusion, *Crit Care Med* 18:585-589, 1990.
66. Grundler W, Weil MH, Rackow EC: Arteriovenous carbon dioxide and pH gradients during cardiac arrest, *Circulation* 74:1071-1074, 1986.
67. Sato Y, Weil MH, Tang W: Tissue hypercarbic acidosis as marker of acute circulatory failure, *Chest* 114: 263-274, 1998.
68. Sato Y, et al: Esophageal PCO_2 as a monitor of perfusion failure during hemorrhagic shock, *J Appl Physiol* 82:558-562, 1997.
69. Dantzker DR: The gastrointestinal tract: the canary of the body? *JAMA* 270:1247-1248, 1993.
70. Gutierrez G: Recent advances in gastric tonometry. In Vincent JL (editor): *Yearbook of intensive care and emergency medicine,* New York, 1994, Springer-Verlag.
71. Alexander CM, Teller LE, Gross JB: Principles of pulse oximetry: theoretical and practical considerations, *Anesth Analg* 68: 368-376, 1989.
72. Scott B, Falk JL: *The appropriate utilization of pulse oximetry in cost effective diagnostic testing in emergency medicine,* Dallas, 1994, American College of Emergency Physicians.

Management of Pain and Anxiety in the Severely Injured Patient

10

JAMES B. JONES AND WILLIAM H. CORDELL

Throughout human history, pain and trauma have been inseparable. One can only imagine the horrible pain caused by swords, spears, arrows, musket balls, and scalpels, before the advent of modern analgesia and anesthesia. Yet, although modern medicine has vastly improved care, injured patients often receive little or no analgesia in the emergency department (ED).

Pain, in general, is under-treated. Furthermore there are certain types of situations, severe, multiple-system trauma being a prime example, where pain control is particularly difficult. The reasons for "oligoanalgesia" are numerous and include the inherently subjective nature of pain and our fear, justified or not, of "missing something." But why would pain control be inadequate in obviously wounded patients, many of whom are screaming and thrashing in agony? Studies show that pain control is rarely a priority in acute trauma management and is especially neglected in children, elderly, and non-English-speaking patients. Even after severely injured patients have been assessed and stabilized they receive little or no pain medications. Thoracostomy tubes and femoral traction are often performed with little or no analgesia. As many as 40% to 60% of patients with long-bone fractures may never receive pain medication in the ED, and the few that do receive too little too late.[1,2,3]

Oligoanalgesia may simply be a reflection of the healthcare profession's general under-treatment of pain, or it may reflect a tacit belief on the part of clinicians that pain is something to be endured. Of course, it is relatively easy to be stoic regarding *someone else's* pain. Compounding the problem is the relative paucity of studies regarding analgesia in severely injured patients in the ED or prehospital phase of care. Therefore much of our approach to pain is extrapolated from experience in the military, surgical anesthesia, post-surgical care, and intensive care settings.

There are important reasons for adequately controlling pain. First, health care is both a technical and an ethical enterprise. "The ethical obligation to manage pain and relieve the patient's suffering is at the core of a healthcare professional's commitment."[1] Second, additional benefits–early mobilization, shorter hospital stay, and reduced costs–may be realized when pain is adequately treated or preempted in severely injured patients.

Pain control in trauma must be individualized. Consider the following two victims. The first is an 18-year-old male with an isolated gunshot wound to the extremity with stable vital signs. The second is a 58-year-old female extricated from a motor vehicle crash (MVC). She presents to the ED with blunt head trauma, multiple rib fractures, and a pneumothorax with an initial blood pressure of 100/60 mmHg. Both patients are awake and screaming in pain. Each will require a different approach to pain control.

This chapter will focus on the initial ED management of pain in victims of trauma. We review available literature, propose a management approach, and point to controversies. Although our focus is the severely injured patient with multiple-system trauma, many of the principles also apply to single-system injuries and "minor trauma." Our approach is listed in Box 10-1.

TERMINOLOGY OF PAIN AND PAIN MANAGEMENT

The terminology and mechanisms underlying the perception of pain have important implications in pain control. Common definitions are listed in Table 10-1.

Pain is an unpleasant sensory and emotional experience arising from actual or potential tissue damage.[8] It is a unique, highly subjective, multidimensional experience encompassing many sensory and affective

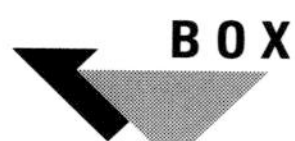

BOX 10-1

Top 10 Principles of Pain Control in Severely Injured Patients

1. **INTEGRATE ANALGESIA INTO PATIENT EVALUATION AND MANAGEMENT.**
   Pain management and anxiety control should be incorporated into trauma resuscitation and care protocols. Pain control requires a skilled approach that merges pharmacologic and non-pharmacologic interventions.

2. **RECOGNIZE AND TREAT COGNITIVE ASPECTS OF PAIN.**
   Pain involves both a physical stimulus, neuroanatomical process, and an emotional reaction. Anxiety frequently accompanies and exacerbates pain in the severely injured patient and must be addressed.

3. **USE SCALES TO MEASURE CHANGES IN PAIN.**
   Pain is the ultimate subjective complaint. Vital signs, physical examination, and appearance of wounds are unreliable in predicting pain. Ghastly looking injuries may be well tolerated in some, whereas other wounds that appear innocuous may be excruciating.[4] Ask patients to rate the intensity of their pain on a 1 to 10 scale "where 10 is the worst pain that can be experienced or imagined." After intervention, have them rescore their pain.

4. **AVOID "OLIGOANALGESIA."**
   Pain in severely injured patients is unlikely to be treated. Concerns for an adverse effect may be real in those with borderline hemodynamic or neurologic status. However, this fear is often unfounded, since medications can be selected and titrated to effect. Physicians also worry that medications will obscure an important finding. Patients should be examined before the administration of analgesics. In the era of the computed tomography (CT) scan, objective tests may be more accurate than physical examination. Under-treatment also occurs because of the inability to objectively measure pain, engrained practice habits, and a relative paucity of research.

5. **BEWARE OF THE "QUIET ONES."**
   Just as the "squeaky wheel get the oil," vocal, agitated patients are seen and treated most quickly. Quiet or unresponsive patients, who cannot "state their case," are treated less urgently. Serious injury, speech or hearing impairment, language barrier, cognitive disorders, and age all impair the treatment of pain.

6. **INDIVIDUALIZE PAIN CONTROL.**
   An individual's response to pain depends on the mechanism, location, and severity of injury. Other factors include the patient's psychological makeup, age, sex, and ethnic background. The agent, dose, and route must be tailored to the individual and titrated to both control pain and minimize side effects.

7. **ANTICIPATE RATHER THAN REACT.**
   Because pain is dynamic, prevention is better than treatment. Without treatment, sensory input from injured tissue reaches spinal cord neurons and intensifies subsequent response.[5] Because "pain begets pain," discomfort is best treated early.[6] For severe pain, analgesics should be administered regularly, continuously, or self-administered rather than on an as-needed basis.

8. **PUT THE PATIENT IN CHARGE.**
   When possible, empower patients to control their own pain, which can be accomplished by Patient Controlled Analgesia (PCA) pumps. This autonomy decreases analgesic needs and improves patient satisfaction. These pumps should find a growing use in emergency departments.

9. **COMBINE THERAPY.**
   Pain control should combine pharmacologic and nonpharmacologic interventions. Pharmacologic options include intravenous opioids, intravenous ketorolac, nerve blocks, or combinations of these. Nonpharmacologic interventions include reassurance, splinting, ice packs, limb elevation, and moving trauma victims off spine boards.

10. **USE A MULTIDISCIPLINARY, TEAM APPROACH.**
    Trauma resuscitation involves a protocol-driven team approach.[7] This same algorithm-driven, team approach lends itself to the management of pain. Pain scales may be included in the trauma flow sheet. Nursing protocols may include routine pain assessment. Care of the trauma patient is a continuum that begins in the prehospital phase and moves to the ED, operating suite, and critical care unit. Treatments started in the early phase must be compatible and synergistic with treatment "downstream."

TABLE 10-1
Common Terminology of Pain and Pain Management

Term	Definition
Pain	An unpleasant sensory and emotional experience arising from actual or potential tissue damage or described in terms of such damage.[8]
Anxiety	Often the primary anticipatory emotion to acute pain. Anxiety will increase pain and physiologic arousal such as heart rate.[12] Reduction of anxiety is termed *anxiolysis* and such agents are called *anxiolytics*.
Sedation	The act or process of calming someone or allaying their activity or excitement. *Sedatives* decrease anxiety, moderate excitement, and calm the recipient.[15]
Hypnosis	A state of altered consciousness induced by suggestion or by pharmacologic agents. *Hypnotics* induce drowsiness and facilitate sleep.[16]
Amnesia	The loss of memory. Drugs that induce amnesia are termed *amnestics*.
Nociception	A response to a noxious stimulus. Because the majority of research on pain is performed on animals, the term *nociception* was proposed for use in studies of pain.[10]
Nociceptors	Afferent receptors detecting and signaling noxious stimuli.[10] Peripheral, nonencapsulated sensory pain fibers that respond selectively to a stimulus that directly damages or threatens to damage tissue and transmit the impulse generated to the central nervous system.
Sensitization	A change in the nociceptor sensitivity and the recruitment of the "sleeping nociceptors."
Hypersensitization	Recruitment of nerve fibers not initially involved in the transmission of the pain signal that results from a prolonged painful stimuli. This phenomenon generally leads to an exaggerated pain response (hyperalgesia).
Hyperalgesia[17]	An altered state of sensibility in which the intensity of pain sensation induced by noxious stimuli is greatly increased. *Primary hyperalgesia* becomes evident within minutes of the injury and is characterized by increased sensitivity to both heat and mechanical stimuli. *Secondary hyperalgesia* has delayed onset and different character in that sensitivity is increased only in response to thermal stimuli.
Allodynia[17]	Refers to a condition in which ordinarily nonnoxious stimulation is perceived as being exquisitely painful.

components.[9] Because the emotional component of the experience is included in the definition, the experience of pain can be studied directly only in humans.[10] *Anxiety* and pain are closely related and often confused. Both can cause an increase in heart and respiratory rate, blood pressure, peripheral vasoconstriction, muscle tension, and pupillary diameter. Both lead to a decrease in gastric motility and blood flow, impaired concentration, and feelings of helplessness and dread.[11] Humans in an acute crisis such as surgery and severe trauma are faced with uncertainty and fear.[12] Warfield and Stein[13] wrote, "Of the myriad of psychologic influences on the perception of pain, anxiety and depression are paramount: They not only greatly intensify suffering but are often easily treatable."

Analgesia is an absence of pain despite a stimulus that is normally hurtful. *Pain relief* and *pain control* occur on a continuum. To control pain implies a lessening of discomfort, whereas pain relief implies obliteration of the suffering. An *analgesic* is an agent that reduces pain. It may be a pharmacologic agent such as an opiate, opioid, or a nonsteroidal, antiinflammatory drug. Nonpharmacologic methods include ice, elevation, splinting, transcutaneous electrical nerve stimulation (TENS), or acupuncture.

Pain can be treated at several sites. These sites include the peripheral terminal of the nociceptive afferent nerve, the central terminal of the primary afferent located within the dorsal horn of the spinal cord, and supraspinal sites. *Peripherally acting agents* modulate the transmission of the painful stimulus to the central nervous system (CNS) by decreasing the activation of primary afferent nerve fibers (nociceptors). This decreases painful input to the spinal cord. Mediators of peripheral nociceptive transmission include bradykinins, prostaglandins, leukotrienes, and substance P.[14] Nonsteroidal antiinflammatory drugs (NSAIDs), for example, modulate pain by inhibiting prostaglandin synthesis. *Centrally acting analgesics*, of which morphine and meperidine are examples, modulate pain in the spinal cord or brain. Peripherally acting agents combined with centrally acting agents provide *balanced analgesia*.

Much confusion exists regarding the terms *opioid*, *opiate*, and *narcotic*. Strictly speaking, an *opiate* is a compound that contains, or is derived from, opium, a milky exudate from the unripened seeds of the poppy plant, ***Papaver somniferum***. Examples of opiates include morphine and codeine. The term *opioid* initially referred to synthetic drugs, not derived from opium, but with morphinelike actions. Examples of opioids include fentanyl and meperidine. Today, the term *opioid* refers to all drugs, natural or synthetic, with morphinelike actions. The term *narcotic*, derived from the Greek word for "stupor," is generally applied to agents that produce narcosis, an insensibility, or stupor. This term is medically obsolete, but will not likely disappear from colloquial use.

BALANCING ACT OF ANALGESIA

Mackersie and Karagianes[18] wrote, "The initial therapeutic goals in the management of the injured patient include (1) preservation of life, (2) preservation of limb, (3) preservation of function, (4) avoidance of complications, and (5) avoidance of diagnostic delay. However, the treatment of discomfort and anxiety is an additional and desirable goal in the management of these patients. The pharmacologic interventions used to accomplish these goals often fall at cross purposes, particularly in the early hospital course, with the therapeutic goals of the trauma surgeon." Because of the high acuity of multiple-trauma patients and the resulting therapeutic "tempo," treatment of pain is given low priority and is frequently overlooked. Pain control in the severely injured is important for many reasons. The first is as part of the compassionate, humanistic approach to patients in pain. The second is to prevent the unexpected, harmful consequences of untreated pain. Such deleterious consequences include increased blood pressure and heart rate, peripheral vasoconstriction, splinting, shallow respirations, decreased cough, and immobility. These effects may lead to serious respiratory complications, including atelectasis and pneumonia.[4] Pain also discourages activity, promoting deep venous thrombosis and deconditioning.[19]

Theoretically, the treatment of pain may have important advantages in diagnosis. Severe pain in one body area may distract the patient (and physician) and prevent recognition of other injuries. Studies show that pain control can facilitate the examination of patients with atraumatic abdominal pain by reducing patient anxiety and relaxing the abdominal musculature.[20-23] However, this phenomenon is not well studied in the trauma victim.

Pathophysiologically, tissue injury and concomitant pain evoke a metabolic response, essential to the maintenance of homeostasis.[14] Pain may also trigger a behavioral response to withdraw from an offending agent. However, once the process of injury has been identified and halted, further pain serves no protective effect. It may only increase anxiety and the stress response, taxing physiologic reserves.

Untreated pain has other deleterious consequences. Release of peripheral mediators such as substance P and serotonin result in marked inflammatory changes that in turn release more inflammatory mediators. A vicious cycle ensues where additional nociceptors immediately adjacent to the injured site are sensitized, resulting in hyperalgesia. Once initiated, these changes may be difficult to control.[14] Preemptive analgesia prevents the activation of peripheral nociceptors and blocks the development of hyperalgesia.

During the resuscitation of severely injured patients, clinicians must balance the need for pain control with other physiologic needs of the patient. These include the ability to monitor the patient's neurologic status and maintain respirations, heart rate, and blood pressure. Many factors must be weighed, including the patient's neurologic and hemodynamic status, his or her rating of pain intensity, the location and extent of injury, chronic underlying illness, and recent consumption of alcohol and drugs. Analgesic regimens in the ED should also be compatible and synergistic with anesthetic agents that will be administered in the operating suite and with analgesic regimens administered in the intensive care unit (ICU).

The emergency physician must choose agents and dosages that will not significantly impair monitoring of the patient, his or her hemodynamic status, or coagulation (Box 10-2). Some argue that narcotic analgesics should not be given to trauma victims for fear of obscuring abdominal tenderness. A convincing counter-argument is that patients in great distress from a femur fracture are likely to have an unreliable abdominal examination. In addition, diagnosis in trauma is not limited to physical findings. Although judicious use of narcotics is unlikely to affect abdominal tenderness, no amount of morphine will sway the results of the abdominal CT.

This balancing act is not unique to the ED. Wheeler[19] noted that the art of pain control is difficult in the ICU setting where patient comfort is balanced against the numerous adverse drug effects. Wheeler wrote, "Unfortunately, concerns over safety often cause nurses and physicians to err on the side of insufficient relief of patient discomfort." He further noted that while patient comfort is a laudable goal, excessive sedation or analgesic use can produce numerous complications. Excessive sedation causes hypotension, gastrointestinal hypomotility, and masks intercurrent illnesses. Pharmacologic obtundation also reduces tidal volume, vital capacity, minute ventilation, and inhibits forceful coughing.

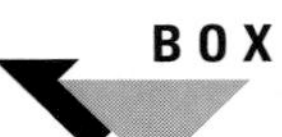

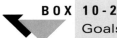

BOX 10-2

Goals of Pain Control Regimens in Severely Injured Patients

THESE REGIMENS *SHOULD* PROVIDE APPROPRIATE SEDATION AND PAIN CONTROL:

- As part of compassionate care
- To prevent deleterious physiologic consequences
- To facilitate a history and physical examination
- During procedures (such as thoracostomy tube placement or dislocation/fracture reduction)
- During rapid sequence intubation
- During traction
- During transport
- To encourage early mobilization (to help prevent deep venous thrombosis and promote muscle tone)
- To encourage deep breathing
- To be compatible or synergistic with agents administered during prehospital care and in the operating room and intensive care unit
- To be as physician and nurse labor-sparing as possible

THESE REGIMENS *SHOULD NOT*:

- Significantly impair neurologic status monitoring
- Impair obtaining a history or performing a physical examination
- Compromise hemodynamic status
- Compromise ventilation
- Impair coagulation
- Produce adverse events

The challenge is equilibrium—adequately controlling pain without causing harm. Relieve anxiety while still permitting serial examinations. Addressing the need for analgesia in severely injured patients, Cantees and Yealy[6] recommended that pharmacologic analgesic agents be given during resuscitation, unless one of three conditions exists: hemodynamic instability, respiratory depression, or profound sedation or coma.

INTEGRATING PAIN CONTROL INTO THE CARE OF THE SEVERELY INJURED PATIENT

Pain control must be integrated into a care process. It must be compatible with evaluation of injuries and, in particular, the detection of occult bleeding. Pain control must account for patient stability and mechanism of injury.

Reassure the Patient

Victims of severe trauma are typically in pain and fearful of dying. They are rushed into a strange environment where crowds of masked people assail them with probing fingers, tubes, and needles. One of the simplest and frequently overlooked components of pain management is reassurance. Physicians and nurses should introduce themselves and inform their patient about what is happening.

Introductions can include reassuring statements such as "We are members of the trauma team and have taken care of thousands of people who have been injured." Patients should be kept informed about what is about to happen: "Other team members will be checking you over. We're going to have to put some IV lines in your arm and a tube into your bladder." The issue of pain control should be addressed: "As we check you over, we're going to give you some pain medicine and ask you if your pain is getting better." The promise of pain relief will greatly increase patient cooperation and decrease their anxiety.

Assess and Monitor the Intensity of Pain

Along with blood pressure, heart rate, respiratory rate, temperature, oxygen saturation, and Glasgow Coma Scale score, the intensity of pain should be considered a vital sign. Pain intensity and relief must be constantly reassessed. Allow the patient to describe his or her pain using a numerical scale, then assess the success or failure of analgesia by rescoring the pain. Because victims of trauma undergoing resuscitation are typically too ill or injured to write, the pain intensity scale is usually verbal. Ask, "On a scale of zero to ten, ten being the worst pain you've ever had and zero being no pain, how bad is your pain right now?" Written pain scales may be employed to assess pain intensity in the intubated, but awake, patient. For children, a visual scale using a happy face versus a crying face may be used.

Consider the Differential Diagnosis of Agitation

The differential diagnosis of agitation is presented in Box 10-3. Agitation or lack of patient cooperation should not be regarded as a "sedative deficiency."[19] When agitation is present, consider correctable causes. First and foremost, CNS hypoxia should be assessed and corrected. Confirm endotracheal tube patency and position, check supplemental oxygen flow, measure oxygen saturation, and verify ventilator couplings and settings. Other causes of agitation in the severely injured patient include shock, hypoglycemia,

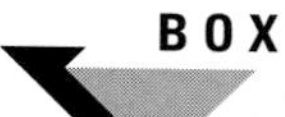

BOX 10-3
Differential Diagnosis of Agitation in the Severely Injured Patient

Shock
CNS hypoxia
Hypoglycemia
Brain injury
Uncontrolled/unidentified pain
Drug ingestion/intoxication

brain injury, uncontrolled pain, alcohol and other drug intoxication, stomach and bladder distention, and "fighting the (endotracheal) tube." Although pain control and sedation are both important, the physician should go through a checklist to search for correctable causes of agitation, and not reflexively sedate.

Control Pain and Anxiety with an Appropriate Pharmacologic Agent or Intervention

Patients in severe pain without hemodynamic instability, respiratory depression, or profound sedation should receive an analgesic agent. There are numerous choices and opinions regarding which agents are most effective and safe. Opioids, particularly morphine and fentanyl, have been the cornerstone of therapy. Other agents include ketorolac and ketamine. Because anxiety and pain coexist, an anxiolytic agent may be employed. No single agent or combination will be effective in all patients or be free of adverse events. The most important agents and routes and methods of administration are discussed in the following section and summarized in Box 10-4.

NONPHARMACOLOGIC INTERVENTIONS

Pain control involves the judicious and skilled use of *both* pharmacologic agents and nonpharmacologic techniques (Box 10-5). Physicians frequently overlook the importance of talking to the trauma victim. We demand, yell, and order, but we rarely provide the reassurance that they so desperately need. Nonpharmacologic interventions include reassurance and communication, early splinting, application of ice, elevation of injured extremities, and prevention of unnecessary movement and shivering. Other nonpharmacologic interventions such as TENS units, music, dimmed lighting, and hypnosis, though important in controlling pain of other origins, are likely to be of limited value in the acute resuscitation of severely injured patients.

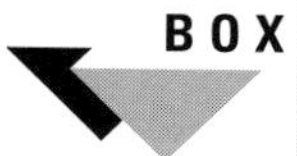

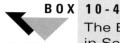

BOX 10-4
The Bottom Line—Pain Control in Severely Injured Patients

GENERAL

- **Early relief.** Pain and anxiety control is important in the early care of severely injured patients.
- **Find a balance.** Analgesia in these patients requires a skillful balancing act. Provide adequate analgesia without worsening the neurologic or hemodynamic status or the ability to examine or monitor the patient.
- **Nonpharmacologic.** Pain control in severely injured patients involves a combination of pharmacologic and nonpharmacologic interventions.
- **Individualize and titrate.** Titrated intravenous analgesia is the best approach to severe pain. Effects are predictable, whereas absorption of oral and intramuscular medications is erratic in the trauma patient.
- **Procedures.** "Routine" procedures such as intravenous and central line insertion, bladder catheterization, and nasogastric tube placement may be very painful to anxious, severely injured patients.
- **Reassess.** Pain control must be monitored as a vital sign.

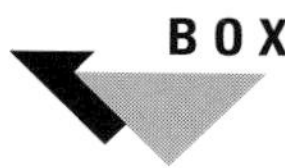

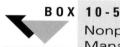

BOX 10-5
Nonpharmacologic Management of Pain

Reassurance and communication
Touch
Elevation
Ice, cold compresses
Early removal of patients from spine boards
Splinting
Prevention of shivering
Transcutaneous electrical nerve stimulation (TENS)
Acupuncture/acupressure

One important yet frequently overlooked method of pain control is the removal of the patient from rigid spine boards as soon as safe and practical. Several studies have associated spine boards with significant patient discomfort and the development of occipital pressure ulcers.[24-27] Accident victims often lie strapped to the hard, flat, unyielding surface of a spine board, unable to turn or roll, for extended periods. Severely injured patients transferred from other facilities may lie on the spine board for hours, resulting in pain and placing them at risk for developing decubitus ulcers.

By the time patients on spine boards are examined, many may have neck and back pain *from* the prolonged immobilization. A spinal clearance policy may reduce the number of spinal films needed in the ED. If physicians are called to the ambulance entrance to evaluate patients on backboards, they may clinically clear their spines and remove the board even before the patient is registered.

OPIOIDS

Fentanyl. Fentanyl, a synthetic opioid, is considered an agent of choice for pain relief during resuscitation.[5] Fentanyl is 80 times more potent than morphine and is dosed in micrograms rather than milligrams. The major advantage of fentanyl in the trauma patient is the lack of histamine-related cardiovascular changes, even after large doses. It has a rapid onset and relatively short duration of action.

Dosing. Fentanyl is titrated intravenously by administering an initial dose of 0.25 to 0.5 μg/kg (50 to 100 μg for adults). This dose can be repeated every 5 to 10 minutes based on reduction of pain intensity, level of alertness, and hemodynamic status.

Adverse Events and Precautions. Fentanyl is primarily active at the μ receptor within the CNS, giving it a more favorable side effect profile than other opioids. Nevertheless, as with all opioids, hypotension, ventilatory depression, and pronounced sedation may occur. Chest wall rigidity following fentanyl administration has been described, but mostly occurs with higher doses (>8 μg/kg).

Morphine. Morphine (MSO_4) was isolated from opium by Sertürner in 1806 and has been widely used to treat pain including traumatic injuries and postsurgical pain.

Dosing. Like fentanyl, morphine is typically administered by IV titration to severely injured patients. One such titration regimen is the administration of a 5 mg loading dose IV followed by 2 to 5 mg increments every 10 minutes in adult patients.

Adverse Events and Precautions. The most notable and concerning side effect associated with the use of MSO_4 in the trauma patient is sedation. Other effects include change in mood and mental clouding. Although these effects are dose-related, it becomes difficult to conduct serial neurologic examinations in the head-injured patient, or extremity examinations in a person whose injury may place him or her at risk for compartment syndrome. Respiratory depression and hypotension are the most serious adverse events when MSO_4 or other opioids are administered to severely injured patients. Morphine directly depresses the central respiratory centers and alters the airway protective measures, which may lead to aspiration. Hypotension, although not considered significant in the recumbent patient, results from direct vasodilatation of the peripheral venous system, leading to a reduced peripheral resistance and an inhibition of the baroreceptor reflexes. This relative hypotension can usually be overcome with fluid administration. MSO_4 and other opioids decrease the secretion of gastric and other digestive enzymes, as well as decreasing peristalsis.

Meperidine. Meperidine is a synthetic analgesic introduced by Eisleb and Schaumann in 1939. Meperidine offers no advantage over morphine and may cause neuromuscular excitability through the accumulation of the metabolite normeperidine. We do not recommend its use in the severely injured patients.

Methods and Routes of Opioid Administration

Intravenous Titration. IV titration is the preferred route of opioid administration for treatment of severe pain. Titration is the technique of administering a loading dose of medication followed by increments until either the desired effect is achieved or clinically significant side effects occur. Such an approach "individualizes" dosing, affords better monitoring, and avoids erratic drug absorption associated with the intramuscular route. Titration of fentanyl and morphine are covered in the previous discussion. These dosing schedules are arbitrary, since an optimal titration regimen has not been well defined. In general, these agents should be titrated to the point of comfort and not necessarily total pain ablation. In the uncommon event hypotension or respiratory depression occur, further incremental doses may be withheld and naloxone and/or IV fluids administered.

Patients who are habituated to narcotics may require many times the suggested dosage for pain control. This increased dosage is particularly true of patients on methadone.

PCA Pumps. Although PCA pumps allow patients to self-titrate opioids and are frequently utilized postsurgery and in hospitalized patients, they are infrequently used in the ED. Barriers to their use include equipment cost and maintenance, lack of familiarity, and pharmacy charges for filling the syringes. Patients given the opportunity to self-administer small opioid doses maintain plasma drug concentrations above that required for analgesia while incurring fewer side effects. Moreover, an enhanced sense of personal control may reduce anxiety and improve analgesia.[28]

Balanced Analgesia. The combination of multiple analgesics is termed *multimodal* or *balanced analgesia*. In practice, this term often means the simultaneous administration of two classes of drugs such as an opioid plus an NSAID. Kehlet and Dahl[29] wrote, "The rationale for this strategy is achievement of sufficient analgesia due to additive or synergistic effects between different analgesics, with concomitant reduction of side effects, due to resulting lower doses of analgesics and differences in side-effect profiles." In discussing the intensive care setting, Wheeler[19] noted that a balanced, multidrug approach maximizes patient comfort and minimizes side effects.

Intraspinal Opioids. The administration of opioids through spinal microcatheters provides effective analgesia and is particularly useful in post-surgical and intensive care phases of care. Because the technique is usually performed by an anesthesiologist, its use in most EDs during trauma resuscitation is limited. It is particularly useful in patients with multiple rib fractures.

Continuous IV Infusion. Continuous IV infusion of analgesics produces better analgesia, but carries the potential risk of accidental overdosage. It requires strict medical supervision.[29] Continuous subcutaneous infusion of MSO_4 has also been studied.[30]

On-Demand and Intermittent Dosing. The traditional approach to analgesia in trauma has been to administer an opioid followed by on-demand (PRN) parenteral injections of opioids. Intermittent dosing regimens may result in insufficient analgesia between doses. The continued pain serves to increase anxiety and stress response. Intermittent dosing is a suboptimal approach for controlling pain in severely injured patients.

Subcutaneous and Intramuscular. Occult shock or poor peripheral profusion results in erratic, unpredictable absorption of opioids given by the subcutaneous or intramuscular routes. In 1943 Beecher[31] reported delayed MSO_4 poisoning in soldiers wounded in Italy in World War II. He attributed this outcome to poor absorption of repeated subcutaneous doses of MSO_4 in wounded men who were wet and chilled or had circulatory impairment. On receiving fluids and being rewarmed, many developed profound respiratory depression from the "seriously rapid absorption of all the morphine injected."

NONOPIOID AGENTS

Ketorolac Tromethamine. In 1989 ketorolac became the first NSAID in the United States to be approved for parenteral use as an analgesic. The IM and IV formulations are identical.

Dosing. In 1995 the manufacturer's prescribing recommendations were changed to an IV dose of 30 mg and IM dose of 60 mg for single-dose injections, and 30 mg for both IV and IM administration of multiple doses. The maximum daily dose must not exceed 120 mg.

Adverse Events and Precautions. Complications most commonly associated with NSAIDs include gastrointestinal upset, bleeding, and renal failure. Results from clinical studies, as well as two epidemiologic surveillance studies show that these complications are relatively uncommon, especially used either as a single dose or administered in recommended doses for less than 5 days.[32,33] Although ketorolac is extensively used preoperatively, intraoperatively, and post-operatively, questions and concerns remain regarding its use in severely injured patients with respect to its effect on platelets. Platelet inhibition from ketorolac tromethamine is a reversible process, unlike the permanent platelet damage that results from aspirin.

Ketamine. Ketamine hydrochloride, a derivative of phencyclidine, is commonly used as a dissociative anesthetic. Its use induces a state of sedation, immobility, amnesia, and marked analgesia. It is often used as an IM injection for procedural sedation in children. Its use in adults is limited by the high incidence of emergence reactions on awakening.

Ketamine Subcutaneous Infusion. Gurnani and colleagues[34] conducted a study in India that compared low-dose ketamine by subcutaneous infusion to intermittent morphine IV in 40 adults who had acute musculoskeletal trauma not requiring immediate surgery.[34] Subjects receiving ketamine had a loading dose of 0.25 mg/kg IV followed by 0.1 mg/kg/hr subcutaneous infusion. The infusion was administered through a 26-gauge cannula placed subcutaneously, preferably on the anterior abdominal wall, and connected via an extension tube (capacity 3.6 ml) to a 20 ml syringe mounted on a syringe pump. The MSO_4 dosing was 0.1 mg/kg IV every 4 hours. Those experiencing inadequate analgesia received morphine 0.3 mg IV only on patient demand. The design was randomized and double-blinded, used a visual analog scale (VAS) scale to assess pain, and a 4-point drowsiness scale to assess sedation. Pain relief was significantly better with the ketamine infusion than with the intermittent IV MSO_4. Subjects receiving ketamine were more awake and alert and none required rescue analgesia. Peak expiratory flow rate improved better with the ketamine infusion. These patients could be more easily mobilized for traction and splinting compared with control subjects. Seven subjects in the MSO_4 group experienced nausea and vomiting while two in the ketamine groups reported pleasant dreams. One patient in the MSO_4 group had to be catheterized for urinary retention.

Adverse Events and Precautions. Ketamine has the potential to increase intracranial pressure and should be avoided in patients with head injuries. There is also some concern about increased eye movement and intraocular pressures when it is administered to patients with ocular trauma, particularly penetrating eye injuries. Laryngospasm may also occur with ketamine use but generally can be managed with positive pressure ventilatory support.

ANXIOLYTICS

Wheeler[19] noted that the ICU is an extremely stressful environment where anxiety is prevalent, pain frequent, and sleep almost impossible. Relief of pain is often neglected while efforts are focused on life-threatening concerns. However, reassurance and titration of benzodiazepines provide safe anxiolysis. Midazolam is used where short duration is desirable, whereas lorazepam has longer effects. Dosages are listed in Box 10-6.

PROCEDURAL SEDATION

Combinations of pharmacologic analgesics, sedatives, and anxiolytics should be used during procedures including joint reduction, long-bone fracture splinting, and thoracostomy tube insertion. The goal is to produce analgesia, amnesia, and light sedation, usually of brief duration, without inducing deep sedation or compromise of airway protective reflexes, ventilation, or hemodynamic status. Fentanyl and midazolam administered by IV titration is a commonly used combination in the ED. Other options include nitrous oxide, propofol, etomidate, and ketamine. Follow the Joint Commission guidelines regarding procedural sedation and the need for pulse oximetry and cardiac monitoring.

Nitrous Oxide. Nitrous oxide is a colorless, odorless gas that produces analgesia in a dose-dependent fashion by affecting cellular membranes within the CNS. It provides amnesia at concentrations of 60%. The Nitronox machine available in most EDs delivers a 50-50 nitrogen-oxygen mixture. Not all EDs have access to necessary equipment and scavenger devices. The patient should be given 100% oxygen in the recovery phase to prevent secondary hypoxia. The safest method of using nitrous oxide is self-administration. Allow the patient to hold the mask over his or her own face, rather than strapping it on or holding it for them. Self-administered nitrous has a fail-safe mechanism that prevents overdose. If patients fall asleep, they drop the mask and stop breathing the agent.

Adverse Events and Precautions. Nitrous oxide is contraindicated in patients with a pneumothorax because of gas expansion in the pleural space. It is also contraindicated in pregnant patients because of its potential teratogenic effects. Other contraindications include pneumocephalus and COPD.

Propofol. The use of propofol in the ED is less common than those agents already discussed. It is classified as a general anesthetic and is used mainly in the operating suite. Anecdotal experience in the ED is confined to minor painful procedures such as suturing and fracture reductions. It can produce anesthesia and recovery as rapidly as thiopental.

Dosing. 2 mg/kg IV followed by a maintenance infusion of 0.1 to 0.2 mg/kg/minute IV infusion.

Adverse Events and Precautions. Because propofol may result in decreased cerebral blood flow, it should not be used in patients with increased intracranial pressure. Propofol may produce a 30% reduction in systemic arterial pressure as a result of vasodilation. Rapid infusion or high dosage produces apnea.

Etomidate. Etomidate is an ultrashort-acting nonbarbiturate hypnotic agent that does not have analgesic properties. Similar to propofol, it provides anesthesia with rapid onset and recovery.

Dosing. 0.3 mg/kg IV bolus induces sleep for 3 to 5 minutes. It has a relatively short initial half-life of 2 to 4 minutes, but a secondary half-life of up to 4 hours, making serial examinations on patients with significant head trauma difficult.

Adverse Events and Precautions. Etomidate has a relatively safe side-effect profile. Cardiovascular and respiratory depression usually do not occur. Involuntary movements may occur. The effect of even a single dose of etomidate has been shown to inhibit the adrenal gland and has resulted in increased mortality when used for prolonged sedation in the ICU setting. However, these are unlikely to be of clinical significance in emergency practice. Like propofol, it can produce apnea or hypoventilation.

REGIONAL ANESTHESIA

Transmission of painful stimuli to the CNS can be blocked by proper use of regional anesthesia.

Intercostal nerve block is an effective but underutilized form of regional anesthesia that is capable of controlling pain associated with rib fractures, chest wall injuries, and flail chest.[37] The neurovascular bundle is approached below the rib, and the nerve anesthetized with a long-acting agent such as bupivacaine. Complications include pneumothorax, hypotension, and systemic toxicity from absorbed anesthetic. Disadvantages include the necessity for multiple and repeated blocks. Femoral nerve block may be useful in controlling pain originating from femoral shaft fractures and injuries of the anterior thigh, knee, and medial aspect of the leg. The nerve is approached just lateral to the femoral artery at the inguinal ligament. Dilworth and MacKellar[38] reported pain control in 245 children with fractured femurs using femoral nerve blocks. A dose of 5 to 7 cc of bupivacaine may give hours of pain relief. This block is safe and effective even in the hands of junior staff.[39]

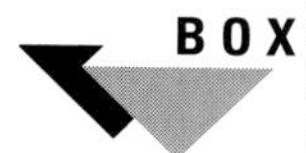

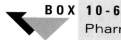

BOX 10-6

Pharmacologic Management of Pain

OPIOIDS

Fentanyl

Administration: IV titration.

Dose: 1 to 2 μg/kg (50 to 100 μg for adults) → repeat every 5 to 10 minutes based on pain intensity, level of alertness, and hemodynamic status.

Comment: Short-acting, titratable, potent, fewer hemodynamic effects than morphine. May cause hemodynamic, ventilatory, or cognitive impairment. Chest rigidity is rare in this dose range.

Morphine

Administration: IV titration.

Dose (adult): 2 to 5 mg q 5 minutes up to pain relief. Patients with severe burns may require 30 mg or more in the first hour.

Comment: Although the gold standard treatment for severe pain control, morphine is associated with more hemodynamic effects than fentanyl and is best reserved for the well-resuscitated patient.

Codeine

Administration: IV titration.

Dose (adult): 5 to 10 mg every 5 minutes up to 30 to 60 mg every 2 to 3 hours.

Comment: Some neurosurgeons prefer to use codeine for pain control in severely injured patients because it produces less sedation than other opioids. PO codeine has many side effects, GI intolerance, and is a poor pain reliever.[35]

Hydrocodone, Oxycodone

Administration: PO.

Dose (adult): 5 to 10 mg every 6 hours. Comment: These medications are often combined with acetaminophen. They are more efficacious than codeine products and have fewer adverse side effects.[36]

NONOPIOIDS

Ketorolac

Administration: IM or IV.

Dose (adult): 30 mg IV every 6 hours (regular dosing) for 5 days maximum; reduce dose to 15 mg if age >65 years or weight <50 kg. Initial IM dose may be 60 mg.

Comment: May be used in combination with opioids ("balanced analgesia" regimen). The only NSAID approved for parenteral administration in the United States. Though widely used pre-operatively, intraoperatively, and post-operatively, concerns still exist regarding worsening hemorrhage (including intracranial) in severely injured patients as a result of inhibition of platelet aggregation. NSAIDs should be routine for burn pain, as they decrease inflammatory mediators. Several studies have suggested that while IV Ketorolac is effective, it offers little advantage over oral NSAIDs.

Ketamine

Administration: Constant intravenous, IM, or subcutaneous infusion.

Dose (adult): Loading dose of 0.25 mg/kg IV subcutaneously followed by 0.1 mg/kg/hr.

Comment: The combination intravenous/subcutaneous regimen is based on a single study of patients with acute musculoskeletal trauma not requiring immediate surgery. It provides significantly better analgesia with fewer adverse events than morphine 0.1 mg/kg IV every 4 hours. However, further study and experience are warranted. Use in setting of increased intracranial pressure contraindicated. Higher dosage causes significant mental status changes and may obscure neurologic deterioration.

ANXIOLYSIS AND/OR SEDATION

Midazolam

Administration: IV titration.

Dose: 0.05 to 0.1 mg/kg

Comment: Short-acting. May cause respiratory depression and obtundation, especially when combined with opioids

Lorazepam

Administration: IV.

Dose (adult): 0.5 to 2 mg every 6 to 8 hours.

Neural Blockade

The use of local anesthetics may provide significant pain relief with minimal systemic effects. Longer acting drugs such as bupivacaine are preferred because of their prolonged effect.

Intercostal Nerve Blocks for Rib Fractures

Femoral Nerve Blocks for Femur Fractures

Sciatic Nerve Blocks

Intrapleural Anesthetics

Intrapleural analgesia involves intermittent boluses or constant infusion of anesthetics into the pleural cavity using an intrapleural catheter. If the patient has a chest tube in place, instill bupivacaine into the chest tube after turning off the suction. By rolling the patient, and placing the gurney in both Trendelenburg and reverse Trendelenburg position, the medication will flow to all parts of the hemithorax. A study by Gabram et al[40] reported that patients with unilateral rib fractures from blunt trauma had improved pulmonary function testing compared with systemic opioid administration. Other studies suggest limited efficacy of this intervention.[41]

CONCLUSION

In 1948 Cornelius Medvei[42] wrote, "The conquest of pain remains, after all, the most important task, the main aim, and the crowning—though yet distant—achievement of every medical man, at the bedside, in the operating theatre, in the laboratory, on the battlefields, and wherever else mankind may suffer." At the beginning of the 21st century, no group of patients in pain treated in the ED is more challenging than those who are severely injured. Emergency physicians and nurses must balance the need to rapidly assess and treat potential life threats with the need to control pain. Pain control is essential for both compassionate and physiologic reasons.

Several steps ensure adequate pain control. First, routinely integrate pain and anxiety needs into treatment protocols. Second, research must settle several controversies. Will administering fentanyl in a victim of trauma with "borderline" hemodynamic status worsen the outcome? Does an analgesic significantly blur the history and physical examination and the ability to monitor the patient? Conversely, does providing adequate analgesia enhance the ability to perform an evaluation? Does ketorolac IV result in clinically significant bleeding?

Finally, all disciplines of health care need to embrace the concept that effective pain control requires interspecialty and interdisciplinary collaboration. Open communication and a team approach is essential to controlling the pain and anxiety that inevitably accompany severe injury.

Exciting new avenues of pain control are on the horizon. New agents such as compounds that modulate cholinergic channels, both peripherally and centrally to produce analgesia (antinociception) are in development.

Despite the potential of the future, the problem of the present is often that pain is treated too little, too late, or not at all. We must continually keep in mind that pain is the number one reason patients seek emergency care and that pain itself is an emergency. We need to not only continue the search for more effective, safer methods of pain control, but constantly improve the education of physicians and nurses who care for patients in pain.

In the past, the treatment of injuries and traumatic pain has been under the purview of military physicians and nurses, anesthesiologists, and surgeons. Over the last two decades, emergency physicians have assumed an increasingly important role in the treatment of severely injured patients and are emerging as leaders and advocates of the treatment, research, and education of the management of acute pain. The advancement of methods and a system of care that lessen or ablate pain in severely injured patients can be one of emergency medicine's greatest legacies.

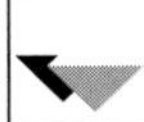

PEARLS & PITFALLS

- Anticipate and prevent pain.
- Assess every conscious patient for pain intensity and reassess after each intervention and at regular intervals.
- Include a numerical pain scale on the trauma flow chart.
- Titrate medications to effect, using the intravenous route.
- Use nonpharmacologic approaches as well. Reassure. Use ice, elevation, and splinting.
- Bupivacaine lasts hours longer than lidocaine.
- Learn and use regional anesthesia such as the femoral nerve block.
- Use a team approach, establish nursing protocols to assess pain along with vital signs.

Acknowledgments

The authors gratefully acknowledge the insights and suggestions provided by James Ducharme, MD; Beverly K Giles, RN; Maureen Misinski, RN; Paul M Paris, MD; George H Rodman, MD; and Donald M Yealy, MD.

REFERENCES

1. Todd KH, Samaroo N, Hoffman JR: Ethnicity as a risk factor for inadequate emergency department analgesia, *JAMA* 269:1537, 1993.
2. Wilson JE, Pendleton JM: Oligoanalgesia in the emergency department, *Am J Emerg Med* 7:620, 1989.
3. Jones JS, Johnson K, McNinch M: Age as a risk factor for inadequate emergency department analgesia, *Am J Emerg Med* 14:157, 1996.
4. Warfield CA: Treating traumatic pain, *Hosp Pract* 21:48M, 48P-48R,48T, 1986.
5. Acute Pain Management Guideline Panel: *Acute pain management: operative or medical procedures and trauma: clinical practice guideline,* Rockville, MD, February, 1992, AHCPR Pub. No. 92-0032, Agency for Health Care Policy and Research, Public Health Service, U.S. Department of Health and Human Services.
6. Cantees K, Yealy DM: Pain management in the trauma patient. In Peitzman AB, et al (editors): *The trauma manual,* Philadelphia, 1998, Lippincott-Raven.
7. Rhodes M: Trauma resuscitation. In Peitzman AB, et al (editors): *The trauma manual,* Philadelphia, 1998, Lippincott-Raven.
8. International Association for the Study of Pain: Pain terms: a list with definitions and notes on usage, *Pain* 6:249, 1979.
9. Prieto E, Geisinger KF: Factor analytic studies of the McGill Pain Questionnaire. In Melzack R (editor): *Pain measurement and assessment,* New York, 1983, Raven Press.
10. Jones SL: Anatomy of pain. In Sinatra RS, et al (editors): *Acute pain: mechanisms & management,* St Louis, 1992, Mosby.
11. Perry SW: Psychological aspects of pain management. In Paris PM, Stewart RD, (editors): *Pain management in emergency medicine,* Norwalk, Conn, 1988, Appleton & Lange.
12. Gil KM: Psychologic aspects of acute pain. In Sinatra RS, et al (editors): *Acute pain: mechanisms & management,* St Louis, 1992, Mosby.
13. Warfield CA, Stein JM: Psychologic factors. In Warfield CA (editor): *Manual of pain management,* Philadelphia, 1991, Lippincott.
14. Aimone LD: Neurochemistry and modulation of pain. In Sinatra RS, et al (editors): *Acute pain: mechanisms & management,* St Louis, 1992, Mosby.
15. Saberski L: Postoperative pain management for the patient with chronic pain. In Sinatra RS, et al (editors): *Acute pain: mechanisms & management,* St Louis, 1992, Mosby.
16. McIlvaine WB: Overview of pediatric analgesia. In Sinatra RS, et al (editors): *Acute pain: mechanisms & management,* St Louis, 1992, Mosby.
17. Raja SN, Meyer RA, Campbell JN: Peripheral mechanisms of somatic pain, *Anesthesiology* 68:571 1988.
18. Mackersie RC, Karagianes TG: Pain management following trauma and burns, *Crit Care Clin* 6:433, 1990.
19. Wheeler AP: Sedation, analgesia, and paralysis in the intensive care unit, *Chest* 104:566, 1993.
20. LoVecchio F, et al: The use of analgesics in patients with acute abdominal pain. *J Emerg Med* 15:775, 1997.
21. Pace S, Burke TF: Intravenous morphine for early pain relief in patients with acute abdominal pain, *Acad Emerg Med* 3:1086, 1996.
22. Arrard AR, et al: Safety of early pain relief for acute abdominal pain, *Br Med J* 305:554, 1992.
23. Zoltie N, Cust MP: Analgesia in the acute abdomen, *Ann Royal Coll Surg Engl* 68:209, 1986.
24. Cordell WH, et al: Pain and tissue-interface pressures during spine-board immobilization, *Ann Emerg Med* 26:31, 1995.
25. Chan D, et al: The effect of spinal immobilization of healthy volunteers, *Ann Emerg Med* 23:48, 1994.
26. Mawson AR, et al: Risk factors for early occurring pressure ulcers following spinal cord injury, *Am J Phys Med Rehabil* 67:123, 1988.
27. Linares HA, et al: Association between pressure sores and immobilization in the immediate post-injury period, *Orthopedics* 10:571, 1987.
28. Portenoy RK: Clinical application of opioid analgesics. In Sinatra RS, et al (editors): *Acute pain: mechanisms & management,* St Louis, 1992, Mosby.
29. Kehlet H, Dahl JB: The value of "multimodal" or "balanced analgesia" in postoperative pain treatment, *Anesth Analg* 77:1048, 1993.
30. Goudie TA, et al: Continuous subcutaneous infusion of morphine for postoperative pain relief, *Anaesthesia* 40:1086, 1985.
31. Beecher HK: Delayed morphine poisoning in battle casualties, *JAMA* 124:1193, 1943.
32. Strom BL, et al: Parenteral ketorolac and risk of gastrointestinal and operative site bleeding: a postmarketing surveillance study, *JAMA* 275:376, 1996.
33. Feldman HI, et al: Parenteral ketorolac: the risk for acute renal failure, *Ann Intern Med* 126:193, 1997.
34. Gurnani A, et al: Analgesia for acute musculoskeletal trauma: low-dose subcutaneous infusion of ketamine, *Anaesth Intensive Care* 24:32, 1996.
35. deCraen AJ, et al: Analgesic efficacy and safety of paracetamol-codeine combinations versus paracetamol alone: a systematic review, *Br Med J* 313:321, 1996.
36. Turturro MA, et al: Hydrocodone versus codeine in acute musculoskeletal pain, *Ann Emerg Med* 20:1100, 1991.
37. Chung KS: Intercostal nerve block. In Sinatra RS, et al (editors): *Acute pain: mechanisms & management,* St Louis, 1992, Mosby.
38. Dilworth NM, MacKellar A: Pain relief for the pediatric surgical patient, *J Pediatr Surg* 22:264, 1987.
39. McGlone R, et al: Femoral nerve block in the initial management of femoral shaft fractures, *Arch Emerg Med* 4:163, 1987.
40. Gabram SG, et al: Clinical management of blunt trauma patients with unilateral rib fractures: a randomized trial, *World J Surg* 19:388, 1995.
41. Short K, et al: Evaluation of intrapleural analgesia in the management of blunt traumatic chest wall pain: a clinical trial, *Am Surgeon* 62:488, 1996.
42. Medvei C: Forward. In Mann RD (editor): *The history of the management of pain: from early principles to present practice,* Carnforth, England, 1988, Parthenon Publishing Group.

PART THREE

MANAGEMENT OF SPECIFIC INJURIES

11 Traumatic Brain Injury

BRIAN J. ZINK AND PATRICIA L. LANTER

Teaching Case

A 29-year-old male skied into a tree. He lost consciousness for 3 minutes, but then awoke and was able to answer questions appropriately. Transport time to the hospital was 65 minutes. His Glasgow Coma Scale (GCS) score was 15 for the first 60 minutes, but suddenly plummeted to 3 and his left pupil became markedly dilated. He was intubated in the ambulance. On arrival to the ED, he was rapidly taken for a computed tomography (CT) scan of the brain. The CT scan showed a large, left temporal, epidural hemorrhage (EDH) with midline shift to the right. He was emergently taken to the operating suite. An intraoperative diagnostic peritoneal lavage (DPL), performed concomitantly with a craniectomy, was negative. After evacuation of the EDH, the patient made a full neurologic recovery and was discharged home after 5 days.

This case demonstrates that patients who initially appear fully alert and awake after head trauma may harbor life-threatening intracranial lesions. Operative intervention is often curative, and the chances for full recovery are excellent for EDH if patients are quickly taken to the operating suite. ■

Humans have evolved into the dominant life form on Earth, largely as a result of the development of our complex brain. Despite a beefy intellect, this spongy organ has a limited capacity to withstand injury. Traumatic brain injury (TBI) results in devastating consequences for patients, families, employers, and healthcare resources.[1,2] In the past decade a new knowledge on TBI has changed medical practice.

EPIDEMIOLOGY

The incidence of TBI varies among populations and is the primary factor in at least one fourth of all trauma deaths. It accounts for approximately 75,000 deaths each year in the United States.[3,4] Nonfatal TBI is a major public health problem, resulting in an estimated 373,000 hospital admissions.[3] The majority of these admitted patients (about 80%) have mild injury, and the remainder is divided between moderate and severe TBI. An estimated 1.6 million patients per year seek medical attention for TBI in the United States, and most are evaluated in an emergency department (ED).[3,4]

Risk Factors for Traumatic Brain Injury

The "typical" TBI patient is an alcohol-intoxicated male in his early twenties who is involved in a motor vehicle crash (MVC). Large epidemiologic studies show a two-fold male predominance. The risk for TBI is highest in the 15- to 24-year-old range, which has twice the incidence compared with the 40- to 50-year-old population. An inverse relationship exists between socioeconomic status and TBI, with alcohol as a major predisposing factor.[3,4] Alcohol intoxication is present in approximately 50% of adults who receive medical attention for this condition.[5-11] Investigators presume that alcohol impairs protective reflexes and increases the likelihood of head trauma.[12]

MVCs are the leading cause of TBI. However, operation of other vehicles is responsible for a significant number of cases, including bicycles, motorcycles, boats, snowmobiles, and all-terrain and farm vehicles. Falls are the next leading cause of TBI and are common in the elderly. Assaults are also an important factor, and gunshot wounds account for about 40% of fatal TBI cases in large U.S. cities.[13]

PATHOPHYSIOLOGY

Despite the rigid cranial vault, the brain is very susceptible to injury. One way of conceptualizing the pathophysiology of TBI is to consider primary and secondary brain injury. Primary brain injury is the physical or functional disruption of brain tissue that results from mechanical forces. Secondary brain injury is brain dysfunction or cellular damage that occurs after the initial insult. Hypoxia and hypotension mediate most of secondary brain injury (Table 11-1).

Cerebral autoregulation provides homeostasis of cerebral blood flow (CBF) in the normal brain. CBF remains relatively constant despite changes in cerebral perfusion pressure (CPP). CPP is calculated by subtracting intracranial pressure (ICP) from the systemic mean arterial pressure (MAP). Cerebral autoregulation is dependent on the integrity of the blood-brain barrier (BBB). The BBB consists of specialized cerebrovascular endothelial cells and continuous tight junctions between these cells that block the passive diffusion of electrolytes, plasma proteins, and other large molecules into the brain extracellular space. Disruption of the BBB by injury forces may impair cerebral autoregulation.

TABLE 11-1
Secondary Injury Factors

INTRINSIC	EXTRINSIC OR IATROGENIC
Elevated ICP	Inadequate fluid or blood resuscitation
Low CBF/CPP	Inadequate oxygen delivery
Systemic hypotension/shock	Over hyperventilation
Reperfusion	Alcohol and other drug intoxication
Hypoventilation/hypoxemia	Nosocomial infections
Brain edema and mass effect	
Brain herniation	
Brain hemorrhage	
Cerebral arterial vasospasm	
Inflammation	
Hyperthermia	
Chronic systemic illness	

Brain shift is the movement of brain tissue because of expanding masses, focal areas of edema, or high ICP. If large hematomas are not evacuated or ICP elevation is not attenuated by compensatory mechanisms, brain tissue may shift and squeeze through the tentorial opening, resulting in brain herniation. Brain herniation may be unilateral uncal transtentorial herniation, central herniation, or transfalxial cingulate herniation, depending on the location of mass lesions or hemorrhages. Brain shift eventually compresses cardiorespiratory centers in the brainstem, leading to respiratory arrest or cardiocirculatory collapse. Brain herniation because of severely elevated ICP is usually a preterminal event.

Ischemia, elevated intracranial pressure, hemorrhage, and the neurochemical injury cascade are all components of secondary brain injury.[14] Extraneous or iatrogenic events can also exacerbate secondary injury. Hypoxia and systemic arterial hypotension are the two most important secondary insults in the early postinjury period. Apnea often occurs immediately after TBI, and respiratory depression may follow. Up to 30% of TBI patients are hypoxic on presentation to the ED.[14,15] Alcohol and other drugs worsen respiratory depression.[10,14,16] Hypoxemia clearly increases mortality.[17-19] Similarly, hypotension aggravates both morbidity and mortality following TBI.[14,15,18,19] Factors such as hemorrhagic shock, decreased cardiac output, neurogenic shock, and drugs all decrease CPP to critically low levels. In areas of the brain that are already affected by traumatic ischemia, a drop in CPP and failure of cerebral autoregulation accelerates ischemia and brain cell necrosis. Other secondary insults include seizures, electrolyte imbalances, hyperthermia, and alcohol and drug intoxication.[14,20]

Alcohol intoxication potentiates injury.[21,22] In animal TBI models ethanol reduces CBF and ventilation in the early postinjury period.[16,22] Intoxicated patients with isolated central nervous system (CNS) injury are more likely to die within the first hour post-injury when compared with sober patients.[10]

Seizures may occur in the acute course of TBI and are relatively common in the convalescent phase of patients with moderate and severe TBI. Focal brain damage may create an epileptogenic focus. These seizures are detrimental in a number of ways. Seizures increase metabolic demands in the brain, and subsequent acidosis and hypoxemia worsen metabolic imbalance. Tonic-clonic movements, breath holding, and hypertension during a seizure can elevate ICP.[14,23]

The pathophysiology of coma remains unknown. The most accepted theory is that TBI-induced coma results from widespread axonal dysfunction that prevents normal communication between neurons. Disconnection of the cerebral cortical centers from each other and from subcortical areas causes unconsciousness.[24] Other influences such as hypoxemia, circulatory shock, expanding hematomas, and markedly elevated ICP can contribute to alterations in consciousness.

Following TBI, neurotransmitters and neurochemical mediators of injury produce an array of cellular responses. It is beyond the scope of this text to provide in-depth discussion of all these potential mediators of brain injury at the microscopic level. However, it should be mentioned that excitatory amino acids such as glutamate and aspartate, oxygen free radicals, nitric oxide, endogenous opioids, acetylcholine, adenosine, catecholamines, and cytokines (e.g., tumor necrosis factor [TNF] and interleukins 1,6, and 8) may all play a role in brain injury.

Pathophysiology of Mild Traumatic Brain Injury

The pathophysiologic changes that occur in mild TBI are not as well studied as those with severe TBI. Large hemorrhages and hematomas, elevated ICP, reduced CBF, and coma are not seen in mild TBI. However, many of the cellular and subcellular processes that are active in severe TBI are probably also operative in mild TBI. These processes include activation of excitatory neurotransmitters and endogenous opioids, and alterations in cerebral energy metabolism. The blood-brain barrier may also be affected by mild TBI. Animal studies suggest that in mild TBI the BBB is not structurally disrupted, but has altered function resulting in temporarily increased vascular permeability. Both serum proteins and neuroactive mediators of injury may leak into the injured brain.

CLINICAL PRESENTATION

Classification of Traumatic Brain Injury

The spectrum of TBI can range from a mild headache, to the patient who presents in flaccid coma. Several classification systems categorize patients, affect triage decisions, direct emergent therapy, predict outcome, and assist research on TBI patients. The Glasgow Coma Scale (GCS) is the best way to classify TBI in the prehospital and ED settings. Teasdale and Jennett[25] developed this scale in 1974 as a simple, quantifiable assessment of the TBI patient with low interobserver variability. The GCS tallies basic neurologic functioning in motor, verbal, and eye-opening categories (Table 11-2). Some special circumstances are important in recording the GCS. Intubated patients are given the motor and eye-opening score followed by the letter *T* (for "tube") to indicate that it is physically impossible for them to speak. If the patient is unable to open his or her eyes as a result of swelling, also note this finding beside the GCS. Document whether the patient was given paralytics before scoring.

Other head injury scales and scoring systems have been proposed, including the Brussels Coma Grades, Grady Coma Grades, Ommaya Scale, Leeds Coma Scale, Innsbruck Coma Scale, and Reaction Level Scale.[26,27] Although some features of these scales may provide an occasional advantage, the GCS remains the most widely used classification system. Related schemes derived from the GCS, include a three-level scale of mild (presenting GCS 13 to 15), moderate (GCS 9 to 12), and severe TBI (GCS 3 to 8), as well as an expanded version, with TBI categories of minimal, mild, moderate, severe, and critical.[3,9,27]

TBI can also be classified in terms of gross pathologic lesions discovered on radiologic studies, surgery, or autopsy. Common pathologic changes include subarachnoid hemorrhage, cerebral contusions, and subdural or epidural hematomas. Diffuse injuries cause neurologic impairment without obvious gross pathology.

Clinical Features of Traumatic Brain Injury

Patients with moderate to severe TBI will present with altered mental status. They may be comatose, obtunded, agitated, or inappropriate. The motor and sensory neurologic examinations of patients with mass lesions may demonstrate focal deficits compared with the symmetric examination of those with diffuse injury. Coma predicts severe injury and correlates with high ICP. Rapid deterioration in the neurologic status may signal an expanding intracerebral hematoma or brain herniation. Many factors obscure the initial evaluation of TBI patients, including hypoxia, shock, and alcohol and drug intoxication.

EPIDURAL HEMATOMA

The classic scenario is an initial loss of consciousness, followed by a "lucid interval" in which consciousness is regained, with subsequent lethargy. Although the patient may be awake on arrival in the ED, deterioration can occur rapidly. EDH frequently occurs from a direct blow to the temporal region and the patient may or may not have an associated skull fracture. The injury disrupts epidural arteries or veins, with the middle meningeal artery as the most commonly affected vessel. EDH caused by venous bleeding is limited by the space between the dura and the skull. However, arterial hemorrhages produce sufficient pressure to herniate the brain. As the hematoma enlarges, the temporal lobe may squeeze over the tento-

TABLE 11-2
The Glasgow Coma Scale

EYE OPENING		
Spontaneously	4	Reticular activating system is intact: patient may not be aware
To verbal command	3	Opens eyes when told to do so
To pain	2	Opens eyes in response to pain
None	1	Does not open eyes to any stimuli
VERBAL RESPONSE		
Oriented-converses	5	Relatively intact CNS Aware of self and environment
Disoriented-converses	4	Well articulated, organized, but patient is disoriented
Inappropriate words	3	Random, exclamatory words
Incomprehensible	2	Moaning, no recognizable words
No response	1	No response or intubated
MOTOR RESPONSE		
Obeys verbal commands	6	Readily moves limbs when told to
Localizes to painful stimuli	5	Moves limb in an effort to remove painful stimuli
Flexion withdrawal	4	Pulls away from pain in flexion
Abnormal flexion	3	Decorticate rigidity
Extension	2	Decerebrate rigidity
No response	1	Hypotonia, flaccid: suggests loss of medullary function or concomitant spinal cord injury

From Biros M: Head trauma. In Rosen P, et al (editors): *Emergency medicine: concepts and clinical practice,* ed 4, St Louis, 1998, Mosby.

rium, compressing the third nerve and causing an ipsilateral fixed and dilated pupil. Tentorial herniation may occur on the opposite side as well, causing either a contralateral or bilateral blown pupil (called Kernohan's notch syndrome). On CT scanning, EDHs are lens-shaped lesions on the surface of the brain (Fig. 11-1). EDH is more common in the second and third decades and is rare in infants and the elderly.

SUBDURAL HEMATOMA

Subdural hematoma (SDH) is six times more common than EDH and has a higher mortality rate. Clinical features vary with the size of the hematoma, the surrounding parenchymal injury, and the rapidity of growth. SDH can be acute, subacute, or chronic. Acute SDH usually results from acceleration/deceleration injuries such as MVCs. In small children and infants with acute SDH and an inconsistent history, child abuse must be suspected. Patients with acute SDH often present with a focal neurologic deficit or depressed mental status. On CT scanning, acute SDHs are high attenuation, crescent-shaped collections of blood usually along the calvarium, but can also be found along the falx or tentorium (Fig. 11-2). Subacute or chronic SDH accumulate more slowly. Patients with these hematomas present with a gradual change in mental status or personality. Elderly patients may exhibit slowly increasing confusion. The initial injury may have occurred days to weeks prior and may be forgotten by the patient and his or her family. On CT scanning, the fluid collections may be isodense, hypodense, or of mixed density depending on the age of the lesion. The unwary physician may overlook these lesions because the blood in isodense subdurals has the same density as surrounding brain. Some large isodense subdurals may demonstrate a mass effect but smaller collections may only efface the sulci on the affected side (Fig. 11-3).

DELAYED TRAUMATIC INTRACRANIAL HEMORRHAGE

Some patients with TBI who do not initially have EDH, SDH, or intracerebral hemorrhage (ICH) will develop a delayed hemorrhage. Delayed traumatic intracranial hemorrhages (DTICH) are more frequent in patients with severe TBI and increase the morbidity and mortality. With the increased and repetitive use of CT scanning, DTICH is now more commonly recog-

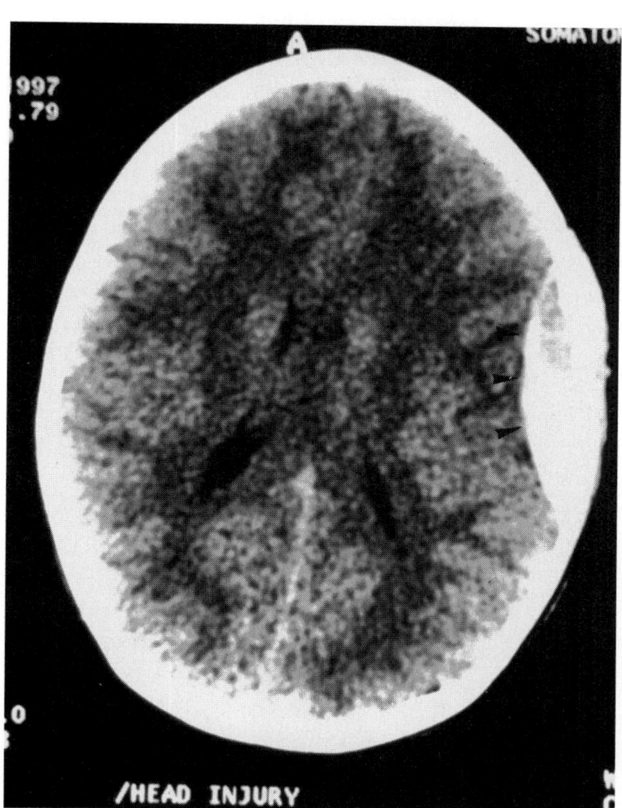

Fig. 11-1 Head CT scan demonstrating an epidural hematoma.

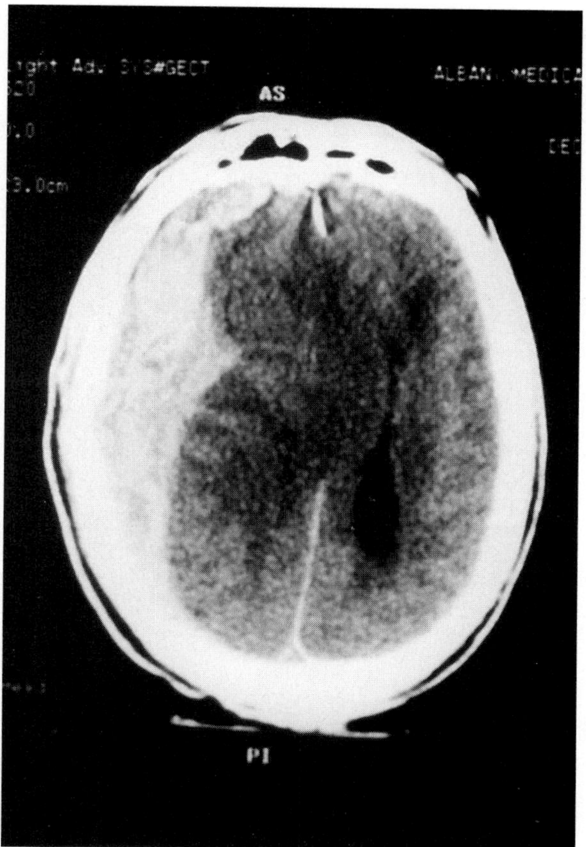

Fig. 11-2 Head CT scan demonstrating an acute subdural hematoma.

nized. Two common scenarios occur with DTICH. The first is the delayed development (hours to days) of an intraparenchymal hemorrhage in an area of the brain that was merely contused. The second is the development of an EDH or SDH in a TBI patient who has a relatively normal initial brain scan. These patients may have minimal symptoms before sudden neurologic deterioration. Factors that may contribute to DTICH are the adherence of the dura mater to the skull (in younger people the dura is less adherent), the presence of skull fractures, systemic arterial hypotension followed by fluid or blood resuscitation, and coagulopathy. This phenomenon explains the sudden neurologic deterioration seen in some severely injured patients whose blood pressure is restored by resuscitation.[28-31] A rate for the development of DTICH as high as 8.5% has been described by some authors.[32] Most lesions are seen within 36 hours postinjury.

SUBARACHNOID HEMORRHAGE

The presentation of these patients depends on the size of the hemorrhage and the coexisting injuries. Patients with traumatic subarachnoid hemorrhage (SAH) have higher morbidity and mortality, regardless of mechanism (i.e., penetrating versus nonpenetrating). One half of these patients have intracranial hematomas. Patients with SAH are more likely to have hypoxia, hypotension, and higher ICP, and are thus at risk for secondary brain injury. As with nontraumatic SAH, cerebral arterial vasospasm in the second or third day postinjury may lead to cerebral ischemia, and worsen outcome. On CT scanning, SAH is identified by high attenuation in the sulci and basal cisterns (Fig. 11-4).[33-35]

CEREBRAL CONTUSION

The patient with isolated cerebral contusions may exhibit altered mental status, but rarely coma. Contusions occur with rapid deceleration injuries such as MVCs and falls, or with direct blows. Contusions typically appear on the tips of frontal and temporal lobes, where the skull base is irregular. On CT scanning, contusions show as areas of punctate hemorrhage (Fig. 11-5). Contusions on the side opposite the impact are known as contrecoup injuries.

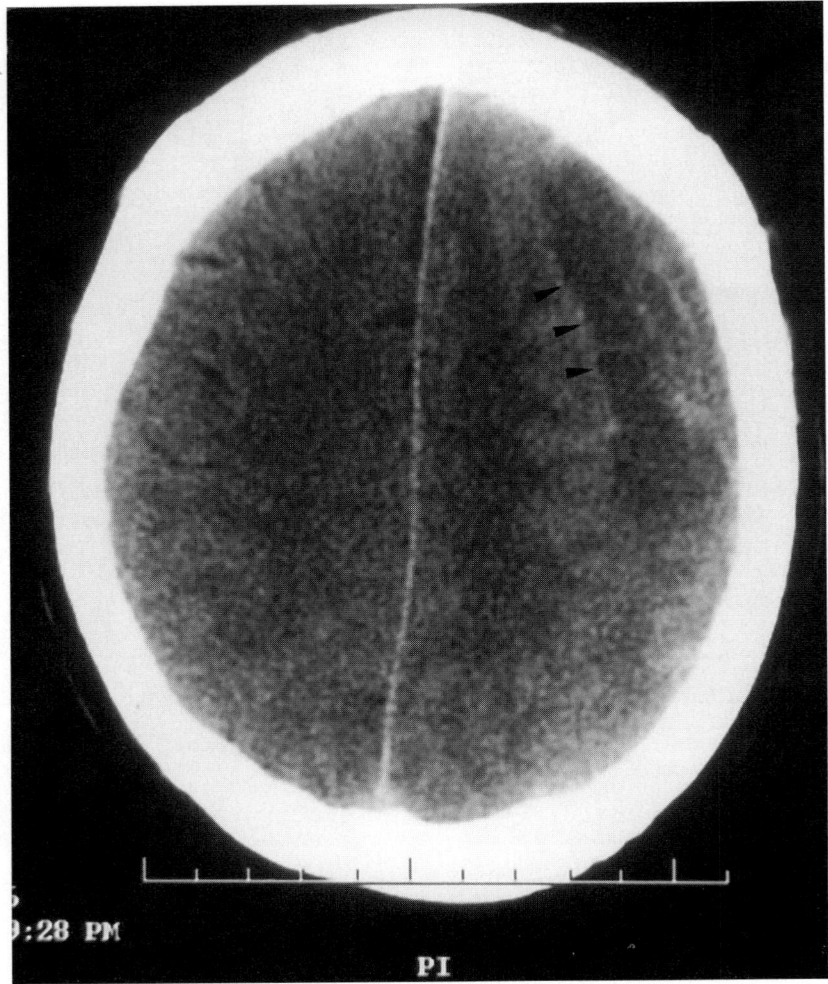

Fig. 11-3 Head CT scan demonstrating a chronic subdural hematoma.

DIFFUSE AXONAL INJURY

Patients who suffer severe diffuse axonal injury (DAI) may be comatose but nonfocal on neurologic examination. The physical examination is typically symmetric, unless there is an associated intracerebral hematoma. The mechanism of injury for DAI is usually rapid acceleration/deceleration. CT scan findings are nonspecific and include blurring of the gray matter/white matter interface, signs of edema, loss of cortical sulci, and obliteration of the ventricles.[36,37] Magnetic resonance imaging (MRI) demonstrates the injury more clearly.

CONCUSSION OR MILD TRAUMATIC BRAIN INJURY

Patients with mild TBI may be harder to classify and diagnose than those with moderate or severe TBI. Mild TBI (concussion) is a traumatically induced physiologic disruption of brain function as manifested by at least one of the following:[38]

1. Any loss of consciousness
2. Any loss of memory for events immediately before or after the accident
3. Any alteration in mental state at the time of the accident (e.g., feeling dazed, disoriented, or confused)
4. Focal neurologic deficit(s) where the severity of the injury does not exceed the following:
    - Loss of consciousness of 30 minutes
    - After 30 minutes, an initial GCS of 13 to 15, and posttraumatic amnesia (PTA) not greater that 24 hours

Patients with mild TBI often have significant memory difficulties, including PTA. Family members may observe changes in the patient's behavior or personality. By definition, patients with mild TBI have a nor-

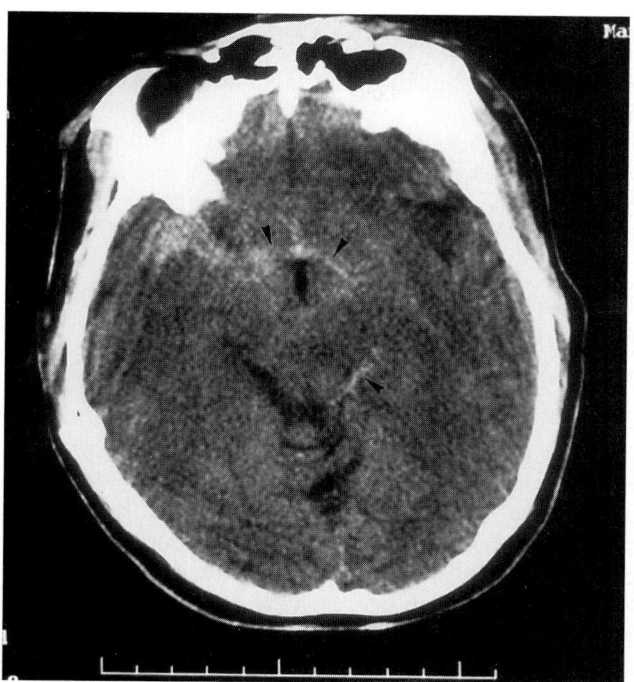

Fig. 11-4 Head CT scan demonstrating a traumatic subarachnoid hemorrhage.

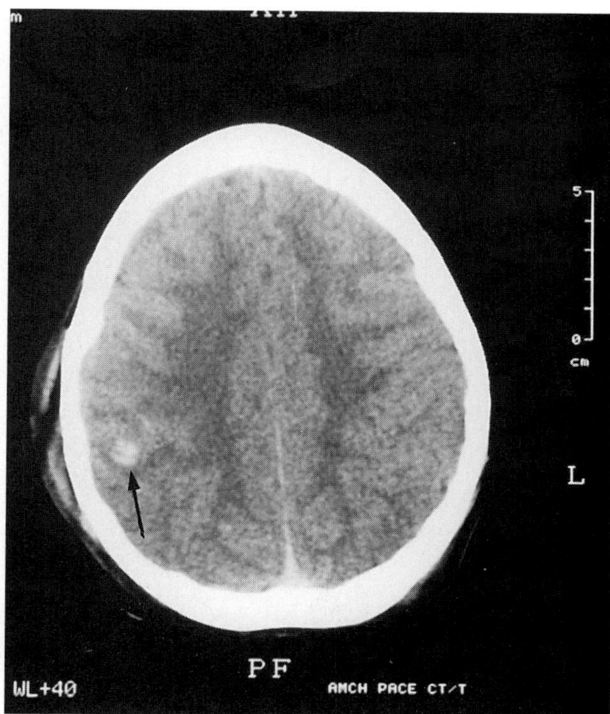

Fig. 11-5 Head CT scan demonstrating a cerebral contusion.

mal brain CT scan; however, other imaging modalities, such as MRI, may demonstrate subtle anatomic abnormalities. Recent studies support the idea that concussions are a mild form of DAI.[37] At least 25% of patients with mild TBI (GCS 13 to 15) develop long-term problems with cognition, memory, headaches, and fatigue. The nonspecific term *postconcussive syndrome* applies to these sequelae.[39-43]

SKULL FRACTURES

Skull fractures result from a direct blow to the calvarium and are present in about 60% of patients with severe TBI.[44,45] They can be divided into linear, depressed, and basilar. Linear skull fractures are usually an incidental CT finding. Hematomas, soft tissue swelling, and point tenderness materialize over the site of impact. A simple closed-linear skull fracture needs no surgical intervention or specific treatment.

A growing skull fracture is an uncommon complication of a linear skull fracture that takes place in children under 2 years of age. The pathogenesis is a tear in the dura mater underneath a diastatic fracture (one that crosses a suture, or has a width of greater than 4 mm) that allows pulsatile tissue in the growing brain to enlarge and erode the surrounding bone. A common, but not universal, finding is a leptomeningeal cyst, a painless, pulsatile swelling. Operative repair of the dural rent is usually curative.[46]

Depressed skull fractures may also have soft tissue swelling over the site of the trauma, and a bony step-off may be palpated. The size and the depth of the fracture may not be obvious on clinical examination secondary to scalp swelling. There are three types of depressed skull fractures: true, flat, and ping-pong ball fractures. The true fracture has a connection with the cranial vault and is the most common type. The flat fracture has a depressed segment without any communication with the cranial vault and is the least common type. The ping-pong ball fracture is a pediatric greenstick fracture of the skull and is discussed in Chapter 33.

Brain CT scanning is the best method for evaluating depressed skull fractures (Fig. 11-6). The mechanism of injury is usually an intense blow to the scalp with an object that has a small surface area. Surgical repair is usually indicated if the inner table of the skull is damaged and the fragment is depressed more than 5 mm.[44]

Basilar skull fractures (BSFs) result from a blow to the parietal, temporal, or occipital area of the skull. The temporal bone is most commonly affected. Since the temporal bone houses the structures of the inner

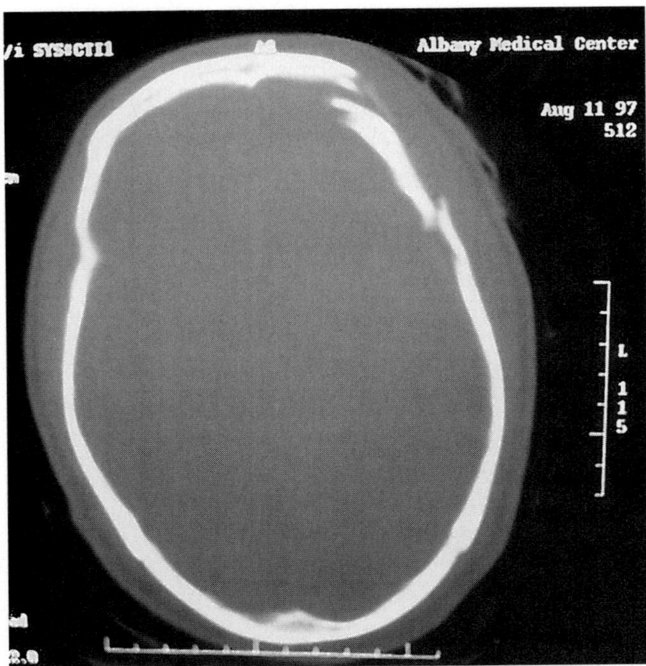

Fig. 11-6 Head CT scan demonstrating a depressed skull fracture.

ear, and is traversed by the facial nerve, hearing and facial function may be impaired. Another complication is leakage of CSF from the nose or ears. Other clinical signs include hemotympanum, ecchymosis over the mastoid area (**Battle's sign**), or periorbital ecchymosis (**"raccoon eyes"**). The development of Battle's sign and raccoon eyes usually takes several hours. BSFs are ill-defined on standard brain CT scans and thin cuts through the region may be needed (Fig. 11-7).

CERVICAL SPINE INJURY

Severe TBI is a risk factor for cervical spine injury. About 7% of patients with severe TBI have an associated cervical spine fracture.[47] Cervical spine injuries may produce neurologic deficits that mimic TBI, such as unilateral hemiparesis.

Differential Diagnosis of Traumatic Brain Injury

The differential diagnosis of TBI is similar to that for any patient with altered mental status. Causes include hypoxia, hypercarbia, hypotension, metabolic abnormalities, alcohol and drug intoxication, and psychogenic causes. Many of these conditions also contribute to secondary brain injury.

Trauma patients have a high incidence of alcohol and drug intoxication, which may obscure the initial evaluation. Other pathologic processes in the trauma patient that may mimic or obfuscate TBI include hypothermia and exposure to chemicals (usually through fires) that may induce coma, such as carbon monoxide or cyanide. Patients may also suffer trauma and present with altered mental status following seizures or hypoglycemic episodes. In these situations, the laboratory or bedside testing may establish a diagnosis.

EMERGENCY DEPARTMENT EVALUATION

History

The initial history in the severe TBI patient is deferred until the primary survey and stabilization is complete. Since most serious TBI patients, and many with moderate or mild TBI, are unable to provide a history, the clinician depends on other sources. Emergency medical service (EMS) providers, the patient's family, and witnesses to the injury provide crucial information. The patient's initial response to injury, an early GCS, and any observed changes are valuable. Determine the speed and deformation in a MVC, use of safety restraints, interior damage to the vehicle, evidence of alcohol or drug use, estimated blood loss, and the estimated time before EMS arrival. For other injuries, information such as the type of weapon or the height of a fall may be helpful. Family members or acquaintances of the patient are usually able to provide essential information regarding the patient's living situation and previous level of function, diseases, medications, and allergies.[35]

Physical Examination of Severe Traumatic Brain Injury Patients

The examination of the severe TBI patient is standard. The primary trauma survey, including an initial GCS, is completed on the patient's arrival to the ED. One of the most critical aspects is evaluation of the airway and oxygenation. Tachypnea and hyperventilation may indicate rising ICP. Coexisting injuries that produce hypoxia include pneumothorax, facial fractures, and rib fractures.

The next step is assessment of the circulation with attention to pulse, blood pressure, and capillary refill. Hypovolemia, hypoxia, hyperthermia, and pain all produce tachycardia. Cushing's response, or hypertension with bradycardia, is an ominous finding that portends brain herniation and death.[48]

NEUROLOGIC EXAMINATION

A single neurologic examination of the TBI patient is of limited value, since it can change very quickly.

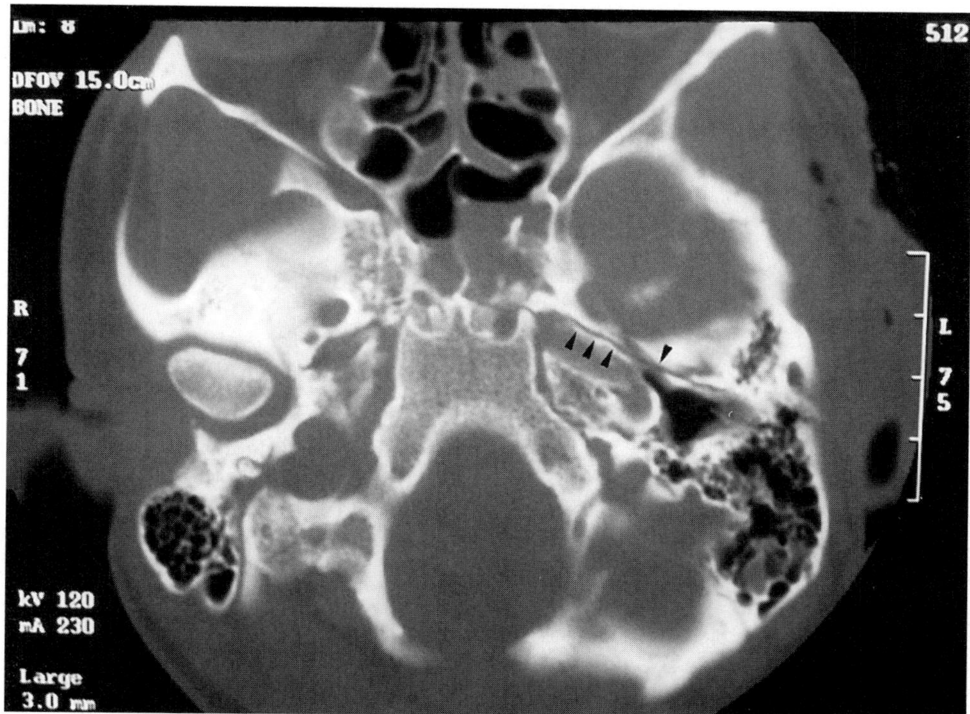

Fig. 11-7 Head CT scan demonstrating a basilar skull fracture.

However, the initial examination provides a baseline to which future examinations are compared. An exhaustive neurologic assessment in the early phases is not always possible or desirable. A directed neurologic examination is more appropriate, including GCS scoring, pupillary and cranial nerve function, motor strength, gross sensory function, and deep tendon reflexes. Flaccidity indicates either severe brain or cervical cord injury.

Cranial nerve sensory and motor deficits may indicate pressure on the trigeminal or facial nerves from mass lesions or skull fractures. The motor, sensory, and reflex examinations of the extremities provide further clues to the presence of focal brain lesions. Comprehensive neurologic evaluation should occur after the patient has been stabilized and the brain CT scan is complete. Repetitive neurologic examinations are the most important part of the clinical assessment of TBI patients.

Special tests may determine the extent of the TBI. In the trauma patient, do not perform the **oculocephalic reflex** or **doll's eye maneuver**. A comatose patient may have a ligamentous injury to the neck despite normal radiographs. A safer test to evaluate brainstem function in the comatose patient is the **oculovestibular reflex** or **cold caloric test**. This test can be performed despite cervical immobilization. First, the ear canals are inspected to verify that the tympanic membranes are intact; 10 ml of ice water is instilled into the ear canal. Nystagmus occurs in awake patients, with the slow movement toward the irrigated ear, and rapid movement toward the midline. (Note: this test is *not* indicated in awake patients, who obviously have an intact brainstem and are likely to vomit.) The rapid movement defines the nystagmus. If the brainstem is intact, but the cortex is injured, the eyes will deviate toward the irrigated side. If brainstem function is absent, no eye movement will occur. Another test of brainstem function is the **corneal reflex**. Patients who have an intact brainstem will blink (cranial nerves V and VII) when the cornea is lightly touched with a wisp of sterile cotton.

Decerebrate posturing is seen as extension of both the arms and legs, with internal rotation of the arms and plantar flexion of the feet. Brainstem lesions result in symmetric decerebrate posturing. **Decorticate posturing** is similar to decerebrate posturing, but with upper extremity flexion. Symmetric decorticate posturing implies bihemispheric lesions.

HEAD AND EYE EXAMINATION

The detailed physical examination in the TBI patient includes an evaluation of the head, with attention to facial and skull fractures, bony asymmetry, and entrance/exit wounds. The ears and nose are inspected for blood and cerebrospinal fluid (CSF) leaks, as well as hemotympanum. When dropped on a paper towel or a bed sheet, CSF mixed with blood forms a double ring or "halo." The central splotch is blood, while the surrounding tint represents CSF. This finding is *not* specific for a CSF leak and will occur with a traumatized runny nose. Unlike CSF, simple rhinorrhea (absent blood) does not contain glucose. Although the bedside glucose tests cannot distinguish CSF from rhinorrhea, standard laboratory glucose can separate the two.

Examination of the eyes may reveal anisocoria. Although herniation *must always be the first consideration,* other causes include a glass eye, ophthalmic drops, direct eye trauma, and hereditary anisocoria. Bilateral fixed and dilated pupils occur in severe brain injury with significant global brain damage. It is important to note that neuromuscular blocking drugs do not affect pupillary function. Rhythmic eye movements or nystagmus may indicate ongoing seizure activity. Eyes may deviate towards a hemisphere that harbors a mass lesion.

Physical Examination of the Mild Traumatic Brain Injury Patient

Classification of mild TBI is partly dependent on historical information. The presence and duration of unconsciousness is significant. Document the length of PTA, since this finding correlates with persistent symptoms and disability. The mild TBI patient has a constellation of symptoms that may include headache, dizziness or vertigo, visual changes, hearing changes, nausea, vomiting, and paresthesias.

The examination of a patient with mild TBI differs from that of a patient with a more severe injury. By definition, the patient is arousable and can speak. The awake state may represent a "lucid interval" and subsequent deterioration may occur. Deficits may occur in recall, naming objects, and insight. Cognitive dysfunction includes short- and long-term memory loss, and information processing is often impaired. Although some investigators feel that formal neuropsychiatric testing is useful, it is not clear which tests are valuable during emergency evaluation.[39,49-51]

A full neurologic examination is mandatory for patients with mild TBI. The sensory examination includes evaluation of the ability to detect pinprick, position, vibration, and light touch. Tests of cerebellar function include balance and tandem walking, having the patient touch the finger to the examiner's finger and back to the nose, and having the patient slide the heel from the knee down the shin. Motor examination includes muscle strength testing of key muscle groups: biceps, triceps, hand grasp, finger extensors, quadriceps, and dorsi- and plantar-flexion of the feet. Strength is graded on a scale from 0 to 5 (Box 11-1).

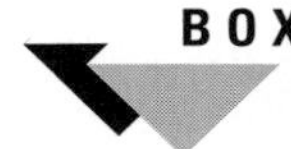

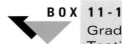

BOX 11-1
Grading of Muscle Strength Testing

0: Flaccid
1: Flickering movement
2: Movement with gravity eliminated
3: Movement against gravity
4: Movement against some resistance
5: Normal strength

Imaging of Traumatic Brain Injury

COMPUTED TOMOGRAPHY

Nowhere has the impact of CT been more important than in the evaluation of TBI. CT provides anatomic and pathologic information used to classify TBI and determine the need for emergent craniotomy. The availability of head CT has reduced morbidity and mortality, as well as the need for surgical exploration.[36,52]

In addition to defining intracranial hemorrhage and hematomas, head CT detects edema and mass effect, cerebral contusions, skull fractures, pneumocephali, and in some cases, cerebral infarctions.[53] With newer machines the imaging time is under 2 minutes. Newer scanners provide high resolution that detects small hemorrhages and edema. CT findings associated with worse outcome include midline shift >5 mm, compression of the cisterns, and high- or mixed-density lesions with a volume of blood >25 ml.[54] Brain edema can be quantified by a technique called tomodensitometry.[55] The initial brain CT scan should be done without intravenous (IV) contrast, since contrast obscures the evaluation of blood. Contrast administration may mimic a posttraumatic SAH.

CT is the cornerstone of the initial evaluation of all severe or moderate TBI patients. It can rapidly detect a surgical lesion and prompt intervention. If CT is not available at the presenting institution, the seriously injured patient should be transferred immediately to a medical center where emergent head CT and neurosurgical back up are available. For patients with mild TBI, selective use of head CT conserves healthcare resources. High-yield criteria have been developed for head CT in mild TBI.[56-62] These criteria recommend head CT for all TBI patients who have a GCS <15, and for those patients with a GCS of 15 who have a history of prolonged unconsciousness (>5 minutes), severe headache, recurrent vomiting, or are alcohol-intoxicated with signs of head trauma. Other trauma care providers recommend brain CT for any patient with evidence of mild TBI who will require general anesthesia for operative repair of other injuries, even if the GCS is 15. Many case reports document subsequent neurologic deterioration requiring surgery in patients classified as low-yield for head CT. The cost/benefit analysis for determining whether or not to perform head CT on mild TBI patients must consider costs of long-term care for missed injury, potential litigation, as well as the cost of hospitalizing mild TBI patients.[58-60,63]

Some authors suggest scanning the upper cervical vertebrae in any patient in coma. Routine imaging of the upper cervical vertebrae may demonstrate fractures undetected by plain films.[64,65] A CT scan of the cervical spine should be obtained for any areas that remain in question after plain radiographs are completed.

CT has some limitations that are more of a concern in the long-term care of the TBI patient than in the ED. CT has low-contrast resolution, so while good at detecting hemorrhages, CT is poor at defining nonhemorrhagic areas such as diffuse axonal shear. This limitation explains the common finding of a TBI patient with a low GCS despite a relatively normal CT.[36] For this reason, the initial brain CT may not correlate with the eventual neurologic outcome. Plain CT also does not define the functional or metabolic status of the brain or provide information on blood flow.

MAGNETIC RESONANCE IMAGING

Magnetic resonance imaging (MRI) is available in most medical centers and better defines nonhemorrhagic lesions. DAI, cortical contusions, subcortical gray matter injury, and brainstem lesions are all readily seen on MRI.[36,66] Unfortunately, MRI cannot predict neurologic outcome in TBI.[36,67]

MRI is not necessary in the emergency management of traumatic brain injury. MRI is less accurate than CT in defining hemorrhages. It is not as convenient, takes longer to perform, is more expensive, and requires special nonferrous monitoring equipment. One study found brain CT required an average time of 2 to 5 minutes, while MRI took 45 minutes.[67] Early MRI findings do not lead to changes in management.

PLAIN RADIOGRAPHS

Skull radiographs have a limited (some say no) place in evaluation of TBI. The presence of a skull fracture does not predict intracranial injury.[58] Radiographs may be of some value in infants suspected of being abused.

Laboratory Testing in Traumatic Brain Injury

Other tests that may assist in the evaluation of TBI include arterial blood gases (ABGs), ethanol levels, drug screens, electrolytes, and a complete blood count. A bedside glucose should be routine for all blunt trauma patients with altered mental status. The physician may assume coma is due to head trauma when in reality a hypoglycemic reaction precipitated the fall or MVC.[68] A bedside test for hypoglycemia will obviate a frantic run to the CT suite.

An ABG provides information on oxygenation, ventilation, and perfusion of the TBI patient. Serum electrolytes are typically normal in trauma patients. Persistent hyperglycemia may adversely affect cerebral metabolism and should be monitored and treated if necessary.[69] Although a blood alcohol level and a drug of abuse screen determines whether or not the patient is intoxicated, these tests do not rule out concurrent TBI. However, a low blood alcohol level is helpful in excluding intoxication as a cause of altered mental status. Altered mental status should be attributed to intoxication in the trauma patient only after other diagnoses have been excluded.

EMERGENCY DEPARTMENT MANAGEMENT

Management concentrates on preventing secondary injury. Early recognition and treatment of hypoperfusion, hypoxemia, and elevated ICP promote good outcomes.[15,17,18] In 1995 the Brain Trauma Foundation published Guidelines for the Management of Severe Head Injury.[70] Using a multidisciplinary, evidence-based approach, these guidelines were the first comprehensive, authoritative review of clinical management of TBI. Much of the following discussion is derived from this source. Fig. 11-8 summarizes the emergency management of the TBI patient.

Airway Management and Ventilation

The pathogenesis of TBI is closely linked to brain oxygenation. In compromised patients prehospital care providers must choose between forced oral intubation, nasotracheal intubation, or assisting ventilation with a bag-valve mask apparatus. The risk of increasing ICP during endotracheal intubation in a nonsedated, nonparalyzed patient must be weighed against the risk of ongoing hypoxia. Other considerations are the likelihood of vomiting, aspiration, and possible cervical spine injury.

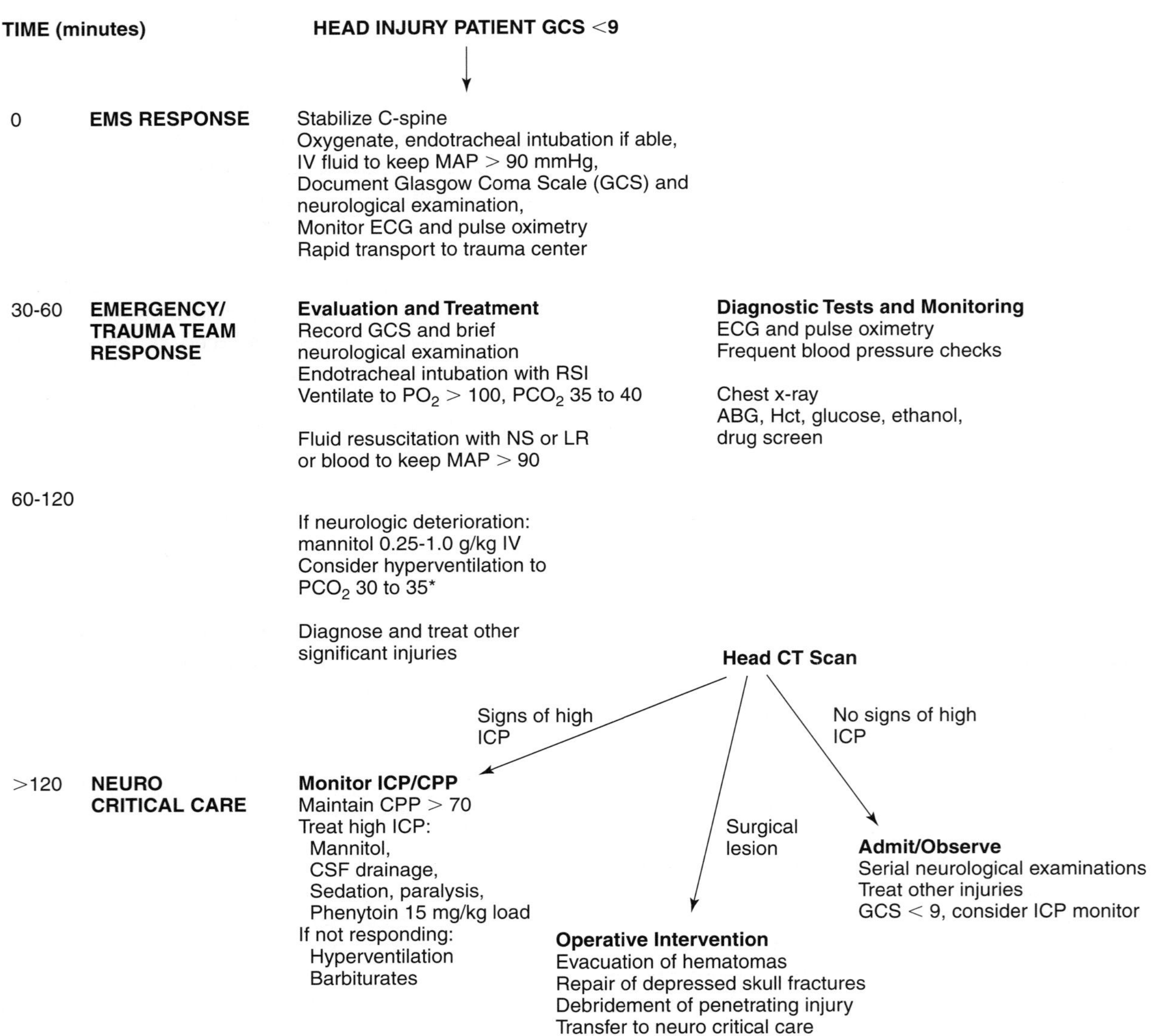

Fig. 11-8 Emergency management of the traumatic brain injury patient.

ENDOTRACHEAL INTUBATION

Endotracheal intubation is the preferred method of maintaining proper oxygenation and protecting the airway from aspiration in patients with serious TBI.[71] Endotracheal intubation is indicated in any patient with a GCS score <9, and perhaps, in any patient who cannot follow commands.[72] TBI patients with a GCS ≥9 may be initially managed without endotracheal intubation if proper oxygenation is ensured, during continuous monitoring of hypoxemia and hypoventilation. The best method for emergency endotracheal intubation in multiple trauma and TBI patients is controversial. In the past decade rapid sequence intubation (RSI) has emerged as the best method for immediate airway control in serious TBI patients.[73-76]

The technique for RSI has been described elsewhere.[76,77] A number of issues require consideration when performing RSI in the TBI patient. A very rapid neurologic examination, noting movement of the extremities and the GCS, should occur before the administration of paralyzing agents. Occasionally, the airway needs of a patient in extremis may take precedence over this examination. Document any focal signs. The selection of paralytic and induction agents for RSI is aimed at rapidly providing good intubating conditions without adversely affecting ICP or cerebral perfusion pressure. Available induction agents that render rapid unconsciousness while maintaining cerebral perfusion and preventing increased ICP include thiopental, etomidate, and fentanyl. Etomidate has the least potential for inducing systemic hypotension and is preferred over thiopental and fentanyl in hemodynamically unstable multiple-trauma patients.[78] Barbiturates may precipitate dangerous hypotension in patients with blood loss.

Most RSI protocols use succinylcholine for paralysis. Although concern has been raised over the risk of increased ICP with succinylcholine, there are no convincing data to substantiate this claim.[76,79] Most induction agents may ablate the transient increase in ICP caused by laryngoscopy. Lidocaine, 1.5 to 2 mg IV push, administered 2 to 3 minutes before succinylcholine may prevent ICP rises resulting from laryngoscopy and succinylcholine, although no controlled studies have been done to support this practice.[76] A small dose of a nondepolarizing agent before succinylcholine may also prevent fasciculations and limit ICP increases during intubation. Although nondepolarizing neuromuscular blockers can be primary agents for emergency intubation, they do not provide rapid intubating conditions, and have a much longer duration of action. The resultant prolonged paralysis makes it difficult to assess the neurologic condition of the TBI patient.[76] However, if patients need to be chemically paralyzed to accomplish the performance of procedures (such as CT scanning), repeat boluses can be given at 30- to 40-minute intervals, assessing neurologic function in between dosing.

TBI is a risk factor for cervical spine injury. The incidence of cervical spine injury in serious TBI patients (GCS ≤8) is around 7%, compared with about 1% to 2% in all multiple-trauma patients.[47] Minimize neck movement during airway management in TBI patients. The current standard of care, based on a limited number of studies, is in-line stabilization of the neck with the patient in a rigid cervical collar. Traction on the neck should be avoided.[80,81] The optimal intubation technique has been debated, with no clear consensus. Clinical series find no detrimental effects when RSI is used in patients with cervical spine injuries.[76,82,83]

After intubation, the focus shifts to oxygenation and ventilation. The level of pO_2 needed to ensure adequate oxygenation is in the range of 100 to 120 torr. It is not known if increasing the inspired oxygen concentration to maintain pO_2 greater than 100 torr is beneficial or detrimental in TBI.

HYPERVENTILATION

The use of mechanical hyperventilation to lower pCO_2 and reduce ICP has long been part of therapy in serious TBI. Hypocapnia decreases ICP through constriction of cerebral vasculature and reduces blood volume in the brain. The converse is also true—increased pCO_2 leads to increased cerebral blood volume. The magnitude of this effect has been reported to be a 4% change in CBF for every 1 mmHg change in pCO_2.[84] Since CBF is one of the main determinants of ICP, lowering CBF will usually lower ICP. Regional differences have been found, with the cerebrum most sensitive to pCO_2 and the cerebellum less responsive.[84,85] The degree of ICP reduction in response to hyperventilation is variable and disappears over time. Within hours, alkalosis induced by hyperventilation stimulates the kidney to excrete bicarbonate and retain hydrogen ions, normalizing blood pH and subsequently CBF.[84,86]

In the past, patients with a GCS of ≤8 were routinely hyperventilated. Studies show that routine hyperventilation leads to worse outcomes in such patients.[87] For this reason, routine use of hyperventilation is no longer indicated in patients with severe TBI. If pCO_2 is decreased below 25 mmHg, CBF may decrease to the point where some regions of the injured brain become ischemic. If pCO_2 falls below 20 mmHg, severe cerebral vasoconstriction can produce widespread ischemia.[70,86]

In the prehospital or ED setting, when the ICP is unknown, the use of hyperventilation can be hazardous. Inadvertent hyperventilation occurs in prehospital transport and during intrahospital or interhospital transfers from overzealous bag-valve mask ventilations. *The BTF Guidelines recommend the use of hyperventilation only if the patient is experiencing herniation or neurologic deterioration that is unresponsive to adequate resuscitation and mannitol.* The pCO_2 should be maintained in the 35 to 40 torr range. If hyperventilation is to be used, the initial target pCO_2 is 30 to 35 torr, and requires frequent monitoring of ABGs or end-tidal CO_2 concentration. Hyperventilation to a pCO_2 below 30 torr is only a last resort for uncontrolled high ICP or impending herniation. The response to hyperventilation depends on the degree of ICP elevation and the time after injury. In general, hyperventilation loses effectiveness within 24 to 48 hours. At this point, the pCO_2 can be slowly normalized. Marked ICP increases may occur with discontinuation of prolonged hyperventilation.[70,85,86,88]

Cardiovascular and Cerebral Resuscitation

The maintenance of CPP above 70 mmHg is a cornerstone of management of TBI.[89] During prehospital and emergency care, ICP is not usually known, so rely on measurement of MAP. In this imperfect situation, MAP should be maintained in the range of 90 to 100 mmHg, allowing adequate CPP even if ICP climbs to 20 to 30 mmHg. Fluid restriction for TBI patients is dangerous, particularly in emergency management.[90,91] Up to 75% of TBI patients have serious injuries to other organ systems that require fluid therapy.[11,15]

INTRAVENOUS FLUID THERAPY

The choice of resuscitation fluid in TBI patients remains controversial. In the acute TBI patient with no evidence of shock, standard IV crystalloid solutions (normal saline or lactated Ringer's solution) provide maintenance requirements. Despite recent literature on hypotensive resuscitation, most resuscitation protocols suggest infusion of 10 to 20 ml/kg of crystalloid, followed by administration of blood if shock persists.[92,93] Unless hypoglycemia is documented, glucose-containing solutions are not recommended for fluid resuscitation in TBI.

Hypertonic Saline. In the TBI patient, concerns over elevated ICP and brain edema have sparked interest in alternative resuscitation fluids, such as hypertonic saline. Hypertonic saline is usually administered as a small bolus of 7.5% saline. In hemorrhagic shock it improves hemodynamics and increases oxygen delivery.[94,95] At the same time, hypertonic saline may cause osmotic shifts in the brain. These shifts can limit edema and decrease ICP.[95] The effects of hypertonic saline are transient,[91] but when combined with dextran, the results are prolonged.[96] The consequences of hypertonic saline on the brain depend on the integrity of the BBB. If the BBB is intact, osmotic shifts occur, and hypertonic saline may be helpful. However, if the BBB is damaged and normal ionic gradients are lost, hypertonic saline does not produce osmotic effects. In this setting, hypertonic saline may exacerbate brain edema by increasing systemic arterial pressure and CBF. At least one animal study has raised concern that hypertonic saline may injure the BBB.[97] Although hypertonic saline may produce desirable changes in the injured brain, more extensive clinical studies are needed.

Blood Products. Blood products are needed in the resuscitation of TBI only if severe hemorrhage or coagulopathy is present. When the hemoglobin drops below 6 to 8 g/dl, cerebral oxygen delivery (DO_2) may be compromised. The brain can increase oxygen extraction if cerebral DO_2 drops, up to a maximum of 70%. The brain's ability to extract oxygen makes it fairly tolerant to anemia, particularly if it develops slowly.[91] In hemorrhagic shock, the drop in CBF to critically low levels is more a factor in reducing DO_2 than is the reduction in hemoglobin. The decision to give blood to TBI patients is based more on other injuries. The emphasis for cerebral resuscitation is to optimize CPP and cerebral DO_2.

Pharmacologic Treatment

A number of pharmacologic agents have shown promise in improving outcome in animal models of TBI. However, to date, the number of pharmacologic agents available to treat TBI in humans is limited. None of these agents modulate the neurochemical response to TBI. Rather, drugs reduce ICP and control clinical consequences such as agitation and seizures.

OSMOTIC AGENTS

Mannitol is the most commonly used osmotically active agent for reducing ICP in TBI patients. Mannitol can favorably affect cerebral perfusion by lowering ICP and increasing MAP.[98,99] The mechanism of action likely involves an immediate effect on cerebral hemodynamics, followed by a delayed effect on brain edema. IV mannitol increases oncotic pressure in the intravascular compartment, leading to a transient rise in central venous pressure and MAP. The hyperosmolar state may stimulate myocardial contractility.[100-102] This early increase in cardiac output, MAP, and thus CPP, does not translate into increased ICP.[48,98,99,103,104] In fact, mannitol lowers ICP, sometimes within minutes of administration. By augmenting CPP, mannitol vasoconstricts the cerebral vasculature and thus reduces cerebral blood volume and ICP.[89,99] Mannitol may also diminish blood viscosity and alter red blood cells. Less viscous blood carries more oxygen.

When administered as a rapid IV infusion or bolus, mannitol reduces ICP by forming an osmotic gradient across the BBB. Brain water moves across this gradient into the intravascular space. The source of brain water includes neurons, glial cells, brain extracellular fluid, and possibly CSF.[105-107] The maximal effect occurs within 30 to 60 minutes. The optimal dose and regimen for mannitol administration is debated. Doses of 0.25 to 1.0 gm/kg effectively lower ICP and doses on the lower end are as effective as higher doses.[108,109] The most commonly recommended regimen is 0.25 to 1.0 gm/kg given every 4 to 6 hours to maintain ICP in a normal range.[107-109]

Because mannitol can produce an osmotic diuresis, patients should be volume resuscitated with blood or crystalloid before administration. If the TBI patient develops deepening coma, new focal neurologic signs, or anisocoria, a presumptive diagnosis of increasing ICP may be made, and mannitol administration is reasonable. Otherwise, mannitol can be deferred until the CT scan result is known and neurosurgical consultation is available.[70]

Serum osmolality increases to 310 to 320 mOsm with a standard dose of mannitol. An increase of at least 10 mOsm is needed to decrease ICP. If ICP is not controlled with these doses, a continuous infusion may be used at 6 gm/hr. However, studies have found a more beneficial effect with bolus dosing as opposed to a continuous infusion. With higher doses or prolonged infusion, a hyperosmolar state will harm other organs. Therefore use of mannitol mandates frequent evaluation of serum osmolality and electrolytes. In the intensive care unit setting, these evaluations are typically done every 4 hours. Serum osmolality exceeding 320 mOsm places the kidneys at increased risk for acute tubular necrosis. In such cases, mannitol should be discontinued and other therapies instituted.[108-110]

Some authors express concern regarding cardiovascular collapse from mannitol-induced diuresis in patients with concurrent hemorrhagic shock. However, numerous animal studies fail to demonstrate this purported deleterious effect. In these studies mannitol actually improved cardiac index and CPP in animals with elevated ICP and hemorrhagic shock.[100,111-113] One study found indirect evidence that IV mannitol maintained or increased CBF while reducing ICP, compared with hyperventilation that simultaneously reduced ICP and CBF.[114] In an animal model of epidural hematoma, mannitol increased regional CBF without leading to changes in tissue edema or cerebral perfusion.[115] Others worry that mannitol may stimulate new bleeding in TBI patients with traumatic SDH. Proponents of this theory hypothesize that as the brain shrinks from mannitol, a previously tamponaded bleed becomes worse. However, mannitol administration does not induce large shifts in brain matter that could initiate new bleeding. Most convincingly, no investigations or case reports have ever been published that demonstrate this hypothetical concern. Although it is clear that definitive care for traumatic SDH with mass effect is emergent craniotomy, mannitol may be used as a temporizing measure in these cases.

DIURETICS

Loop diuretics have been used as adjuncts to mannitol in reducing brain water and ICP.[116-118] Furosemide decreases total body water and may secondarily reduce brain water content, leading to decreased ICP. Furosemide may also decrease the formation of CSF. The theoretic advantage of using furosemide in conjunction or alternately with mannitol is that furosemide can accentuate mannitol's effect by generating a gradient at the distal renal tubules.[119] This combination achieves a prolonged reduction of ICP, making a hyperosmolar state less likely. The usual dose of furosemide is 10 to 20 mg IV bolus. In the emergency management of TBI, the addition of furosemide to mannitol is probably not necessary unless mannitol alone is not effective, or a marked hyperosmolar state occurs early.

STEROIDS

The use of steroids for TBI has been debated for over two decades.[120] The most recent clinical trials show no benefit of steroids in severe TBI patients (i.e., patients presenting with a GCS ≤8).[121-125] Although steroids can lessen cerebral edema in other situations, they do not reduce edema associated with TBI. Possible disadvantages include increased infections (especially pneumonia), altered fluid and glucose balance, and adrenocortical suppression. The BTF Guidelines recommend *against* the use of glucocorticoids in the severe TBI patient.[70]

SEDATIVE/HYPNOTICS

Many severe TBI patients are agitated, combative, and restless. Straining and resisting the ventilator can lead to dangerous increases in ICP. Nursing care and physiologic monitoring can be very difficult in this setting. Intravenous sedative/hypnotic agents may reduce agitation and limit ICP spikes. Although TBI patients may be comatose, they perceive pain as demonstrated by hemodynamic and ICP changes when painful stimuli occur. Pain medication should be provided to TBI patients, especially those with concurrent painful injuries. Opiate agents such as morphine and fentanyl may be used in bolus doses or as infusions. Fentanyl may have less hemodynamic effects than morphine and has a much shorter half-life, making it a better agent.[126]

Benzodiazepines control agitation and are commonly used as sedative agents for TBI patients. These agents act on brain GABA receptors to stimulate the activity of inhibitory neurons. They have minimal hemodynamic effects, but may induce respiratory depression. Benzodiazepines do not directly reduce ICP. In the emergency setting midazolam is a good choice for managing agitation in TBI patients.[127] With long-term use, benzodiazepines produce prolonged obtundation.

Although the effects of both opiates and benzodiazepines can be rapidly reversed by administration of specific receptor antagonist agents (naloxone and flumazenil, respectively), this practice is dangerous in the TBI patient. Stimulation of the CNS results, increasing ICP and agitation. Sedative/hypnotic agents should be slowly tapered to prevent this rebound phenomenon.[128]

Although barbiturates have been advocated for use in TBI, clinical trials have not demonstrated improved outcome.[129-131] Barbiturates are sometimes used to induce a deep coma in severe TBI. One study showed that pentobarbital limited ICP spikes in severe TBI.[128,132] In the ED however, barbiturates are not usually indicated and do not provide any clear benefits.[128] Barbiturate-induced coma in an intensive care unit is a last resort after other measures to control high ICP have failed.[70]

Propofol is a newer IV sedative/hypnotic with CNS depressant effects similar to barbiturates, but with a short duration of action. Propofol infusion provides deep sedation in TBI patients who are monitored in an ICU setting. Recovery from the sedative effects is faster than with the benzodiazepines. Unfortunately, propofol produces dose-dependent hemodynamic and respiratory depression, and is not recommended for the hemodynamically unstable.[128,133]

PARALYTIC AGENTS

Neuromuscular blockers (NMBs) are often used to prevent otherwise uncontrollable straining movements. The rationale for use is that excessive motor activity leads to increased MAP and thus ICP. The use of nondepolarizing NMBs such as vecuronium, pancuronium, and atracurium to provide continuous paralysis has become standard.[76] In the ED neuromuscular blockade can hasten diagnostic and therapeutic maneuvers, and in particular, CT scanning. Unfortunately these agents conceal changes in neurologic examination. Vecuronium, atracurium, mivacurium, and rocuronium in standard doses induce paralysis for 20 to 40 minutes. The duration of paralysis varies with the agent, dose, and hemodynamic state of the patient. Pancuronium has a longer duration of action, usually greater than 1 hour, and often causes tachycardia.

Recent authors question the use of continued paralysis for TBI patients in the ICU.[134,135] A retrospective study found that routine early paralysis of TBI patients was associated with longer ICU stays and increased pneumonia.[134] Short-term paralysis during the ED management of TBI patients has not been demonstrated to have adverse effects. At this point in time, there is no contraindication to short-term paralysis in the ED.

ANTICONVULSANTS

The BTF guidelines suggest that anticonvulsants are an *option* that may prevent *early* posttraumatic seizures in patients at high risk. High risk includes those patients with:

1. GCS score <10
2. Cortical contusion
3. Depressed skull fracture
4. Subdural hematoma
5. Epidural hematoma
6. Intracerebral hematoma
7. Penetrating head wound
8. Seizure within 24 hours of injury

Both phenytoin and carbamazepine prevent early posttraumatic seizures; however, there is no evidence that they improve outcome following head injury. Seizure activity in the acute TBI patient is treated the same as in the nontrauma patient. Intravenous benzodiazepines are first-line agents. Lorazepam (2 to 4 mg IVP) or diazepam (5 mg IVP) may be used every 5 minutes until the seizure stops or to a maximum of 8 to 10 mg for lorazepam or 20 mg for diazepam. Beyond these doses, additional benzodiazepines are unlikely to be effective, and another agent should be considered. Benzodiazepines cause dose-dependent respiratory depression, which may prompt the need for intubation. In the hemodynamically unstable patient, benzodiazepines may cause cardiovascular depression. If benzodiazepines are not effective in stopping seizures, barbiturates are the next line of treatment.

Phenytoin may prevent further seizures and is administered as soon as possible after the seizure starts. Intravenous loading of phenytoin (15 mg/kg) must be given no faster than 50 mg/min, limiting its usefulness in the acute situation. In a TBI patient with frequent seizures or status epilepticus, more rapid loading may be achieved by using fos-phenytoin.[23,136] Phenytoin is often administered prophylactically for serious TBI patients, especially if a focal lesion is identified on CT scan. Other than the potential for transient hypotension during infusion, phenytoin administration has no known adverse effects in TBI patients.

Surgical Treatment

Emergency craniotomy provides definitive care for significant traumatic epidural and subdural hematomas. Forty percent of TBI patients who are not able to follow commands (GCS ≤9) have an intracranial hematoma and many need emergent surgery.[17,60,124] A study of patients with acute SDH found an inverse relationship between length of time to operation and mortality. Comatose patients who were operated on within 4 hours after injury had a significantly better outcome.[137] Failure to promptly diagnose and treat EDH may also lead to disaster. Patients with EDH do better than those with SDH, mostly because EDH is less commonly associated with parenchymal injuries.

The indications for surgery in TBI include a large expanding mass lesion (EDH, SDH, focal contusion, or intracerebral hemorrhage), a penetrating injury, a significantly depressed skull fracture, or clinical deterioration in a patient with a mass lesion. Emergency craniotomy has two main benefits. The first is to remove the mass and the second is to clean and débride contaminated penetrating wounds. Standard surgical technique for SDH and EDH includes an initial small craniotomy for immediate removal of clot, followed by a larger craniectomy flap to completely evacuate the hematoma and control bleeding.[138]

Although it is imperative to obtain a rapid brain CT scan in the severely injured TBI patient, the scan may conflict with other needs. The decision to undertake emergent CT scanning before emergent laparotomy depends on a case-by-case appraisal of clinical circumstances. Chapter 19 discusses the priorities in management for patients with both intracranial and intraabdominal injuries.

EMERGENCY BURR HOLE

On very rare occasions an emergency craniotomy or burr hole may be indicated in a decompensating TBI patient.[139,140] The indications include a rapidly deteriorating patient who is herniating, a relative certainty of an expanding EDH or SDH, and an expected long delay in neurosurgical care. In this situation a physician familiar with the technique of emergency craniotomy may prevent death. In most circumstances, impending herniation is signaled by dilatation of the pupil on the same side as the mass lesion. Other measures to reduce ICP should be first attempted, including mannitol and hyperventilation. If these measures fail, a burr hole may be the only alternative.

The emergency burr hole is placed in the temporal region on the same side as the dilated pupil. The landmark for the initial incision is a point approximately 6 cm anterior and 6 cm superior to the tragus of the ear. Make the initial vertical incision through the scalp superior to the superficial temporal artery, to avoid excessive hemorrhage. Once the galea is incised, a rotary drill or twist drill is used to make a hole in the skull. Both the outer and inner tables must be traversed before the dura is visible. If an EDH is present, frank arterial hemorrhage or clot will be encountered above the dura and must be suctioned. If an SDH is present, it appears as a blue mass beneath the bulging dura. In this case, the dura can be incised with a scalpel and subdural blood drained or suctioned. If an initial "dry" hole is made, drill additional burr holes superiorly to the original in the frontal and parietal regions of the ipsilateral skull. If these secondary holes do not reveal hematoma, reevaluate the diagnosis. If impending herniation appears likely, a burr hole can tap the contralateral skull. Cover the burr hole with a sterile, nonocclusive bandage before patient transfer.[139,140]

Monitoring

Prevention of secondary brain injury is a major goal of emergency management of TBI. Factors that produce secondary injury may be most active in the first hours after injury and may be iatrogenic. Careful monitoring of the TBI patient can identify the threats.[72,141] Monitoring can range from frequent checks of vital signs, neurologic examination, and GCS to measurement of ICP with an intraventricular catheter. The complexity of monitoring should increase with the severity of brain injury.

BASIC MONITORING

Prehospital and ambulance data recording and monitoring is an integral part of early management. In the prehospital setting, it is possible to perform serial GCS and vital signs, pulse oximetry, and cardiac monitoring. In the ED, monitoring is expanded to include temperature, automated blood pressure readings, serial ABGs, continuous oxygen saturation measurement, and urine output. Portable devices to measure blood glucose are useful. The use of an arterial catheter to continuously measure systemic blood pressure can calculate MAP. This port can also be used for serial blood draws. End-tidal CO_2 measurement can assess the effects of mechanical ventilation. The need for a central line is based more on the patient's other injuries and co-morbid disease than on the head trauma. An elderly TBI patient with circulatory shock may require central hemodynamic monitoring with a pulmonary artery thermodilution catheter.

INTRACRANIAL PRESSURE MONITORING

Effective management of increased ICP lowers mortality and morbidity from TBI.[14,89,99,141-143] In severe TBI patients, continuous monitoring of ICP and CPP is an essential element of care. Monitoring of ICP with an intraventricular catheter was pioneered in the mid 1960s.[144] The main issues involve identification of patients who will benefit from ICP monitoring, choosing a monitoring method and system, and deciding if monitoring should be initiated in the emergency setting. Severe TBI patients are likely to have increased ICP and may benefit most from early ICP monitoring. In general, patients with a GCS score of ≤8 who have abnormalities on initial head CT scan are the best candidates. In patients who have higher GCS scores, or who have minimal findings on initial CT scan, the decision regarding ICP monitors can be difficult. One study found that subsequent ICP elevation was more likely to occur in TBI patients who had "normal" CT scans when the age was over 40 years, systolic blood pressure was <90 on admission, or motor posturing was present. These investigators recommend ICP monitoring for patients who have all three of these characteristics.[145]

Common methods to monitor ICP include ventriculostomy or placement of fiberoptic catheters intraparenchymally. Ventriculostomy has the advantage of being able to drain off CSF. Hemorrhage is a possible complication, since many TBI patients are coagulopathic from release of brain tissue thromboplastin. Candidates for ICP monitor placement should have coagulation studies evaluated before placement. Another major complication is infection and is directly proportional to the time the catheter is left in place.[142,146,147]

The decision to monitor ICP in the ED must be made on a case-by-case basis. The benefits of having continuous data on CPP and ICP must be weighed against the delay that the procedure introduces. In the unstable multiple-trauma patient with TBI, it may be best to expedite the ED work-up. Prompt transfer to the ICU allows for definitive monitoring.

CUTTING EDGE
Cerebral Oxygenation and Brain Tissue PO_2 Monitoring

Although ICP monitoring has become standard for severe TBI patients, ICP and CPP alone provide little information on CBF or brain metabolic function. Other methods include jugular venous oxygen saturation (SvO_2) monitoring. Jugular SvO_2 readings below 50% are associated with cerebral ischemia. A falling SvO_2 indicates inadequate cerebral perfusion.[148]

Brain tissue pO_2 monitoring awaits final approval for use in the United States but has been used in other countries. A probe placed in the brain parenchyma contains an oximetric electrode capable of measuring adjacent tissue pO_2. Brain tissue pO_2 levels correlate well with regional CBF, and falling tissue pO_2 may indicate cerebral ischemia.[149,150] If a combination ICP/tissue pO_2 catheter becomes available, it is conceivable that this type of monitoring could be placed in the ED.

Other Cerebral Monitoring Methods

The search for clinically feasible, noninvasive methods for assessing CBF and elevated ICP has intensified over the past decade. **Transcranial Doppler sonography** (TCDS) has the potential to measure cerebral hemodynamics. With this technique, an ultrasound probe placed over thin areas of the cranium detects blood velocity in underlying vessels. By adjusting the depth of insonation, Doppler ultrasound provides an indirect measure of flow through the target vessel. TCDS may assess large reductions in blood flow to an area of the brain. For instance, in patients with large traumatic SDH, TCDS flow signals may be significantly lower on the side of the hematoma.[151-153] Transcranial Doppler studies may also evaluate cerebral autoregulation and the responsiveness to hyperventilation. TCDS can detect vasospasm in patients with nontraumatic subarachnoid hemorrhage[147,151,152] and has also been investigated in TBI patients.[154] TCDS may also provide clues to traumatic dissection of the carotid artery. Although no studies have been reported on the use of TCDS in the ED care of TBI patients, the portable and noninvasive nature of this technique makes it attractive for emergency use.

A promising method for assessing CBF in the ED is stable **xenon-enhanced computed tomography** (Xe-CT). TBI patients studied within 3 hours after injury with this technique demonstrated regional areas of decreased CBF.[155-159] Other methods for assessing CBF using radioactive compounds with portable imaging devices or **single photon emission CT** (SPECT) scanning have been described. SPECT with technetium-99m hexamethylpropyleneamine oxime (HMPAO) imaging reliably measures gross regional CBF, but does not provide anatomic detail or spatial resolution.[36,160,161] **Contrast-enhanced magnetic resonance perfusion imaging** may be better than SPECT Tc-99m HMPAO imaging for correlating blood flow changes with anatomic injury.[36,160,162]

The **Kety-Schmidt nitrous oxide saturation method** is another way of assessing CBF in patients with severe TBI. The technique can be done at the bedside but is fairly labor intensive and cannot measure regional blood flow differences.[163] Although information on CBF is desirable, most centers are not routinely assessing this parameter. Hopefully, technologic advances in the next decade will make it possible to acutely image the injured brain to evaluate anatomic injury, CBF, and metabolic changes.

Monitoring to Asses Brain Death

A subset of severe TBI patients may lose brain function in the early postinjury period. In these patients, determination of "brain death" guides further management, including organ procurement. Brain death can be defined clinically as the absence of spontaneous respiration and brainstem reflexes in a normothermic patient. In the setting of trauma, brain death is usually the result of severe intracranial hypertension with diffuse brain ischemia and cessation of CBF. The apnea test is used in many centers. In hospitals where TCDS is available, it may also assist in brain death determination. Just before brain death, the transcranial ultrasound signal becomes increasingly pulsatile, and then is no longer detectable when CBF ceases.[147] Xe-CT is also a useful method for documenting that CBF is absent, but this technology is not universally available.[159] A traditional method for determining brain death is with an electroencephalogram (EEG) that shows no brain electrical activity.

DISPOSITION

Since it is clear that all severe TBI patients require admission to the hospital, the main issues with disposition center around transfer and definitive care. TBI patients require specialized care. Care is best delivered in a medical center with trained neurocritical care providers and comprehensive monitoring and imaging. The effects of secondary injury begin soon after TBI. Therefore the expeditious transfer of a severe TBI patient to such a facility plays a crucial role. The primary role of prehospital providers and physicians at transferring hospitals is to carefully guard against hypoxemia and hypotension. The severe TBI patient should be endotracheally intubated and adequately resuscitated before transfer. One mistake frequently made by smaller hospitals is delay in transfer. All patients with severe TBI require neurosurgical evaluation regardless of the CT scan. A comatose trauma victim should probably not have a CT scan if that hospital does not have a neurosurgeon, unless (1) there is a potential for delayed transfer, in this situation an EP may need to perform a burr hole for a large EDH or SDH; or (2) the patient needs urgent laparotomy before transfer and has lateralizing findings on neurologic examination.

Disposition decisions are much more complicated in less severely injured patients. These patients have continued altered mental status (GCS <15), an abnormal head CT, or persistent neurologic findings following ED evaluation. For such patients, prolonged observation or hospitalization for frequent neurologic examinations is appropriate. Patients with a mild TBI, GCS of 15, a normal head CT, and a normal neurologic examination may be discharged from the ED to the care of a responsible adult. Patients with a normal CT and a normal discharge neurologic examination are unlikely to experience neurologic deterioration. Some researchers feel that the significant incidence of neuropsychiatric deficits following mild TBI mandates follow-up in a brain rehabilitation setting for further testing and management of continuing problems.[164] However, studies have not determined who is likely to benefit from this referral. Until these data are available, patients who demonstrate persistent memory deficits, behavioral change, headaches, dizziness, and visual or hearing changes in the ED should be referred for further care. On discharge from the ED, the patient with mild TBI should be given a list of warning signs for more severe TBI, and should be discharged under the care of a competent adult who can observe the patient for the next day (Fig. 11-9).[39-41,43,61]

SUGGESTED CLINICAL PATHWAYS

The Brain Trauma Foundation Guidelines for the Management of Severe Head Injury include two algorithms that apply directly to emergency care. The first is on initial resuscitation and the second on treatment of intracranial hypertension. Adaptations of these algorithms are presented in Fig. 11-8. The management of mild TBI is summarized in Fig. 11-9. TBI is usually one component of serious injuries in the multiple-trauma patient. The approach to the TBI patient is multidisciplinary, extending from paramedical providers to emergency physicians, trauma surgeons, neurosurgeons, other surgical subspecialists, and finally to rehabilitation specialists. Although physicians must function as a coordinated team, nurses provide the majority of bedside management of TBI. Improvements in TBI outcome over the past two decades are largely attributable to specially trained critical care nurses who can effectively manage the dynamic changes that occur in a seriously ill trauma patient. It is imperative that providers who are trained in management of TBI educate those who are not yet aware of the advances outlined in the BTF Guidelines.

CONTROVERSIES AND FUTURE DIRECTIONS

Some of the classic controversies in TBI management have recently been laid to rest, including the role of hyperventilation and the use of steroids. Recently a debate has emerged over whether TBI patients are best managed by carefully controlling ICP or by maintaining CPP at a desirable level. A number of studies are ongoing to address this issue. Preliminary results suggest that use of IV fluids alone to maintain CPP may result in an increase in ARDS.[165]

Studies on the treatment of TBI with moderate hypothermia are nearly completed, and the preliminary data suggest that cooling patients with isolated severe TBI to approximately 32° C for 24 hours postinjury may improve outcome.[166] Whether hypothermia could be successfully used in TBI patients with multiple trauma remains to be determined.

The ideal resuscitation fluid for the TBI patient also remains controversial. Hypertonic saline has been advocated for at least a decade, but no large studies prove it superior to standard IV fluids. Artificial blood

History

- Name, age, sex, race, occupation
- Mechanism of injury
- Time of injury
- Loss of consciousness immediately after injury
- Subsequent level of alertness
- Amnesia: retrograde, anterograde
- Headache: mild, moderate, severe
- Seizures

General examination to exclude systemic injuries

Limited neurological examination

Cervical spine and other radiographs as indicated

Blood alcohol level and urine toxic screen

Computed tomography (CT) scan of the head in all patients except completely asymptomatic and neurologically normal patients is ideal

Observe in/admit to hospital
- No CT scanner available
- Abnormal CT scan
- All penetrating head injuries
- History of loss of consciousness
- Deteriorating level of consciousness
- Moderate to severe headache
- Significant alcoholic/drug intoxication
- Skull fracture
- Cerebral spinal fluid leak rhinorrhea or otorrhea
- Significant associated injuries
- No reliable companion at home
- Unable to return promptly
- Amnesia

Discharge from hospital
- Patient does not meet any of the criteria for admission
- Discuss need to return if any problems develop and issue a "warning sheet"
- Schedule follow-up clinic visit, usually within 1 week

Fig. 11-9 Management of mild traumatic brain injury. (From Valadka AB, Narayan RK: Emergency room management of the head-injured patient. In Narayan RK, et al [editors]: *Neurotrauma*, New York, 1996, McGraw-Hill.)

products such as stroma-free hemoglobin are in clinical studies and have potential to ensure adequate oxygen delivery to the injured brain during shock.[167]

Preliminary studies in the 1980s and early 1990s found a number of agents with neuroprotective effects, igniting optimism.[168] Phase II clinical trials hinted that agents such as nimodipine, a calcium channel blocker, and the free radical scavenging agent PEG-superoxide dismutase (PEG-SOD) would show benefit.[169] Optimism has been replaced by disappointment, since nimodipine, PEG-SOD, tirilazad mesylate (a 21-amino-steroid with antioxidant effects), and selfotel, an NMDA receptor blocker, provided no benefit in multicenter, double-blind, Phase III clinical trials.[168,170-172] The reasons for the discrepancy between preclinical and clinical performance have been debated. One consideration is that animal brain injury models do not adequately simulate the pathophysiology of human TBI.

Given that the pathogenesis of TBI is multifactorial, it may be naive to think that single-drug therapy can significantly improve outcome. Multiple-drug treatment with a "neuroprotective cocktail" may offer a way to block various injury pathways.[173] However, the logistics of industry-sponsored clinical trials are not conducive to multiple-drug trials.

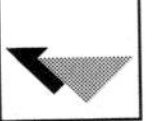

PEARLS & PITFALLS

- ◆ Avoid hypoxemia and hypotension in the early resuscitation of the TBI patient.
- ◆ Intubate the TBI patient with GCS <9 early in his or her ED course.
- ◆ Avoid pCO_2 levels below 35 torr unless signs of neurologic deterioration or herniation are seen.
- ◆ Pharmacologic treatment in the emergency setting should include the judicious use of mannitol, sedatives, and anticonvulsants.

- If paralytic agents must be used in the early management of TBI, select drugs and dosages to allow for neurologic checks at least every 30 minutes.
- Do not assume that mental status changes are due to intoxication since the risk of SDH and severe TBI may be increased in the alcoholic patient.
- Charts should reflect repeat neurologic examinations, management decisions, the role of consultants, and the disposition of the patient.

REFERENCES

1. Bennett BR, Jacobs LM, Schwarz RJ: Incidence, cost and DRG-based reimbursement for traumatic brain injured patients: a 3-year experience, *J Trauma* 29:556-565, 1989.
2. Van Zomeren AH and Saan RJ: Psychological and social sequelae of severe head injury. In Braakman R (editor): *Handbook of clinical neurology,* New York, 1990, Elsevier.
3. Kraus JF, et al: Epidemiology of brain injury. In Narayan RK, Wilberger JE, Povlishock JT (editors): *Neurotrauma,* New York, 1996, McGraw-Hill.
4. Kraus JF, et al: The incidence of acute brain injury and serious impairment in a defined population, *Am J Epidemiol* 119:186-201, 1984.
5. Brismar B, Engstrom A, Rydberg U: Head injury and intoxication: a diagnostic and therapeutic dilemma, *Acta Chir Scand* 149:11-14, 1983.
6. Edna TH: Alcohol influence and head injury, *Acta Chir Scand* 148: 209-212, 1982.
7. Gurney JG, et al: The effects of alcohol intoxication on the initial treatment and hospital course of patients with acute brain injury, *J Trauma* 33:709-713, 1992.
8. Jagger J, et al: Effect of alcohol intoxication on the diagnosis and apparent severity of brain injury, *Neurosurgery* 15:303-306, 1984.
9. Rimel R, et al: Moderate head injury: completing the clinical spectrum of brain trauma, *Neurosurgery* 11:344-351, 1982.
10. Zink BJ, Maio RF, Chen B: Alcohol, central nervous system injury, and time to death in fatal motor vehicle crashes, *Alcohol Clin Exp Res* 20:1518-1522, 1996.
11. Zink BJ: Traumatic brain injury, *Emerg Med Clin North Am* 14: 115-150, 1996.
12. Honkanen R, Smith G: Impact of acute alcohol intoxication on patterns of non-fatal trauma: cause-specific analysis of head injury effect, *Injury* 22:225-229, 1991.
13. Jennett B, Frankowski RF: The epidemiology of head injury. In Braakman R (editor): *Handbook of clinical neurology,* New York, 1990, Elsevier.
14. Doberstein CE, Hovda DA, Becker DP: Clinical considerations in the reduction of secondary brain injury, *Ann Emerg Med* 22:993-997, 1993.
15. Miller JD: Assessing patients with head injury, *Br J Surg* 77:241-242, 1990.
16. Zink BJ, Feustel PJ: Effects of ethanol on respiratory function in traumatic brain injury, *J Neurosurg* 82:112-118, 1995.
17. Becker DP: Common themes in head injury. In Becker DP, Gudeman SK (editors): *Textbook of head injury,* Philadelphia, 1989, Saunders.
18. Miller JD: Changing patterns in acute management of head injury, *J Neurol Sci* 103(suppl):S33-S37, 1991.
19. Shackford SR, et al: Epidemiology and pathology of traumatic deaths occurring at a level I trauma center in a regionalized system: the importance of secondary brain injury, *J Trauma* 29: 1392-1397, 1989.
20. Neil-Dwyer G, Cruickshank JM, Doshi R: The stress response in subarachnoid hemorrhage and head injury, *Acta Neurochir* (suppl) 47:102-110, 1990.
21. Waller PF, et al: The potentiating effects of alcohol on driver injury, *JAMA* 256:1461-1466, 1986.
22. Zink BJ, Maio RF: Alcohol use and trauma, *Acad Emerg Med* 1:171-174, 1994.
23. Bleck TP: Seizures, *Baillieres Clin Neuro* 5:565-576, 1996.
24. Povlishock JT: Pathobiology of traumatically induced axonal injury in animals and man, *Ann Emerg Med* 22:980-986, 1993.
25. Teasdale G, Jennett B: Assessment of coma and impaired consciousness: a practical scale, *Lancet* 2:81-84, 1974.
26. Frowein RA, Firsching R: Classification of head injury. In Braakman R (editor): *Handbook of clinical neurology,* New York, 1990, Elsevier.
27. Stein SC: Classification of head injury. In Narayan RK, Wilberger JE, Povlishock JT (editors): *Neurotrauma,* New York, 1996, McGraw-Hill.
28. Brown FD, Mullan S, Duda EE: Delayed traumatic intracerebral hematomas, *J Neurosurg* 48:1019-1022, 1978.
29. Cohen TI, Gudeman SK: Delayed traumatic intracranial hematoma. In Narayan RK, Wilberger JE, Povlishock JT (editors): *Neurotrauma,* New York, 1996, McGraw-Hill.
30. Ferrera PC, Mayer DM: Delayed presentation of an epidural hematoma, *Am J Emerg Med* 15:76-78, 1997.
31. Gudeman SK, et al: The genesis and significance of delayed traumatic intracerebral hematoma, *Neurosurgery* 5:309-312, 1979.
32. Roberson FC, et al: The value of serial computerized tomography in the management of severe head injury, *Surg Neurol* 12: 161-167, 1979.
33. Greene KA. et al: Impact of traumatic subarachnoid hemorrhage on outcome in nonpenetrating head injury. Part II: Relationship to clinical course and outcome variables during acute hospitalization, *J Trauma* 41:964-971, 1996.
34. Morris GF, Marshall LF: A new practical classification of traumatic subarachnoid hemorrhage. Tenth International Symposium on Intracranial Pressure and Neuromonitoring in Brain Injury, Williamsburg, VA, 1997.
35. White, RJ, Likavec, MJ: The diagnosis and initial management of head injury, *N Engl J Med* 327:1507-1511, 1992.
36. Gentry LR: Imaging of closed head injury, *Radiology* 191:1-17, 1994.
37. Mittl RL, et al: Prevalence of MR evidence of diffuse axonal injury in patients with mild head injury and normal head CT findings, *Am J Neuroradiol* 15:1583-1589, 1994.
38. Mild Traumatic Brain Injury Committee of the Head Injury Interdisciplinary Special Interest Group of the American Congress of Rehabilitation Medicine: Definition of mild traumatic brain injury, *J Head Trauma Rehab* 8:86-87, 1993.
39. Binder LM: A review of mild head trauma. Part II: Clinical implications, *J Clin Exp Neuropsychol* 19:432-457, 1997.
40. Kibby MY, Long CJ: Minor head injury: attempts at clarifying the confusion, *Brain Injury* 10:159-186, 1996.
41. Levin HS, et al: Neurobehavioral outcome following minor head injury: a three-center study, *J Neurosurg* 66:234-243, 1987.
42. Macciocchi SN, et al: Neuropsychological functioning and recovery after mild head injury in collegiate athletes, *Neurosurgery* 39:510-514, 1996.

43. Rimel RW, et al: Disability caused by minor head injury, *Neurosurgery* 9:221-228, 1981.
44. Graham DI: Neuropathology of head injury. In Narayan RK, Wilberger JE, Povlishock JT (editors): *Neurotrauma,* New York, 1996, McGraw-Hill.
45. Olshaker JS, Whye DW: Head trauma, *Emerg Med Clin North Am* 11:165-186, 1993.
46. Muhonen MG, Piper JG, Menezes AH: Pathogenesis and treatment of growing skull fractures, *Surg Neurol* 43:367-373, 1995.
47. Hills MW, Deane SA: Head injury and facial injury: is there an increased risk of cervical spine injury? *J Trauma* 34:549-554, 1993.
48. Mendelow AD: Clinical examination in traumatic brain damage. In Braakman R (editor): *Handbook of clinical neurology,* New York, 1990, Elsevier.
49. Cattelani R, et al: Post-concussive syndrome: paraclinical signs, subjective symptoms, cognitive functions and MMPI profiles, *Brain Injury* 10:187-195, 1996.
50. Kelly JP, Rosenberg JH: Diagnosis and management of concussion in sports, *Neurology* 48:575-580, 1997.
51. Malec JF: DSM-IV postconcussional disorder: recommendations, *J Neuropsych Clin Neurosci* 8:113-114, 1996.
52. Johnson MH, Lee SH: Computed tomography of acute cerebral trauma, *Radiol Clin North Am* 30:325-352, 1992.
53. Eisenberg HM, et al: Initial CT findings in 753 patients with severe head injury: a report from the NIH Traumatic Coma Data Bank, *J Neurosurg* 73:688-698, 1990.
54. Marshall LF, Marshall SB, Klauber MR: The diagnosis of head injury requires a classification based on computed axial tomography, *J Neurotrauma* 9(suppl 1):S287-S292, 1992.
55. Tjuvajev J, et al: Correlations between brain oedema volume on CT and CSF dynamics in severely head injured patients, *Acta Neurochir* 51(suppl):305-307, 1990.
56. Borczuk P: Predictors of intracranial injury in patients with mild head trauma, *Ann Emerg Med* 25:731-736, 1995.
57. Madden C, et al: High-yield selection criteria for cranial computed tomography after acute trauma, *Acad Emerg Med* 2:248-252, 1995.
58. Masters SJ, et al: Skull x-ray examinations after head trauma: recommendations by a multidisciplinary panel and validation study, *N Engl J Med* 316:84-91, 1987.
59. Miller EC, Derlet RW, Kinser D: Minor head trauma: is computed tomography always necessary? *Ann Emerg Med* 27:290-294, 1996.
60. Miller EC, Holmes JF, Derlet RW: Utilizing clinical factors to reduce head CT scan ordering for minor head trauma patients, *J Emerg Med* 15:453-457, 1997.
61. Stein SC, Ross SE: Minor head injury: a proposed strategy for emergency management, *Ann Emerg Med* 22:1193-1196, 1993.
62. Valadka AB, Narayan RK: Emergency room management of the head-injured patient. In Narayan RK, Wilberger JE, Povlishock JT (editors): *Neurotrauma,* New York, 1996, McGraw-Hill.
63. Holmes JF, Baier ME, Derlet RW: Failure of Miller criteria to predict significant intracranial injuries in patients with GCS score of 14 after minor head trauma, *Acad Emerg Med* 4:788-792, 1997.
64. Link TM, et al: Substantial head trauma: value of routine CT examination of the cervicocranium, *Radiology* 196:741-745, 1995.
65. Kirshenbaum KJ, et al: Unsuspected upper cervical spine fractures associated with significant head trauma: role of CT, *J Emerg Med* 8:183-198, 1990.
66. Sklar EM, et al: Magnetic resonance applications in cerebral injury, *Radiol Clin North Am* 30:353-366, 1992.
67. Ogawa T, et al: Comparative study of magnetic resonance and CT scan imaging of cases of severe head injury, *Acta Neurochir* 55(suppl):8-10, 1992.
68. Luber SD, et al: Acute hypoglycemia masquerading as head trauma: a report of four cases, *Am J Emerg Med* 14:543-547, 1996.
69. Robertson CS, et al: The effect of glucose administration on carbohydrate metabolism after head injury, *J Neurosurg* 74:43-50, 1991.
70. Bullock R, et al: Guidelines for the management of severe head injury: Brain Trauma Foundation, *Eur J Emerg Med* 3:109-127, 1996.
71. Winchell RJ, Hoyt DB: Endotracheal intubation in the field improves survival in patients with severe head injury, *Arch Surg* 132:592-597, 1997.
72. Gentleman D, et al: Guidelines for resuscitation and transfer of patients with serious head injury, *Br Med J* 307:547-552, 1993.
73. Nakayama DK, et al: The use of drugs in emergency airway management in pediatric trauma, *Ann Surg* 216:205-211, 1992.
74. Redan JA, et al: The value of intubating and paralyzing patients with suspected head injury in the emergency department, *J Trauma* 31:371-375, 1991.
75. Rotondo MF, et al: Urgent paralysis and intubation of trauma patients: is it safe? *J Trauma* 34:242-246, 1993.
76. Walls RM: Rapid-sequence intubation in head trauma, *Ann Emerg Med* 22:1008-1013, 1992.
77. Morris IR: Pharmacologic aids to intubation and the rapid sequence induction, *Emerg Med Clin North Am* 6:753-768, 1988.
78. Harris CE, et al: Effects of thiopentone, etomidate and propofol on the haemodynamic response of tracheal intubation, *Anaesthesia* 43(suppl):32-36, 1988.
79. Warner DS, Todd MM: Anesthetic agents and the nervous system. In Crockard A, Hayward R, Hoff JT (editors): *Neurosurgery: the scientific basis of clinical practice,* ed 2, Oxford, 1992, Blackwell Scientific.
80. Bivins HG, et al: The effect of axial traction during orotracheal intubation of the trauma victim with an unstable cervical spine, *Ann Emerg Med* 17:25-29, 1988.
81. Turner, LM: Cervical spine immobilization with axial traction: a practice to be discouraged, *J Emerg Med* 7:385-386, 1989.
82. Scannell G, et al: Orotracheal intubation in trauma patients with cervical fractures, *Arch Surg* 128:903-905, 1993.
83. Wright SW, Robinson GG II, Wright MB: Cervical spine injuries in blunt trauma patients requiring emergent endotracheal intubation, *Am J Emerg Med* 10:104-109, 1992.
84. Cold GE: Cerebral blood flow in acute head injury: the regulation of cerebral blood flow and metabolism during the acute phase of head injury, and its significance for therapy, *Acta Neurochir* 49(suppl):1-64, 1990.
85. Turner E, et al: Metabolic and hemodynamic response to hyperventilation in patients with head injuries, *Intens Care Med* 10:127-132, 1984.
86. Havill JH: Prolonged hyperventilation and intracranial pressure, *Crit Care Med* 12:72-74, 1984.
87. Muizelaar JP, et al: Adverse effects of prolonged hyperventilation in patients with severe head injury: a randomized clinical trial, *J Neurosurg* 75:731-739, 1991.
88. Heffner JE, Sahn SA: Controlled hyperventilation in patients with intracranial hypertension: application and management, *Arch Intern Med* 143:765-769, 1983.
89. Rosner MJ, Daughton S: Cerebral perfusion pressure management in head injury, *J Trauma* 30:933-941, 1990.
90. Scalea TM, et al: Resuscitation of multiple trauma and head injury: role of crystalloid fluids and inotropes, *Crit Care Med* 22:1610-1615, 1994.

91. Sutin KM, Ruskin KJ, Kaufman BS: Intravenous fluid therapy in neurologic injury, *Crit Care Clin* 8:367-408, 1992.
92. Jorden RC: Multiple trauma. In Rosen P, Barkin RM (editors): *Emergency medicine: concepts and clinical practice,* ed 3, St Louis, 1992, Mosby.
93. Kline JA: Shock. In Rosen D, et al (editors): *Emergency medicine: concepts and clinical practice,* ed 4, St Louis, 1998, Mosby.
94. Schmoker JD, Zhuang J, Shackford SR: Hypertonic fluid resuscitation improves cerebral oxygen delivery and reduces intracranial pressure after hemorrhagic shock, *J Trauma* 31:1607-1613, 1991.
95. Wade CE, et al: Individual patient cohort analysis of the efficacy of hypertonic saline/dextran in patients with traumatic brain injury and hypotension, *J Trauma* 42(5 suppl):S61-65, 1997.
96. Maningas PA, et al: Hypertonic saline-dextran solutions for the prehospital management of traumatic hypotension, *Am J Surg* 157:528-533, 1989.
97. Gunnar W, et al: Head injury and hemorrhagic shock: studies of the blood-brain barrier and intracranial pressure after resuscitation with normal saline solution, 3% saline solution and dextran-40, *Surgery* 103:398-407, 1988.
98. Muizelaar JP, Lutz HA, Becker DP: Effect of mannitol on ICP and CBF and correlation with pressure autoregulation in severely head-injured patients, *J Neurosurg* 61:700-706, 1984.
99. Rosner MJ, Coley I: Cerebral perfusion pressure: a hemodynamic mechanism of mannitol and the postmannitol hemogram, *Neurosurgery* 21:147-156, 1987.
100. Israel S, et al: Hemodynamic effect of mannitol in a canine model of concomitant increased intracranial pressure and hemorrhagic shock, *Ann Emerg Med* 17:560-566, 1988.
101. Willerson JT, et al: Influence of hypertonic mannitol on ventricular performance and coronary blood flow in patients, *Circulation* 51:1095-1100, 1975.
102. Wise BL, Chater N: The value of hypertonic mannitol solution in decreasing brain mass and lowering cerebrospinal-fluid pressure, *J Neurosurg* 19:1038-1043, 1962.
103. Abou-madi M, et al: Does a bolus of mannitol initially aggravate intracranial hypertension? *Br J Anaesth* 59:630-639, 1987.
104. Auer LM, Haselsberger K: Effect of intravenous mannitol on cat pial arteries and veins during normal and elevated intracranial pressure, *Neurosurg*ery 21:142-146, 1987.
105. Brown FD, et al: Detailed monitoring of the effects of mannitol following experimental head injury, *J Neurosurg* 50:423-432, 1979.
106. Nath F, Galbraith S: The effect of mannitol on cerebral white matter water content, *J Neurosurg* 65:41-43, 1986.
107. Takagi H, et al: The mechanism of ICP reducing effect of mannitol. In Ishii S, Nagai H, Brock M (editors): *Intracranial pressure V,* New York, 1983, Springer Verlag.
108. Marshall LF, et al: Mannitol dose requirements in brain-injured patients, *J Neurosurg* 48:169-172, 1978.
109. Smith HP, et al: Comparison of mannitol regimens in patients with severe head injury undergoing intracranial monitoring, *J Neurosurg* 65:820-824, 1986.
110. Moran JL: Latent and manifest hyperosmolar states—two consequences of osmotherapy for head injury, *Anaesth Intens Care* 10:365-369, 1982.
111. Freshman SP, et al: Hypertonic saline (7.5%) versus mannitol: a comparison for treatment of acute head injuries, *J Trauma* 35: 344-348, 1993.
112. Mendelow AD, et al: Effect of mannitol on cerebral blood flow and cerebral perfusion pressure in human head injury, *J Neurosurg* 63:43-48, 1985.
113. Oppido PA, et al: Brain oedema and intracranial hypertension treatment by GLIAS, *Acta Neurochir* 55(suppl):40-42, 1992.
114. Fortune JB, et al: The effect of hyperventilation, mannitol, and ventriculostomy drainage on cerebral blood flow after head injury, *J Trauma* 39:1091-1097, 1995.
115. Dempsey RJ, Kindt G: Experimental augmentation of cerebral blood flow by mannitol in epidural intracranial masses, *J Trauma* 22:449-454, 1982.
116. Cottrell JE, et al: Furosemide and mannitol-induced changes in intracranial pressure and serum osmolality and electrolytes, *Anesthesiology* 47:28-30, 1977.
117. Pollay M, et al: Effect of mannitol and furosemide on blood-brain osmotic gradient and intracranial pressure, *J Neurosurg* 59:945-950, 1983.
118. Wilkinson HA, Rosenfeld SR: Furosemide and mannitol in the treatment of acute experimental intracranial hypertension, *Neurosurgery* 12:405-410, 1983.
119. Roberts PA, et al: Effect on intracranial pressure of furosemide combined with varying doses and administration rates of mannitol, *J Neurosurg* 66:440-446, 1987.
120. Galicich JH, French LA: The use of dexamethasone in the treatment of cerebral edema resulting from brain tumors and brain surgery, *Am Pract Dig Treat* 12:169-174, 1961.
121. Braakman R, et al: Megadose steroids in severe head injury: results of a prospective double blind clinical trial, *J Neurosurg* 58:326-330, 1983.
122. Cooper PR, et al: Dexamethasone and severe head injury: a prospective double-blind study, *J Neurosurg* 51:307-316, 1979.
123. Dearden NM, et al: Effect of high-dose dexamethasone on outcome from severe head injury, *J Neurosurg* 64:81-88, 1986.
124. Miller JD, Leech P: Effects of mannitol and steroid therapy on intracranial volume-pressure relationships in patients, *J Neurosurg* 42:274-281, 1975.
125. Saul T, et al: Steroids in severe head injury: a prospective randomized clinical trial, *J Neurosurg* 54:596-600, 1981.
126. Chudnofsky CR, et al: The safety of fentanyl use in the emergency department, *Ann Emerg Med* 18:635-639, 1989.
127. Wright SW, et al: Midazolam in the emergency department, *Am J Emerg Med* 8:97-100, 1990.
128. Chiolero RL, de Tribolet N: Sedatives and antagonists in the management of severely head-injured patients, *Acta Neurochir* 55(suppl):43-46, 1992.
129. Marshall LF, Smith RW, Shapiro HM: The outcome with aggressive treatment in severe head injuries: acute and chronic barbiturate administration, *J Neurosurg* 50:26-30, 1979.
130. Rockoff MA, Marshall LF, Shapiro HM: High-dose barbiturate therapy in humans: a clinical review of 60 patients, *Ann Neurol* 6:194-199, 1979.
131. Ward JD, et al: Failure of prophylactic barbiturate coma in the treatment of severe head injury, *J Neurosurg* 62: 383-388, 1985.
132. Eisenberg HM, et al: High-dose barbiturate control of elevated intracranial pressure in patients with severe head injury, *J Neurosurg* 69:15-23, 1988.
133. Herregods L, Mergaert C, Rolly G: Comparison of effects of 24-hour propofol or fentanyl infusions on intracranial pressure, *J Drug Dev* 2(suppl):99-100, 1989.
134. Hsiang JK, et al: Early, routine paralysis for intracranial pressure control in severe head injury: is it necessary? *Crit Care Med* 22:1471-1476, 1994.
135. Prough DS, Joshi S: Does early neuromuscular blockade contribute to adverse outcome after acute head injury? *Crit Care Med* 22:1349-1350, 1994.
136. Biros MH: Anticonvulsants. In Barsan WG, Jastremski MS, Syverud SA (editors): *Emergency drug therapy,* Philadelphia, 1991, Saunders.

137. Seelig JM, et al: Traumatic acute subdural hematoma: major mortality reduction in comatose patients treated within four hours, *N Engl J Med* 304:1511-1518, 1981.
138. Johnson DL, Duma C, Sivit C: The role of immediate operative intervention in severely head-injured children with a Glasgow Coma Scale score of 3, *Neurosurgery* 30:320-324, 1992.
139. Andrews BT, Pitts LH: *Traumatic transtentorial herniation and its management,* Mt. Kisco, NY, 1991, Futura Publishing.
140. Lang RG: Emergency drainage of traumatic intracranial hematomas. In Roberts JR, Hedges JR (editors): *Clinical procedures in emergency medicine,* ed 2, Philadelphia, 1991, Saunders.
141. Ghajar J, Hariri RJ: Management of pediatric head injury, *Pediatr Clin North Am* 39:1093-1125, 1992.
142. Kasoff SS, et al: Aggressive physiologic monitoring of pediatric head trauma patients with elevated intracranial pressure, *Pediatr Neurosci* 14:241-249, 1988.
143. Saul TG, Ducker TB: Effect of intracranial pressure monitoring and aggressive treatment on mortality in severe head injury, *J Neurosurg* 56:498-503, 1982.
144. Lundberg H, Troupp H, Lorin H: Continuous recording of the ventricular fluid pressure in patients with severe acute traumatic brain injury, *J Neurosurg* 22:581-590, 1965.
145. Narayan RK, et al: Intracranial pressure: to monitor or not to monitor? A review of our experience with severe head injury, *J Neurosurg* 56:650-658, 1982.
146. Mayhall CG, Archer NH, Lamb VA: Ventriculostomy-related infection: a prospective epidemiologic study, *N Engl J Med* 310: 553-559, 1984.
147. Unwin DH, Giller CA, Kopitnik TA: Central nervous system monitoring: what helps, what does not, *Surg Clin North Am* 71:733-747, 1991.
148. Sheinberg M, et al: Continuous monitoring of jugular venous oxygen saturation in head-injured patients, *J Neurosurg* 76:212-217, 1992.
149. Dings J, Meixensberger J, Roosen K: Brain tissue pO_2-monitoring: catheter stability and complications, *Neurol Res* 19:241-245, 1997.
150. Kiening KL, et al: Brain tissue pO_2-monitoring in comatose patients: implications for therapy, *Neurol Res* 19:233-240, 1997.
151. Aaslid R, Markwalder TM, Nornes H: Noninvasive transcranial Doppler ultrasound recording of flow velocity in basal cerebral arteries, *J Neurosurg* 57:769-774, 1982.
152. Cardoso ER, Kupchak JA: Evaluation of intracranial pressure gradients by means of transcranial Doppler sonography, *Acta Neurochir* 55(suppl):1-5, 1992.
153. Shigemori M, et al: Monitoring of severe head-injured patients with transcranial Doppler (TCD) ultrasonography, *Acta Neurochir* 55(suppl):6-7, 1992.
154. Weber M, Grolimund P, Seiler RW: Evaluation of posttraumatic cerebral blood flow velocities by transcranial Doppler ultrasonography, *Neurosurgery* 27:106-112, 1990.
155. Bouma GJ, et al: Ultra-early evaluation of regional cerebral blood flow in severely head-injured patients using xenon-enhanced computerized tomography, *J Neurosurg* 77:360-368, 1992.
156. Bouma GJ, Muizelaar JP: Evaluation of regional cerebral blood flow in acute head injury by stable xenon-enhanced computerized tomography, *Acta Neurochir* 59(suppl):34-40, 1993.
157. Marion DW, Bouma GJ: The use of stable xenon-enhanced computed tomographic studies of cerebral blood flow to define changes in cerebral carbon dioxide vasoresponsivity caused by a severe head injury, *Neurosurgery* 29:869-873, 1991.
158. Stringer WA, et al: Hyperventilation-induced cerebral ischemia in patients with acute brain lesions: demonstration by xenon-enhanced CT, *Am J Neuroradiol* 14:475-484, 1993.
159. Yonas H, Pindzola RP, Johnson DW: Xenon/computed tomography cerebral blood flow and its use in clinical management, *Neurosurg Clin North Am* 7:605-616, 1996.
160. Bullock R, et al: Early post-traumatic cerebral blood flow mapping: correlation with structural damage after focal injury, *Acta Neurochir* 55(suppl):14-17, 1992.
161. Goncalves JM, et al: HM-PAO spect in head trauma, *Acta Neurochir* 55(suppl):11-13, 1992.
162. Meixensberger J: Xenon 133—CBF measurements in severe head injury and subarachnoid haemorrhage, *Acta Neurochir* 59(suppl):28-33, 1993.
163. Robertson C: Measurements of cerebral blood flow and metabolism in severe head injury using the Kety-Schmidt technique, *Acta Neurochir* 59(suppl):25-27, 1993.
164. Cicerone KD, et al: Neuropsychological rehabilitation of mild traumatic brain injury, *Brain Injury* 10:277-286, 1996.
165. Robertson CS, et al: Prevention of secondary insults after head injury, Tenth International Symposium on Intracranial Pressure and Neuromonitoring in Brain Injury, Williamsburg, VA, 1997.
166. Marion DW, et al: Treatment of traumatic brain injury with moderate hypothermia, *N Engl J Med* 336:540-546, 1997.
167. Rabinovici R, et al: Hemoglobin-based oxygen-carrying resuscitation fluids, *Crit Care Med* 23:801-804, 1995.
168. Doppenberg EM, Bullock R: Clinical neuro-protection trials in severe traumatic brain injury: lessons from previous studies, *J Neurotrauma* 14:71-80, 1997.
169. Muizelaar JP, et al: Improving the outcome of severe head injury with the oxygen radical scavenger polyethylene glycol conjugated superoxide dismutase: a phase II trial, *J Neurosurg* 78:375-382, 1993.
170. Bullock R, et al: Failure of the competitive NMDA antagonist selfotel (CGS 19755) to improve outcome after severe head injury: results of Phase III trials (abstract), Tenth International Symposium on Intracranial Pressure and Neuromonitoring in Brain Injury, Williamsburg, VA, 1997.
171. Davis SM, et al: Termination of acute stroke studies involving selfotel treatment, *Lancet* 349:32, 1997.
172. Young B, et al: Effects of pegorgotein on neurologic outcome of patients with severe head injury, *JAMA* 276:538-543, 1966.
173. Faden AI: Comparison of single and combination drug treatment strategies in experimental brain trauma, *J Neurotrauma* 10:91-100, 1993.

12 Spinal Cord Injuries

PETER C. FERRERA AND DAVID B. MARKOWITZ

Teaching Case

A 94-year-old woman struck the back of her head on a glass pane while in a restaurant. She arrived without a standard cervical collar in place. She had no focal deficits on arrival to the emergency department (ED). While waiting for radiographs of her cervical spine, she became agitated and began to move on her stretcher. The woman became dyspneic, unresponsive, and flaccid. After intubation, cervical spine radiographs showed a C5/6 fracture-dislocation. She was begun on the methylprednisolone protocol. Her family requested that the patient not be resuscitated in case of a cardiac arrest. She was placed in a Roto-Rest bed and admitted to the intensive care unit. A cervical magnetic resonance image (MRI) obtained on the sixth hospital day showed cord edema from C4 to C7. She ultimately developed pneumonia and was provided comfort care. She died on the tenth hospital day.

In a busy ED it becomes difficult to oversee the activities of every patient. This patient did not have an appropriate cervical collar and movement of her neck either exacerbated or caused the underlying cord injury, resulting in respiratory arrest. Because their spine is osteoarthritic, the elderly are especially prone to spinal cord injury (SCI), since osteophytes impinge on the cord. Properly immobilize the spines of patients with potential cervical spine injury. Rapid sequence intubation and chemical paralysis may be necessary to protect the patient from self-harm. ■

Few injuries are as devastating as those affecting the spinal cord. Young adults and adolescents have the highest prevalence of SCI and often suffer permanent disability. Hospitalization and rehabilitation costs for the victims are enormous, and the emotional damage to the patients and their families immeasurable. The emergency physician (EP) must detect or exclude SCI and minimize further damage to the cord. Ultimately, most cord-injured patients are best treated at a major trauma center with the expertise to facilitate recovery.

EPIDEMIOLOGY

Although spinal cord injuries are relatively infrequent, there are approximately 10,000 to 14,000 new cases annually in the United States, representing 2.6% of the patients enrolled in the Major Trauma Outcome Study.[1-3] Motor vehicle crashes (MVCs), falls, and penetrating wounds are the three leading causes, in descending order of frequency.[1,3,4] Patients between 15 and 24 years of age, primarily males, have the highest incidence, followed by patients older than 55 years.[3,4] Greater than half of all patients with SCI retain some degree of sensory or motor function and therefore have incomplete injuries.[5] Overall mortality for SCI is approximately 17%, although in patients with isolated SCI this rate is only 6.9%.[1] The cost of caring for these patients is astronomic, since continued rehabilitation and lost wages from disability continue throughout their lifetimes. The average inpatient hospitalization costs in 1987 for patients with SCI ranged from $50,000 to $90,000 per person for paraplegics and $170,000 to $250,000 for high-level tetraplegics.[3]

PATHOPHYSIOLOGY

There are three basic types of nerve injuries.[6] **Neuropraxia** is the mildest form, resulting from stretching or contusion of nerve roots. This stretching transiently impedes conduction of nerve impulses through intact axons. Recovery from neuropraxia typically occurs within 6 weeks postinjury.[6] The intermediate type of injury is **axontmesis**, in which the axons lose continuity but the endoneurial tubes remain intact. In this case, recovery is determined by axonal regeneration. The most severe form of injury is **neurotmesis**, whereby the nerve is completely severed and regeneration typically does not occur. Most patients display a mixed-injury pattern.

Damage to the spinal cord occurs by both a direct mechanism and by secondary changes. Impact from bone fragments, vertebral dislocations, and herniated discs produce direct injury,[7] and the cord may sustain varying degrees of laceration, including complete transection. Secondary insults arise from damage to the microcirculation, biochemical changes, and electrolyte disturbances.[7] Hemorrhages, which develop within the cord, are often progressive and disrupt the microcirculation.[7] Vasospasm and intravascular thrombosis lead to ischemic damage.[7] Accumulation of the excitatory neurotransmitter glutamate results in elevated intracellular calcium, which injures cells via proteases and lipases.[7] Lipid peroxidation and free radical formation are other potential secondary insults. These mechanisms provide the theoretic basis for corticosteroids in the treatment of SCI.[7]

CLINICAL PRESENTATION

Patients with SCI may present with subtle neurologic deficits or grossly obvious paralysis. Cervical cord injuries may result in insidious respiratory compromise, which ultimately interferes with oxygenation and causes hypoxemia. Priapism, which is an abnormal penile erection, is frequently seen.

Depending on the level and severity of the injury, systemic manifestations may include bradycardia and hypotension, which may persist for months.[7] A combination of diminished sympathetic tone and unopposed vagal effects on the heart leads to this **neurogenic shock**.[7] However, hypotension with a systolic blood pressure <80 mmHg is rarely due to SCI alone, and other causes such as hemorrhage must be excluded.

The patient with suspected SCI must undergo meticulous testing of motor and sensory function in the various essential muscle groups, which serve as a baseline for subsequent examinations. Severity of injury is qualified as **tetraplegia**, **paraplegia**, or **incomplete paralysis** or **sensory loss**. There are 28 dermatomes (Fig. 12-1), and sensory function is graded as 0, 1, and 2, representing absent, impaired, or normal sensation, respectively. The motor examination tests key muscles in 10 paired myotomes (Table 12-1) and is graded on a scale from 0 to 5 (Table 12-2).[8]

The neurologic level is defined as the most caudal spinal cord segment on both sides of the body with normal sensory and motor function.[8] Incomplete lesions show either partial sensory or motor function distal to the injury and include the phenomenon of sacral sparing.[8] **Sacral sparing** is an important finding wherein the perineal reflexes such as the **anal wink** and **bulbocavernosus** remain intact. Sacral sparing in an otherwise paralyzed patient implies chance of recovery. The grading system of Frankel et al (Table 12-3)[9] has been replaced by the American Spinal Injury Association (ASIA) Impairment Scale (Table 12-4).

Spinal (Neurogenic) Shock

Spinal shock accompanies physiologic or anatomic transection or near-transection of the spinal cord immediately following trauma.[10] A period of flaccid paralysis and absence of reflexes below the neurologic injury characterizes spinal shock. Although the complete pathophysiology of spinal shock is unknown, decreased blood pressure or hypotension may occur from loss of sympathetic tone to the legs and venous pooling with low thoracic lesions; from venous pooling in the legs and splanchnic beds with upper thoracic lesions; and from loss of cardiovascular intrinsic sympathetic tone with cervical lesions.[10] Spinal shock is known as "warm shock," since the skin may feel warm from peripheral vasodilatation, in contrast to the often "cool and clammy" presentation of hemorrhagic shock. Twenty to thirty percent of patients with spinal shock require pressors because of frank hypotension.[10] The bladder becomes areflexic, causing urinary retention.[11] Spinal shock is rare in patients with injury levels lower than T6.

Spinal shock may last for days to weeks, and its resolution is evidenced by the return of a bulbocavernosus reflex, anal wink, or other muscle spindle reflexes.[10,12] The bulbocavernosus reflex is tested by tugging on the Foley catheter, or by squeezing the tip of the penis or pushing on the clitoris, while keeping another finger in the rectum; a positive reflex consists of a rectal sphincter contraction.

Partial Cord Syndromes

CENTRAL CORD SYNDROME

Of the partial cord syndromes, central cord syndrome (CCS) is the most common.[13] In CCS, motor dysfunction is greater in the upper extremities than in the lower extremities, and many patients demonstrate urinary retention and varying degrees of sensory loss.[14] When recovery occurs, lower extremity function returns first, then bladder function, and finally upper extremity strength.[14] The most common mech-

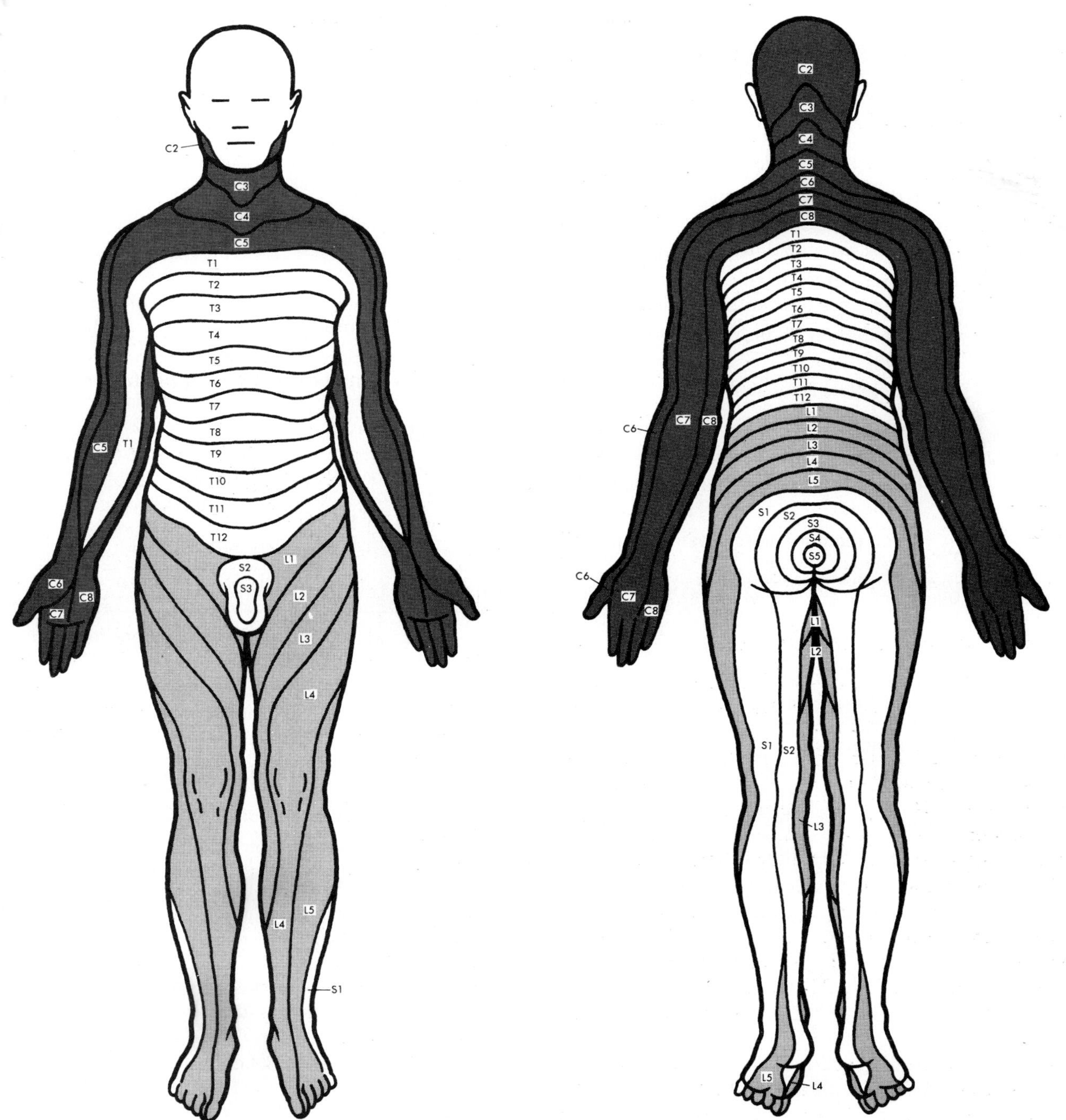

Fig. 12-1 Dermatomes of each spinal segment. (From Hockberger RS, et al: Spinal injuries. In Rosen P, et al [editors]: *Emergency medicine: concepts and clinical practice,* ed 4, St Louis, 1998, Mosby.)

anism of injury is severe hyperextension of the neck, often associated with arthritis of the cervical spine.

The pathogenesis of the CCS is controversial. Classic teaching describes a somatotopic organization to the spinal cord, wherein the medial portions of the corticospinal tract (the tract subserving motor function) contain the neurons serving the upper extremities.[15] However, some researchers refute this theory for lack of neuroanatomic evidence.[15] They propose that the corticospinal tract is more vital for upper than

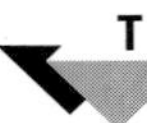

TABLE 12-1
Key Muscles for Testing Motor Function

CORD LEVEL	MUSCLES
C5	Elbow flexors (biceps, brachialis)
C6	Wrist extensors (extensor carpi radialis longus and brevis)
C7	Elbow extensors (triceps)
C8	Finger flexors to the middle finger (flexor digitorum profundus)
T1	Small finger abductors (abductor digiti minimi)
L2	Hip flexors (iliopsoas)
L3	Knee extensors (quadriceps)
L4	Ankle dorsiflexors (tibialis anterior)
L5	Long toe extensors (extensor hallucis longus)
S1	Ankle plantarflexors (gastrocnemius, soleus)

Adapted from Ditunno JF Jr, et al: *Paraplegia* 32:70-80, 1994.

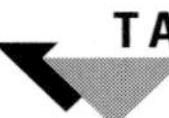

TABLE 12-2
Muscle Strength Grading

GRADE	MUSCLE STRENGTH
0	Flaccid
1	Contraction
2	Active movement with gravity eliminated
3	Active movement against gravity
4	Active movement against moderate resistance
5	Active movement against full resistance

TABLE 12-3
Frankel et al Classification of Spinal Cord Injuries

GRADE	LESION
A	Motor and sensory complete below the level of injury
B	Motor complete, sensory incomplete below level of injury
C	Motor useless
D	Motor useful, with occasional ability to ambulate
E	Recovered; no weakness or sensory loss; abnormal reflexes possibly present

TABLE 12-4
ASIA Impairment Scale

GRADE	LESION
A	Motor and sensory complete below the level of injury
B	Motor complete, some sensation preserved below neurological level with sacral sparing
C	Preserved motor function with majority of key muscles below the neurological level having a muscle grade less than 3
D	Preserved motor function with majority of key muscles below the neurological level having a muscle grade greater than or equal to 3
E	Normal motor and sensory function

Adapted from Ditunno JF Jr, et al: *Paraplegia* 32:70-80, 1994.

for lower extremity function. For this reason, leg movement tends to be preserved because other descending tracts assist locomotor function.

The differential diagnosis of the patient presenting with traumatic upper extremity weakness includes **Bell's cruciate paralysis** and **bilateral brachial plexus injury**.[14,16] The proposed mechanism of Bell's cruciate paralysis is compression of the cervicomedullary junction between the odontoid and foramen magnum.[14,16] Bell theorized that the fibers supplying the upper and lower extremities separate in the pyramidal decussation, with the upper extremity fibers being more cephalad.[16]

A variant of the CCS is the "**burning hands syndrome**" in which patients complain of burning dysesthesias of the hands.[17,18] This phenomenon may be caused by contusion of the spinothalamic tract.

BROWN-SEQUARD SYNDROME

Spinal cord hemisection, resulting in ipsilateral motor and dorsal column dysfunction with contralateral loss of pain and temperature sensation, characterizes the **Brown-Sequard syndrome** (BSS). The patient is paralyzed on the side of the injury and a pinprick feels dull on the side opposite the injury. Less commonly appreciated, there is also ipsilateral hyperesthesia distal to the level of injury.[19] BSS comprises only 2% to 4% of all spinal injuries.[20] The pure form of this syndrome is in fact rare, and most cases are actually **Brown-Sequard-plus syndromes** (BSPS).[21,22] In this situation, there is asymmetric paraplegia with hypalgesia more pronounced on the stronger side. Both BSS and BSPS have favorable outcomes, including ambulation and bowel and bladder continence.[22]

ANTERIOR CORD SYNDROME

Anterior SCI is uncommon and results in preserved dorsal column function (i.e., proprioception, vibration, and light touch) with impaired motor function and altered pain and temperature sensation.[8,23] Causative factors include compression of the anterior cord by displaced bone fragments, a herniated disc, or direct destruction of the anterior portion of the cord or its blood supply.[13,23] Flexion "tear-drop" fractures are frequently associated with this syndrome.[13] Thoracic aorta injuries may disrupt blood supply to the anterior cord and produce this complex.

POSTERIOR CORD SYNDROME

Isolated injury to the posterior spinal cord is extremely rare. This lesion results in destruction of the functions of light touch, vibration, and proprioception, which are controlled by the dorsal columns.[3] Ambulation becomes difficult because of impaired proprioception.[3]

CAUDA EQUINA SYNDROME

Trauma rarely injures the cauda equina, the lumbosacral nerve roots below the tip of the spinal cord.[24,25] In typical cases of cauda equina syndrome (CES), the patient complains of unilateral or bilateral sciatica, bowel and bladder incontinence, bilateral lower extremity weakness, and hypesthesia or analgesia in the saddle distribution (i.e., genital and anal region).[24-27] This lesion is a surgical emergency, and the EP should immediately consult the appropriate specialist.[24,26] Patients who undergo decompression within 24 to 48 hours after onset of symptoms have a better outcome than those with late intervention.[24-26] Permanent bladder and rectal dysfunction may occur with surgical delay.[25]

EMERGENCY DEPARTMENT EVALUATION

History

Ascertain the details of the event leading up to the injury. Ask the patient if he or she had or has any numbness, weakness, or paresthesias. Neck or back pain is frequently associated with cord injuries. A prior history of cervical or rheumatoid arthritis increases the risk of upper cord injury in the presence of relatively minor trauma.

Physical Examination

Test all appropriate dermatomes and muscle groups for sensation and function. Recognize the big "skip" area in sensation associated with cervical injuries (since the dermatomes of the cervical roots run down the arms, the chest dermatomes "jump" from C4 to T2). Therefore pinprick testing of the chest is normal in the upper chest but then suddenly disappears with cervical SCI. Application of a tuning fork or a buzzing beeper to the feet or hands will test vibratory function. Testing of the sacral roots, rectal tone, and perineal reflexes such as the anal wink and bulbocavernosus gives important prognostic information. Priapism is an ominous finding associated with permanent paralysis.

Because complete cord injuries obliterate sensation, the physical examination is compromised. A soft, nontender abdomen may hide a ruptured spleen, and a major pelvic fracture is painless. The EP may easily overlook a femur fracture unless the extremity is carefully stressed. For these reasons, cord-injured patients need frequent reexaminations.

Diagnostic Studies

Although plain-film radiography and computed tomography (CT) are invaluable for fractures, dislocations, and ligamentous instability, these tests are blind to the spinal cord. **Magnetic resonance imaging** is the definitive modality for assessing cord injury. In patients with obvious neurologic deficits, make plans to obtain a spinal MRI of the suspected segments as soon as possible. Findings on MRI that suggest severe injury include cord compression by hemorrhage or herniated discs (Fig. 12-2), epidural hemorrhage (Fig. 12-3), increased cord signals (Figs. 12-4 and 12-5), or cord transection.[2,28] The main contraindications to MRI is hemodynamic instability, the presence of pacemakers, aneurysm clips, or metallic foreign bodies imbedded in the eye or spinal cord, since these substances may either malfunction or move in the magnetic field.[3]

In general, injury to one level of the spinal column predicts a 5% to 6% chance of there being a second noncontiguous spinal column injury. Therefore the entire spine will ultimately need to be imaged, initially by plain films.

EMERGENCY DEPARTMENT MANAGEMENT

Once the patient is stabilized, attention may proceed to evaluation and management of the injured spine. During resuscitation, the patient with potential SCI requires spinal immobilization. All patients with hy-

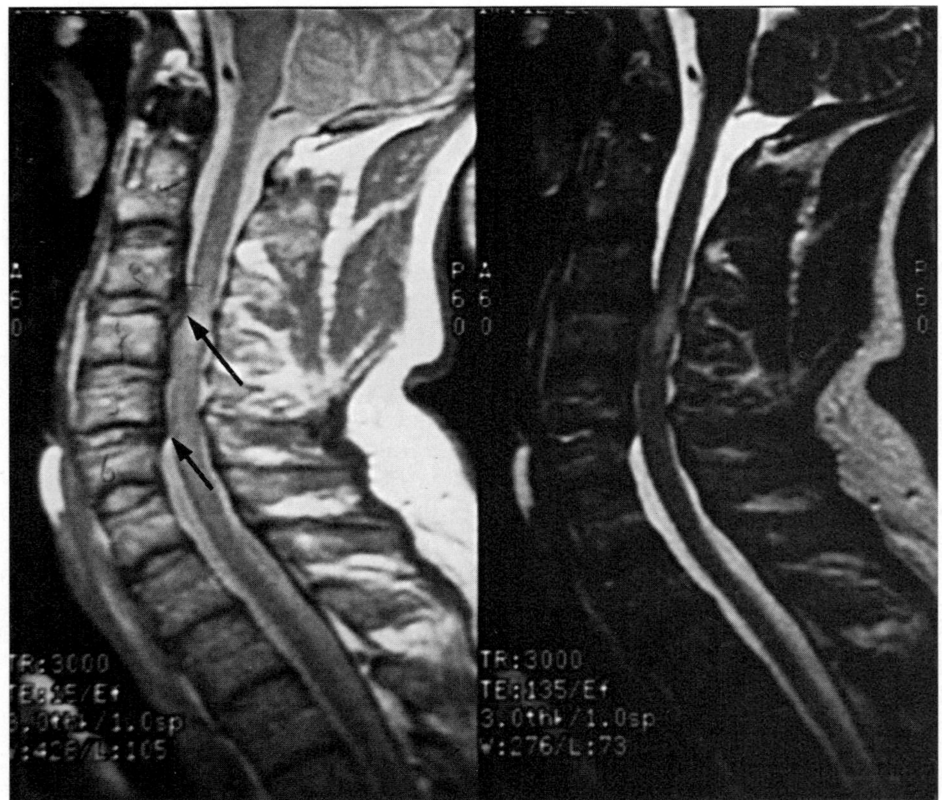

Fig. 12-2 Sagittal MRI shows herniated discs at C3/4 and C5/6 levels *(arrows)*, resulting in cord compression and spinal cord contusion.

potension and cord injury require objective evaluation for hemorrhage into the thoracic, intraabdominal, or pelvic cavities. Never assume hypotension is due to spinal shock until hemorrhage is excluded.

Patients with low cord lesions, C4-C6, may present with normal respirations. However, such patients are at risk for delayed respiratory decompensation, since swelling of the cord may compromise diaphragm function. Serial measurements of pulmonary function, such as negative inspiratory force (NIF) or forced vital capacity may identify impending respiratory failure and the need for endotracheal intubation.

If the patient is initially evaluated in a nontrauma center, consider prompt transfer to a level I trauma center. Immobilization with Gardner-Wells tongs and closed reduction of fracture-dislocations may be required, therefore mandating urgent orthopedic or neurosurgic consultation.[3] Early decompressive surgery has not been shown to unequivocally improve outcome following SCI.[29-32] The primary goal of operative fixation is to restore spinal alignment.[33]

Some authorities promote aggressive management of blood pressure to maximize spinal perfusion.[29] They use volume and pressors to maintain a mean arterial pressure of >85 mmHg. The majority of their patients treated in this fashion improved neurologically within 6 to 12 months.

Methylpredinsolone

In the past, acute SCI management and treatment had been limited to bone realignment or other measures to prevent complications.[34] In the mid 1970s, attention focused on secondary injury. A number of pharmacologic agents were used, hoping to halt progressive spinal impairment.[35] Until 1990 no drug demonstrably improved neurologic function when given early during the injury phase.

In May 1990 Bracken et al[36] published the second National Acute Spinal Cord Injury Study (NASCIS II). They evaluated the efficacy and safety of methylprednisolone (MP) and naloxone in patients with acute spinal cord injury. The rigorous methodology included a randomized multicenter, double-blind, placebo-controlled design. They administered MP as a bolus of 30 mg/kg of body weight, followed by infusion at 5.4 mg/kg per hour for 23 hours. The researchers compared the admission neurologic examination with a standardized examination performed at 6 weeks and 6 months. Patients treated with MP within

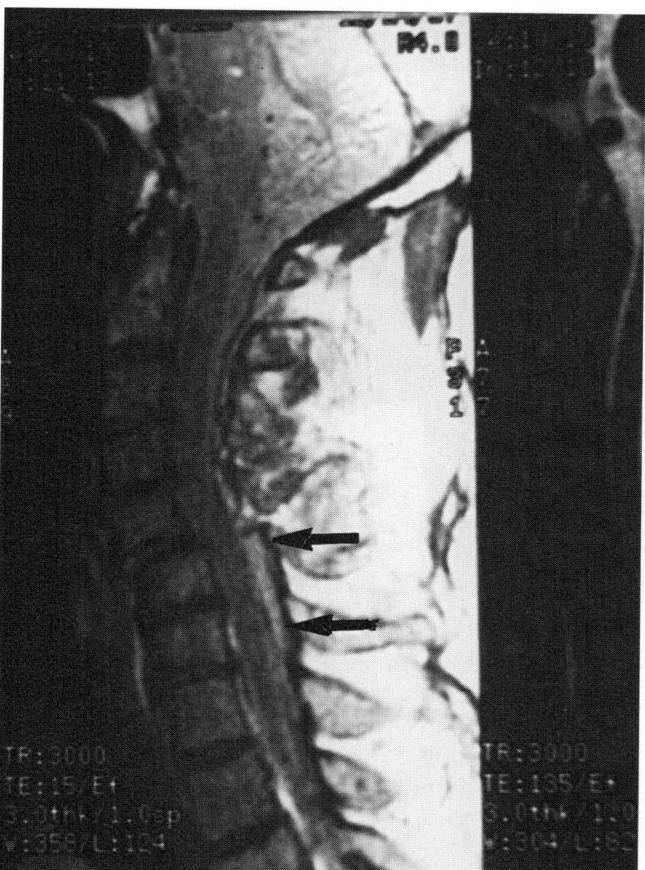

Fig. 12-3 Sagittal MRI shows spinal epidural hemorrhage from C4 to T1 *(arrows)*.

8 hours of injury showed improved motor and sensory function, compared with placebo or naloxone. The apparent benefit of MP was lost if given after 8 hours.

The current dosage of MP follows the study protocol: a loading dose of 30 mg/kg over 15 minutes is followed by an infusion of 5.4 mg/kg/hr over 23 hours. The infusion is placed in 230 cc D_5W and run at 10 cc/hr.

The proposed mechanisms of action include (1) enhancement of blood flow to the cord; (2) inhibition of free radical-induced lipid peroxidation, thereby preventing destruction of neurofilament cell membranes; and (3) limitation of the breakdown of arachidonic acid, which otherwise leads to vasospasm of the cord vessels.[36,37]

Before the publication of NASCIS II, the National Institutes of Health disseminated the study results, instructions, and drug administration protocols to all physicians.[38] The media trumpeted the results with great fanfare.[38] Because of this attention, the administration of MP to patients with SCI became the current standard of care in the United States.[38] Because of medical, legal, and financial reasons, no well-designed studies have attempted to validate the findings of NASCIS II. Despite this lack of validation, some consider it legally unwise to withhold MP from patients with SCI.

Several retrospective studies compared neurologic outcomes of patients receiving the NASCIS II protocol with historical controls who did not receive MP. These studies show no significant difference in neurologic outcomes between these populations.[34,38,39]

Penetrating SCI were excluded from NASCIS II.[40,41] Two studies reviewed the efficacy of MP in patients with penetrating SCI. One retrospective study concluded that MP did not significantly improve the functional outcomes of patients with spinal injuries resulting from gunshot wounds.[41] An earlier retrospective study arrived at the same conclusion, and noted that MP therapy for penetrating SCI may actually impair neurologic recovery.[40]

Currently, a third multicenter randomized trial, NASCIS III, is underway.[35] All study patients receive a bolus of MP followed by either a standard or prolonged infusion. One group will receive 10 mg/kg/day of tirilazad mesylate, a potent lipid peroxidation inhibitor, for 48 hours in addition to the initial MP bolus.

SPECIAL CONSIDERATIONS

Pediatric Cases

Pediatric cases of SCI occur much less frequently than in adults, with a reported annual rate of 18 cases per 1 million.[42] This figure represents 0.65% to 9.47% of all cases of SCI.[43,44] Motor vehicle crashes remain the leading cause of SCI among children, followed by falls and sports-related injuries.[42,45-47] Injuries resulting from pedestrian-MVCs are frequently seen in children less than 10 years of age.[45,48-50] Sports-related trauma, especially diving, occurs more often in adolescents than in younger children.[46]

Injuries involving the skull base to the C2 spinal level are more likely in children up to 8 years of age compared with older children and adults.[43-46,50,51] High-cord injury results in apnea, cardiac arrest, or severe hypotension, and the few survivors sustain hypoxic brain injury.[52]

Although adults and adolescents tend to suffer lower cervical injuries, the young child's relatively large head elevates the neck fulcrum to C2-C4. In addition, the horizontal orientation of the facet joints is more pronounced in the child's upper cervical segments.[44,53] Although neurologic outcome is poor for patients with complete lesions, patients with central cord lesions or Brown-Sequard syndrome often have

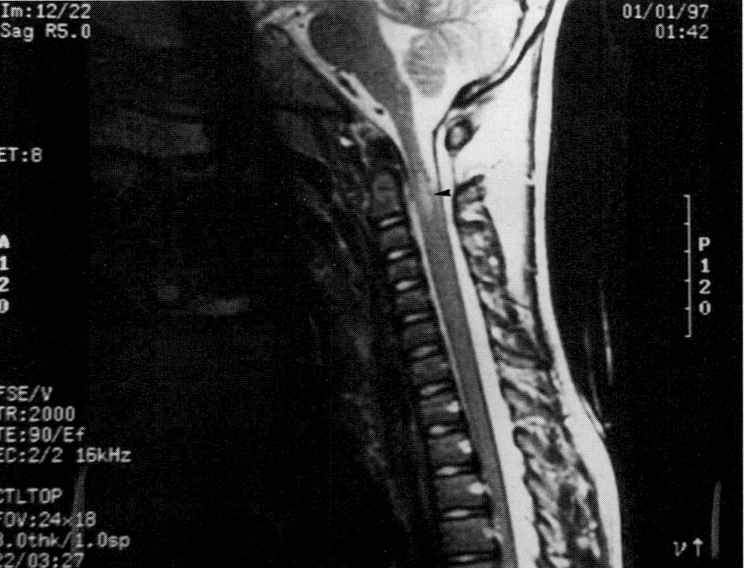

Fig. 12-4 Sagittal MRI shows spinal cord hyperintensity at C2 level *(arrowhead)* in a patient with the Brown-Sequard syndrome.

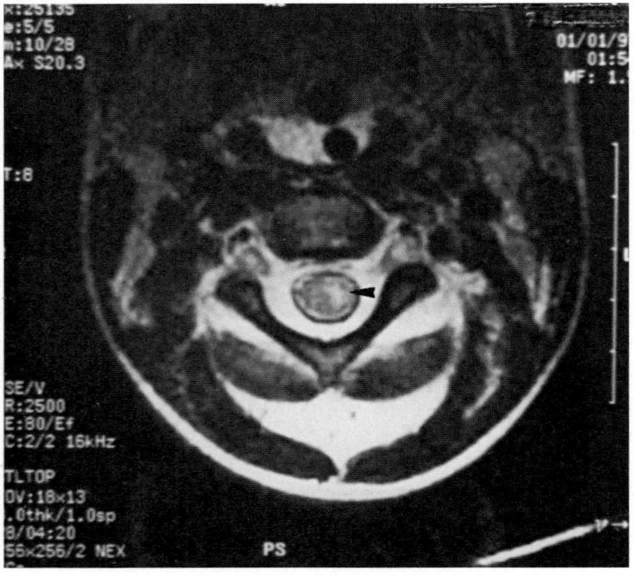

Fig. 12-5 Axial magnetic resonance imaging shows spinal cord hyperintensity at C2 level *(arrowhead)* in a patient with the Brown-Sequard syndrome.

good recovery.[48] Similar to adults, spinal surgery does not improve outcome in those with either complete or incomplete lesions.[48]

SCIWORA SYNDROME

Some children have spinal cord injury without radiologic abnormality, the so-called **SCIWORA syndrome**.[53] This term indicates the lack of bony abnormalities seen on plain radiographs or by CT scanning in the face of neurologic deficits. The presentation ranges from transient neurologic symptoms to complete paralysis.

The rate of SCIWORA ranges from 4% to 67% of all pediatric SCI, but is rare in adults.[53-56] As a result of the elasticity of their spinal cords, children <8 years of age are more susceptible than older children.[45,54,55] Beyond 8 years of age, the spine is less mobile as it stiffens and becomes stronger.[55] Younger children are also prone to this injury because of their relatively larger head size, horizontally oriented facets, and poorly developed neck muscles.[45,55] Spinal cord ischemia and infarction may contribute to the development of SCIWORA.[53,55]

Patients who present with complete injuries in the setting of SCIWORA have a poor prognosis,[42,53,55] whereas those with mild deficits usually do well.[53] Most patients with SCIWORA have positive MRI findings,[42,54] which correlate with outcome. Patients with a normal MRI have an excellent prognosis and usually recover,[55,57] whereas major cord hemorrhage or transection portends poor results.[57]

If the initial injury goes undiagnosed, SCIWORA may become recurrent and lead to neurologic deterioration. Causes of deterioration include spinal instability or continued spinal cord ischemia.[55] Flexion and extension views should be obtained in verbal patients with transient neurologic symptoms to exclude subluxation.[55]

Penetrating Spinal Cord Injuries

Gunshot wounds (GSW) are currently the third leading cause of SCI, with an estimated 50 cases per 1 million persons annually.[58] Over the past 25 years, the

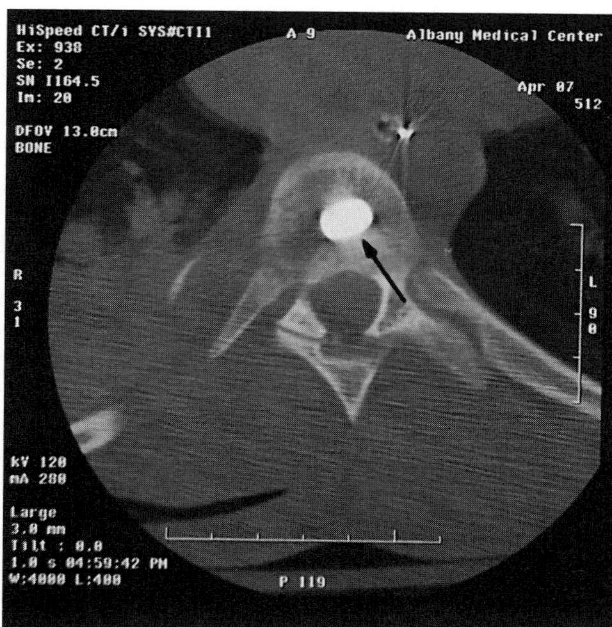

Fig. 12-6 Axial computed tomography shows a bullet lodged in T8 *(arrow)*, resulting in paraplegia.

number of SCIs caused by firearms has risen dramatically, and urban centers are much more likely to encounter penetrating injuries than rural hospitals.[59] Ethnic minority groups suffer the most firearm-induced spinal injuries, and men greatly outnumber women.[59,60] Patients who are stabbed are more likely to have functional recovery from their spinal injuries than their counterparts who are shot.[61]

Unlike wartime injuries, civilian GSWs are secondary to low-velocity handguns, which inflict significantly less damage than military weaponry.[58,62] Twenty-five to seventy percent of these patients have associated systemic injuries that take precedence over the cord injury.[4,60]

Most neurologic deficits are due to direct damage by the bullet. However, secondary projectiles created when the bullet strikes the vertebral column, or a cavitation effect caused by the kinetic energy of the bullet, also produce injury.[4,58,62] In addition, spinal cord ischemia from damaged spinal arteries and systemic hypotension may also result in SCI.[4]

Obtain plain radiographs only after the patient is stabilized. Radiographs are helpful to assess for fractures, bone, and bullet fragments. However, extrapolating the bullet's trajectory from radiographs is a hazardous endeavor. The bullet may ricochet off bone and settle far from the cord.[4] CT scanning better defines bony destruction and the presence of fragments in the spinal canal (Fig. 12-6). Although MRI is the imaging modality of choice following blunt SCI, its use is contraindicated by the presence of bullet shards.[4]

Although penetrating injuries may lead to meningitis, cerebrospinal fluid leak, and spinal osteomyelitis, these complications are rare.[58] Bony instability is also unusual after penetrating injuries.[4,63] Cases of transperitoneal violation are best managed by irrigation of the missile tract and antibiotic therapy without the need for laminectomy or removal of intracanal bullet fragments.[58] Patients with bullet fragments retained in the spinal canal usually do well if the bullet is left in place.[63] Although a theoretic concern, lead intoxication has not been seen with retained intracanal fragments.[63-65]

Neurologic recovery depends on the initial injury rather than the intervention, and surgery rarely improves outcome.[60,65-67] One exception involves patients sustaining bullet wounds at the T12 through L4 level. The reasons cited for improved outcome with bullet removal at the thoracolumbar level include: (1) the large number of nerve roots within the cauda equina that can be compressed by a bullet; and (2) the ability of axons to regenerate within intact nerve roots.[68] Although management is conservative in most cases,[64] patients who deteriorate may also require spinal decompression.[4,63,66,67] Patients with initially complete lesions usually have poor outcomes, but those with incomplete lesions usually regain ambulation.[65] Corticosteroids are not indicated in patients sustaining penetrating SCI.[4,40,41] Antibiotics, usually a second- or third-generation cephalosporin, should be administered, since these wounds are at risk for infection.[4]

Spinal Cord Concussion

Although SCI often leads to permanent neurologic disability, a small percentage of patients with motor or sensory dysfunction recover rapidly and completely. This phenomenon of transient paralysis is known as **spinal cord concussion** (SCC).[69,70] In a review of approximately 500 patients with cord injury, Ducker et al[71] found that while 85% of the injuries remained permanent and complete, approximately 3% of patients fully recovered. To make the diagnosis, the concussion must resolve within 48 to 72 hours and be consistent with the level of injury.[69,70] Congenital spinal fusion and spinal stenosis predispose to SCC.[70,72-74] Patients often recover within 2 to 3 hours, and some deficits resolve within 15 minutes.[69,70,72,74,75]

In contrast to cerebral concussion, where the synapses are the site of injury, in SCC injury occurs within the axons.[76-78] One theory suggests that axonal permeability to sodium is altered following injury.[78] The cell membrane develops a new resting potential that inhibits sodium influx at the start of an action potential and leads to paralysis. Motor function returns when the normal membrane physiology is restored.

As in all cases of spinal cord deficit, plain radiographs are needed to rule out associated vertebral fractures. Obtain an MRI soon after the injury to evaluate possible spinal hemorrhage. In the early phase of SCI, it is impossible to predict neurologic recovery. Therefore all injured patients presenting with neurologic deficits from blunt trauma should receive the methylprednisolone protocol.

OVERALL PROGNOSIS

Functional recovery may follow spinal injury. However, if paralysis continues for days after resolution of spinal shock, complete recovery is unlikely.[79] Only 1% to 4% of patients with complete lesions and no perianal sensation at 48 hours postinjury recover.[12,13,80,81] However, some researchers believe that neurologic status at 72 hours better predicts long-term outcome.[82]

Sacral sparing on the initial examination (e.g., intact perianal sensation, toe flexion, anal sphincter control) is an auspicious sign.[6,12,83] Sparing may be a result of preserved white matter in the cervical spinal cord, which promotes resolution of paralysis.[83] Patients with sensory or sacral sparing often improve over the ensuing year.[32,39,79,84,85]

Patients who sustain Frankel or ASIA C & D injuries usually recover ambulation without surgical or pharmacologic treatment.[84,85] Upper extremity muscles with some function in the first 72 hours postinjury exhibit earlier recovery than paralyzed muscles.[5] The overwhelming majority of patients less than 50 years of age with CCS and partial muscle strength in at least one lower extremity usually walk within 6 months of injury.[5] However, patients older than 50 years of age have a worse prognosis.[5]

Patients with partial cord syndromes vary in outcome. A BSS injury often improves despite complete transection of the ipsilateral tract.[86] Recovery begins within 24 to 48 hours after injury and continues over months to years.[86,87] Contralateral motor recovery tends to appear earlier than ipsilateral function.[87] Extensor function may recover sooner than flexor function, and proximal muscles before distal muscles.[86] Patients with an anterior cord syndrome have the worst prognosis of incomplete cord syndromes, and the potential for functional ambulation is limited.[12,13]

After SCI, the patient is at risk for infectious complications. The most common complications include urinary tract infection, pneumonia, and infected pressure sores.[88,89] Pneumonia has surpassed urinary tract infection as the leading cause of death in the patient with SCI.[89] Patients with SCI do not have typical symptoms associated with these infections and may complain of vague back or abdominal discomfort, incontinence, malaise, or increased spasticity.[88]

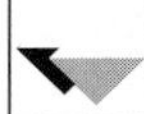

PEARLS & PITFALLS

- ◆ The most important goals in the management of the patient with SCI are to prevent further damage to the cord, while excluding other potential life-threatening injuries.
- ◆ Do not assume that hypotension is due to SCI until hemopneumothorax, hemoperitoneum, or pelvic bleeding has been excluded.
- ◆ Patients with lesions at C4 or C5 are at risk for delayed respiratory failure from cord edema. Consider serial measurements of pulmonary function while in the ED.
- ◆ Corticosteroids in blunt SCI may prevent secondary injury. Give methylprednisolone as a bolus of 30 mg/kg of body weight, followed by infusion at 5.4 mg/kg per hour for 23 hours as soon as possible after injury.
- ◆ Patients less than 8 years old are at risk for high cervical injuries. Young children may have neurologic deficits without obvious fractures or dislocations, a condition known as SCIWORA.
- ◆ Patients with partial cord syndromes and those with sacral sparing have a good chance for functional recovery.
- ◆ A small subset of patients with initial paraplegia or tetraplegia will regain complete function within 72 hours; a condition referred to as spinal cord concussion. Patients who remain with complete SCI after 72 hours rarely recover.

REFERENCES

1. Burney RE, et al: Incidence, characteristics, and outcome of spinal cord injury at trauma centers in North America, *Arch Surg* 128:596-599, 1993.
2. Kalfas I, et al: Magnetic resonance imaging in acute spinal cord trauma, *Neurosurgery* 23:295-299, 1988.
3. Slucky AV, Eismont FJ: Treatment of acute injury of the cervical spine, *Instr Course Lect* 44:67-80, 1995.
4. Jallo GI: Neurosurgical management of penetrating spinal injury, *Surg Neurol* 47:328-330, 1997.
5. Ditunno JF Jr, Graziani V, Tessler A: Neurological assessment in spinal cord injury, *Adv Neurol* 72:325-333, 1997.

6. Waters RL, et al: Motor and sensory recovery following incomplete tetraplegia, *Arch Phys Med Rehabil* 75:306-311, 1994.
7. Tator CH: Update on the pathophysiology and pathology of acute spinal cord injury, *Brain Pathol* 5:407-413, 1995.
8. Ditunno JF Jr, et al: The international standards booklet for neurological and functional classification of spinal cord injury, *Paraplegia* 32:70-80, 1994.
9. Frankel HL, et al: The value of postural reduction in the initial management of closed injuries of the spine with paraplegia and tetraplegia, *Paraplegia* 7:179-192, 1969.
10. Atkinson PP, Atkinson JL: Spinal shock, *Mayo Clin Proc* 71:384-389, 1996.
11. Watanabe T, Rivas DA, Chancellor MB: Urodynamics of spinal cord injury, *Urol Clin North Am* 23:459-473, 1996.
12. Stauffer ES: Diagnosis and prognosis of acute cervical spinal cord injury, *Clin Orthop Rel Res* 112:9-15, 1975.
13. Bosch A, Stauffer ES, Nickel VL: Incomplete traumatic quadriplegia: a ten-year review, *JAMA* 216:473-478, 1971.
14. Maroon JC, et al: Central cord syndrome, *Clin Neurosurg* 37:612-621, 1991.
15. Levi AD, Tator CH, Bunge RP: Clinical syndromes associated with disproportionate weakness of the upper versus the lower extremities after cervical spinal cord injury, *Neurosurgery* 38:179-183, 1996.
16. Bell HS: Paralysis of both arms from injury of the upper portion of the pyramidal decussation: "Cruciate paralysis," *J Neurosurg* 33:376-380, 1970.
17. Maroon JC: 'Burning hands' in football spinal cord injuries, *JAMA* 238:2049-2051, 1977.
18. Wilberger JE, Abla A, Maroon JC: Burning hands syndrome revisited, *Neurosurgery* 19:1038-1040, 1986.
19. Aminoff MJ: Brown-Sequard and his work on the spinal cord, *Spine* 21:133-140, 1996.
20. Rumana CS, Baskin DS: Brown-Sequard syndrome produced by cervical disc herniation: case report and literature review, *Surg Neurol* 45:359-361, 1996.
21. Koehler PJ, Endtz LJ: The Brown-Sequard syndrome: true or false? *Arch Neurol* 43:921-924, 1986.
22. Roth EJ, et al: Traumatic cervical Brown-Sequard and Brown-Sequard-plus syndromes: the spectrum of presentations and outcomes, *Paraplegia* 29:582-589, 1991.
23. Schneider RC: The syndrome of acute anterior spinal cord injury, *J Neurosurg* 12:95-122, 1955.
24. Shapiro S: Cauda equina syndrome secondary to lumbar disc herniation, *Neurosurgery* 32:743-746, 1993.
25. Dinning TA, Schaeffer HR: Discogenic compression of the cauda equina: a surgical emergency, *Aust N Z J Surg* 63:927-934, 1993.
26. Sayegh FE, et al: Functional outcome after experimental cauda equina compression, *J Bone Joint Surg* 79-B:670-674, 1997.
27. Coscia M, Leipzig T, Cooper D: Acute cauda equina syndrome: diagnostic advantage of MRI, *Spine* 19:475-478, 1994.
28. Fox JL, et al: Central spinal cord injury: magnetic resonance imaging confirmation and operative considerations, *Neurosurgery* 22:340-346, 1988.
29. Vale FL, et al: Combined medical and surgical treatment after acute spinal cord injury: results of a prospective pilot study to assess the merits of aggressive medical resuscitation and blood pressure management, *J Neurosurg* 87:239-246, 1997.
30. Vaccaro AR, et al: Neurologic outcome of early versus late surgery for cervical spinal cord injury, *Spine* 22:2609-2613, 1997.
31. Waters RL, et al: Effect of surgery on motor recovery following traumatic spinal cord injury, *Spinal Cord* 34:188-192, 1996.
32. Asazuma T, et al: Management of patients with an incomplete cervical spinal cord injury, *Spinal Cord* 34:620-625, 1996.
33. Botel U, Glaser E, Niedeggen A: The surgical treatment of acute spinal paralysed patients, *Spinal Cord* 35:420-428, 1997.
34. George ER, et al: Failure of methylprednisolone to improve the outcome of spinal cord injuries, *Am Surg* 61:659-663, 1995.
35. Bracken MB: Pharmacological treatment of acute spinal cord injury: current status and future projects, *J Emerg Med* 11:43-48, 1993.
36. Bracken MB, et al: A randomized, controlled trial of methylprednisolone or naloxone in the treatment of acute spinal-cord injury, *N Engl J Med* 322:1405-1411, 1990.
37. Hall ED: The neuroprotective pharmacology of methylprednisolone, *J Neurosurg* 76:13-22, 1992.
38. Gerhart KA, et al: Utilization and effectiveness of methylprednisolone in a population-based sample of spinal cord injured persons, *Paraplegia* 33:316-321, 1995.
39. Merry WH, et al: Functional outcome after incomplete spinal cord injuries due to blunt injury, *Injury* 27:17-20, 1996.
40. Prendergast MR, et al: Massive steroids do not reduce the zone of injury after penetrating spinal cord injury, *J Trauma* 37:576-579, 1994.
41. Levy ML, et al: Use of methylprednisolone as an adjunct in the management of patients with penetrating spinal cord injury: outcome analysis, *Neurosurgery* 39:1141-1148, 1996.
42. Manary MJ, Jaffe DM: Cervical spine injuries in children, *Pediatr Ann* 25:423-428, 1996.
43. Birney TJ, Hanley EN: Traumatic cervical spine injuries in childhood and adolescence, *Spine* 14:1277-1282, 1989.
44. Ruge JR, et al: Pediatric spinal injury: the very young, *J Neurosurg* 68:25-30, 1988.
45. Hadley MN, et al: Pediatric spinal trauma: review of 122 cases of spinal cord and vertebral column injuries, *J Neurosurg* 68:18-24, 1988.
46. McGrory BJ, et al: Acute fractures and dislocations of the cervical spine in children and adolescents, *J Bone Joint Surg* 75A:988-995, 1993.
47. Anderson JM, Schutt AH: Spinal injury in children: a review of 156 cases seen from 1950 through 1978, *Mayo Clin Proc* 55:499-504, 1980.
48. Kewalramani LS, Tori JA: Spinal cord trauma in children: neurologic patterns, radiologic features, and pathomechanics of injury, *Spine* 5:11-18, 1980.
49. Kewalramani LS, Kraus JF, Sterling HM: Acute spinal-cord lesions in a pediatric population: epidemiological and clinical features, *Paraplegia* 18:206-219, 1980.
50. Nitecki S, Moir CR: Predictive factors of the outcome of traumatic cervical spine fracture in children, *J Pediatr Surg* 29:1409-1411, 1994.
51. Evans DL, Bethem D: Cervical spine injuries in children, *J Pediatr Orthop* 9:563-568, 1989.
52. Bohn D, et al: Cervical spine injuries in children, *J Trauma* 30:463-469, 1990.
53. Pang D, Wilberger JE Jr: Spinal cord injury without radiographic abnormalities in children, *J Neurosurg* 57:114-129, 1982.
54. Matsumura A, et al: Magnetic resonance imaging of spinal cord injury without radiologic abnormality, *Surg Neurol* 33:281-283, 1990.
55. Kriss VM, Kriss TC: SCIWORA (Spinal cord injury without radiographic abnormality) in infants and children, *Clin Pediatr* 35:119-124, 1996.
56. Hachen HJ: Spinal cord injury in children and adolescents: diagnostic pitfalls and therapeutic considerations in the acute stage, *Paraplegia* 15:55-64, 1977.
57. Grabb PA, Pang D: Magnetic resonance imaging in the evaluation of spinal cord injury without radiographic abnormality in children, *Neurosurgery* 35:406-414, 1994.

58. Kihtir T, et al: Management of transperitoneal gunshot wounds of the spine, *J Trauma* 31:1579-1583, 1991.
59. Waters RL, Adkins RH: Firearm versus motor vehicle related spinal cord injury: preinjury factors, injury characteristics, and initial outcome comparisons among ethnically diverse groups, *Arch Phys Med Rehabil* 78:150-155, 1997.
60. Simpson RK Jr, Venger BH, Narayan RK: Treatment of acute penetrating injuries to the spine: a retrospective analysis, *J Trauma* 29:42-46, 1989.
61. Velmahos GC, et al: Changing profiles in spinal cord injuries and risk factors influencing recovery after penetrating injuries, *J Trauma* 38:334-337, 1995.
62. Yoshida GM, Garland D, Waters RL: Gunshot wounds to the spine, *Orthop Clin North Am* 26:109-116, 1995.
63. Kupcha PC, An HS, Cotler JM: Gunshot wounds to the cervical spine, *Spine* 15:1058-1063, 1990.
64. Wigle RL: Treatment of asymptomatic gunshot injuries to the spine, *Am Surg* 55:591-595, 1989.
65. Aarabi B, et al: Comparative study of functional recovery for surgically explored and conservatively managed spinal cord missile injuries, *Neurosurgery* 39:1133-1140, 1996.
66. Heiden JS, et al: Penetrating gunshot wounds of the cervical spine in civilians: review of 38 cases, *Neurosurgery* 42:575-579, 1975.
67. Hammoud MA, Haddad FS, Moufarrij NA: Spinal cord missile injuries during the Lebanese civil war, *Surg Neurol* 43:432-437, 1995.
68. Waters RL, Adkins RH: The effects of removal of bullet fragments retained in the spinal canal: a collaborative study by the National Spinal Cord Injury Model System, *Spine* 16:934-939, 1991.
69. Zwimpfer TJ, Bernstein M: Spinal cord concussion, *J Neurosurg* 72:894-900, 1990.
70. Del Bigio MR, Johnson GE: Clinical presentation of spinal cord concussion, *Spine* 14:37-40, 1989.
71. Ducker TB, Lucas JT, Wallace CA: Recovery from spinal cord injury, *Clin Neurosurg* 30:495-513, 1983.
72. Rathbone D, Johnson G, Letts M: Spinal cord concussion in pediatric athletes, *J Pediatr Orthop* 12:616-620, 1992.
73. Scher AT: Spinal cord concussion in rugby players, *Am J Sports Med* 19:485-488, 1991.
74. Torg JS, et al: Neurapraxia of the cervical spinal cord with transient quadriplegia, *J Bone Joint Surg* 68A:1354-1370, 1986.
75. Ferrera PC, Hayes ST, Triner WR: Spinal cord concussion in previously undiagnosed osteogenesis imperfecta, *Am J Emerg Med* 13:424-426, 1995.
76. Parkinson D: The biomechanics of concussion, *Clin Neurosurg* 29:131-145, 1982.
77. Parkinson D, Del Bigio M, Jell RM: Spinal cord concussion, *Surg Neurol* 16:347-349, 1981.
78. Kobrine AI: The neuronal theory of experimental traumatic spinal cord dysfunction, *Surg Neurol* 3:261-264, 1975.
79. Waters RL: Functional prognosis of spinal cord injuries, *J Spinal Cord Med* 19:89-92, 1996.
80. Bohlman HH: Acute fractures and dislocations of the cervical spine, *J Bone Joint Surg* 61A:1119-1142, 1979.
81. Waters RL, et al: Recovery following complete paraplegia, *Arch Phys Med Rehabil* 73:784-789, 1992.
82. Brown PJ, et al: The 72-hour examination as a predictor of recovery in motor complete quadriplegia, *Arch Phys Med Rehabil* 72:546-548, 1991.
83. Katoh S, El-Masry WS: Motor recovery of patients presenting with motor paralysis and sensory sparing following cervical spinal cord injuries, *Paraplegia* 33:506-509, 1995
84. Katoh S, et al: Neurologic outcome in conservatively treated patients with incomplete closed traumatic cervical spinal cord injuries, *Spine* 21:2345-2351, 1996.
85. Alander DH, Parker J, Stauffer ES: Intermediate-term outcome of cervical spinal cord-injured patients older than 50 years of age, *Spine* 22:1189-1192, 1997.
86. Little JW, Halar E: Temporal course of motor recovery after Brown-Sequard spinal cord injuries, *Paraplegia* 23:39-46, 1985.
87. Taylor RG, Gleave JR: Incomplete spinal cord injuries with Brown-Sequard phenomena, *J Bone Joint Surg* 39B:438-450, 1957.
88. Montgomerie JZ: Infections in patients with spinal cord injuries, *Clin Infect Dis* 25:1285-1992, 1997.
89. Hartkopp A, et al: Survival and cause of death after traumatic spinal cord injury: a long-term epidemiological survey from Denmark, *Spinal Cord* 35:76-85, 1997.

13 Vertebral Injuries

STACY WEEKS JANDREAU AND MICHAEL A. GIBBS

The diagnosis of vertebral injury remains one of the most daunting challenges to emergency physicians (EPs) and trauma teams. Multiply-injured patients may have few signs of vertebral fracture, yet can suffer devastating neurologic sequela. Emergency physicians must be expert at protection and evaluation of the spine.

EPIDEMIOLOGY

Up to 12,000 new spinal injuries occur annually in the United States.[1-3] The cost of supportive care may approach 1 to 5 million dollars over the lifetime of the patient.[4] More significantly, the personal and family impact of lost function cannot be measured.

Cervical spine injuries occur in 5% to 6% of trauma patients, whereas fractures of the thoracolumbar spine occur in 2% to 3%. Motor vehicle crashes (MVCs) are responsible for 85% of vertebral injuries; major contributors include speeding, alcohol, and failure to use restraints. One in every 300 MVC victims suffers a spinal injury and that occurrence soars to 1 in every 14 if the occupant is ejected. About 14% of spinal injuries result from falls and 1% from "miscellaneous" causes, such as diving accidents, assaults, sports injuries, and missile injuries.[3]

Spinal injury is predominantly a disease of young adults. Since males, particularly adolescents and young adults, engage in high-risk behaviors, they are also the predominant victims of traumatic injuries.[2,3,5,6] The male-to-female ratio of spinal injuries is approximately 3 to 1.[3]

A variety of associated injuries occur in patients with spinal fractures. Young adults with fractures of the thoracic spine are likely to have multisystem and, in particular, chest injuries resulting from the high forces involved. Children with a seatbelt sign and lumbar fracture are likely to suffer concomitant small bowel injury.[7]

CLINICAL PRESENTATION

Because the clinical presentation of vertebral injury can be subtle, it is often overshadowed by other injuries. Several researchers have investigated correlations of vertebral injury.[8-11] These studies demonstrate that pain, tenderness, or neurologic deficit most reliably predict fractures.

Suspicion for vertebral injuries must begin in the prehospital setting. Before 1980 the majority of patients with spinal *cord* injury arrived in the emergency department (ED) with complete deficits. During the ensuing decade, educational and technical advances resulted in standard protocols for spinal immobilization in the prehospital setting.

Recently, a number of centers have studied whether paramedics and EPs agree on the need for spinal immobilization in a given patient. The results of these studies suggest that the groups disagree in a substantial subset of patients.[12,13] For this reason, most prehospital systems continue a policy of immobilizing many blunt trauma patients despite a low likelihood of spinal injury.

Many patients with unstable vertebral fractures are neurologically intact on arrival, and as many as 60% of identified spinal cord injuries are incomplete. However, inappropriate manipulation during ED evaluation and resuscitation may result in neurologic impairment. Of those patients who sustain cervical spine injury, 39% to 47% have an associated spinal deficit.[14-16] Unfortunately, between 5% and 10% of these patients deteriorate neurologically after the initial resuscitation. Once the patient is placed on the trauma stretcher, the EP must evaluate and diagnose spinal injuries without causing further damage to the cord.

EMERGENCY DEPARTMENT EVALUATION

Initial Stabilization

As with all patients suffering significant trauma, the EP must first identify and manage injuries that pose an immediate threat to life. Cervical fractures rarely fall into this category. After airway patency, hemodynamic stability, and adequate ventilation are ensured, attention is directed to the spinal and neurologic examination.

If urgent airway management is needed, *do not* waste time obtaining a cross-table-lateral cervical spine radiograph before intubation. This single view is inadequate to exclude injury; even under optimum conditions it will miss 15% of cervical fractures. Waiting for the radiograph squanders precious time and gives the operator a false sense of security when the film is interpreted as "normal." Assume that all patients have cervical injury, and maintain in-line stabilization at all times during airway management.[17]

Many authorities debate the safety of oral intubation in the presence of cervical spine injury. Historically this issue divides both practitioners and scholars alike.

One theory argues that manipulation of the airway during direct laryngoscopy might displace unstable elements, resulting in spinal cord injury. This largely theoretic premise was widely accepted for years and led to blind nasotracheal intubation as an airway maneuver of choice in the multiply-injured trauma patient. In the situation where nasotracheal intubation was not possible, proponents recommended surgical cricothyroidotomy.[18-20]

The countervailing position held that oral endotracheal intubation is safe even in the presence of cervical spine injury, given meticulous immobilization of the cervical spine throughout the process of intubation. Although there are no randomized controlled trials to settle this debate, an increasing body of literature argues in favor of oral intubation with spinal stabilization.[17]

Several series demonstrate that properly performed rapid sequence intubation (RSI) with in-line cervical immobilization is safe in the presence of proven cervical spine injury.[17-22] However, there are several caveats to oral intubation in the presence of a possible or known spinal injury.

1. Emergency physicians must perform laryngoscopy and intubation in an atraumatic manner. RSI is favored over awake oral intubation or intubation with sedation alone because it allows for immediate airway control and eliminates the risk of patient movement during laryngoscopy. A recent review demonstrates that neuromuscular blockade reduces the risk of complications during emergency intubation.[23]
2. An assistant maintains precise cervical immobilization throughout the intubation sequence. This individual's sole responsibility is manual immobilization of the spine. Ideally, this person should stand at the side rather than the head of the bed to give the intubator unimpeded access to the airway.
3. When the emergency physician believes the intubation will be difficult or impossible, he or she should consider an alternative technique. The technique employed (e.g., laryngoscopy with sedation, fiberoptic intubation, blind nasotracheal intubation, or cricothyroidotomy) depends on the clinical scenario and the experience of the operator.

History and Physical Examination

A thorough history, when available, can provide clues regarding vertebral injury. Apparently minor injuries must not dissuade the physician from performing a complete primary and secondary survey. Emergency physicians should routinely question the victim, prehospital providers, and witnesses about the incident to help focus further diagnostic and therapeutic efforts. A history of pain in the neck or back, numbness, or weakness (even transient) may herald vertebral injury. Certain concurrent medical conditions may predispose to spinal injury. Patients with advanced rheumatoid arthritis may suffer rupture of the posterior odontoid ligament, whereas those with Down syndrome may develop atlantooccipital dislocations. The history of isolated use of a lap belt (without a shoulder harness) increases the risk of a lumbar spine fracture, particularly a horizontal fracture through the body of L1-3 (Chance fracture).

Patients with a lower thoracic or any lumbar fracture may develop abdominal distention from an associated ileus. Such patients may also complain of pain in the back with abdominal palpation.

Once the EP has managed any immediate life threats (all the while *assuming* a spinal injury), they can then assess the spine and spinal cord. Gently roll the patient while stabilizing the cervical spine, and carefully palpate the entire vertebral column from occiput to sacrum. Look for ecchymosis, focal tenderness, or obvious deformity. The EP must distinguish midline vertebral tenderness from paravertebral muscular tenderness. When there is doubt, employ a low threshold for spinal radiography.

A detailed and precise neurologic examination is critical in the evaluation of the patient with a possible spinal injury. Serial examination is of equal importance to identify and document evolving neurologic pathology. The American Spinal Injury Association (ASIA) has established guidelines for motor and sensory evaluations.[24] In the awake, interactive patient assess light-touch sensation by dermatome to localize the most cephalad extent of the spinal injury. Pain sensation determines contralateral spinothalamic tract function. Measure motor function, which indicates ipsilateral corticospinal tract integrity, on a 0 to 5 scale. The dorsal columns control proprioception and vibration in the distal extremities. Testing these functions differentiates between a complete lesion and an anterior cord syndrome. Rectal tone, sacral sensation, and bowel and bladder function deserve special attention to avoid missing injuries to the conus medullaris and cauda equina. The presence of these functions may help distinguish between complete versus incomplete cord injury.[24,25]

Spinal shock may eliminate all spinal function and reflexes for the first 24 to 48 hours following injury. Reversal of spinal shock is heralded by the return of the bulbocavernosus reflex. To assess this reflex, insert a finger in the rectum and feel for sphincter contractions in response to a standard stimulus. A quick tug on a Foley catheter, pinching the glans in a male, or pressing on the clitoris in a female should provoke an anal "wink."

Indications for Cervical Radiography

The failure to obtain indicated radiographs is the most common reason for missed cervical spine fracture. The recommended indications for cervical spine radiography have evolved considerably during the past decade. Until recently the American College of Surgeons recommended cervical radiography in "any patient with major blunt trauma."[26] Some physicians obtain films on all patients immobilized by paramedics, relinquishing this important medical decision. Although this approach would appear sensitive for fracture, it comes at the expense of a tremendous number of negative radiographs. In an era of rational use of resources, universal imaging of the cervical spine is both impractical and inefficient. Universal radiographic screening may result in false-positive films, some related to congenital bony abnormalities, and unnecessary interventions. In addition to the obvious financial implications, this approach also results in needless exposure to radiation and potential delays in patient evaluation and treatment. Recent evidence suggests that in many cases, the EP can clinically identify patients at low risk for cervical injury.

Ten published case series, with a combined total of over 30,000 patients detailed low-risk clinical criteria for cervical spine injury.* In these studies there were *no* cervical spine fractures in alert patients without spinal tenderness who were neurologically intact, not intoxicated, and who did not suffer from other severely painful injuries. Based on the cited literature, cervical spine radiography is mandatory in blunt trauma patients who have the following:

1. Posterior midline tenderness: midline cervical tenderness on palpation (although a few studies used the criteria of cervical *pain*)
2. Altered mental status because of brain injury, intoxication, or metabolic derangement
3. Neurologic deficits
4. Distracting injuries: considered severe enough to "distract" patients from cervical spine pain or tenderness

In patients without these clinical findings, cervical radiography can be safely deferred. Similar criteria have been successfully used in children.[32,33] In the recently published National Emergency X-Radiography Utilization Study (NEXUS) these criteria were prospectively validated in a cohort of 27,389 low-risk patients at 22 academic and nonacademic emergency departments.[31] Only 15 fractures (0.05%) were missed, of which 1 (0.004%) required surgical intervention. None of the injuries were unstable. Trials demonstrate that the interrater reliability of these criteria is substantial. Admittedly the criteria are somewhat subjective: in particular, the assessment of what constitutes a distracting injury.[34] A fractured finger may be distracting for some patients, whereas others remain conversational despite a broken femur. Two studies examined low-risk clinical criteria for the assessment of the thoracolumbar spine with similar positive results.[35,36] A consensus statement by the American College of Radiology supports this clinically-driven approach.[37]

In contrast, scientific scrutiny does not support the old dictum that "any patient with an injury above the clavicles" needs cervical imaging. Several studies demonstrate little, if any, relationship between head injury and facial injury and cervical spine injury. Patients with these injuries should be evaluated as all other victims of blunt trauma. However, altered mental status as a result of head trauma is a clear indication for cervical radiography.[38-42] There is also a growing body of literature that cervical radiography can be safely deferred in patients with isolated gunshot wounds to the head, provided the missile trajectory does not traverse the neck.[43,44]

---

*References 1, 2, 8, 10, 11, 27-31.

Numerous researchers have debated whether or not there is such a thing as an asymptomatic spinal injury.* Though a few case reports describe clinically occult spinal injuries,[6,45-50] these reports have significant flaws.[1-2,5,51] An excellent review by Saddison et al[52] revealed that the injuries described were not truly asymptomatic. Several of the cited patients did have cervical pain or tenderness; those without clinical findings of spinal injury were either brain-injured, were under the influence of drugs or alcohol, or were victims of severe multisystem trauma.

Indications for Thoracolumbar Radiography

The clinical indications for thoracic and lumbar films are less well-studied than for cervical radiography. However, a standard approach uses the same clinical indicators as those governing C-spine injuries. Most research demonstrates that a patient who is awake and alert without concomitant distracting injuries *and* has no clinical evidence of a thoracolumbar fracture does not require plain films of the dorsal spine.[53-55]

However, all told, these studies comprise less than 600 patients examined in a retrospective fashion. In one study, the authors emphasized that the absence of back pain does not exclude significant thoracolumbar injury.[56] Based on a retrospective study of 167 patients, they suggest the following criteria for thoracolumbar films:

1. Trauma patients with back pain or tenderness
2. A fall greater than 10 feet
3. Ejection from a car or motorcycle traveling at 50 miles per hour or greater
4. Glasgow Coma Score of ≤8
5. Neurologic deficit

At least in children, plain films appear a more sensitive screen for lumbar fractures than even thin-slice CT scan. In one study, CT missed nearly 60% of pediatric lumbar fractures diagnosed on plain films.[57]

Plain Film Radiograph Selection

Aside from failure to obtain *indicated* radiographs, the most common etiology of missed cervical spine fractures is failure to obtain *adequate* radiographs. In a review of 32,000 blunt trauma patients Davis et al[58] found delayed diagnosis or missed diagnosis of cervical spine injuries in 34 of 740 patients (4.6%). More than 70% of these injuries were unstable, and major neurologic consequences occurred in 29%. In the majority of cases, missed fractures were the result of inadequate radiographs.

*References 1-3, 5, 8-11, 25.

HOW MANY VIEWS?

In many centers the cervical spine is "cleared" using a cross-table lateral view (CTL) alone. This approach is a mistake. A CTL alone is inadequate to rule out cervical injury, because of an unacceptably low sensitivity between 57% and 85%.[59-61] The addition of the anterior-posterior view (AP) and open-mouth odontoid view (OMO) increases the sensitivity to 99%.[62] For this reason, obtain at least three views in all cases where cervical radiography is needed for victims of trauma. The issue of whether oblique views should be routine remains controversial. Some authors believe that oblique views are essential because they provide superior visualization of the posterior column (pedicles, articular pillars, neural foramina, and lamina).[63] Although some studies have found that the oblique view demonstrates certain fractures not detected on the three-view series,[64] others fail to demonstrate a benefit of the five-view series over the three-view series.[65] Although there is no consensus in the literature concerning the necessity for routine oblique radiographs in cervical trauma, these views may help evaluate poorly visualized areas of the posterior column. In addition, the supine oblique views provide excellent definition of the cervicothoracic junction and may be used in conjunction with the often inadequate swimmer's view to visualize this area.[66,67] It is reasonable to order the oblique views selectively if a three-view series suggests pathology or is inadequate.

Indications for flexion-extension films lack rigorous study. In neurologically intact patients with persistent neck pain and/or tenderness despite normal plain radiographs, flexion and extension views may demonstrate ligamentous injury.[68] It is essential that the patient be alert and cooperative, since the patient must actively move his or her neck and stop movement immediately with increased pain. Manipulation of the neck by the physician or radiology technologist to overcome spasm is contraindicated. Flexion-extension views are often inadequate in the acute setting because muscle pain and spasm prevent the patient from relaxing. In this situation, follow-up films may be required to exclude ligamentous injury. In the obtunded or uncooperative patient with normal radiographs, dynamic fluoroscopy through the full range of flexion and extension may rule out ligamentous injury.[69] However, this study is rarely ordered by the EP and is best deferred until after transfer to an in-patient bed. When a cervical spine cannot be cleared because of an alteration in mental status or intubation, apply a soft cervical collar pending follow-up evaluation.

Computed Tomography

The role of computed tomography (CT) in the evaluation of cervical trauma has grown substantially. Most of the current radiology and trauma literature supports the use of CT as an adjunct to plain films in the patients with the following:

1. Negative cervical spine radiographs but persistent neck pain or neurologic dysfunction
2. Suspicious abnormality on the plain films
3. Inadequate visualization of the cervicothoracic junction
4. CT is also helpful to further evaluate injuries diagnosed initially by plain film radiography[16,70-72]

In addition, several authors have suggested that patients with severe brain injury who are undergoing cranial tomography should have CT imaging extended from the skull base to C3, since this area is difficult to visualize in the intubated patient. Link et al[73] evaluated 202 intubated patients with significant traumatic brain injury using a standard imaging protocol that included CT cuts to the top of C3. They found that plain film radiographs alone would have missed 11 of 28 patients with a C1 or C2 fracture, and 8 of 9 patients with occipital condyle fractures.

Magnetic Resonance Imaging

Magnetic resonance imaging (MRI) plays an increasing role in evaluation of spinal cord injury. Advantages include lack of ionizing radiation, multiplanar imaging capabilities, and, most importantly, the ability to delineate soft tissue structures such as the intervertebral disks, ligamentous structures, and spinal cord.[74,75] MRI is indicated for the following:

1. Complete or incomplete neurologic deficits
2. Deterioration of neurologic function
3. Suspicion of ligamentous injury despite negative plain films[74]
4. MRI is also useful to identify spinal cord injuries in patients without associated vertebral fracture (e.g., central cord syndrome, Spinal Cord Injury without Radiographic Abnormalities [SCIWORA])

Notable disadvantages of MRI include a prolonged acquisition time, limited availability, and several contraindications, including patients with pacemakers, ferromagnetic aneurysm clips, metallic fragments in the spinal cord, and claustrophobia.

An algorithm for the radiologic evaluation of the cervical spine is presented in Fig. 13-1.

Radiograph Interpretation

Another major cause of missed cervical spine trauma is a failure to diagnose injury despite adequate radiographs. To avoid this error, emergency physicians must become expert in cervical plain film interpretation, and follow a diagnostic protocol when reading the films. A number of authors advocate an "ABCs" approach to the interpretation, "A" refers to *adequacy* and *alignment*, "B" refers to *bony integrity*, "C" refers to the *cartilage* and "S" describes the *soft tissue structures*.[45,76-78] Using this standard approach helps avoid missed injuries.

Cervical Spine Radiography

LATERAL VIEW

An *adequate* lateral film should visualize all seven cervical vertebrae, as well as the top of the first thoracic vertebrae. Because pulling on a patient's arms may be painful or impossible in those with upper extremity fractures, pushing down on the patient's shoulders from above using a pair of crutches may be useful. If caudal traction on the upper extremities is insufficient, obtain a swimmer's view or supine oblique views. When these views fail to define the cervicothoracic junction, obtain a CT scan.

Alignment. The alignment of the cervical column in the lateral view is determined by four normally smooth lordotic curves (Fig. 13-2), which can be created by visually connecting the following:

1. Anterior vertebral bodies from C1 through T1
2. Posterior cervical vertebral bodies
3. Spinolaminar line
4. Tips of the spinous processes

Evaluate these four lines for their smoothness and their integrity; any step-off, subluxation, or disruption is abnormal and may represent an injury. A step-off greater than 2 mm is abnormal (Fig. 13-3).[45] Though displacement can occur as a result of degenerative changes, muscle spasm, previous injury, or positioning, in the setting of trauma, assume that it represents an injury and order further radiographic evaluation. It is imperative to examine the space between the anterior surface of the dens and the posterior surface of the anterior arch of C1, the "predental space." This space should measure less than 3 mm in an adult and less than 5 mm in a child less than 8 years old.[76,77]

Loss of the normal lordosis on the lateral view may also represent an abnormality. Though this finding usually represents muscle spasm or a normal variant, it can also result from fractures, dislocations, and acute disc herniation. Give special consideration to the line created by the spinous processes. Normally the tips of the processes should converge to a point behind the neck, and the space between each process should be nearly equidistant. Widening of the space ("fanning") is a possible sign of a ruptured posterior ligamentous complex. (Fig. 13-4).[76,77]

When a vertebral body is displaced in an anterior direction, measure the amount of displacement. If the width of anterior displacement is less than one half the width of the vertebral body, it represents a dislo-

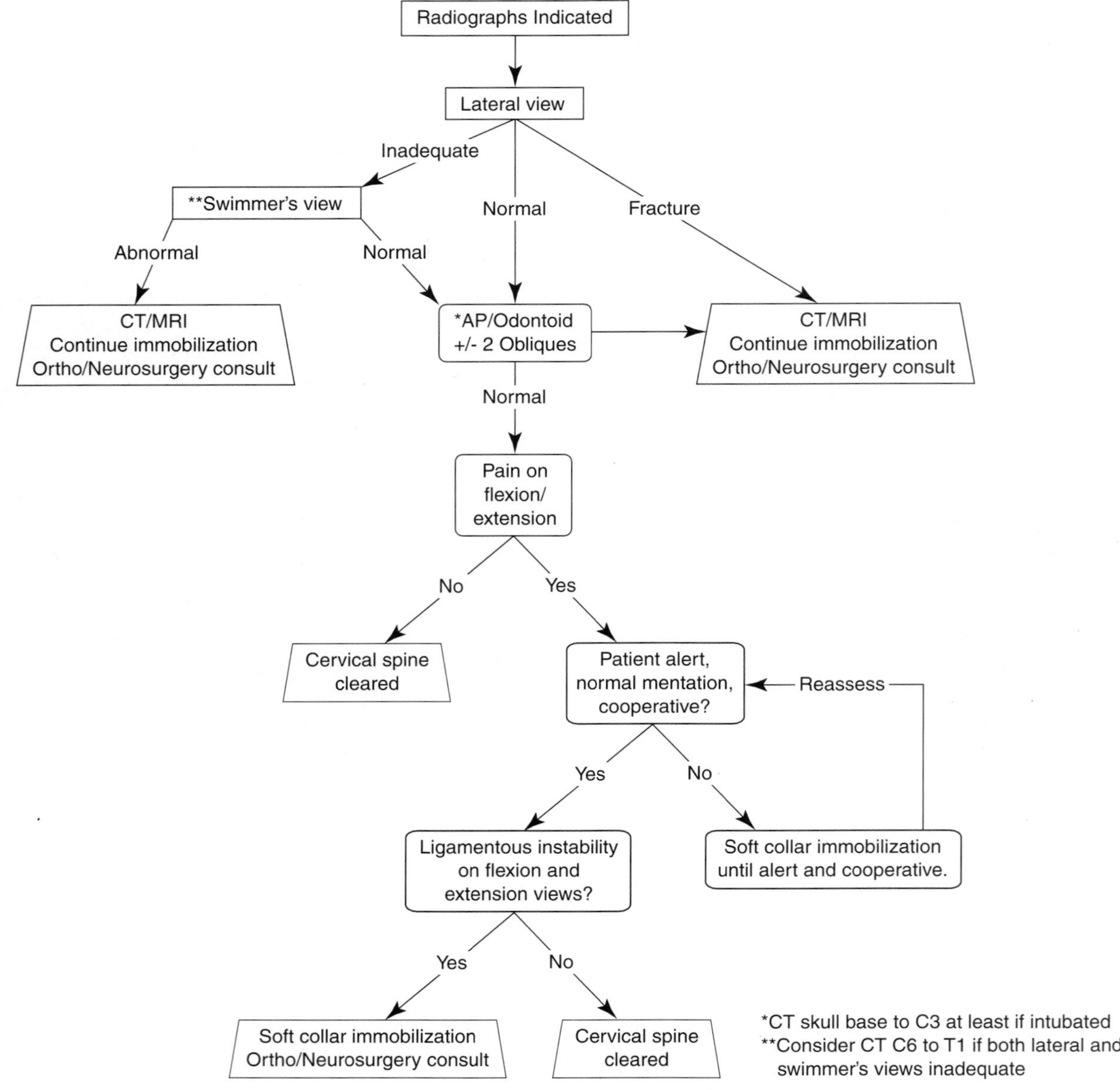

Fig. 13-1 Algorithm for cervical spine clearance.

cation of a single facet; if greater than one half, the injury is a bilateral facet dislocation, an unstable injury. In a bilateral facet dislocation, radiologic signs include fanning, narrowing of the intervertebral disc space, and soft tissue edema. Although similar findings are seen with a unifacet dislocation, a "bow-tie" sign is also present when a single facet is displaced. This sign demonstrates both facet surfaces on the lateral view.[76,77]

Bones. After evaluating the alignment on the lateral radiograph, the next step is to examine the individual bones. In a systematic manner, examine each of the vertebrae following the cortical surfaces, noting the shape and height. Loss of height, cortical breaks, or wedging of the vertebrae implies a fracture. The height of the anterior vertebral body should be no less than 3 mm smaller than the posterior height. An important structure is the "ring" of C2 located at the bottom half of this vertebra. A break in this ring is an important clue to a type III dens fracture.[79] Some additional findings that are nontraumatic in nature include osteophytes and vertebral body degeneration. Though these lesions can sometimes alter the appearance of the disc spaces, they are often seen in multiple areas and are typically the result of degenerative changes.[45]

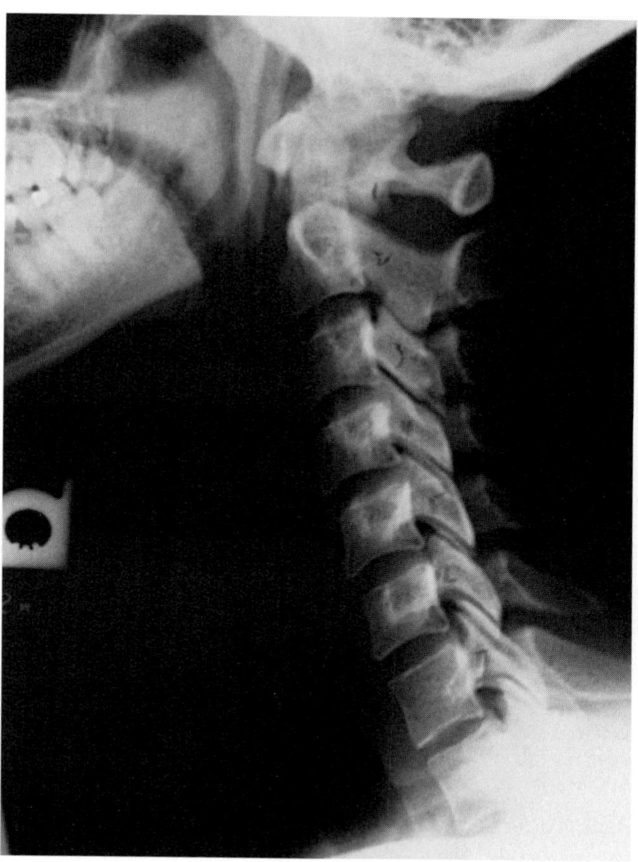

Fig. 13-2 Normal appearance of lateral cervical spine.

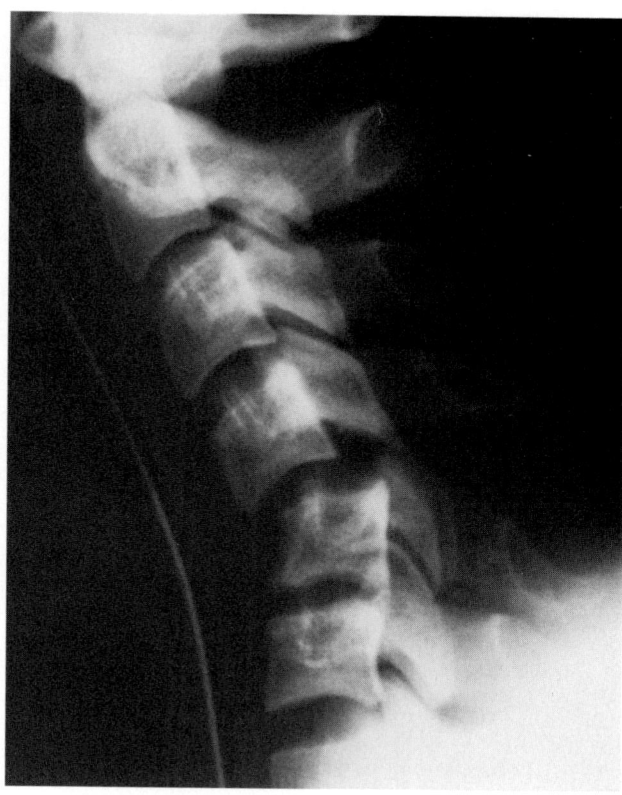

Fig. 13-3 Abnormal alignment of C4/5 level following direct strike to neck.

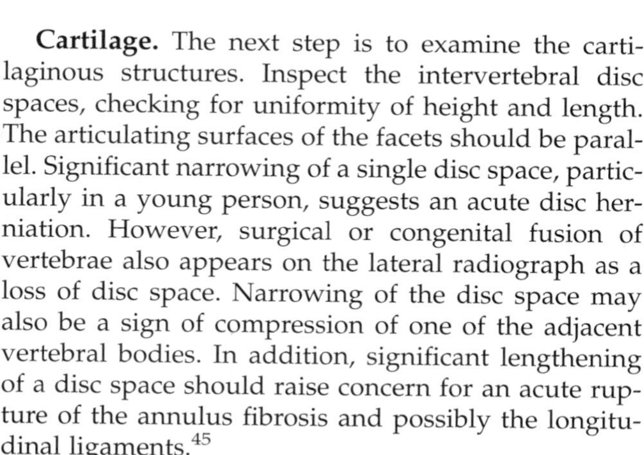

Cartilage. The next step is to examine the cartilaginous structures. Inspect the intervertebral disc spaces, checking for uniformity of height and length. The articulating surfaces of the facets should be parallel. Significant narrowing of a single disc space, particularly in a young person, suggests an acute disc herniation. However, surgical or congenital fusion of vertebrae also appears on the lateral radiograph as a loss of disc space. Narrowing of the disc space may also be a sign of compression of one of the adjacent vertebral bodies. In addition, significant lengthening of a disc space should raise concern for an acute rupture of the annulus fibrosis and possibly the longitudinal ligaments.[45]

Soft Tissues. Finally, the lateral radiograph images the soft-tissue spaces; the prevertebral soft tissue depicts the important retropharyngeal space. In the trauma setting, widening of the prevertebral soft tissue suggests cervical injury, particularly indicative of C1 and C2 fractures. In an adult, the normal width of the soft tissue space at the level of C1-C4 is less than or equal to 5 mm; and at C5-T1, 21 mm or less. Hemorrhage, free air, infections, foreign bodies, and tumors can also cause an abnormal widening of this space. Occasionally a widening of the soft tissue space may be the only sign of injury on the lateral radiograph.[45]

ANTEROPOSTERIOR VIEW

The anteroposterior (AP) view of the cervical spine is required to adequately view the cervical spine. The AP view should include C3 to T1, since the occiput and mandible obscure the first two cervical vertebrae. Note the alignment of the vertebral bodies and the spinous processes; the spinous processes should define a straight line down the middle of the vertebral bodies. Unifacet dislocation and fractures of the lateral articulating surface can cause malalignment of the spinous processes—producing an irregular line, with rotation of the process to the side of the injury.[76,77]

Inspect each vertebra for any abnormal step-off or breaks in the integrity of the cortical surface. In addition, examine the body for any abnormal lucencies or

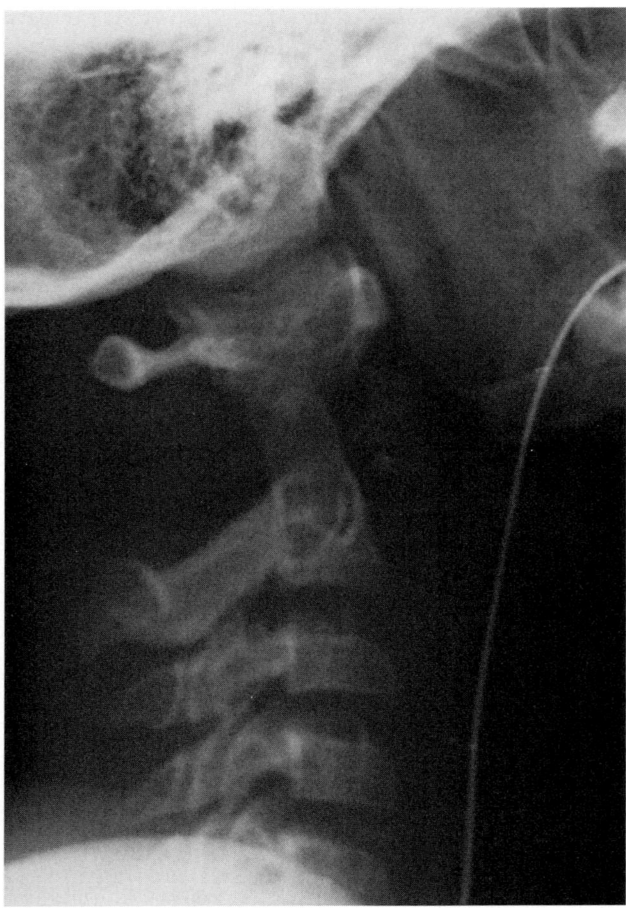

Fig. 13-4 Widely separated C1 and C2 vertebrae (atlantoaxial dislocation) in a pedestrian-motor vehicle crash.

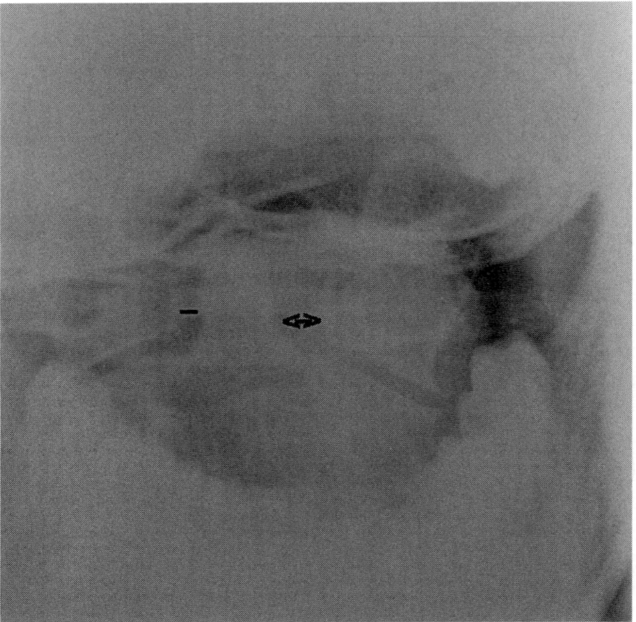

Fig. 13-5 The lateral tilt sign of an odontoid fracture. Note varying distances of the lateral masses with respect to the dens.

densities, indicating possible fractures. The intervertebral joint spaces and the paravertebral soft tissue should be uniform and undisrupted.

ODONTOID VIEW

This view identifies fractures of the dens and the ring of C1 (Jefferson's fractures). Again, use an ABCs approach, and alignment is especially important. The dens should be perpendicular to the lateral masses of C1, with uniform space on each lateral side. An important radiographic sign of odontoid fracture is the lateral tilt sign; this sign may be the only evident radiographic abnormality on plain film (Fig. 13-5).[80-82] Thomeier et al,[80] in a retrospective series, showed that a tilt of more than five degrees from the perpendicular (a dens angle of less than 85 degrees) usually indicates a fracture of the dens. When this sign is present, perform a CT scan of the odontoid process.

Shadows from overlying teeth or underlying bone may mislead the physician into diagnosing a fracture (Mach effect). A common mistake involves interpreting a vertical split in the dens as an injury; in most cases, this split is caused by the airspace between the upper central incisors projected onto the dens. Close inspection may identify the overlapping teeth. The bottom of the central incisors or the ring of the foremen magnum may also cast a horizontal shadow on the dens.

Examine both the relationships and the cortices of the odontoid process and the lateral masses of the atlas. Fractures may present as an asymmetry or disruptions in the cortex. Finally, assess the joint spaces for symmetry; the articulating surfaces should be parallel. The paravertebral soft tissue should not demonstrate any overlying shadows within the soft tissue in the odontoid view.[76,77]

SUPPLEMENTAL VIEWS

As mentioned previously, many facilities rely on three views to radiographically clear the cervical spine, whereas others use a five-view series. The two additional views usually consist of left and right lateral obliques (Fig. 13-6). These views focus on the facets and the intervertebral foramina. If these views are not part of the standard series, they should supplement the initial three-view series if a fracture or dislocation of the facets or foramina is suspected.

Finally, flexion and extension views can be used in the evaluation of the cervical spine in the trauma pa-

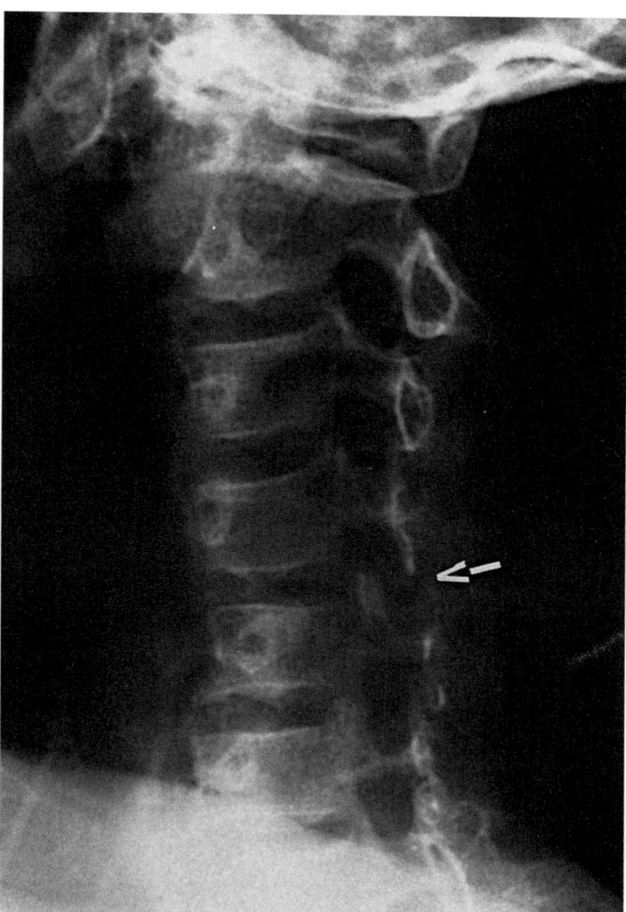

Fig. 13-6 Oblique view shows jumped facet of C4 on C5.

tient once fractures have been excluded by the previous radiographic series. The criteria used to evaluate stability based on flexion/extension radiographs are not universally accepted. White et al[83] suggested that as much as 3.5 mm of horizontal displacement can be normal. Lewis et al[84] suggested a more conservative approach, accepting some false-positive error, using 2 mm of horizontal displacement as their criteria. Most authorities suggest that an angulation of 16 degrees or more indicates instability.[83,84]

Flexion-extension films are neither 100% sensitive nor specific.[84] False-negative results occur if cervical spasm limits mobility of the neck, thus masking an underlying ligamentous injury. When spasm limits adequate flexion and extension, the studies must be judged indeterminate.

PEDIATRIC CONSIDERATIONS

Cervical spine fractures are infrequent in children; fewer than 1% occur in patients less than 12 years of age. In contrast to adults, where most injuries occur in the lower cervical vertebrae, the majority of pediatric cervical injuries involve the occipital-atlantoaxial segments.[85,86] Several anatomic factors predispose to this pattern: (1) a proportionally heavier head and a higher fulcrum of flexion; (2) more lax ligaments, which permit increased mobility at C1-C2; (3) unfused physes; and (4) horizontally inclined articular facets that facilitate sliding.[87]

There are also a number of anatomic characteristics unique to the pediatric cervical spine that may mimic injury. These characteristics include the following:

1. Pseudosubluxation at either C2-C3 or C3-C4
2. Anterior wedging of vertebral bodies (especially C3 and C4)
3. Secondary ossification centers that may mimic avulsions
4. Variable interspinous distances
5. Widening of the predental space (up to 5 mm)
6. Lateral displacement of the lateral masses of C1 on C2.

These normal variants can make the interpretation of pediatric cervical spine radiographs particularly difficult.

Pseudosubluxation involves up to 3 mm of anterior displacement of C2 on C3 or C3 on C4 and may occur up to age 12 (see Chapter 33). It should not be associated with soft-tissue swelling or disruption of the spinolaminar line. The EP should use the lateral film to draw a straight line through the spinolaminar junctions of C1, C2, and C3. A straight line (Swischuck's line) indicates the subluxation is physiologic and not traumatic. Soft-tissue swelling on the lateral film is frequent in children, since the loose tissues balloon outwards with expiration. Timing the film to inspiration results in normalizing of the prevertebral width.

Thoracolumbar and Sacral Spine Radiography

The standardized approach to radiographic evaluation applies to the thoracic, lumbar, and sacral spines. Here, the standard radiographs include the AP and the lateral views. Oblique films are occasionally useful in cases of suspected lumbar pedicle fracture, in which the "Scotty dog" profile of the vertebra demonstrates a "broken neck." Regarding the thoracic spine, widening of the paraspinous stripe in the AP film suggests a thoracic fracture. This same "mediastinal" hematoma associated with a thoracic spine injury may mimic an aortic disruption on CXR. If an abnormality is suspected based on the plain films, obtain a CT scan that includes a vertebra above and below the area in question. MRI is useful in cases of spinal cord impingement, depending on the stability of the patient

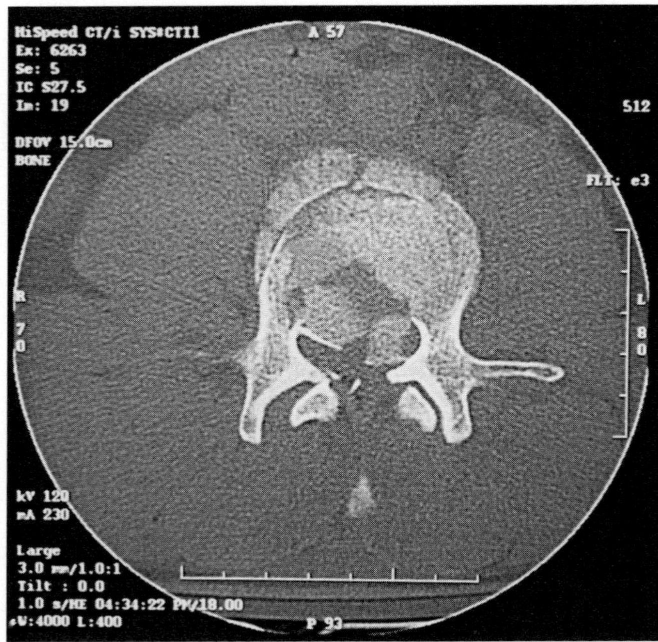

Fig. 13-7 Axial computed tomography scan showing L3 burst fracture.

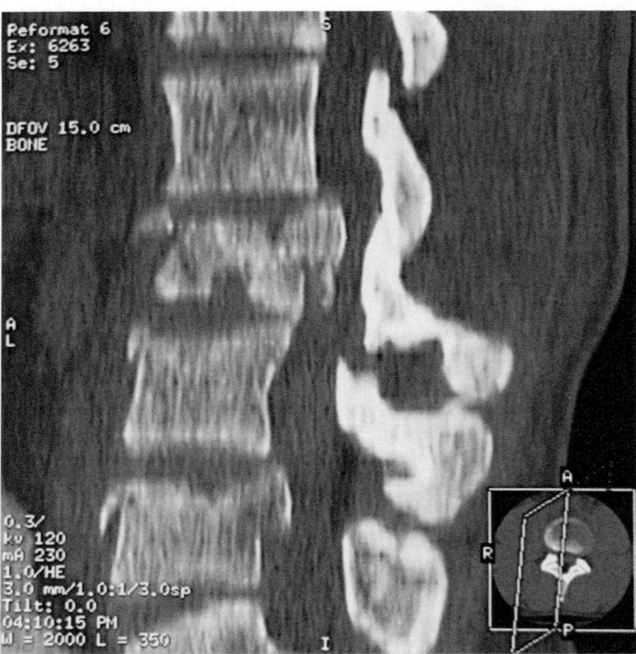

Fig. 13-8 Sagittal computed tomography scan shows L3 burst fracture.

and the presence of concomitant injuries. Most injuries to the dorsal spine occur at the thoracolumbar junction and involve T11 through L2.

SPECIFIC VERTEBRAL FRACTURES

Compression/Burst Fractures

Several specific fractures involve the vertebral bodies in trauma. Compression fractures result from axial loading forces. Such injuries demonstrate loss of vertebral body height, as well as an increased density of the vertebrae.[88] Compression fractures are most common in the lumbar spine, but also occur in the lower cervical or thoracic vertebrae. In children, a wedging of C3 and occasionally one of C4 can be a normal result of incomplete ossification,[89] making determination of vertebral injury difficult. If there is any question regarding a traumatic compression fracture, CT is indicated.

Burst fractures are also the result of axial loading and are similar to compression fractures (Figs. 13-7 and 13-8). However, burst fractures produce fragments that can impinge on the spinal canal, occasionally necessitating surgical reduction. Burst fractures are diagnosed by the loss of cortical integrity, fracture fragments, and lucencies through the body.[45]

Burst fractures of the lumbar spine can be appreciated on the AP film by a widening of the pedicles. The "eyes" of the vertebra appear widened, and do not align with the pedicles above or below the injury.

Teardrop Flexion/Hyperextension Fractures

There are two radiographic presentations referred to as teardrop fractures, each with a different mechanism. The *hyperextension* teardrop fracture, which may be either stable or unstable, is characterized by a triangular fragment displaced from the anterior-inferior corner of the C2 vertebral body.[45,84] It is usually not associated with ligamentous instability and occurs much less frequently than its counterpart, the hyperflexion teardrop fracture. The *hyperflexion* teardrop is characterized by a triangular fracture fragment from the anterior-inferior aspect of the vertebral body, associated with posterior ligamentous damage (Fig. 13-9).[90] Flexion teardrop fractures are also associated with a fracture line that traverses the vertebral body.

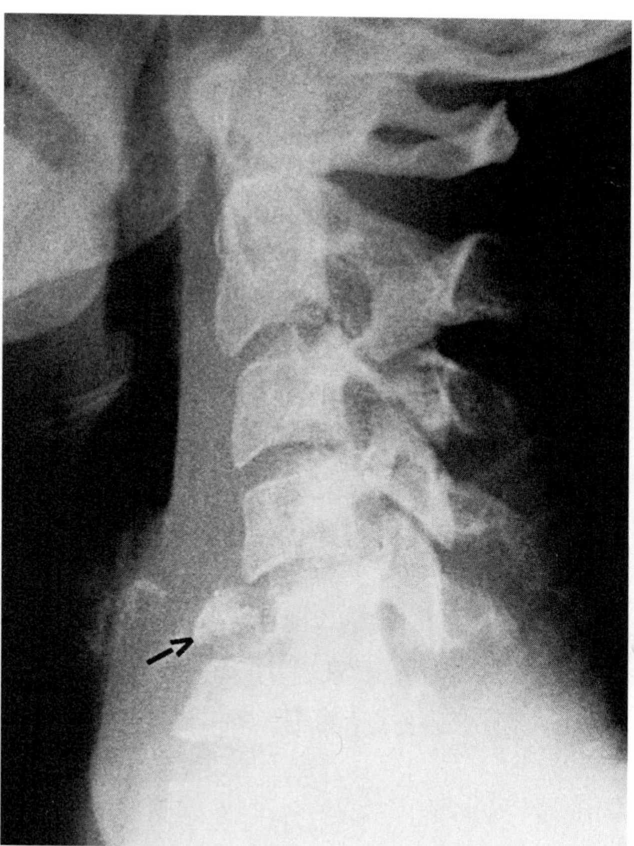

Fig. 13-9 Flexion teardrop fracture of C5.

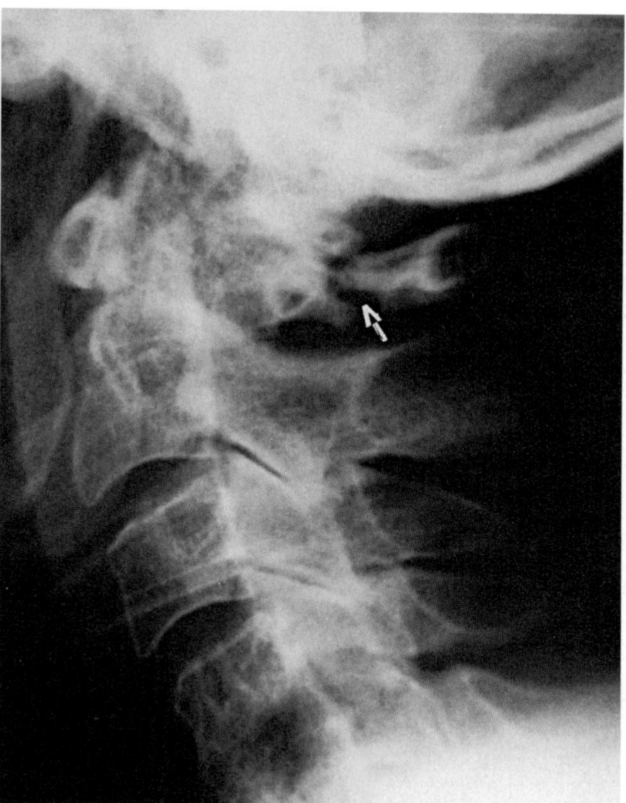

Fig. 13-10 Lateral radiograph shows Jefferson fracture.

In contrast to the hyperextension teardrop fracture, the hyperflexion teardrop is always unstable.[45,88]

Jefferson Fracture

Jefferson burst fractures are unstable injuries involving both the anterior and posterior arches of C1.[88] On the lateral radiograph (Fig. 13-10) lucencies through the cortex may indicate fractures, but the presence of soft-tissue swelling anterior to the body is more frequent. The Jefferson fracture is best viewed through the open mouth odontoid (Fig. 13-11), notable for the lateral displacement of both lateral masses. As many as one third of all Jefferson fractures are associated with fractures of C2.[76,77] CT is very useful in defining this injury (Fig. 13-12).

Posterior C1 Body Fracture

In contrast to the Jefferson's fracture, fractures of the posterior arch of C1 are hyperextension injuries, resulting from compression of the posterior arch between the spinous processes of C2 and the occiput.[88] These fractures may be visualized on the lateral or the obliques, but often require CT evaluation. With this injury, there is no involvement of the anterior arch of C1 and no lateral displacement of the lateral masses, as in Jefferson fractures.

Hangman's Fracture

The Hangman's fracture is a fracture of the pedicle of C2, and occurs as the result of hyperextension (Fig. 13-13).[45] This injury results in a rotatory instability, which can lead to spinal cord injury. However, since the spinal cord at this level occupies only one third of the diameter of the spinal canal, Hangman's fractures rarely yield neurologic deficits. The Hangman's fracture is frequently associated with subluxation of C2 on C3.[88]

Clay Shoveler's Fracture

The "clay shoveler's" fracture is an avulsion of a spinous process and usually involves C6 through T3. Statistically, the most common site is C7.[45] It was originally recognized in men who snapped off the bony process during ditch digging. When throwing the wet

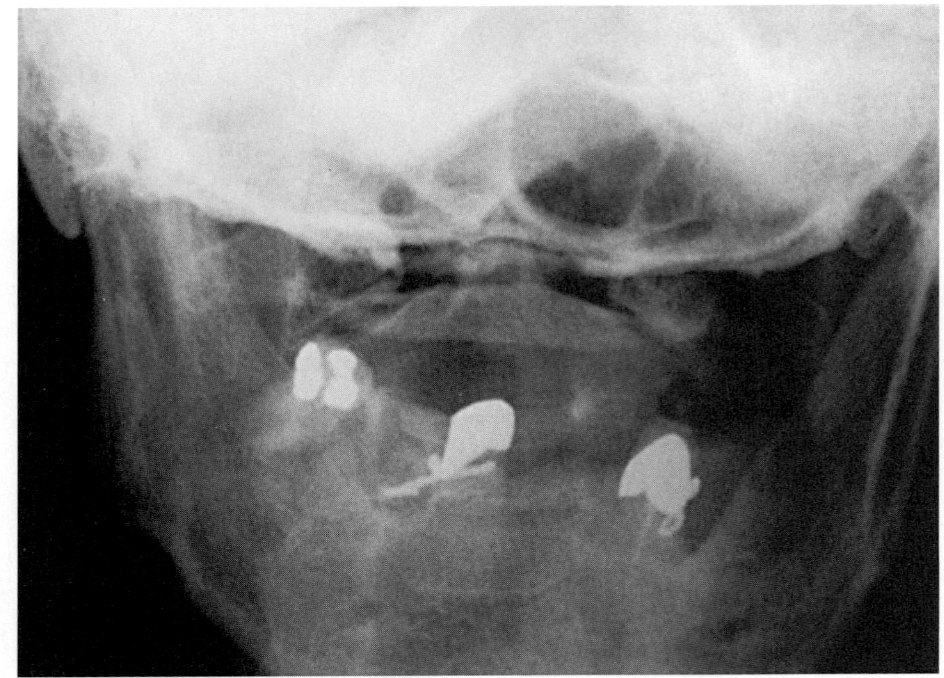

Fig. 13-11 Odontoid view shows widening of C1 lateral masses, indicative of a Jefferson fracture.

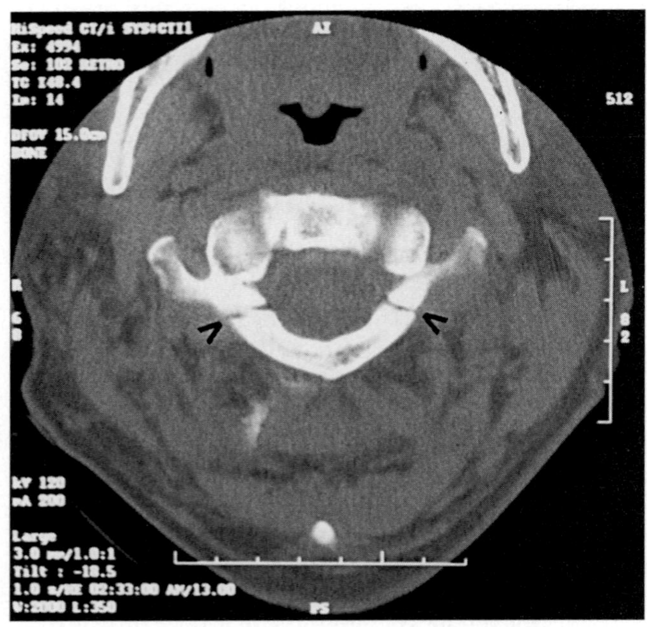

Fig. 13-12 Computed tomography shows posterior element fracture of C1 (Jefferson fracture).

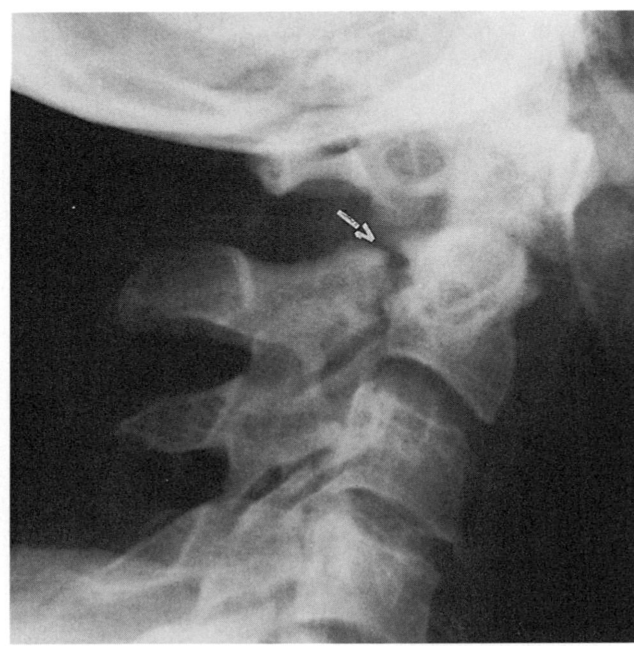

Fig. 13-13 Lateral radiograph shows Hangman's fracture.

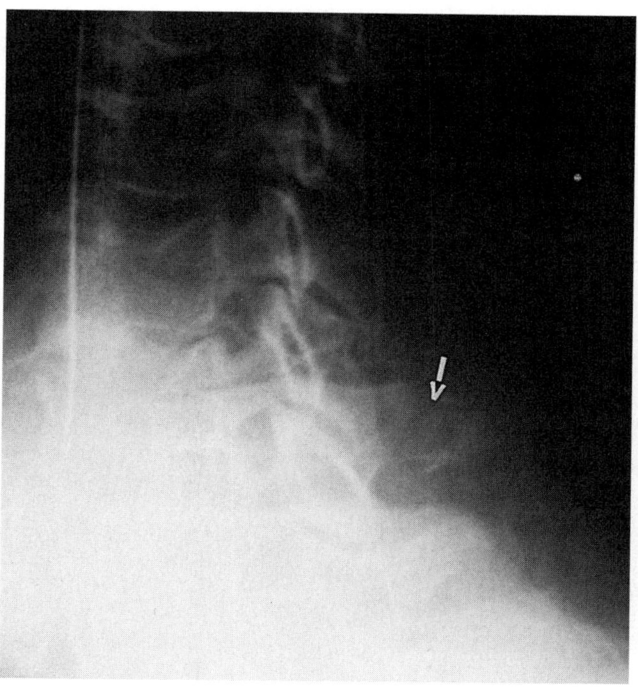

Fig. 13-14 C7 clay shoveler's fracture.

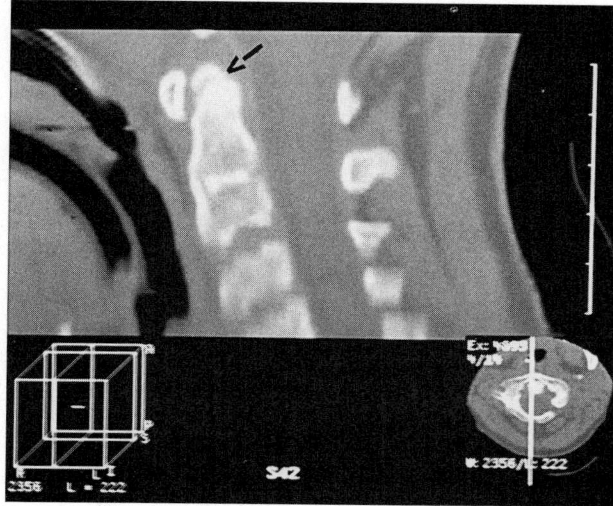

Fig. 13-15 Sagittal computed tomography scan shows type I odontoid fracture.

clay off the shovel, a forcible contraction of the rhomboids and other muscles can break the bone beneath the muscular attachment. Most injuries now occur as the result of hyperextension (Fig. 13-14). This fracture is one of the most commonly missed cervical spine fractures, usually because of failure to adequately visualize the cervicothoracic junction. Fortunately, the clay shoveler's fracture is a stable injury.

Odontoid Fractures

The odontoid (dens) fracture is an unstable injury that produces a lucency through the dens or an abnormal predental space on the lateral radiograph. The predental space should normally measure less than 3 mm in an adult and be symmetric without angulation. The most commonly used classification of dens fractures is that of Alfred and d'Alonzo.[90] In this system, a fracture through the tip of the dens is a type I (Fig. 13-15). The type I fracture is very rare and is usually clinically insignificant. A type II fracture (Fig. 13-16) traverses the dens at the junction between the dens and the central body of C2. This unstable injury is much more common than a type I.[90] Type III dens fractures (Fig. 13-17) involve the vertebral body of C2, below the junction of the dens and the axis. Because type II fractures carry a worse prognosis, it is helpful to make a determination of the classification.[31] Though plain

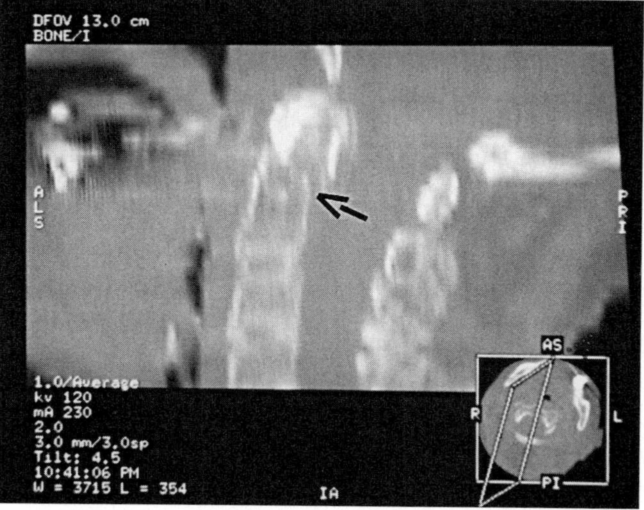

Fig. 13-16 Sagittal computed tomography scan shows type II odontoid fracture.

films alone usually provide the diagnosis, a CT is usually obtained to determine of the extent of injury.

Atlantooccipital Dislocation

The most dramatic of all cervicospinal injuries is undoubtedly atlantooccipital dislocation (AOD). This in-

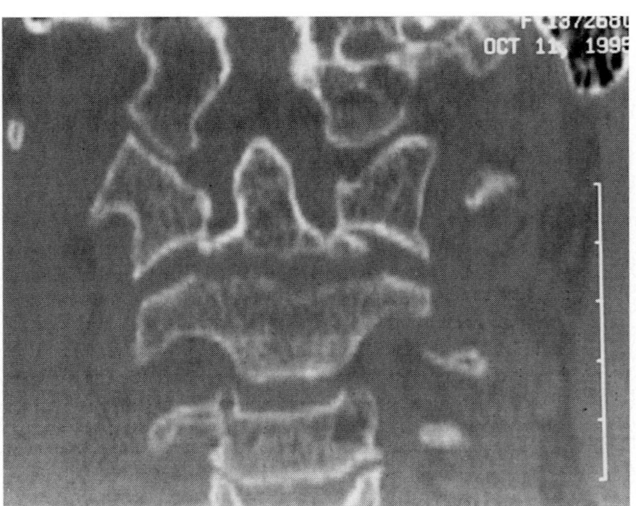

Fig. 13-17 Coronal computed tomography scan shows type III odontoid fracture.

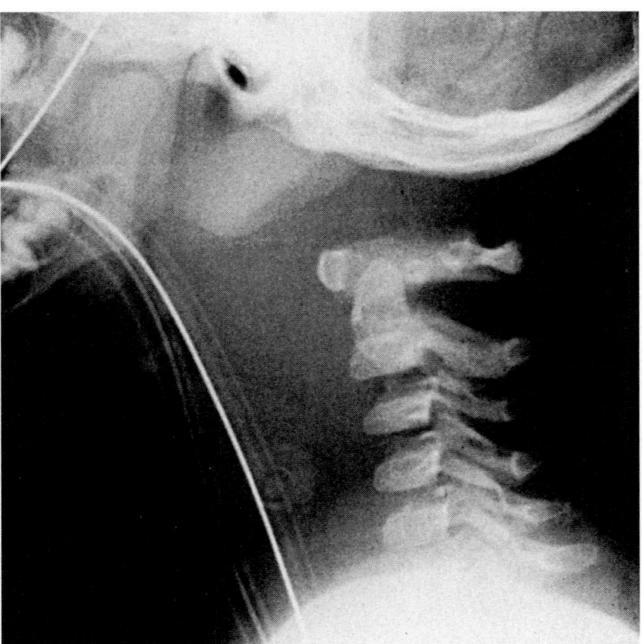

Fig. 13-18 Atlantooccipital dislocation.

jury is mostly seen in infants and young children as a result of a relatively large cranial mass and poorly developed neck musculature. Because these injuries are usually associated with spinal cord transection at the level of C1, they are typically fatal and usually diagnosed at autopsy.[90,91] However, several centers report cases of AOD in patients who survived.[91,92] A cross-table lateral cervical spine radiograph is usually adequate to make the diagnosis (Fig. 13-18). Normally, a line drawn along the clinoid should intersect the tip of the dens; in a patient with an atlantooccipital dislocation, this line bypasses the odontoid.

EMERGENCY DEPARTMENT MANAGEMENT

Once a diagnosis of a cervical spine fracture has been made, continue to protect the spinal cord from further injury. A spine board, cervical collar, and/or headblocks are frequently employed. A spinal vacuum splint is used in some centers and is more comfortable than the hard spine board. It may be prudent to reassess the neurologic examination for subtle signs of injury.

Whenever a spinal fracture is identified, image the entire spine, since 5% to 20% of spinal fractures are multiple.[90,93,94] For this reason, the identification of a single fracture should prompt a search for injury at other levels.

Whether or not the injury to the cervical spine is stable or unstable is important to determine. This information helps direct the management by the orthopedist or neurosurgeon and plays an important part in the patient's prognosis. If there is clinical evidence for associated spinal cord involvement, administer corticosteroids according to the accepted protocol (see Chapter 12).

DISPOSITION

Early consultation with an orthopedic surgeon or neurosurgeon is warranted. Definitive management involves prolonged spinal immobilization, which may necessitate surgical reduction and fusion, internal fixation devices such as the Harrington rod, or external fixation devices such as Gardner-Wells tongs, traction, or a stabilization vest. The surgical consultant decides on these interventions. If local expertise is unavailable, arrange for transfer to an appropriate referral center.

Most patients who sustain trauma to the neck or back are discharged from the ED. Give these patients both verbal and written instructions regarding symptoms that necessitate immediate return. These indications include worsening pain; pain unrelieved by analgesics; the development of numbness, weakness, or paresthesias; or incontinence.

On discharge prescribe adequate analgesics, and give instructions regarding the appropriate level of activity for the patient to assume at home.

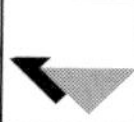

PEARLS & PITFALLS

- The failure to obtain indicated radiographs is the most common reason for missed cervical spine fracture.
- Assume that all patients have cervical injury, and maintain in-line stabilization at all times during airway management.
- A single lateral view is inadequate to exclude injury; under optimum conditions it will miss 15% of cervical fractures.
- Oblique views provide good visualization of the cervicothoracic junction.
- Consider computed tomography imaging from the skull base to C3 in patients with severe brain injury.
- Clearing the spine in a patient with altered mental status involves more than a negative film. In such cases, apply a soft cervical collar pending serial examinations as the patient awakens. In the comatose patient, the accepting physician may order fluoroscopic-guided flexion-extension films.
- Five to twenty percent of spinal fractures are multiple. The identification of a single fracture should prompt a search for injury at other levels.
- Pseudosubluxation is common in younger children. A straight line incorporating the spinolaminar junction of C1, C2, and C3 demonstrates the finding is physiologic.
- Soft-tissue swelling is also common in children. A film timed to inspiration may normalize the film.

REFERENCES

1. Velmahos GC, et al: Radiographic cervical spine evaluation in the alert asymptomatic blunt trauma victim: much ado about nothing? *J Trauma* 40:768-773, 1996.
2. Bachulis BL, et al: Clinical indications for cervical spine radiographs in the traumatized patient, *Am J Surg* 153:473-477, 1987.
3. Ringenberg BJ, et al: Rational ordering of cervical spine radiographs following trauma, *Ann Emerg Med* 17:792-796, 1988.
4. Bracken MB: Pharmacologic treatment of acute spinal cord injury: current status and future projects, *J Emerg Med* 1:43-48, 1993.
5. Fischer RP: Cervical radiographic evaluation of alert patients following blunt trauma, *Ann Emerg Med* 13:905-907, 1984.
6. Walter J, Doris PE, Shaffer MA: Clinical presentation of patients with acute cervical spine injury, *Ann Emerg Med* 13:512-515, 1984.
7. Sivit CJ, et al: Safety-belt injuries in children with lap-belt ecchymosis: CT findings in 61 patients, *Am J Roentgenol* 157:111-114,1991.
8. Kreipke DL, et al: Reliability of indications for cervical spine films in trauma patients, *J Trauma* 29:1438-1439, 1989.
9. Saddison D, Vanek VW, Racanelli JL: Clinical indications for cervical spine radiographs in alert trauma patients, *Am Surg* 57:366-369, 1991.
10. Roberge RJ, Wears RC: Evaluation of neck discomfort, neck tenderness, and neurologic deficits as indicators for radiography in blunt trauma victims, *J Emerg Med* 10:539-544, 1992.
11. Roberge RJ, et al: Selective application of cervical spine radiography in alert victims of blunt trauma: a prospective study, *J Trauma* 28:784-788, 1988.
12. Brown LH, Gough JE, Simonds WB: Can EMS providers adequately assess trauma patients for cervical spinal injury? *Prehosp Emerg Care* 2:33-36,1998.
13. Meldon SW, et al: Out-of-hospital cervical spine clearance: agreement between emergency medical technicians and emergency physicians, *J Trauma* 45:1058-1061,1998.
14. Kraus JF: A comparison of recent studies on the extent of the head and spinal cord injury problem in the United States, *J Neurosurg* 53:S35-43, 1980.
15. Riggins RS, Kraus JF: The risk of neurologic damage with fractures of the vertebrae, *J Trauma* 17:126-133, 1977.
16. Borock EC, et al: A prospective analysis of a two-year experience using computed tomography as an adjunct for cervical spine clearance, *J Trauma* 31:1001-1005, 1991.
17. Bivins HG, et al: The effect of axial traction during orotracheal intubation of the trauma victim with an unstable cervical spine, *Ann Emerg Med* 17:25-29, 1988.
18. Shatney CH, et al: The safety of orotracheal intubation in patients with unstable cervical spine fracture or high spinal cord injury, *Am J Surg* 170:676-679, 1995.
19. Crosby ET, Lui T: The adult cervical spine: implications for airway management, *Can J Anaesth* 37:77-93, 1990.
20. Suderman VS, Crosby ET, Lui A: Elective oral tracheal intubation in cervical spine-injured adults, *Can J Anaesth* 39:516-517, 1992.
21. Rhee KJ, et al: Oral intubation in the multiply injured patient: the risk of exacerbating spine cord damage, *Ann Emerg Med* 19:511-514, 1990.
22. Walls RM: Airway management in the blunt trauma patient: how important is the cervical spine? *Can J Surg* 35:27-34, 1992.
23. Li J, et al: Complications of emergency intubation with and without paralysis, *Am J Emerg Med* 17:141-143,1999.
24. Ditunno JF Jr, et al: The international standards booklet for neurological and functional classification of spinal cord injury, *Paraplegia* 32:70-80, 1994.
25. Jacobs LM, Schwartz R: Prospective analysis of acute cervical spine injury: a methodology to predict injury, *Ann Emerg Med* 15:44-49, 1986.
26. Subcommittee on Advanced Trauma Life Support of the American College of Surgeons Committee on Trauma: *Advanced trauma life support manual: student manual,* ed 5, Chicago, 1993, American College of Surgeons.
27. Roth BJ, et al: Roentgenographic evaluation of the cervical spine: a selective approach, *Arch Surg* 129:643-645, 1994.
28. Mirvis SE, et al: Protocol-driven radiographic evaluation of suspected cervical spine injury: efficacy study, *Radiol* 170:831-834, 1989.
29. McNamara R, Heine E, Esposito B: Cervical spine injury and radiography in alert, high-risk patients, *J Emerg Med* 8:177-182, 1990.
30. Hoffman JR, et al: Low-risk criteria for cervical-spine radiography in blunt trauma: a prospective study, *Ann Emerg Med* 21: 1454-1460, 1992.
31. Hoffman JR, et al: Selective cervical spine radiography of blunt trauma victims: results of the National Emergency X-radiography Utilization Study (NEXUS), *Acad Emerg Med* 6:451, 1999.

32. Rachesky I, et al: Clinical prediction of cervical spine injuries in children, *Am J Dis Child* 141:199-201, 1987.
33. Orenstein JB, Klein BL, Ochsenschlager DW: Delayed diagnosis of pediatric cervical spine injury, *Pediatrics* 89:1185-1188, 1992.
34. Mahadevan S, et al: Interrater reliability of cervical spine injury criteria in patients with blunt trauma, *Ann Emerg Med* 31:197-201, 1998.
35. Terrigrino CA, et al: Selective indications for thoracic and lumbar radiography in blunt trauma, *Ann Emerg Med* 26:126-129, 1995.
36. Samuels LE, Kerstein MD: 'Routine' radiographic evaluation of the thoracolumbar spine in blunt trauma patients: a reappraisal, *J Trauma* 34:85-89, 1993.
37. American College of Radiology: *Appropriateness criteria for imaging and treatment decisions,* Reston, VA, 1995, American College of Radiology.
38. Hills MW, Deane SA: Head injury and facial injury: is there an increased risk of cervical spine injury? *J Trauma* 34:549-553, 1993.
39. Williams J, et al: Head, facial and clavicular trauma as a predictor of cervical-spine injury, *Ann Emerg Med* 21:719-722,1992.
40. Soicher E, Demetriades D: Cervical spine injuries in patients with head injuries, *Br J Surg* 78:1013-1014, 1991.
41. Sinclair D, et al: A retrospective review of the relationship between facial fractures, head injuries, and cervical spine injuries, *J Emerg Med* 6:109-112, 1988.
42. O'Malley KF, Ross SE: The incidence of injury to the cervical spine in patients with craniocervical trauma, *J Trauma* 28:1467-1478, 1988.
43. Kaups KL, Davis JW: Patients with gunshot wounds to the head do not require cervical spine immobilization and evaluation, *J Trauma* 44:865-867, 1998.
44. Chong CL, Ware DN, Harris JH: Is cervical spine imaging indicated in gunshot wounds to the cranium? *J Trauma* 44:501-502, 1998.
45. 1Williams CF, Bernstein TW, Jelenko C 3rd: Essentiality of the lateral cervical spine radiograph, *Ann Emerg Med* 10:198-204, 1981.
46. 1Cox GR, Barish RA: Delayed presentation of unstable cervical spine injury with minimal symptoms, *J Emerg Med* 9:123-127, 1991.
47. 1Webb KB, et al: Hidden flexion injury of the cervical spine, *J Bone Joint Surg* 58B:322-327, 1976.
48. Maull KI, Sachatello CR: Avoiding a pitfall in resuscitation: the painless cervical fracture, *South Med J* 70:477-478, 1977.
49. Bresler MJ, Rich GH: Occult cervical spine fracture in an ambulatory patient, *Ann Emerg Med* 11:440-442, 1982.
50. Walter J, Doris PE, Shaffer MA: Clinical presentation of patients with acute cervical spine injury, *Ann Emerg Med* 13:512-511, 1984.
51. Gatrell CB: "Asymptomatic" cervical injuries: a myth? (letter), *Am J Emerg Med* 3:263-265, 1985.
52. Saddison D, Vanek VW, Racanelli JL: Clinical indicators for cervica spine radiography in alert patients, *Am Surg* 57:366-369, 1991.
53. Durham RM, et al: Evaluation of the thoracic and lumbar spine after blunt trauma, *Am J Surg* 170:681-684,1995.
54. Meldon SW, Moettus LN: Thoracolumbar spine fractures: clinical presentation and the effect of altered sensorium and major injury, *J Trauma* 39:1110-1114, 1995.
55. Samuels LE, Kerstein MD: "Routine" radiologic evaluation of the thoracolumbar spine in blunt trauma patients: a reappraisal, *J Trauma* 34:85-89,1993.
56. Frankel HL, et al: Indications for obtaining surveillance thoracic and lumbar spine radiographs, *J Trauma* 37:673-676,1994.
57. Glass RB, et al: Lumbar spine injury in a pediatric population: difficulties with computed tomographic diagnosis, *J Trauma* 37:815-819,1994.
58. Davis JW, et al: The etiology of missed cervical spine injuries, *J Trauma* 34:342-346, 1993.
59. Blahd WH, Iserson KV, Bjelland J: Efficacy of the posttraumatic cross table lateral view of the cervical spine, *J Emerg Med* 2:243-249, 1985.
60. Shaffer MA, Doris PE: Limitations of the cross table lateral view in detecting cervical spine injuries: a retrospective analysis, *Ann Emerg Med* 10:508-513, 1981.
61. Streitweiser DR, et al: Accuracy of standard radiographic views in detecting cervical spine fractures, *Ann Emerg Med* 12:538-541, 1983.
62. MacDonald RL, et al: Diagnosis of cervical spine injury in motor vehicle crash victims: how many x-rays are enough? *J Trauma* 30:392-397, 1990.
63. Doris PE, Wilson RA: The next logical step in the emergency radiographic evaluation of cervical spine trauma: the five-view trauma series, *J Emerg Med* 3:371-385, 1985.
64. Turetsky DB, et al: Technique of use of supine oblique views in acute cervical spine trauma, *Ann Emerg Med* 22:685, 1993.
65. Freemyer B, et al: Comparison of five-view and three-view cervical spine series in the evaluation of patients with cervical trauma, *Ann Emerg Med* 18:818, 1989.
66. Nichols CG, Young DH, Schiller WR: Evaluation of cervicothoracic junction injury, *Ann Emerg Med* 16:640-642, 1987.
67. Davis JW: Cervical injuries–perils of the swimmer's view: case report, *J Trauma* 29:891-893, 1989.
68. Lewis LM, et al: Flexion-extension views in the evaluation of cervical-spine injuries, *Ann Emerg Med* 20:117-121, 1991.
69. Davis JW, et al: Clearing the cervical spine in obtunded patients: the use of dynamic fluoroscopy, *J Trauma* 39:435-438, 1995.
70. Tehranzadeh J, et al: Efficacy of limited CT for nonvisualized lower cervical spine in patients with blunt trauma, *Skeletal Radiol* 23:349-352, 1994.
71. Ross SE, et al: Clearing the cervical spine: initial radiologic evaluation, *J Trauma* 27:1055-1059, 1987.
72. Clark CR, White AA 3rd: Fractures of the dens: a multicenter study, *J Bone Joint Surg* 67-A:1340-1348, 1985.
73. Link TM, et al: Substantial head trauma: value of routine CT examination of the cervicocranium, *Radiology* 196: 741-745, 1995.
74. Orrison WW, et al: Magnetic resonance imaging evaluation of acute spinal trauma, *Emerg Radiol* 2:120-128, 1995.
75. Rizzolo SJ, Vaccaro AR, Cotler JM: Cervical spine trauma, *Spine* 19:2288-2298, 1994.
76. Driscoll PA, Ross R, Nicholson DA: ABC of emergency radiology: cervical spine. I, *BMJ* 307:785-789, 1993.
77. Driscoll PA, Ross R, Nicholson DA: ABC of emergency radiology: cervical spine. II, *BMJ* 307:855-859, 1993.
78. Jackson FE, et al: The Achilles's neck and vulnerable vertebrae, *Emerg Med* 9:22-41, 1977.
79. Van Hare RS, Yaron M: The ring of C2 and evaluation of the cross-table lateral view of the cervical spine, *Ann Emerg Med* 21:733-735,1992.
80. Thomeier WC, Brown DC, Mirvis SE: The laterally tilted dens: a sign of subtle odontoid fracture on plain radiography, *Am J Neuroradiol* 11:605-608, 1990.
81. Weir DC: Roentgenographic signs of cervical injury, *Clin Orthop Rel Res* 109:9-17, 1975.
82. Southwick WO: Management of fractures of the dens (odontoid process), *J Bone Joint Surg* 62A:482-486, 1980.
83. White AA 3rd, et al: Biochemical analysis of clinical stability in the cervical spine, *Clin Orthop Rel Res* 109:85-95, 1975.

84. Lewis LM, et al: Flexion-extension views in the evaluation of cervical-spine injuries, *Ann Emerg Med* 20:117-121, 1991.
85. Ehara S, el-Khoury GY, Sato Y: Cervical spine injury in children: radiologic manifestations, *Am J Roentgen* 151:1175-1178, 1988.
86. Lui T, et al: C1-C2 fracture dislocations in children and adolescents, *J Trauma* 40:408-411, 1996.
87. Orenstein JB, et al: Age and outcome in pediatric cervical spine injury: 11-year experience, *Pediatr Emerg Care* 10:132-137, 1994.
88. Kaye JJ, Nance EP Jr: Cervical spine trauma, *Orthop Clin North Am* 21:449-462, 1990.
89. Swischuk LE, Swischuk PN, John SD: Wedging of C-3 in infants and children: usually a normal finding and not a fracture, *Radiology* 188:523-526, 1993.
90. Clark CR, et al: Radiographic evaluation of cervical spine injuries, *Spine* 13:742-747, 1988.
91. Bohlman HH: Acute fractures and dislocations of the cervical spine: an analysis of three hundred hospitalized patients and review of the literature, *J Bone Joint Surg* 61A:1119-1142, 1979.
92. Ferrera PC, Bartfield JM: Traumatic atlanto-occipital dislocation: a potentially survivable injury, *Am J Emerg Med* 14:291-296, 1996.
93. Vaccaro AR, et al: Noncontiguous injuries of the spine, *J Spinal Disord* 5:320-329, 1992.
94. Calenoff L, et al: Multiple level spinal injuries: Importance of early recognition, *AJR* 665-669, 1978.

Maxillofacial Trauma

14

JENNIFER L. ISENHOUR AND STEPHEN A. COLUCCIELLO

One of the most important and frequently encountered injuries in the emergency department (ED) is maxillofacial trauma. The injuries have the potential for serious and rapid decompensation as a result of airway compromise. The emergency physician (EP) must address life threats, diagnose both facial and associated injuries, and orchestrate needed consultants. Specialties involved in the care of patients with facial trauma may include otolaryngology (ENT), ophthalmology, plastic surgery, oral and maxillofacial surgery, neurosurgery, and trauma surgery.

Up to 60% of patients with significant facial injuries sustain trauma to other organ systems. The often disfiguring and grotesque nature of maxillofacial trauma can potentially distract the EP from addressing these sometimes occult threats.

This chapter will enable the EP to quickly diagnose, prioritize, and stabilize patients with maxillofacial trauma. To accomplish this goal, the EP must develop a systematic and sophisticated physical examination (PE) coupled with judicious use of imaging studies and aptly timed intervention. Although EPs capably manage most facial injuries, we must remain aware of which patients require consultation and admission.

ETIOLOGY/INCIDENCE

Historically, up to 50% of facial injuries result from motor vehicle crashes (MVCs). However, during the last 30 years 70% of severe facial trauma in urban centers have been with associated assaults.[1,2] Falls and MVCs, especially in the elderly and very young population, comprise a majority of the remainder of injuries.[3]

The incidence of these injuries varies as to geographic location. Urban centers continue to see a significantly larger percentage of penetrating injuries and assaults, resulting in midface and zygoma fractures. The community hospital treats primarily nasal and mandibular injuries related to both MVCs and sporting and recreational mishaps.[1,2]

Unfortunately, the incidence of facial trauma related to domestic violence, elder abuse, and pediatric nonaccidental trauma continues to rise.[4] Recent studies show that as many as 25% of female patients sustaining facial trauma are the victims of domestic violence.[5] This percentage increases to 30% when there is an associated orbital fracture.[6]

ANATOMY

Knowledge of facial anatomy is imperative in diagnosing facial fractures. Bony damage is based primarily on mechanism of injury and age of the patient (Figs. 14-1 and 14-2). Several buttresses and arches stabilize the face both vertically and horizontally.[7] Laterally, the zygomatic-maxillary buttresses provide vertical stability. Medially, the frontal processes of the maxilla support the vertical face. The zygomatic-maxillary arches and hard palate create a horizontal foundation.[8] Each of these areas is linked by sutures, which create a predictable pattern of injury in trauma. With this knowledge, the EP can target palpation to the vulnerable buttresses and sutures.

Other important structures and attachments occur at the sutures linking the sphenoid wings, pterygoid plates, and zygomatic arches. These structures lie behind the maxilla and attach the face to the skull. Disruption of these structures creates the classic Le Fort facial injuries.[9] Finally, the orbit presents a complex array of seven bones: the maxilla, zygoma, frontal, sphenoid, palatine, ethmoid, and lacrimal. Throughout these bones lie orbital fissures that carry vital nerves, such as the optic nerve. It is easy to comprehend that injury to any of the orbital structures can compress the nerve and endanger vision.

ASSOCIATED INJURIES

Several of the facial bones are delicate, such as the nose, and may shatter in a minor altercation. How-

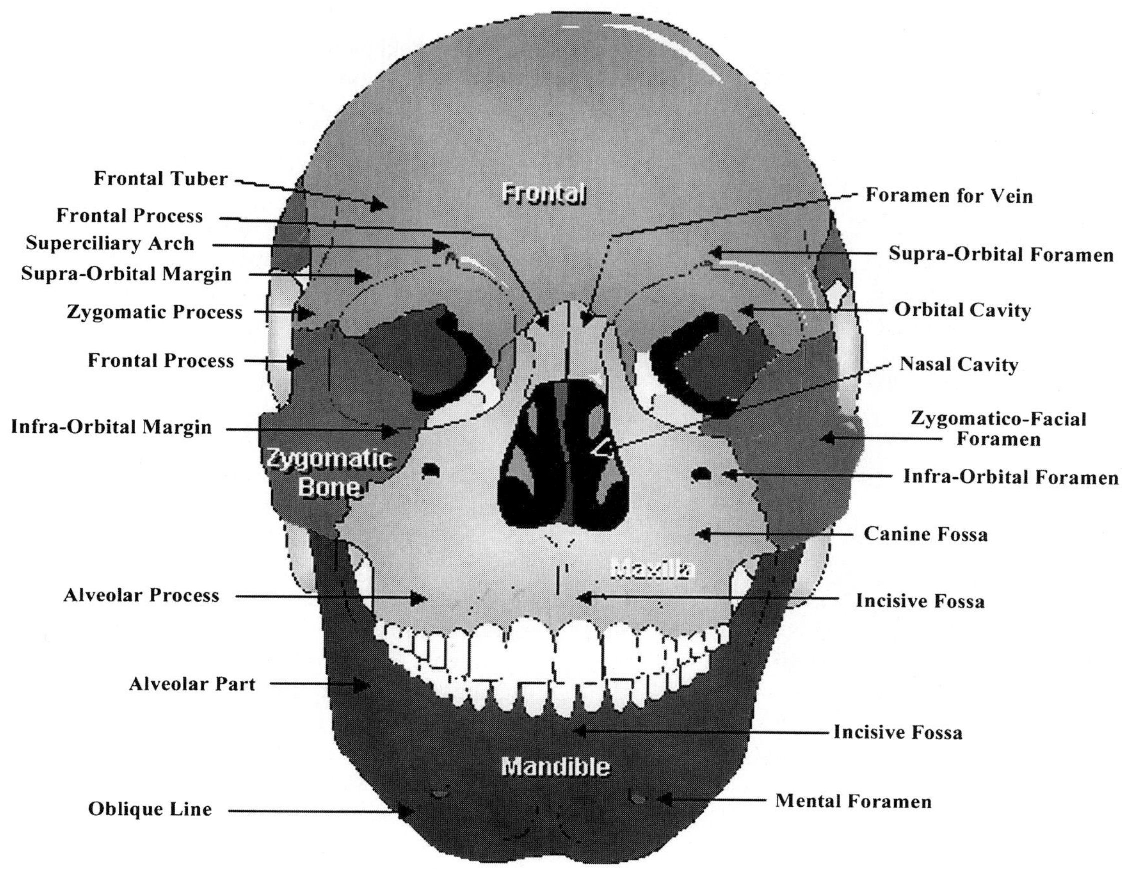

Fig. 14-1 Facial anatomy.

ever, others require significant force to fracture, such as the maxilla and mandible. When such a formidable bone is broken, the emergency physician must suspect associated injuries to the brain, cervical spine (C-spine), major vessels, and eyes. [10,11] Some studies show that up to 20% to 50% of patients with facial trauma have concomitant brain injury; this percentage is even higher in young children.[12-14] Brain injury is more likely in patients suffering upper or midface fractures, since considerable force is necessary to disrupt these bones.[15]

Several studies claim that associated C-spine trauma is rare, occurring in only 1% to 4% of patients with significant facial trauma.[12,16,17] However, EPs must remain suspicious of this injury and exclude it by clinical or radiographic means in any patient with serious facial trauma. Of interest, one recent study linked severe facial trauma with carotid injury.[18]

Ocular injury is an obvious concern for patients with facial trauma. As many as 30% of patients with periorbital fractures may suffer associated ocular trauma.[1,19,20] Periorbital fractures may entrap extraocular muscles or even penetrate the globe itself. The Le Fort fractures and zygoma fractures are the injuries that most often result in blindness.[21] Although most blindness occurs with penetrating ocular injury, any patient with extraocular muscle dysfunction or decreased visual acuity needs to be evaluated by an ophthalmologist emergently. It is easy to overlook serious eye injuries in patients with altered mental status, and serial ocular examinations or consultation may be helpful in those with periorbital fractures.

Finally, the EP must remember not to overlook the devastating psychologic consequences facial trauma brings with it. Posttraumatic stress disorder, as well as severe depression, occurs in almost one third of patients.[22] Offer referrals to the appropriate psychologic services.

EMERGENCY DEPARTMENT EVALUATION

ABCs

Although initial trauma care always begins with the airway, nowhere is airway management more important than with facial trauma. Airway management is of central concern and begins with basic airway maneuvers in the prehospital phase. Medics must re-

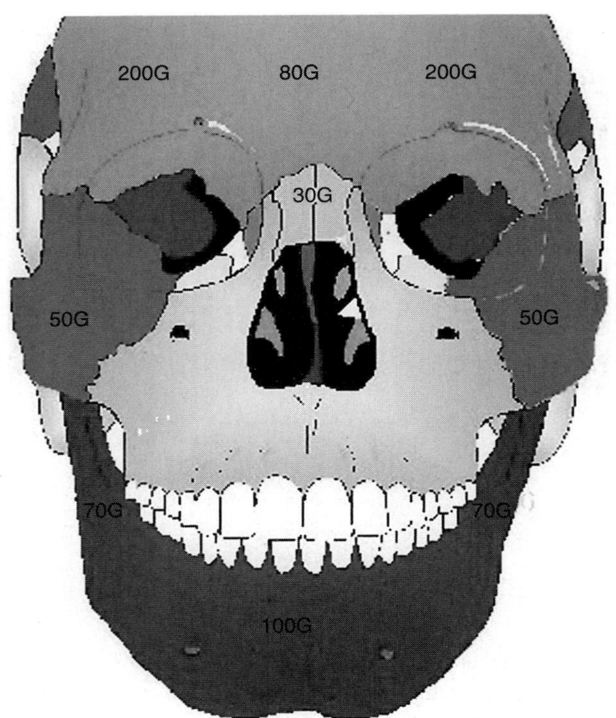

Fig. 14-2 Fracture G forces required.

move foreign bodies and clear the oropharynx of bloody secretions. The airway can easily be occluded by the patient's tongue. Jaw-thrusts with C-spine immobilization or a modified chin-lift can clear this obstruction.

Once in the ED, control of the airway is paramount. If patients are alert and their C-spines can be cleared sufficiently, allow them to sit up and use a Yankauer or tonsil tip suction to clear blood from the airway. If patients cannot perform this task and the airway continues to be compromised, the steps to intubation must be initiated. If the tongue obstructs the airway despite a chin lift or jaw thrust (which may occur with mandibular fractures), grasp the tongue with a towel clip or gauze pad, or place a silk suture through it and lift it out of the hypopharynx.[23]

Intubation in the patient with facial injury can be challenging. Nasotracheal intubation should be avoided in these patients, since intracranial intubation is possible if the cribriform plate is fractured.[24] Some cite that these injuries are so rare that the nasotracheal approach is acceptable.[25] However, most authorities believe that EPs have become so adept at orotracheal intubation that it remains the preferred route.[24] In addition, nasotracheal intubation may precipitate even more hemorrhage, leading to further airway compromise.

The rapid sequence induction (RSI) method of orotracheal intubation is perhaps best modified for use in these patients. Often the patient with significant deformity of the mandible or lower maxilla will be difficult to ventilate with a bag-valve-mask in case of a failed airway attempt. If possible, avoid the use of paralytics in this situation. Patients with unstable jaws may undergo "awake intubation." In this case, the patient receives sedation with a benzodiazepine, droperidol, or an induction agent that minimally reduces respiratory drive, and orotracheal intubation is attempted.

If time and patient stability permit, the emergency physician may be creative during intubation. Fiberoptic intubation in a semiprone position allows the patient to maintain a clear airway until it is secured with an endotracheal tube (ETT).[26] Other less often used airway adjuvants include the Bullard laryngoscope, laryngeal mask airway, and the pharyngeal-esophageal airway (Combitube). Additional temporizing measures include percutaneous transtracheal jet ventilation or retrograde intubation.

The EP must always be prepared for the need for emergent cricothyroidotomy in the patient with facial injuries, especially if the EP elects to paralyze a patient with a ruined face. "Prepared" means an open cricothyroidotomy tray at the bedside with scalpel loaded, tracheostomy tube at hand, and Betadine on the patient's neck.

Once the airway and breathing are stabilized, the EP must assess circulation. In patients with facial injury there is a potential for uncontrolled hemorrhage. However, most facial injuries do not result in hemodynamic collapse and shock.[27] Avoid blind clamping of vessels; many vessels run in close proximity to vital structures, such as the facial nerve and parotid duct. Direct pressure controls most bleeding. In case of massive nasopharyngeal bleeding, packing of the nasal passages is necessary. Anterior packs alone will rarely stop severe hemorrhage; tamponade posterior bleeding with a large Foley catheter balloon filled with water or with a commercially available nasal balloon device.[28] Occasionally with Le Fort fractures, severe bleeding may require packing the pharynx once an ETT is in place. Manual reduction of the severely displaced midface fractures by grasping the anterior hard palate and realigning the fragments may also temporize the bleeding.[29,30]

Finally, after assessing the ABCs, conduct a thorough secondary survey with close attention to other possible life-threatening injuries to the head, chest, abdomen, and pelvis.[31]

History

Elicit an AMPLE history (allergies and tetanus status, medications, past medical history, last meal, and events surrounding the injury) from the patient whenever possible. Remember that emergency medical services personnel, family members, and bystanders may provide crucial information about the mechanism, timing, and severity of the injury. Specific questions for assessing the severity of facial injury include (1) "How is your vision?" (eye involvement); (2) "Is any part of your face numb?" (facial nerve injury); and (3) "Are your teeth meeting normally?" (alignment of the face).

Elaborate on the initial questions and ask about diplopia and pain with extraocular movement. Monocular diplopia suggests injury to the cornea, lens dislocation, or retinal damage. Binocular diplopia points to extraocular muscle or nerve injury. Painful eye movement should prompt careful inspection of the globe and orbit.

Finally, continue to be suspicious about abuse. If medics did not transport the patient from an MVC, ask about the possibility of domestic violence. Although men are victims of domestic violence, women, children, and elderly are at greater risk. Abused women often have a "cover story" for facial trauma, such as "I ran into a door" or "I fell down some stairs" (see Chapter 36). Patients are more likely to reveal the truth when directly questioned by the treating physician. Keep in mind that more than 50% of children presenting with face, head, mouth, and neck trauma may be victims of abuse.[4] Tears of the frenulum of the upper lip may occur with forced feeding of infants. Address the potential for elder abuse in geriatric trauma.

Physical Examination

Begin with a global approach. Inspect the patient's face and skull from all angles, since subtle changes can indicate particular injury patterns (e.g., elongation in the frontal plane suggests a high-grade Le Fort fracture). Get a view from above, looking for enophthalmos and exophthalmos, and from below, looking for any asymmetries. Test the muscles of facial expression (have the patient smile, frown, raise his or her eyebrows, and close his or her eyes tightly). Fractures of the temporal bone may produce a posttraumatic Bell's palsy. Look for ecchymosis suggesting underlying bony disruption, such as the periorbital ecchymosis (raccoon's eyes) or mastoid ecchymosis (Battle's sign) found with basilar skull fracture. These findings are rare on initial evaluation, but evolve over time.

Most facial fractures are diagnosed on physical examination alone, especially in the awake, mentating patient.[32] Simultaneously palpate each side of the patient's face to note subtle changes in symmetry. Feel the entire face for bony crepitus, step-offs, subcutaneous emphysema, and tenderness. An anatomically perceptive physician targets the bony sutures, especially those of the infraorbital rim and zygomatic-frontal junction (located on the superior-lateral aspect of the orbit), noting any disruption. Use the intraoral palpation test to differentiate tenderness of the soft tissues of the cheek from true bony pain. Place a gloved finger on the lateral aspect of the upper molars along the buccal mucosa and underneath the zygomatic arch to palpate for collapse and tenderness. To assess facial stability, grasp the hard palate/maxillary arch and rock it back and forth. Simultaneously palpating the midface during maxillary manipulation will disclose Le Fort fractures with better sensitivity than plain radiographs.[33]

Finally, a careful neurologic examination of the cranial nerves is crucial. Anesthesia of the upper lip and maxillary teeth suggests injury to the infraorbital nerve, often secondary to a blowout fracture or isolated infraorbital rim fracture.[34] Sensory loss of the lower lip and lower teeth may occur with mandibular fractures. Although many patients with facial anesthesia suffer only nerve contusions that resolve spontaneously, numbness suggests bony injury.

ORBITS

A thorough eye examination is imperative in the patient sustaining facial trauma. This key element must be conducted as soon as possible during the patient's evaluation, since edema only increases and may render many aspects of the examination impossible. A good approach is to evaluate the eye from the outside in.

Begin by inspecting the orbits for any asymmetries, enophthalmos, or exophthalmos. Look for any ecchymosis suggestive of occult basilar skull fracture (i.e., raccoon eyes). Palpate each of the orbits in its entirety, feeling for any step-offs, crepitus, or emphysema. Inspect the eyelids, noting any lacerations, especially those involving the medial canthus or tarsal plate. A plastic surgeon or ophthalmologist should repair such high-risk injuries.

Measure the distance between the medial canthi. This distance is normally 35 to 40 mm.[35] Any increase **(telecanthus)** appears as a flattened nasal bridge and suggests serious orbital and naso-ethmoid-orbital (NEO) injury. Increase in the interpupillary distance **(hypertelorism)** occurs when the orbits are fractured and blown apart, usually resulting in blindness.[36]

Test the muscles of extraocular motion. Remember that paralysis of upward gaze causing binocular diplopia may occur with infraorbital muscle entrapment secondary to fracture of the orbital floor or zygoma. To determine true entrapment, the EP may employ the **forced duction test**, or defer the test to an ophthalmologist. This test involves topically anesthetizing the eye, grasping the sclera and pulling upwards towards the supraorbital rim. If the eye still does not move, there is true entrapment.

Next observe the inner structure of the eye. Look at the sclera for lateral hemorrhages, seen with zygoma fractures, or imbedded foreign bodies. Perform a fluorescein test to detect corneal abrasions and lacerations. A slit lamp will demonstrate lens dislocation and provide information regarding the anterior chamber. Examine the anterior chamber for loss of normal depth, which can occur in globe ruptures, and traumatic hyphema, which can result in vision loss.

Look at the shape of the pupil. A single irregular pupil suggests globe penetration or corneal laceration. Test the reactivity of the pupil with the swinging flashlight test. A **Marcus-Gunn pupil** is noted when a pupil first dilates rather than constricts when exposed to a swinging light. This sign suggests optic nerve or retinal damage and mandates immediate ophthalmologic consultation.[37]

Finally, documentation of visual acuity using the standard Snellen chart is paramount.[19] If the patient cannot discern the letters on the chart, determine the ability to count fingers; at the very least, ascertain light perception. Loss of visual acuity requires immediate ophthalmologic consultation, since emergency decompression of the optic nerve may prevent permanent blindness.

NOSE

Again, begin with inspection for any asymmetry. Remember that edema may obscure subtle nasal deviation. Gently palpate the nasal bridge for crepitus, step-off, or emphysema. Examine the nasal septum for deviation or hematoma, a bluish bulging mass that is soft to palpation with a cotton swab.

Check any nasal drainage for the presence of cerebrospinal fluid (CSF) suggesting violation of the skull base. The halo or double-ring sign occurs when CSF mixed with blood is dropped onto a sheet or paper towel. However, this test is not specific for the presence of CSF, since simple rhinorrhea mixed with blood will produce a similar effect.[38] The best way to differentiate the two is the presence of glucose in CSF. Rhinorrhea (in the absence of blood) will not contain glucose. Unfortunately, the bedside glucometer cannot distinguish between CSF and rhinorrhea, and thus it must be sent to the laboratory, making this test quite impractical.[39,40] Dogma holds that appearance of a double-ring sign, in the presence of facial trauma, suggests CSF leak and should prompt further evaluation for basilar skull fracture.

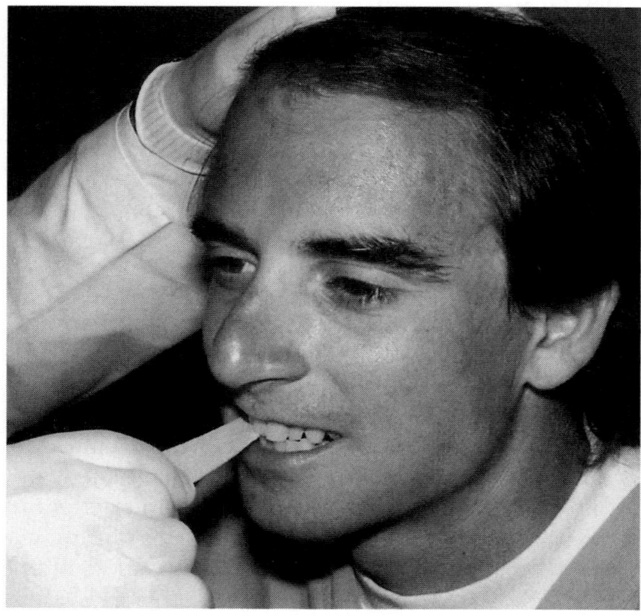

Fig. 14-3 Tongue blade test.

MOUTH

Observe for any jaw deviation suggestive of temporomandibular joint (TMJ) dislocation or fracture of a condyle. The chin will point away from a dislocation and towards a fracture. Have the patient open and close his or her mouth to determine malocclusion. Patients with mandibular or maxillary fractures will likely complain that their "teeth don't meet right." Any trismus or inability to close the mouth raises the possibility of a Le Fort or zygoma fracture. In both cases, bone fragments may impinge on the masseter muscle or coronoid process of the mandible.

The intraoral examination should identify the presence of any hematomas. Have the patient lift his or her tongue, since a sublingual hematoma is pathognomonic of a mandible fracture. Observe for any dental fracture or avulsions. Any lacerations or bleeding around teeth near a mandible fracture renders the fracture open, mandating intravenous antibiotics.

Finally, test for jaw stability. The mandibular condyles are best palpated by placing a finger in the external auditory canal and pressing down while the patient opens and closes his or her mouth. The **tongue blade test** is a sensitive and easily performed bedside test to detect mandibular fractures (Fig. 14-3).[41] Have the patient bite down on a tongue depressor and then twist the blade. In the presence of a mandible fracture, the patient will reflexively open his or her mouth; however, the patient with an intact mandible should break the blade. A recent study demonstrated that this test is 95% sensitive and almost 65% specific for mandibular fracture.[42]

EARS

Begin by observing the pinna for any trauma. The EP should drain a subperichondral hematoma and apply a pressure dressing to prevent reaccumulation of blood and subsequent deformity of the pinna.[43] Be sure to look behind the pinna for mastoid ecchymosis (Battle's sign) seen with basilar skull fractures. Examine inside the ear for any canal lacerations or CSF leak. A purple, (not red or silvery) tympanic membrane (TM) represents a hemotympanum and suggests basilar skull fracture. Fractures of the mandibular condyles may also rupture the TM.

Radiology

Diagnostic radiology comes after stabilization and management of life-threats. Only after these issues are managed should further testing be conducted.[44]

Physical examination may be more important than radiographic studies. In a 1997 study,[32] 90% of clinically significant fractures were diagnosed on physical examination alone. On the other hand, physical examination has its limits, since 17% of patients who underwent plain film radiography and computed tomography (CT) had management of their fractures altered based on the radiographic findings. The timing of radiographic studies is problematic. Certainly, in the hemodynamically or neurologically unstable patient facial imaging may be deferred for days. But what about the patient with isolated facial trauma and a suspicious physical examination? Many patients can be referred for outpatient CT scans and further management. However, some argue that if patients know their definitive diagnosis based on a facial CT scan at the time of ED discharge, they are more likely to keep follow-up appointments.

PLAIN-FILM RADIOGRAPHS

These films serve as a good screening examination for patients with facial trauma. The films are best viewed by examining for bony symmetry, suture lines, and lucencies. Air-fluid levels in the sinuses after trauma are highly suggestive of fracture. Subcutaneous emphysema is also visualized on these films.[45]

Physical examination will guide the specific view or radiograph ordered. An occipitomental view **(Water's view)** (Fig. 14-4) best visualizes the orbital rims, infraorbital floors, maxilla, and maxillary sinuses. The submentovertex **(jug-handle)** view scrutinizes the zygomatic arches and skull base. A posterior-anterior radiograph **(Caldwell view)** (Fig. 14-5) best evaluates the frontal bones and sinuses, the orbits, and the mandibular symphysis. In general, the standard three-view facial and skull series includes the Water's view, Caldwell view, and a lateral (to evaluate the sinuses).[46]

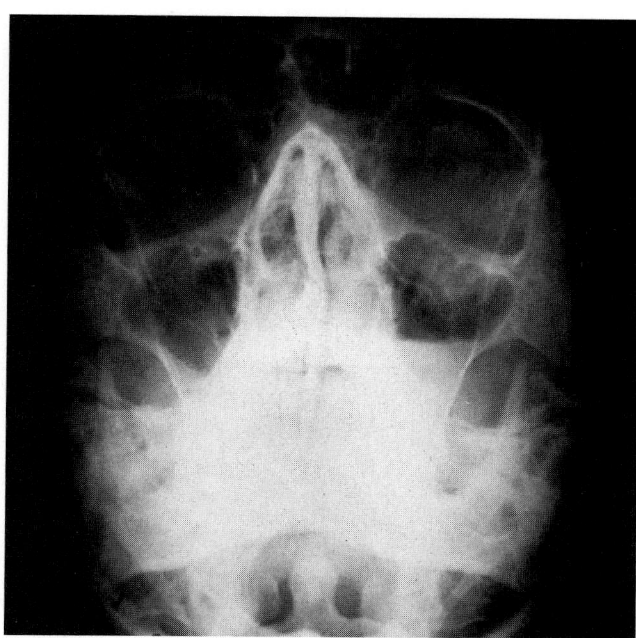

Fig. 14-4 Water's view radiograph.

In certain situations, specialized views can be helpful. These views include the **Towne's view** (35° caudad anterior-posterior) for the zygoma and mandibular rami. For mandible fractures, consider a **Panorex** (180° of the mandible and maxilla), or the **oblique mandible** to evaluate the mandibular condyles/rami and base of the skull.

COMPUTED TOMOGRAPHY

For patients with known or highly suspected periorbital or midface fractures, CT scanning is the most desirable test (Fig. 14-6).[47] In addition, CT permits evaluation of the globe and orbital fissures. In addition to the standard axillary views, specialized cuts through the face include coronal, sagittal, parasagittal, and thin-slice sections. CT three-dimensional reconstruction is superior to standard two dimensional CT in patients with tripod and complex maxillary fractures.[48,49] When ordering a CT, consider the plane of the suspected fracture, and include CT slices at 90 degrees to that plane. For instance if the medial orbital

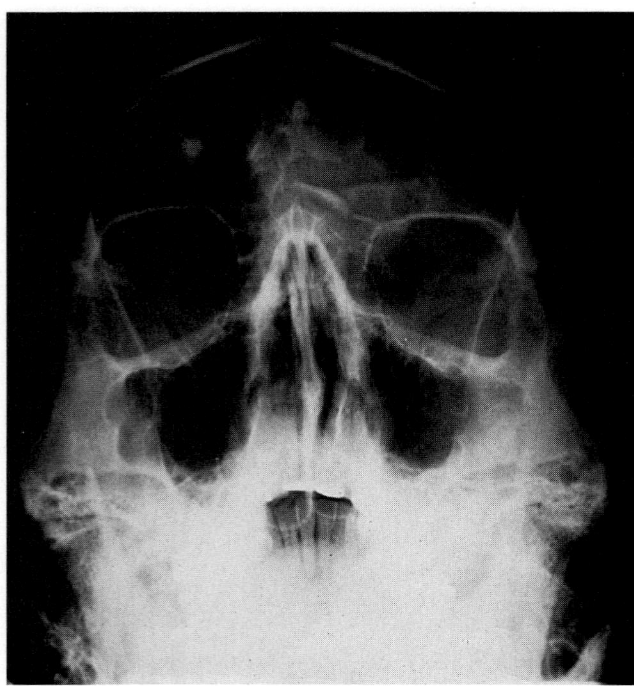

Fig. 14-5 Fracture seen on Caldwell view of radiograph.

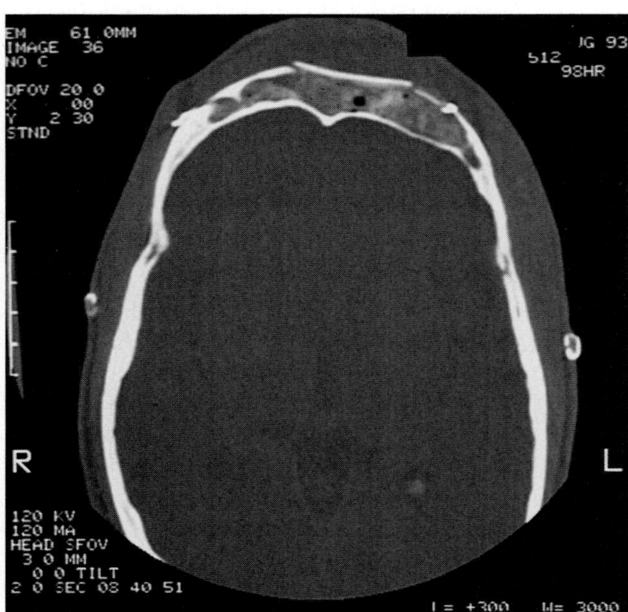

Fig. 14-6 Computed tomography scan of frontal bone fracture.

wall is at risk, order an axial CT; to best view the orbital floor, obtain a coronal CT.

If a patient who suffers multisystem trauma requires a brain CT scan, consider a screening facial CT. Approximately 10% of these patients will have occult facial fractures.[15] Remember that facial scans should be delayed until patients are hemodynamically and neurologically stable.

MAGNETIC RESONANCE IMAGING

The final radiologic modality available in facial trauma is magnetic resonance imaging (MRI). This study is best employed by the consultant to evaluate soft tissue and nerve injuries, especially the optic nerve and potential retrobulbar hematoma. MRI is much less sensitive in diagnosing fractures and thus is rarely useful in the ED setting.[50-52]

RADIOGRAPHIC CONTROVERSIES

Some authorities argue that a facial CT should be the first and only diagnostic test for significant facial fractures. However, plain films continue to play a significant role in emergency care.[47,53,54] In patients with low suspicion or minor injury a $100 to $200 plain film may be all that is required for ruling out consequential fractures compared with approximately $900 for full series facial CT.

Alternatively, a limited view facial CT scan (e.g., only an injured orbit) costs as little or less than a plain film, and ultimately provides more information.[55] Also, many of the plain radiographs described previously require a cooperative patient with a "cleared" C-spine for correct positioning. Therefore, in some patients, plain radiographs may be impossible to obtain, leaving CT as the only and best option.

SPECIFIC FRACTURES

Frontal Bone/Frontal Sinus Fractures

MECHANISM

These fractures are usually the result of a direct blow to the head with a blunt object, such as a lead pipe or brick. Because of their prominent skull, children are likely to suffer these injuries.

PHYSICAL EXAMINATION

Palpate the area, especially along the supraorbital rims, for any crepitance, bony step-offs, or emphysema. Do a thorough ocular examination checking for ptosis, enophthalmos, or paralysis of upward gaze. Check for CSF leaks from the wound, suggesting intracranial violation. Finally, assess forehead sensation, which may be lost with injury to the supraorbital or supratrochlear nerves.

ADJUVANT TESTS

Perform a plain-film Caldwell view for any patient with a suspicious mechanism or PE findings. If there are hard physical findings such as bony step-off or emphysema, CT scanning is the diagnostic gold standard.

COMPLICATIONS

These fractures are often associated with disruption of the posterior table of the sinuses and intracranial injury.[56] Dural tears and orbital roof injury may lead to brain impairment or blindness.[57] Late-developing cranial empyemas (collections of pus between the brain parenchyma and skull) may occur with dural tears, whereas mucopyoceles (collections of pus and mucus) appear if fractures block sinus drainage.[28]

TREATMENT AND DISPOSITION

Consult a neurosurgeon or an otolaryngologist for all patients with depressed fractures, open fractures, or those with posterior table involvement. Surgical repair and intravenous antibiotics may be required.[44] For other patients managed on an outpatient basis, consultation with the appropriate specialist to determine follow-up and antibiotic choice is reasonable.

There is much controversy concerning the use of antibiotics. Some physicians believe that prophylactic antibiotics promote the growth of resistant organisms. However, most practitioners use a first-generation cephalosporin, amoxicillin/clavulanate, erythromycin, or trimethoprim/sulfamethoxazole to cover common sinus pathogens.[19] Advise these patients to avoid nose-blowing, which will increase subcutaneous emphysema.

Orbital Floor (Blowout) Fractures

MECHANISM

Orbital floor fractures are the most common of the orbital fractures. When a blunt object, such as a ball or fist, strikes the globe, increased intraorbital pressure may rupture the delicate floor.[28,58] Intraorbital contents, such as muscle or even the globe, may herniate through the breech. Direct blows to the orbital rim may also produce a blowout fracture.

PHYSICAL EXAMINATION

Observe the patient for any enophthalmos, sunken globe, or proptosis, which develop in severe injuries, and palpate for any bony step-off. Subcutaneous emphysema suggests fracture into a sinus.[59] Check for diplopia on upward gaze, remembering to employ the forced duction test if necessary.[60] Despite traditional teaching, diplopia will most often be the result of direct muscle injury and *not* true entrapment.[55] Because blowout fractures often injure the infraorbital nerve, test the maxillary teeth and upper lip for anesthesia.[59]

ADJUVANT TESTING

Plain-film Water's view is often useful to diagnose orbital floor fractures. One author suggests that this view is all that is required except in patients with a clinical indication for surgery (i.e., >2 mm enophthalmos and/or persistent diplopia).[61] Often a "hanging teardrop" sign is seen when orbital fat herniates into the maxillary sinus, and an air-blood level is common in patients with this injury. A fragment of bone protrudes into the sinus, appearing on the radiograph as an "open bomb-bay door" sign.[62] Plain radiographs are also good in detecting metallic foreign bodies.[46]

If a blowout fracture is detected during PE or by plain-film radiography, an orbital CT scan with coronal sections is needed to better define the fracture. One study showed that 33% of periorbital emphysema, 10% of fractures, and up to 70% of complex fractures are only seen on CT.[62] CT scanning is best done while the patient is still in the ED, since patients with orbital fractures historically have poor follow-up.[63] However in a busy ED with limited CT resources, compliant patients may return for this study at a later date. Determine local practices, since some plastic surgeons delay repair of the orbital floor for weeks to months.

COMPLICATIONS

Ocular injury occurs in 10% to 25% of blowout fractures. Binocular diplopia resulting from direct muscle injury usually resolves in up to 82% of injuries, whereas true inferior rectus entrapment may require surgical intervention.[64] Malignant emphysema and/or retrobulbar hematoma is a surgical emergency requiring emergent lateral canthectomy to decrease intraocular pressure and preserve optic nerve function. Canthectomy is a procedure that EPs should perform only after consultation with an ophthalmologist. Anesthetize then crush the lateral canthus with a hemostat (to decrease bleeding) and then incise it with scissors.[65] The lids will spring apart and intraocular pressure should dramatically decline.

Perhaps the most significant complication of blowout fracture is an associated NEO injury, which occurs in 10% to 71% (see the following discussion).

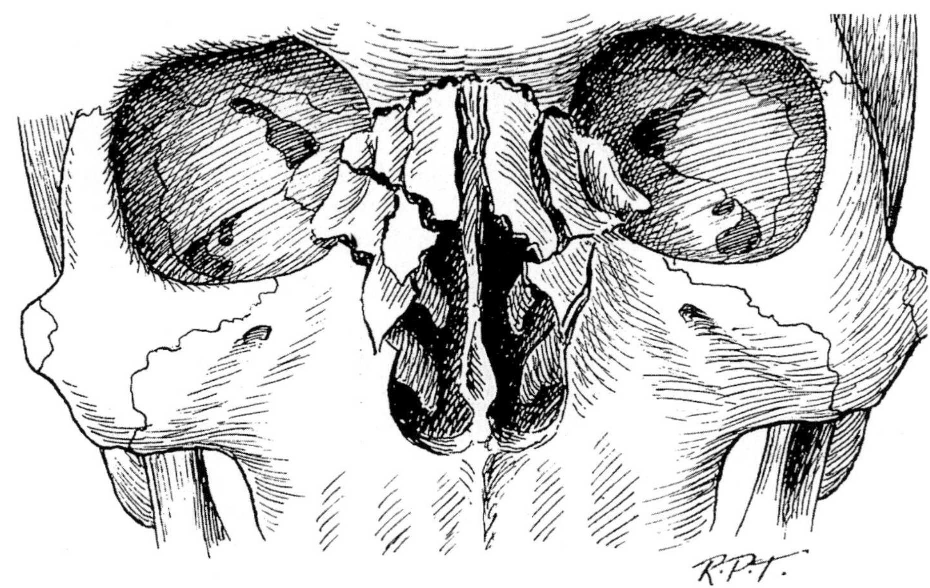

Fig. 14-7 Naso-ethmoid-orbital fracture.

TREATMENT AND DISPOSITION

Consult with a maxillofacial surgeon to arrange for follow-up. The timing and even need for repair of these fractures is controversial.[44,66,67] Absolute surgical intervention is indicated for severe ocular trauma, significant enophthalmos, persistent diplopia, and true extraocular muscle entrapment.

Once again, most consultants suggest antibiotics that cover sinus pathogens (ampicillin, amoxicillin, erythromycin, trimethoprim/sulfamethoxazole or a first-generation cephalosporin).[68] Also, remind patients to refrain from blowing their nose.

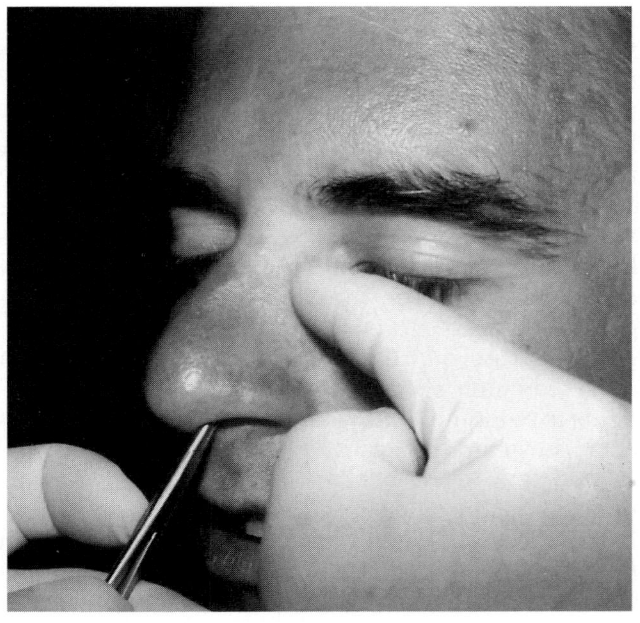

Fig. 14-8 Intranasal palpation test.

Naso-Ethmoid-Orbital Injuries

MECHANISM

Naso-ethmoid-orbital injuries result from high-energy blows to the bridge of the nose or medial orbital wall (Fig. 14-7).[69] A blow from a fist is usually inadequate to rupture these structures; common mechanisms include a bat to the face or an MVC.

PHYSICAL EXAMINATION

Often these patients demonstrate pain with extraocular muscle movement and epiphora (tears continuously spilling over the lids). Measure the intercanthal distance to determine the presence of telecanthus (>35 mm to 40 mm). To the physician, the intercanthal distance appears greater than the width of the patient's orbit.

In patients with suspicious injury (especially those with tenderness over the medial canthus) consider the intranasal palpation test (Fig. 14-8).[70] Anesthetize the nasal passage on the side of the injury with topical cocaine or xylocaine. Insert a hemostat into the naris and press laterally along the medial orbital rim (intranasal palpation) while simultaneously palpating the ipsilateral medial canthus with the other hand (extranasal palpation). Movement of the bone indicates an NEO injury. Check the nares for CSF leakage.

ADJUVANT TESTS

If the PE is suggestive of NEO injury, a facial CT is required, since plain films are insensitive.[71] Thin axial slices through the medial orbital wall may be necessary.[35,72]

COMPLICATIONS

Patients with NEO injury frequently have lacrimal disruption and dural tears. The medial canthal ligament may rupture, and medial rectus muscle can become entrapped. Most importantly, these patients are at risk of developing malignant periorbital emphysema and bilateral blindness.[8]

TREATMENT AND DISPOSITION

All patients with this injury need to be evaluated by a maxillofacial surgeon and admitted for repair. Most physicians begin antibiotics to cover sinus pathogens.[11]

Nasal Fractures

MECHANISM

The nose is the most common facial bone fractured. Blunt force, most often from a punch to the face, creates this injury.

PHYSICAL EXAMINATION

Allow the patient to look in a mirror and assess any cosmetic deformity. Palpate the nasal bridge for crepitance and step-offs and have the patient breathe through each naris separately and assess for any obstruction. Inspect the septum for any hematomas or deviation.

ADJUVANT TESTS

Nasal radiographs do not determine management of a nasal fracture. In addition, these films have a high false-negative and false-positive rate.[11,73-76] Only 50% of nasal fractures heal by ossification and thus the remainder are visible on radiographs for life. Although many patients expect a radiograph, straightening of a nasal deformity does not require x-rays, nor does the mere presence of a fracture mandate intervention. Because unmet expectations may lead to patient frustration, explain why films were not ordered, and reassure patients with nasal deformity that a specialist will fix their nose.

COMPLICATIONS

Cosmesis and airway obstruction are the two key issues and should prompt referral to a maxillofacial surgeon.[77] Some patients will also have significant epistaxis associated with their nasal fracture, which is best managed with direct pressure and packing. On rare occasions, the EP or consultant may need to acutely reduce a severely displaced nose to achieve hemostasis.

Septal hematomas require drainage in the ED. In theory, drainage prevents infection and subsequent nasal septum necrosis with saddle deformity, although there are few cases in the literature to support this assumption.[28,78] Anesthetize the nasal mucosa topically, then incise the hematoma along its inferior aspect with a #11 blade. Once the hematoma is evacuated, the nose should be packed to oppose the perichondrium to the septal cartilage and prevent reaccumulation of blood. These patients require prompt follow-up in 2 to 3 days with a maxillofacial surgeon or reevaluation in the ED.[78]

TREATMENT AND DISPOSITION

Treat patients with an isolated nasal fracture on an out-patient basis. The presence of open nasal fractures requires covering exposed bone with skin, but does not otherwise change treatment. Osteomyelitis of the nasal bone is almost unknown. If a septal hematoma was drained and packed, begin antibiotics covering sinus pathogens and establish an appointment for recheck in 2 to 3 days. For patients who have significant deformity with minimal edema, the EP may reduce the nose by hand and apply a Denver splint. Patients with significant edema should be reevaluated by a maxillofacial surgeon in 5 to 7 days for adults or 3 to 5 days for children (ossification occurs faster in pediatric patients).[79] Have patients elevate the head of the bed, use topical decongestants such as phenylephrine, and apply ice to the nose to reduce swelling. Again, patients should avoid blowing their nose.

Zygomatic Arch Fractures

MECHANISM

Injuries to the zygomatic arch are the third most common facial fracture (after nasal and mandible fractures) and result from a direct blow to the side of the face.

PHYSICAL EXAMINATION

Look from above and below to determine any enophthalmos and/or malar flattening. Palpate the zygomatic arch intraorally for any step-offs or crepitus. Inspect the sclera for associated subconjunctival hemorrhages, which may accompany a tripod fracture. Look for an open bite.

ADJUVANT TESTS

Usually only the plain radiograph jug-handle view is required for this isolated injury, and CT scanning is unnecessary.[1,80]

COMPLICATIONS

Most complications are cosmetic if the injury goes unrepaired, and the patient develops a "flat face" on the side of the fracture. Occasionally, the patient will have an open bite secondary to the fracture fragment impinging on the coronoid process.

TREATMENT AND DISPOSITION

Arrange for outpatient follow-up with a maxillofacial surgeon. Closed versus open reduction depends on the degree of depression of the fracture fragment.[1,80]

Zygomaticomaxillary Complex (Tripod) Fractures

MECHANISM

The tripod fracture is the most serious of all the zygoma fractures, involving the infraorbital rim, diastasis of the zygomatic-frontal suture, and disruption of the zygomatic-temporal junction. This fracture complex results from a forceful blow to the temple and cheek (Fig. 14-9).

PHYSICAL EXAMINATION

Observe closely for eye "tilt" secondary to the bony fragment dropping and pulling the lateral canthus down.[81] Lateral subconjunctival hemorrhages, lateral orbital edema, and periorbital ecchymosis may also appear. Test for infraorbital anesthesia.[82] Ipsilateral epistaxis may be present.

ADJUVANT TESTS

Often these fractures are apparent on plain-film Water's view. Air-fluid levels in the sinuses are usually detected on Caldwell view. However, these fractures require facial CT scanning for complete evaluation and delineation of orbital floor injury (Fig. 14-10).

COMPLICATIONS

Trismus or open bite secondary to masseter muscle or coronoid impingement by the fracture is common.[81] Binocular diplopia, from extraocular muscle entrapment, and lateral canthal ligament disruption are also frequently encountered.[1] Look for associated globe injury and be sure to evaluate visual acuity.

TREATMENT AND DISPOSITION

All patients with a tripod fracture require admission and evaluation by a maxillofacial surgeon for open reduction and internal fixation of the fragments.

Maxillary (Le Fort) Fractures

MECHANISM

Le Fort fractures result from high-energy forces, usually following high-speed MVCs resulting in multisystem trauma.[11] **Le Fort type I** is a transverse fracture

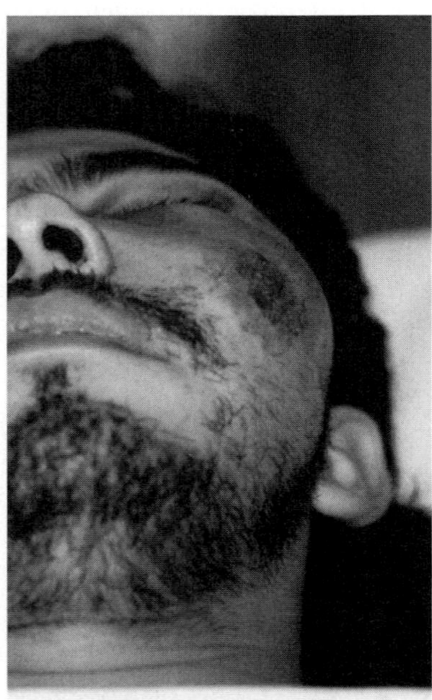

Fig. 14-9 Patient with a zygomatic tripod fracture.

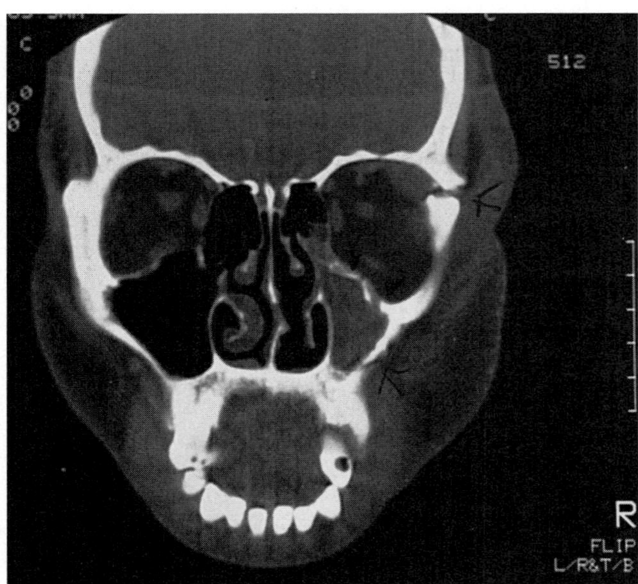

Fig. 14-10 Coronal computed tomography scan of zygomatic tripod fracture.

separating the hard palate from its bony frame. **Le Fort type II** is a pyramidal fracture involving the central maxilla and palate. **Le Fort type III** is effectively a craniofacial disruption with fractures extending from the frontozygomatic sutures, orbits, and nasoethmoidal regions (Fig. 14-11).[83,84] A **Le Fort type IV** is a Le Fort III fracture with concurrent frontal bone fracture.[33] Usually there are "mixed" fractures on either side (e.g., a low-grade Le Fort fracture on one side with a higher grade on the other).[11]

PHYSICAL EXAMINATION

Airway assessment and control is of the utmost importance in these patients. Once the airway has been secured, assess for midface mobility by grasping the hard palate and "rocking" it back and forth. Remember that impacted or greenstick fractures may be immobile.[33] Check for malocclusion and dental trauma. Test extraocular muscles and look for facial elongation and periorbital ecchymosis (raccoon eyes). Since these fractures have a high incidence of blindness, assess visual acuity in cooperative patients. Examine any nasal drainage for the presence of CSF.

ADJUVANT TESTS

Once the patient's airway is secured and other life-threats have been addressed, a facial CT scan is the diagnostic test of choice. Plain radiographs are of little benefit in these patients. If the patient has significant other injuries such as an intracranial hematoma or hemoperitoneum, delay facial CT until they stabilize.

COMPLICATIONS

Airway compromise is the number one complication seen with these fractures.[29] Significant hemorrhage from fracture displacement often occurs. If bleeding is severe, manual closed reduction while in the ED may be necessary. For uncontrolled hemorrhage, intubate the patient and pack the nose with both anterior and posterior packs. In rare circumstances, angiographic embolization may be required to stem the bleeding. Blindness is a significant concern in patients with Le Fort type III injuries. Finally, because these facial fractures are the result of high-energy transfers, the EP must always suspect other dangerous injuries.

TREATMENT AND DISPOSITION

All patients with a Le Fort fracture should be admitted for operative fixation and treatment of their associated injuries.[85,86]

Mandibular Fractures

MECHANISM

The mandible is the second most commonly injured facial bone. Multiple fractures occur >50% of the time as a result of the ring shape of the mandible.[3,34,86]

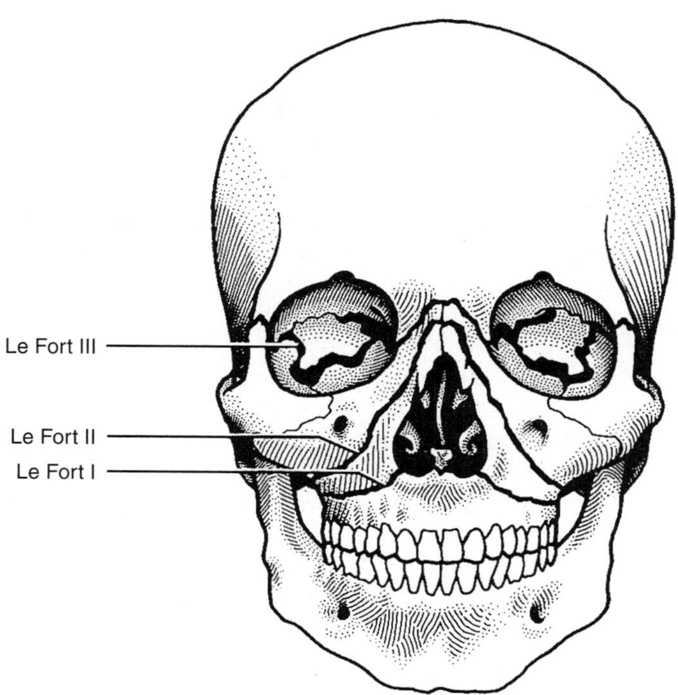

Fig. 14-11 Le Fort classification system. (From Cantrill S: Facial trauma. In Rosen P, et al [editors]: *Emergency medicine: concepts and clinical practice,* ed 4, St Louis, 1998, Mosby.)

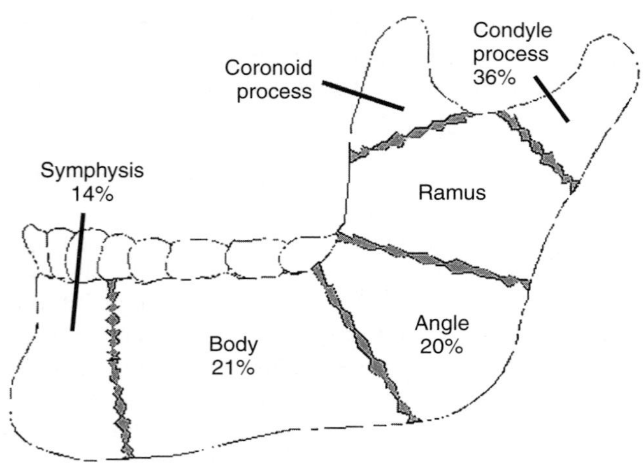

Fig. 14-12 Mandible fracture location.

Patients usually sustain these fractures following a direct blow to or fall onto the chin.

PHYSICAL EXAMINATION

Usually a good history and thorough PE can detect all mandible fractures. The most common site for a fracture is the condyle (approximately 35%) followed by the body and angle of the mandible (20%) (Fig. 14-12).[11]

Observe for any jaw deviation (chin towards a fracture, away from a dislocation) or deformity. Check for malocclusion, pain, or crepitus with jaw movement. It is important to detect intraoral lacerations, since an open fracture is managed differently than a closed one. Sublingual ecchymosis accompanies most fractures, whereas mandibular nerve damage produces anesthesia of the lower lip. Finally, perform the tongue blade test as earlier described. A patient who can break the tongue blade usually does not have a mandibular fracture.[42]

ADJUVANT TESTS

Further tests are rarely necessary in patients with normal occlusion and a negative tongue blade test. For those patients with an abnormal PE, the best views of the mandible are the Panorex and Towne's view (to look at the condyles). If these views are negative, but clinical suspicion of a fracture is high, a CT scan of the condyles is warranted.[87]

COMPLICATIONS

Again, airway management is paramount, since the tongue can occlude the pharynx as it loses its normal attachment to the mandible. Significant dental trauma and bleeding can also occur. Transmission of forces through the condyles may result in temporal bone fracture and rupture of the tympanic membrane.

TREATMENT AND DISPOSITION

All open fractures must be admitted for IV antibiotics and operative fixation. The drug of choice for these fractures is penicillin, but clindamycin or a first-generation cephalosporin may also be used.[88] A Barton's bandage, an elastic bandage wrapped around the patient's jaw and head, provides some comfort, and prevents jaw mobility. Patients with closed fractures may be discharged for outpatient management after consultation with a maxillofacial surgeon. They, too, may benefit from a Barton's bandage and may drink blended meals through a straw until follow-up. Adequate pain medication is essential for these agonizing fractures.

Temporomandibular Joint (TMJ) Dislocation

MECHANISM

Tempromandibular joint (TMJ) dislocation results from blunt trauma to the jaw or following seizures or excessive mouth opening or yawning. The condyle becomes "locked" anterior to the glenoid fossa and masseter muscle spasm prevents it from relocating. This injury rarely occurs in children unless there is a concurrent fracture.

PHYSICAL EXAMINATION

The chin deviates away from the dislocation if it is unilateral and juts forward in bilateral dislocations. The bite is always off. Palpate for a preauricular depression (Fig. 14-13).

ADJUVANT TESTS

If the dislocation is the result of trauma, obtain plain radiographs (Panorex and Towne's). If it is spontaneous or recurrent, no films are needed.

TREATMENT AND DISPOSITION

Emergency physicians can easily reduce TMJ dislocations.[89] Give the patient a benzodiazepine for muscle relaxation and/or anesthetize the masseter muscle with local anesthetic. Stand behind the seated patient and place gloved- and gauze-wrapped thumbs on the posterior molars or mandibular ridges. Push down on the molars and upwards and forward on the mandibular symphysis to direct the condyles backward and downward into the glenoid fossa; a rocking motion is often helpful. Following reduction, apply a Barton's bandage. The patient can be discharged home on a

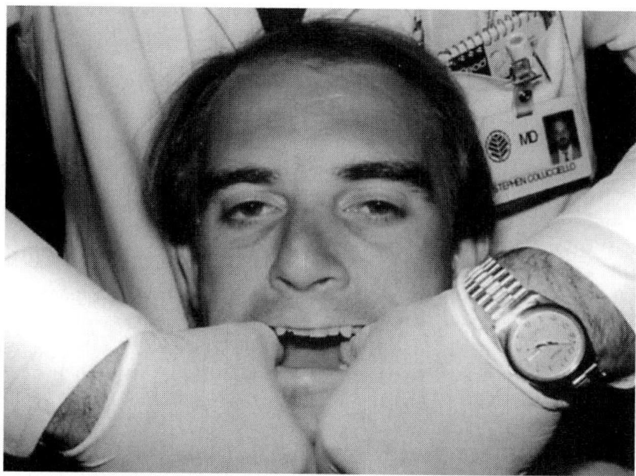

Fig. 14-13 Reduction of temporomandibular joint dislocation.

liquid diet with follow-up in several days. Caution the patient not to overuse the jaw for several days, since repeat dislocation is frequent.

OTHER CONCERNS

Superior Orbital Fissure Syndrome

Several facial fractures, especially frontal and orbital fractures, can occur in close proximity to where vital nerves exit the skull. The oculomotor and ophthalmic divisions of the trigeminal nerve are especially vulnerable as they course along the supraorbital fissure. If the supraorbital rim is fractured, bone fragments can compress these vital structures within the canal, resulting in ptosis, paralysis of extraocular muscles, and periorbital anesthesia.[90] If the optic nerve is compressed (the orbital apex syndrome), blindness can ensue.[84] A thorough ophthalmologic examination, including a test for visual acuity and the swinging light maneuver, should detect this injury and prompt immediate ophthalmologic consultation.

Penetrating Facial Trauma

Penetrating trauma is often more devastating than blunt trauma. Up to one third of patients with penetrating trauma will have significant complications.[91] Shotgun blasts are particularly detrimental and have a high incidence of blindness resulting from globe violation.

Airway compromise arises earlier and more rapidly, requiring emergent intubation and increasing the incidence of cricothyroidotomy. Penetrating trauma also endangers the brain. Not only is the brain parenchyma at risk, but there is the possibility of cavernous sinus fistulas and involvement of the great vessels. Zone III injuries to the carotids are common, and many patients require angiography.[92]

Finally, the risk of infection soars, especially when the missile violates the intraoral cavity.[93] Administer IV antibiotics such as penicillin, clindamycin, or a first-generation cephalosporin to cover oral flora.[94]

Pediatric Injury

The approach to pediatric facial injury is driven by a number of anatomic and developmental concerns.[95,96] Fracture patterns differ amongst these small patients. Their prominent frontal bone is fractured more frequently than that of adults.[97] Children under the age of 6 years have poorly developed sinuses, which leave the bones of the midface relatively strong and resistant to fracture.[98-100] For this reason, young children almost never suffer maxillary fractures. As their sinuses pneumatize, the facial buttress weakens, and Le Fort fractures increase. By 12 to 16 years of age, adolescents have injury patterns similar to adults.

Associated injuries are more common and difficult to assess in the pediatric patient. As a result of the prominent skull, up to 60% of children with facial fractures have concurrent intracranial injury,[98,101,102] Also, cervical injuries usually occur at C1-C3 rather than the lower injuries seen in adults. Even if C-spine radiographs are normal, the pediatric patient remains susceptible to spinal cord injury without radiographic abnormality (SCIWORA) (see Chapter 12).

Airway control can be quite challenging in these patients. The incidence of subglottic stenosis and tracheomalacia precludes the use of cricothyroidotomy in children less than 12 years old. If oral intubation fails, percutaneous transtracheal jet ventilation may provide a bridge to formal tracheotomy in the operating suite.

Children less than 5 years old are at increased risk for serious cosmetic disfigurement after facial trauma, since growth may become asymmetric after a fracture. Especially concerning are subcondylar fractures of the jaw and displaced nasal fractures. Facial deformity, micrognathia, and ankylosis of the TMJ can result unless a maxillofacial surgeon promptly intervenes. Children begin to form callus in approximately 1 week, rendering later correction of the fracture more difficult, if not impossible.[99,103,104] Thus all pediatric patients need urgent follow-up (within 3 to 5 days) following significant facial trauma.

The astute EP must consider the possibility of nonaccidental trauma. Any child with an unexplained skull fracture, torn frenulum, or facial bruising warrants further investigation.[97] In such cases, examine the patient fully undressed and order a radiographic skeletal series to rule out occult fracture.

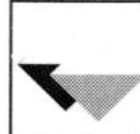

PEARLS & PITFALLS

- Airway compromise is the greatest life threat in patients with isolated facial trauma.
- Stabilize the patient before any ancillary tests and consider associated injuries.
- Ask the patient about visual complaints, facial anesthesia, and if their teeth meet normally since the injury.
- Physical examination must include palpation and inspection of the face, plus an eye evaluation and intraoral examination.
- The intranasal palpation, tongue blade, and swinging flashlight tests may provide important information.
- CT scans in a plane 90 degrees to suspected injury provide definitive assessment of facial fractures. They are best used for periorbital fractures (including tripod fractures), as well as Le Fort injuries. Patients with frontal sinus fractures may also benefit from this study.
- Obtain consultation for decreased vision, tripod fractures, Le Fort fractures, open mandible fractures, NEO injuries, and pediatric fractures.
- Be wary of possible domestic violence, elder abuse, and nonaccidental pediatric trauma.

REFERENCES

1. Covington DS, et al: Changing patterns in the epidemiology and treatment of zygoma fractures: 10-year review, *J Trauma* 37:243-248, 1994.
2. Scherer M, et al: An analysis of 1,423 facial fractures in 788 patients at an urban trauma center, *J Trauma* 29:388-390, 1989.
3. Hussain K, et al: A comprehensive analysis of craniofacial trauma, *J Trauma* 36:34-47, 1994.
4. Jessee SA: Physical manifestations of child abuse to the head, face and mouth: a hospital survey, *ASDC J Dent Child* 62:245-249, 1995.
5. Ochs HA, Neuenschwander MC, Dodson TB: Are head, neck and facial injuries markers of domestic violence? *J Am Dent Assoc* 127:757-761, 1996.
6. Hartzell KN, Botek AA, Goldberg SH: Orbital fractures in women due to sexual assault and domestic violence, *Ophthalmology* 103:953-957, 1996.
7. Manson PN, Hoopes JE, Su CT: Structural pillars of the facial skeleton: an approach to the management of Le Fort fractures, *Plast Reconstr Surg* 66:54-64, 1980.
8. Markowitz BL: Complex facial fractures-organization of treatment, *Trauma Quar* 9:102-113, 1992.
9. Merriman S, Sargent LA: Anatomy of the face, *Trauma Quar* 9:9-19, 1992.
10. Nakhgevany KB, LiBassi M, Esposito B: Facial trauma in motor vehicle accidents: etiological factors, *Am J Emerg Med* 12: 160-163, 1994.
11. Cantrill, SV: Facial trauma. In Rosen P, et al (editors): *Emergency medicine: concepts and clinical practice*, ed 4, St Louis, 1998, Mosby.
12. Williams J, et al: Head, facial, and clavicular trauma as a predictor of cervical-spine injury, *Ann Emerg Med* 21:719-722, 1992.
13. Haug RH, et al: Cervical spine fractures and maxillofacial trauma, *J Oral Maxillofac Surg* 49:725-729, 1991.
14. Conforti PJ, Haug RH, Likavec M: Management of closed head injury in the patient with maxillofacial trauma, *J Oral Maxillofac Surg* 51:298-303, 1993.
15. Rehm CG, Ross SE: Diagnosis of unsuspected facial fractures on routine head computerized tomographic scans in the unconscious multiply injured patient, *J Oral Maxillofac Surg* 53: 522-524, 1995.
16. Haug RH, et al: A review of 100 closed head injuries associated with facial fractures, *J Oral Maxillofac Surg* 50:218-222, 1991.
17. Hills MW, Deane SA: Head injury and facial injury: is there an increased risk of cervical spine injury? *J Trauma* 34:549-554, 1993.
18. Marciani RD, Israel S: Diagnosis of blunt carotid injury in patients with facial trauma, *Oral Surg Oral Med Oral Pathol Oral Radiol Endod* 83:5-9, 1997.
19. Smith RG: Maxillofacial injuries. In Harwood-Nuss A, et al (editors): *The clinical practice of emergency medicine*, Philadelphia, 1996, Lippincott-Raven.
20. Pelletier CR, et al: Assessment of ocular trauma associated with head and neck injuries, *J Trauma* 44:350-354, 1998.
21. Zachariades N, Papavassiliou D, Christopoulos P: Blindness after facial trauma, *Oral Surg Oral Med Oral Pathol Oral Radiol Endod* 81:34-37, 1996.
22. Bisson JI, Shepherd JP, Dhutia M: Psychological sequelae of facial trauma, *J Trauma* 43:496-500, 1997.
23. Bavitz JB, Collicott PE: Bilateral mandibular subcondylar fractures contributing to airway obstruction, *Int J Oral Maxillofac Surg* 24:273-275, 1995.
24. Walls RM: Blind nasotracheal intubation in the presence of facial trauma: is it safe? *J Emerg Med* 15:243-244, 1997.
25. Rosen CL, et al: Blind nasotracheal intubation in the presence of facial trauma, *J Emerg Med* 15:141-145, 1997.
26. Neal MR, Groves J, Gell IR: Awake fiberoptic intubation in the semi-prone position following facial trauma, *Anaesthesia* 51: 1053-1054, 1996.
27. Subcommittee on Advanced Trauma Life Supportof the American College of Surgeons Committee on Trauma: *Advanced trauma life support*, ed 6, Chicago, 1998, American College of Surgeons.
28. Converse JM: *Surgical treatment of facial injuries*, Baltimore, 1974, Williams & Wilkins.
29. Thompson JN, Gibson B, Kohut RI: Airway obstruction in Le Fort fractures, *Laryngoscope* 97(3 Pt1):275-279, 1987.
30. Crawley WA: Initial assessment and emergency treatment of maxillofacial injuries, *Trauma Q* 9:20-26, 1992.
31. Piotrowski WP: The primary treatment of frontobasal, and midfacial fractures in patients with head injuries, *J Oral Maxillofac Surg* 50:1264-1268, 1992.
32. Thai KN, et al: The role of computed tomographic scanning in the management of facial trauma, *J Trauma* 43:214-217, 1997.
33. Hehmann RJ, Sargent LA: Maxillary fracture, *Trauma Q* 9:67-75, 1992.
34. Robeson MC, Smith DJ Jr: Maxillofacial area. In Moore EE, et al (editors): *Early care of the injured patient*, ed 4, Toronto, 1990, Decker.

35. Sanderov B, Viccellio P: Fractures of the medial orbital wall, *Ann Emerg Med* 17:973-976, 1988.
36. Markowitz BL, et al: High-energy orbital dislocations: the possibility of traumatic hypertelorbitism, *Plast Reconstr Surg* 88:20-28, 1991.
37. Joondeph BC: Blunt ocular trauma, *Emerg Med Clin North Am* 6:147-167, 1988.
38. Dula DJ, Fales W: The 'ring' sign: is it a reliable indicator for cerebrospinal fluid? *Ann Emerg Med* 22:718-720, 1993.
39. Steedman DJ, Gordon M: CSF rhinorrhoeae: significance of the glucose oxidase strip test, *Injury* 18:327-328, 1987.
40. Beckhardt RN, Setzen M, Carras R: Primary spontaneous cerebrospinal fluid rhinorrhea, *Otolaryngol Head Neck Surg* 104:425-432, 1991.
41. Brentnall E: Spatula test for fracture of the mandible, *Aust Fam Physic* 21:1007, 1992.
42. Alonso LL, Purcell TB: Accuracy of the tongue blade test in patients with suspected mandibular fracture, *J Emerg Med* 13:297-304, 1995.
43. Reil B, Kranz S: Traumatology of the maxillo-facial region in childhood, *J Maxillofac Surg* 4:197-200, 1976.
44. Thaller SR, Kawamoto HK: Care of maxillofacial injuries: survey of plastic surgeons, *Plast Reconstr Surg* 90:562-567, 1992.
45. Harris JH, et al: An approach to mid-facial fractures, *Crit Rev Diagn Imaging* 21:105-132, 1984.
46. Lustrin ES, et al: Radiologic assessment of trauma and foreign bodies of the eye and orbit, *Neuroimaging Clin North Am* 6:219-237, 1996.
47. Kassel EE, Noyek AM, Copper PW: CT in facial trauma, *J Otolaryngol* 12:2-15, 1983.
48. Ohkawa M, et al: The role of three-dimensional computed tomography in the management of maxillofacial bone fractures, *Acta Med Okayama* 51:219-225, 1997.
49. Ray CE, et al: Applications of three-dimensional CT imaging in head and neck pathology, *Radiol Clin North Am* 31:181-194, 1993.
50. Ilankovan V, et al: A comparison of imaging techniques with surgical experience in orbital injuries: a prospective study, *J Craniomaxillofac Surg* 19:348-352, 1991.
51. Roden DT, Savino PJ, Zimmerman RA: Magnetic resonance imaging in orbital diagnosis, *Radiol Clin North Am* 26:535-545, 1988.
52. Gentry LR: Facial trauma and associated brain damage, *Radiol Clin North Am* 27:435-446, 1989.
53. Berardo N, Leban SG, Williams FA: A comparison of radiographic treatment methods for evaluation of the orbit, *J Oral Maxillofac Surg* 46:844-849, 1988.
54. Finkle DR, et al: Comparison of the diagnostic methods used in maxillofacial trauma, *Plast Reconstr Surg* 75:32-41, 1985.
55. Sargent LA: Internal orbital fractures, *Trauma Q* 9:94-101, 1992.
56. Lee KF: High resolution computed tomography of facial trauma associated with closed head injury. In Toombs BD, Sandler CN (editors): *Computed tomography in trauma*, Philadelphia, 1987, Saunders.
57. Martello JY, Vasconez HC: Supraorbital roof fractures: a formidable entity with which to contend, *Ann Plast Surg* 38:223-227, 1997.
58. Nguyen PN, Sullivan P: Advances in the management of orbital fractures, *Clin Plast Surg* 19:87-98, 1992.
59. O'Hare TH: Blow-out fractures: a review, *J Emerg Med* 9:253-263, 1991.
60. Holt GR, Holt JE: Management of orbital trauma and foreign bodies, *Otolaryngol Clin North Am* 21:35-52, 1988.
61. Bhattacharya J, Moseley IF, Fells P: The role of plain radiography in the management of suspected orbital blow-out fractures, *Br J Radiol* 70:29-33, 1997.
62. Birrer RB, Robinson T, Papachristos P: Orbital emphysema: how common, how significant? *Ann Emerg Med* 24:1115-1118, 1994.
63. Stewart MG, Chen AY: Factors predictive of poor compliance with follow-up care after facial trauma: a prospective study, *Otolaryngol Head Neck Surg* 117:72-75, 1997.
64. al-Qurainy IA, et al: Diplopia following midfacial fractures, *Br J Oral Maxillofac Surg* 29:302-307, 1991.
65. Jordan DR, et al: Orbital emphysema: a potentially blinding complication following orbital fractures, *Ann Emerg Med* 17: 853-855, 1988.
66. Mathog RH: Management of orbital blow-out fractures, *Otolaryngol Clin North Am* 24:79-91, 1991.
67. Levin LM, Kademani D: Clinical considerations in the management of orbital blow-out fractures, *Compendium of Continuing Education in Dentistry* 18: 593, 596-598, 600, 1997.
68. Silver HS, et al: Severe orbital infection as a complication of orbital fracture, *Arch Otolaryngol Head Neck Surg* 118:845-848, 1992.
69. Heine RD, et al: Naso-orbital-ethmoid injury: report of a case and review of the literature, *Oral Surg Oral Med Oral Pathol* 69:542-549, 1990.
70. Paskert JP, Manson PN: The bimanual examination for assessing instability in naso-orbitoethmoidal injuries, *Plast Reconstr Surg* 83:165-167, 1989.
71. Nolasco FP, Mathog RH: Medial orbital wall fractures: classification and clinical profile, *Otolaryngol Head Neck Surg* 112:549-556, 1995.
72. Leipziger LS, Manson PN: Nasoethmoid orbital fractures: current concepts and management principles, *Clin Plast Surg* 19: 167-193, 1992.
73. Logan M, O'Driscoll K, Masterson J. The utility of nasal bone radiographs in nasal trauma, *Clin Radiol* 49:192-194, 1994.
74. Illum P: Legal aspects in nasal fractures, *Rhinology* 29:263-266, 1991.
75. Nigam A, et al: The value of radiographs in the management of the fractured nose, *Arch Emerg Med* 10:293-297, 1993.
76. Clayton MI, Lesser TH: The role of radiography in the management of nasal fractures, *J Laryngol Otol* 100:797-801, 1986.
77. Constant E: Trauma to the face. In Schwartz GR (editor): *Principles and practice of emergency medicine*, ed 4, Baltimore, 1999, Williams & Williams.
78. Ginsburg CM: Nasal septal hematoma, *Pediatr Rev* 19:142-143, 1998.
79. Renner GJ: Management of nasal fractures, *Otolaryngol Clin North Am* 24:195-213, 1991.
80. Rohrich RJ, Hollier LH, Watumull D: Optimizing the management of orbitozygomatic fractures, *Clin Plast Surg* 19:149-165, 1992.
81. Rumsey C, Sargent LA: Zygomatic fractures, *Trauma Q* 9:76-85, 1992.
82. Prendergast ML, Wildes TO: Evaluation of the orbital floor in zygoma fractures, *Arch Otolaryngol Head Neck Surg* 114:446-450, 1988.
83. Le Fort R: Etude experimentale sur les fractures de le machoire superieure, *Rev Chir* 23:208, 1901.
84. Pathria MN, Blaser SI: Diagnostic imaging of craniofacial fractures, *Radiol Clin North Am* 27:839-853,1989.
85. Davidoff G, et al: The spectrum of closed-head injuries in facial trauma victims: incidence and impact, *Ann Emerg Med* 17:6-9, 1988.

86. Robertson BC, Manson PN: Concepts in mandibular fractures, *Trauma Quar* 9:54-66, 1992.
87. Horowitz I, Abrahami E, Mintz SS: Demonstration of condylar fractures of the mandible by computed tomography, *Oral Surg Oral Med Oral Pathol* 54:263-268, 1982.
88. Beck RA, Blakeslee DB: The changing picture of facial fractures: 5-year review, *Arch Otolaryngol Head Neck Surg* 115:826-829, 1989.
89. Luyk NH, Larsen PE: The diagnosis and treatment of the dislocated mandible, *Am J Emerg Med* 7:329-335, 1989.
90. Unger JM: Orbital apex fractures: the contribution of computed tomography, *Radiology* 150:713-717, 1984.
91. Chen AY, Stewart MG, Raup G: Penetrating injuries of the face, *Otolaryngol Head Neck Surg* 115:464-470, 1996.
92. Dolin J, et al: The management of gunshot wounds to the face, *J Trauma* 33:508-514, 1992.
93. Belfer RA, Ochsenschlager DV, Tomaski SM: Penetrating injury to the oral cavity: a case report and review of the literature, *J Emerg Med* 13:331-335, 1995.
94. Wallick K IV, Davidson P, Shockley L: Traumatic carotid cavernous sinus fistula following a gunshot wound to the face, *J Emerg Med* 15:23-29, 1997.
95. Kaban LB: Diagnosis and treatment of fractures of the facial bones in children, *J Oral Maxillofac Surg* 51:722-729, 1993.
96. Gussack GS, et al: Pediatric maxillofacial trauma: unique features in diagnosis and treatment, *Laryngoscope* 97:925-930, 1987.
97. Worlock P, Stower M, Barbor P: Patterns of fractures in accidental and non-accidental injury in children: a comparative study, *Br Med J* 293:100-102, 1988.
98. McGraw BL, Cole RR: Pediatric maxillofacial trauma: age-related variations in injury, *Arch Otolaryngol Head Neck Surg* 116:41-45, 1990.
99. VanderKolk CA: Pediatric facial fractures, *Trauma Q* 9:132-140, 1992.
100. Anderson PJ, Poole MD: Orbital floor fractures in young children, *J Craniomaxillofac Surg* 23:151-154, 1995.
101. Kenna MA: Maxillofacial trauma. In Touloukian RJ (editor): *Pediatric trauma*, St Louis, 1990, Mosby.
102. Dufresne CR, Manson PN, Iliff NT: Early and late complications of orbital fractures, *Clin Plast Surg* 15:239-253, 1988.
103. Hunter JG: Pediatric maxillofacial trauma, *Pediatr Clin North Am* 39:1127-1143, 1992.
104. Crockett DM, Mungo RP, Thompson RE: Maxillofacial trauma, *Pediatr Clin North Am* 36:1471-1494, 1989.

Ocular Trauma

15

WILLIAM H. SHOFF AND SUZANNE M. SHEPHERD

Significant visual loss resulting from ocular trauma has affected over 1 million Americans.[1] Fortunately, recent advances in ophthalmologic therapy and ocular microsurgery can now save vision that previously would have been lost to trauma.[2,3] The emergency physician (EP) must recognize those conditions that menace sight and initiate treatment and consultation to minimize visual impairment. Although EPs provide comprehensive care for most of the common eye complaints seen in the emergency department (ED), they must also recognize indications for referral.[4-6]

Consider all eye injuries a threat to vision until history and physical examination exclude serious trauma. Some serious conditions present with minimal signs and symptoms, such as damage to the optic nerve, lens, retina, or globe integrity.[2] Documentation of the examination, especially visual acuity (VA), is essential to avoid both medical and legal peril.

Although two studies show that EPs satisfactorily manage 97% to 99% of all ophthalmologic problems,[5,7] they often falter in documentation. In one study, EPs recorded acuity in only 56% of cases, fluorescein evaluation in 85%, corneal examination in 85%, and eye movement in 90%.[7] By comparison, ophthalmologists charted the same parts of the examination in 95% or more of the cases. Documenting a systematic eye examination is essential to the management and follow-up of the patient with ocular trauma.

EPIDEMIOLOGY AND ETIOLOGY

Eye complaints comprise 3% to 10% of the annual 100 million ED visits in the United States.[5,6,8] Over 2 million ocular injuries occur each year either at home, during sports, in accidents outside the home, or in the workplace.[9] As many as 60,000 patients are admitted to the hospital,[10] while 50,000 lose some degree of sight.[9] Males account for 70% to 85% of cases.[11-13]

Three groups account for over 80% of ocular injuries: children, young adults, and the elderly. The important locations for children are at home, during play, and while participating in organized sports. For young adults, motor vehicle crashes (MVCs), assaults, and workplace accidents are the leading causes, whereas falls predominate in the elderly.

The estimated annual cost in the United States for ocular trauma includes 227,000 days of hospital care for a total between $175 and $200 million.[14] The personal and financial costs of eye injury are enormous. In 90% of cases, the injury could have been prevented or lessened by wearing protective lenses.[9]

PATHOPHYSIOLOGY

Trauma to the globe and surrounding tissues occurs by four mechanisms: abrasion, blunt force, penetrating object, and burns. Abrasions and other wounds of the cornea and conjunctiva may produce a retained foreign body (FB). Blunt force and penetrating objects can yield multiple simultaneous injuries. Ocular burns involve heat, chemicals, ultraviolet (UV) radiation, infrared (IR) radiation, and electricity. The potential for multiple and clandestine injuries is high, and frequently the extent of ocular damage is not apparent at the time of presentation. Any trauma to the eye may produce inflammation in the **uveal tract** (iris, ciliary body, and choroid). This inflammation is designated **uveitis** or **anterior uveitis.**[15] **Acute traumatic iritis** involves the iris, whereas traumatic **iridocyclitis** refers to both the iris and ciliary body. **Posterior uveitis** involves the vitreous, retina, choroid, or any combination of posterior structures.[15] Injury may also occur to the **zonular fibers**, the structures holding the lens to the ciliary body.

Any of these conditions generates white cells and protein in the anterior chamber.[15-17] This **anterior chamber reaction**, or "flare" as it is sometimes called, occurs in 2% to 18% of eye trauma.[18,19] If the white cell reaction is sufficiently large for the white cells to layer out, it is called a **hypopyon** (pus in the anterior chamber).

Abrasive Trauma

Abrasions of the cornea usually involve only the epithelium, which is 5 to 6 cells thick. Healing occurs by a leading edge of aggregated epithelial cells and usually takes 12 to 36 hours depending on the extent of the abrasion.[20] Any corneal wound risks bacterial infection, which increases with the depth of the wound. This risk is amplified by an FB, as seen in contact lens–related corneal abrasions. These abrasions are prone to *Pseudomonas* infections.[20] Another FB complication is the deposition of a rust ring when the FB contains iron. The deposit usually occurs after the FB is present for more than a few hours. Minor or major trauma may induce **subconjunctival hemorrhages**. These superficial hemorrhages do not threaten vision and are not associated with decreased visual acuity.

Blunt Trauma

Trauma to the orbit by blunt force or a penetrating object can produce multiple injuries because of the close proximity of vital structures. These structures include eight orbital bones, seven muscles, six cranial nerves, five major foramina, four paraorbital sinuses, three different types of glands, two eyelids, and the globe itself.[21]

The orbital bones in the floor and medial wall are paper thin (0.5 mm), making them the most common sites for **blowout fractures**.[21,22] There are two postulated mechanisms for these fractures: (1) a sudden rise in pressure within the orbit from compression of the globe, and (2) direct transmission of force through the orbital rim and subsequent buckling of the orbital floor.[21] Ophthalmoplegia occurs when the muscles are entrapped or contused. The inferior rectus muscle is most commonly involved, producing diplopia on upward gaze. The infraorbital nerve traverses the floor of the orbit and is readily contused or lacerated, producing numbness of the ipsilateral facial cheek and upper lip. Fractures of the orbital roof can potentially breech the cranial vault. **Tripod**, **Le Fort II**, and **Le Fort III** fractures also involve the orbit and are described elsewhere in this text.

Since the orbit has a volume of only 35 ml, any force sufficient to cause a fracture delivers significant energy to the entire contents. The globe is injured in 5% to 10% of blowout fractures.[23] Overall, facial fractures have been associated with a 12% to 29% incidence of ocular injury.[24,25] In two studies, blindness occurred in 6% to 14% of individuals.[24,25]

Blunt or penetrating trauma, with or without associated fractures, may produce bleeding, air, or both in the orbit or the globe. Vision-threatening increases in pressure, both intraorbitally and intraocularly, may ensue. Blowout fractures leak air (**orbital emphysema**) into the skin or the orbit. If the air becomes trapped in the orbit (one-way valve created by fracture fragment) and cannot be released, **orbital compartment syndrome** results, leading to a marked increase in intraorbital pressure and threatening vision by three mechanisms: optic nerve ischemia, central retinal artery occlusion, and increased intraocular pressure (IOP) (Box 15-1).[26]

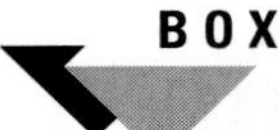

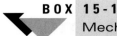

BOX 15-1
Mechanisms of Visual Loss with Orbital Compartment Syndrome

Optic nerve ischemia
Central retinal artery occlusion
Increased intraocular pressure

Another cause of increased intraorbital pressure is **retrobulbar** (i.e., behind the globe) **hemorrhage**.[17] Hemorrhage may also occur within the globe in the anterior chamber (hyphema), the vitreous, or the retina. **Hyphema** results from tearing of small vessels in the ciliary body and iris.[27] The blood is absorbed through the trabecular meshwork over a period of 1 to 10 days. On occasion resorption is blocked by clots obstructing the canal of Schlemm or by rebleeding. Obstruction of the canal of Schlemm increases IOP and may ultimately cause acute glaucoma and corneal blood staining. Rebleeding occurs within several days in 4% to 37% of cases.[27-29] **Vitreous** and **retinal hemorrhages** result from tearing of retinal or choroidal vessels, avulsion of the optic nerve head, and detachment of the retina or vitreous.

The concussive and traction forces associated with trauma contuse, rupture, and stretch the contents of the orbit and globe, producing a multitude of injuries. The nature of these injuries varies with their location. The globe can be ruptured, and the weakest points are at the attachment of the extraocular muscles, the limbus (corneoscleral junction), and the equator of the globe.[27,30] The globe can be dislocated from the socket, putting tension on the optic nerve and threatening its viability.

The optic nerve may be injured (**traumatic optic neuropathy**) along its course by direct or indirect means. Examples of a direct mechanism are fracture fragments, hematoma, or penetrating FB. Examples of an indirect mechanism include blunt head trauma, blunt ocular trauma, or fractures not involving the optic canal.[17,25] The choroid, retina, and vitreous may detach, bleed, or tear. A high-speed missile can rupture the retina and choroid in the absence of penetration, while leaving the sclera intact.[17,21] With this injury there is associated hemorrhage, significant retinal damage, and decreased vision.

Damage to the retina may be more limited with the occurrence of **commotio retina**, also known as retinal contusion, retinal edema, or Berlin's edema. Commotio retina is typically a contrecoup injury (i.e., occurring on the contralateral side of the globe in relation to the point of impact) with disruption of the photoreceptors and retinal blood flow. This latter finding distinguishes commotio retina from occlusion of the central retinal artery in which there is no inner retinal flow.[21] Healing of commotio retina occurs in 1 to 2 weeks, and vision is spared, unless the macula is involved. When the macula is damaged, the thin, capillary-free fovea may necrose, leading to macular edema and ultimately visual loss.

The lens can be subluxed or dislocated by stretching or disrupting the zonular fibers. If the lens capsule is ruptured by concussive forces or by penetrating trauma, cataract formation may result. When the normally dehydrated environment of the lens is violated, the stromal cells absorb fluid and swell, forming a cataract over days to months.[27] In addition, the swollen lens can obstruct the outflow of aqueous humor, leading to acute glaucoma.[27]

Concussive and traction injuries of the anterior segment of the eye produce several injuries. A common sequela includes **traumatic glaucoma** secondary to bleeding, inflammation, and scarring. These injuries occur because of hydraulic forces, causing the tissues to yield to the incompressible intraocular fluids.[20] Multiple structures are vulnerable to rupture, including disruption at the site of attachment of the ciliary body to the scleral spur, and the attachment of the ora serrata to the retina (**retinal dialysis**). Other structures injured include the ciliary body (angle recession), the peripheral iris (**iridodialysis,** traumatic separation of the iris root from the ciliary body), the pupil, the trabecular meshwork, and the zonular fibers. The iris responds to injury either by constriction resulting from irritation or contusion, or dilation caused by small tears. A rent in the iris will distort the pupil rendering it teardrop-shaped, with the narrow end pointing to the iris defect.

Penetrating Trauma

Because of the close proximity of structures, all lacerations and penetrating injuries around the eyes raise important concerns. The EP must consider the depth of the wound, injury to underlying structures, a retained FB, and associated injuries outside the orbit.

Intraocular FBs can produce varying degrees of inflammatory reactions. Copper, iron, steel, vegetable matter, and wood produce severe reactions, whereas aluminum, nickel, mercury, and zinc create mild reactions. Carbon, coal, glass, gold, lead, plaster, plastic, platinum, porcelain, rubber, silver, and stone are inert. Because iron, nickel, and steel are magnetic, using magnetic resonance imaging (MRI) to evaluate these injuries is problematic.[16,17,27] Intraocular FBs predispose to **endophthalmitis** (infection within the globe), which can devastate an eye in short order. *Bacillus cereus* is the worst offender and elaborates enzymes and toxins that permit an explosive infection, which leads to loss of the eye in less than 24 hours.[20]

Burns

Ocular burns vary depending on the type of energy delivered: heat, chemical, UV, IR, or electrical.

THERMAL BURNS

Thermal burns of the globe are rare,[31,32] since the eye is protected by **Bell's phenomenon**, a reflex upward globe rotation and lid blinking in response to a noxious stimulus.[27] Light from the thermal object travels at 300,000 meters per second and reaches the eye faster than the thermal energy, allowing Bell's phenomenon to protect the globe.[31]

Most burns to the globe involve the corneal epithelium and occur secondary to hot ashes, lighted matches, spitting grease, boiling liquids, and steam, particularly from a car radiator. These burns heal in a few days.[32]

CHEMICAL BURNS

Alkali burns cause devastating damage to the eye because they penetrate deep within the globe via liquefaction necrosis. Alkalis are strong bases found in many household and industrial products, and these burns are relatively common. On contact, cell membranes loosen as a result of fat saponification. If the damage is severe, the epithelium sloughs, exposing the stroma of the cornea and leading to endothelial destruction.[33] Further penetration increases the pH of the anterior chamber, injuring adjacent tissues including the trabecular meshwork, iris, lens, and ciliary body.[34] The cornea takes on a white appearance (marbleization), and IOP rises secondary to shortening of collagen fibers in the cornea and sclera.[35] Debris fills the anterior chamber, and a strong inflammatory response ensues, choking the chamber angle and leading to glaucoma. Further damage to the ciliary body may culminate in ocular atrophy (**phthisis bulbi**). Ulceration of the eye is seen during the repair phase.[33] Restoration of vision is never guaranteed in patients with even moderately severe injury.[33]

Unlike alkali burns, **acid burns** are less likely to cause extensive damage. Strong acids precipitate proteins, which form a barrier to further penetration (coagulation necrosis).[17] Still, the coagulation necrosis, produced by certain strong acids, can be severe.[17]

ULTRAVIOLET BURNS

Ultraviolet (UV) radiation causes an acute, diffuse, symmetric **superficial punctate keratitis** (**SPK**) of the corneal epithelium beginning 6 to 12 hours after exposure. The sources include welder's arcs, tanning salons, and the sun. Because of this time delay from injury, many patients with UV keratitis present to the ED at night. Important considerations with sun exposure are reflection, particularly from water, rocks, or snow, and altitudes above 8000 feet (snow blindness).[21] Prolonged exposure can damage the retina, particularly the fovea. The visual disturbance can develop 1 to 2 days after exposure.[36]

INFRARED BURNS

Infrared (IR) radiation burns were more common in the days of metal furnace stokers. Today, glass blowers with improper goggles are at risk. These workers may form cataracts after years of exposure.[21]

ELECTRICAL BURNS

Electrical energy is rarely delivered directly to the eye. However, indirect eye damage can occur in association with electrical injury of the head. Cataracts develop 6 to 12 months after exposure in 9% of patients experiencing significant electrical injuries about the head, particularly lighting strikes.[37]

TABLE 15-1
Signs and Symptoms or Ocular Injuries

INJURY	SYMPTOMS	SIGNS
Corneal abrasion	Pain, FB sensation, photophobia, halos, blurred vision	Hyperemia, fluorescein uptake, possible FB
Subconjunctival hemorrhage	None	Flat hemorrhage
Blowout fracture	Diplopia, pain, ipsilateral cheek numbness	Enophthalmos, globe displacement, orbital rim tenderness
Retrobulbar hemorrhage	Pain, blurred vision, diplopia	APD, chemosis, proptosis
Traumatic optic neuropathy	Decreased vision	APD, red desaturation
Globe rupture	Blurred vision, pain	Low IOP, deep or shallow AC, poor visual acuity, abnormal pupil
Intraocular FB	Blurred vision, pain or no pain, diplopia	Escape of AC fluid, abnormal pupil, AC cells
Traumatic iritis	Blurred vision, pain, photophobia, tearing	Miosis, mydriasis, AC cells/flare
Traumatic cataract	Blurred vision, glare from lights, reduced color vision	Decreased VA, lens opacity, reduced red reflex, indistinct retina
Lens luxation/subluxation	Blurred vision, monocular diplopia	Decreased VA, displaced lens
Hyphema	Pain, blurred vision	AC red cells, decreased VA
Commotio retina	Blurred vision	Retinal edema, scattered hemorrhages
Retinal detachment	Blurred vision, flashes of light, floaters	Decreased VA, gray retina
Chemical conjunctivitis	Pain, burning, photophobia	Hyperemia, mild decreased VA
Alkali/acid burns	Pain, blurred vision, photophobia	AC reaction, chemosis, corneal edema or opacification
Ultraviolet keratitis	Pain, burning, photophobia	AC reaction, hyperemia, SPK
Endophthalmitis	Blurred vision, pain	Hyperemia, AC cell/flare, decreased VA, hypopyon
Sympathetic ophthalmia	Pain, blurred vision	Iris edema, uveal inflammation

FB, Foreign body; *APD,* afferent pupillary defect; *IOP,* intraocular pressure; *AC,* anterior chamber; *VA,* visual acuity; *SPK,* superficial punctate keratitis.

EMERGENCY DEPARTMENT EVALUATION

History

Eye symptoms direct attention to the globe and may include blepharospasm (involuntary lid closure), blurred vision, eye pain, and discharge from the eye. Other patients complain of flashes of light and floaters, which suggest retinal involvement. Patients with anterior globe problems are likely to have an FB sensation, halos, photophobia, or tearing. Periorbital symptoms direct attention to the orbit and surrounding tissues and may include bruising, deformity, epistaxis, laceration, numbness, pain, and swelling.

In some instances symptoms may be absent, but the history suggests an eye injury. For example, a history that something struck the eye while the patient was using a hammer to strike metal raises the possibility of an intraocular metallic FB. Because of the ruinous consequences of a missed intraocular FB, routinely ask about "metal hitting metal" exposures. Table 15-1 lists signs and symptoms for specific ocular injuries.

Physical Examination

In suspected globe rupture, do not apply external pressure to the eye before definitive management by an ophthalmologist. A ruptured globe is suggested by VA limited to light perception (or worse), asymmetric anterior chamber depth, hemorrhagic chemosis (Fig. 15-1), hyphema (Fig. 15-2), a tear-shaped pupil (Fig. 15-3), IOP <5 mmHg, or penetrating trauma. Protect the orbit from contact by a guard (metal, plastic, or one fashioned with a paper or Styrofoam cup), and obtain immediate ophthalmologic consultation.[38,39]

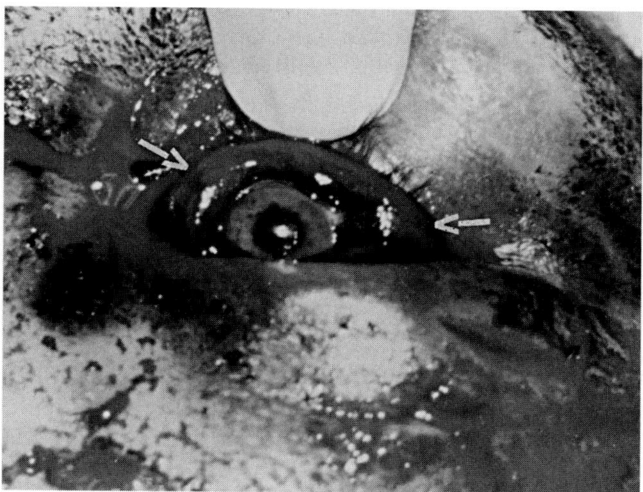

Fig. 15-1 Severe left hemorrhagic chemosis *(arrows)*.

SEVEN ASPECTS OF THE EMERGENCY DEPARTMENT EYE EXAMINATION

1. Visual Acuity. *Document VA as soon as possible because it the most important predictor of visual outcome.* A VA should be recorded for every patient with ocular injury, unless he or she is unconscious or hemodynamically unstable.

The best VA is recorded for each eye beginning with the worse eye. If the patient has poor vision or wears corrective lenses, measure the corrected vision. Vision can be corrected by having the patient look through one of several devices: a multiple pinhole disc, a piece of paper with a hole punched in it using an 18-gauge needle, or a hand-held ophthalmoscope. The patient can look through the ophthalmoscope and spin the focusing wheel until he or she can best visualize the Snellen chart.

If the patient is unable to read the chart, record finger counting at a specified distance, or failing that, the presence or absence of light perception. Use a hand-held chart or a newspaper to measure VA in patients who are unable to stand. For patients who can cooperate but do not read, use an "E" chart.[4,17,21]

For suspected malingering, the physician must be both crafty and neuroanatomically astute. Patients with cortical blindness will still maintain a pupillary light response. The best way to determine malingering or hysteric blindness (which are separate entities) is by the presence of an **optokinetic reflex**. A strip of paper with alternating black and white vertical bars is passed rapidly back and forth in front of the patient's eyes. A blind patient will have no response, but malingerers and those with hysteric blindness will either demonstrate nystagmus with this maneuver or close their eyes.

Sometimes a physician who suspects malingering will suddenly jab at a patient's eyes to see if he or she blinks. This technique is problematic in two ways. First, a blind person may blink when he or she feels

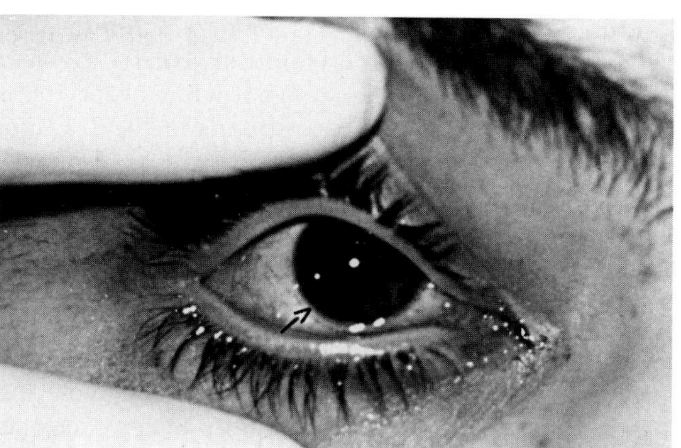

Fig. 15-2 Right hyphema *(arrow)*.

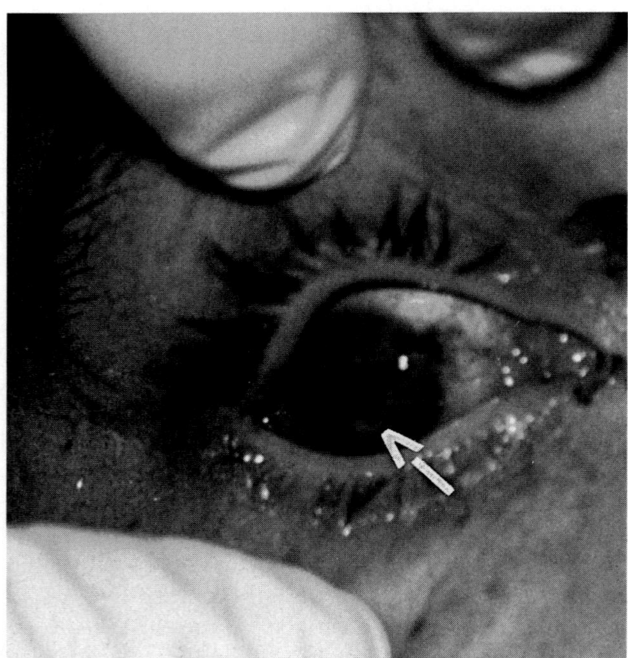

Fig. 15-3 Tear-shaped left pupil and escape of aqueous fluid *(arrow)* after penetrating injury. The apex of the tear points superomedially.

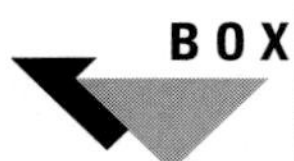

BOX 15-2
Causes of Ptosis

Third nerve palsy
Contusion of levator palpebrae
Horner's syndrome
- Traumatic dissection of carotid artery
- Basilar skull fracture involving carotid sheath
- Cervical spine fracture/dislocation
- Brainstem trauma

the rush of air on their cornea, and second, the physician may misjudge the distance to the eye and add injury to insult.

The examination of children deserves special consideration. For newborns the optokinetic reflex demonstrates that the patient is not blind and corresponds to a visual acuity of about 20/400.[17,21] By 6 weeks the infant can fixate with some smooth pursuit. By 10 to 12 weeks infants fixate with accurate smooth pursuit (fix and follow).[17] Use a colorful toy, parent's face, or your face as the object to follow. Do not use a light. Move the object slowly from side to side. Test one eye at a time by occluding the other eye with a patch.[17] Be sure that distracting sounds are not the cause of eye or head movement. For infants older than 6 months, use a light or toy as the object. Hold the object 1 to 3 feet from the infant's eyes, then move it while observing if the child tracks. Tracking corresponds to 20/40 vision if there is a steady fixation on the light as it moves, 20/100 vision if there is an unsteady fixation, and worse than 20/400 vision if there is no fixation.[4] For the cooperative child from 3 to 6 years of age, use Allen pictures.[17] Initially show the pictures up close to avoid confusion. Normal VA at 3 years is 20/40, at 4 to 5 years is 20/30, and at 6 years and older is 20/20.[17]

2. Examination of the Lids and Orbit. Note the location and depth of any laceration. Several aspects of lid injury determine complications including canthal injuries, violation of the tarsal plate, and injuries to the canaliculi, which drain tears from the eye. Determine if an upper lid laceration penetrates the tarsal plate or the muscle layer, or if it is through-and-through. Such injuries require consultation and may involve injury to the globe. Lacerations of the lid margins are prone to complications and should be referred to a surgical subspecialist for repair. The medial third of the lids contains the canaliculi. Damage to these canaliculi results in epiphora (tears overflowing the lids).

Note the presence of proptosis, which suggests a retroorbital hemorrhage, or enophthalmos, which may accompany a blowout fracture or globe rupture. Ptosis is associated with a third nerve palsy, Horner's syndrome, or contusion of the levator palpebrae (Box 15-2). Horner's syndrome (miosis, ptosis, and anhydrosis) occurs with traumatic dissection of the carotid artery, basilar skull fracture that includes the carotid sheath, fracture-dislocation of the cervical spine, and brainstem trauma.[17]

Palpate the orbital rim and zygoma, noting point tenderness, step-off, and subcutaneous emphysema. Subcutaneous emphysema is pathognomonic of a fracture into the nasal antrum or a sinus.

Inspect the skin about the eyes for FBs or lacerations. Remove superficial FBs at the time of examination. FB impalement of the eye requires immediate ophthalmologic consultation. If there is a periorbital laceration, check the wound for fat. Fat protruding from such a wound signifies penetration of the orbital septum, and increases the likelihood of globe perforation.

3. Examination of the Anterior Segment (Sclera, Conjunctiva, Cornea, Anterior Chamber, Iris, and Lens). If the eyes are swollen shut, try to examine them as early as possible since continuing edema will make evaluation increasingly difficult. Use lid retractors or bent paper clips to pry the eyelids open (an assistant is required). Lid retractors are preferred, since the bent paper clips may shed flecks of zinc plating into the eye. Double eversion of the lids, lifting them out and away from the globe while simultaneously folding them in half, allows detection of most superficial ocular FBs. Inspect for FBs, such as glass from shattered windshields. Evert the upper eyelid to look for FBs, which can be removed in a similar manner after anesthetic drops. Remove a contact lens as soon as it is identified. **Remember that fluorescein dye permanently stains soft contact lenses.** Document the presence of a subconjunctival hemorrhage.

Inspect the cornea using a flashlight. Any alteration from the usual crisp light reflex represents a corneal abnormality.[39] Note any gross corneal FBs, hyphema, or limbal erythema. Limbal injection (erythema) is a vascular flush circling the outer border of the cornea and is found with traumatic iritis or keratitis.[4,39]

When possible, perform a slit-lamp examination. Emergency physicians should be proficient in the operation of a slit-lamp microscope, since it will often illuminate pathologic conditions invisible to the naked eye. Use the slit-lamp to check the cornea for FBs and abrasions. A high-power examination may reveal a hyphema or signs of iritis (cell and flare reaction). The slit-lamp may also display a globe laceration or leaking vitreous.

To inspect the cornea for abrasions, moisten a fluorescein strip with anesthetic drops and apply the fluorescein to the inferior conjunctival sac. Then examine the eye with a slit-beam or full-blue beam directed at an oblique angle across the cornea. Abrasions will glow as bright green dye adheres to the abrasion. The dye remains attached with eyelid blinking. If a slit-lamp examination cannot be performed, use a Wood's lamp or an ophthalmoscope at positive 10 to 12 diopters.

To inspect the cornea for FBs, direct a slit-beam or full-beam of white light at an oblique angle to the cornea and move the beam to view the entire cornea. FBs appear as bright objects against a dark background.

To observe suspended cells in the anterior chamber, direct a tall and narrow bright beam of white light at a very oblique angle into the anterior chamber. Suspended cells sparkle as they float into the path of the light. Direct a bright slit-beam of white light at 90° to observe flare. **Flare** will appear like car headlights shining into a fog. Cell, flare, or both indicate anterior chamber reaction (e.g., iritis or hyphema).

Test the globe for leaking aqueous humor using **Seidel's test**. Apply a drop of fluorescein to a potential site of perforation. Under the white light the fluorescein is diluted by the aqueous and appears as a green (dilute) stream within the dark-orange (concentrated) dye.[16] Under the blue light the leak appears as a swirling stream of green dye within a background of green.

The iris is inspected under the slit-lamp using a full-white beam for any irregularity suggesting **iridodialysis** or sphincter tear.[17] Grossly inspect the lens for displacement and opacification (traumatic cataract).

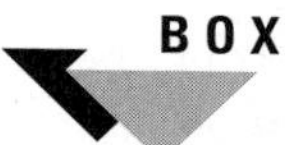

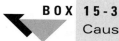

BOX 15-3

Causes of Pupillary Dilation

- Intracranial mass lesions compressing the third cranial nerve
- Posttraumatic mydriasis caused by damage to the pupilloconstrictor fibers
- Pharmacologic blockade with atropinelike medications
- Adie's tonic pupil (denervation injury to the ciliary ganglion)

4. Examination of the Pupils. Normal pupils are equal, round, and reactive to light. An abnormality may be acutely related to the trauma or may be a result of a past disease or injury. The patient or his or her family may be aware of a prior pupillary abnormality. Alternatively, look at the patient's picture on his or her driver's license. Magnification with an ophthalmoscope provides photographic evidence of an old pupillary abnormality.

Look for pupillary irregularity. A teardrop-shaped pupil suggests globe rupture, with the apex of the teardrop pointing toward the rupture.[4] Document the presence of anisocoria, which has variously been defined as >0.3 mm,[21] >0.5 mm,[40] and 1.0 mm.[4] If the pupils are briskly reactive and the degree of anisocoria is similar under conditions of light and dark, the anisocoria is physiologic.[17] If the anisocoria is more pronounced in the dark, the smaller pupil is abnormal and traumatic **Horner's syndrome** is likely.[17] If the anisocoria is more pronounced in the light, the larger pupil is abnormal and third nerve damage is a major concern.[17]

Pupillary dilation may occur with intracranial mass lesions compressing the third cranial nerve, posttraumatic mydriasis caused by damage to the pupilloconstrictor fibers, or as a result of pharmacologic blockade with atropinelike medications. Pharmacologic blockade cannot be overcome by instillation of pilocarpine; however, pupillary dilation caused by third nerve compression can be reversed by pilocarpine. **Adie's tonic pupil** is a dilated pupil, which occurs secondarily to denervation (injury to the ciliary ganglion). However, the pupil will still react to a near object but then slowly redilates when fixating on a far object. Box 15-3 lists causes of pupillary dilatation.

The **Marcus Gunn** or **"swinging flashlight"** examination is an important test of visual function. It is extremely sensitive to visual loss. The test is positive in many conditions that interrupt the visual pathways: optic nerve damage, efferent cranial nerve III injury, glaucoma, iris incarceration, massive internal derangement of the eye, optic chiasm/tract damage, retinal detachment, traumatic mydriasis, or vitreous hemorrhage.[16,17,25] An eye that demonstrates a Marcus Gunn pupil is said to have a **relative afferent pupillary defect (RAPD)**. To test for a RAPD with the swinging-light test, begin by observing pupillary symmetry and size in ambient light. Then swing a bright light on the unaffected eye. When the light strikes the unaffected eye, both pupils constrict. Then swing the light to the affected eye. When the light strikes the affected eye, both pupils paradoxically dilate. A pupil that dilates during the swinging flashlight test demonstrates an afferent pupillary defect. Repeating the test is as easy as swinging the flashlight between the pupils. Even with subtle optic nerve injury, after a few alternations of the light the constriction of the normal eye contrasts dramatically with the dilatation of the abnormal eye.

5. Examination of Extraocular Motion. Conduct this part of the examination after excluding the possibility of globe rupture.[25] Check the six cardinal positions of gaze: up and right, down and right, up and left, down and left, right, and left.[21,41] For infants, use keys, lights, or toys and follow the dictum of "one toy, one look" for each direction of gaze.[4] If the patient complains of diplopia, determine if the double vision is monocular or binocular by repeating the test with each eye closed. **Binocular diplopia** occurs when the coordinated movement of the eyes is disrupted, as in a cranial nerve palsy, orbital floor fracture with muscle entrapment, extraocular muscle contusion, or retrobulbar hemorrhage.[4,16,25] **Monocular diplopia** (double vision with one eye closed or covered) indicates corneal irregularity, dislocated lens, iridodialysis, or retinal detachment.[16,27] Only after pathology is ruled out can malingering, hysteria, or anxiety be considered an etiology.

6. Examination of the Posterior Segment (Vitreous, Retina, and Optic Nerve). Perform direct ophthalmoscopy without dilating the pupil. Absence of the red reflex or inability to visualize the macula or optic disc suggests cataract, hyphema, lens rupture, retinal detachment, or vitreous hemorrhage.[25] Look at the optic disc, noting atrophy, avulsion, or swelling. Test the visual field of each eye by confrontation.

Perform a test for RAPD (see the previous discussion). If the pupils are nonreactive or irregular, use relative brightness or red desaturation to assess optic nerve functon.[17] To test for **relative brightness**, shine a bright light into the normal eye along the visual axis and assign the brightness of this light a value of 100%.

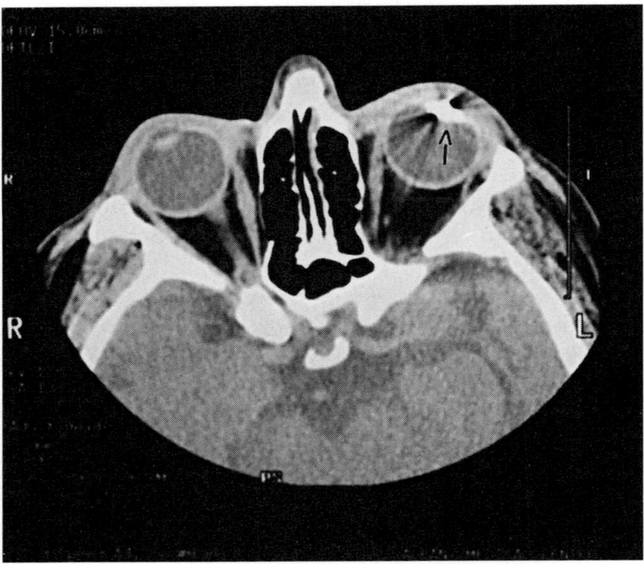

Fig. 15-4 Computed tomography scan of left intraocular foreign body *(arrow)*.

Then shine the same light into the affected eye along the visual axis and ask the patient to make a comparison on the same scale. Normally, they should be equivalent.

Testing for **red desaturation** is performed using any bright-red object. Ask the patient to view the object with each eye, while the other eye is covered, and compare the two images. With optic nerve damage, the object appears gray or washed out to the damaged eye versus the unaffected eye. This evaluation is sufficient for the emergency evaluation of the posterior segment.[4,21]

7. Measuring Intraocular Pressure. Normal intraocular pressure (IOP) for a person under age 40 is 12 mmHg (range 10 to 20 mmHg).[42] The pressure increases by 1 mmHg for each decade thereafter.[42] After trauma, increased IOP (>22 mmHg) suggests acute glaucoma secondary to angle recession, hyphema, lens dislocation, lens swelling, ruptured globe, suprachoroidal hemorrhage, or retrobulbar hemorrhage.[16,17] If the IOP is <5 mmHg, strongly consider a diagnosis of globe rupture.[38]

Diagnostic Studies

Imaging studies are occasionally helpful for evaluating orbital and ocular trauma, especially when there is an inconclusive history and physical examination despite repeated evaluation, evidence of periorbital fractures, or depressed mental status.[17,43] Computed tomography (CT) scanning is the study of choice, using both axial and coronal cuts. Other studies useful in

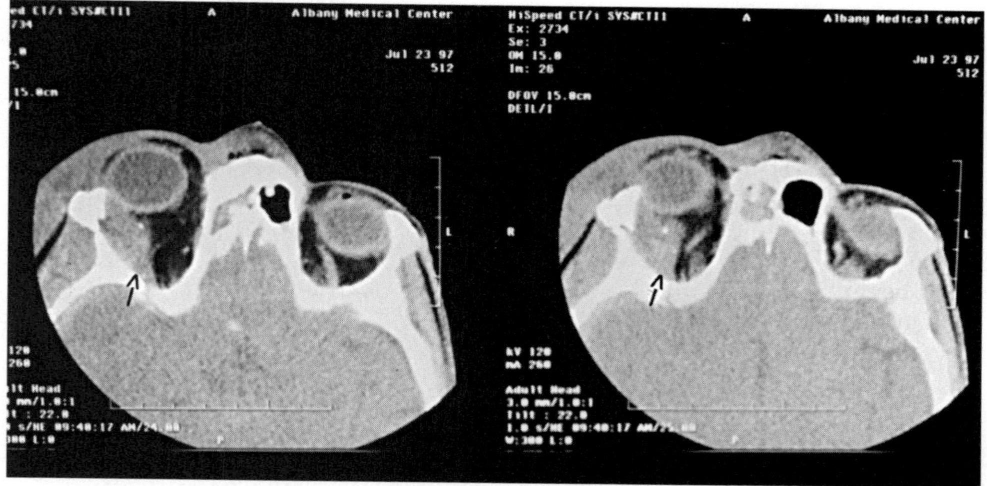

Fig. 15-5 Computed tomography scan of right retroorbital hemorrhage *(arrows).*

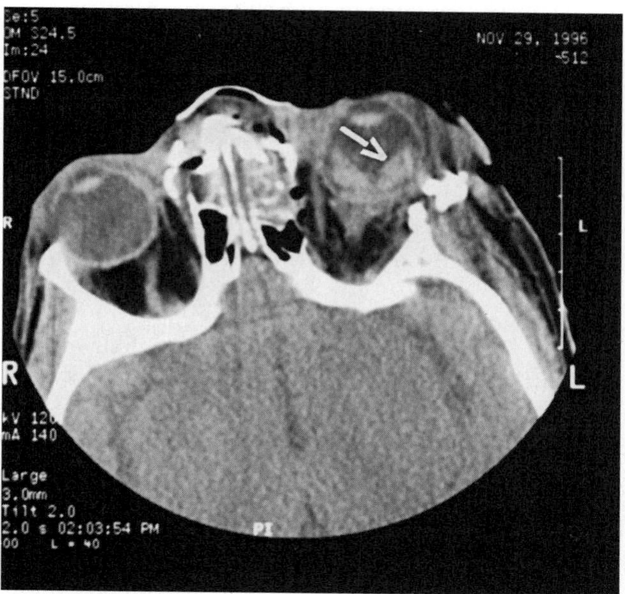

Fig. 15-6 Computed tomography scan of left intraocular hemorrhage *(arrow).*

the acute setting include MRI, ultrasound (US), and plain radiographs.

The optimal CT scan of the orbit employs 1.5 to 2.0 mm axial sections and 2.0 to 4.0 mm coronal sections using spiral CT scanning. Spiral scanning is faster, uses less radiation, and provides higher quality reconstructions than conventional CT.[17] CT detects choroidal detachment, fractures, intraocular FBs (Fig. 15-4); retroorbital or intraocular hemorrhage (Figs. 15-5 and 15-6); lens dislocation (Fig. 15-7); globe rupture (Fig. 15-8); bony intraorbital fragments (Fig. 15-9); and evaluates impaled orbital FBs (Fig. 15-10).[11,43]

Foreign body detection deserves additional comment. The limits of resolution vary with the size and composition of the FB.[44-47] The minimum resolution is 0.6 mm^3 for steel and copper and 1.5 mm^3 for aluminum and glass. Plastic and cement are hypodense, whereas wood is radiolucent, making all three of these materials difficult to detect by CT scanning.

MRI can be a useful adjunct for soft tissue evaluation *in the absence of metallic FBs.* Currently, MRI has two major limitations that will likely change with advancement of technology—availability and motion artifact. MRI can detect choroidal detachment, old hemorrhage, subperiosteal hemorrhage, and vitreous hemorrhage.[17,43]

In experienced hands, US provides useful information regarding orbital trauma. Because the transducer must be applied to the eyelids, globe, or both, suspected ruptured globe is a relative contraindication to US. Ultrasound can detect choroidal rupture, FBs ($\geq$0.2 mm diameter), fractures (considerably limited compared with CT scan), orbital hemorrhage/hematoma, retinal detachment, ruptured globe, and vitreous hemorrhage.[17,43]

Plain films are less useful than the other modalities. In the absence of CT scan and MRI, they can be used to screen for metallic FBs, fractures, and sinus injury.[17]

EMERGENCY DEPARTMENT MANAGEMENT

There are two traumatic eye emergencies that must trigger immediate action:

1. **Chemical burns:** The eye must be irrigated immediately with saline or other neutral solution

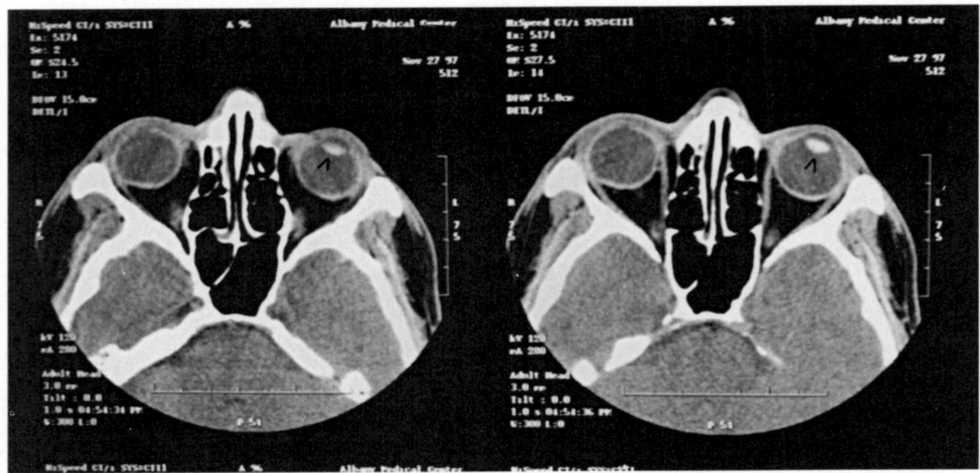

Fig. 15-7 Computed tomography scan of right lens dislocation. Note normal appearance and position of left lens *(arrowheads).*

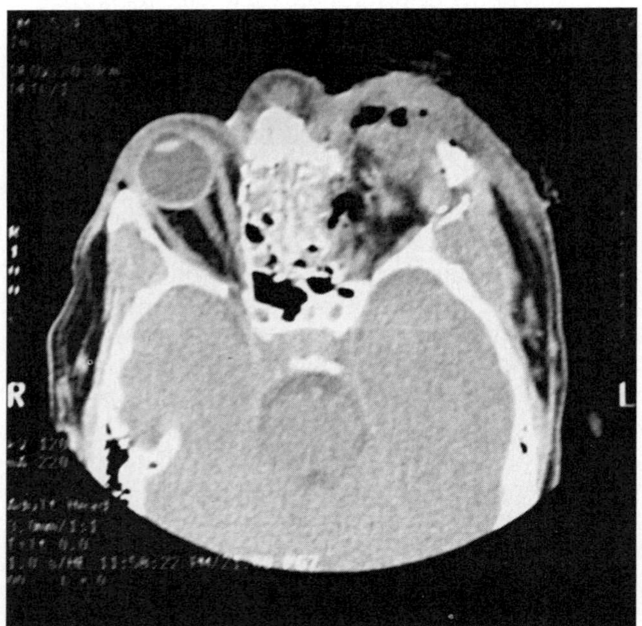

Fig. 15-8 Computed tomography scan of left globe rupture.

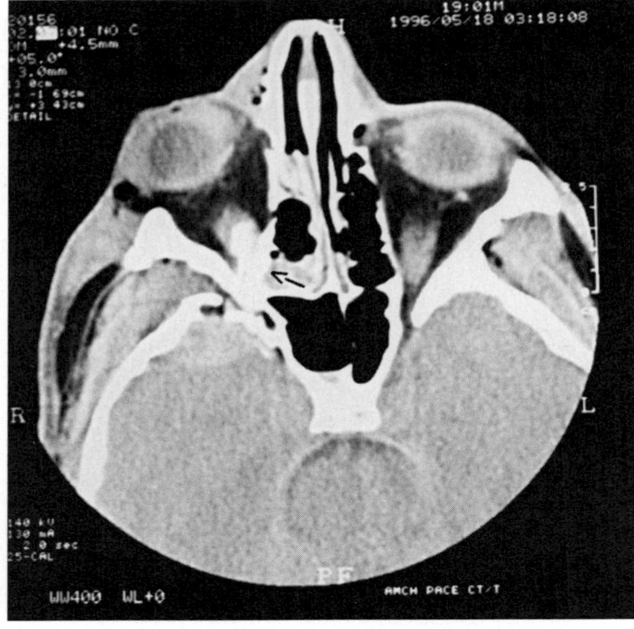

Fig. 15-9 Computed tomography scan of bony fragment endangering right optic nerve *(arrow).*

continuously for 30 minutes *before completion of triage or registration.*

2. **Traumatic endophthalmitis:** This condition is seen as acute pain and inflammation out of proportion to the penetrating eye trauma. The onset of signs and symptoms is often not at the time of presentation (as early as 1 day and a mean of 4 days after the injury).[48,49] The symptoms include blurred vision (100%) and pain (75%). The signs include conjunctival hyperemia (100%), anterior cell and flare (100%), decreased vision to 5/200 or worse (90%), cells and opacities in the vitreous (90%), hypopyon (85%), eye redness (85%), and decreased red reflex (75%). Consult an ophthalmologist immediately because the patient will need intravitreal antibiotics.[17]

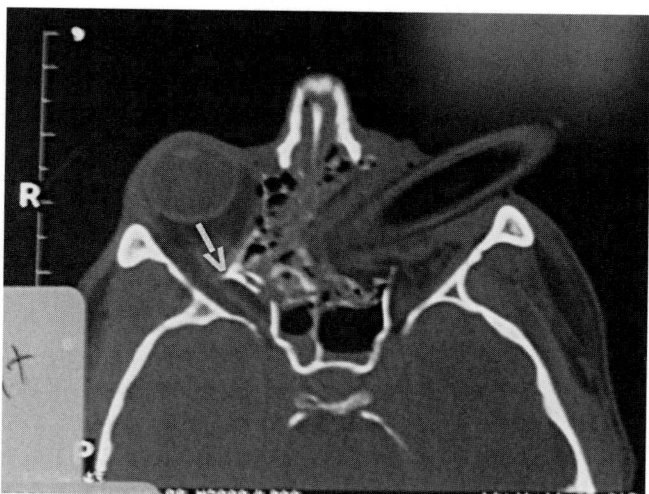

Fig. 15-10 Computed tomography scan of large wooden object impaling left orbit, causing bony fragments to impinge on right optic nerve *(arrow)*.

Specific Ocular Injuries

CORNEAL ABRASION (WITH OR WITHOUT FOREIGN BODY)

Patients with corneal abrasions usually complain of something striking the eye. It is important to distinguish between a low-speed particle (dropped in, blew in) and a high-speed particle (shot, propelled, metal striking metal). High-speed particles can perforate the globe. The symptoms of corneal abrasion include blepharospasm, blurred vision, eye pain, FB sensation, photophobia, tearing, and seeing halos around lights. A tiny abrasion, even in the absence of an FB, produces an FB sensation. Symptoms usually develop within minutes after the trauma.

Physical examination shows a red eye with mildly swollen eyelids. VA may be mildly decreased. On slit-lamp examination, an abrasion is highlighted by fluorescein, a FB may or may not be present, and a mild anterior chamber reaction is sometimes noted. Be sure to remove any contact lens, if present, before fluorescein instillation, since this agent permanently stains soft contact lenses.[15]

In assessing the abrasion, note the size (in mm), shape (round, linear), and location (e.g., 4 o'clock position). It is important to note whether there is penetration of the anterior chamber. In 80% of cases, intraocular FBs enter the eye through the cornea.[50] An FB under the upper eyelid can produce linear scratches of the cornea with blinking (the **"ice rink" sign**). Document extraocular motility and pupillary reaction. With a low-speed, low-mass particle, insignificant trauma, and a clear anterior chamber, the IOP need not be measured.

Management

1. Instill anesthetic drops (2 drops, 20 seconds apart and additional drops as necessary). Do not send patients home with topical anesthetics, since abrasions may become worse, since further injury may occur in the insensate eye.
2. Remove any FBs from cornea, either by gentle irrigation with saline solution or by careful use of a moistened cotton-tipped applicator or 25-gauge needle (under slit-lamp microscope).
3. Remove FB rust ring. Assuming the FB did not penetrate any deeper than the corneal epithelium, the rust ring extrudes over 2 to 3 days. At this time, it can be readily removed using an ophthalmic burr or spud. Manage the remaining corneal defect as a corneal abrasion.
4. Dilate the eye. A **cycloplegic** (1 to 2 drops of homatropine 2% or cyclopentolate 2%) may be instilled, depending on the size of the abrasion, to reduce posterior synechiae formation (adhesions between iris and lens), ciliary muscle spasm, and photophobia.[15] Instruct the patient to use sunglasses in bright light. It is not necessary to give a prescription for a cycloplegic. Give the patient a note stating which cycloplegic was used, its concentration, and the number of drops instilled. *Do not use atropine drops in the eye, since accommodation may be affected for up to 2 weeks.*
5. Patching the eye is *not* necessary. Multiple studies show that eye patches offer no benefit in the treatment of corneal abrasions, either in terms of healing or pain.[51-53] If the physician elects to patch the eye, instill an antibiotic ointment before patching and instruct patients not to drive or operate machinery, since their depth perception will be altered.
6. Antibiotics. Prescribe an antibiotic ointment (e.g., sulfacetamide, erythromycin, tobramycin) to be taken 2 to 3 times a day or drops 4 times a day until the eye is no longer red.[16] Avoid neomycin-containing compounds, since these agents are more likely to cause an allergic conjunctivitis.
7. Prescribe analgesics. Use a nonsteroidal antiinflammatory (NSAID) medication daily for 3 days coupled with a prescription for a narcotic-containing analgesic (4 to 6 pills).
8. Provide follow-up. Provide follow-up on corneal abrasions until vision returns to normal and all signs and symptoms clear. Make the next appointment for 24 to 36 hours, either in the ED or in an ophthalmologist's office. With each follow-up visit, the guidelines for evaluation

and management are the same as with the initial visit. Because minor abrasions are rarely problematic, some physicians suggest follow-up only if there is pain or visual symptoms that persist for more than 2 days.

9. Prognosis: Excellent.

CONJUNCTIVAL/SUBCONJUNCTIVAL FOREIGN BODY

Patients with ocular FBs do not always report a history of something striking the eye. The symptoms are eye pain, FB sensation, and tearing. The VA is usually unaffected unless there was significant trauma. An associated corneal injury may be present. Anesthetize the eye with proparacaine or tetracaine and look for exposed white scleral tissue. The wound may be obscured by hemorrhage.

Seidel's test can provide additional information. However, a negative Seidel's test does not exclude scleral penetration. Suspicion of penetration warrants an immediate ophthalmologic consultation. Shield the eye from any further contact. Note that iron-containing FBs leave a deposit (**rust ring**) after being on the cornea for 2 or more hours.

Management

1. After instillation of a topical anesthetic, remove FBs from any of the following possible locations: superior fornix (evert the upper eyelid), bulbar conjunctiva, or inferior fornix.
2. Evaluate for corneal abrasion.
3. Prescribe a topical antibiotic. If there is any conjunctival injection, prescribe a topical antibiotic to be taken until the eye is no longer red.[16]
4. If the FB is removed completely and there is no corneal abrasion or conjunctival wound/inflammation, there is no need for follow-up.
5. If there is any residual FB or suspicion thereof, refer the patient to an ophthalmologist within 24 to 72 hours.
6. Prognosis: Excellent.

CONJUNCTIVAL LACERATION

A laceration of the conjunctiva is of minimal consequence, since the conjunctiva provides no structural support to the eye.

Management. Exclude the possibility of scleral injury.

ISOLATED SUBCONJUNCTIVAL HEMMORHAGE

A subconjunctival hemorrhage appears flat and involves a sector of the bulbar conjunctiva with no break in the conjunctival membrane (Fig. 15-11); otherwise, the eye examination is normal. There is no complaint of eye pain. The hemorrhage(s) may be a manifestation of a more severe process, such as traumatic asphyxia or scleral rupture.

Management

1. Because the hemorrhage usually clears within 14 days, no specific treatment is necessary for an isolated subconjunctival hemorrhage.
2. Prescribe artificial tears for mild irritation.
3. Follow-up is necessary only if the hemorrhage does not resolve or if there are recurrent hemorrhages.
4. Prognosis: Excellent.

BLOWOUT FRACTURES

The four most common mechanisms producing blowout fractures are falls, assaults, MVCs, and sports-related injuries.[22,23] Complaints may be minor and the physical findings subtle.[22] Perhaps the most common presentation includes periorbital subcutaneous emphysema (identifying rupture into a sinus) and point tenderness of the orbital rim or maxilla. Several other signs suggest a blowout fracture: diplopia, enophthalmos, and inferior displacement of the globe.[4,16,21,22] Additional stigmata include ipsilateral numbness of the cheek and the upper lip from infraorbital nerve damage, periorbital ecchymosis, and periorbital swelling.

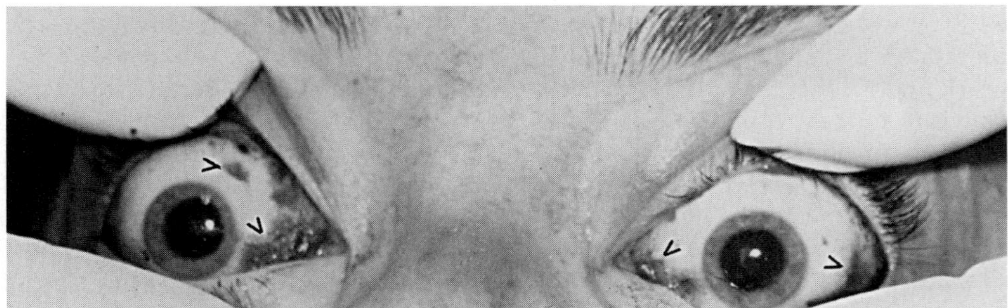

Fig. 15-11 Bilateral subconjunctival hemorrhages *(arrowheads).*

Fracture of the orbital floor can lead to gaze paralysis secondary to damage of either the inferior rectus or the inferior oblique muscle, including muscle entrapment, contusion, or hematoma.[21,22] Enophthalmos is also associated with fracture, but is rarely present on ED evaluation. It might be masked by exophthalmos secondary to orbital edema, hematoma, or inflammation.[21]

Plain radiographs have been used to screen for this fracture. Suggestive findings are an air-fluid level in the maxillary sinus, a positive "teardrop sign" (orbital contents herniated into the maxillary sinus), and a visible fracture of the orbit floor (Fig. 15-12). False-negative (3% to 60%) and false-positive (46%) radiographs have been reported.[22,54] Orbital floor fractures do not typically involve the orbital rim, but might when there is an associated tripod fracture.[21] The imaging study of choice is CT scanning of the orbits with axial and coronal cuts (Fig. 15-13). Further discussion of imaging of facial fractures is in Chapter 14.

Fracture of the medial orbital wall, the **lamina papyracea** of the ethmoid sinus, occurs secondary to blows to the orbit or bridge of the nose.[17,21,22] Epistaxis is often present.[21,22] Rarely, the medial rectus muscle is damaged,[21] and enophthalmos can occur.[17,21] The nasolacrimal system might be injured because of its proximity, leading to epiphora, lacrimal sac mucocele, or dacryostenosis.[21]

Because of the heavy bone structure, fracture of the supraorbital roof is uncommon.[55] It is associated with central nervous system injury, dural tear with cerebrospinal fluid leak, frontal sinus fracture, intracranial bleeding, and intracranial FB.[17,21,55] Many of these fractures are open.[55] Damage to the superior rectus or superior oblique muscle occurs infrequently.[17]

Management

1. Exclude injury to the globe, which occurs in 5% to 10% of blowout fractures.[27]
2. Some authors suggest a nasal decongestant spray for use over the next 10 to 14 days.
3. Some authorities recommend an antibiotic (e.g., amoxicillin/clavulanate) to be taken for 10 to 14 days. (There is no evidence-based data on this topic.)
4. Avoid sneezing or nose blowing.
5. Apply ice packs, 15 minutes on/15 minutes off, as needed, to reduce swelling during the first 48 hours.
6. Contact a plastic surgeon, otolaryngologist, or maxillofacial surgeon to arrange follow-up in case of need for surgical repair.
7. Contact an ophthalmologist to arrange for a complete outpatient evaluation within 36 hours.
8. Inpatient management is indicated with severe injuries such as intraocular hemorrhage, ruptured globe, severe facial deformity, traumatic glaucoma, and violation of the cranial vault.
9. Prognosis: Most asymptomatic and symptomatic (enophthalmos, diplopia, and infraorbital hypes-

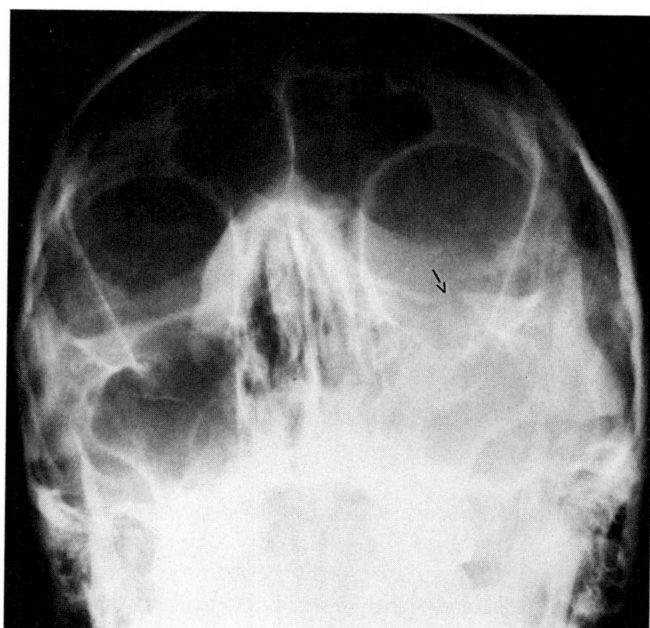

Fig. 15-12 Plain radiograph of left orbital blowout fracture *(arrow)*. Note opacification of left maxillary sinus.

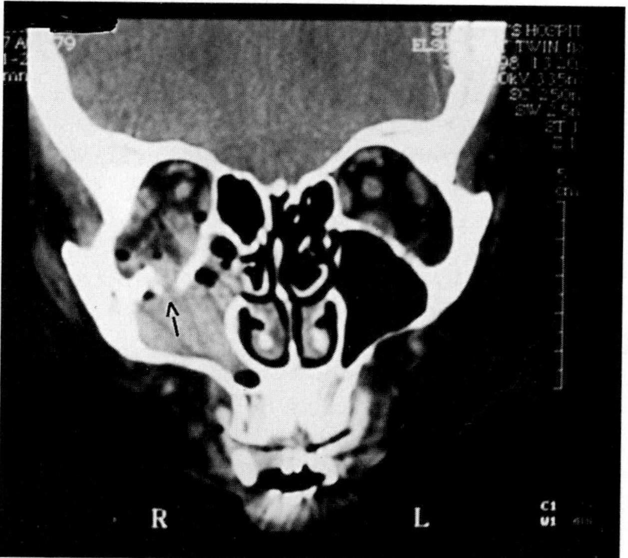

Fig. 15-13 Coronal computed tomography scan of right orbital blowout fracture *(arrow)*.

thesia) blowout fractures have a good prognosis without surgery.[23] Surgical repair, when indicated, can be delayed for 10 to 14 days.

OTHER FACIAL FRACTURES

Midface fractures (Le Fort II or III) are associated with serious and blinding ocular injuries.[56] Any type of ocular injury may be associated with a Le Fort fracture. Fractures of the mandible and nasal bone are associated with temporary injuries, including corneal abrasion, decreased ocular motility, retinal edema, and subconjunctival hemorrhage.[56]

RETROBULBAR HEMORRHAGE

Retrobulbar hemorrhage is rare after trauma and develops within the first 24 hours.[17,21] The patient complains of pain, and the VA is decreased. There may be diplopia, nausea, and vomiting. Signs vary with severity and include afferent pupillary defect, dystopia (malposition of the eye), elevated or decreased IOP, hemorrhagic chemosis (diffuse, bloody scleral edema), impaired ocular motility, and proptosis. Retrobulbar hemorrhage may develop slowly (hours) or rapidly (minutes) after injury. If vision is threatened, emergency decompression of the retroorbital space is essential.

Management

1. Obtain immediate ophthalmologic consultation for any suggestion of retrobulbar hemorrhage.
2. Look for signs of threatened vision: RAPD, red desaturation, reduced relative brightness, or deteriorating VA.
3. If developing slowly over hours and vision is not threatened, manage retrobulbar hemorrhage conservatively as follows:
   - Elevate the head.
   - Apply ice packs.
   - Administer acetazolamide 500 mg IV.
   - Administer mannitol (20%) 1 to 2 g/kg IV over 45 minutes.
   - Instill timolol 0.5% q30 minutes times 2.
   - Avoid coagulation-altering medications.
   - Reassess VA, IOP, and pupillary responses q30 minutes.[16]
4. If the hemorrhage/hematoma develops rapidly (over minutes) or vision is threatened, emergency decompression of the retrobulbar space by lateral canthotomy and cantholysis may be vision-saving.
   - Anesthetize the lateral canthal area with 2% lidocaine with 1:100,000 epinephrine.
   - Place a hemostat horizontally on the lateral canthus tissue extending out to the orbital rim and clamp it for 1 minute.
   - Release the clamp and cut the compressed tissue for 1 cm into the canthus using sterile scissors.
   - Separate the skin and conjunctival tissue, exposing the inferior arm of the lateral canthal tendon.
   - Cut the tendon with a vertical incision using sterile scissors.[16,17]
5. Admit for ophthalmologic management.
6. Prognosis: Guarded; potential for irreversible visual loss.

TRAUMATIC OPTIC NEUROPATHY

Traumatic optic neuropathy (TON) results from injury to the optic nerve anywhere along its course and can be produced by trauma to the eye, orbit, or head. Typically the patient experiences an acute decrease in vision, a RAPD, red desaturation, and sluggish pupils.[17,25] The eye itself may not be red or swollen. The optic disc usually appears normal, but is occasionally edematous depending on the location of the injury.[17]

Management

1. With suspected TON, shield the eye from further contact and obtain ophthalmologic consultation immediately.
2. Be aware that the treatment of TON is still controversial. In a recent meta-analysis, patients receiving some form of treatment (high-dose corticosteroids, surgical decompression, or both) were found to have better outcomes than patients who did not receive any treatment.[57] However, neither surgery nor corticosteroids had an advantage over one another.
3. Prognosis: Guarded.

RUPTURE OF THE GLOBE SECONDARY TO BLUNT TRAUMA

The globe is ruptured in about 1.1% to 3.5% of the trauma cases.[38,58] Ruptures usually occur at the weakest points: the insertions of ocular muscles, the limbus, and the equator. Rupture may also occur at the site opposite the impact.[27,30] The conjunctiva is often intact.[30] Certain clinical signs offer clues to rupture. In the presence of ocular hemorrhage (hyphema, hemorrhagic chemosis, or severe vitreous hemorrhage), any *one* of the following four signs has a 100% sensitivity and 98.5% specificity of predicting rupture:[38]

1. An abnormally deep or shallow anterior chamber
2. IOP of 5 mmHg or less
3. Media opacity preventing a clear view of the fundus
4. VA showing light perception only or worse

When assessing for globe rupture, perform the IOP only if the other measures are negative to avoid pressure on the globe. When associated with rupture, hyphemas often contain clot, and the hemorrhagic chemosis is usually circumferential.[27] EPs can readily identify several of these signs and make an expectant diagnosis of ruptured globe.

Management

1. Shield the eye from further contact as soon as rupture is suspected. Use an eye shield, paper cup, or Styrofoam cup, secured by tape.
2. Do a CT scan to exclude intraocular FBs and confirm the diagnosis of rupture.
3. Consult an ophthalmologist immediately.
4. Do not remove or manipulate a penetrating object.
5. Get the patient prepared for the operating suite.
6. Give systemic antibiotics for prophylaxis, principally against *Bacillus* species (particularly, *B. cereus*), *Staphylococcus epidermidis, Streptococcus* species, gram-negative organisms, and *Staphylococcus aureus,* as follows:
   - Gentamicin 3 mg/kg q24h (pediatric, 2.5 mg/kg q8h) IV
   - Vancomycin 1 gm q12h (neonates, 15 mg/kg initial dose, then 10 mg/kg q8h; infants/children, 10 mg/kg q6h) IV; or clindamycin 600 mg q12h (pediatric, 20 mg/kg/24h, divided in 3 or 4 doses) IV[20,59-63]
7. Administer antiemetics to minimize vomiting, which will increase the IOP and extrude more intraocular contents.
8. Admit for ophthalmologic management.
9. Prognosis: Guarded.

LACERATIONS AND OTHER PENETRATING TRAUMA

Penetrating ocular trauma may be difficult to diagnose. Any penetrating wound in proximity to the eye necessitates evaluation for orbital injury. If there is overt penetration, document VA, shield the eye from further contact, and consult an ophthalmologist immediately. Do not remove or manipulate any penetrating object.

Isolated lacerations of the conjunctiva are benign. Any laceration of the sclera, or full thickness rent of the cornea, is treated as a penetrating eye injury. Eyelid lacerations may be simple or complex (Fig. 15-14). The EP can repair simple eyelid lacerations, those involving only the skin. An ophthalmologic consultation is warranted with complex lacerations (e.g., through-and-through wound, exposed orbital fat, and damage to underlying structures such as the globe, nasolacrimal system, muscle, or tarsal plate).

The lacrimal portion of the nasolacrimal drainage system is located in the medial canthal area and extends 5 to 7 mm laterally in the lids. Medially, the canaliculi merge into a common canaliculus (~1 mm long), which then enters the vertical nasal portion (~24 mm high) of the excretory system at a point 4 mm from its apex.[20] Be aware of this underlying structure when assessing lacerations near the medial canthus of the eye.

To determine injury to the canaliculi, cannulate the punctum with a 6-0 Prolene suture (the suture material, *not* the needle). If the suture exits the wound, the duct is damaged. A less invasive method of determining integrity of the ductal system is to instill fluorescein in the eye and use a Wood's lamp to ascertain the presence of dye in the wound.

Some penetrating injuries are easily overlooked unless a careful evaluation is performed.[64] Three clinical scenarios increase the chances of penetrating eye trauma.[64]

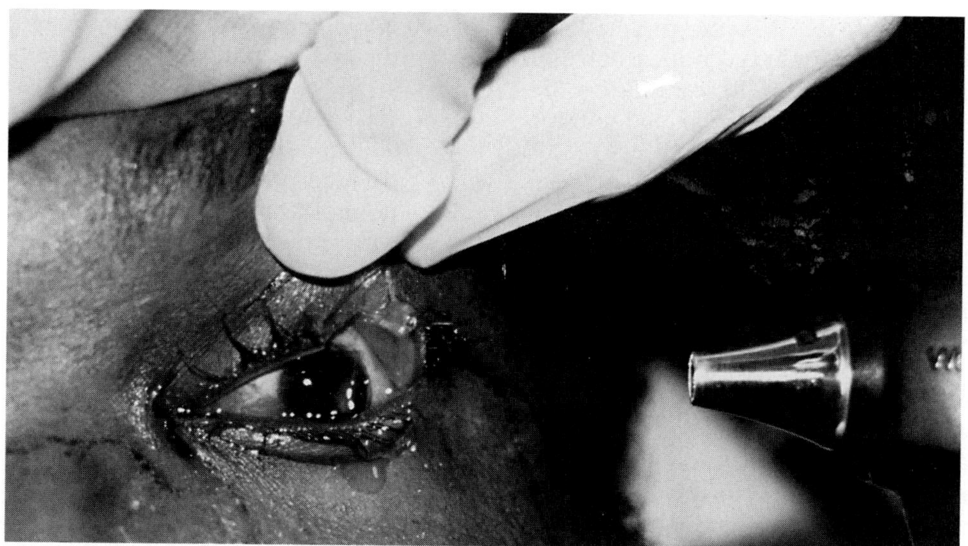

Fig. 15-14 Left upper eyelid laceration through the lid margin, associated with penetrating corneal injury with escape of aqueous material.

1. A patient with a history of something striking the eye while hammering metal on metal
2. A child with a vague history of something sharp being near the eye who indicates pain in the eye
3. A patient with head trauma and eyes swollen shut. When the eyes are swollen shut after head trauma, the eyelids must be retracted to examine the globe

Management

Simple Laceration of Eyelid

1. Exclude injury to the globe and other underlying structures.
2. Close the wound with single interrupted skin sutures of 6-0 or 7-0 nylon. Remove sutures in 5 days.
3. Unless there was minimal trauma to the eye, contact an ophthalmologist to arrange for outpatient ophthalmologic evaluation.

Complex Laceration of Eyelid

1. Obtain immediate ophthalmologic consultation.
2. If globe rupture is suspected, treat as outlined in the previous section. If globe rupture is not suspected, administer cefazolin 1 gm IV (pediatrics, age 1 month and older, 25 mg/kg) and ensure tetanus status.[63]

INTRAOCULAR AND INTRAORBITAL FOREIGN BODY

About 80% of all intraocular FBs enter the eye through the cornea.[50] When there is a history of something striking the cornea, consider a diagnosis of penetrating FB. Metal splinters from hammering metal and glass splinters from shattering glass can penetrate the eye painlessly.[65] The resulting intraocular FB may remain asymptomatic or produce an inflammatory reaction and endophthalmitis. FBs secondary to grinding often do not penetrate the eye because of small size and low momentum and usually go no further than the cornea and conjunctiva.[64] CT scanning is the imaging study of choice for intraocular and intraorbital FBs.

TRAUMATIC IRITIS

Any trauma to the eye may produce inflammation in the anterior segment. Symptoms include blurred vision, pain, photophobia, and tearing, which vary from mild to relentless, depending on the severity of the injury. VA is usually mildly decreased, but in some instances the decrement is profound. Pain from ciliary muscle spasm is exacerbated by light directly striking the injured eye (**photophobia**) and the uninjured eye (**consensual photophobia**). Because this contraction of the ciliary muscle exacerbates eye pain, patients may also complain of pain on accommodation (e.g., it hurts to read). The pupil is smaller (**traumatic miosis**) and more sluggish than the unaffected eye. After several hours, the pupil may dilate (**traumatic mydriasis**). The bulbar conjunctiva is injected, particularly the limbus, and the globe is tender. Slit-lamp evaluation reveals cells in the anterior chamber and a positive flare. Rarely, with a severe reaction, there is hypopyon.

Management

1. Instill a cycloplegic.
2. Prescribe NSAIDs to be taken daily for 3 days coupled with a narcotic analgesic to provide analgesia.
3. Instruct the patient to wear sunglasses.
4. Obtain an ophthalmologic consultation within 24 hours. The ophthalmologist may suggest ocular steroids during phone consultation.[16]
5. Prognosis: Excellent. This condition should clear over a week.

TRAUMATIC GLAUCOMA AND ANTERIOR SEGMENT TISSUE INJURY

Tearing of tissues of the anterior segment produces bleeding, inflammation, lens displacement, lens capsule rupture, and subsequent scarring. Any of these injuries can give rise to glaucoma. If the pupil is torn, a "second pupil" appears and monocular diplopia can occur. In the ED, the IOP may be low, and an elevation in the pressure may not occur for months or years. Conversely, the IOP may be elevated (>22 mmHg) soon after the injury (within hours). Hyphema is present in varying degrees. Slit-lamp examination may reveal tears in the iris or a displaced lens.

Management

1. Shield the eye from further contact.
2. Consult an ophthalmologist immediately.
3. Administer medications that decrease the production of aqueous humor.
   - Topical ophthalmic β-blocker: timolol 0.25% or 0.5%, 1 drop bid. Their use is relatively contraindicated in patients who have asthma, emphysema, congestive heart failure, and heart block.
   - Carbonic anhydrase inhibitors: acetazolamide 250 mg po q6h (pediatric, 8 to 30 mg/kg/24h divided q6-8h); 500 IM or IV repeated in 2 to 4 hours PRN (pediatric, 5 to 10 mg/kg q6h).[63]
   - Mannitol: 1.5 to 2 g/kg/dose IV over 30 minutes.
4. An ophthalmologist should direct the administration of miotics, such as pilocarpine. Although these agents may improve the outflow of aqueous humor, they can worsen the glaucoma secondary to vasocongestion.[21]
5. Prognosis: Guarded.

TRAUMATIC CATARACT

Lens opacities (**cataracts**) can occur after blunt or penetrating trauma with or without violation of the lens capsule. Cataracts develop in hours to months, and violation of the capsule accelerates the process. Cataracts are also associated with lightning injuries. Symptoms include blurred vision, glare from lights (particularly headlights), and reduced color vision. Signs include decreased VA, indistinct retina, lens opacity, and reduced red reflex.

Management

1. Shield the eye from further contact.
2. Consult an ophthalmologist immediately.
3. Be aware that, ultimately, treatment may involve surgical removal if vision is significantly affected.

LENS LUXATION/SUBLUXATION

The lens may be displaced minimally, producing myopia, or displaced sufficiently that only the edge remains in the visual axis, producing monocular diplopia. The major complaint is blurred vision. Signs include asymmetry of the anterior chamber, decreased VA, and visualization of the displaced lens. The iris or lens may quiver after rapid eye movement, and vitreous may protrude into the anterior chamber. The IOP may rise, causing glaucoma.

Management

1. Shield the eye from further contact.
2. Consult an ophthalmologist immediately.
3. Note that treatment is indicated emergently if secondary glaucoma develops as a result of pupillary block. In this instance, a mydriatic cycloplegic is indicated to permit aqueous egress from the posterior chamber.[66]
4. Surgery is required for complete dislocations.

HYPHEMA

Disruption of tissue in the anterior chamber produces hyphema of varying degrees. The typical symptoms are blurred vision and pain. The amount of bleeding can be grossly quantitated as microscopic (cells floating in the anterior chamber by slit-lamp), grade I (less than 33% of the chamber filled with blood), grade II (33 to 50% full), grade III (50% to 90% full), and 100% ("**eight ball**" hyphema). There may be associated traumatic iritis. The VA is variously affected. The IOP may be elevated above 30 mmHg. Patients with sickle cell disease or sickle cell trait are at increased risk of rebleeding and subsequent complications.

Management

1. Shield the eye from further contact.
2. Consult an ophthalmologist immediately.
3. Admit for ophthalmologic management.
4. Have the patient rest quietly in the ED with the head of the bed elevated to 30 degrees.
5. Avoid NSAIDs.
6. Administer ophthalmologic atropine 1% at the direction of an ophthalmologist.
7. Administer aminocaproic acid (50 mg/kg q4h po, maximum 30 g/24h) at the direction of an ophthalmologist. Avoid with coagulopathies, hematuria, pregnancy, and renal failure. Use caution in the presence of cardiovascular, cerebrovascular, and hepatic diseases.[16]
8. Prescribe an antiemetic.
9. Prescribe narcotic analgesia.
10. Treat increased IOP.
11. Cooperative patients with microscopic hyphemas can sometimes be managed as outpatients. Patients who are discharged from the ED require daily ophthalmologic evaluation for several days. Discuss care with an ophthalmologist before discharging the patient from the ED. Instruct the patient to return immediately for increased pain or decreased vision.

POSTERIOR SEGMENT TRAUMA

Posterior segment trauma may be asymptomatic or show nonspecific symptoms, such as blurred vision and pain. A curtain of darkness, flashes of light, and floaters all incriminate the posterior segment, but do not localize the injury to a specific tissue. Important signs are blurring of fundus detail, decreased VA, and an RAPD. If RAPD testing cannot be performed, relative brightness testing and red desaturation are suitable, but cruder, alternatives. Findings may not be apparent on direct funduscopy performed in the ED even with dilation. Dilated indirect funduscopy by an ophthalmologist is usually needed to identify these findings.

Management. All signs and symptoms pointing to posterior segment trauma mandate an immediate ophthalmologic consultation.

CHEMICAL CONJUNCTIVITIS

All chemical exposures of the eye mandate immediate irrigation by the patient at the site of exposure and irrigation by prehospital personnel. Irrigation must continue in the ED even if the eye was lavaged before arrival. Identify the chemical(s) involved and establish the pH of the agent. If necessary, contact the local poison control center for assistance in identifying the chemical(s) in the agent and for recommendations regarding specialized treatment. The symptoms are a burning sensation, pain, and photophobia. After the irrigation is completed, check the conjunctival pH and perform an ophthalmologic examination. The signs of mild injury are conjunctival hyperemia and decreased VA (usually mild). With a more extensive injury, the eye may display chemosis and subconjunctival hemorrhage. There may be associated first-degree periorbital skin burns. The vessels of the conjunctiva, limbus, and episclera are intact in minor chemical burns.

Management

1. Instill anesthetic drops.
2. Before irrigation, remove FBs with a moistened cotton-tipped applicator. Calcium hydroxide tends

to cake and may be easier to remove if the applicator is moistened with 10% EDTA.
3. Irrigate the eye immediately with saline solution or Ringer's lactate for 30 minutes. A Morgan lens, which is a contact lens hooked to IV tubing, is an effective and convenient means of irrigation.
4. Check the pH by touching a piece of litmus paper or the pH tab of a urinary dipstick to the inferior fornix 5 minutes after completion of the irrigation. Repeat irrigation until the pH is between 7.0 and 7.4.
5. After the irrigation is completed, perform an ophthalmologic examination.
6. Treat elevated IOP.
7. If the burn constitutes a mild irritation with mild hyperemia and an otherwise normal examination, after irrigation, treat the eye with an antibiotic ointment twice daily until it is no longer red.
8. Arrange for follow-up. Refer to an ophthalmologist within 24 hours as needed. Patients with minor exposures such as gasoline and household bleach generally do well.

CHEMICAL CONJUNCTIVITIS BY ALKALI OR ACID BURNS

An alkali or acid burn can devastate the eye. Immediate irrigation with saline or Ringer's lactate solution is imperative. Continue the irrigation until the pH of the eye is between 7.0 and 7.4. Blurred vision, severe pain, and severe photophobia are common symptoms. The signs involve anterior chamber reaction, chemosis, reddened or whitened eye, corneal edema or opacification, and vessel loss or ischemia (conjunctiva, limbus, and episclera). A red eye demonstrates good vascularity, whereas a white "marble-eye" is a grim prognostic sign.

The degree of injury is best characterized using the Hughes classification,[67] which relates early clinical findings to prognosis:

Grade I	Good prognosis Corneal epithelial damage No ischemia
Grade II	Good prognosis Cornea hazy but iris details seen Ischemia of less than one third of limbus
Grade III	Guarded prognosis Total loss of corneal epithelium Stromal haze blurring iris details Ischemia of one third to one half of limbus (whitening of the limbus)
Grade IV	Poor prognosis Cornea opaque, obscuring view of iris or pupil Ischemia of more than one half of limbus

Management

1. Instill anesthetic drops.
2. Consult an ophthalmologist immediately.
3. Irrigate the eye immediately with saline solution or Ringer's lactate for 30 minutes. Consider the use of a Morgan lens. Alkali burns may benefit from longer irrigation using many liters of saline.
4. Check the pH by touching a piece of litmus paper or the pH tab of a urinary dipstick to the inferior fornix 5 minutes after completion of the irrigation. Repeat irrigation until the pH is between 7.0 and 7.4.
5. Treat elevated IOP.
6. If the injury is severe, admit for ophthalmologic management.
7. If the injury is mild to moderate, manage on an outpatient basis as follows:
   - Follow the guidelines under Chemical Burns previously discussed.
   - Refer immediately to the ophthalmologist as an outpatient.

ULTRAVIOLET KERATITIS

The most common source of UV exposure is from a welder's arc. The exposure need only be momentary if the patient is not wearing protective eye gear. Symptoms develop 6 to 12 hours later. Indoor sunbathing with a sunlamp without protective eyewear can also expose the individual's eyes to UV light. The symptoms are burning sensation, pain, and photophobia. Examination may reveal anterior chamber reaction (cell and flare), conjunctival hyperemia, decreased VA, SPK, and a swollen eyelid.

Management

1. Instill anesthetic drops.
2. Instill a cycloplegic.
3. Instill antibiotic ointment.
4. Prescribe a narcotic analgesic
5. Recheck in the ED or refer to an ophthalmologist in 24 hours.
6. Prognosis: Excellent.

THERMAL BURNS

First, classify the eyelid burn as partial-thickness (first or second degree) or full-thickness (third degree). These injuries are managed as burns in other parts of the body. Some authorities avoid the use of silver sulfadiazine on the face, since sunlight may precipitate the silver, resulting in tattooing. Antibiotic ointment is a good alternative dressing, and an ophthalmic ointment is safe for the lids and periorbital tissues.

SPECIAL CONSIDERATIONS

Airbag-Induced Eye Injuries. Airbags commonly induce chemical keratitis (secondary to sodium hydroxide combustion product and noncombusted, aerosolized sodium azide). The airbag can cause a plethora of other ocular injuries that encompass nearly every orbital structure.[68-71] Management depends on the particular injury.

Dog Bites. Over half of the severe dog bites that occur to the face involve children.[20] This high frequency has been attributed to the child's short stature, inexperience with dogs, and propensity of dogs to bite the face.[72] Be aware of underlying injuries, since dogs' jaws can exert a force of 200 to 450 psi, which can puncture sheet metal.[73] A thorough eye examination is necessary and may need to be performed under anesthesia. The value of systemic antibiotics is controversial in this condition, but they are frequently prescribed.

Golf-Related Eye Injuries. Golf balls and golf club heads fit within the orbital rim, allowing their full energy to be transmitted to the globe. As a result, there is a high incidence of globe rupture and lens expulsion/luxation/subluxation. Other reported injuries include blowout fracture, multiple retinal tears, retinal detachment, and traumatic cataract.[74,75] In two series, 9 of 17 eyes required enucleation.[74,75] Racquetballs, paddleballs, handballs, and champagne corks also fit neatly within the orbital rim.

Nylon Line Lawn Trimmer–Related Eye Injuries. Nylon line trimmers operate at speeds of 6000 to 14,000 rpm. Projectiles may fly 30 feet and can include nylon cord, metal, rock, and wire fragments. These missiles may penetrate the eye or produce blunt trauma resulting in anterior chamber reaction, corneal injury, hyphema, iris tear, and rupture of lens capsule.[76] Always look for a retained FB with these injuries. Similar risks have been documented with power mowers.[77]

Domestic Violence. Domestic violence (DV) is a major cause of injuries to women, particularly involving the head and neck. The injuries may not be reported as secondary to DV because of isolation, fear, poor self-esteem, or a desire to protect the perpetrator. In one series, 6 of 19 consecutive women with orbital fractures referred to a university ophthalmology service were victims of DV or sexual assault.[78] Eliciting a history of DV requires a sensitive approach (see Chapter 36).

Super Glue (Cyanoacrylate) Injury. With cyanoacrylate eye injury, the eyelids are typically sealed partially or completely. There may be a corneal abrasion secondary to hardened glue. Usually no long-term morbidity is seen.[79] Petroleum-based ophthalmic ointments will rapidly dissolve the glue. If the lids remain glued in the ED, allow the patient to reapply the ointment several times an hour. The patient can be discharged with instructions to apply frequently at home and return the following day for a recheck.

Sympathetic Ophthalmia. Sympathetic ophthalmia is an autoimmune response that occurs in an uninjured eye, following penetrating trauma to the other eye. It leads to photophobia, inflammatory changes, and even visual loss.

The incidence of sympathetic ophthalmia is 0.2% after penetrating eye injury.[20] About 65% of cases begin between 2 and 8 weeks after the insult, and 90% occur within 1 year (range of 5 days to decades).[20] The signs and symptoms in the sympathetic eye begin as a mild anterior uveitis that progresses over time to anterior and posterior uveitis. In about 5% of the cases, only the posterior uveitis is evident (blurred vision, floaters, pain, photophobia, and possible redness).[16,20] The condition of the injured eye (exciting eye) may worsen at the same time.[20] Treatment regimens include cycloplegics, systemic steroids, and possibly immunosuppressants such as cyclosporine A.[66] On occasion the ophthalmologist may need to enucleate the injured eye.

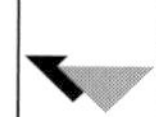

PEARLS & PITFALLS

- Document a visual acuity for every patient with ocular injury, unless they are unconscious or hemodynamically unstable.
- Ask about possible domestic violence in women with ocular trauma.
- Suspect penetrating ocular injuries in metal-striking-metal injuries.
- Perform immediate copious irrigation for dangerous chemical exposures before doing a full eye examination.
- Perform the eye examination as early as possible, since progressive lid edema may prohibit visualization of the globe.
- Shield all suspected globe ruptures and penetrating eye injuries from further damage.
- In 80% of cases, intraocular FBs enter the eye through the cornea.
- Intraocular FBs predispose to endophthalmitis.
- CT scanning is the most useful radiologic study for ocular injuries.
- In 90% of cases, the injury could have been prevented or lessened by wearing protective lenses.
- Topical anesthetics must never be used *except* for diagnostic purposes. Do not send patients home with topical anesthetics.
- Consider narcotic analgesics for patients discharged with corneal abrasions, iritis, and keratitis.

- In general, avoid patching eyes. If the eye is patched, the patient must not drive or operate machinery, since depth perception is lost.

REFERENCES

1. Life Site. National Society to Prevent Blindness. Schaumberg, IL (800-221-3004), 1998.
2. Hague S, Cooling RJ: Ocular trauma, *Practitioner* 232:181-184, 1988.
3. DeJuan E Jr, Sternberg P Jr, Michels RG: Penetrating ocular injuries: types of injuries and visual results, *Ophthalmology* 90:1318-1322, 1983.
4. Hander JA, Ghezzi KT: General ophthalmologic examination, *Emerg Med Clin North Am* 13:521-538, 1995.
5. Clancy MJ, Hulbert M: A study of the eye care provided by an accident and emergency department, *Arch Emerg Med* 8:122-124, 1991.
6. Edwards RS: Ophthalmic emergencies in a district general hospital casualty department, *Br J Ophthalmol* 71:938-942, 1987.
7. Flitcroft DI, et al: Who should see eye casualties? A comparison of eye care in an accident and emergency department with a dedicated eye casualty, *J Accid Emerg Med* 12:23-27, 1995.
8. American College of Emergency Physicians, 1994, statistical data.
9. Impact Protection and Polycarbonate Lenses. Prevent Blindness America. Schamburg, IL, 1995.
10. Tielsch JM, Parver L, Shankar B: Time trends in the incidence of hospitalized ocular trauma, *Arch Ophthalmol* 107:519-23, 1989.
11. Schein OD, et al: The spectrum and burden of ocular injury, *Ophthalmology* 95:300-305, 1988.
12. Zagelbaum BM, et al: Urban eye trauma: a one-year prospective study, *Ophthalmology* 100:851-856, 1993.
13. Dunn ES, et al: The epidemiology of ruptured globes, *Ann Ophthalmol* 24:405-410, 1992.
14. Tielsch JM, Parver LM: Determinants of hospital charges and length of stay for ocular trauma, *Ophthalmology* 97:231-237, 1990.
15. Palay DA, Krachmer JH (editors): *Ophthalmology for the primary care physician,* St Louis, 1997, Mosby.
16. Cullom RD Jr, Chang B: *The Wills eye manual,* Philadelphia, 1994, Lippincott-Raven.
17. MacCumber MW (editor): *Management of ocular injuries and emergencies,* Philadelphia, 1998, Lippincott-Raven.
18. McCannel CA, et al: Causes of uveitis in the general practice of ophthalmology, *Am J Ophthalmol* 121:35-46, 1996.
19. Rothova A, et al: Clinical features of acute anterior uveitis, *Am J Ophthalmol* 103:137-145, 1987.
20. Shingleton BJ, Hersh PS, Kenyon DR (editors): *Eye trauma,* St Louis, 1991, Mosby.
21. Catalano RA: *Ocular emergencies,* Philadelphia, 1992, Saunders.
22. O'Hare TH: Blow-out fractures: a review, *J Emerg Med* 9:253-263, 1991.
23. Catone GA, Morrissette MP, Carlson ER: A retrospective study of untreated orbital blow-out fractures, *J Oral Maxillofac Surg* 46:1033-1038, 1988.
24. Jabaley ME, Lerman M, Sanders HJ: Ocular injuries in orbital fractures: a review of 119 cases, *Plast Reconstr Surg* 56:410-418, 1975.
25. Gossman MD, Roberts DM, Barr CC: Ophthalmic aspects of orbital injury: a comprehensive diagnostic and management approach, *Clin Plast Surg* 19:71-85, 1992.
26. Jordan DR, et al: Orbital emphysema: a potentially blinding complication following orbital fractures, *Ann Emerg Med* 17:853-855, 1988.
27. Linden JA, Renner GS: Trauma to the globe, *Emerg Med Clin North Am* 13:581-605, 1995.
28. Kearns P: Traumatic hyphema: a retrospective study of 314 cases, *Br J Ophthalmol* 75:137-141, 1991.
29. Bloom JN: Traumatic hyphema in children, *Pediatr Ann* 19:368-375, 1990.
30. Joondeph BC: Blunt ocular trauma, *Emerg Med Clin North Am* 6:147-167, 1988.
31. Lipshy KA, Wheeler WE, Denning DE: Ophthalmic thermal injuries, *Am Surg* 62:481-483, 1996.
32. Vajpayee RB, et al: Contact thermal burns of the cornea, *Can J Ophthalmol* 26:215-218, 1991.
33. Pfister RR, Koski J: Alkali burns of the eye: pathophysiology and treatment, *South Med J* 75:417-422, 1982.
34. Paterson CA, Pfister RR, Levinson RA: Aqueous humor pH changes after experimental alkali burns, *Am J Ophthalmol* 79: 414-419, 1975.
35. Paterson CA, Pfister RR: Intraocular pressure changes after alkali burns, *Arch Ophthalmol* 91:211-218, 1974.
36. Tso MO, LaPiana RG: The human fovea after sungazing, *Trans Am Acad Ophthalmol Otolaryngol* 79:788-795, 1975.
37. Van Johnson E, Kline LB, Skalka HW: Electrical cataracts: a case report and review of the literature, *Ophthalmic Surg* 18:283-285, 1987.
38. Kylstra JA, Lamkin JC, Runyan DK: Clinical predictors of scleral rupture after blunt ocular trauma, *Am J Ophthalmol* 115: 530-535, 1993.
39. Shingleton BJ: Eye injuries, *N Engl J Med* 325:408-413, 1991.
40. Rose GE, Pearson RV: Unequal pupil size in patients with unilateral red eye, *Br Med J* 302:571-572, 1991.
41. DegowinEL, Degowin RL: *Bedside diagnostic examination,* ed 2, London, 1969, Macmillan.
42. Martin XD: Normal intraocular pressure in man, *Ophthalmologica* 205:57-63, 1992.
43. Lustrin ES, et al: Radiologic assessment of trauma and foreign bodies of the eye and orbit, *Neuroimaging Clin North Am* 6:219-237, 1996.
44. Lindahl S: Computed tomography of intraorbital foreign bodies, *Acta Radiol* 28:235-240, 1987.
45. Topilow HW, Ackerman AL, Zimmerman RD: Limitations of computerized tomography in the localization of intraocular foreign bodies, *Ophthalmology* 91:1086-1091, 1984.
46. Kadir S, Aronow S, Davis KR: The use of computerized tomography in the detection of intra-orbital foreign bodies, *Comput Tomogr* 1:151-156, 1977.
47. Tate E, Cupples H: Detection of orbital foreign bodies with computed tomography: current limits, *Am J Radiol* 137:493-495, 1981.
48. Brinton GS, et al: Posttraumatic endophthalmitis, *Arch Ophthalmol* 102:547-550, 1984.
49. Alfaro DV, et al: Paediatric post-traumatic endophthalmitis, *Br J Ophthalmol* 79:888-891, 1995.
50. Coleman DJ, et al: Management of intraocular foreign bodies, *Ophthalmology* 94:1647-1653, 1987.
51. Patterson J, et al: Eye patch treatment for the pain of corneal abrasion, *South Med J* 89:227-229, 1996.
52. Kirkpatrick JN, Hoh HB, Cook SD: No eye pad for corneal abrasion, *Eye* 7:468-471, 1993.
53. Flynn CA, D'Amico F, Smith G: Should we patch corneal abrasions? A meta-analysis, *J Fam Pract* 47:264-270, 1998.
54. Crikelair GF, et al: A critical look at the "blowout" fracture, *Plast Reconstr Surg* 49:374-379, 1972.

55. Martello JY, Vasconez HC: Supraorbital roof fractures: a formidable entity with which to contend, *Ann Plast Surg* 38:223-227, 1997.
56. Holt JE, Holt GR, Blodgett JM: Ocular injuries sustained during blunt facial trauma, *Ophthalmology* 90:14-18, 1983.
57. Cook MW, et al: Traumatic optic neuropathy: a meta-analysis, *Arch Otolaryngol Head Neck Surg* 122:389-392, 1996.
58. Joseph E, et al: Predictors of blinding or serious eye injury in blunt trauma, *J Trauma* 33:19-24, 1992.
59. Davey RT Jr, Tauber WB: Posttraumatic endophthalmitis: the emerging role of *Bacillus cereus* infection, *Rev Infect Dis* 9:110-123, 1987.
60. Hemady R, et al: Bacillus-induced endophthalmitis: new series of 10 cases and review of the literature, *Br J Ophthalmol* 74:26-29, 1990.
61. Weber DJ, et al: In vitro susceptibility of *Bacillus* spp. to selected antimicrobial agents, *Antimicrob Agents Chemother* 32:642-645, 1988.
62. *Physician's Desk Reference,* ed 52, Montvale, NJ, 1998, Medical Economics Company.
63. Benitz WE, Tatro DS: *The pediatric drug handbook,* ed 2, St Louis, 1988, Mosby.
64. Gregory-Roberts J: Pitfalls in penetrating eye injuries, *Med J Aust* 157:398-399, 1992.
65. Lubeck D: Penetrating ocular injuries, *Emerg Med Clin North Am* 6:127-146, 1988.
66. Pavan-Langston D: Burns and trauma. In Pavan-Langston D (editor): *Manual of ocular diagnosis and therapy,* ed 3, New York, 1991, Little, Brown.
67. Hughes WF Jr: Alkali burns of the eye. II. Clinical and pathologic course, *Arch Ophthalmol* 36:189-214, 1942.
68. Smally AJ, et al: Alkaline chemical keratitis: eye injury from airbags, *Ann Emerg Med* 21:1400-1402, 1992.
69. Larkin GL: Airbag-mediated corneal injury, *Am J Emerg Med* 9:444-446, 1991.
70. Duma SM, et al: Airbag-induced eye injuries: a report of 25 cases, *J Trauma* 41:114-119, 1996.
71. Vichnin MC, et al: Ocular injuries related to air bag inflation, *Ophthalmic Surg Lasers* 26:542-548, 1995.
72. Beck AM, Loring H, Lockwood R: The ecology of dog bite injury in St Louis, Missouri, *Public Health Rep* 90:262-267, 1975.
73. Chambers GH, Payne JF: Treatment of dog-bite wounds, *Minn Med* 52:427-430, 1969.
74. Burnstine MA, Elner VM: Golf-related ocular injuries, *Am J Ophthalmol* 121:437-438, 1995.
75. Mieler WF, et al: Golf-related ocular injuries, *Arch Ophthalmol* 113:1410-1413, 1995.
76. Lubniewski A, Olk RJ, Grand MG: Ocular dangers in the garden: a new menace–nylon line lawn trimmers, *Ophthalmology* 95:906-910, 1988.
77. Barsky D: Eye injuries due to power lawn mowers, *Arch Ophthalmol* 64:385-387, 1960.
78. Hartzell KN, Botek AA, Goldberg SH: Orbital fractures in women due to sexual assault and domestic violence, *Ophthalmology* 103:953-957, 1996.
79. McLean CJ: Ocular superglue injury, *J Accid Emerg Med* 14:40-41, 1997.

16 Neck Injury

ROBERT M. DUCHYNSKI

TEACHING CASE

A 28-year-old helmeted man was riding a dirt bike when he crashed into a low-hanging branch and was thrown off the motorcycle. His friends brought him to a local hospital, where he complained of anterior neck pain, right knee pain, and back pain.

He told the physician he heard a "whooshing sound" in his right ear, but the ear was normal on examination. His left pupil was larger than his right but both reacted to light. The right lid seemed "droopy" but the physician attributed this finding to early swelling. He was alert and oriented to person, place, and time, and his vital signs were stable. Further evaluation revealed a small ecchymosis to the neck and swelling of both knees. He had no evidence of neurologic injury. The patient was discharged after plain radiographs of his cervical spine were normal.

One week later the patient presented to the same emergency department (ED) with left hemiparesis. Brain computed tomography (CT) scanning suggested ischemic stroke (Fig. 16-1). Subsequent Doppler ultrasound of the carotid arteries showed a right internal carotid artery dissection, and angiography revealed an occlusion distal to the bifurcation (Fig. 16-2). The patient was admitted to the intensive care unit, where his mental status declined. Repeat CT scanning showed a dense ischemic stroke (Fig. 16-3). He was declared brain dead on hospital day five.

The evaluation and management of patients with anterior neck trauma is one of the most challenging scenarios facing the emergency physician (EP). These patients can present with life-threatening hemorrhage, a "nightmare" airway, or be entirely asymptomatic. There is considerable controversy in management of the asymptomatic or minimally symptomatic patient with anterior neck trauma.

ANATOMY

The many vital organs packed within a small area portend significant morbidity in case of trauma. These organs include vascular, respiratory, digestive, and central nervous system structures. In many instances, they may be only several millimeters from the skin. Unlike the chest, where the heart and lung are protected by the ribs, the anterior neck is completely vulnerable. One of the most significant anatomic boundaries of the neck is the platysma, a thin muscle layer that lies between the skin of the anterior neck and the investing fascia.

The investing fascia is divided into two layers, a superficial layer encompassing the platysma and the deep cervical fascia.

The neck is divided into three anatomic zones (Fig. 16-4) that are important in management.[1] **Zone I** extends from the clavicle to the cricoid cartilage,[1-4] although a previous classification system used the sternal notch to mark the upper boundary.[5-7] **Zone II** continues from the cricoid cartilage to the angle of the mandible, and **zone III** lies above the angle of the mandible.[1] Structures found within zone I include the trachea, esophagus, common carotid artery, internal jugular vein, thyroid gland, and cervical nerve roots. Zone II contains the common carotid artery, internal jugular vein, larynx, and esophagus. Zone III includes the internal and external carotid arteries, oropharynx, cranial nerves, and salivary glands.

The neck is also divided into anterior and posterior triangles by the sternocleidomastoid muscle (SCM) (Fig. 16-5). The anterior triangle is in front of the SCM and the posterior triangle rests posteriorly. The anterior triangle contains the more vital structures and is injured more often.[4,6] Injuries to the posterior triangle often breach the chest or spine.[4]

There are several anatomic differences between

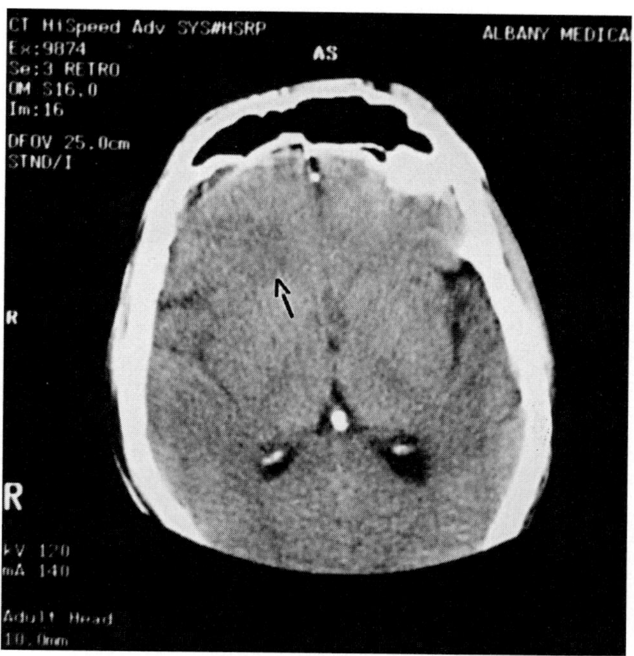

Fig. 16-1 Computed tomography scan of the brain with possible early infarction of the right frontal lobe in the middle cerebral artery distribution *(arrow)*.

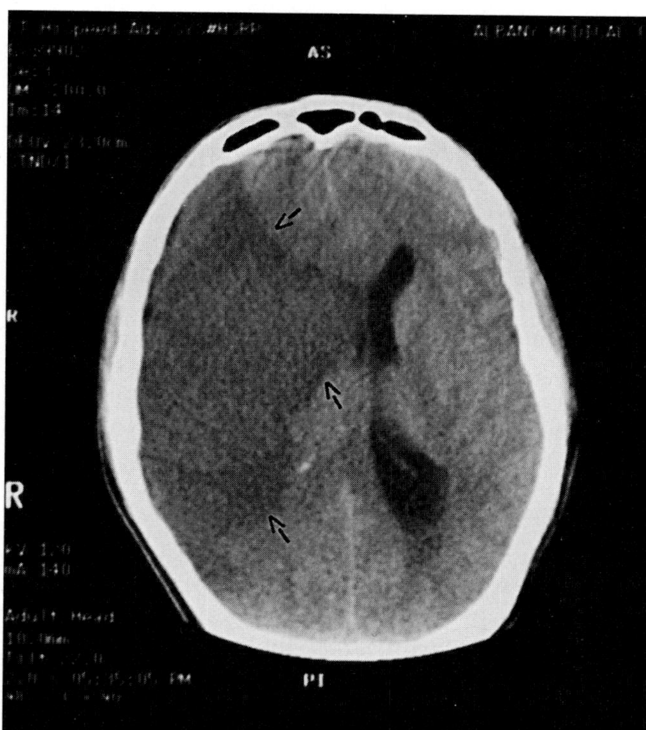

Fig. 16-3 Computed tomography scan now showing a larger area of infarction of the right hemisphere consistent with right middle cerebral artery or right internal carotid artery occlusion *(arrows)*.

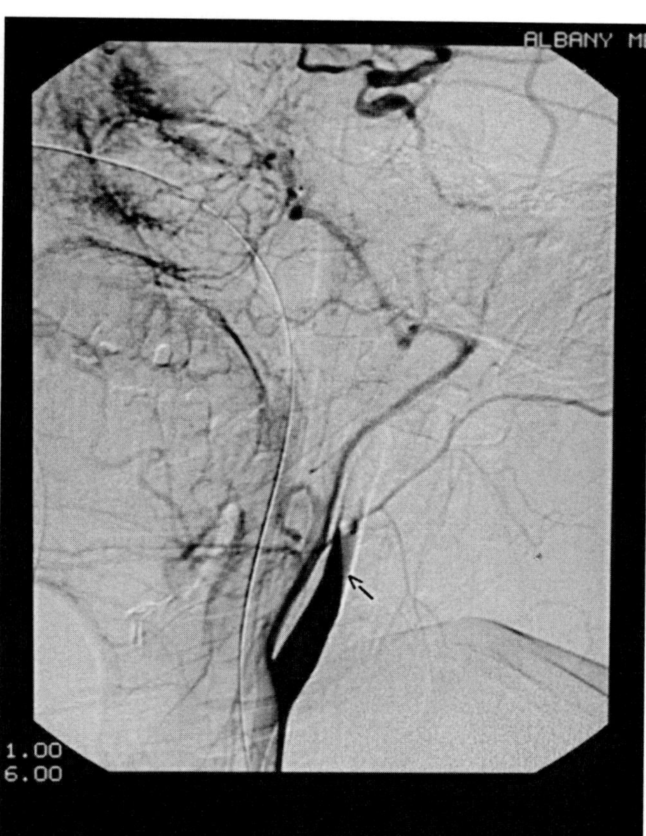

Fig. 16-2 Carotid angiography showing an extracranial right internal carotid artery occlusion 3 cm distal to the bifurcation of the common carotid artery *(arrow)*.

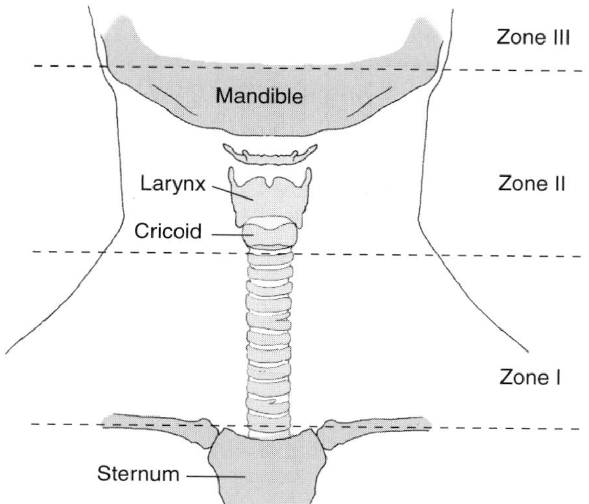

Fig. 16-4 Zones of the neck.

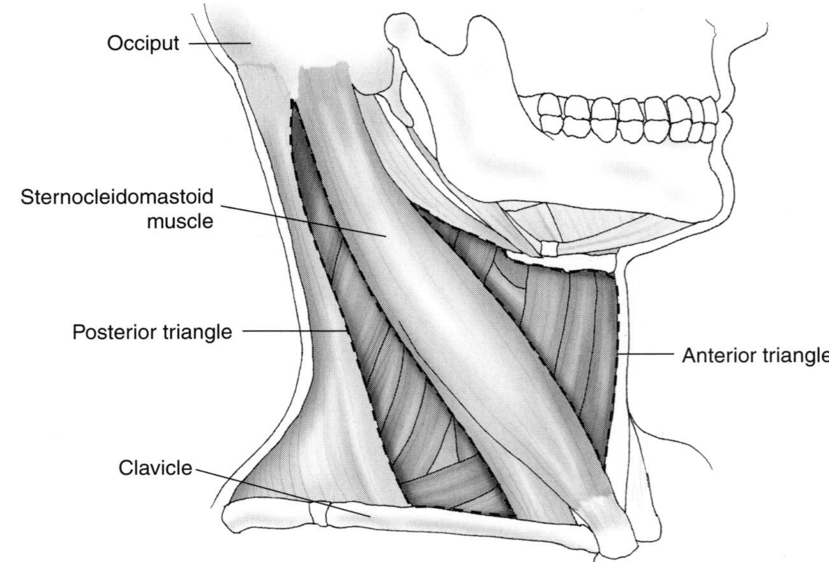

Fig. 16-5 Anterior and posterior triangles of the neck.

children and adults. In children, the larynx is higher and better protected,[8] and children are prone to subglottic stenosis, making cricothyroidotomy contraindicated.

PENETRATING ANTERIOR NECK INJURY

Epidemiology

Penetrating neck trauma constitutes about 5% to 10% of all trauma and is most often caused by stabbing or gunshot wounds (GSWs). The relative incidence of stabbings versus GSWs varies according to the city.[6,9] Males outnumber females by approximately four to one.[9] Most injuries are to zone II.[4,10]

Mortality has decreased significantly over the past century. Mortality from penetrating neck trauma during the Civil War was 15%.[11] Recent statistics now place it around 4%.[2] Death and disability result from exsanguination, airway compromise, stroke, or spinal cord injury.[12]

Vascular structures are most often injured, followed by a nearly equal distribution of laryngotracheal and pharyngoesophageal trauma.[2-4,6] Among vascular injuries, venous outnumber arterial.[3,4] The common carotid artery is the most common arterial injury, followed by the subclavian,[2,4] whereas the vertebral artery is well protected by the spine and rarely injured.[2,4]

Clinical Presentation

Presentation can range from the completely asymptomatic to the moribund patient in marked respiratory distress. It is useful to consider presentations in light of the underlying organ injury.

VASCULAR INJURIES

Patients with significant vascular injuries present with shock, pulsatile or expanding hematoma, respiratory distress, absent pulses, bruits, or hemorrhage.

Carotid Injuries. Carotid injuries include tears that can lead to ischemia of the ipsilateral brain. Ischemia may be caused by disruption, dissection, or intimal tears that later embolize. Such patients exhibit a profound neurologic deficit on the contralateral side. If a neck hematoma from a carotid injury expands rapidly, it may compress the airway, leading to marked respiratory distress. Vascular injuries in zone I can also produce a hemothorax.

Venous Injuries. In general, venous injuries present in a less dramatic fashion. On the other hand, large lacerations involving the jugular venous system can generate an air embolism. Such patients are tachypneic, tachycardic, and hypotensive.[1,6,8]

RESPIRATORY TRACT INJURIES

Injuries to the respiratory tract can cause cough, subcutaneous emphysema, dyspnea, and stridor. Other signs and symptoms include hoarseness, hemoptysis, and dysphonia; pain along the cricoid and thyroid cartilage; and partial or complete airway obstruction. Pneumothorax and respiratory distress are common following a zone I injury.

NEUROLOGIC INJURIES

Direct neurologic deficits result from injury to cranial nerves, peripheral nerves, or the spinal cord, whereas ischemic deficits arise from vascular injuries. Patients with spinal cord injury may have spinal shock, diaphragmatic breathing, priapism, decreased anal tone, or peripheral deficits. Hoarseness may result from vagal or recurrent laryngeal nerve injury, as well as mechanical trauma to the larynx. On occasion, damage to the facial nerve produces a traumatic Bell's palsy, whereas hypoglossal nerve injury deviates the tongue. Elevated hemidiaphragm and dyspnea occur with phrenic nerve dysfunction. Brachial plexus injuries, depending on the nerve or root involved, yield an assortment of upper extremity sensory and motor deficits.

An unusual injury is seen with the involvement of the sympathetic chain. Such patients may present with a Horner's syndrome comprised of the classic triad of ptosis, miosis, and anhydrosis on the involved side. Because the sympathetic chain is anatomically wed to the carotids, suspect arterial injury in patients with Horner's syndrome.[1,8,10]

AERODIGESTIVE TRACT INJURIES

Aerodigestive tract injuries (esophagus and oropharynx) are notoriously occult. Some patients may exhibit subcutaneous emphysema, hematoma, or tracheal deviation. Others will have pain on swallowing or hematemesis. Findings on chest radiograph include pneumomediastinum, retropharyngeal air, or a wide mediastinum. Auscultation of the chest may reveal a "**Hamman's crunch**." This sound has been compared with that of a heavy man walking in fresh snow. The "crunch" occurs with each beat of the heart.

Emergency Department Evaluation and Management

PRIMARY SURVEY

Airway Management. Managing the airway is the most crucial emergency intervention for patients with anterior neck trauma. Ten percent of such patients present with respiratory distress.[13] Clear foreign bodies and dentures then suction blood and emesis. All patients require 100% oxygen. Some authorities recommend a slight Trendelenburg position to prevent air embolism,[4] although this maneuver has not been studied in a prospective fashion. Immobilize the cervical spine in patients with neurologic deficits and those in whom the missile trajectory jeopardizes the cord. Cervical collars may be difficult to apply as a result of swelling and can obscure bleeding. Sandbags and tape immobilization on a backboard, without a cervical collar, may be necessary.[11-14]

In one series of penetrating neck trauma, one quarter of patients required an emergency airway. Some authors have suggested several indications for definitive airway control, including:

- Inadequate ventilation
- Progressive cervical swelling
- Extensive subcutaneous emphysema
- Stridor
- Altered mental status[2,4,14]

Delays in airway management may allow an expanding hematoma to obscure or distort anatomy, which makes intubation or surgical airway difficult or impossible. However, not every patient with penetrating neck trauma requires intubation. Fully 40% of patients with penetrating neck trauma were never intubated during their hospital stay.[14] Stable patients who show no respiratory distress and no expansion of the neck hematoma may have their airway followed clinically without the need for intubation.

When deciding on the optimal approach to controlling the airway, the EP should consider both the patient's particular circumstances and his or her own expertise. Options for airway management include awake orotracheal intubation, fiberoptic nasotracheal intubation, orotracheal intubation with rapid sequence induction, cricothyrotomy, tracheostomy, and percutaneous transtracheal jet ventilation.[15] Avoid blind nasotracheal intubation, since the blind probing may produce massive hemorrhage from injured soft tissues or airway compromise.[10] Furthermore, blind nasotracheal intubation is also difficult in patients with distorted anatomy.[15]

Awake Intubation. Although paralytic agents often facilitate intubation, their use in penetrating neck trauma can be dangerous. It may be difficult or impossible to intubate patients with distorted anatomy. If intubation fails in a paralyzed patient, this same distorted anatomy may prevent effective bag-valve-mask ventilation. For this reason, consider awake intubation in patients with penetrating neck trauma especially in the presence of a significant cervical hematoma. The use of agents such as ketamine or droperidol may enhance patient cooperation. If time permits, anesthetize the airway by allowing the patient to breathe nebulized 4% lidocaine. If paralytic agents are chosen, the EP must prepare for immediate back-up cricothyrotomy. Preparation in this case involves sterilizing the neck with iodine solution, opening the cricothyrotomy tray, and ensuring that the scalpel and tracheostomy tube are available. If possible, recruit a second physician to perform the surgical airway should orotracheal intubation fail.

Although some recommend fiberoptic nasotracheal intubation, this technique is far easier to recommend than accomplish. Bleeding frequently makes visualization impossible despite suctioning.

Surgical Solutions. Some advocate a tracheostomy in patients with laryngotracheal disruption. However, even in the hands of an experienced surgeon, a tracheostomy usually takes 5 minutes or more to accomplish. A dying patient cannot spare these minutes. One approach is an attempt at awake oral intubation. Should endotracheal intubation fail, the choice of a surgical airway is between formal tracheostomy or cricothyrotomy. *If time permits*, tracheostomy is preferred over cricothyrotomy in patients with laryngeal trauma. However, patients in extremis are best served by an emergent cricothyrotomy by the EP.[13-15]

Percutaneous Transtracheal Jet Ventilation. Percutaneous transtracheal jet ventilation (PCTV) is another useful alternative for patients with distorted anatomy who cannot be intubated orally. It is a technique of choice in children under 8 years of age in whom cricothyroidotomy may be difficult and fraught with both acute and delayed complications. A large bore catheter placed through the cricothyroid membrane provides up to 1 hour of ventilation until tracheotomy can be performed.[13,15]

Open Trachea. Some patients present with complete tracheal transection, and the airway may be visible through the wound. In such cases, grasp the trachea with a towel clip or hemostats and insert a tube directly through the wound into the trachea.[2,4,16]

Breathing, Circulation, and Disability. Complete the primary survey in the usual fashion. Look for signs of tension pneumothorax on chest examination and control active external bleeding with direct pressure. Avoid blind clamping that may injure important structures.[6] Bleeding from the subclavian vessels is resistant to external pressure and difficult to access via thoracotomy. If a surgeon is not immediately available to take the patient to the operating room, a Foley catheter placed in the wound and inflated with normal saline may control life-threatening hemorrhage.[17]

All patients with penetrating neck injury require large-bore intravenous (IV) access. For patients with zone I injuries, at least one IV line should be placed in the opposite extremity. Uncontrolled intrathoracic hemorrhage from a zone I injury may require an emergent thoracotomy for control of bleeding.[4] Perform a brief neurologic examination, including level of consciousness, pupillary size and responsiveness, and motor and sensory function of all four extremities.

SECONDARY SURVEY

After completion of the primary survey and initial stabilization, completely expose the patient to perform the secondary survey. At this time obtain a focused history. Emergency medical services personnel may provide crucial information, including initial vital signs, reports of hypotension, and the response to prehospital therapy. Inquire as to the wounding agent and amount of blood at the scene. Ask the patient about pain and its location. In particular, determine if there is pain with breathing, talking, or swallowing. Determine if the patient has hemoptysis, hematemesis, changes in voice, and weakness or numbness.

Perform a complete physical examination with particular attention to the head, neck, and chest. Locate and classify the injury by zone. Do not completely rely on the entrance and exit wounds to suggest trajectory, since a bullet may veer from tumble or ricochet off the spine. Wound exploration should be limited to determine whether the platysma has been violated. *If the platysma is lacerated, call a surgeon.* Avoid blind probing, which may dislodge a clot and increase bleeding.[3,4,13]

Perform several simple tests in the conscious and stable patient.

- Ask the patient to speak. An abnormal voice mandates laryngoscopy.
- Ask the patient to cough. Hemoptysis requires bronchoscopy.
- Have the patient swallow his or her saliva or sips of water. Pain on swallowing suggests esophageal injury.
- Listen for a bruit over the carotids. A glove placed over the stethoscope head protects it from blood.

Obtain soft tissue lateral and anterioposterior radiographs to look for subcutaneous air, bullet fragments, and changes to the airway. All patients need a chest radiograph to rule out pneumothorax, pneumomediastinum, abnormal aortic contour, and hemothorax. Cervical spine radiographs are indicated in those with an altered mental status, neurologic deficit, and victims of gunshot wounds.

The placement of a nasogastric tube (NGT) is controversial. By emptying the stomach, the risk of aspiration is decreased. However, NGT placement may also dislodge a clot and worsen hemorrhage.[2-4,17] The decision to place a NGT varies between trauma centers, and the decision making should be shared with the surgeon who will care for the patient subsequently.

FURTHER EVALUATION AND TREATMENT

The choice of diagnostic studies depends on the history, physical examination, and stability of the patient (Fig. 16-6). Patients in shock and those with hard signs of carotid injury need immediate surgical intervention.[3,18,19] Violation of the platysma requires surgical consultation and selective imaging studies depending on the zone transgressed.

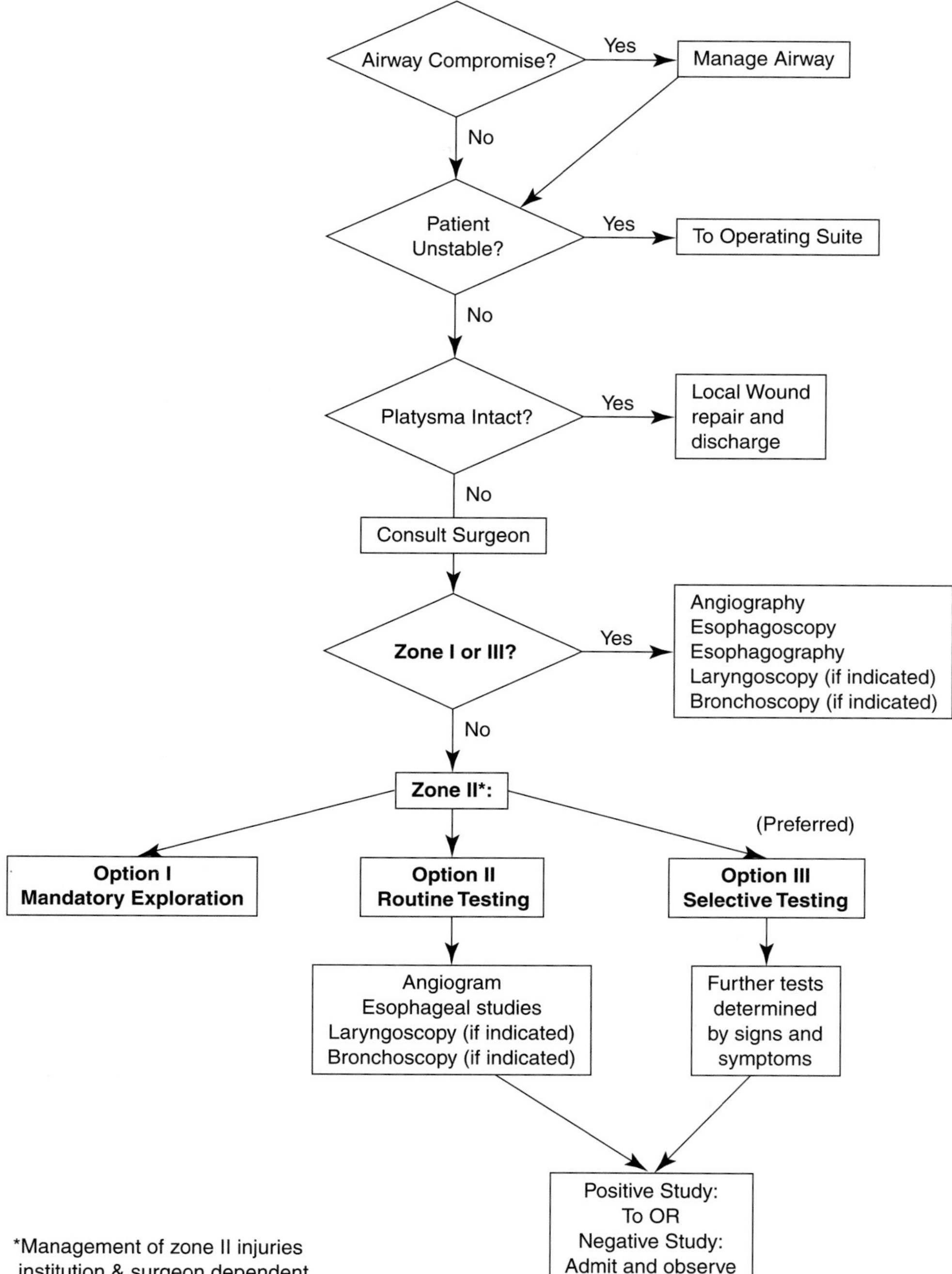

Fig. 16-6 Management of penetrating neck injuries.

Zones I and III. Surgical exploration of zones I and III is difficult because it is difficult for the surgeon to obtain vascular control. For this reason, mandatory operation is reserved for the patient with clear signs of serious injury. Testing may be *selective* (based on physical findings or symptoms) or *routine* (everyone is tested). Although some centers suggest testing be reserved for symptomatic patients, most centers liberally study patients with zone I or III injuries. Angiography is routine in most centers. Even completely asymptomatic patients may require angiography since physical signs are insensitive to zones I and III vascular injuries.[1,3,6,20-22] Color-flow Doppler (CFD) may be a reasonable alternative to formal angiography.[23,24]

Zone II Injuries. There are three widely differing approaches to management of zone II injuries, mandatory exploration, routine testing, and selective testing. Mandatory exploration results in an operation for *all* patients whose wound violates the platysma. Proponents argue that mandatory exploration reduces missed injuries and has little morbidity.[1,9,11,19] Although this strategy dominated surgical practice for years, it has fallen from favor in many trauma centers.

During the 1980s, many centers abandoned mandatory exploration in favor of routine testing. *In this strategy, patients with hard signs of aerodigestive, neurologic, or vascular injury still go directly to the operating suite with few or no preoperative studies.* Asymptomatic or minimally symptomatic patients undergo routine testing. Studies include angiography to rule out vascular injury; laryngoscopy and bronchoscopy for respiratory trauma; and esophagoscopy and/or swallow studies to evaluate aerodigestive injuries. We refer to this constellation of tests as ABEL (angiography, bronchoscopy, esophagoscopy/esophagography, and laryngoscopy).

Selective testing differs from routine testing in that all tests are not ordered in every patient. Instead, tests are selected based on the patient's symptoms or physical examination. All patients with altered mental status or inability to follow commands are always tested, since their examination is unreliable.

Current practice tends to favor selective testing. Proponents argue that the selective approach results in fewer negative explorations and lower costs while detecting all serious injuries.[2,3,6,25-27] Proponents of mandatory surgical exploration argue that extensive testing, including angiography, esophagoscopy, and panendoscopy, are more expensive than a negative surgical exploration.[19,28-30] They believe that patients with negative explorations have shorter hospital stays and use fewer resources than those undergoing mandatory ABEL.[12,19]

The literature provides data that can support all these positions. Proponents of mandatory angiography cite the low sensitivity of physical examination in detecting vascular injuries.[5,9,28,30,31] Those authors who champion a selective approach note that injuries that require operation occur only in patients with positive clinical findings.[2,18,32-37] All agree that patients who are difficult to assess, such as those who are intoxicated or unconscious, should be thoroughly tested.

For the EP the decisions regarding management of zone II injuries is best left to consensus-driven institutional protocols. The approach to penetrating neck trauma, whether mandatory exploration, routine testing, or selective testing, must be made in conjunction with the surgeon assuming care. Selective testing is only safe in level I or II trauma centers where there is continuing availability of the operating suite, ancillary testing, and adequate personnel to perform serial examinations.[2,3,6,17,25,35,38]

Vascular Injuries. A four-vessel angiogram is sensitive for arterial injury, but cannot provide information regarding venous trauma unless an arteriovenous fistula is present. Signs of carotid injury include shock, active bleeding, expanding hematoma, neurologic deficit in the carotid distribution, a bruit or thrill, and a "machinery" murmur. Patients with shock, pulse deficit, and a rapidly expanding hematoma, require immediate exploration in the operating suite. Hemorrhage alone does not portend carotid injury, since bleeding may occur from muscular arteries.[19] Patients with stable hematomas and those unable to cooperate with clinical assessment may benefit from angiography. The asymptomatic patient may be imaged or observed based on local practice and clinical suspicion.

In several studies the physical examination alone predicts the need for angiography.[33,36] Although less than 2% of patients with negative physical examinations did have carotid injury on angiography, none of these lesions required surgery. Of course, others have found opposite results. In Sclafani et al's[21] retrospective series, physical examination was only 80% sensitive and 60% specific for arterial injuries, and angiography was recommended for asymptomatic patients. Because transcervical wounds (i.e., those wounds that cross the midline) and shotgun wounds are considered high risk for vascular injury, some centers suggest routine angiography for these types of injuries.

Some centers use duplex ultrasonography with CFD instead of angiography for the evaluation of penetrating neck injuries. In a study by Ginzburg et al,[24] this technology was 100% sensitive and 85% specific for lesions needing operation. These authors recommend angiography only for those patients with a positive ultrasound. Other investigations validate this approach and show that CFD is sensitive for significant injury and is much faster than angiography, with less morbidity and less cost.[39] The combination of physical examination and CFD has been shown to be effective in excluding significant injuries.[23]

Pharyngoesophageal Injuries. Because delays in diagnosis and repair of esophageal injuries are associated with rocketing mortality,[19,40,41] all patients with signs or symptoms referable to the esophagus should be explored or tested. Pain on swallowing water or saliva is a sensitive sign. Data are inconclusive regarding the need to study asymptomatic patients. In a review by Weigelt et al[29] the sensitivity of physical examination for esophageal injury was only 80%. In contrast, Demetriades et al[18] found in a prospective study that physical examination reliably excluded esophageal injury.

In the stable patient, objective testing may prevent the need for surgical exploration even in the presence of suspicious signs. One series showed that only 36% of patients with subcutaneous emphysema required an operation.[32] The choice of objective tests includes rigid esophagoscopy, flexible esophagoscopy, barium swallow, and gastrografin swallow. Some authorities suggest that a water-soluble agent such as gastrografin should be used for esophagography, since it is less toxic to the mediastinum than barium (Fig. 16-7). In addition, barium may interfere with subsequent endoscopy. On the other hand, in the patient with altered mental status, water-soluble agents are more toxic if aspirated. Because water-soluble agents are less accurate than barium, some authorities suggest that a negative gastrografin study requires a confirmatory barium swallow.[29,40,41]

Controversy also exists regarding the role of esophagoscopy. Some studies show rigid endoscopy as more sensitive than flexible, but the rigid scope increases the risk of perforation and need for general anesthesia.[3,29] A patient suspected of esophageal injury may undergo numerous sequential testing, usually starting with a gastrografin swallow, followed by a barium swallow, and finally endoscopy, assuming that each study is negative.

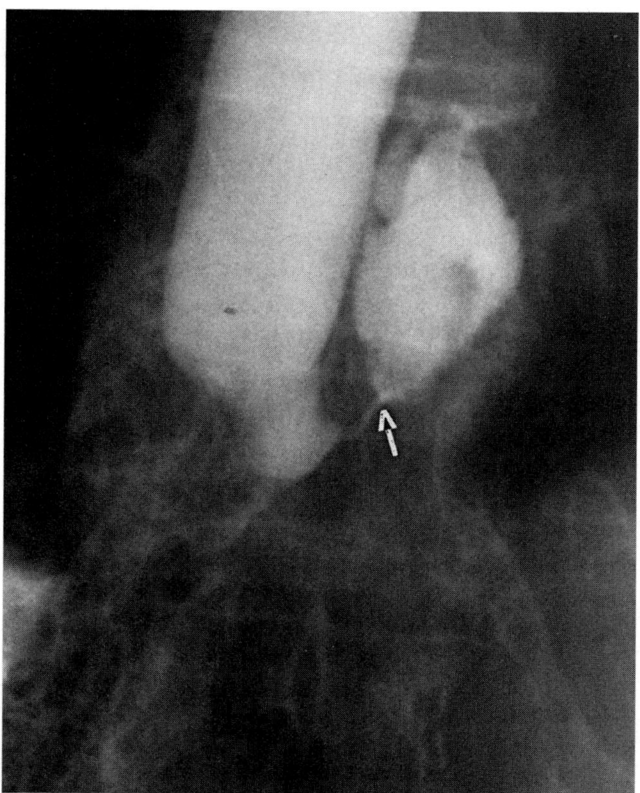

Fig. 16-7 Esophagram showing extravasation and indicating an esophageal injury in a victim of penetrating trauma *(arrow).*

Respiratory Injuries. A change in voice, subcutaneous air, hemoptysis, or respiratory difficulties should prompt airway evaluation.[3,14] Asymptomatic patients without signs of respiratory tract injuries can be observed with or without testing depending on local practice. Studies include direct or indirect laryngoscopy, fiberoptic bronchoscopy, and CT scanning of the airway. Patients with known esophageal injury also require evaluation of the respiratory tract. Conversely, patients with respiratory tract injury must be examined for associated esophageal injury.[17,42]

CONTROVERSIES AND CUTTING EDGE

In the past, all patients with penetrating injuries to zones I and III underwent angiography. Recent data indicate that patients with zone I and III injuries who remain asymptomatic may not require ancillary studies. In one study, 21 asymptomatic patients with zone III injuries were observed without complication or missed injuries.[35] Demetriades et al[23] concluded that neither asymptomatic zone I *nor* zone III injuries require further study. In their series, 82 asymptomatic patients with injuries to zone I or III had no clinically significant injuries if the physical examination was normal (negative predictive value of 100%). All *symptomatic* zone I and III injuries require evaluation of the esophagus and arteries.

DISPOSITION

Consult a surgeon for all patients with injuries that violate the platysma. Unstable patients with severe signs or symptoms need immediate operation. Many stable patients are admitted for a minimum of 24 hours observation. Some surgeons may explore these neck wounds in the operating suite and discharge the patient if the wound proves superficial.

If the platysma is not violated, patients may be safely discharged as long as they have no significant associated injury. Use standard wound care for the superficial neck injuries. Wounds less than 12 hours old and not grossly contaminated may be sutured, but high-risk wounds may be left open to heal by secondary intention. Give tetanus toxoid as indicated.

BLUNT ANTERIOR NECK INJURY

Etiology and Demographics

Blunt trauma to the anterior neck is relatively rare[43,44] and usually results from the so-called "padded dash syndrome" associated with a motor vehicle crash (MVC).[45] This syndrome occurs in the unrestrained, or minimally restrained (lap belt only), front seat occupant in a head-on MVC. On impact, the victim's head moves forward and strikes the windshield while his or her body is held to the seat. This mechanism extends the neck, and exposes the larynx and trachea to the steering wheel or the dashboard.[44-47] The introduction of the shoulder harness in the late 1960s offered some protection against this injury.[45,48,49] Other mechanisms of injury include bicycling accidents where the rider falls forward onto the handlebars, hanging, and strangulation. A particularly lethal mechanism is the "clothesline" injury, where the rider of a motorcycle, snowmobile, or bicycle runs into an unseen wire or tree limb.[46,47,50]

A force applied to the larynx compresses it against the relatively immobile cervical spine. Blunt laryngotracheal injuries can range from soft-tissue edema and ecchymosis to mucosal lacerations, vocal cord avulsion, and arytenoid joint subluxation. Other patterns include recurrent laryngeal nerve damage, fractures of the thyroid and cricoid cartilages, and complete laryngotracheal separation.[47]

Hyperextension and concomitant lateral flexion of the neck stretches the carotid artery. This mechanism can produce rupture of the intima, clot formation, or dissection. Other vascular injuries include pseudoaneurysms and thromboses. Direct trauma to the carotid can occur when a child falls with an object in his or her mouth.[51] Carotid and vertebral injuries may follow coughing, nose blowing, yoga, sports activities, chiropractic manipulation, and neck turning.[51] Fibromuscular dysplasia, Marfan syndrome, syphilis, atherosclerosis, and hypertension-induced intimal thickening all predispose the patient to vascular injury.[51]

Blunt esophageal injuries are rare and are likely associated with laryngotracheal trauma. However, the mortality of a missed esophageal perforation is extremely high.

Clinical Presentation

In blunt trauma, neck injuries are rarely seen in isolation.[46,50] They are often associated with significant wounds that include closed head injury, neck and face fractures, as well as chest and abdominal trauma.[46,47] As with penetrating neck trauma, patients with blunt trauma range from completely asymptomatic to moribund.[50,52] *The absence of soft tissue injuries does not rule out underlying trauma.* Significant injuries to the larynx and carotid arteries occur with minimal soft tissue findings.[50,52]

Patients with injuries to the trachea and larynx can present with subcutaneous emphysema, hoarseness, dysphagia, hemoptysis, or respiratory difficulty.[46,47,50,52,53] Injuries to the laryngotracheal complex include avulsion of the cords, dislocation of the arytenoid cartilage, and disruption of thyroepiglottic ligament. Others may suffer tracheal laceration, mucosal edema, laryngotracheal separation, or vocal cord paralysis.[44] Those with esophageal injury can present similarly.[46]

Blunt carotid or vertebral artery injuries are often unrecognized on admission.[51] Patients who are initially asymptomatic may develop focal or global neurologic deficits hours to months later. Carotid deficits are often straightforward and isolated to the ipsilateral cerebrum. Thus patients often present with aphasia, contralateral hemiplegia, or sensory loss.[51,54-57] Patients with carotid injury may display a **Horner's syndrome** (injury to the sympathetic chain, which winds around the carotid). Auscultation for bruits over the carotid artery in any patient with blunt anterior neck injury is required.

Patients with vertebral artery trauma pose a clinical conundrum. They may complain of vague brainstem symptoms of visual changes, nausea, and vertigo. More puzzling, clinical findings are not referable to the side of injury. Because clot in a vertebral artery must pass through the basilar artery on its way to the brain, emboli from the right vertebral artery can travel to either the right or left posterior circulation. The initial clot can go right while the subsequent clot flows left, jumbling the clinical picture. Patients may have a variety of cranial nerve deficits, or changes in mental status.[51,54,55,57]

Posttraumatic carotid-cavernous fistula can present with audible bruits, exophthalmos, and pulsation of the orbit. Others with this condition may exhibit chemosis, diplopia, visual disturbances, headache, and paresthesias of the face and scalp.[51]

Emergency Department Management

PRIMARY SURVEY

Blunt trauma presents a challenge to airway management. Such patients may suffer airway edema, bleeding, and laryngeal fractures, all of which distort landmarks. Endotracheal intubation and cricothyrotomy may be difficult or impossible. Patients with complete laryngotracheal transection pose additional risks. If such patients are paralyzed with neuromuscular blockade, intubation may be rendered impossible. In the neurologically intact patient, neck muscles support the airway and hold severed ends in alignment. When these muscles relax, the conduit to the lung is lost. If a patient with tracheal disruption is pharmacologically paralyzed, the endotracheal tube will exit the proximal end of a disrupted trachea, and abut the soft tissues of the neck.[58] Patients with blunt anterior neck injury are also more likely to sustain cervical spine trauma.

Any patient in respiratory distress or who is unable to protect his or her airway requires intubation. Prolonged delays in obtaining or protecting the airway may result in progressive hematoma and edema, making intubation difficult and obscuring landmarks for surgical access.[46] Patients who are not intubated early must be carefully monitored for signs of progressive respiratory distress. Consider calling anesthesia for backup in those patients with the potential for distorted anatomy. If the patient requires transfer, secure a problematic airway before transport to a trauma center.

Some authorities believe that endotracheal intubation is the best approach in blunt neck trauma.[44,47] Others contend that it is dangerous, often unsuccessful and instead recommend tracheostomy.[48,50,53,58-60] In emergency practice, this issue is often moot. Endotracheal intubation is immediately life-saving, whereas tracheostomy requires special expertise and precious minutes to perform. Unless a surgeon is *present at the bedside,* tracheostomy is not the airway of choice in those with marked distress. While some debate whether distortion of external landmarks is a *relative* contraindication for cricothyrotomy,[44] this procedure is frequently indispensable. Nasotracheal intubation should be avoided.[46]

Patients with stridor and those with distorted external landmarks may benefit from awake intubation.[52] Preparation is essential to anticipate managing the airway in patients already exhibiting stridor. Place a tracheostomy tube by the bedside and use the techniques previously described.

Breathing is the next priority. Pneumothorax, hemothorax, and pulmonary contusion are common in patients with blunt neck trauma. Tension pneumothorax is the most life-threatening of these conditions and should be diagnosed and treated on clinical grounds. The combination of hypotension, respiratory distress, and unilateral decreased breath sounds should prompt immediate needle thoracentesis and tube thoracostomy.

Blunt neck injury alone rarely presents with shock. However, other injuries such as traumatic aortic injury or hemothorax frequently accompany blunt neck trauma. Assess blood pressure, pulses, and obtain IV access.

Neurologic examination is also important in blunt neck injuries. In addition to searching for signs of intracranial and spinal injury, examine the brachial plexus.

SECONDARY SURVEY

Perform the secondary survey after initial stabilization of the patient. If possible, detail the accident, past medical history, and interview the medics. Specifically determine loss of consciousness, weakness, numbness, neck pain, dysphagia, trouble speaking, shortness of breath, and chest pain. Patients with significant blunt neck trauma require chest, as well as cervical spine, radiographs. The placement of a nasogastric tube is less controversial than in patients with penetrating neck trauma.

Further Evaluation and Treatment

VASCULAR INJURY

Suspect blunt injury to the carotid or vertebral arteries in any patient with a neurologic deficit and a normal CT scan.[51,54,55] These injuries are often initially missed, and patients may develop signs or symptoms months after injury. Most patients with vertebral artery injury or dissection have significant posterior neck pain and occipital headache. Patients with vertebral artery injury may have vague complaints, referable to the posterior circulation, involving vision, gait, or coordination.

Consider a four-vessel angiogram for (1) neurologic findings incompatible with CT scan findings, (2) monoplegia or hemiplegia with normal mental status, (3) signs or complaints of severe cervical trauma with an abnormal neurologic examination (particularly brainstem findings), or (4) basilar skull fracture with persistent alteration of mental status.[51] Magnetic resonance angiography (MRA) may also play a role.[61]

Treatment options for blunt arterial injury remain the purview of the specialist. Interventions may include simple observation, anticoagulation, ligation of the artery, extracranial bypass, or arterial reconstruction.[51,57] In the presence of major cardiac instability or coma, surgical treatment is contraindicated.[51,57,61] Consult the neurosurgeon or the vascular surgeon to determine the need for heparin.[55,57,61] Anticoagulation may prevent propagation or development of a thrombus within the injured vessel. Anticoagulation is more often used with distal lesions that are inaccessible to surgical repair.[57] Many patients with blunt neck trauma are at risk for hemorrhagic complications, particularly those with intracranial lesions. Surgery is generally reserved for minimally symptomatic or asymptomatic patients.[57,61]

PHARYNGOESOPHAGEAL INJURY

There is a close association with esophageal and laryngotracheal injuries. Any patient with signs of one should be evaluated for the other.[50,53]

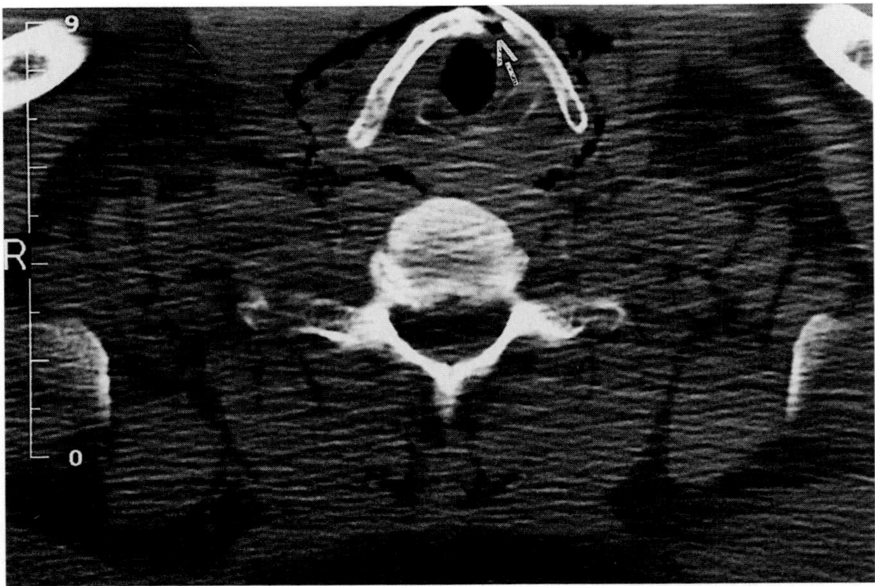

Fig. 16-8 Computed tomography scan of the neck showing a thyroid cartilage fracture *(arrow).*

RESPIRATORY TRACT (LARYNGOTRACHEAL) INJURY

Patients with serious laryngotracheal injuries may have minimal symptoms and trauma to other regions often obscures neck findings.[46,62] Patients with suspected injuries of the respiratory tract require either direct or fiberoptic laryngoscopy.* Endoscopy may reveal edema, mucosal lacerations, hematomas, exposed cartilage, cord disruption, and abnormal landmarks. Laryngeal trauma is well imaged by CT scanning. If patients with hoarseness or subcutaneous air do not require immediate operation or intubation, they may undergo CT scanning of the larynx to identify fractures or dislocations (Fig. 16-8).[43,59,65] Some authors recommend CT scanning for all patients suspected of laryngotracheal injury.[53,63] Indications for surgery include hematemesis, hemoptysis, exposed cartilage, cord paralysis, displaced fractures, or significant mucosal injury.[59] Early treatment will decrease complications and improve outcomes,† whereas delayed repair can lead to infection, distortion of the airway, and increased scarring.[52] All patients should receive humidified oxygen, voice rest, and elevation of the head of the bed if possible. The decision to use antibiotics, steroids, and gastric acid blockers are controversial and should be made in conjunction with the admitting physician.[44,53,56]

*References 48, 52, 53, 58, 59, 63, 64.

†References 48, 50, 53, 59, 64, 66, 67.

Disposition

Any patient with signs or symptoms of laryngotracheal, esophageal, or arterial injury should be observed or admitted. Some authorities suggest at least 24 hours of observation regardless of the results of the diagnostic studies.[46] Asymptomatic patients with a negative evaluation may be safely discharged. All discharged patients must return immediately for any worsening. Patients with significant laryngotracheal injury require a head and neck surgeon, which may require transfer from smaller hospitals. Always protect the airway of such patients before transfer if there are signs of respiratory distress (Fig. 16-9).

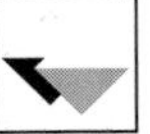

PEARLS & PITFALLS

Penetrating Trauma

- All penetrating neck injuries that violate the platysma need surgical consultation.
- Exploration deep to the platysma should be done in the operating suite by a surgeon.

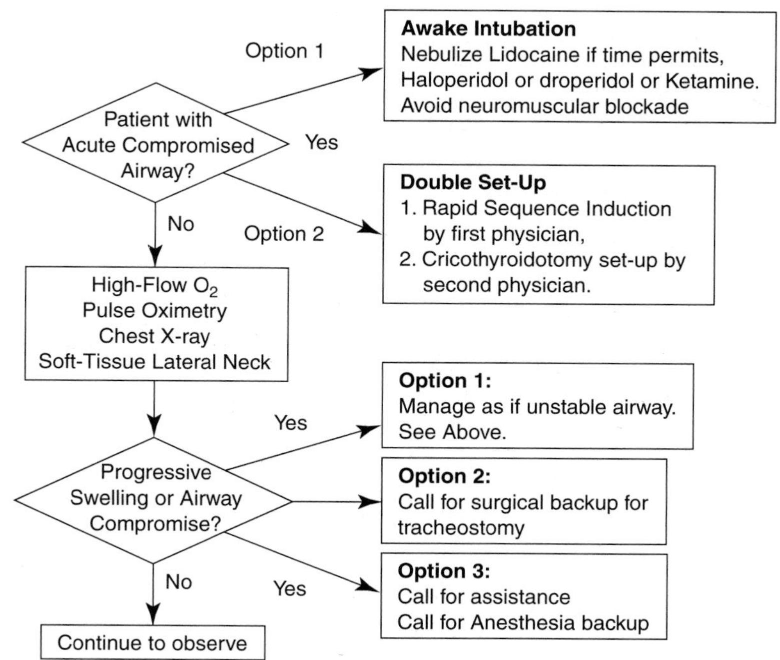

Fig. 16-9 Airway management in blunt trauma.

- Aggressively manage the airway in patients with distress or expanding hematoma. Consider awake intubation and calling for anesthesia backup.
- Avoid blind nasotracheal intubation.
- Zone I and zone III penetrating neck injuries may require angiography, esophagoscopy, esophagography, and laryngoscopy.
- Zone II penetrating neck injuries may be managed by surgical exploration or selectively with diagnostic testing. Angiography and triple endoscopy are often reserved for those with suspicious physical findings.
- Any patient who cannot cooperate with a clinical examination, such as the intoxicated or comatose, needs surgery or an objective test.
- Delay in recognition of esophageal injury leads to increased morbidity and mortality.
- Ask the stable patient to cough and to swallow water or his or her saliva. Listen to the patient's voice for hoarseness and auscultate his or her carotid arteries for bruits.
- Transcervical wounds (those that cross the midline) and shotgun wounds are "high risk." More aggressive testing may be indicated for patients not requiring surgery.

Blunt Trauma

- Suspect blunt vascular injury in a patient with a normal brain CT scan and abnormal neurologic findings.
- Blunt vascular injuries may present with delayed symptoms hours to months after injury.
- Tracheostomy is useful in patients with laryngeal fracture. However, patients in distress require immediate endotracheal intubation or cricothyroidotomy.
- In patients with a compromised airway, consider awake intubation. (Consider nebulized lidocaine, intravenous droperidol, and/or ketamine.)
- CT scanning is an excellent way to image blunt laryngeal injury.

REFERENCES

1. Roon AJ, Christensen N: Evaluation and treatment of penetrating cervical injuries, *J Trauma* 19:391-396, 1979.
2. McConnell DB, Trunkey DD: Management of penetrating trauma to the neck, *Adv Surg* 27:97-127, 1994.
3. Asensio JA, et al: Management of penetrating neck injuries: the controversy surrounding zone II injuries, *Surg Clin North Am* 71:267-296, 1991.
4. Carducci B, Lowe RA, Dalsey W: Penetrating neck trauma: consensus and controversies, *Ann Emerg Med* 15:208-215, 1986.

5. Bishara RA, et al: The necessity of mandatory exploration of penetrating zone II neck injuries, *Surgery* 100:655-660, 1986.
6. Miller RH, Duplechain JK: Penetrating wounds of the neck, *Otolaryngol Clin North Am* 24:15-29, 1991.
7. Narrod JA, Moore EE: Initial management of penetrating neck wounds: a selective approach, *J Emerg Med* 2:17-22, 1984.
8. Balkany TJ, et al: The management of neck injuries. In Zuidema GD, Rutherford RB, Ballinger WF, (editors): *The management of trauma,* ed 4, Philadelphia, 1985, Saunders.
9. Markey JC Jr., Hines JL, Nance FC: Penetrating neck wounds: a review of 218 cases, *Am Surg* 41:77-83, 1975.
10. Campbell WH, Cantrill SV: Neck trauma. In Rosen P, et al (editors): *Emergency medicine: concepts and clinical practice,* ed 3, St Louis, 1992, Mosby.
11. Fogelman MJ, Stewart RD: Penetrating wounds of the neck, *Am J Surg* 91:581-593, 1956.
12. Thal ER, Meyer DM: Penetrating neck trauma, *Curr Prob Surg* 29:1-56, 1992.
13. Sankaran S, Walt AJ: Penetrating wounds of the neck: principles and some controversies, *Surg Clin North Am* 57:139-150, 1977.
14. Eggen JT, Jorden RC: Airway management, penetrating neck trauma, *J Emerg Med* 11:381-385, 1993.
15. Shearer VE, Giesecke AH: Airway management for patients with penetrating neck trauma: a retrospective study, *Anesth Analg* 77:1135-1138, 1993.
16. Pate JW: Tracheobronchial and esophageal injuries, *Surg Clin North Am* 69:111-123, 1989.
17. Demetriades D, et al: Complex problems in penetrating neck trauma, *Surg Clin North Am* 76:661-683, 1996.
18. Demetriades D, et al: Evaluation of penetrating Injuries of the neck: prospective study of 223 patients, *World J Surg* 21:41-48, 1997.
19. Apffelstaedt JP, Muller R: Results of mandatory exploration for penetrating neck trauma, *World J Surg* 18:917-919, 1994.
20. Flint LM, et al: Management of major vascular injuries in the base of the neck: an 11-year experience with 146 cases, *Arch Surg* 106:407-412, 1973.
21. Sclafani SJ, et al: The role of angiography in penetrating neck trauma, *J Trauma* 31:557-562, 1991.
22. Jurkovich GJ, et al: Penetrating neck trauma: diagnostic studies in the asymptomatic patient, *J Trauma* 25:819-822, 1985.
23. Demetriades D, et al: Penetrating injuries of the neck in patients in stable condition: physical examination, angiography, or color flow Doppler imaging, *Arch Surg* 130:971-975, 1995.
24. Ginzburg E, et al: The use of duplex ultrasonography in penetrating neck trauma, *Arch Surg* 131:691-693, 1996.
25. Golueke PJ, et al: Routine versus selective exploration of penetrating neck injuries: a randomized prospective study, *J Trauma* 24:1010-1014, 1984.
26. Sofianos C, et al: Selective surgical management of zone II gunshot injuries of the neck: a prospective study, *Surgery* 120:785-788, 1996.
27. O'Donnell VA, Atik M, Pick RA: Evaluation and management of penetrating wounds of the neck: the role of emergency angiography, *Am J Surg* 138:309-313, 1979.
28. Noyes LD, McSwain NE Jr., Markowitz IP: Panendoscopy with arteriography versus mandatory exploration of penetrating wounds of the neck, *Ann Surg* 204:21-31, 1986.
29. Weigelt JA, et al: Diagnosis of penetrating cervical esophageal injuries, *Am J Surg* 154:619-622, 1987.
30. Meyer JP, et al: Mandatory versus selective exploration for penetrating neck trauma: a prospective assessment, *Arch Surg* 122: 592-597, 1987.
31. McCormick TM, Burch BH: Routine angiographic evaluation of neck and extremity injuries, *J Trauma* 19:384-387, 1979.
32. Demetriades D, Charalambides D, Lakhoo M: Physical examination and selective conservative management in patients with penetrating injuries of the neck, *Br J Surg* 80:1534-1536, 1993.
33. Atteberry LR, et al: Physical examination alone is safe and accurate for evaluation of vascular injuries in penetrating zone II neck trauma, *J Am Coll Surg* 179:657-662, 1994.
34. Menawat SS, et al: Are arteriograms necessary in penetrating zone II neck injuries, *J Vasc Surg* 16:397-400, 1992.
35. Mansour MA, et al: Validating the selective management of penetrating neck wounds, *Am J Surg* 162:517-521, 1991.
36. Beitsch P, et al: Physical examination and arteriography in patients with penetrating zone II neck wounds, *Arch Surg* 129:577-581, 1994.
37. Hall JR, Reyes HM, Meller JL: Penetrating zone-II neck injuries in children, *J Trauma* 31:1614-1617, 1991.
38. Ordog GJ: Penetrating neck trauma, *J Trauma* 27:543-554, 1987.
39. Fry WR, et al: Duplex scanning replaces arteriography and operative exploration in the diagnosis of potential cervical vascular injury, *Am J Surg* 168:693-695, 1994.
40. Bladergroen MR, Lowe JE, Postlethwait RW: Diagnosis and recommended management of esophageal perforation and rupture, *Ann Thorac Surg* 42:235-239, 1986.
41. Richardson JD, et al: Unifying concepts in treatment of esophageal leaks, *Am J Surg* 149:157-161, 1985.
42. Grewal H, et al: Management of penetrating laryngotracheal injuries, *Head Neck* 17:494-502, 1995.
43. Gold SM, et al: Blunt laryngotracheal trauma in children, *Arch Otolaryngol Head Neck Surg* 123:83-87, 1997.
44. Gussack GS, Jurkovich GJ, Luterman A: Laryngotracheal trauma: a protocol approach to a rare injury, *Laryngoscope* 96: 660-665, 1986.
45. Butler RM, Moser FH: The padded dash syndrome: blunt trauma to the larynx and trachea, *Laryngoscope* 78:1172-1182, 1968.
46. Mace SE: Blunt laryngotracheal trauma, *Ann Emerg Med* 15:836-842, 1986.
47. Kadish H, Schunk J, Woodward GA: Blunt pediatric laryngotracheal trauma: case reports and review of the literature, *Am J Emerg Med* 12:207-211, 1994.
48. Yen PT, et al: Clinical analysis of external laryngeal trauma, *J Laryngol Otol* 108:221-225, 1994.
49. Stack. BC Jr, Ridley MB: Arytenoid subluxation from blunt laryngeal trauma, *Am J Otolaryngol* 15:68-73, 1994.
50. Reece GP, Shatney CH: Blunt injury of the cervical trachea: review of 51 patients, *South Med J* 81:1542-1548, 1988.
51. Sanzone AG, Torres H, Doundoulakis SH: Blunt trauma to the carotid arteries, *Am J Emerg Med* 13:327-330, 1995.
52. Camnitz PS, Shepherd SM, Henderson RA: Acute blunt laryngeal and tracheal trauma, *Am J Emerg Med* 5:157-162, 1987.
53. Bent JP, Silver JR, Porubsky ES: Acute laryngeal trauma: a review of 77 patients, *Otolaryngol Head Neck Surg* 109:441-449, 1993.
54. Stringer WL, Kelly DL Jr: Traumatic dissection of the extracranial internal carotid artery, *Neurosurgery* 6:123-130, 1980.
55. Watridge CB, Muhlbauer MS, Lowery RD: Traumatic carotid artery dissection: diagnosis and treatment, *J Neurosurg* 71:854-857, 1989.
56. Frantzen E, Jacobsen HA, Therkelsen J: Cerebral artery occlusions in children due to trauma to the head and neck, *Neurology* 11:695-700, 1961.
57. Pretre R, et al: Blunt carotid artery injury: difficult therapeutic approaches for an under recognized entity, *Surgery* 115:376-381, 1994.
58. Schaefer SD: The acute management of external laryngeal trauma: a 27-year experience, *Arch Otolaryngol Head Neck Surg* 118:598-604, 1992.

59. Fuhrman GM, Stieg FH III, Buerk CA: Blunt laryngeal trauma: classification and management protocol, *J Trauma* 30:87-92, 1990.
60. Snow JB Jr: Diagnosis and therapy for acute laryngeal and tracheal trauma, *Otolaryngol Clin North Am* 17:101-106, 1984.
61. Bok AP, Peter JC: Carotid and vertebral artery occlusion after blunt cervical injury: the role of MR angiography in early diagnosis, *J Trauma* 40:968-972, 1996.
62. Cozzi S, et al: Difficult diagnosis of laryngeal blunt trauma, *J Trauma* 40:845-846, 1996.
63. Bent JP, Porubsky ES: The management of blunt fractures of the thyroid cartilage, *Otolaryngol Head Neck Surg* 110:195-201, 1994.
64. Cherian TA, Rupa V, Raman R: External laryngeal trauma: analysis of thirty cases, *J Laryngol Otol* 107:920-923, 1993.
65. Schaefer SD, Brown OE: Selective application of CT in the management of laryngeal trauma, *Laryngoscope* 93:1473-1475, 1983.
66. Leopold DA: Laryngeal trauma: a historical comparison of treatment methods, *Arch Otolaryngol* 109:106-112, 1983.
67. Ford HR, Gardner MJ, Lynch JM: Laryngotracheal disruption from blunt pediatric neck injury: impact of early recognition and intervention on outcome, *J Pediatr Surg* 30:331-334, 1995.

17 Blunt Chest Trauma

CARLO L. ROSEN AND RICHARD E. WOLFE

TEACHING CASE

A 50-year-old woman was the unrestrained driver in a rollover motor vehicle crash (MVC). The paramedics found her outside of the car. She was unresponsive and underwent orotracheal intubation in the field. On arrival to the emergency department (ED), she had a blood pressure of 142/80 mmHg, a heart rate of 120 beats per minute, and abrasions on her chest and abdomen. She was minimally responsive and did not move her left side to painful stimulus. The initial supine chest radiograph demonstrated a widened mediastinum. The patient underwent head, abdomen, and chest computed tomography (CT) scans that demonstrated an epidural hematoma, a high-grade splenic laceration, and an aortic injury with mediastinal hematoma. The patient was taken to the operating suite and underwent a splenectomy and craniotomy with decompression of her epidural hematoma. While in the operating suite, an arterial line was placed and an esmolol drip was started to maintain a systolic blood pressure of 110 mmHg. After the operation, an aortogram was obtained, which demonstrated an aortic injury at the isthmus. She was taken back to the operating suite for repair of the aorta. After 2 weeks in the hospital she was discharged to a rehabilitation hospital where she made a successful recovery. ■

Blunt chest trauma (BCT) ranges from dramatic injuries to silent killers that present with minimal findings. A sequenced diagnostic approach is essential to successful management. The emergency physician (EP) must recognize and treat time-sensitive emergencies such as tension pneumothorax. The next challenge is to identify the 15% of patients with chest trauma who require surgical intervention.[1] The EP must possess an understanding of the pathophysiology of the different chest injuries and be able to prioritize the necessary studies and emergency procedures. Although chest trauma can be life threatening, most patients who reach the hospital alive will survive with minimal sequelae. The majority of patients who survive the initial insult (85%) can be managed nonoperatively with emergency procedures such as airway management and thoracostomy tube placement.[1] However, most patients with severe chest trauma have associated injuries that require immediate management. Prioritization of interventions both diagnostic and therapeutic becomes especially important. The primary causes of death in these patients are hemorrhagic shock, ventilation failure, and pump failure resulting from cardiogenic or mechanical shock. Box 17-1 lists the variety of blunt chest injuries discussed in this chapter.

EPIDEMIOLOGY

Chest trauma accounts for an estimated 16,000 deaths a year and causes 20% of all trauma deaths. The majority of these injuries are due to MVCs. Chest injuries are the second most common cause of all trauma deaths, after head trauma.[1]

Types of Injury

The incidence of different types of blunt chest injuries depends on the study population and how the injuries are defined. For instance, the reported incidence of blunt myocardial injury ranges widely, from 3% to 75% of all patients with BCT.[2-5] This difference relates to variations in definition, since there is no gold standard for myocardial injury short of autopsy. The most common injury after BCT is rib fracture, occurring in 56% of patients with chest trauma, followed by pneumothorax (PTX) in 40% and pulmonary contusion in 35% of patients. Flail chest occurs in 13% of patients,

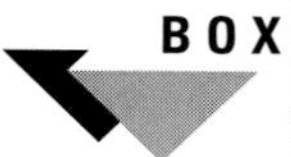

BOX 17-1
Injuries Following Blunt Chest Trauma

CARDIOVASCULAR
Myocardial concussion
Myocardial contusion
Cardiac rupture
Air embolus
Traumatic aortic injury
Aortic fistula
Great vessel injury
Traumatic asphyxia

PULMONARY
Tracheal tear
Bronchial tear
Pneumothorax
Pneumomediastinum and subcutaneous emphysema
Hemothorax
Lung lacerations
Pulmonary contusion
Acute respiratory distress syndrome

CHEST WALL
Rib fractures
Flail chest
Sternal fractures
Thoracic spine fractures

DIAPHRAGMATIC GASTROINTESTINAL
Esophageal injuries

whereas injury to the heart and great vessels occurs in 5% of patients with significant chest trauma.[6] Reports of great vessel injuries range from 4% to 17%.[7] As many as 1% to 6% of all patients with multiple trauma may sustain a diaphragmatic injury.[6,8-11] The incidence of air embolism is 4% after major chest trauma,[12] whereas tracheobronchial injury occurs in 2% of patients with significant chest trauma.[6] Blunt cardiac rupture is a devastating injury, reported in 0.3% to 0.5% of blunt trauma patients admitted to a trauma center.[13,14]

Mortality

A major cause of *immediate* trauma deaths (before arrival to the hospital) is BCT. The most common cause of scene mortality following an MVC or fall is traumatic aortic injury (TAI). Aortic injury accounts for up to 15% of MVC fatalities.[15-17] Seventy-five to ninety percent of patients with TAI die before the arrival of prehospital care providers.[18,19] Between 80% and 90% of deaths caused by blunt cardiac trauma also occur in the prehospital setting and are usually a result of cardiac rupture or dysrhythmias (most commonly ventricular fibrillation).[20] Blunt myocardial injury accounts for up to 15% of all patients who die after major chest trauma.[2,21]

Associated Injuries

Associated injuries occur in 66% to 80% of patients with chest trauma and usually involve the head, abdomen, pelvis, and extremities.[1,6] Certain high-energy injuries such as TAI and diaphragmatic rupture are likely to occur in conjunction with multisystem trauma. Eighty percent of patients with diaphragmatic hernia after blunt trauma have associated injuries, including splenic lacerations (48%), rib fractures (52%), pelvic fractures (52%), and long bone (48%) fractures.[8] Abdominal (35%) and orthopedic (49%) injuries constitute the most frequent concomitant trauma requiring operation.[22]

PATHOPHYSIOLOGY

Most severe injuries associated with BCT are caused by either direct compressive forces or a sudden deceleration. Direct compressive forces damage the chest wall, resulting in rib fractures, flail chest, sternal fractures, or thoracic spine fractures or injure the underlying structures. "Deep" injuries include pulmonary contusion, blunt myocardial injury, esophageal injury, diaphragmatic rupture, and lung laceration. Traumatic asphyxia results from compressive forces. Compression of the thorax causes reflux of the cardiac blood into the superior veins of the head and neck, resulting in capillary rupture and the characteristic petechial lesions.

Deceleration produces traction on vessels as in the case of aortic injury or the trachea in the case of tracheobronchial disruption. Disruption occurs near points of anatomic fixation; most aortic injuries occur near the ligamentum arteriosum, whereas 80% of tracheobronchial injuries occur within 2.5 cm of the carina.[23,24]

Another general mechanism of injury includes the displacement of bony fragments, resulting in damage to other structures. Rib fractures may produce hemothoraces (HTXs) or pneumothoraces (PTXs), or may lacerate abdominal viscera.

CLINICAL PRESENTATION

The clinical presentation of BCT varies from an asymptomatic patient without external signs of trauma to one in severe respiratory distress or shock. Some patients with life-threatening injuries may appear clinically well on arrival to the ED. To diagnose and manage the "silent killers" that result from BCT, the EP must recognize subtle findings on physical examination or diagnostic studies. Nearly half of all patients with TAI,[25,26,27] and up to one third of patients with myocardial contusion,[2,28,29] have no external signs of trauma.

EMERGENCY DEPARTMENT MANAGEMENT

Prehospital Considerations

The primary stabilization of these patients begins with early, aggressive airway management. Needle decompression of the chest is indicated in any patient who has clinical evidence of tension PTX. Potential indications include imminent or full cardiac arrest from blunt torso trauma. If a tension PTX is suspected, then needle-chest decompression should precede intubation.

Once the airway is secured and breathing stabilized, the prehospital providers should focus their attention on the treatment of shock. Although the benefit of immediate aggressive fluid resuscitation of patients with penetrating torso trauma has been questioned,[30] at present there are no clinical studies to suggest that BCT patients should not undergo prehospital fluid resuscitation. Military anti-shock trousers (MAST) have been shown to have no survival benefit in patients with chest trauma and play no role in the management of these patients.[31-33]

Primary Survey

AIRWAY

On arrival, the EP should reassess the "ABCs." Indications for airway management include airway obstruction, failure of ventilation, coma, profound shock, and hypoxia (PaO_2 <60 mmHg on room air at sea level or <80 on 100% oxygen). In the ED, anticipate the future course of the patient's treatment in making airway decisions. An unstable multitrauma patient who will require CT and other radiologic procedures may require intubation to avoid respiratory decompensation while out of the department. Patients with pulmonary contusion or flail chest require high-flow oxygen and, in severe cases, intubation. Elderly patients with a significant pulmonary contusion or flail injury may benefit from early intubation to decrease their work of breathing and maximize oxygenation.[25,34,35]

Rapid sequence intubation (RSI) has become the most widely used and recommended airway technique in the ED for trauma patients.[36,37] Patients who decompensate immediately after intubation may have venous air embolism.[38]

BREATHING

The need for emergent chest decompression should be determined *before obtaining any radiographic studies.* Tension PTX requires chest decompression via needle thoracostomy or tube thoracostomy; needle decompression is theoretically helpful when tension PTX is suspected and the thoracostomy kit is not immediately available (see Chapter 51). Specific indications include shock or profound respiratory distress in a patient with unilateral decreased breath sounds or subcutaneous emphysema. The technique involves the placement of a 14-gauge angiocatheter into the pleural space. The needle should be inserted *over* the fifth rib at the midaxillary line or over the second rib in the midclavicular line.[39] The catheter should be left in place until tube thoracostomy is performed.

If a patient suspected of having a simple PTX or HTX is hemodynamically stable without respiratory distress *and* chest radiography is immediately available, then tube thoracostomy can be delayed until the radiograph is performed. In patients with BCT and suspected HTX, a large chest tube (36 to 40 French) should be placed to allow drainage of blood and clots. The tube should be inserted over the top of the rib at the fifth intercostal space (midaxillary line) to avoid the neurovascular bundle. A gloved finger should be used to extend the opening in the skin and verify the absence of adhesions and position within the thorax. The tube is then advanced superiorly and posteriorly until all holes are within the pleural cavity.[40] In patients with suspected diaphragmatic injury, a finger sweep should be performed once inside the thoracic cavity to prevent placement of the tube into bowel. If the tube can be twisted smoothly without resistance after insertion, it is not kinked. Patients with a large HTX that is not adequately drained by the first chest tube or those with a persistent air leak may require a second chest tube.

CIRCULATION

The initial management of shock includes ensuring intravenous (IV) access with two large-bore lines followed by the administration of crystalloid, then blood as needed.[39] Although excessive fluid resuscitation is often considered to be dangerous in patients with pulmonary contusion, there are little data to support this belief. In patients with massive HTX, autotransfusion of blood removed via tube thoracostomy can reduce the need for stored-blood transfusion. Prior preparation and training of the ED staff in autotransfusion techniques can streamline this procedure.[41]

Central line placement with central venous pressure (CVP) monitoring can help guide fluid management and provides rapid clues to cardiac tamponade. A CVP of greater than 15 cm H_2O suggests tamponade.[42] The CVP line can also be used for rapid fluid administration.

Secondary Survey

HISTORY

Historical information obtained from medics and the patient can help the EP direct the ED evaluation. For instance, a rapid deceleration or high-speed impact is associated with aortic disruption. In a recent study, MVCs caused 81% of TAI; of these, the accident was head-on impact in 72%, side impact in 24%, and rear impact in only 4%.[43] The driver and any ejected occupant are at greater risk for aortic trauma than a restrained passenger.

The history of damage to the steering wheel is also significant. Direct compressive force to the anterior chest is a common precipitant of blunt myocardial injury, as well as flail chest and rib fractures. The reported mechanism for blunt diaphragmatic injuries are MVCs in 86% of patients, auto-pedestrian accidents in 4%, falls in 3%, motorcycle crashes in 3%, and crush injuries in 3%.[9,44]

Symptoms may be absent or minimal in patients with altered mentation from alcohol, drugs, or head injury. Patients with distracting injuries and those with spinal cord damage may not complain of chest pain or shortness of breath despite notable pathologic conditions. Some victims of trauma with normal mentation remain asymptomatic despite having life-threatening injuries.

Chest pain is one of the most common features of BCT. In the case of PTX or HTX, pneumomediastinum, and rib or sternal fractures, pain is likely pleuritic. Patients with myocardial contusion or air embolus may have anginalike chest pain, which can radiate to the back, abdomen, or arms. Pain from TAI is often interscapular or retrosternal.[45,46] Chest or neck pain that increases with swallowing or neck flexion characterizes esophageal injury.[25,47] Although dysphagia often indicates either TAI or esophageal injury, subcutaneous air in the neck from any cause may precipitate this complaint.

Abdominal pain is frequent in patients with chest trauma. Pain may signal injury to abdominal viscera, in particular, the liver or spleen. Those with diaphragmatic herniation can also present with upper abdominal pain. Some patients with PTX or HTX may have pleuritic pain referred to the upper abdomen.

The second most common *symptom* is dyspnea, which can be caused by hypoxia, ventilatory insufficiency, or shock. Causes of hypoxia include pulmonary contusion, tracheobronchial injury, PTX, and HTX. Mechanical problems such as tension PTX or a flail chest may produce ventilatory insufficiency. Traumatic aortic injury may also cause dyspnea as a result of concomitant hemothorax or shock.

PHYSICAL EXAMINATION

Vital Signs. The *clinical signs* of BCT begin with vital signs, which should include pulse oximetry (the "fifth" vital sign). Signs of shock such as hypotension and tachycardia are evidence of hemorrhage, cardiac tamponade, venous air embolus, or tension PTX. Hemodynamic collapse or cardiac arrest immediately after intubation is characteristic of venous air embolus or tension PTX.[12]

Tachycardia is common in blunt myocardial injury, present in 41% of patients.[48] An irregular heart rate may occur in patients who develop atrial fibrillation from blunt myocardial injury or in those with a preexisting dysrhythmia.

Numerous injuries may cause hypotension in the patient with chest trauma. Although patients with TAI may be hypotensive on presentation, associated injuries are usually responsible for hemodynamic instability unless a massive hemothorax is present. Isolated aortic injury rarely results in hypotension, until patients suffer free rupture into the chest or, rarely, the pericardium. Pulsus paradoxus (a drop in systolic blood pressure of greater than 10 mmHg during inspiration) may be present in patients with cardiac tamponade after cardiac rupture.[49] However, this finding is difficult to appreciate in patients who are in shock.

Hypertension is rare after trauma, but TAI is one of the few causes. Patients with isolated TAI frequently are hypertensive. Less commonly, patients with TAI may have the pseudocoarctation syndrome (hypertension in the upper extremities and weak or absent pulses in the lower extremities).[25]

An increased respiratory rate is a sensitive, yet nonspecific marker of chest injury, indicating shock, hypoxia, or ventilatory insufficiency. Causes include PTX, HTX, pulmonary contusion, flail chest, TAI, blunt myocardial injury, and pericardial tamponade. Perform continuous pulse oximetry on all patients with significant BCT. Decreasing oxygen saturation may precede clinical decompensation and is one of the first abnormal signs in patients with tension PTX, before other changes in vital signs.[50]

Skin. Hypoxia from any cause may produce cyanosis. Other skin findings after BCT include the deep violet color of the skin of the head and neck in patients with traumatic asphyxia or venous obstruction caused by neck or mediastinal injury.[51]

Head and Neck. Other head and eye findings in patients with traumatic asphyxia include subconjunctival petechial hemorrhages, retinal edema, and facial edema.[12,52] Use an ophthalmoscope to look for bubbles in the retinal vessels in patients who might have air embolism.[12]

On examination of the neck, jugular venous distension (JVD) indicates life-threatening chest trauma. JVD occurs with tension PTX, cardiac tamponade, venous air embolism, blunt myocardial injury, congestive heart failure, and tricuspid valve rupture. Neck veins may remain flat despite any of these conditions, as a result of associated hemorrhagic shock.

Subcutaneous emphysema in the neck suggests PTX, pneumomediastinum, or a tear in the tracheobronchial tree and is best felt at the root of the neck. Swelling at the base of the neck, diminished carotid pulses, and neck bruits can accompany TAI. Stridor is a sign of upper airway obstruction or compression of the laryngeal nerve, which can occur in patients with TAI.[25,26] Tracheal deviation is a late sign of tension PTX.

Heart and Lungs

Inspection. Chest inspection may reveal ecchymosis, chest wall deformities, and abnormal chest wall movement. Flail chest is defined as the presence of three or more ribs fractured in two or more places, resulting in a freely mobile segment. The EP may overlook the flail segment if not assiduous in the examination, or in the conscious patient who is splinting. Indeed, 31% of these injuries remain unrecognized during the first 6 hours after injury.[53]

Palpation and Percussion. On palpation of the chest, subcutaneous emphysema may be present, indicating the presence of an underlying PTX or tracheobronchial injury.[54-56] Chest wall tenderness is routine in patients with rib fractures, which may be associated with underlying lung or abdominal injury. The chest should be gently compressed in both the lateral and anteroposterior directions to elicit localized pain and crepitus, and to determine chest wall stability. Both decreased tactile fremitus and dullness to percussion can occur with HTX, whereas unilateral hyperresonance usually indicates PTX.

Auscultation. Although decreased breath sounds usually signify PTX, HTX, or unilateral bronchial disruption, splinting results in a similar disparity. Another cause of unilateral loss of breath sounds is mainstem intubation. Since nearly all mainstem intubations involve the right mainstem, this condition results in decreased breath sounds on the left. To confirm proper placement of the endotracheal tube, the EP should ensure that the tube is no deeper than 21 cm in women or 23 cm in men, measured from the teeth.[57]

Patients with pulmonary contusion can have rales or diminished breath sounds, whereas bowel sounds in the chest suggest diaphragmatic herniation.[58,59]

Cardiac auscultation is difficult in the tumult of the trauma room. Patients with cardiac tamponade may have muffled heart sounds. Murmurs may provide important clues to injury, but without access to prior medical records, it is usually impossible to distinguish a new significant murmur from a chronic one. However, certain trauma-associated murmurs are unique. Turbulent blood flow across an aortic injury causes a harsh systolic cardiac murmur over the precordium or posterior intrascapular area, heard in as many as 26% of patients with TAI.[42,45] In patients with venous air embolism, air in the right atrium generates a "mill-wheel" cardiac murmur.[60-63] Although patients with cardiac valvular injuries can have either systolic or diastolic murmurs, a complete rupture of a papillary muscle may remain silent. A Hamman's crunch (crepitus heard during systole on auscultation of the heart) indicates air in either the pericardium or mediastinum.

Emergency Interventions

PERICARDIOCENTESIS

In the setting of trauma, pericardiocentesis is primarily a therapeutic rather than a diagnostic procedure. It may be falsely negative as a result of clotted blood in the pericardial sac. The primary indication is for decompression of pericardial tamponade in the setting of cardiac rupture. Another potential use of this technique is for aspiration of air from the pericardial sac in patients with tension pneumopericardium.[53] The technique involves the subxiphoid insertion of a 6-inch needle pointing towards the left shoulder at a 45° angle. If a pericardiocentesis needle is not available, a lumbar puncture needle can be used (see Chapter 51). A positive pericardiocentesis is an indication for operative thoracotomy. If the patient is in arrest, then emergency department thoracotomy is indicated.

EMERGENCY DEPARTMENT THORACOTOMY

Although resuscitative thoracotomy is primarily indicated in patients in extremis or arrest after penetrating chest trauma, recent data suggest a potential role in the management of BCT as well.[64] There are several potential benefits of performing ED thoracotomy. The initial goal of the procedure is to relieve pericardial tamponade via pericardotomy and then inspect the heart for cardiac injuries. Aortic cross-clamping increases coronary and cerebral perfusion in cases of gross hemorrhage, whereas cross-clamping the pulmonary hilum can control pulmonary exsanguination. The lungs can be inspected for injuries

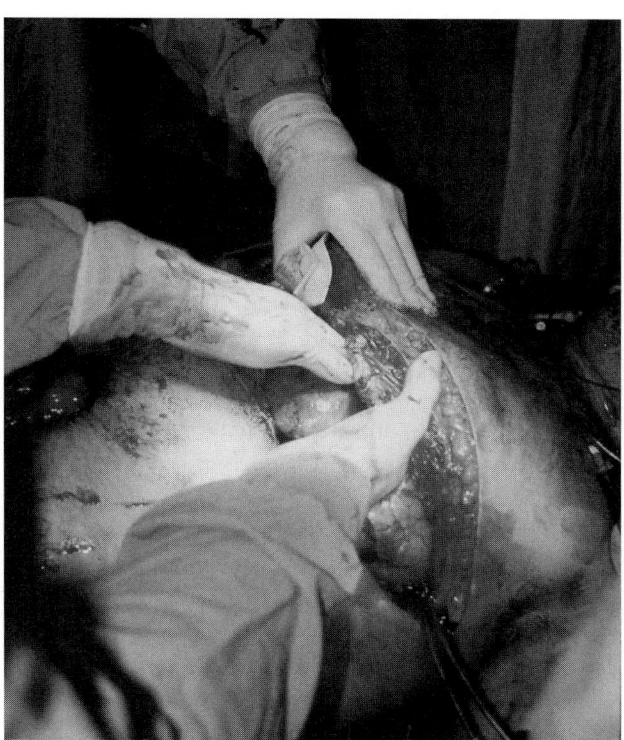

Fig. 17-1 Left thoracotomy.

during cardiac massage.[65] Finally, open-chest cardiopulmonary resuscitation with cardiac massage (Fig. 17-1) is more effective in generating cardiac output and coronary perfusion pressure than closed chest compressions.[42,66-69]

Factors associated with improved survival after ED thoracotomy include the presence of vital signs in the field, penetrating trauma, sinus rhythm or ventricular fibrillation on arrival to the ED, and pericardial tamponade.[70-72] However, in the largest series of resuscitative thoracotomy patients (950 patients), the rate of survival to discharge with good neurologic outcome was only 1% for all blunt trauma patients. The survival for patients with BCT was 2% (two patients), but one patient had significant neurologic sequelae. Based on these results, the authors recommend that ED thoracotomy for blunt trauma patients only be performed in those patients who have vital signs in the field and arrest in the ED or in patients who lose vital signs en route but have cardiac electrical activity in the ED.[64] Even with these caveats, the prognosis for blunt trauma arrest is grim. The negative aspects of ED thoracotomy such as cost, resource utilization, and risk of HIV transmission to healthcare personnel must be weighed against the remote benefits. The main risk is blood exposure to the healthcare workers performing the procedure. The estimated cost per life saved for ongoing medical care after ED thoracotomy ranges from $93,175 in a study published in 1994[72] to $140,811 in a report in 1991.[73] However, these figures may exaggerate the potential benefit of ED thoracotomy since they are based mostly on patients with *penetrating* trauma.

Another potential indication for ED thoracotomy is suspected venous air embolism, which may occur in patients with blunt lacerations of the lung parenchyma. Definitive treatment involves thoracotomy with aspiration of the ventricles to remove the air.[74] To prevent further embolization of air, the hilum on the side of the lung injury can be clamped. Thoracotomy for suspected air embolism should be performed in the ED only if the patient is moribund and immediate transport to the operating suite is impractical.

EMERGENCY DEPARTMENT EVALUATION

Laboratory Tests

HEMOGLOBIN/HEMATOCRIT

Few laboratory tests are helpful in the work-up of patients with BCT. Order a hematocrit in all major trauma patients, although recognize that the initial value may be falsely normal because of the lag between acute hemorrhage and anemia. Fluid resuscitation and intravascular fluid shifts may alter the hematocrit and diminish the utility of serial hematocrits.

CARDIAC ENZYMES

See the following section on myocardial injury.

Electrocardiography

Electrocardiography (ECG) is the best initial test available in the ED for patients with suspected blunt myocardial injury. Any patient with external evidence of precordial trauma, such as ecchymoses or contusions, sternal tenderness, or radiographic evidence of sternal fracture may benefit from an ECG. Furthermore, an ECG should be performed on any patient with ischemic-type chest pain.

Conduction system abnormalities are important findings in patient with possible myocardial injury. Right bundle branch block occurs more frequently than left bundle branch block and advanced heart block is an ominous sign. Nonspecific ST and T-wave changes are common.[75]

The incidence of clinically significant dysrhythmias in blunt myocardial injury is overestimated. Most life-threatening dysrhythmias occur within 24 hours of trauma,[76] and premature ventricular tachycardias or premature atrial tachycardias are the most common findings.[77,78] Other dysrhythmias such as atrial fibril-

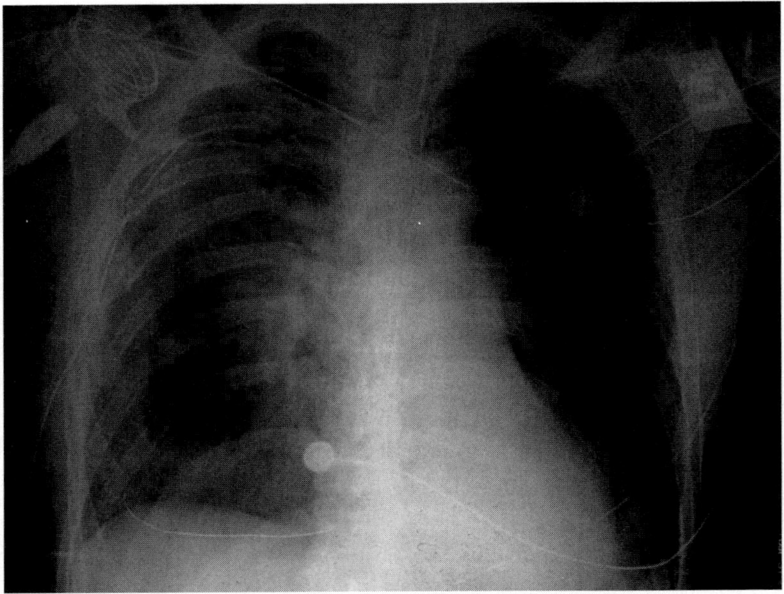

Fig. 17-2 Chest radiograph illustrating right flail chest.

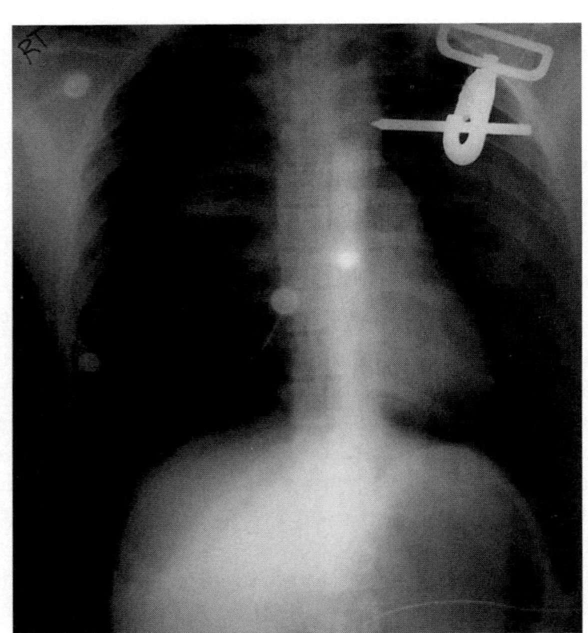

Fig. 17-3 Chest radiograph of bilateral pneumothoraces.

lation, atrial flutter, ventricular tachycardia, or ventricular fibrillation are less common.

The dysrhythmias in patients with BCT may also result from other causes such as hypoxia, intracranial injury, hypovolemia, or electrolyte abnormalities. Electrical alternans is a rare finding sometimes seen in patients with pericardial tamponade.

Although the ECG is the best initial test for myocardial injury, it is neither sensitive nor specific. Although the right heart is usually injured, the ECG is insensitive for right heart damage.[77] In a recent study of 17 patients with myocardial injury, the ECG was abnormal in 12 patients. Two of the patients had a normal ECG, and three had sinus tachycardia.[76]

Plain-Film Radiographs

The supine chest radiograph (CXR) should be the initial ancillary study ordered in the patient with BCT. The CXR may demonstrate rib fractures, flail chest (Fig. 17-2), sternal fractures, PTX (Fig. 17-3), pulmonary contusion (Fig. 17-4), pneumomediastinum, pneumopericardium (Fig. 17-5), or HTX. It may also show findings consistent with TAI (Fig. 17-6) or diaphragmatic hernia (Fig. 17-7). In patients with a widened mediastinum on a supine CXR, obtain an upright CXR if clinically feasible. Almost 40% of patients with an abnormal mediastinum on supine CXR have a normal mediastinum on an upright chest radiograph.[79] The upright CXR has a sensitivity of 79% for detecting serious chest injuries, whereas the supine CXR is 58% sensitive for chest pathology.[80] Both pneumothorax and hemothorax are best appreciated on an upright film. Although the diagnosis of tension PTX should be clinical, many cases are diagnosed by CXR

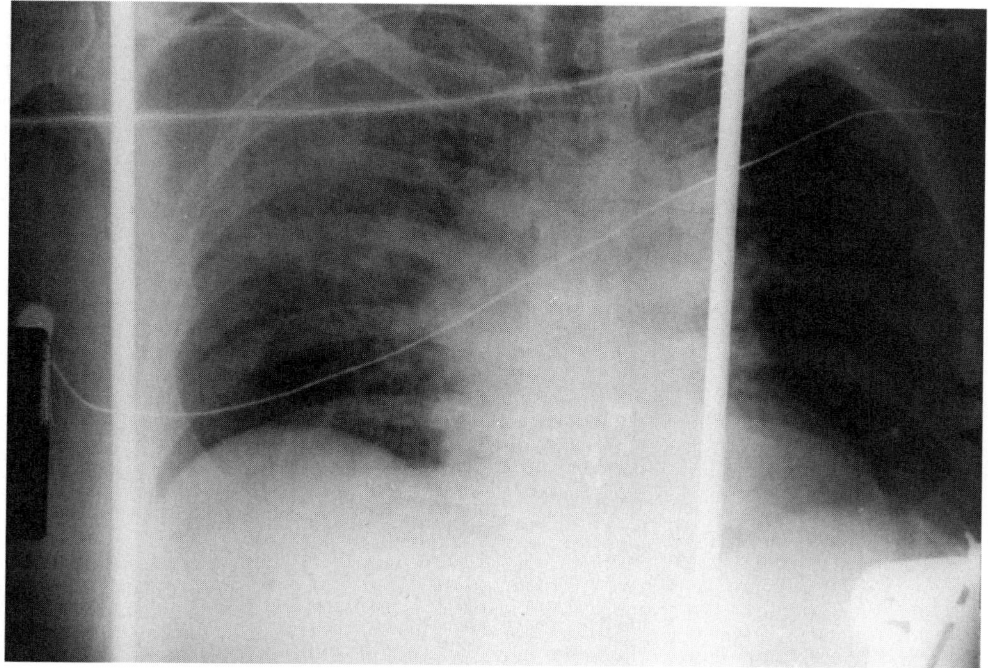

Fig. 17-4 Chest radiograph of right pulmonary contusion.

(Fig. 17-8). The lateral view or specific sternal views are beneficial only if sternal fracture is suspected.

The radiographic findings of pulmonary contusion, which may be present initially or within 4 to 6 hours of the injury, include areas of opacification that range from patchy alveolar infiltrates to frank consolidation. Plain-film radiography is not as sensitive as CT for diagnosing pulmonary contusion (Fig. 17-9). In the acute setting, CXR detects 23% to 38% of pulmonary contusions; however, those seen on plain films are more likely to be clinically significant.[81,82]

The most common radiographic finding of ruptured diaphragm is an elevated hemidiaphragm. CXR findings consistent with the diagnosis of diaphragmatic injury include a stomach bubble or intestinal air in the chest. Placing a nasogastric tube before obtaining a chest film may reveal a tube curled in an intrathoracic stomach. Diaphragmatic rupture is often associated with PTX, atelectasis, or pleural thickening.[83,59] However, at least 15% of patients with diaphragmatic injury have a normal CXR.[59]

Although the cardiac silhouette may provide clues to myocardial rupture, cardiac injury is almost never diagnosed on a plain film. Suggestive findings include pneumopericardium and a widened cardiac silhouette.

The initial CXR is important in the diagnosis of TAI. The most sensitive sign is the widened mediastinum. A widened mediastinum is defined as >6 cm at the level of the aortic knob on the posteroanterior view and >8 cm on the supine anteroposterior view.[84] The sensitivity of CXR for detecting aortic injury based on the finding of a widened mediastinum ranges from 50% to 92%. The specificity is low (10%) since there are other causes of a widened mediasti-

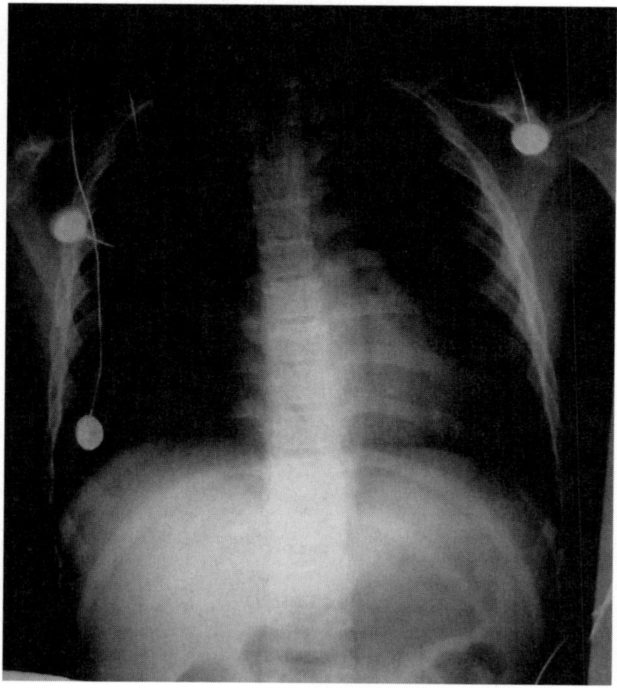

Fig. 17-5 Chest radiograph of pneumopericardium.

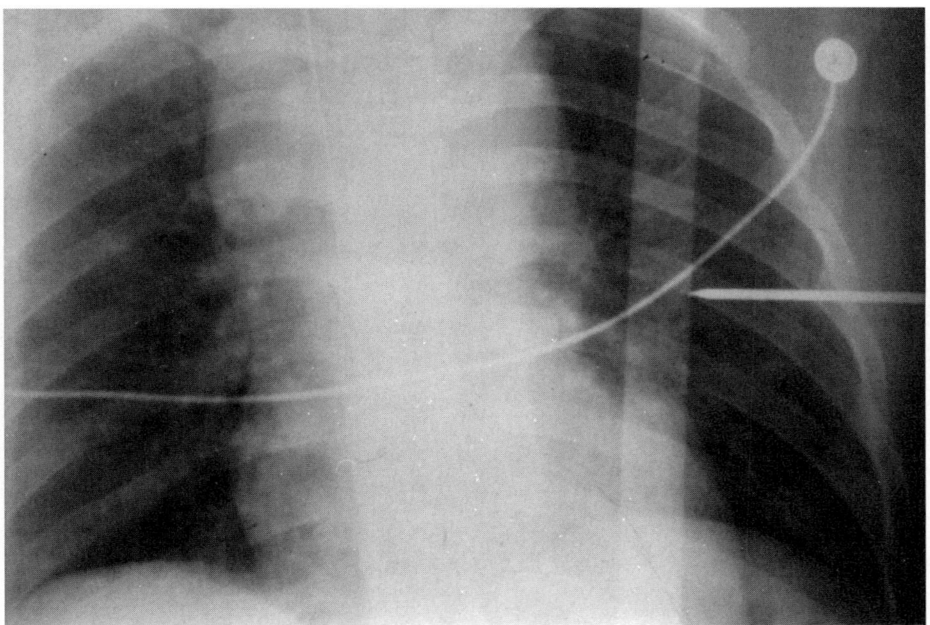

Fig. 17-6 Chest radiograph of wide mediastinum.

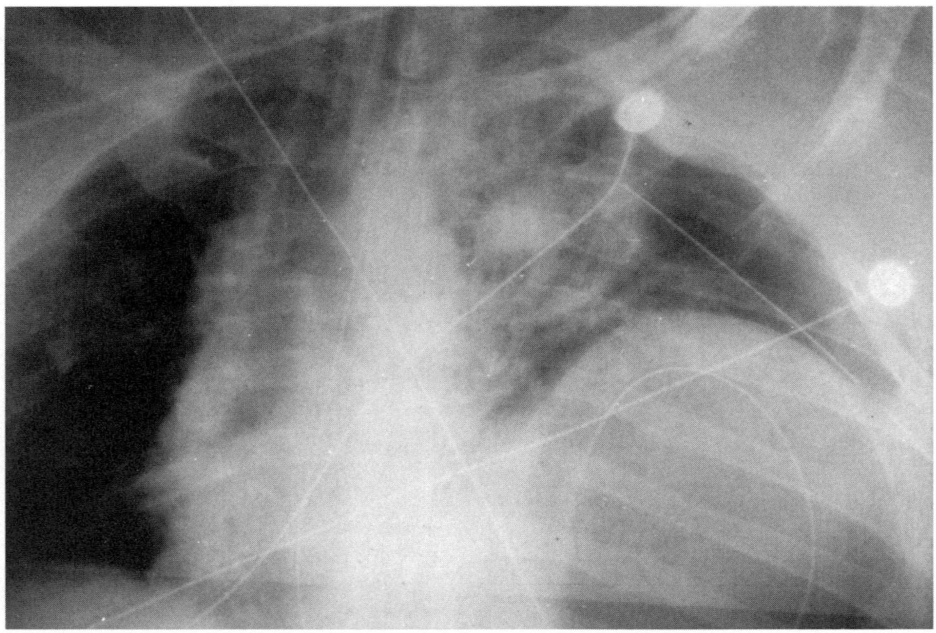

Fig. 17-7 Chest radiograph of left diaphragmatic rupture.

num, such as the technical limitations of the supine CXR, spinal fractures, rib fractures, sternal fractures, or pulmonary contusions.[27,45,79,85-92] There is wide variation in the normal width of the mediastinum with inspiration versus expiration and with the supine versus the erect position.[93]

Other findings on CXR suggestive of a TAI are obliteration of the aortic knob, tracheal deviation to the right, left apical pleural cap, elevation and rightward deviation of the right mainstem bronchus, depression of the left mainstem bronchus, deviation of the nasogastric tube to the right (Fig. 17-10), left HTX,

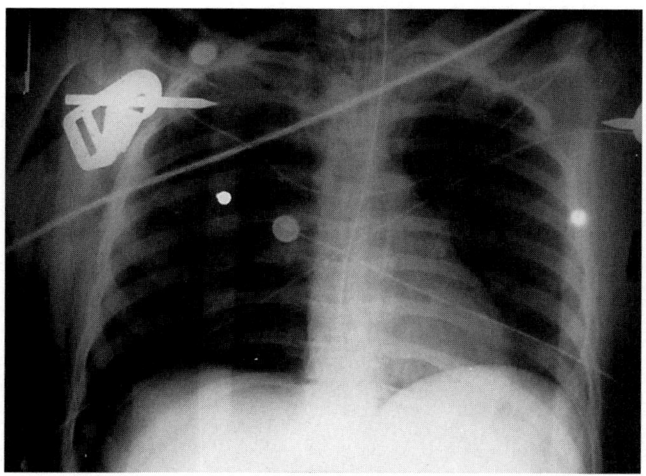

Fig. 17-8 Chest radiograph illustrating right deep sulcus, right pneumothorax, and mediastinal shift to the left.

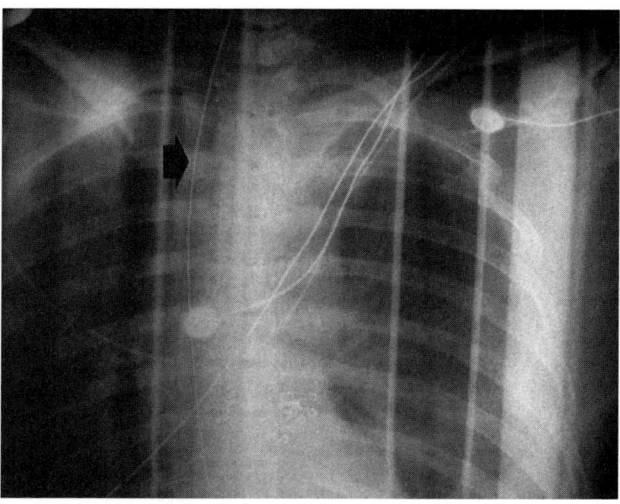

Fig. 17-10 Chest radiograph shows deviation of nasogastric tube to the right *(arrowhead).*

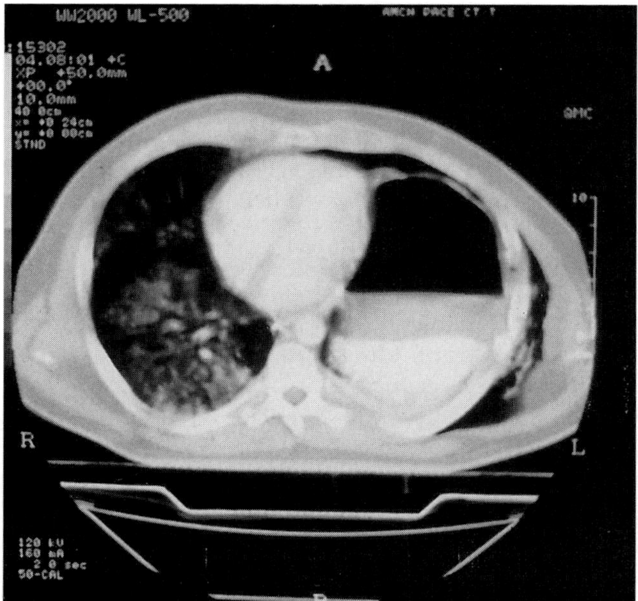

Fig. 17-9 Computed tomography of right pulmonary contusion and left ruptured hemidiaphragm.

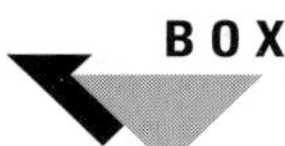

BOX 17-2

Chest Radiographic Findings Suggesting Traumatic Aortic Injury

- Widened mediastinum
- Obliteration of the aortic knob
- Tracheal deviation to the right
- Left apical pleural cap
- Elevation and rightward deviation of the right mainstem bronchus
- Depression of the left mainstem bronchus
- Deviation of the nasogastric tube to the right
- Left hemothorax
- Obliteration of the space between the pulmonary artery and the aorta
- Widened paratracheal stripe
- Sternal fractures
- Upper rib fractures
- Thoracic spine fractures

obliteration of the space between the pulmonary artery and the aorta, and a widened paratracheal stripe.[79] Box 17-2 summarizes the chest radiographic findings for TAI.

A recent multicenter study of 274 patients with aortic injury found that 7% had a normal initial CXR.[43] A normal chest film is less reassuring in the elderly. In one study, two thirds of patients with TAI who were over 65 years of age had a normal mediastinum on CXR.[86] In spite of these limitations, the initial CXR and the mechanism of injury often determine the need to further evaluate the aorta. Specifically, any patient

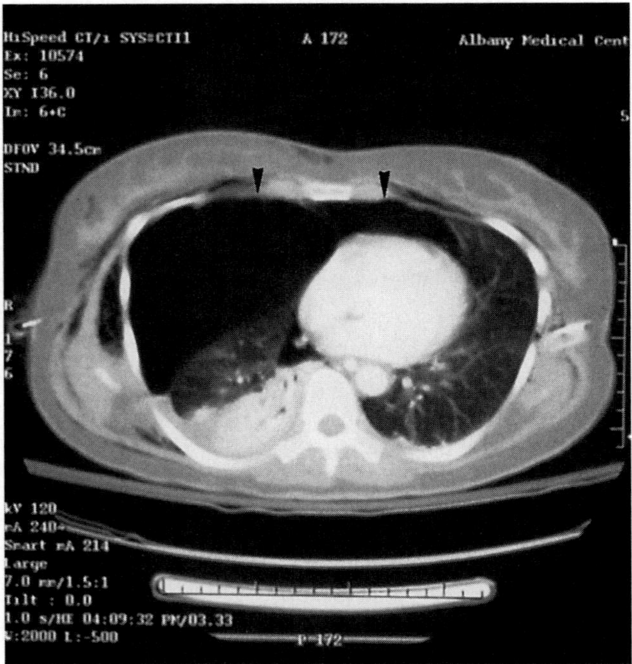

Fig. 17-11 Computed tomography of bilateral pneumothoraces *(arrowheads).*

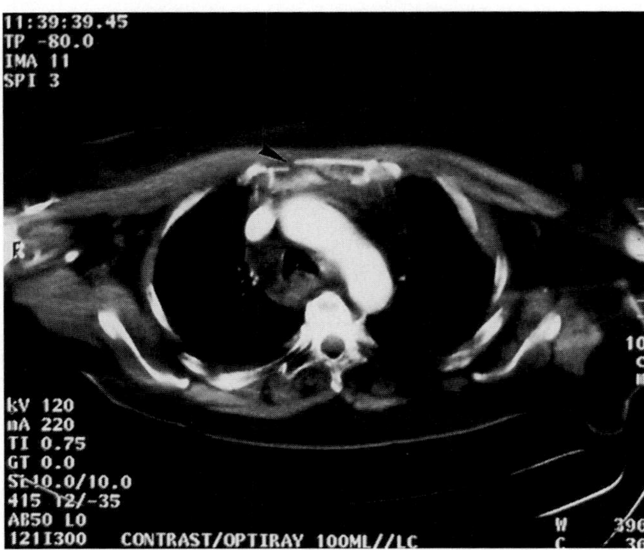

Fig. 17-12 Computed tomography of sternal fracture *(arrowhead).*

with a suggestive finding on CXR such as a widened mediastinum or one of the other findings described previously or a significant deceleration mechanism (fall from a height or head-on impact MVC) should undergo further testing with helical chest CT, TEE, or aortography.

Computed Tomography

The primary indication for chest CT is suspected TAI. After the CXR, helical chest CT has become the initial screening study of choice for this condition. Helical CT is rapid and can image the abdomen and head in the multitrauma patient. The helical CT (as opposed to older generation technology) has significantly improved the efficiency and speed with which aortic injuries are detected.[43,94,95]

Computed tomography can also be used to detect other chest injuries. It provides more specific information and may be more sensitive for other injuries such as pulmonary contusion, diaphragmatic injury (Fig. 17-9), PTX (Fig. 17-11), HTX, rib fractures, and sternal fractures (Fig. 17-12) than CXR. Bowel and other abdominal contents may be seen in the chest as a result of diaphragm herniation, and CT evidence of pulmonary contusion may also prompt cautious use of intravenous fluids. Chest CT is sensitive for hemopericardium and provides an alternative when echocardiography is not available. In one recent study, the sensitivity, specificity, and accuracy for detecting hemopericardium in stable patients were 100%, 97%, and 97%, respectively.[96] Chest CT demonstrates 3 to 4 times as many abnormalities than do plain films of the chest.[97,98] However, in the acute setting, this additional information may be superfluous, since it rarely changes management.

Trupka et al[97] performed a prospective study to examine the role of IV contrast–enhanced CT of the chest in 103 patients with BCT. Chest CT demonstrated important findings in 65% of patients, including pulmonary contusions in 32%, PTX in 26%, and HTX in 20%. Many of these injuries were not apparent on the CXR. In 41% of patients, there was a change in management based on the CT result, including tube thoracostomy placement in 30%. The authors concluded that CT should be used early in the evaluation of patients with severe injuries and suspected chest trauma. However, this study did not examine whether or not the changes in management were justified. Furthermore, the mere presence of a PTX (as opposed to a clinically significant PTX) prompted chest tube insertion. This fact is emphasized by another study regarding the utility of routine chest CT in blunt torso trauma, which found its utility minimal.[98]

The management implication of a PTX detected only by CT has been studied. Patients who are receiving positive pressure ventilation or who will be transferred to another hospital are at risk of developing a tension PTX and should undergo tube thoracostomy.[99] Other studies show that not all pneumothoraces seen on CT require tube thoracostomy.[100,101]

Chest CT is valuable to answer a specific question, such as whether or not there is a mediastinal hematoma or a posterior clavicular dislocation. Computed tomography is an excellent study to evaluate suspected posterior sternoclavicular dislocation. However, its use as a routine test to detect other injuries such as rib fractures and even pulmonary contusions is not indicated, since in most cases it does not lead to a change in management.

The disadvantages of chest CT involve time constraints (including transport, set-up, and expert interpretation), expense, and the need to move the patient to an environment where monitoring and resuscitation are problematic. In general, CT is not an accurate test for diaphragmatic herniation. Finally, there is an associated risk of dye reaction.

The primary finding on chest CT suggestive of TAI is mediastinal hematoma, which is nonspecific. Numerous injuries produce mediastinal hematoma including sternal, spinal, and rib fractures. Only 25% to 30% of patients with mediastinal hematoma actually have an aortic injury.[102,103] Direct evidence of the aortic injury, such as an intimal flap (Fig. 17-13) or vessel contour abnormality, may be seen on CT. However, this finding is not as common as mediastinal hematoma. Atherosclerotic disease or a prominent ductus diverticulum may cause false-positive results.

Chest CT has a sensitivity of 74% to 100% and a specificity of 23% to 100% for detecting TAI; the worst performances were found in older generation machines.[43,94,102-105] More recent studies utilizing helical CT report sensitivities and negative predictive values of 100%.[95,106] When interpreted by a radiologist experienced in reading helical chest CTs, this technique can decrease aortography by 67%.[104]

The finding of mediastinal hematoma by CT usually mandates aortography. If the CT scan is indeterminate, then aortography should be performed to rule out TAI. However, in the face of a diagnostic helical CT (actual visualization of an intimal flap), a cardiothoracic surgeon may proceed directly to operation. If the helical scan of the aorta and mediastinum is completely normal and clinical suspicion is low, then no further testing is necessary. Whenever the physician continues to suspect aortic injury, the patient should proceed directly to aortography.

Three-dimensional CT angiography can also be used to detect TAI.[107] Multiple thin cuts are taken through the aorta during the injection of iodinated contrast, and three-dimensional reconstructions are then produced. CT angiography may not be more accurate than axial helical CT for detecting TAI.[105] However, in certain circumstances, CT angiography may help define the aortic injury already detected by helical CT. Although CT angiography has not replaced traditional aortography, the advantages of this new technique are that it is faster and can be performed in the radiology suite as other CTs are acquired.

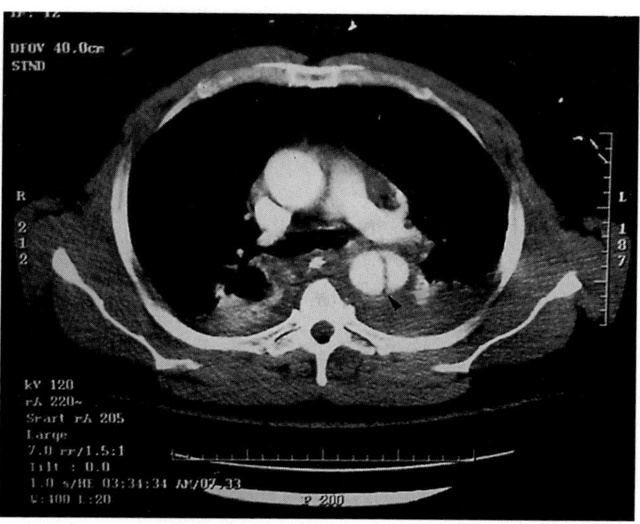

Fig. 17-13 Computed tomography of traumatic aortic intraluminal defect *(arrowhead).*

Transthoracic Echocardiography

In the emergency department, the main use of transthoracic echocardiography (TTE) is for the diagnosis of pericardial tamponade in an unstable patient with myocardial rupture. Bedside echocardiography (ECHO) is an extension of the FAST examination (Focused Assessment for the Sonographic Examination of the Trauma Patient) and can be performed with a high degree of accuracy by the EP or surgeon. In a recent study, bedside ECHO proved 98% sensitive and 100% specific for tamponade.[108] Bedside ultrasonography (US) can also rapidly detect HTX. In a study of 240 patients by Ma and Mateer,[109] emergency department US was 96% sensitive, 100% specific, and 100% accurate for HTX. Although the initial CXR provides this diagnosis, an US examination can identify both intraperitoneal hemorrhage and HTX within minutes of a patient's arrival.

Emergency department TTE has no role in hemodynamically stable patients with suspected myocardial contusion since it has not been shown to predict clinically significant complications.[4,110-112] Furthermore, one third of portable TTEs for blunt myocardial injury are uninterpretable.[113] Transthoracic echocardiography also cannot be used to rule out aortic injury.

The classic findings for pericardial tamponade on TTE are pericardial fluid and diastolic collapse of the right ventricle or atrium. Another ultrasonographic indication is a negative "sniff test" (the failure of the inferior vena cava to contract with a deep inspiration).

Transesophageal Echocardiography

The primary use of transesophageal echocardiography (TEE) after BCT is to detect aortic injury in the unstable patient. Specially trained physicians can perform TEE in the trauma resuscitation room to provide detailed images of the descending aorta and aortic isthmus. If a multiply-injured patient requires immediate cranial or abdominal surgery, TEE is performed in the operating suite concurrent with laparotomy or craniotomy.

Transesophageal echocardiography has multiple advantages over helical CT and aortography, since it does not require moving the patient out of the ED, nor does it necessitate contrast administration. In addition to the transport and contrast issues, the other major advantage of this technique is time. TEE can significantly decrease the time to surgical repair of the aorta compared with patients who undergo aortography. In one recent report, the mean study time for TEE was 27 minutes versus 76 minutes for aortography.[114] When TEE demonstrates an aortic injury, the next step depends on whether the cardiothoracic surgeon is willing to operate based on the results. In many cases, an obvious intimal flap on the TEE spurs operative repair without the need for additional studies.

Transesophageal echocardiography requires considerable operator expertise and is contraindicated in patients with unstable cervical spine injuries or esophageal injury. In the ED, its use is limited to detection of TAI, since TTE is much faster and easier to obtain when evaluating for pericardial tamponade. TEE is more sensitive for blunt myocardial injury, valvular disruption, and pericardial effusion than TTE, although it is more invasive and is not as readily available.[113,115]

Research proves that not only can TEE accurately detect TAI,[113,114,116-119] but in certain circumstances it may actually be superior to aortography.[114] Several prospective studies report sensitivities from 91% to 100% and specificities from 88% to 100%.[113,116-119] In patients with TAI, TEE demonstrates the actual aortic wall flap and periaortic hematoma better than CT. However, TEE may miss injuries to the midascending aorta and aortic arch branches.[65] As the technique becomes more widely available, it may supplant aortography in certain cases.

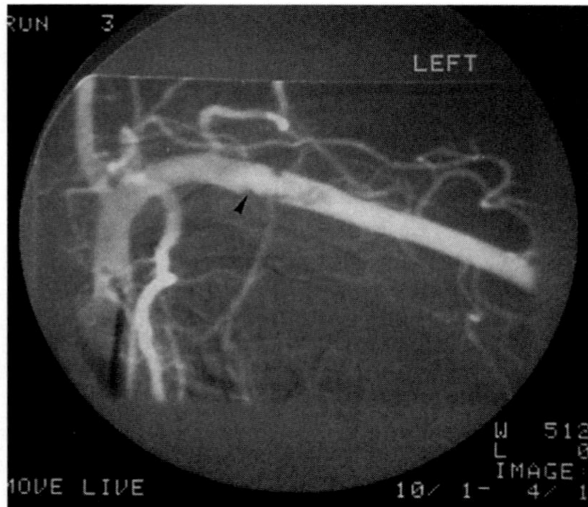

Fig. 17-14 Angiogram illustrating left subclavian artery injury *(arrowhead).*

Intravascular Ultrasound

Intravascular ultrasonography is a new technique that utilizes an intraarterial transducer. It can be used to image the descending aorta and exclude mural injury, yet it does not provide adequate images of the ascending aorta and brachiocephalic arteries.[120-122] It is unlikely to become an important test for TAI.

Magnetic Resonance Imaging

Magnetic resonance imaging (MRI) is another diagnostic modality available for detecting aortic injuries after BCT. Because it takes considerable time to perform and is not always available, it is usually not performed in the setting of acute trauma. Furthermore, the difficulties in monitoring patients during the MRI confine its use to hemodynamically stable patients. However, it can detect diaphragmatic injuries and aortic injuries that are not well defined by CT.[8,59,123]

Aortography

Aortography remains the "gold standard" for detecting aortic injury, although CT and TEE are replacing it in many patients. Aortography precisely localizes the aortic rupture and defines multiple aortic tears that might otherwise be missed intraoperatively. Aortography is more sensitive than TEE or CT for the detection of injuries to the aortic arch branches, which occur in 19% of patients (Fig. 17-14).[124] It defines both aortic and coronary anatomy, which may assist in operative decisions.[124] Positive findings on aortography include pseudoaneurysm of the isthmus (Fig. 17-15), lateral bulging of the aorta, or a linear-filling defect caused

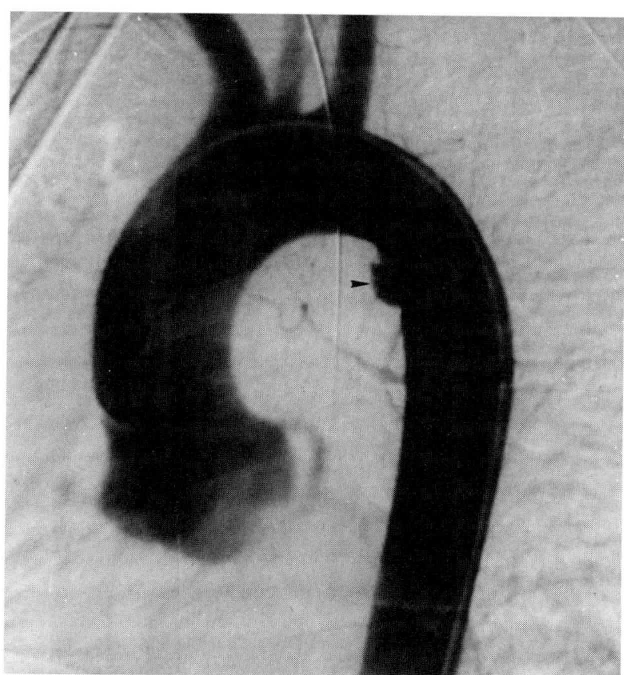

Fig. 17-15 Aortogram of traumatic pseudoaneurysm *(arrowhead).*

by the torn intima and media. It may also demonstrate injury to the great vessels arising from the arch, which occurs in 1% of patients with aortic injury.[124]

There are obviously difficulties involved in studying the accuracy of aortography, since the only true gold standards are operative reports and autopsy results. The reported sensitivity of aortography is 73% to 100% and the specificity is 99%.[119,125] A false-positive study can occur in patients with atherosclerotic plaque or prominent ductus diverticulum (Fig. 17-16). The false-negative rate is also as high as 15% and results from poor opacification, inadequate projections, thrombosis of the pouch, or small tears.[126]

The major disadvantages include the approximately 90 minutes it takes to perform and the need to move a potentially unstable patient into an unsafe environment. It also requires significant technical support and manpower not readily available at all hours. The other limitation of using aortography is that only 10% actually are positive.[90] There is a significant dye load associated with the test. The associated morbidity and the low positive rate raise the question of safety. In the setting of acute trauma, aortography has a morbidity of 3% to 10%, even in patients without TAI.[127]

With the recent use of TEE and CT to screen patients for TAI, the rate of positive aortograms should

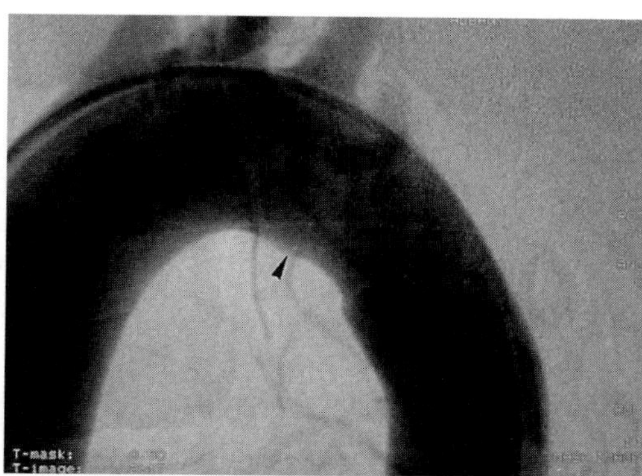

Fig. 17-16 Aortogram of ductus diverticulum *(arrowhead).*

increase. In certain patients, aortography should be ordered as the first imaging study, rather than spending time obtaining other less definitive studies such as CT. If the clinical suspicion is high based on a widened mediastinum on CXR or other plain radiographic abnormalities, or if the patient has a high-speed deceleration mechanism with suggestive clinical findings, then aortography is indicated. Any patient with mediastinal hematoma by CT or equivocal TEE results must undergo aortography to define the injury. In patients with intracranial hemorrhage, intraperitoneal hemorrhage, or major pelvic injuries, aortography should be delayed to address these other life-threatening injuries first.

Bronchoscopy

Bronchoscopy is indicated in any patient with suspected tracheobronchial injury. Such patients may include those with subcutaneous emphysema without an underlying PTX or those with a persistent air leak despite multiple chest tubes.[128] It is also indicated in patients with significant atelectatic segments and those with bronchial foreign bodies (Fig. 17-17).

Esophagoscopy

Esophagoscopy (rigid or flexible) is indicated in patients with clinical evidence (odynophagia) or CXR findings suggestive of an esophageal injury. It may be used as an adjunct to esophagram.[25,47]

In a recent small study, flexible endoscopy or esophagogastroduodenoscopy (EGD) was used as the primary diagnostic tool in 31 patients with suspected esophageal injury, 7 of whom had blunt trauma. The overall sensitivity for esophageal injury was 100% and specificity was 96%.[129]

Esophagram

The esophagram may be more sensitive for esophageal injury than esophagoscopy. It should be performed with water-soluble contrast medium (gastrografin), which is less irritating to the mediastinum in case the contrast leaks through a tear. Some authorities suggest that a negative gastrografin study requires a subsequent barium swallow, which is purported to be more sensitive. Contrast extravasation into the mediastinum or pleural cavity suggests esophageal injury (Fig. 17-18).[25,47,130]

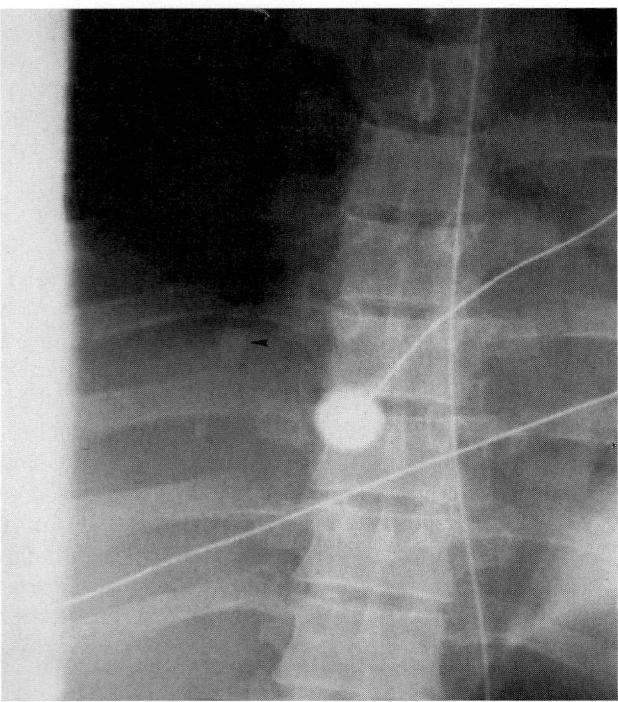

Fig. 17-17 Chest radiograph illustrating right bronchial tooth *(arrowhead)*.

Laparoscopy

In trauma patients, laparoscopy is primarily used in patients with penetrating trauma to the abdomen or lower chest. However, some centers employ it in the evaluation of blunt trauma. Laparoscopy appears a reliable means to detect diaphragmatic injury. The technique permits direct visualization of the diaphragm and is useful in those who have equivocal results with other diagnostic tests.[131]

Thoracoscopy

Fiberoptic thoracoscopy is occasionally employed by surgeons to detect diaphragmatic injury,[132,133] although it is rarely used as the initial study. Thoracoscopy can also evacuate residual hemothoraces days to weeks after trauma.[134] In two case reports, video-assisted thoracoscopy diagnosed and treated patients with pleuropericardial rupture (herniation of the heart through a pericardial tear).[135,136]

SPECIFIC INJURIES

Pneumothorax and Hemothorax

Pneumothoraces and hemothoraces are among the most common thoracic injuries. Primary causes of hemothoraces include lung parenchymal lacerations or injury to an intercostal vessel or internal mammary artery. Bleeding from lung parenchymal injury is usually brief, whereas persistent bleeding is most often

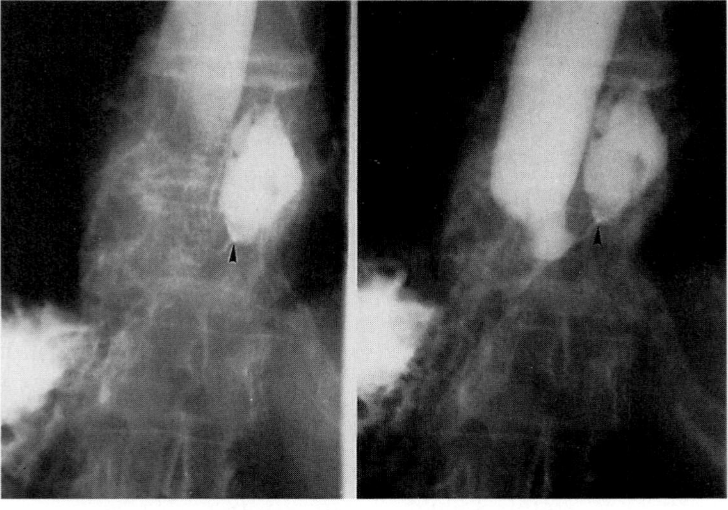

Fig. 17-18 Esophagram of extravasation *(arrowheads)*.

from disruption of an intercostal vessel or the internal mammary artery.[137]

A simple PTX is air in the pleural space that does not communicate with the atmosphere or distort the mediastinum. The two possible mechanisms include laceration of the pleura or lung parenchyma by a fractured rib and compression of the chest against a closed glottis that ruptures the alveoli.

In a tension PTX, air accumulates under pressure. This phenomenon shifts the mediastinum and compresses the contralateral lung and great vessels. Clinically, tension PTX causes hypotension and marked respiratory distress. The development of a tension PTX requires a "one-way" valve type of injury to the lung (i.e., air enters with inspiration but does not exit with expiration). It occasionally occurs with spontaneous breathing, but is more likely in those who undergo bag-valve-mask or mechanical ventilation. Positive pressure ventilation can convert a simple PTX to a tension PTX. As the intrapleural pressure increases, the lung collapses, the mediastinum shifts, and venous return is impaired. Tension pneumothorax increases the central venous pressure, decreases cardiac output, and ultimately produces cardiovascular collapse.[34,138]

Operative Thoracotomy: Hemothorax

The definitive treatment of major intrathoracic bleeding is operating suite thoracotomy. Indications include the following:

1. An initial tube thoracostomy output greater than 20 cc/kg or 1500 cc
2. Continuing blood loss greater than 7 cc/kg/hour for 3 to 4 hours
3. Continuing blood loss greater than 300 cc/hour for 3 to 4 hours[34,137,138]
4. Persistent hypotension despite adequate volume replacement
5. Lack of lung reexpansion
6. Increasing hemothorax on chest radiograph despite tube thoracostomy[137]

Other injuries that require immediate operative intervention are tracheobronchial disruption, esophageal injury, and traumatic diaphragmatic hernia.

Pulmonary Contusion and Flail Chest

Pulmonary contusion is defined as traumatic lung parenchymal damage with edema and hemorrhage without lung laceration. This injury is characterized by localized edema, microhemorrhage, and extravasation of blood into the interstitial and alveolar spaces.[34,139] Arteriovenous shunting causes hypoxia and respiratory failure. Respiratory failure develops with progression of the hemorrhage, and radiographic findings may be present on admission or take hours to develop.[34,140]

Severe compression of the chest wall with or without rib fractures causes a pulmonary contusion. In children, the rib cage is more compliant and transmits significant force to the lungs, resulting in a lung contusion without rib fractures.

Flail chest is another injury resulting from extreme chest compression. It is defined as three or more ribs fractured at two or more places, resulting in a freely moving segment of chest wall. Paradoxical chest wall movement occurs as the flail segment moves inward with inspiration and outward during expiration.[25,139] In the conscious patient who is splinting, the flail segment may not be immediately apparent, which explains why 31% of these injuries are not recognized within the first 6 hours after injury.[53] The flail segment disrupts the mechanics of breathing, prevents lung inflation, and produces significant ventilatory compromise and hypoxia. However, the underlying pulmonary contusion, not the mechanical disruption of the chest wall, causes the respiratory insufficiency.[25]

Certain patients with BCT require special interventions—often after the initial resuscitation. In patients with pulmonary contusion, aggressive chest physiotherapy is indicated. However, there is no proven benefit to steroids or prophylactic antibiotics. Patients with flail chest also require aggressive chest physiotherapy and analgesia once admitted to the hospital. Pain-management techniques include nerve blocks of the intercostal nerves, intrapleural local anesthetics administered via the chest tube, and epidural or systemic analgesia (see Chapter 10 on pain management techniques). If the patient is hypoxic or hypercarbic, intubation is indicated. There is no clear benefit from rib belts or other methods of rib stabilization.[25,34,35] Although not well studied for patients with pulmonary contusion or flail chest, continuous positive airway pressure (CPAP) mask ventilation and other forms of noninvasive ventilation may help avoid intubation. The reported mortality rate for patients with flail chest is 20% and depends on the presence of associated injuries.[6]

Blunt Myocardial Injury

There are several proposed mechanisms for blunt myocardial injury. The most accepted explanation is direct force to the chest wall, compressing the heart between the sternum and the thoracic spine (or an elevated diaphragm).[77] However, deceleration may also play a role. With a sudden stop experienced in a high fall or MVC, the heart swings forward and strikes the sternum. Factors such as the phase of the cardiac cycle may also play a role in injury. During end-diastole or early systole the heart becomes rigid and is less capable of diffusing energy. In a dog model, contusion produces a transient fall in coronary artery blood flow, causing global ischemia and transient dysrhythmias. In dogs, the decrease in coronary blood flow occurs within two minutes after impact and normalizes after 20 minutes.[42,141]

Even low-speed MVCs can produce myocardial injury. In one study, blunt myocardial injury occurred in patients in MVCs at speeds of 20 to 35 mph, and many patients had no external evidence of chest trauma.[142]

Blunt myocardial injury represents a spectrum of cardiac damage.[77] A *myocardial concussion* (commotio cordis) results from a direct blow to the chest causing brief dysrhythmia, hypotension, loss of consciousness (LOC), or sudden death. A blow to the chest from a baseball or hockey puck can cause myocardial concussion, which may lead to sudden death.[142-146] Myocardial concussion is a stun response, without cellular injury or permanent damage. However, echocardiography may demonstrate transient wall motion abnormalities and the patient can experience symptoms such as brief palpitations or syncope.

Myocardial contusion is a more severe injury in which red blood cells extravasate into the muscle wall and myocardial necrosis may occur. Hemorrhage is usually located in the anterior wall of the right atrium or ventricle and is primarily subendocardial but occasionally transmural.[147] Unlike myocardial infarction, a sharp margin defines the injured and uninjured tissue. Edema, polymorphonuclear infiltration of the myocardium, and necrosis may result in cardiac dysfunction. Lacerations of the endocardium or epicardium may produce hemopericardium or mural thrombi.[77] Necrosis of the wall of the heart may lead to scarring or weakening of the wall and development of a ventricular aneurysm; delayed ventricular rupture can occur weeks after injury.[148]

Myocardial infarction is the most severe form of injury seen in patients who survive to ED arrival. It originates from injury to the coronary arteries or from severely contused myocardium.[42,149]

MORBIDITY AND MORTALITY

The overall mortality rate after blunt myocardial injury ranges from 0% to 27%.[4,28,78,150] This wide variation is due to the difficulty in diagnosing and defining this injury. The rate of deaths directly caused by myocardial injury in patients who reach the ED alive is very low. The incidence of significant complications requiring treatment is 2.6% to 4.5% in a recent metaanalysis.[48] The most common complication is dysrhythmia (present in approximately 75% of patients with complications), followed by pump failure.[48] The mortality rates are hard to define because of the different inclusion criteria used in various studies and because of the lack of a gold standard for diagnosis. The mortality rate is 2% for patients admitted to "rule out" blunt myocardial injury[5] and 7% for patients with blunt myocardial injury determined by gated cardiac scintigraphy.[151] Hemodynamically stable patients admitted to rule out blunt myocardial injury have an even lower mortality rate (0.8%).[3] The morbidity and mortality in these patients is usually due to associated injuries. The long-term sequelae after this type of injury are minimal. In one study, there were no long-term effects on cardiac function as determined by ejection fraction 1 year after injury in patients with blunt myocardial injury initially defined by cardiac scintigraphy.[152]

APPROACH TO SUSPECTED BLUNT MYOCARDIAL INJURY

Electrocardiography. Patients with blunt chest trauma and an abnormal ECG should be admitted for further monitoring. Additional studies in the ED are only indicated based on the hemodynamic stability of the patient. A patient with an injury pattern on the ECG consistent with a myocardial infarction should undergo echocardiography as an inpatient.

Several recent studies have investigated the value of the initial ECG findings in the ED for predicting complications and subsequent lethal dysrhythmias. A recent retrospective study of 184 pediatric patients with blunt cardiac injury reported that complications requiring treatment did not occur in patients with a normal ECG in the ED.[153] Fildes et al[154] prospectively studied 74 hemodynamically stable patients, less than 55 years of age, without coronary artery disease who had a normal initial ECG. None of these patients had associated injuries requiring surgery, and none of them developed a cardiac complication. Furthermore, in a recent meta-analysis of 41 articles including 1210 patients prospectively studied and 2471 patients retrospectively studied, the incidence of complications requiring treatment was negligible in patients with a normal ECG.[48] Even in patients with an abnormal ECG the incidence of clinically significant contusion is very low. In one study of 336 patients with BCT, 138 of whom had myocardial contusion, the patients who developed complications requiring treatment were older than 60 years, had more than three rib fractures, pulmonary contusions, flail chest, major vascular injury, or other severe associated injuries.[150] The incidence of complications requiring treatment was 6% (19 patients) and was not predicted solely by an abnormal ECG in the ED. Since clinically significant complications are negligible in patients with a normal ECG, the ECG can be used as a screening test in asymptomatic patients. If it is normal and there are no other associated significant injuries, then the patient can be discharged from the ED.

Cardiac Enzymes. Physicians historically used cardiac enzymes, specifically the CK-MB, to detect blunt myocardial injury. Although a handful of early studies suggested that CK-MB greater than 5% could screen for myocardial injury in the ED,[28,155] more recent studies demonstrate that cardiac enzymes are unreliable in blunt chest trauma. They do not correlate with outcome or other diagnostic test results and do not predict complications.[4,5,75,110,156] CK-MB is a nonspecific test and is usually elevated after major skeletal muscle injury.

In a recent metaanalysis of blunt myocardial injury, a normal CK-MB in the ED correlated with the absence of cardiac complications.[48] However, most studies contradict this finding. Most trials show that CK-MB does *not* correlate with echocardiographic findings or the results of other tests used to demonstrate myocardial injury.[4,156] Another recent investigation of 359 patients with BCT documented that cardiac enzyme elevation was never the sole predictor of complications in those with blunt myocardial injury.[76]

There are several recent reports on the use of troponin I and T for detecting blunt myocardial injury. Although the studies on troponin I demonstrated 100% sensitivity and specificity for predicting echocardiographic abnormalities, available studies *do not* suggest a strong correlation between troponin levels and complications in patients with myocardial injury.[157-160]

Based on the literature, cardiac enzyme determination has either a limited or no role in the evaluation of patients with BCT. The patient who gives a history compatible with cardiac ischemia *before* the traumatic event may require a standard cardiac evaluation.

Echocardiography. The routine use of TTE as a screening test in young stable patients with suspected blunt myocardial injury who do not have major thoracic or extrathoracic trauma is not supported in the literature.[4,110-112] Although some authors recommend its use in combination with CK-MB and ECG to identify patients with "significant" myocardial contusions, abnormal findings do not predict clinically significant complications. In the ED, TTE appears to be useful only in the management of patients with myocardial decompensation to identify cardiac rupture, pericardial tamponade, or valvular disruption. A patient with an abnormal TTE suggestive of valvular disruption may be a candidate for TEE to further define the injury before surgery.

The most common finding in patients with blunt myocardial injury is right ventricular free wall dyskinesia or other wall motion abnormalities. Patients with blunt myocardial injury may have small pericardial effusions, usually 1 to 2 weeks after injury, but these are usually not clinically significant and are self-limiting. TTE may be used to detect other less common complications of blunt myocardial injury such as pericardial tamponade, valvular rupture, intraventricular thrombus, pericardial effusion, and ventricular aneurysm. In the hemodynamically stable patient with suspected blunt myocardial injury, TTE findings do not necessarily predict patient outcome. In a recent meta-analysis of 25 prospective studies (2210 patients) and 16 retrospective studies (2471 patients) the results for TTE were not congruent between the retrospective and prospective studies.[48] For the prospective studies, an abnormal TTE did not correlate with complications. However, for the retrospective and combined analyses, an abnormal TTE predicted complications.

Treatment. Treatment of dysrhythmias associated with blunt myocardial injury is seldom required in the ED, and prophylactic antidysrhythmic therapy is not indicated. If dysrhythmias do occur, they should be treated in the same manner as nontraumatic dysrhythmias. The chest pain is usually refractory to nitroglycerin and responds to analgesics.

Cardiac Rupture and Valve Dysfunction

Patients with myocardial rupture usually present in extremis, with hypotension and tachycardia.[14] Cardiac rupture is rare and usually results in immediate death. Survivors usually have right- or left-sided atrial rupture. The right ventricle is most commonly involved.[14,161-164] Blunt cardiac rupture accounts for 5% of traumatic deaths resulting from highway accidents in the United States.[161]

Blunt injury to the cardiac valves is rare. There are isolated reports of acute valvular dysfunction after chest trauma. Patients may exhibit a loud murmur, precipitous congestive heart failure, or impressive pulsatile neck veins depending on the injured valve. Echocardiography may be helpful.

The survival rates for patients with cardiac rupture depend on the chamber ruptured and the presence or absence of vital signs on presentation. The overall survival is hard to define, since the denominator of all patients with cardiac rupture is unknown, since many of these patients die in the field. The mortality rates range from 50% to 85%.[13,14,162,165,166] As of 1989 there were only 61 reported cases of survivors in English-language literature. Patients with prehospital cardiac arrest or who arrest immediately after arrival to the ED have a 100% mortality rate.[165] If vital signs are present in the ED, the survival rate for cardiac rupture is much higher (48% to 50%).[13,165] The survivors have injury to the right atrium (59%), right ventricle (20%), or left atrium (18%). There are at least four cases of patients surviving left ventricular rupture.[162]

Cardiac Tamponade

Cardiac tamponade is rare after BCT. It can occasionally occur with myocardial rupture and an intact pericardial sac. The pressure-volume relationship in the minimally distensible pericardium means that small increases in volume result in large pressure gradients. The hemorrhage within the pericardial sac prevents diastolic filling of the heart and results in reduced stroke volume, cardiac output, and systolic blood pressure.[167,168] At a critical point, the patient declines precipitously. As a compensatory measure, heart rate and total peripheral resistance increase.[169] Central venous pressure usually rises from mechanical obstruction to right atrial filling, although hemorrhage in another body compartment may obscure this phenomenon. Beck's triad defines the classic findings in cardiac tamponade (hypotension, muffled heart sounds, and JVD). However, these findings are absent in the majority of patients and may be hard to detect in a noisy trauma room.[42] If the patient is hypovolemic from other bleeding sources, then JVD is absent. Patients are usually tachycardic and may be hypotensive. Bedside ECHO can be used to make the diagnosis of cardiac tamponade. (See earlier section on TTE.) If the patient is unstable, then an attempt at pericardiocentesis can be made. The patient in cardiac arrest should undergo left lateral thoracotomy with incision of the pericardial sac to decompress the tamponade. Definitive treatment is operative thoracotomy with repair of the cardiac injury.

Traumatic Aortic Injury

The aorta is most often injured in the descending portion distal to the left subclavian artery at the ligamentum arteriosum. More than 90% of aortic injuries occur at this site.[43,45,170,171] Other sites of disruption include the aortic arch in 4% of patients, ascending aorta in 3%, and distal descending aorta at the diaphragm in 0.3%.[43]

Researchers propose several mechanisms of TAI. The first proposed mechanism is based on the fact that the descending aorta is fixed at the isthmus. With deceleration, the mobile aortic arch swings forward, shearing the aorta at this point.[15,42,172]

According to the "osseous pinch" model, the aorta is pinched between the sternum, first rib, and medial clavicles anteriorly and the vertebral column posteriorly. Shearing forces cause injury to the aorta. This mechanism has recently been confirmed with a skeletal model, an animal model, as well as by computed tomography (CT).[173,174]

Injury to the ascending aorta may occur through a slightly different mechanism. With rapid deceleration, the heart is displaced into the posterior left chest, causing a shearing stress just above the aortic valve. In addition, a sudden increase in intraaortic pressure with compression of the chest also results in laceration of the ascending aorta.[42] Injury to the ascending aorta is frequently associated with involvement of the coronary ostia and occlusion of the coronary arteries.

Patients with TAI may present with dramatic multisystem injury or with few signs of external trauma. Some exhibit hoarseness from laryngeal nerve compression as a result of hemorrhage. Decreased pulses in the lower extremities can result from the pseudocoarctation syndrome in patients with TAI, or they may be caused by generalized hypovolemic shock.[45,26,175] Neurologic deficits can be present in patients with TAI and usually manifest as lower extremity paralysis.[45]

For patients with TAI who survive to the ED, 30% die within 6 hours and another 20% die within 24 hours if prompt diagnosis and management do not occur.[25,176] For patients with TAI, the survival rate for those who make it to surgery is 75% to 86%.[6,22,175,177-180] The mortality rates depend on the type of operative procedure performed, the presence of vital signs on presentation, age, and the presence of associated injuries. In one series mortality rates were 100% for patients who arrived in the ED in cardiac arrest or with a systolic blood pressure ≤90 mmHg and 34% for patients who arrived hemodynamically stable.[181] In a recent study,[182] the survival rate for stable patients was 72%. Co-morbidities, especially coronary artery disease and increasing age, were associated with mortality, whereas a delay to operative repair of greater than 4 hours was not associated with an increased mortality. The use of β-blocking agents and normalization of systolic blood pressure was associated with an increased survival.

MEDICAL MANAGEMENT

The treatment of TAI begins in the ED. In up to 95% of patients, associated orthopedic, intraperitoneal, and intracranial injuries are present that require operative intervention and delay repair of the aorta.[22] Many authorities suggest pharmacologic control of blood pressure is necessary in cases of delayed repair.[106,175] Although anecdotal reports of medical management appear compelling, no randomized controlled trials have put this theory to test.

The goal of medical therapy is to decrease the shearing forces on the wall of the aorta and prevent free rupture. The dual considerations are reducing both intraluminal pressure and the rate of rise of the aortic pressure wave (dP/dt). Treatment should begin with β-blocking agents to lower the systolic blood pressure to 100 mmHg. A short-acting titratable agent such as esmolol is preferred since it can be easily turned off in case of hypotension. The dose includes a 500 μ/kg bolus followed by a maintenance drip of 50 μ/kg/min to 200 μ/kg/min. Other β-blocking agents may be used such as labetalol or propranolol. Some centers use esmolol as the sole agent for medical management of TAI. In other trauma centers, nitroprusside is employed to maintain the desired blood pressure after the β-blocking agent is started. Overaggressive blood pressure control (below 100 mmHg) should be avoided.

SURGICAL MANAGEMENT

The definitive management of traumatic aortic injuries is operative repair. There are several techniques available. The clamp and sew technique involves clamp exclusion of the injured aorta and direct repair. This approach does not require cardiopulmonary bypass or pumps, and avoids heparinization. Bypass techniques provide distal aortic perfusion during the repair, and require heparinization. Newer centrifugal pumps allow distal perfusion, but do not require heparinization.[43,177,183,184] For patients who undergo TAI repair, the overall postoperative paraplegia rate is 0% to 20%, and is associated with an aortic cross-clamp time of greater than 30 minutes.[43,181,185]

Esophageal Injuries

Blunt injury to the esophagus is rare after chest trauma. The lower third of the esophagus is the most common location.[25] Blunt injuries to the upper esophagus usually result from trauma to the neck and are associated with laryngotracheal injuries and cervical spine fractures.[186,187]

Clinical findings that suggest an esophageal injury include evidence of PTX, left-sided pleural effusion, food particles in the chest tube drainage, or chest tube bubbles that are continuous during inspiration and expiration. Patients may have pain with swallowing, and the EP may observe Hamman's crunch on chest auscultation. The diagnosis is made by esophagoscopy or esophagography. After esophageal injury, the mortality rate is 18% and increases significantly if the diagnosis is delayed.[188] Esophageal injuries require expeditious surgical repair.

Diaphragm Injuries

The most common cause of diaphragmatic injury is a direct blow to the upper abdomen or lower chest. Up to 72% to 88% of diaphragmatic injuries resulting from blunt trauma occur on the left side.* The left side of the diaphragm is more prone to injury because it is not protected by the liver. The left posterolateral area is the weakest part of the diaphragm and therefore the most common site of rupture and herniation.

The mechanism of injury determines the size of the disruption. After penetrating trauma, the hole is usually 2 to 2.6 cm; after blunt trauma, the defect in the diaphragm is considerably larger, between 5 and 15 cm.[8,9,47] After the injury, the peritoneal-pleural pressure gradient maintains the rent. Failure to repair the injury results in delayed herniation of abdominal contents into the chest.[47,191]

Delay in diagnosis is common and occurs in 18% to 69% of patients.[8,9,44] Misdiagnosis occurs because of attention to associated injuries and because many ruptures are not recognized on the chest radiograph or CT. Overlooked injuries may present weeks to years later when abdominal contents herniate into the chest.

There are three phases of diaphragmatic injury. The *acute phase* begins with injury and ends after the initial recovery from other associated trauma. In the *acute phase* patients may have decreased breath sounds on the side of the injury; bowel sounds may be heard in the chest. If the diagnosis is not made, then the patient progresses into the *latent phase*, characterized by intermittent visceral herniation of any abdominal structure through the defect. Patients complain of nausea, vomiting, belching, and vague postprandial abdominal pain that is better with sitting or standing. Common organs that herniate include the liver on the right and the colon, stomach, small bowel, and spleen on the left. This phase may last months to years until the *obstructive phase* occurs. This phase is characterized by incarceration of the abdominal organs, with intestinal obstruction and ischemia.[58] Patients are ill-appearing and have significant abdominal pain, vomiting, and abdominal tenderness.[25] Another complication of diaphragmatic rupture is a tension viscero-thorax, which occurs when bowel or other abdominal organs herniate into the chest, causing an increase in intrapleural pressure and shift of the mediastinum with hemodynamic collapse.[192,193]

The mortality rates for diaphragmatic injury vary depending on the series. Many of the reports include penetrating diaphragmatic injury cases. The mortality

*References 9, 44, 83, 58, 189, 190.

rate ranges from 7% to 18% and may even be higher after blunt trauma as a result of the presence of associated injuries.[8,190] Complications may occur in up to 64% of patients with blunt diaphragmatic injury and include intraabdominal abscess and pneumonia.[8]

Traumatic Asphyxia

During the initial phase of resuscitation, traumatic asphyxia is an infrequent but dramatic finding. This condition is caused by a crush to the chest and upper abdomen, resulting in a surge of cardiac blood to the superior veins and increasing pressure and stasis in the head and neck capillaries.[51]

Up to one third of patients with traumatic asphyxia have a loss of consciousness, although intracranial hemorrhage is rare.[51] Retinal hemorrhage and edema may also occur.[52] Although the course is self-limited, the presence of traumatic asphyxia suggests more serious chest wall and pulmonary injuries.[51]

Venous Air Embolism

A rare cause of profound shock and cardiac arrest after BCT is venous air embolism. This phenomenon most often occurs with multiple rib fractures or a tracheobronchial tear that results in a bronchopulmonary venous fistula.[74] Cardiovascular compromise results when air enters the coronary arteries causing myocardial ischemia and infarction, or when air enters the heart causing ventricular outflow obstruction.[63] The first clue to air embolism is usually sudden decompensation after a patient is intubated.

Mental status changes and hemoptysis may also be present in patients with air embolus. Some demonstrate a "machinery-type" murmur on cardiac auscultation, whereas funduscopic examination may reveal air bubbles in the retinal vasculature. If air is suspected on the right side of the heart, then the patient should be placed in the left lateral decubitus position to trap air in the right atrium. A central line can be placed for aspiration of air. A patient with air suspected on the left side of the heart should be placed in the Trendelenburg position to prevent air from embolizing to the brain. In the case of unilateral chest trauma, selective intubation of the uninjured lung may decrease further embolization. Because of the tracheal-bronchial angle, right mainstem intubation is easily accomplished by simply advancing the endotracheal tube. Left mainstem intubation usually requires a fiberoptic scope and perhaps the expertise of an anesthesiologist. In patients with air embolism who undergo ED thoracotomy, air bubbles may be seen in the coronary vessels.[12,74] Patients with air embolism after blunt trauma have an 80% mortality. This high mortality rate may be a result of associated nonthoracic injuries.[74]

Pneumodiastinum

Pneumomediastinum has many causes, including pharyngeal tears, esophageal rupture, tracheobronchial injury, and PTX.[34,194] In all of these cases, air tracks into the mediastinum. In rare cases, positive pressure ventilation may produce a tension pneumomediastinum or tension pneumopericardium. In general, pneumomediastinum is a benign phenomenon as long as esophageal injury is not the cause.

Sternal Fractures and Upper Rib Fractures

Older literature suggested an association between certain fractures and underlying chest injury. Physicians believed that scapular and first rib fractures indicated an aortic injury, whereas sternal fractures were invariably associated with myocardial contusion. The management implications of these fractures have changed in recent years. Newer studies demonstrate that the mere presence of these injuries does not predict TAI or blunt cardiac injury and *in isolation* does not mandate extensive diagnostic evaluation.[195-199]

Patients with scapular, first, and second rib fractures require a targeted diagnostic evaluation. In such patients, the function of the brachial plexus should be tested and an arterial brachial index should be performed to evaluate integrity of the vasculature. The chest film should be closely examined for signs of aortic injury. Patients with sternal fractures should undergo electrocardiography to look for evidence of blunt myocardial injury. However, the presence of sternal fracture alone does not predict the presence of myocardial injury and does not require admission or extensive work-up of the heart.[196,199]

Pediatric Cases

The incidence of chest trauma in children presenting to a pediatric trauma center is less than 5%. However, pediatric trauma patients with chest trauma have mortality rates that range from 11% to 40% compared with less than 2% for children without thoracic injuries.[200,201] Children with injury to the heart or great vessels have the highest mortality rates (75%). Pulmonary contusion carries a mortality rate of 33%.[201]

The majority of chest trauma in children is due to blunt mechanisms, and only 20% of these injuries require surgery. The most common mechanisms include pedestrian accidents, MVCs, and assaults, whereas the most common injuries are pulmonary contusion and rib fractures, followed by PTX and HTX. The incidence of injury to the heart or great vessels is low (7.7%).[201]

The main difference in chest anatomy between adults and children concerns the increased chest wall compliance in children. Consequently, forces are transmitted to the underlying structures such as the lung, causing pulmonary contusion without rib fractures. Rib fractures are less common in children (32% in one series), as is flail chest (1% incidence).[201]

Blunt cardiac injuries are rare in children but can result from MVCs; most patients have associated injuries.[202] Pediatric patients with suspected blunt myocardial injury who are hemodynamically stable in the ED with a normal ECG are at low-risk for developing cardiac dysrhythmias, shock, or dying during hospitalization and do not require intensive care unit (ICU) admission. Pediatric patients who present in shock or with serious dysrhythmias or premature ventricular contractions require ICU monitoring. Unstable patients with suspected cardiac injury should undergo echocardiography to evaluate chamber function and wall motion.[153]

TAI is rare in children, and the reported incidence is 0.064%.[203,204] The most common mechanism is MVC followed by auto-pedestrian accidents. Associated injuries are common. In one series, 100% of patients with TAI had a pulmonary contusion, 50% had pelvic or long bone fractures, and 17% had blunt myocardial injury. The diagnostic approach is similar to that of adult patients, and CXR findings resemble those in adults.[204]

OVERALL PROGNOSIS

The associated morbidity and mortality rates from BCT are approximately 36% and 18%, respectively.[1,6,139] The overall prognosis depends on the type of injury and the presence of associated trauma. (See various sections on specific injuries.)

The presence of three or more rib fractures is associated with a higher mortality rate (4% versus 0.9%) and an increased risk of associated injuries compared with patients with fractures of one or two ribs.[205]

DISPOSITION

Admission criteria for patients with BCT depend on several factors, including the severity of known chest injuries, premorbid illness, age, and associated injuries. Patients with PTX, HTX, pulmonary contusion, flail chest, pneumomediastinum, TAI, and evidence of blunt myocardial injury should be admitted.[205] Some centers will admit patients with three or more rib fractures for observation, especially if the patient is older or has underlying pulmonary disease. Elderly patients with multiple displaced rib fractures are at risk for delayed HTX. In general, certain conditions in isolation do not require extensive evaluation. For instance, an isolated sternal fracture or rib fractures do not mandate studies for myocardial contusion or aortic injury, and do not require admission.[199]

The admission criteria for patients with suspected blunt myocardial injury remain controversial. However, new data suggest that mechanism alone should not dictate admission criteria, since mechanism is neither reliable nor cost effective. Indications for admission include persistent severe chest pain or an abnormal ECG. Patients with minimal chest tenderness and sinus tachycardia can be observed for 4 to 6 hours until the tachycardia resolves, then discharged. Patients less than 55 years old who are stable and asymptomatic without major injuries and have a normal ECG (or no new changes) can be discharged from the ED. Even young patients with an abnormal ECG are unlikely to develop complications, and usually require only 24 hours of monitoring in a telemetry unit. Unstable patients with major chest trauma require ICU admission. Patients with any dysrhythmias or hemodynamic instability in the ED should be admitted to an ICU or telemetry bed.[48,76,150,206]

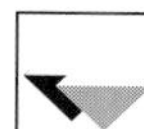

PEARLS & PITFALLS

Resuscitation

- Tube thoracostomy should be performed before chest radiography in patients with a clinical presentation suggestive of tension pneumothorax.
- Early airway management is especially important in the elderly or hemodynamically unstable patient.

Diagnostic Studies

- The chest radiograph should be the initial ancillary study ordered in the patient with BCT since it determines the need for further diagnostic studies and procedures.
- If possible, an upright film should be obtained to carefully evaluate the mediastinum.

Suspected Cardiac Injury

- Stable patients suspected of blunt myocardial injury who are less than 55 years of age, have no significant associated injuries, and have a normal ECG can be discharged from the ED.

- Cardiac enzymes, troponin, and echocardiography should not be used in the ED to predict which patients will develop significant complications after blunt myocardial injury.

Suspected Aortic Injury

- Helical computed tomography of the chest is highly sensitive for traumatic aortic injury and can be used to rule out the diagnosis in many patients.
- TEE can be used to evaluate the aorta in the unstable patient.
- Blood pressure should be controlled with β-blocking agents and nitroprusside in patients with TAI.

Frequently Missed Injuries

- The diagnosis of diaphragmatic rupture and TAI can be easily missed in the presence of associated trauma.

REFERENCES

1. LoCicero J III, Mattox KL: Epidemiology of chest trauma, *Surg Clin North Am* 69:15-19, 1989.
2. Feghali NT, Prisant LM: Blunt myocardial injury, *Chest* 108: 1673-1677, 1995.
3. Dubrow TJ, et al: Myocardial contusion in the stable patient: what level of care is appropriate? *Surgery* 106:267-274, 1989.
4. Frazee RC, et al: Objective evaluation of blunt cardiac trauma, *J Trauma* 26:510-520, 1986.
5. Wisner DH, Reed WH, Riddick RS: Suspected myocardial contusion: triage and indications for monitoring, *Ann Surg* 212:82-86, 1990.
6. Dougall AM, et al: Chest trauma: current morbidity and mortality, *J Trauma* 17:547-553, 1977.
7. Pretre R, Chilcott M: Blunt trauma to the heart and great vessels, *N Engl J Med* 336:626-632, 1997.
8. Meyers BF, McCabe CJ: Traumatic diaphragmatic hernia: occult marker of serious injury, *Ann Surg* 218:783-790, 1993.
9. Wise L, et al: Traumatic injuries to the diaphragm, *J Trauma* 13:946-950, 1973.
10. Drews JA, Mercer EC, Benfield JR: Acute diaphragmatic injuries, *Ann Thorac Surg* 16:67-78, 1973.
11. Troop B, Myers RM, Agarwal NN: Early recognition of diaphragmatic injuries from blunt trauma, *Ann Emerg Med* 14:97-101, 1985.
12. Swanson J, Trunkey D: Failed diagnosis: pitfalls in chest trauma, *Top Emerg Med* 10:81-88, 1988.
13. Fulda G, et al: Blunt traumatic rupture of the heart and pericardium: a ten-year experience (1979-1989), *J Trauma* 31:167-173, 1991.
14. Martin TD, et al: Blunt cardiac rupture, *J Trauma* 24:287-290, 1984.
15. Feczko JD, et al: An autopsy case review of 142 nonpenetrating (blunt) injuries of the aorta, *J Trauma* 33:846-849, 1992.
16. Greendyke RM: Traumatic rupture of the aorta: special reference to automobile accidents, *JAMA* 195:527-530, 1966.
17. Sutorius DJ, Schreiber JT, Helmsworth JA: Traumatic disruption of the thoracic aorta, *J Trauma* 13:583-590, 1973.
18. White CS, Mirvis SE: Pictorial review: imaging of traumatic aortic injury, *Clin Radiol* 50:281-287, 1995.
19. Williams JS, et al: Aortic injury in vehicular trauma, *Ann Thorac Surg* 57:726-730, 1994.
20. Nirgiotis JG, Colon R, Sweeney MS: Blunt trauma to the heart: the pathophysiology of injury, *J Emerg Med* 8:617-623, 1990.
21. DeMuth WE Jr, Baue AE, Odom JA Jr: Contusions of the heart, *J Trauma* 7:443-455, 1967.
22. Lee RB, Stahlman GC, Sharp KW: Treatment priorities in patients with traumatic rupture of the thoracic aorta, *Am Surg* 58:37-43, 1992.
23. Relland JY, Miller DM, Carberry DM: Traumatic rupture of tracheobronchial tree, *NY State J Med* 73:1291-1295, 1973.
24. Payne WS, De Remee RA: Injuries of the trachea and major bronchi, *Postgrad Med* 49:152-158, 1971.
25. Jackimczyk J: Blunt chest trauma, *Emerg Med Clin North Am* 11:81-96, 1993.
26. Weiss JP, et al: Traumatic rupture of the thoracic aorta, *Emerg Med Clin North Am* 9:789-804, 1991.
27. Kram HB, et al: Diagnosis of traumatic thoracic aortic rupture: a ten-year retrospective analysis, *Ann Thorac Surg* 47:282-286, 1989.
28. Healey MA, Brown R, Fleiszer D: Blunt cardiac injury: is this diagnosis necessary? *J Trauma* 30:137-146, 1990.
29. Snow N, Richardson JD, Flint LM Jr: Myocardial contusion: implications for patients with multiple traumatic injuries, *Surgery* 92:744-750, 1982.
30. Bickell WH, et al: Immediate versus delayed fluid resuscitation for hypotensive patients with penetrating torso injuries, *N Engl J Med* 331:1105-1109, 1994
31. Chang AK, et al: MAST 96, *J Emerg Med* 14:419-424, 1996.
32. Mattox KL, et al: Prospective MAST study in 911 patients, *J Trauma* 29:1104-1111, 1989.
33. Mattox KL, et al: Prospective randomized evaluation of antishock MAST in post-traumatic hypotension, *J Trauma* 26:779-786, 1986.
34. Vukich DJ, Markovchick V: Thoracic trauma. In Rosen P, et al (editors): *Emergency medicine: concepts and clinical practice,* ed 4, St Louis, 1998, Mosby.
35. Wilson RF, Murray C, Antonenko DR: Nonpenetrating thoracic injuries, *Surg Clin North Am* 57:17-36, 1977.
36. Walls RM: Airway management, *Emerg Med Clin North Am* 11:53-60, 1993.
37. Barton ED, et al: Emergency department intubation of trauma patients, *Acad Emerg Med* 5(abstract):457, 1998.
38. Ho AM, Ling E: Systemic air embolism after lung trauma, *Anesthesiology* 90(2):564-575, 1999.
39. American College of Surgeons Committee on Trauma: *Advanced trauma life support for doctors,* ed 6, Chicago, 1997, American College of Surgeons.
40. Miller KS, Sahn SA: Chest tubes, indications, technique, management and complications, *Chest* 91:258-264, 1987.
41. Jorden RC: Penetrating chest trauma, *Emerg Med Clin North Am* 11:97-106, 1993.
42. Markovchick V, Wolfe RE: Cardiovascular trauma. In Rosen P, et al (editors): *Emergency medicine: concepts and clinical practice,* ed 4, St Louis, 1998, Mosby.
43. Fabian TC, et al: Prospective study of blunt aortic injury: multicenter trial of the American Association for the Surgery of Trauma, *J Trauma* 42:374-383, 1997.
44. Sharma OP: Traumatic diaphragmatic rupture: not an uncommon entity-personal experience with collective review of the 1980's, *J Trauma* 29:678-682, 1989.

45. Symbas PN, et al: Traumatic rupture of the aorta, *Ann Surg* 178:6-12, 1973.
46. Mirvis SE, et al: Imaging diagnosis of traumatic aortic rupture: a review and experience at a major trauma center, *Invest Radiol* 22:187-196, 1987.
47. Kanowitz A, Markovchick V: Esophageal and diaphragmatic trauma, In Rosen P, et al (editors): *Emergency medicine: concepts and clinical practice,* ed 4, St Louis, 1998, Mosby.
48. Maenza RL, Seaberg D, D'Amico F: A meta-analysis of blunt cardiac trauma: ending myocardial confusion, *Am J Emerg Med* 14:237-241, 1996.
49. Spodick DH: Pathophysiology of cardiac tamponade, *Chest* 113:1372-78, 1998.
50. Barton ED, et al: The pathophysiology of tension pneumothorax in ventilated swine, *J Emerg Med* 15:147-153, 1997.
51. Moore JD, Mayer JH, Gago O: Traumatic asphyxia, *Chest* 62: 634-636, 1972.
52. Heurer GJ: Traumatic asphyxia; with special reference to its ocular and visual disturbances, *Surg Gynecol Obstet* 36:686-696, 1923.
53. Blair E, Topuzlu C, Davis JH: Delayed or missed diagnosis in blunt chest trauma, *J Trauma* 11:129-145, 1971.
54. Loop FD, Groves LK: Esophageal perforations, *Ann Thorac Surg* 10:571-587, 1970.
55. McCartney J, Dobrow J, Hendrix TR: Boerhaave syndrome, *Johns Hopkins Med J* 144:28-33, 1979.
56. Flynn AE, et al: Esophageal perforation, *Arch Surg* 124:1211-1214, 1989.
57. Roberts JR, Spadafora M, Cone DC: Proper depth placement of oral endotracheal tubes in adults prior to radiographic confirmation, *Acad Emerg Med* 2:20-24, 1995.
58. Grimes OF: Traumatic injuries of the diaphragm: diaphragmatic hernia, *Am J Surg* 128:175-181, 1974.
59. Guth AA, Pachter HL, Kim U: Pitfalls in the diagnosis of blunt diaphragmatic injury, *Am J Surg* 170:5-9, 1995.
60. Orebaugh SL: Venous air embolism: clinical and experimental considerations, *Crit Care Med* 20:1169-1177, 1992.
61. O'Quin RJ, Lakshminarayan S: Venous air embolism, *Arch Intern Med* 142:2173-2176, 1982.
62. Brunicardi FC, et al: Air embolism during pulsed saline irrigation of an open pelvis fracture: case report, *J Trauma* 29:700-701, 1989.
63. Azimuddin K, Porter J: Survival after cardiac arrest from documented venous air embolism, *J Trauma* 44:398-400, 1998.
64. Branney SW, et al: Critical analysis of two decades of experience with postinjury emergency department thoracotomy in a regional trauma center, *J Trauma* 45:87-95, 1998.
65. Rosenthal MA, Ellis JI: Cardiac and mediastinal trauma, *Emerg Med Clin North Am* 13:887-902, 1995.
66. Crumpton KL, Shockley LW: Emergency department thoracotomy: rationale, indications, technique, and pitfalls, *Emerg Med Rep* 17:245-252, 1996.
67. Bircher N, Safar P, Stewart R: A comparison of standard, "MAST"-augmented, and open-chest CPR in dogs: a preliminary report, *Crit Care Med* 8:147-152, 1980.
68. Boczar ME, et al: A technique revisited: hemodynamic comparison of closed- and open-chest cardiac massage during human cardiopulmonary resuscitation, *Crit Care Med* 23:498-503, 1995.
69. DeBehnke DJ, Angelos MG, Leasure JE: Comparison of standard external CPR, open-chest CPR, and cardiopulmonary bypass in a canine myocardial infarct model, *Ann Emerg Med* 20:754-760, 1991.
70. Kavolius J, Golocovsky M, Champion HR: Predictors of outcome in patients who have sustained trauma and who undergo emergency thoracotomy, *Arch Surg* 128:1158-1162, 1993.
71. Cogbill TH, et al: Rationale for selective application of emergency department thoracotomy in trauma, *J Trauma* 23:453-460, 1983.
72. Esposito TJ, et al: Reappraisal of emergency room thoracotomy in a changing environment, *J Trauma* 31:881-887, 1991.
73. Mazzorana V, et al: Limited utility of emergency department thoracotomy, *Am Surg* 60:516-521, 1994.
74. Yee ES, Verrier ED, Thomas AN: Management of air embolism in blunt and penetrating thoracic trauma, *J Thorac Cardiovasc Surg* 85:661-668, 1983.
75. Gunnar WP, et al: The utility of cardiac evaluation in the hemodynamically stable patient with suspected myocardial contusion, *Am Surg* 57:373-377, 1991.
76. Biffl WL, et al: Cardiac enzymes are irrelevant in the patient with suspected myocardial contusion, *Am J Surg* 168:523-527, 1994.
77. Tenzer ML: The spectrum of myocardial contusion: a review, *J Trauma* 25:620-627, 1985.
78. Potkin RT, et al: Evaluation of noninvasive tests of cardiac damage in suspected cardiac contusion, *Circulation* 66:627-631, 1982.
79. Schwab CW, et al: Aortic injury: comparison of supine and upright portable chest films to evaluate the widened mediastinum, *Ann Emerg Med* 13:896-899, 1984.
80. Hehir MD, Hollands MJ, Deane SA: The accuracy of the first chest x-ray in the trauma patient, *Aust N Z J Surg* 60:529-532, 1990.
81. Karaaslan T, et al: Traumatic chest lesions in patients with severe head trauma: a comparative study with computed tomography and conventional chest roentgenograms, *J Trauma* 39: 1081-1086, 1995.
82. Schild HH, et al: Pulmonary contusion: CT vs. plain radiograms, *J Comput Assist Tomogr* 13:417-420, 1989.
83. Bekassy SM, Dave KS, Ionescu MI: Spontaneous and traumatic rupture of the diaphragm: long-term results, *Ann Surg* 177:320-324, 1973.
84. Kirshner R, Seltzer S, D'Orsi C, DeWeese JA: Upper rib fractures and mediastinal widening: indications for aortography *Ann Thorac Surg* 35(4):450-4, 1983.
85. Ayella RJ, et al: Ruptured thoracic aorta due to blunt trauma, *J Trauma* 17:199-205, 1977.
86. Gundry SR, et al: Indications for aortography in blunt thoracic trauma: a reassesment, *J Trauma* 22:664-671, 1982.
87. Gundry SR, et al: Assessment of mediastinal widening associated with traumatic rupture of the aorta, *J Trauma* 23:293-299, 1983.
88. Hanschen S, Snow NJ, Richardson JD: Thoracic aortic rupture in patients with multisystem injuries, *South Med J* 75:653-656, 1982.
89. Mirvis SE, et al: Value of chest radiography in excluding traumatic aortic rupture, *Radiology* 163:487-493, 1987.
90. Richardson JD, Wilson ME, Miller FB: The widened mediastinum: diagnostic and therapeutic priorities, *Ann Surg* 211:731-736, 1990.
91. Seltzer SE, et al: Traumatic aortic rupture: plain radiographic findings, *AJR* 137:1011-1014, 1981.
92. Sturm JT, Olson FR, Cicero JJ: Chest roentgenographic findings in 26 patients with traumatic rupture of the thoracic aorta, *Ann Emerg Med* 12:598-600, 1983.
93. Lee FT Jr, et al: Reevaluation of plain radiographic findings in the diagnosis of aortic rupture: the role of inspiration and positioning on mediastinal width, *J Emerg Med* 11:289-296, 1993.
94. Biquet JF, Dondelinger RF, Roland D: Computed tomography of thoracic aortic trauma, *Eur Radiol* 6:25-29, 1996.

95. Gavant ML, et al: Blunt traumatic aortic rupture: detection with helical CT of the chest, *Radiology* 197:125-133, 1995.
96. Nagy KK, et al: Computed tomography screens stable patients at risk for penetrating cardiac injury, *Acad Emerg Med* 3:1024-1027, 1996.
97. Trupka A, et al: Value of thoracic computed tomography in the first assessment of severely injured patients with blunt chest trauma: results of a prospective study, *J Trauma* 43:405-411, 1997.
98. Smejkal R, et al: Routine initial computed tomography of the chest in blunt torso trauma, *Chest* 100:667-669, 1991.
99. Enderson BL, et al: Tube thoracostomy for occult pneumothorax: a prospective randomized study of its use, *J Trauma* 35: 726-730, 1993.
100. Wolfman NT, et al: Occult pneumothorax in patients with abdominal trauma: CT studies, *J Comput Assist Tomogr* 17:56-59, 1993.
101. Bridges KG, et al: CT detection of occult pneumothorax in multiple trauma patients, *J Emerg Med* 11:179-186, 1993.
102. McLean TR, Olinger GN, Thorsen MK: Computed tomography in the evaluation of the aorta in patients sustaining blunt chest trauma, *J Trauma* 31:254-256, 1991.
103. Richardson P, et al: Value of CT in determining the need for angiography when findings of mediastinal hemorrhage on chest radiographs are equivocal, *AJR* 156:273-279, 1991.
104. Fisher RG, et al: Arteriography and the fractured first rib: too much for too little? *AJR* 138:1059-1062, 1982.
105. Gavant ML, et al: CT aortography of thoracic aortic rupture, *AJR* 166:955-961, 1996.
106. Fabian TC, et al: Prospective study of blunt aortic injury: helical CT is diagnostic and antihypertensive therapy reduces rupture, *Ann Surg* 227:666-676, 1998.
107. Schnyder P, et al: Helical CT angiography for traumatic aortic rupture: correlation with aortography and surgery in five cases, *J Thorac Imag* 11:39-45, 1996.
108. Plummer D: The sensitivity, specificity, and accuracy of ED echocardiography *Acad Emerg Med* 2(abstract):339-340, 1995.
109. Ma OJ, Mateer JR: Trauma ultrasound examination versus chest radiography in the detection of hemothorax, *Ann Emerg Med* 29:312-315, 1997.
110. Miller FB, Shumate CR, Richardson JD: Myocardial contusion: when can the diagnosis be eliminated? *Arch Surg* 124:805-807, 1989.
111. Beggs CW, et al: Early evaluation of cardiac injury by two-dimensional echocardiography in patients suffering blunt chest trauma, *Ann Emerg Med* 16:542-545, 1987.
112. Hiatt JR, Yeatman LA Jr, Child JS: The value of echocardiography in blunt chest trauma, *J Trauma* 28:914-922, 1988.
113. Chirillo F, et al: Usefulness of transthoracic and transesophageal echocardiography in recognition and management of cardiovascular injuries after blunt chest trauma, *Heart* 75:301-306, 1996.
114. Kearney PA, et al: Use of transesophageal echocardiography in the evaluation of traumatic aortic injury, *J Trauma* 34:696-701, 1993.
115. Shapiro MJ, et al: Cardiovascular evaluation in blunt thoracic trauma using transesophageal echocardiography (TEE), *J Trauma* 31:835-839, 1991.
116. Vignon P, et al: Role of transesophageal echocardiography in the diagnosis and management of traumatic aortic disruption, *Circulation* 92:2959-2968, 1995.
117. Vignon P, et al: Routine transesophageal echocardiography for the diagnosis of aortic disruption in trauma patients without enlarged mediastinum, *J Trauma* 40:422-427, 1996.
118. Smith MD, et al: Transesophageal echocardiography in the diagnosis of traumatic rupture of the aorta, *N Engl J Med* 332:356-362, 1995.
119. Buckmaster MJ, et al: Further experience with transesophageal echocardiography in the evaluation of thoracic aortic injury, *J Trauma* 37:989-995, 1994.
120. Williams DM, et al: The role of intravascular ultrasound in acute traumatic aortic rupture, *Semin Ultrasound CT MRI* 14:85-90, 1993.
121. Read RA, et al: Intravascular ultrasonography for the diagnosis of traumatic aortic disruption: a case report, *Surgery* 114: 624-628, 1993.
122. Williams DM, et al: Acute traumatic aortic rupture: intravascular US findings, *Radiology* 182:247-249, 1992.
123. Hughes JP, Ruttley MS, Musumeci F: Case report: traumatic aortic rupture: demonstration by magnetic resonance imaging, *Br J Radiol* 67:1264-1267, 1994.
124. Ahrar K, et al: Angiography in blunt thoracic aortic injury, *J Trauma* 42: 665-669, 1997.
125. Sturm JT, Hankins DG, Young G: Thoracic aortography following blunt chest trauma, *Am J Emerg Med* 8:92-96, 1990.
126. Frattori R, Celleti F, Bertaccini P, et al: Delayed surgery of traumatic aortic rupture: role of magnetic resonance imaging, *Circulation* 94(11):2865-2870, 1996.
127. Kram HB, Wohlmuth DA, Appel PL, et al: Clinical and radiographic indications for aortography in blunt chest trauma, *J Vasc Surg* 6(2):168-176, 1987.
128. Hara KS, Prakash UB: Fiberoptic bronchoscopy in the evaluation of acute chest and upper airway trauma, *Chest* 96:627-630, 1989.
129. Flowers JL, et al: Flexible endoscopy for the diagnosis of esophageal trauma, *J Trauma* 40:261-266, 1996.
130. Berry BE, Ochsner JL: Perforation of the esophagus: a 30-year review, *J Thorac Cardiovasc Surg* 65:1-7, 1973.
131. Zantut LF, et al: Bilateral diaphragmatic injury diagnosed by laparoscopy, *Rev Paul Med* 111:430-432, 1993.
132. Spann JC, Nwariaku FE, Wait M: Evaluation of video-assisted thoracoscopic surgery in the diagnosis of diaphragmatic injuries, *Am J Surg* 170:628-630, 1995.
133. Simon RJ, Ivatury RR: Current concepts in the use of cavitary endoscopy in the evaluation and treatment of blunt and penetrating truncal injuries, *Surg Clin North Am* 75:157-174, 1995.
134. Graeber GM, Jones DR: The role of thoracoscopy in thoracic trauma, *Ann Thorac Surg* 56:646-648, 1993.
135. Hermansson U, Konstantinov I, Traff S: Lung injury with pleuropericardial rupture successfully treated by video-assisted thoracoscopy: case report, *J Trauma* 40:1024-1025, 1996.
136. Thomas P, et al: Diagnosis by video-assisted thoracoscopy of traumatic pericardial rupture with delayed luxation of the heart: case report, *J Trauma* 38:967-970, 1995.
137. Webb WR: Thoracic trauma, *Surg Clin North Am* 54:1179-1192, 1972.
138. Oreskovich MR, Carrico CJ: Trauma: management of the acutely injured patient. In Sabiston DC (editor): *Textbook of surgery,* ed 13, Philadelphia, 1986, Saunders.
139. Shorr RM, et al: Blunt thoracic trauma: analysis of 515 patients, *Ann Surg* 206:200-205, 1987.
140. Cohn SM: Pulmonary contusion: review of the clinical entity, *J Trauma* 42:973-979, 1997.
141. Baxter BT, et al: Graded experimental myocardial contusion: impact on cardiac rhythm, coronary artery flow, ventricular function and myocardial oxygen consumption, *J Trauma* 28: 1411-1417, 1988.

142. Doty DB, et al: Cardiac trauma: clinical and experimental correlations of myocardial contusions, *Ann Surg* 180:452-460, 1974.
143. Maron BJ, et al: Survival following blunt chest impact-induced cardiac arrest during sports activities in young athletes, *Am J Cardiol* 79:840-841, 1997.
144. Janda DH, et al: Blunt chest impacts: assessing the relative risk of fatal cardiac injury from various baseballs, *J Trauma* 44:298-303, 1998.
145. Crown LA, Hawkins W: Commotio cordis: clinical implications of blunt cardiac trauma, *Am Fam Physician* 55:2467-2470, 1997.
146. Link MS, et al: An experimental model of sudden death due to low-energy chest-wall impact (commotio cordis), *N Engl J Med* 338:1805-1811, 1998.
147. DeMuth WE Jr, Zinsser HF Jr: Myocardial contusion, *Arch Intern Med* 115:434-442, 1965.
148. Silver GM, et al: Ventricular aneurysms and blunt chest trauma, *Chest* 63:628-631, 1973.
149. Van Schil P, et al: Subocclusion of the left anterior descending artery following blunt chest trauma, *Eur Heart J* 9:1361-1362, 1988.
150. Cachecho R, Grindlinger GA, Lee VW: The clinical significance of myocardial contusion, *J Trauma* 33:68-71, 1992.
151. Sutherland GR, et al: Frequency of myocardial injury after blunt chest trauma as evaluated by radionuclide angiography, *Am J Cardiol* 52:1099-1103, 1983.
152. Sturaitis M, et al: Lack of significant long-term sequelae following traumatic myocardial contusion, *Arch Intern Med* 146: 1765-1769, 1986.
153. Dowd MD, Krug S: Pediatric blunt cardiac injury: epidemiology, clinical features and diagnosis, *J Trauma* 40:61-67, 1996.
154. Fildes JJ, et al: Limiting cardiac evaluations in patients with suspected myocardial contusion, *Am Surg* 61:832-835, 1995.
155. King RM, et al: Cardiac contusion: a new diagnostic approach utilizing two-dimensional echocardiography, *J Trauma* 23:610-614, 1983.
156. Keller KD, Shatney CH: Creatine phosphokinase-MB assays in patients with suspected myocardial contusion: diagnostic test or test of diagnosis? *J Trauma* 28:58-63, 1988.
157. Adams JE III, et al: Improved detection of cardiac contusion with cardiac troponin I, *Am Heart J* 131:308-312, 1996.
158. Ferjani M, et al: Circulating cardiac troponin T in myocardial contusion, *Chest* 111:427-433, 1997.
159. Fulda GJ, et al: An evaluation of serum troponin T and signal-averaged electrocardiography in predicting electrocardiographic abnormalities after blunt chest trauma, *J Trauma* 43: 304-310, 1997.
160. Ognibene A, et al: Cardiac troponin I in myocardial contusion, *Clin Chem* 44:889-890, 1998.
161. Calhoon JH, et al: Management of blunt rupture of the heart, *J Trauma* 26:495-501, 1986.
162. Pevec WC, Udekwu AO, Peitzman AB: Blunt rupture of the myocardium, *Ann Thorac Surg* 48:139-142, 1989.
163. Griffith GL, et al: Right atrial rupture due to blunt chest trauma, *South Med J* 77:715-716, 1984.
164. Parmley LF, Manion WC, Mattingly TW: Nonpenetrating traumatic injury of the heart, *Circulation* 18:371-396, 1958.
165. Brathwaite CE, et al: Blunt traumatic cardiac rupture: a 5-year experience, *Ann Surg* 212:701-704, 1990.
166. Mattox KL, et al: Logistic and technical considerations in the treatment of the wounded heart, *Circulation* 51/52(suppl I): I210-I214, 1975.
167. Sharp JR, et al: Hemodynamics during induced cardiac tamponade in man, *Am J Med* 29:640-646, 1960.
168. Stein L, Shubin H, Weil MH: Recognition and management of pericardial tamponade, *JAMA* 225:503-506, 1973.
169. Shoemaker WC: Algorithm for early recognition and management of cardiac tamponade, *Crit Care Med* 3:59-63, 1975.
170. Turney SZ, et al: Traumatic rupture of the aorta: a five-year experience, *J Thorac Cardiovasc Surg* 72:727-734, 1976.
171. Kirsh MM, et al: The treatment of acute rupture of the aorta: a 10-year experience, *Ann Surg* 84:308-316, 1976.
172. Parmley LF, et al: Nonpenetrating traumatic injury of the aorta, *Circulation* 17:1086-1101, 1958.
173. Mattox KL: Red River anthology, *J Trauma* 42:353-368, 1997.
174. Crass JR, et al: A proposed new mechanism of traumatic aortic rupture: the osseous pinch, *Radiology* 176:645-649, 1990.
175. Warren RL, et al: Acute traumatic disruption of the thoracic aorta: emergency department management, *Ann Emerg Med* 21:391-396, 1992.
176. Schepens MA, Van Cauwelaert PA, Gerard YE: Acute traumatic disruption of the thoracic aorta, *Acta Chir Belg* 89:189-195, 1989.
177. Kim FJ, et al: Trauma surgeons can render definitive surgical care for major thoracic injuries, *J Trauma* 36:871-876, 1994.
178. Pate JW: Traumatic rupture of the aorta: emergency operation, *Ann Thorac Surg* 39:531-537, 1985.
179. Merrill WH, et al: Surgical treatment of acute traumatic tear of the thoracic aorta, *Ann Surg* 207:699-706, 1988.
180. Hess PJ, et al: Traumatic tears of the thoracic aorta: improved results using the Bio-Medicus pump, *Ann Thorac Surg* 48:6-9, 1989.
181. Frick EJ, et al: Outcome of blunt thoracic aortic injury in a Level I trauma center: an 8-year review, *J Trauma* 43:844-851, 1997.
182. Camp PC, Shackford SR, Western Trauma Association Multicenter Group: Outcome after blunt traumatic thoracic aortic laceration: identification of a high-risk cohort, *J Trauma* 43:413-422, 1997.
183. McCroskey BL, et al: A unified approach to the torn thoracic aorta, *Am J Surg* 162: 473-476, 1991.
184. Read RA, et al: Partial left heart bypass for thoracic aorta repair: survival without paraplegia, *Arch Surg* 128:746-752, 1993.
185. Clark DE, et al: Blunt aortic trauma: signs of high risk, *J Trauma* 30:701-705, 1990.
186. Niezgoda JA, McMenamin P, Graeber GM: Pharyngoesophageal perforation after blunt neck trauma, *Ann Thorac Surg* 50:615-617, 1990.
187. Krekorian EA: Laryngopharyngeal injuries, *Laryngoscope* 85: 2069-2085, 1975.
188. Splener CW, Benfield JR: Esophageal disruption from blunt and penetrating external trauma, *Arch Surg* 111:663-667, 1976.
189. Meads GE, Carroll SE, Pitt DF: Traumatic rupture of the right hemidiaphragm, *J Trauma* 17:797-801, 1977.
190. Hood RM: Traumatic diaphragmatic hernia, *Ann Thorac Surg* 12:311-324, 1971.
191. Morley JE: Traumatic diaphragmatic rupture, *S Afr Med J* 48: 325-328, 1974.
192. Ordog GJ, Wasserberger J, Balasubramaniam S: Tension gastrothorax complicating post-traumatic rupture of the diaphragm, *Am J Emerg Med* 2:219-221, 1984.
193. Cameron EW, Mirvis SE: Ruptured hemidiaphragm: unusual late presentation, *J Emerg Med* 14:53-58, 1995.
194. Nowak R, Tomlanovich MC: Subcutaneous emphysema, *JACEP* 6:269-272, 1977.
195. Thompson DA, et al: The significance of scapular fractures, *J Trauma* 25:974-977, 1985.
196. Hills MW, Delprado AM, Deane SA: Sternal fractures: associated injuries and management, *J Trauma* 35:55-60, 1993.

197. Lee J, et al: Noncorrelation between thoracic skeletal injuries and acute traumatic aortic tear, *J Trauma* 43: 400-404, 1997.
198. Gouldman JW, Miller RS: Sternal fractures: a benign entity? *Am Surg* 63:17-19, 1997.
199. Chiu WC, D'Amelio LF, Hammond JS: Sternal fractures in blunt chest trauma: a practical algorithm for management, *Am J Emerg Med* 15:252-255, 1997.
200. Sivit CJ, Taylor GA, Eichelberger MR: Chest injury in children with blunt abdominal trauma: evaluation with CT, *Radiology* 171:815-818, 1989.
201. Peclet MH, et al: Thoracic trauma in children: an indicator of increased mortality, *J Pediatr Surg* 25:961-965, 1990.
202. Bromberg BI, et al: Recognition and management of nonpenetrating cardiac trauma in children, *J Pediatr* 128:536-541, 1996.
203. Lowe LH, et al: Traumatic aortic injuries in children: radiologic evaluation, *AJR* 170:39-42, 1998.
204. Spouge AR, et al: Traumatic aortic rupture in the pediatric population: role of plain film, CT and angiography in the diagnosis, *Pediatr Radiol* 21:324-328, 1991.
205. Lee RB, et al: Three or more rib fractures as an indicator for transfer to a level I trauma center: a population-based study, *J Trauma* 30:689-694, 1990.
206. Baxter BT, et al: A plea for sensible management of myocardial contusion, *Am J Surg* 158:557-562, 1989.

18 Penetrating Chest Trauma

VINCENT N. MOSESSO, Jr.

INTRODUCTION AND EPIDEMIOLOGY

Chest injuries cause about one quarter of trauma deaths in the United States[1] and contribute to nearly 50% of all trauma-related mortality.[2] Overall mortality is estimated to be 10%.[3] Immediate deaths are caused by vascular or cardiac penetration, whereas early deaths (within the first few hours) most commonly result from hemorrhage, pericardial tamponade, tension pneumothorax (PTX), or airway obstruction.[4] Late deaths ensue from acquired respiratory distress syndrome (ARDS), multiorgan system failure, sepsis, and missed injuries. Although the mortality from blunt chest trauma is greater than penetrating trauma, penetrating injury more frequently requires an operation.

The emergency physician (EP) can initially manage the vast majority of patients with penetrating chest trauma, as only 15% require an operation. However, when a patient remains unstable after initial interventions, the EP should consult a surgeon immediately or arrange transfer to a trauma center.[2]

PATHOPHYSIOLOGY

Penetrating chest trauma (PCT) comprises a broad spectrum of injuries and severity (Table 18-1). The clinical consequences depend on mechanism, location, associated injuries, and underlying illness. Many organs are at risk in PCT. In addition to the intrathoracic contents, other endangered structures include the diaphragm, intraperitoneal viscera, retroperitoneal space, and neck.

Life-threatening injuries either produce massive hemorrhage, compromise gas exchange, or interfere with cardiac filling. Direct injury to the esophagus, thoracic duct, diaphragm, and bony structures also occurs but is usually not immediately life threatening.

Air exchange depends both on the patency of the airway and on the ability to generate negative intrapulmonary pressure. In the uninjured person, chest expansion creates a negative intrapleural pressure during inspiration. Penetrating trauma may disrupt the chest wall, pleural linings, or large airways and compromise respirations.

Intraabdominal Injury

Stab wounds below the nipple line anteriorly and the inferior tip of the scapula posteriorly may injure the diaphragm and intraabdominal structures. Gunshot wounds (GSW) can penetrate all body regions regardless of point of entry. High-velocity projectiles in particular can easily traverse the entire body. For example, if the victim was diving away from the gunman, a bullet entering the buttocks may lodge in the neck.[5,6]

Mediastinal Injury

Any stab wound between the midclavicular lines and between the clavicle and subxiphoid area endangers the mediastinum (Fig. 18-1). Gunshot wounds can violate the mediastinum regardless of their point of entry.

MECHANISM OF INJURY

Mechanism may be categorized as low, medium, or high velocity. Low-velocity forces include impalement, such as stab wounds and pneumatic nail guns. These forces disrupt only those structures penetrated. Medium-velocity injuries result from most handguns and air-powered pellet guns, whereas rifles, military weapons, and close-range shotgun blasts yield high-velocity projectiles. Medium- and high-velocity agents produce injury both in the permanent cavity and in a temporary cavity as a result of tissue stretching and compression (see Chapter 40).

TABLE 18-1
Thoracic Injuries in 755 Patients

INJURY	NUMBER
Hemothorax	190
Hemopneumothorax	184
Pneumothorax	144
Diaphragmatic rupture	121
Open hemopneumothorax	95
Pulmonary contusion	50
Open pneumothorax	24
Rib fracture	
<2	16
>2	13
Subcutaneous emphysema	14
Bilateral pneumothorax	9
Open bilateral hemopneumothorax	13
Pneumomediastinum	6
Thoracic wall lacerations	4
Bilateral hemopneumothorax	3
Open bilateral pneumothorax	3
Sternal fracture	3
Bilateral diaphragmatic rupture	2

From Inci I, et al: *World J Surg* 22(5):439, 1998.

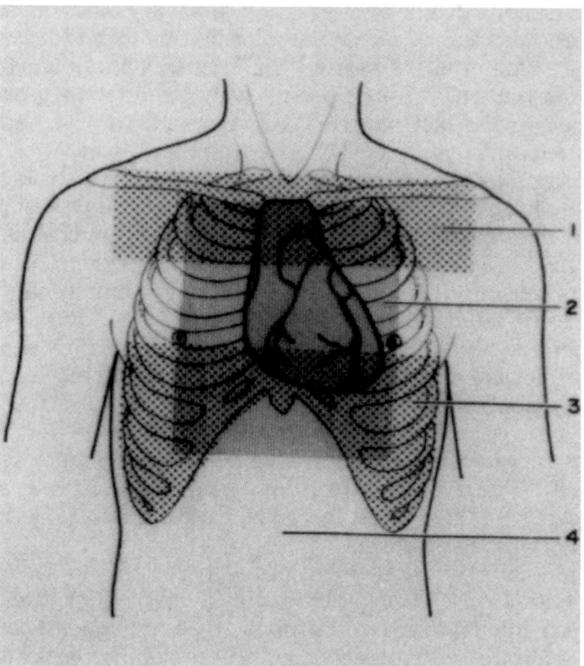

Fig. 18-1 Transmediastinal penetrating trauma and anatomic risk areas. *1,* Great vessels; *2,* precordial; *3,* thoracoabdominal; *4,* abdominal. (From Ferrada R, Garcia A: Penetrating torso trauma. In Maull KI et al (editors): *Advances in trauma and critical care,* vol 8, St Louis, 1993, Mosby.)

CLINICAL PRESENTATION

Clinical presentation may range from asymptomatic to moribund, and patients with similar entrance sites and mechanisms can suffer vastly different injuries. Eight percent of patients with PCT develop acute respiratory failure in the emergency department (ED), usually resulting from shock or hemothorax (HTX). Wilson[5] reported that patients with acute respiratory distress on arrival in the ED requiring intubation correlated with a mortality rate >50%.

HISTORY

Obtain information from the patient and paramedics regarding the mechanism and time of injury. The medics should report prehospital examination including vital signs and the patient's response to any therapy given. A history of prehospital hypotension is particularly important. Although details regarding the offending instrument are routine, such as the length of the knife or caliber of the handgun, potentially lethal internal injury can occur with a "short" knife or "small" gun. Shortness of breath, palpitations, abdominal pain, and light-headedness are all significant symptoms. The single most informative question is "How is your breathing?" If the patient is unable to answer this question, immediate interventions are generally necessary.

PHYSICAL EXAMINATION

Vital Signs

Although tachycardia and hypotension frequently accompany shock, patients may have normal or near-normal vital signs despite significant blood loss. Maneuvers such as measurement of the pulsus paradoxus and the arterial brachial index supply additional information. Pulsus paradoxus is a difference in systolic blood pressures between inspiration and expiration resulting from respirophasic changes in cardiac filling, ventricular septal movement, and subsequent cardiac output. During normal inspiration, a 10-point drop in systolic pressure is normal, whereas larger differences may indicate pericardial tamponade. Use the arterial brachial index (ABI) (see Chapter 30) to detect vascular injury. If the ABI ratio is less than 0.90, the EP must evaluate for vascular injury. Another useful maneuver is comparison of the blood pressures in each arm; a difference in systolic pressure greater than 20 mmHg is suspicious for injury to a great vessel.

Bullet Holes and Stab Wounds

Although these patients usually present with obvious chest wall injury, it is important to search for occult wounds. Remove the patient's clothing, look in the axilla, and examine the back. Gunshot wounds in these locations often go unnoticed, particularly in the event of multiple projectiles.

Certainly, the EP should determine the location and apparent trajectory of penetrating chest wounds. However, potential trajectories may be deceiving. Bullets may tumble and ricochet off bones and mislead the physician regarding the extent of injury. Entrance and exit wounds cannot always be distinguished, and some entrance wounds are larger than the corresponding exit wound. Counting the number of bullet holes may account for the number of missiles remaining in the body. An odd number of holes usually implies retained bullets (although an even number of holes may represent an entry plus an exit wound or two entry wounds).

Neck

The neck examination may reveal jugular veins that distend on inspiration. Venous distention reflects impaired right ventricular filling and suggests a developing tension PTX or pericardial tamponade (Kussmaul's sign). However, jugular distention is often absent despite these conditions in the hypovolemic patient. Tracheal deviation, often considered a hallmark of tension PTX, is rarely seen in clinical practice.

Chest

The lung examination is important to detect abnormal or unequal breath sounds and evaluate the adequacy of air exchange. Palpate the chest and base of the neck for subcutaneous emphysema and look for sucking chest wounds. Auscultation of the heart may reveal muffled heart tones in patients who have pericardial tamponade. Clear heart sounds found early in the resuscitation may later become obscured by accumulating blood in the pericardium.

Abdomen

Stab wounds to the low chest, and gunshot wounds to any part of the torso, jeopardize abdominal viscera. Although tenderness to abdominal palpation is an important finding, the abdomen may remain soft despite serious injury.

EMERGENCY DEPARTMENT EVALUATION AND MANAGEMENT OF UNSTABLE PATIENTS (Fig. 18-2)

Airway

The EP's initial concern is the airway. Indications for emergency endotracheal intubation include apnea, profound shock, and inadequate ventilation. All patients with penetrating trauma require supplemental oxygen. Severe bronchial or unilateral pulmonary injury may require selective intubation of the opposite mainstem bronchus. A persistent PTX that will not resolve with placement of a second chest tube is likely caused by a bronchial injury. Intubation of the right mainstem bronchus is simple (in the adult, just push the tube further into the lung). Intubation of the left mainstem bronchus is technically difficult and is best performed by an anesthesiologist using a double-lumen tube and an intubating bronchoscope. Even though the initial chest film may be normal—*patients intubated for PCT are likely to develop a PTX once positive pressure ventilation is begun.*

Breathing

One of the most frequent mistakes in treatment of PCT involves a radiographic approach to the tension pneumothorax (PTX). A chest radiograph is not indicated in patients who display clinical signs of this condition. Patients in shock who have tracheal deviation and unilateral decreased breath sounds require immediate chest decompression. Decompression may be accomplished by a large-bore needle inserted at the second intercostal space, midclavicular line, or more definitively, by a tube thoracostomy (see Chapter 51). If the needle approach is initially chosen, tube thoracostomy must follow (Fig. 18-3).

Large defects of the chest wall, which create a sucking chest wound, compromise respiration. If the chest hole is two thirds the diameter of the trachea or larger, air preferentially passes through the wound instead of the airway. Cover the wound with an occlusive dressing and leave one corner untaped. This maneuver serves as a flutter valve to release pleural air and prevents insufflation of outside air. Patients with sucking chest wounds require a tube thoracostomy through a separate incision. *Do not place the chest tube through the wound, since this action may precipitate empyema.*

All patients with PCT require an early chest radiograph (although those with a tension PTX need the film after chest decompression). It is most helpful to obtain an upright chest film. An upright chest film more clearly demonstrates HTX, which is seen as a sometimes-diffuse haze on a supine film, but as a clearly defined meniscus on an upright study. A PTX may be imperceptible on a supine film, since the air

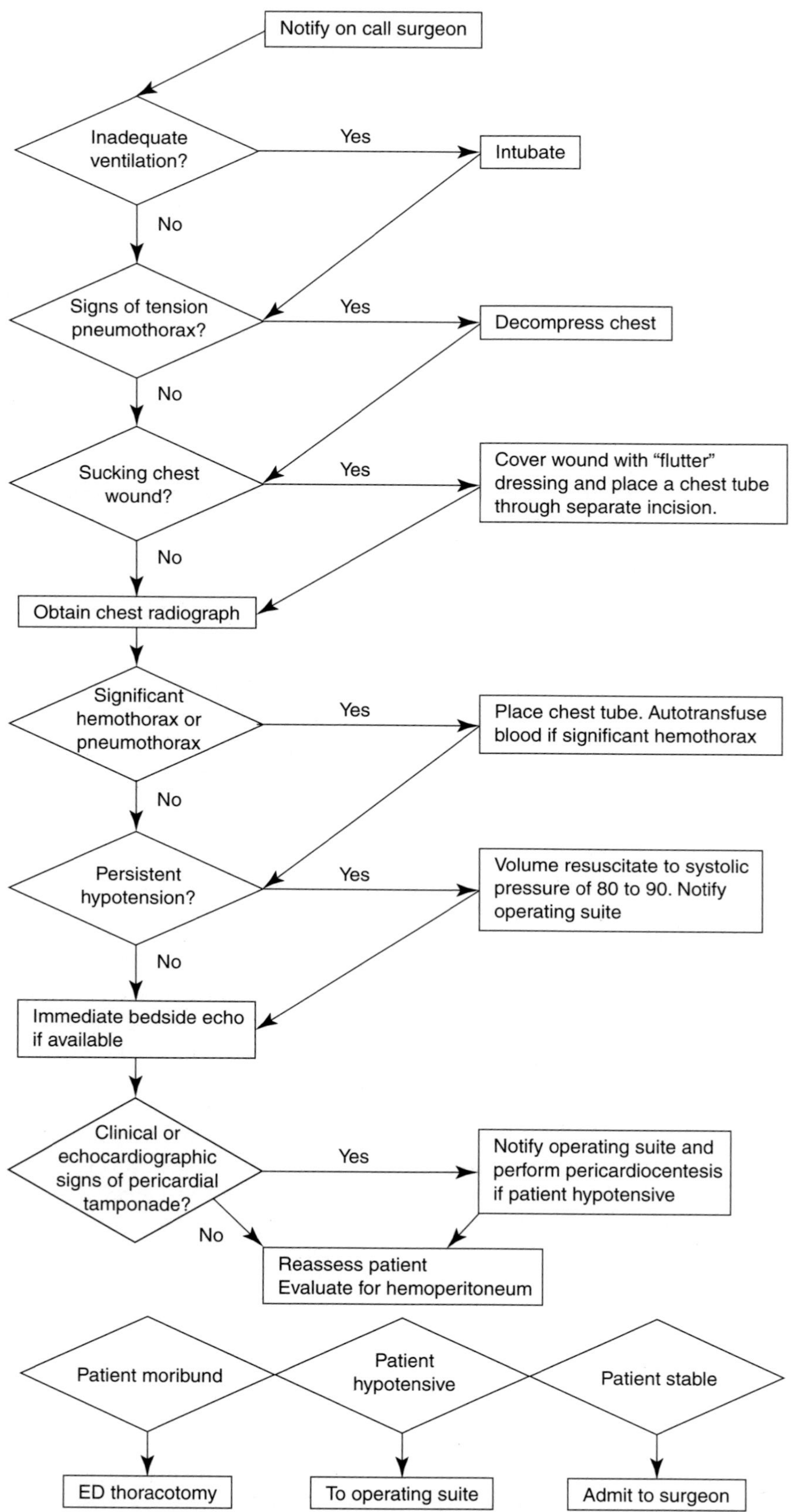

Fig. 18-2 Algorithm for management of penetrating chest trauma in the unstable patient.

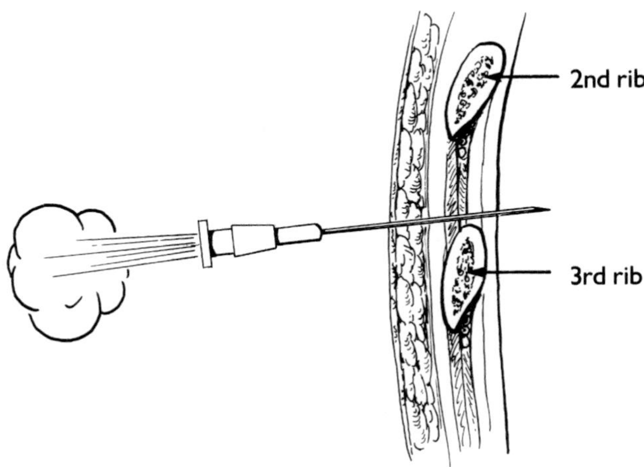

Fig. 18-3 Pneumothorax needle decompression. (From Dunmire S, Paris P: *Atlas of emergency procedures,* Philadelphia, 1994, Saunders.)

rises anteriorly toward the sternum. A PTX is best seen on an upright film since the air ascends to the apices. On occasion, an expiratory film shows a PTX invisible on an inspiratory study.

Circulation

Once the airway and breathing have been stabilized, assess circulatory status. Hypoperfusion may be due not only to blood loss but also to impaired cardiac filling. Both tension PTX and cardiac tamponade decrease venous supply to the heart, producing shock. Prompt decompression of cardiac tamponade results in good survival.[6] ED echocardiography can rapidly identify pericardial effusion. Therapeutic pericardiocentesis, even with removal of as little as 10 to 20 cc, may improve hemodynamic status.

Once tension PTX has been excluded or treated, patients with hypotension or other signs of shock require volume resuscitation, surgery, or both. The amount and rapidity of volume resuscitation is a contentious issue. Some data suggest that volume resuscitation before surgical control of bleeding may worsen outcomes in penetrating torso trauma.[7] For this reason, some authorities would suggest little or no volume resuscitation in the ED in favor of rapid transport to the operating suite (see Chapter 8). However, this restrictive approach to fluid administration is currently confined to a few urban trauma centers.

Most authorities suggest the administration of 1 to 2 liters of crystalloids to the hypotensive patient. This approach may improve hemodynamics even in the face of pericardial tamponade. Avoid over-aggressive fluid loading, which could lead to interstitial and alveolar edema.

When performing fluid resuscitation, start at least two large-bore (16 gauge or larger) intravenous (IV) lines and infuse IV fluids under pressure with large tubing if the patient is in shock. Consider that central venous access may be useful for both fluid resuscitation (using 8.5 French catheters) and to measure central venous pressure. An elevation in CVP may indicate a pericardial tamponade and may be the only early clue to this diagnosis when ultrasound is unavailable. Some authorities suggest lines be placed both above and below the diaphragm in unstable patients; however, there is no empiric data to support this approach.

Failure to respond to initial crystalloid fluid should prompt early blood transfusion and a second notification of the surgeon. Autotransfusing the patient's own blood from the chest tube drainage system is ideal. Type-specific or emergency uncrossedmatched blood may be indicated depending on the patient's response to therapy. Uncontrolled, persistent chest hemorrhage necessitates thoracotomy.

If the patient remains in shock despite volume resuscitation, consider the following:[4]

- ◆ Ongoing hemorrhage into the chest, abdomen, or retroperitoneum
- ◆ Tension pneumothorax
- ◆ Cardiac tamponade
- ◆ Neurogenic shock from a high-cord injury
- ◆ Cardiogenic shock

Monitoring

Many patients with PCT benefit from cardiac monitoring. However, dysrhythmias are rarely the cause of hemodynamic instability in such patients. Direct injury to the heart can lead to hemodynamically significant ventricular dysrhythmias. These conduction disturbances may be treated with antidysrhythmics such as lidocaine in the usual fashion. Other antidysrhythmics such as procainamide, bretylium, ß-blockers, and calcium channel blockers may produce hypotension. Pulseless electrical activity (PEA) should suggest tension PTX, cardiac tamponade, or profound shock.

Pulse oximetry provides important information regarding hypoxia. However, pulse oximetry cannot determine adequacy of ventilation, which is a clinical assessment that may be aided by arterial blood gas analysis.

RESUSCITATIVE THORACOTOMY

The duration of arrest significantly influences mortality. Durham et al[8] found no survivors in intubated patients who were in arrest for 10 minutes or longer and nonintubated patients arrested for greater than

5 minutes. Thoracotomy (see Fig. 51-4) is indicated in the ED for the following:

- Patients who arrest after arrival in the ED
- Patients who had signs of life at the scene but arrested en route to the hospital (who undergo less than 10 minutes of cardiopulmonary resuscitation)
- Moribund patients who have signs of life present but no, or barely detectable, blood pressure
- Patients who remain unstable despite intubation, adequate tube thoracotomies, and volume resuscitation

The EP is most likely to save a patient with a resuscitative thoracotomy if the patient has a gunshot wound or stab wound to the heart. Release of a pericardial tamponade is the primary goal of ED thoracotomy.

Before opening the chest, intubate the patient, ventilate with 100% oxygen, and establish intravenous access. Benefits of ED thoracotomy include the following:

- Release of pericardial tamponade (central goal)
- Control of exsanguinating hemorrhage either by direct vascular compression or proximal clamping
- Direct cardiac massage
- Cross-clamping of the descending aorta
- Control of massive air leak by clamping pulmonary hilum

DIAGNOSTIC MODALITIES

Ultrasonography

Bedside ultrasonography (US) can rapidly assess abnormal fluid collections and is the subject of many recent studies. The FAST (Focused Assessment for the Sonographic examination of the Trauma patient) examination includes evaluation of the thorax and abdomen and can be completed within 5 minutes (Fig. 18-4).[9] Use US in patients with thoracic trauma to detect pleural and pericardial effusions.

Both EPs and trauma surgeons successfully employ transthoracic echocardiography (TTE) in the diagnosis of pleural effusions.[10-14] Sisley et al[15] reported a 97.5% sensitivity and 99.7% specificity for pleural effusions that were present in 40 of 360 patients studied. Bedside US is particularly helpful for the patient who must remain immobilized in the supine position. Chest films are insensitive to small to moderate blood collections in this situation. Not only was US more sensitive than portable CXR (92.5% sensitivity for chest films), US was much faster (1.3 versus 14.2 minutes). Ma and Mateer[16] also reported similar sensitivity and specificity for bedside ultrasonography performed by EPs when compared with chest radiography. Ultrasonography is not only more rapid than chest radiography, it reveals smaller fluid collections:

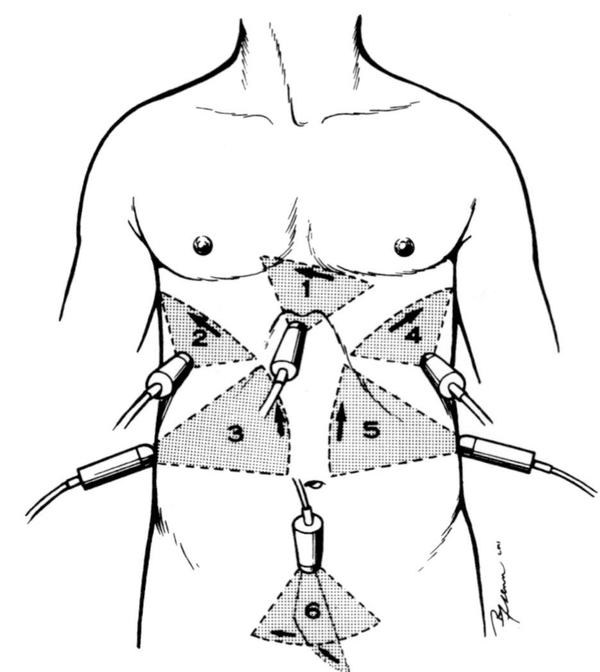

Fig. 18-4 Rapid trauma ultrasound examination. Areas 2 and 4 were used to identify free fluid in the pleural cavities. (From Ma OJ, Mateer JR: *Ann Emerg Med* 29: 313, 1997.)

Ultrasound	20 ml[10]
Upright chest x-ray	50 to 100 ml[23]
Supine chest x-ray	175 ml[9]

Despite its utility in diagnosing HTX, the most valuable use of US in victims of PCT is to identify a pericardial effusion (Fig. 18-5). In the first published report of emergency physicians' use of US in the evaluation of trauma patients, Plummer et al[10] reported on bedside TTE in 49 patients with penetrating cardiac injuries. Ultrasound decreased time to diagnosis and transfer to the operating suite from 42 to 15 minutes compared with retrospective controls. Survival improved from 57% to 100%. Ma and Mateer[16] found that EPs had a 100% sensitivity and 99% specificity for identifying free pericardial fluid, (although only 6 of 245 patients had positive findings). In a recent review, Mattox and Wall[17] write, "ultrasonography at the subxiphoid site should immediately replace sub-xiphoid pericardiotomy for the majority of patients."

Despite the rapidly available information provided by US, chest radiography remains indispensable in assessing trauma patients. Ultrasonography should be seen as complementary to, and not a replacement for, chest radiography.

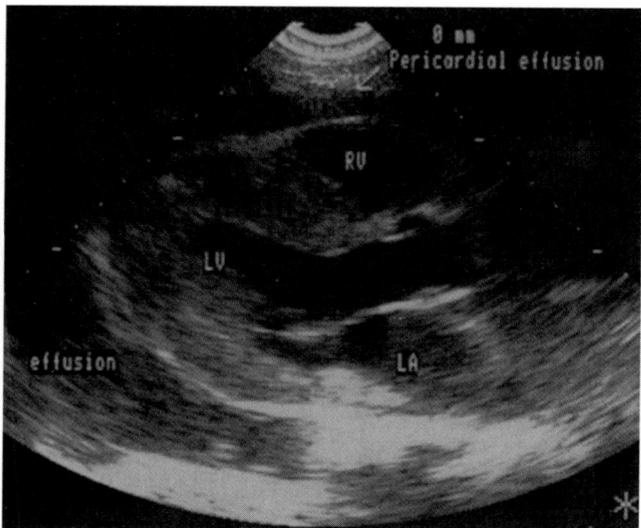

Fig. 18-5 Circumferential pericardial effusion visualized in the parasternal long-axis view of the heart, both posteriorly (posterior to LV) and anteriorly (anterior to RV). *LA*, Left atrium; *LV*, left ventricle; *RV*, right ventricle. (Courtesy of Diku Mandavia, MD. In Chan D: *Emerg Med Clin North Am* 16:194, 1998.)

Transesophageal echocardiography (TEE) is emerging as a useful means of detecting cardiac and aortic injuries. This technique requires greater training and experience than TTE and is usually performed by cardiologists and anesthesiologists. Transesophageal echocardiography can be particularly helpful in the 15% to 20% of trauma patients who cannot be evaluated by TTE resulting from anatomic variations or other traumatic injuries.[18] The presence of subcutaneous air (frequent in PCT) significantly degrades the US images during TTE. The high-frequency transducer gives TEE better image quality and resolution than TTE. Transesophageal echocardiography can image the entire thoracic aorta from the aortic valve to the diaphragm.[11,18] It is a bedside study that is more rapid, less expensive, and associated with less morbidity than aortography. However, the sensitivity for aortic injury varies widely in different studies, likely as a result of differences in operator experience. In one potential strategy, TEE would be the initial test, and aortography reserved for those with a negative US.

Advanced Generation Computed Tomography

EPs should be aware that newer models of computed tomography (CT) equipment are considerably faster and more sophisticated than their predecessors. The role of helical CT is well established in patients with blunt chest and abdominal trauma. However, further study is required to better define the place of new generation CT in PCT.

Laparoscopy

Laparoscopy is generally thought of for use in intraabdominal disorders. However, laparoscopy can diagnose and repair diaphragmatic disruption after penetrating wounds to the lower thorax.[19-21] Despite its sensitivity to diaphragmatic injury, laparoscopy can miss injury to both hollow and solid abdominal organs. Thus if peritoneal penetration is discovered, most authors recommend conversion to laparotomy. The EP should be aware of the potential for tension PTX formation in patients with diaphragmatic tears undergoing laparoscopy as a result of the need for abdominal insufflation. Surgeons can use the laparoscope to perform a diagnostic pericardial window.[22]

EMERGENCY DEPARTMENT EVALUATION AND MANAGEMENT OF STABLE PATIENTS

Many patients with PCT present to the ED in relatively stable condition. Despite their initially benign condition, careful assessment is warranted to determine the true extent of injury (Fig. 18-6). Initial evaluation and management for all patients with potential chest wall penetration include the following:

- Chest radiograph
- Vascular access
- Pulse oximetry
- ECG monitoring

Peripheral Chest Wounds

Peripheral wounds are lateral to the midclavicular line; stab wounds that enter far from the mediastinum are less likely to reach vital structures. However, the trajectory of gunshot wounds may endanger distant organs.

Although stab wounds to the abdomen are usually explored with impunity, avoid probing stab wounds to the chest. Exploration may produce PTX or hemorrhage. Serial clinical examinations and a chest film are sufficient to exclude significant injury in most victims of peripheral stab wounds. Patients with no evidence of mediastinal or abdominal penetration and who have normal chest radiographs should be observed for several hours.

Patients who remain clinically stable for 4 hours with a normal repeat chest radiograph, normal oxygen saturation, and hematocrit may be safely discharged. A repeat chest film at 3 hours after hospital arrival is sensitive to detect delayed PTX.[23]

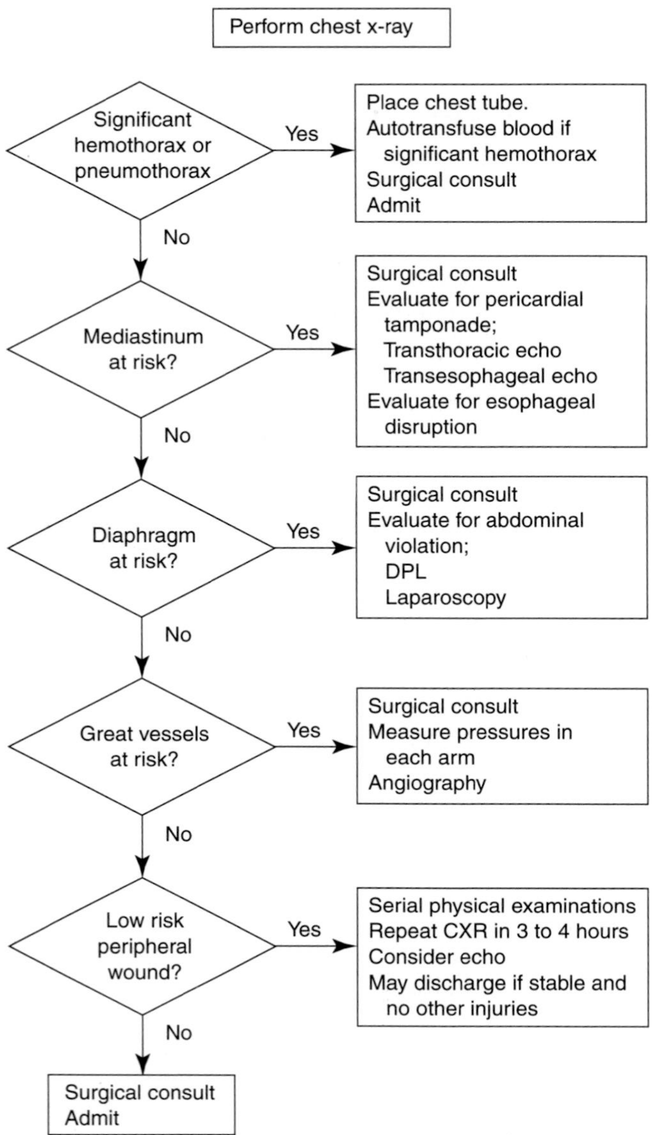

Fig. 18-6 Algorithm for management of penetrating chest trauma in a stable patient.

Patients who are discharged must be given follow-up instructions to return immediately for shortness of breath, fever, hemoptysis, dizziness, increased pain, or any worsening whatsoever. Determine the need for tetanus prophylaxis. There is no evidence to suggest that antibiotic administration benefit such patients.

Inferior Wounds

Low-chest wounds have the potential to perforate the diaphragm and damage intraabdominal structures. Consider thoracoabdominal trauma in any stab wounds that enter the chest below the nipple anteriorly or the scapula posteriorly. Any gunshot wounds with a trajectory towards the abdomen place the patient at risk.

There is no clear consensus on the evaluation of such wounds. At minimum, perform serial abdominal examinations to detect increasing abdominal pain or tenderness. Diagnostic peritoneal lavage (DPL) remains another alternative. However, reduced red cell criteria must be used. One study found that a DPL yielding 5000 red blood cells per ml results in an 87.5% sensitivity and 96.6% specificity for diaphragmatic injury.[24]

Laparoscopy is very accurate in evaluating abdominal consequences of low chest wounds. One study found that laparoscopy never missed an injury. Another study on laparoscopy showed it had a negative predictive value of 100% and a positive predictive value of 89.4%.[25]

CT for the evaluation of low chest wounds is best reserved for patients with posterior injuries (see the following discussion).

LOWER POSTERIOR WOUNDS

Wounds to the posterior chest endanger both retroperitoneal and intraperitoneal structures. These injuries are often clinically occult and during the early stages of evaluation patients may have no abdominal tenderness. If a bullet's trajectory appears to traverse the abdomen, or the patient has a tender abdomen after either a stab wound or GSW to the flank or back, laparotomy is the safest approach.

In the stable patient with minimal or no abdominal findings, a variety of approaches may detect retroperitoneal or intraperitoneal injury. Triple-contrast CT using oral, intravenous, and rectal contrast provides useful information. However the CT scan best determines wound trajectory and depth of penetration; *it is less accurate in demonstrating injury*. If a CT scan demonstrates an intraperitoneal bullet trajectory, the patient must be explored.[26-31] Other authorities believe CT scans are unnecessary in back and flank wounds and trust serial examinations to detect injury (see Chapter 20).

Intravenous pyelography may be falsely negative in retroperitoneal penetrating trauma. If the physician suspects injury to the ureters based on wound trajectory or the presence of hematuria, triple-contrast CT or exploration is indicated.[32]

Central (Trans-Mediastinal) Wounds

Wounds whose trajectory suggests mediastinal involvement place the patient at high risk for serious

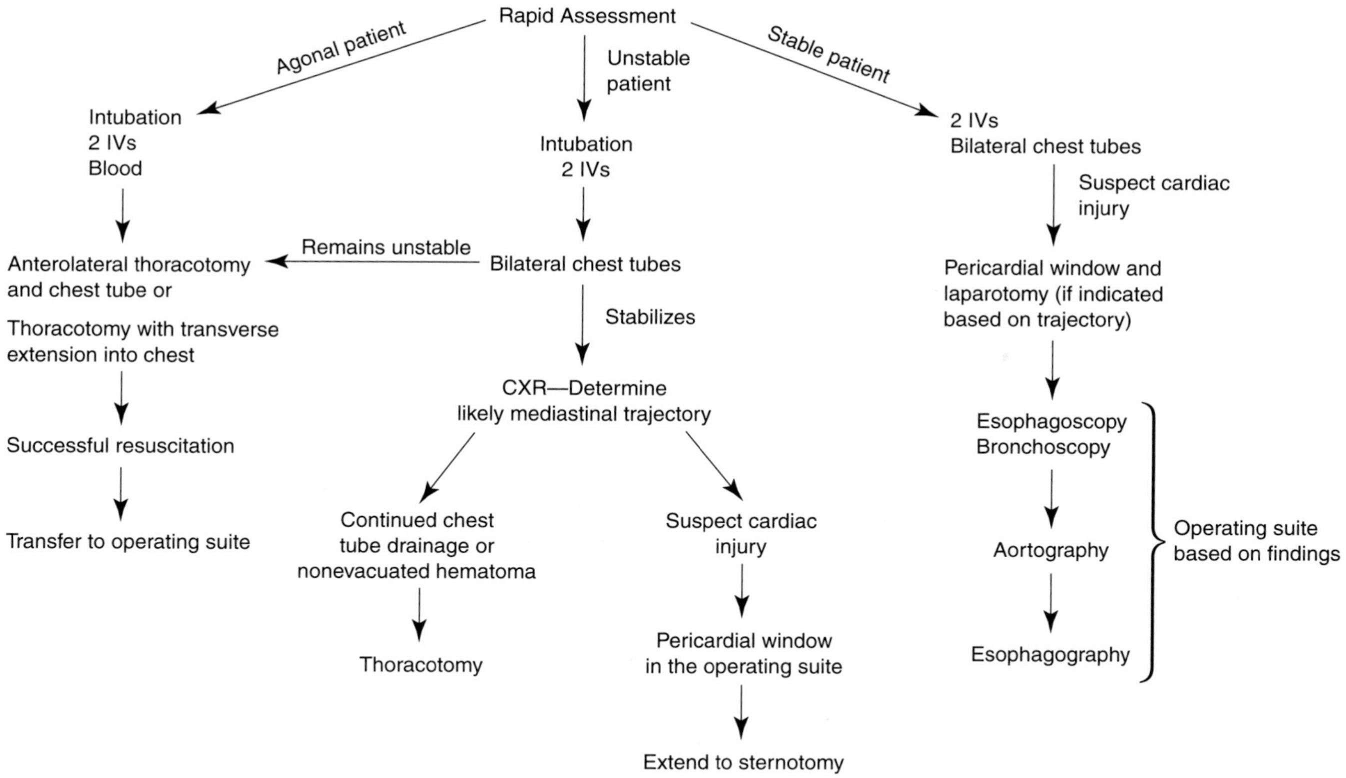

Fig. 18-7 Transmediastinal gunshot wound. (*CXR,* Chest x-ray; *OR,* operating room.) (From Peitzman A, et al: *The trauma manual,* 1998, Lippincott-Raven.)

injury. All such patients require close and repeated observation.

The work-up of asymptomatic patients with wounds that endanger the mediastinum varies widely among trauma centers. An aggressive approach may include routine operation to perform a pericardial window or to directly visualize the great vessels. The operative approach may be combined with or replaced by esophagoscopy, bronchoscopy, and angiography. Either esophagography or esophagoscopy alone may miss up to 40% of esophageal injuries but together have greater than 90% sensitivity.

Other centers utilize observation alone. Echocardiography is becoming an important modality to evaluate possible mediastinal injury. A comprehensive approach for patients with this injury is presented[10,33] (Fig. 18-7).

Impaled Objects

The EP should resist the temptation to remove an impaled object in the ED, since it may be tamponading vascular structures. Instead, it is best to stabilize the object and consult a surgeon for operative removal. However, prehospital care providers or the EP may need to dislodge some transfixed objects to transport or resuscitate the critically injured.

PNEUMOTHORAX

The parietal pleura closely adheres to the interior chest wall, whereas the visceral pleura sticks to the outside surface of the lungs. The right and left pleural spaces do not communicate and are virtual spaces containing a small amount of fluid under negative pressure. The cells lining the pleurae slowly resorb gases to generate the vacuum critical for ventilation.

Simple Pneumothorax. A simple pneumothorax does not communicate to the atmosphere through an opening in the chest wall. Small penetrating wounds can occasionally seal off and result in a simple PTX. A simple PTX can become a tension PTX if a continuing pleural leak leads to increased pressure in the pleural cavity.

Pneumothorax can be graded as small (15% or less of pleural cavity), moderate (15% to 60%), and large (greater than 60%).[34,35] Variations in patient size and radiographic technique make estimates of percent collapse inexact.

Clinical Presentation. Respiratory distress may be minimal or profound, depending on size, and decrease in breath sounds and hyperresonance to percussion may be subtle. Subcutaneous emphysema is an important clue, but not all patients with this finding have a demonstrable PTX.

Management. The chest radiograph is essential. The upright film, when tolerated, is most accurate. Look for a pleural line with loss of vascular markings distal to this line. One clue to PTX on a supine film is the "deep sulcus sign," which darkens the superior border of the diaphragm and produces a deep costophrenic sulcus on the involved side. When possible, obtain an erect chest radiograph after the patient has been sitting upright for several minutes. In patients with indeterminate radiographs, an expiratory chest film may accentuate the pleural line.

CT scanning is very sensitive (perhaps overly sensitive) for PTX. PTX seen only on CT scan has been termed *occult* and, in asymptomatic patients, does not necessarily require a chest tube. In patients with PCT, there is no need for a chest CT in the presence of a normal chest x-ray.[35,36]

Asymptomatic patients with small PTXs may be admitted and observed without tube thoracostomy provided they do not require positive pressure ventilation and are hemodynamically stable.

Most patients with traumatic PTX on CXR should receive tube thoracostomy, especially those with the following indications:

- Moderate to large PTX
- Respiratory distress
- Associated HTX or other significant injuries
- Bilateral PTX
- Positive pressure ventilation
- Air medical transport
- Prolonged ground transport

Chest Tube Placement (see Chapter 51). Tube thoracostomy (see Fig. 51-3) is a painful procedure. A moribund patient may need little or no pain medicine. Here, the emphasis is on rapid decompression of the chest. In patients who are not dying, pain control is an important part of the procedure. A local anesthetic such as lidocaine anesthetizes the skin, chest wall, and intercostal muscles.

There is considerable controversy regarding the need for antibiotics in patients who undergo tube thoracostomy in the emergency department. Several studies indicate that an antistaphylococcal drug, such as a first- or second-generation cephalosporin, decreases infectious complications such as wound infection, pneumonia, and empyema.[37,38]

After placement of the chest tube, reassess the patient both radiographically and clinically. Persistent PTX may be caused by a mechanical problem such as improper tube positioning, leak at the chest wall or at a connection in the collecting system, or inadequate suction. A continuing air leak may also occur with disruption of the bronchus or a large pulmonary laceration. A second chest tube should be placed if the persistent PTX cannot otherwise be corrected. PTX persisting after insertion of two chest tubes on high suction is an indication for thoracotomy in the operating suite.

Open Pneumothorax and Sucking Chest Wound. Open or communicating PTX indicates a connection between the pleural space and the atmosphere. A sucking chest wound occurs when a large defect pulls air through the chest wall, thereby decreasing airflow through the trachea and causing severe respiratory distress. A one-way valve effect may cause a tension PTX.

Clinical Presentation. The degree of respiratory compromise varies greatly, depending on the size of the wound, concomitant injury, and baseline status.

Management. Cover the sucking wound with an occlusive dressing to prevent entrainment of air. Tape three sides of the dressing and leave the fourth untaped to provide a flutter valve effect. The dressing should allow escape of air from the wound during exhalation, preventing tension PTX. Never pack the wound, since the gauze may be sucked into the chest cavity. After the dressing is in place, insert a chest tube as soon as possible. Once the tube is in place, tape the occlusive dressing on the fourth side.

Tension Pneumothorax. In tension pneumothorax, the intrapleural pressure rises to the point that it prevents airflow into the ipsilateral lung and compresses mediastinal structures (Fig. 18-8). This distortion limits venous return to the heart and compromises ventilation in the opposite lung. Blood pressure plummets. Positive pressure ventilation, either after intubation or following bag-valve mask, often converts a simple PTX into a tension PTX.

Clinical Presentation. Tension PTX is an immediately life-threatening condition leading to severe hypotension and respiratory embarrassment. *Tension PTX is a clinical and not a radiographic diagnosis.* Patients will be short of breath and often in shock. They exhibit agitation and restlessness, tachycardia, hypotension, decreased mental status, and other signs of hypoxemia. Some patients present in cardiac arrest, usually with PEA. Breath sounds are absent or diminished on the side of the injury, and the ipsilateral chest may be distended and immobile with hyperresonance to percussion. Although jugular venous distension may be an important clue, it is frequently absent in patients who have lost significant amounts of blood. Tracheal deviation away from the affected side is more often described in textbooks than seen in the trauma room.

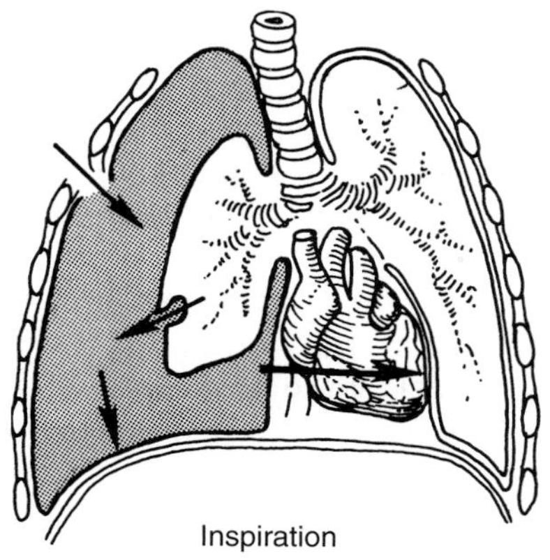

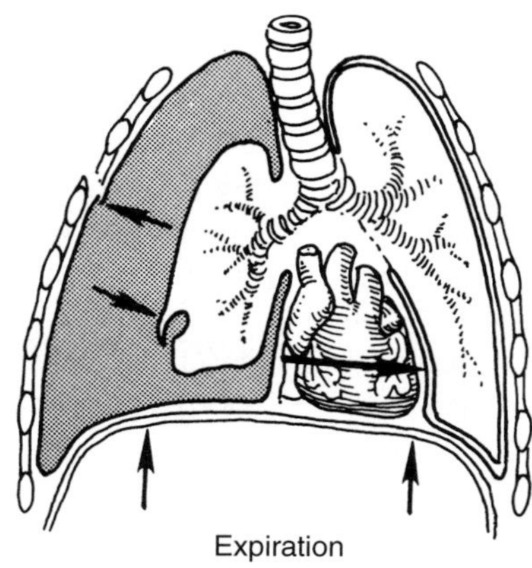

Fig. 18-8 Tension pneumothorax. There are right pneumothorax under tension, total collapse of right lung, and shift of mediastinal structures to left. (From Rosen P, et al: *Emergency medicine: concepts and clinical practice,* ed 4, St Louis, 1998, Mosby.)

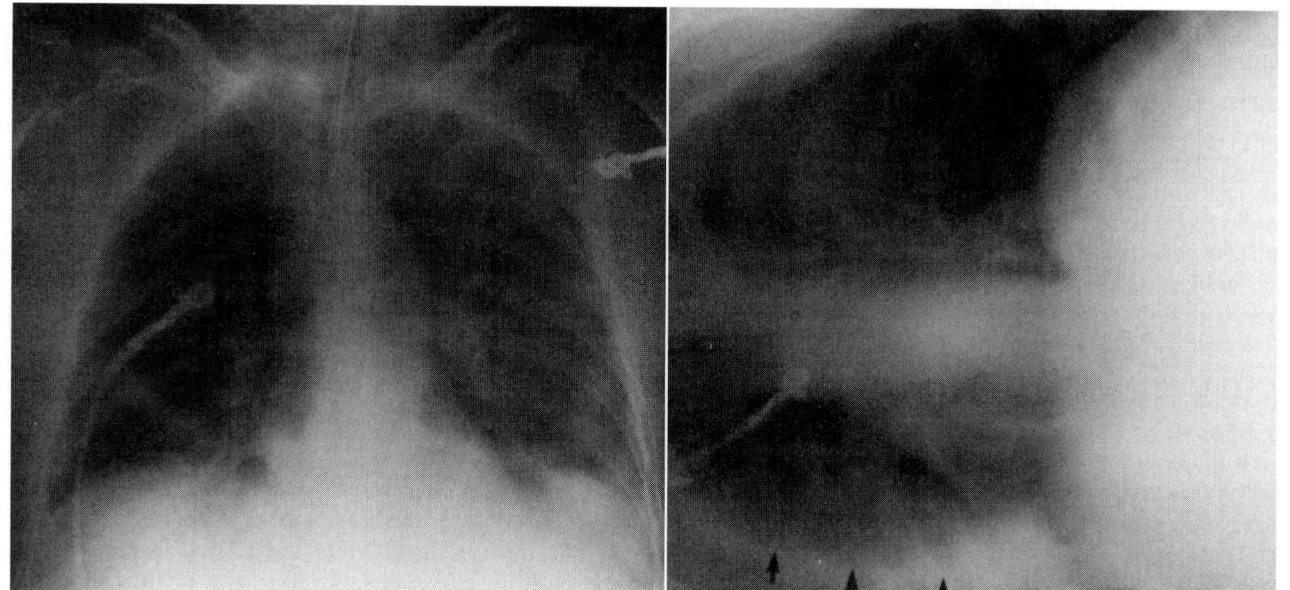

Fig. 18-9 **A,** Supine AP chest radiograph of an intubated multiple-trauma patient. Although there is a suggestion of generally increased opacity of the left lung field compared with the right, it is impossible to determine whether this is due to hemothorax or parenchymal injury. **B,** Left lateral decubitus chest radiograph of the same patient. Note the layering of the left hemothorax *(arrows),* which is now clearly visible. (From Rosen P, et al: *Diagnostic radiology in emergency medicine,* St Louis, 1992, Mosby.)

Management. Radiotherapy cannot cure a tension PTX. It must be managed with a chest tube and not a chest film. A 14-gauge or larger needle placed in the midclavicular line over the second rib may rapidly decompress the chest. Two needles may be better than one. Tube thoracostomy is curative.

HEMOTHORAX

Hemothorax, the accumulation of blood in the pleural space, is a common complication of PCT (Fig. 18-9). The pleural cavity can hold up to 3 liters of blood, and massive HTX can cause hemorrhagic shock. A large HTX will also impair ventilation.

Massive HTX is usually due to arterial hemorrhage from the systemic circulation, most commonly the intercostal and internal mammary arteries. Disruption of the great vessels also results in extensive hemorrhage. Fortunately, most HTXs are caused by lung parenchymal injury. In these cases, the low pressure of the pulmonary circulation, the compressive effect of HTX, and the high concentration of thromboplastin in the lung promote early clotting and hemostasis. A quarter of patients with hemothorax have an associated PTX.[39]

Clinical Presentation. Patients with massive HTX may present in hemorrhagic shock and significant respiratory distress. Breath sounds are decreased on the involved side, and there is dullness to percussion. Diagnosis is usually made by chest radiography. Obtain an erect film if the patient is clinically stable. About 250 to 300 cc of fluid on an erect radiograph blunts the costophrenic angle. Supine films may be misleading, and a liter of blood may appear as a subtle haze in the hemithorax. Bedside US quickly and reliably detects HTX.[40,41]

Management. Not all patients with HTX require chest tubes. Those with slight blunting of the angle and those patients with HTX seen only on CT may be observed. Tube thoracostomy is usually indicated when the volume is estimated to be at least 300 cc or concomitant PTX is present. Large hemothoraces that are left undrained may impair ventilation and provide a nidus for infection over the short term, and, over time, may lead to pleural adhesions and chronic chest complaints.

In the adult patient, it is important to use a large-diameter chest tube (36 to 40 French) to ensure adequate drainage. A small tube may "clot off" and stop functioning. Indications for thoracotomy include >1500 cc of blood on placement of the chest tube or ongoing hemorrhage of >200 cc per hour for 4 hours.

Use autotransfusion devices in patients with large HTX. A cell-saver decreases the risk of coagulopathy associated with autotransfusion. Transfused blood is the most easily available and safest means of transfusion but is frequently under used.

CARDIAC INJURIES

Penetrating cardiac injury can result from knives, ice picks, GSWs, impalement, and industrial accidents such as with high-powered nail guns (Fig. 18-10). In one series, 90% of victims were male, 75% were less than age 35, and overall mortality of patients arriving at the hospital exceeded 50%.[42] Ventricular injuries are more common than atrial, and the right side is involved more often than the left (Table 18-2).[43] Although laceration of a coronary artery occurs in about 5% of cases, the injury is often distal and rarely leads to significant myocardial ischemia. Injury to papillary muscles, valve leaflets, and the septum are also rare, although one author reports this complication in 20% of patients who arrested after penetrating truncal trauma. Positive pressure ventilation and open thoracotomy increase the likelihood of air embolization.

About 80% to 90% of stab wounds and 20% of gunshot wounds lead to cardiac tamponade.[43] Although

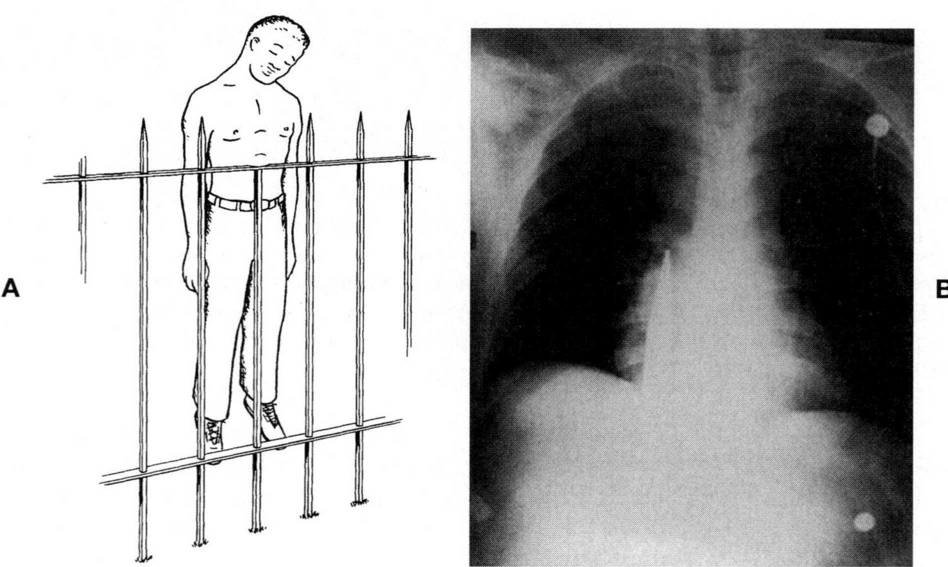

Fig. 18-10 **A,** A middle-aged man was impaled on a wrought-iron fence after falling from a roof. An alert paramedical team had the presence of mind to cut the man free from the iron fence, leaving the iron in place within the patient. **B,** A radiograph on arrival at the emergency department revealed the iron point passing toward the heart. Subsequent exploration revealed the iron had pierced the diaphragm and the right ventricle. The patient survived and was discharged after removal and repair of his right ventricle. (From Brown J, Grover FL: *Chest Surg Clin North Am* 7:316, 1997.)

tamponade is itself a life-threatening complication, it is also protective. In fact, most patients who survive penetrating cardiac trauma live because tamponade prevents exsanguination. The pericardium is nonelastic, and accumulation of as little as 80 cc of blood creates an increase in pericardial pressure, elevating end-diastolic pressure and compromising venous return. As pericardial and end-diastolic pressure rise and stroke volume drops, right- and left-side pressures begin to equalize, and cardiac output falls precipitously.[43,44]

Clinical Presentation. Suspect cardiac injury in patients with stab wounds medial to the midclavicular line and in any patient with a gunshot wound to the trunk. Bullet trajectories are frequently unpredictable, and the distance traveled inside the body can be considerable.

The diagnosis of cardiac tamponade is challenging, since signs and symptoms are unreliable. Beck's triad of hypotension, elevated jugular venous pressure, and muffled heart tones occur in only one third of patients. Suspect tamponade in all patients with hypotension, particularly if there is no other obvious cause. Other clinical findings include pulsus paradoxus (>10 mmHg drop in blood pressure during inspiration) and Kussmaul's sign (increase in neck vein distension during inspiration). However, these findings are present in only a minority of patients, since significant blood loss obliterates both signs. Another finding of cardiac injury is a new murmur, which may be best appreciated after volume resuscitation.[45]

Some patients may demonstrate intermittent hypotension as a result of episodic spontaneous decompression of a pericardial tamponade. This phenomenon is important to recognize, since these patients are likely to survive if treated quickly. Expected survival after cardiac injury in patients who arrive in the ED with signs of life is 70% for gunshot wounds and 85% for stab wounds.[5]

TABLE 18-2
Distribution of Penetrating Cardiac Injury

LOCATION	FREQUENCY (%)
Right ventricle	43
Left ventricle	34
Right atrium	16
Left atrium	7

From Brown J, Grover FL: *Chest Surg Clin North Am* 7:325, 1997.

Management. Patients with significant respiratory distress or severe shock need endotracheal intubation and volume resuscitation. For patients not in extremis, a less aggressive approach is indicated.

Rapidly obtain a chest film, unless the patient has signs of a tension PTX. An upright film is more sensitive for HTX or small PTX than a supine view. Chest radiography shows most foreign bodies, such as retained bullets or other missiles. Foreign bodies which appear blurred and overlie the heart may be intracardiac. However, *a chest radiograph is normal in cases of acute pericardial tamponade.* Unlike medical causes of tamponade, the cardiac silhouette appears normal during rapid blood accumulation within the pericardial sac. In stable patients who have suffered a GSW, place a marker at the presumed entry site before obtaining a chest radiograph. By lining the marker up with the bullet, the physician can obtain some notion of the bullet's trajectory. However, internal tumble and ricochet can render this technique fallible.

A number of diagnostic techniques help manage the patient with PCT. The ECG may reveal cardiac dysrhythmias; in the rare cases of proximal coronary artery disruption, an acute injury pattern may be present. A central line is occasionally useful to measure central venous pressure (CVP), since patients with tamponade and an adequate vascular volume have an elevated value. The CVP will be falsely high if the patient is receiving fluids through a second central line, or if an intubated patient is undergoing positive end-expiratory pressure (PEEP). Echocardiography is a rapid, noninvasive, and accurate test for pericardial fluid with a sensitivity of a least 95%.[10,43] Prompt cardiac US accelerates other interventions in a relatively stable patient. A bedside echocardiogram performed by the emergency physician may reveal significant pericardial fluid. Experienced operators may also appreciate valvular injury and septal lacerations. Pericardiocentesis (Fig. 51-6) can be both diagnostic and therapeutic, although some centers report a false-negative rate of 80% and false-positive rate of 33%.[45] Fortunately, removal of as little as 10 cc may result in significant clinical improvement. This procedure should be reserved for patients who have significant hemodynamic compromise without other likely etiology. Complications of pericardiocentesis include penetration of ventricles, laceration of a coronary vessel, ventricular fibrillation, PTX, and puncture of mediastinal structures.

Rapid thoracotomy (preferably in the operating suite) is crucial for patients who are hypotensive. Prompt transfer to a trauma center is warranted if thoracotomy cannot be done locally. If US is unavailable, an experienced surgeon can perform a pericardial window in the hemodynamically stable patient suspected of tamponade or cardiac injury. Patients who arrive in agonal condition or who arrest after having signs of life in the field should undergo ED thoracotomy. Patients without a pulse in the field who arrive lifeless to the ED have such low likelihood of survival that ED thoracotomy is not warranted.

GREAT VESSEL INJURIES

The great vessels of the chest include the aorta and its major branches at the arch (subclavian, innominate, and carotids), and the major pulmonary arteries. The primary venous conduits include the superior and inferior vena cava and their main tributaries, as well as the pulmonary veins. Damage to vascular structures depends on the specific location and degree of vessel disruption—arterial injuries being more rapidly fatal. High-velocity gunshot wounds are most devastating, but low-velocity injury can also lead to exsanguination. Simple stab wounds without significant twisting or back-and-forth movement of the blade is often sealed off by the adventitial layer of the vessel and by surrounding tissue. On the other hand, a close-range shotgun blast may lead to massive vascular destruction. Injury to a blood vessel may also result in thrombosis and embolization of the missile or air. Late complications include arteriovenous fistulas and false aneurysms.

Clinical Presentation. Patients with vascular injury may present with a wide array of findings. Although uncontrolled hemorrhage produces shock, other patients have serious but occult injury. A contained mediastinal hematoma may compress the superior vena cava, resulting in a suffused face and engorgement of veins in the neck and arms. Hematomas may constrict or distort the airway. Measure the blood pressure in each arm, since asymmetry may accompany vascular injury. A bruit can signify vascular injury, in particular an arteriovenous fistula or false aneurysm. Consider the possibility of intravascular embolization of bullets. On radiographs, the presence of a "fuzzy" foreign body may indicate it is intravascular and pulsating due to arterial flow.

Management. Resuscitation of hypotensive patients should proceed in the usual fashion. First, treat patients with signs of tension PTX by decompressing the chest. Patients in extremis or with profound shock that persists despite volume resuscitation should undergo thoracotomy. After the chest is opened, vascular bleeding in the superior mediastinum and supraclavicular area can be controlled by direct finger pressure to the vessel, vascular clamp, or packing below and above the clavicle. A vascular clamp applied to the pulmonary hilum controls massive pulmonary bleeding.

Because of their location, wounds to the subclavian vessels are very difficult to control with a left lateral thoracotomy (the standard approach for an ED thoracotomy). If a surgeon is unavailable and the patient is exsanguinating, the EP may use a Foley catheter balloon to tamponade a subclavian bleed. Insert the catheter directly into the periclavicular wound and inflate the balloon with saline. This heroic intervention is indicated only for the patient in extremis while awaiting arrival of a surgeon or transport to a trauma center (see Chapter 16).

Patients with severe vascular injuries often present with massive HTX. Patients who are hypotensive (with blood pressure generally above 70 mmHg) should be volume resuscitated to maintain pressure in the 80 to 100 mmHg range and promptly taken to the operating theater for diagnostic and therapeutic procedures. There is growing evidence to suggest that large-volume fluid resuscitation in an attempt to normalize blood pressure leads to increased hemorrhage and worse clinical outcome. Patients who remain moribund require ED thoracotomy unless the surgeon and operating suite are immediately available.[7,33,46]

Air embolism can produce a sudden change in mental status, other acute neurologic deficits, unexplained hypotension, or respiratory distress. Patients who arrest immediately after intubation may suffer from air embolism.

Air embolism most commonly occurs on the venous side, leading to occlusion of the right ventricular outflow track. Air visualized in the coronary arteries on CXR is diagnostic. Treat air embolism by placing the patient on his or her left side with his or her head down (combination of left lateral recumbent and Trendelenburg positions). One hundred percent oxygen promotes resorption of the emboli. Selective intubation of the uninjured lung may decrease further emboli. Immediate thoracotomy is necessary to diagnose and manage the etiology of the hypotension. In the ED, needle aspiration of the heart may restore circulation in case of near arrest.

If the wound trajectory endangers the great vessels, patients with no or minimal symptoms still require evaluation for vascular injury. Although the arterial brachial index is theoretically helpful, most studies have confirmed its value only in penetrating trauma *distal* to the chest. Chest radiograph may reveal HTX or mediastinal hematoma (Fig. 18-11). Arteriography has been the traditional standard for determining a major vessel injury (Fig. 18-12). However, this approach is time consuming and presents the patient with a heavy contrast load. Although use of CT scanning, transesophageal echocardiography, and other modalities are increasing, none has yet replaced angiography.

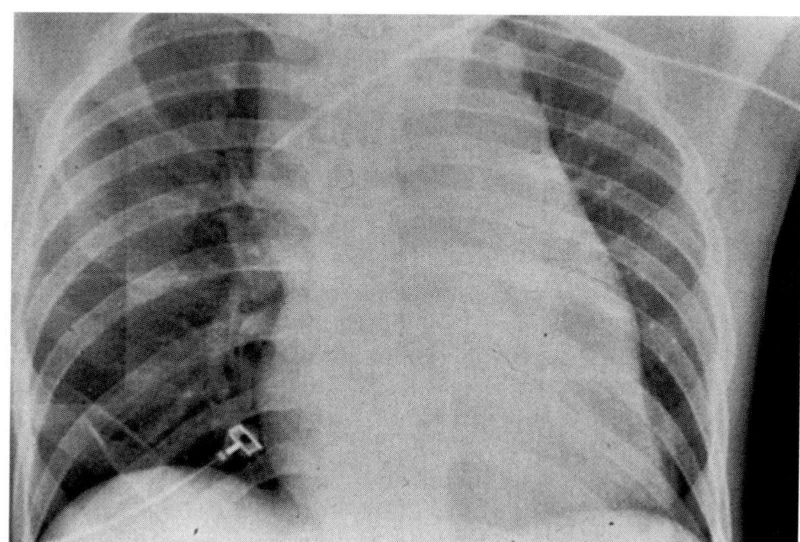

Fig. 18-11 Mediastinal hematoma in hypotensive patient with stab wound to the ascending aorta. (From Feliciano D: *Chest Surg Clin North Am* 7:316, 1997.)

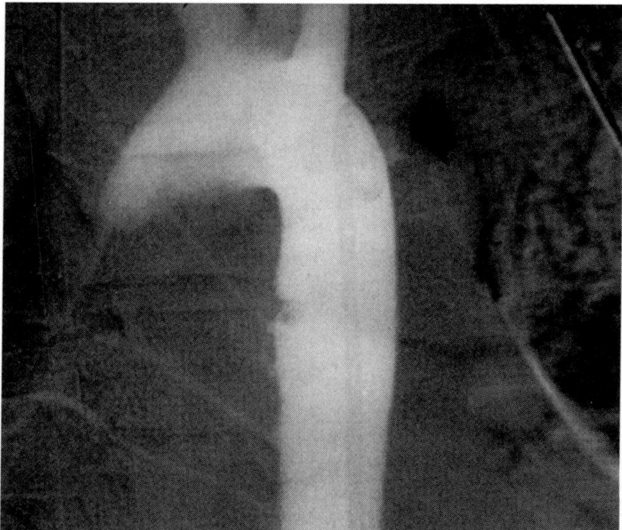

Fig. 18-12 Aortogram of hemodynamically stable patient with through-and-through gunshot wound to the descending thoracic aorta. Arrow demonstrates extravasation at the more proximal injury. (From Feliciano D: *Chest Surg Clin North Am* 7:316, 1997.)

TRACHEOBRONCHIAL INJURIES

These injuries range from the insignificant to profound, including disruption of the cervical trachea. Most patients with major tracheobronchial injury die immediately at the scene. Concurrent injury to the esophagus and other mediastinal structures is common.

Tracheobronchial injury occurs in about 2% to 9% of all victims of penetrating thoracic injury; three fourths involve the cervical trachea, and one fourth the thoracic trachea and bronchi.[4,47] Thus even busy urban trauma centers see only 2 to 4 cases each year.

Most severe penetrating trauma to the airway is from gunshot wounds of the upper chest. Tracheal injuries from stab wounds usually occur in the cervical trachea since the bony thorax protects deeper airway structures. Injury may be caused by direct impact or from sheer of the membranous portion of the trachea. Thoracic tracheobronchial injuries often leak into the pleural space, mediastinum, or lung parenchyma. The most devastating is the intrapleural lesion, which produces massive air leak. Mediastinal rupture is often limited in volume and may go undetected initially. Intraparenchymal injuries tend to seal spontaneously.

Clinical Presentation. Patients with tracheobronchial disruption usually display significant airway distress. Other signs include hemoptysis and subcutaneous emphysema of the neck or supraclavicular region. Hypoxemia and cyanosis are frequent, as are PTX and pneumomediastinum, which may be surmised by Hamman's crunch (the harsh crunch of mediastinal air that syncopates with the cardiac rhythm). Some patients are hoarse or have dysphagia. An important clue to tracheo-bronchial injury is a persistent PTX despite a functioning chest tube. A persistent air leak results in ceaseless bubbling of the water seal chamber directly connected to the chest tube.

Ninety percent of patients with tracheobronchial disruption have some radiographic abnormality, including the following[47]:

- Pneumothorax
- Pneumomediastinum
- Deep cervical emphysema (radiolucent line along prevertebral fascia)

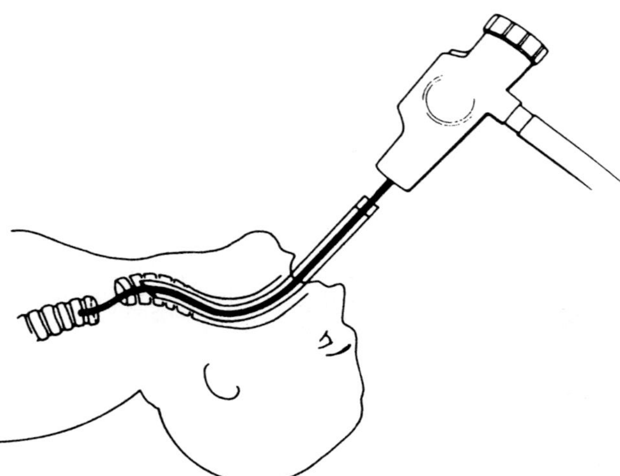

Fig. 18-13 Technique of Grover et al for orotracheal intubation guided by fiberoptic bronchoscopy. (From Lee R: *Chest Surg Clin North Am* 7:286, 1997.)

- Peribronchial air
- "Dropped or fallen lung" (lung apex rests at level of hilum)
- Abnormal location of distal end of endotracheal tube or unusual roundness of orotracheal tube balloon

Management. Initial care is dependent on the degree of injury. Many patients require immediate intubation of the airway and mechanical ventilation. Orotracheal intubation should always be attempted unless massive maxillofacial trauma precludes this approach. With open cervical disruptions, direct placement of a tube into the trachea is appropriate. Closed cervical and intrathoracic tracheal disruptions present the clinician with an imposing challenge. Rapid sequence intubation using neuromuscular blockers is contraindicated in patients suspected of tracheal disruption, since the paratracheal muscles are the only structures that keep the severed ends aligned. Paralysis may make intubation impossible. A flexible bronchoscope can visualize the disrupted end of the trachea. This approach allows an endotracheal tube to slide over the bronchoscope through the vocal cords and into the lower tracheal segment (Fig. 18-13).[47] In general, avoid cricothyroidotomy or tracheostomy to prevent further anatomic disruption of the airway. However, in life-threatening situations, airway control should be obtained in the most expeditious and reliable manner possible. Selective intubation of the noninjured lung may be necessary in cases of bronchial disruption.

Patients in severe distress usually require tube thoracostomy and, if in extremis, open thoracotomy. These injuries often present with massive air leaks requiring more than one chest tube under high suction. Associated vascular injuries are common.

Once the patient is hemodynamically stable, bronchoscopy definitively assesses the airway. Unless an operation is planned, esophagoscopy is also recommended. A surgeon should repair all disruptions of the airway to prevent persistent PTX, empyema, and mediastinitis.

DIAPHRAGMATIC INJURIES

Diaphragmatic disruption is frequently missed in penetrating injury. Penetrating trauma occurs on the left more frequently than on the right, a fact attributed to frontal assaults by right-handed perpetrators. Penetrating diaphragmatic injuries tend to be smaller than blunt traumatic disruptions (2 cm versus >10 cm),[48] and because penetrating defects tend to be relatively small, they are notoriously occult. Associated defects rarely lead to acute herniation of abdominal organs or anatomic displacement of the diaphragm as occurs in blunt trauma. However, because of the continuous pressure gradient across the diaphragm and its constant motion, diaphragmatic rents do not heal spontaneously. Thus patients present with delayed complications such as bowel herniation and strangulation, months to years after injury.

Acute displacement through a large tear or gradual herniation with subsequent strangulation can lead to marked increase in intrathoracic pressure creating what Wilson[5] refers to as "tension enterothorax." The most common abdominal organ to herniate is the stomach. There is a 25% to 40% mortality rate associated with diaphragmatic tears, primarily because of the severity of associated injuries.[4]

Clinical Presentation. There is no specific sign or symptom associated with penetrating diaphragm injury. Recognition is based on a penetrating wound whose trajectory or angle crosses the diaphragm. Most clinical findings are due to associated injury in either the abdomen or chest. Chest radiography is probably diagnostic in only 25% of patients.[6] Demonstration of abdominal viscera in the chest with or without nasogastric tube placement is convincing evidence of diaphragmatic violation. Suggestive findings include diaphragmatic elevation, haziness of the diaphragm, massive lower lobe atelectasis, and pleural effusion.

If a patient with PCT requires a chest tube, the physician has a unique opportunity to diagnose diaphragm injury. By placing a gloved finger in the thoracostomy wound before tube insertion, the physician can palpate tears in the diaphragm, depending on the location of the wound and the length of the physician's finger. Routinely feel the diaphragm during

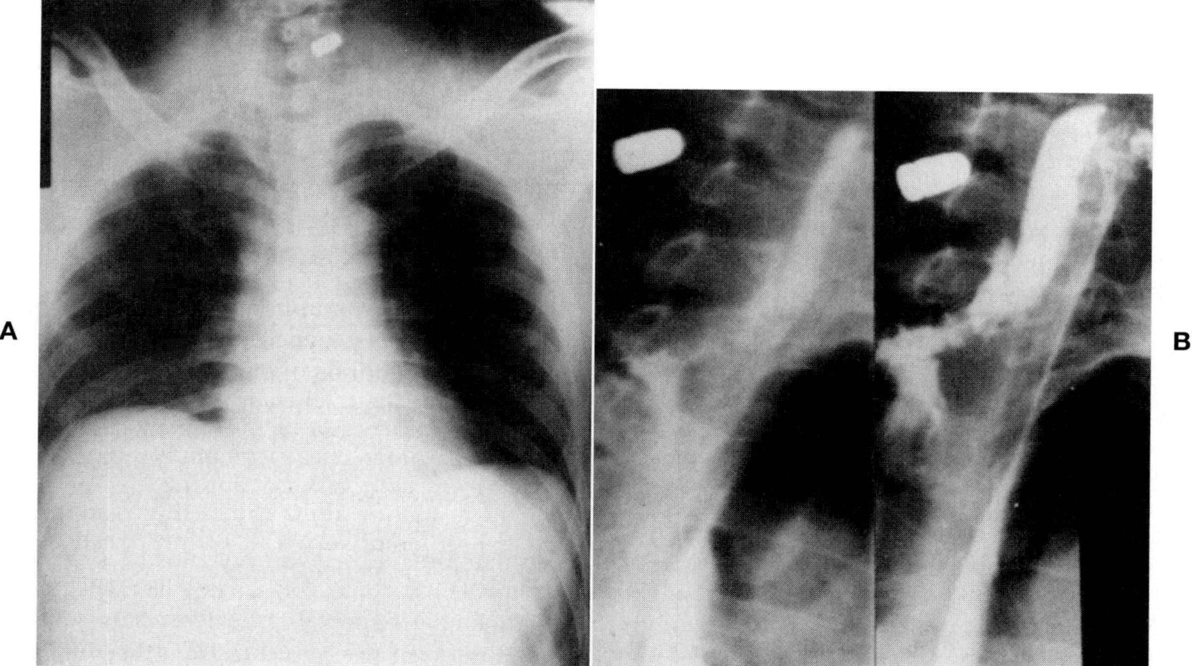

Fig. 18-14 Perforation of the esophagus. **A,** Chest radiograph showing swelling, subcutaneous emphysema, and a missile in the lower neck region in a patient with a bullet wound of the lower neck. **B,** Admission esophagogram shows extravasation of the radiopaque material. (From Symbas PN, et al: *Ann Thorac Surg* 13:552, 1972.)

chest tube insertion. A digital exploration before tube insertion also ensures there are no abdominal structures present in the chest.

Management. The key to management of this injury is recognition. Clinical examination is rarely diagnostic, and chest radiography is frequently nonspecific. Contrast studies are occasionally helpful. Diagnostic peritoneal lavage with adjusted criteria, such as a red blood cell count of 5000 cells/mm^3, is helpful. Lavage fluid that comes out the chest tube is diagnostic of a communication between the abdomen and chest. Methylene blue added to a second lavage aliquot (once the first sample is sent for analysis) might clarify the diagnosis. CT scanning is not reliable, since the injury is often in the same plane as the imaging beam. Magnetic resonance imaging (MRI) has been reported to be accurate in a small series of cases,[49] and laparoscopy and thoracoscopy are useful tools.

Because these injuries do not heal spontaneously, a surgeon must perform a formal repair, usually by laparotomy (and occasionally thoracotomy).

ESOPHAGUS

Disruption of the esophagus is an extremely serious, but fortunately rare, injury. Disruptions of the esophagus leak saliva and other oral and enteral contents into the loose areolar tissues of the neck and mediastinum. The inoculated bacteria produce a rapidly spreading local infection and often sepsis. Mortality is 25% if treated within 12 hours and rises to 50% if treatment is delayed by 24 hours.[5,33]

Clinical Presentation. Esophageal injury may be masked either by other injuries or by the paucity of early signs and symptoms. Perforation of the cervical esophagus usually results in pain, particularly odynophagia. Other findings include dysphagia, hoarseness, and subcutaneous emphysema. Patients may resist flexion and extension of the neck and complain of respiratory distress. Those with intrathoracic perforation have chest pain, subcutaneous emphysema of the supraclavicular area or neck, and dyspnea. Auscultation can reveal a mediastinal crunch. Tachycardia, fever, and increasing respiratory distress develop in hours.[50]

Management. Because many esophageal injuries are initially occult, patients who have trajectories suggestive of esophageal involvement should receive full evaluation. Chest radiographic findings include subcutaneous emphysema, mediastinal emphysema, PTX, pleural effusion, mediastinal widening, retroesophageal air, and prevertebral soft tissue swelling.

To diagnose esophageal disruption, most authors recommend esophagography as the initial test of choice. Water-soluble contrast agents, such as meglumine diatrizoate (Gastrografin), produce less inflammation in the mediastinal tissue than barium, should the contrast leak from an injured esophagus. However, a barium study is more sensitive, and if aspirated, barium produces a less severe pneumonitis than Gastrografin. For this reason some authorities suggest that the first study be performed with Gastrografin and that, if this study is negative, a repeat esophagography be performed with dilute barium (Fig. 18-14).[51]

If esophagography is negative, most authors recommend subsequent esophagoscopy. Although esophagoscopy alone finds only 60% of injuries, the two tests combined have a sensitivity of at least 90%.[4] CT scanning may reveal complications such as air, fluid, or abscesses in the soft tissues of the neck and mediastinum, but is not reliable for primary diagnosis.

Once the diagnosis is made, the patient will require surgery. Nasogastric intubation and evacuation of gastric contents is recommended. Administer broad-spectrum antibiotics active against oral flora, including anaerobes and gram-negative rods.

Definitive management depends in part on the age of the injury. Primary repair may be possible within the first 6 hours after injury, but older injuries usually require temporary esophageal diversion. All cases require wide debridement and drainage.

MEDICO-LEGAL ISSUES

Forensics

Penetrating trauma to the chest often results from interpersonal violence, unintentional injury, or industrial mishaps—mechanisms that often trigger criminal or tort legal proceedings. Thus EPs must be particularly careful in their documentation. Describe wounds in terms of size (by actual measurement when possible) and precise anatomic location, and note relationships to standard anatomic landmarks. Drawings are very effective.

Particular care should be taken in describing gunshot wounds. Entrance and exit wounds may be difficult to discern; instead of the terms *exit* or *entry* wounds, use the term *wound* without these descriptors. Document the presence of wadding, thermal burns, or gunpowder (traumatic tattooing).

Exercise caution when describing radiographic findings. It is better to report "radio-opaque foreign body" or "missile" with a description of the size and shape. Radiographic size of the bullet cannot determine actual caliber.

Maintain the "chain of evidence." Keep any retrieved bullets for police and handle them with rubber-covered instruments. Also, carefully document transfer of the bullet from the victim's body, preferably directly to or in the presence of a law enforcement officer.

Documentation

Documentation of patient condition is also very important. Patients who are in extremis or unstable are often transferred to a trauma center or the operating suite. Such patients often lack a detailed secondary survey. However, even in these cases, careful reporting of certain findings can be critical to criminal, civilian, and even malpractice litigation.

Particularly important items to record include moribund status and any spontaneous movement, particularly of the four extremities. The mechanism of injury, prehospital information, the history and physical examination, and initial diagnostic studies, which prompted early transfer, are key elements. Documentation of the patient's critical condition can explain why the physician "overlooked" less life-threatening injuries.

SUMMARY

The thorax houses the organs of life of the human body. Patients with penetrating injuries to the chest can present moribund or in stable condition with occult but potentially lethal injuries. In the unstable patient early consultation with a surgeon is essential, whereas in the dying patient, diagnosis and resuscitation are nearly simultaneous. The stable patient requires serial physical examinations combined with CXR and sometimes other imaging modalities.

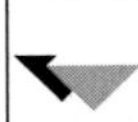

PEARLS & PITFALLS

Pneumothorax

- Act! Don't test. Clinically manage patients with evidence of tension pneumothorax–they need a chest tube, not a chest x-ray.
- Upright films. Obtain an upright film when possible. A small pneumothorax is often hidden on a supine film.
- Chest tube before transport. Patients with pneumothorax who require prolonged transport should receive a chest tube before leaving the transferring hospital.
- Never clamp a chest tube. Leaving the clamp in place may result in tension pneumothorax.

- Think ahead. Perform tube thoracostomy in patients with even small pneumothorax who require positive pressure ventilation or air-medical transport.
- Patients intubated for penetrating chest trauma are likely to develop a pneumothorax once positive pressure ventilation is begun.

Hemothorax

- Beware supine films. Physicians often miss HTX on supine film.
- Beware small tubes. A small chest tube is inadequate to drain HTX.
- Manage blood loss. Autotransfuse blood collected from the chest tube using proper equipment.
- Call a surgeon. Patients with significant chest bleeding need thoracotomy.

Cardiac Injuries

- Look for small-caliber wounds, especially in the back or axilla.
- Do not underestimate the potential of a stab wound to cause cardiac injury.
- Do not assume a trajectory based only on location of entrance and exit wounds.
- Do not expect to find Beck's triad in cardiac tamponade.
- A chest radiograph will be normal in cases of acute pericardial tamponade.

Great Vessel Injuries

- Search for great vessel injury.
- Promptly manage massive HTX.

REFERENCES

1. Rosen P: General principles of trauma. In Harwood-Nuss AL, et al (editors): *The clinical practice of emergency medicine,* ed 2, Philadelphia, 1996, Lippincott-Raven.
2. Calhoon JH, Trinkle JK: Pathophysiology of chest trauma, *Chest Surg Clin North Am* 7:199-211, 1997.
3. Committee on Advanced Trauma Life Support of the American College of Surgeons Committee on Trauma: *Advanced trauma life support for doctors instructor course manual*, ed 6, Chicago, 1997, American College of Surgeons.
4. Peitzman AB, et al: *The trauma manual,* Philadelphia, 1998, Lippincott-Raven.
5. Wilson RF: Thoracic trauma. In Tintinalli JE, Ruiz E, Krome RL (editors): *Emergency medicine: a comprehensive study guide,* ed 4, New York, 1996, McGraw-Hill.
6. Jorden RC: Penetrating chest trauma, *Emerg Med Clin North Am* 11:97-106, 1993.
7. Bickell WH, et al: Immediate versus delayed fluid resuscitation for hypotensive patients with penetrating torso injuries, *N Engl J Med* 331:1105-1109,1994.
8. Durham LA, et al: Emergency center thoracotomy: impact of pre-hospital resuscitation, *J Trauma* 32:775-779, 1992.
9. Melanson SW, Heller M: The emerging role of bedside ultrasonography in trauma care, *Emerg Med Clin North Am,* 16:165-189, 1998.
10. Plummer D, et al: Emergency department echocardiography improves outcome in penetrating cardiac injury, *Ann Emerg Med* 21:709-712, 1992.
11. Chan D: Echocardiography in thoracic trauma, *Emerg Med Clin North Am* 16:191-207, 1998.
12. Ma OJ, et al: Prospective analysis of a rapid trauma ultrasound examination performed by emergency physicians, *J Trauma* 38: 879-885, 1995.
13. Mayron R, et al: Echocardiography performed by emergency physicians: impact on diagnosis and therapy, *Ann Emerg Med* 17:150-154, 1988.
14. Rozycki GS, et al: Prospective evaluation of surgeons' use of ultrasound in the evaluation of trauma patients, *J Trauma* 34: 516-526, 1993.
15. Sisley AC, et al: Rapid detection of traumatic effusion using surgeon-performed ultrasonography, *J Trauma* 44:291-297, 1998.
16. Ma OJ, Mateer JR: Trauma ultrasound examination versus chest radiography in the detection of hemothorax, *Ann Emerg Med* 29:312-315, 1997.
17. Mattox KL, Wall MJ Jr: Newer diagnostic measures and emergency management, *Chest Surg Clin North Am* 7:213-226, 1997.
18. Johnson SB, Kearney PA, Smith MD: Echocardiography in the evaluation of thoracic trauma, *Surg Clin North Am* 75:193-205, 1995.
19. Brandt CP, Priebe PP, Jacobs DG: Potential of laparoscopy to reduce nontherapeutic trauma laparotomies, *Am Surg* 60:416-420, 1994.
20. Livingston DH, et al: The role of laparoscopy in abdominal trauma, *J Trauma* 33:471-475, 1992.
21. Smith RS, et al: Laparoscopic evaluation of abdominal trauma: a preliminary report, *Contemp Surg* 42:13-18, 1993.
22. McMahon DJ, et al: Laparoscopic transdiaphragmatic diagnostic pericardial window in the hemodynamically stable patient with penetrating chest trauma, *Surg Endosc* 11:474-475, 1997.
23. Kerstein KJ: Role of three hour roentgenogram of the chest in penetrating and nonpenetrating injuries of the chest, *Surg Gyn OB* 175:249-253,1992.
24. Merlotti GJ: Peritoneal lavage in penetrating thoraco-abdominal trauma, *J Trauma* 28:17-23, 1988.
25. Ivatury RR, et al: Laparoscopy in the evaluation of the intrathoracic abdomen after penetrating injury, *J Trauma* 33:101-109, 1992.
26. Chihombori A, et al: Role of diagnostic techniques in the initial evaluation of stab wounds to the anterior abdomen, back, and flank, *J Natl Med Assoc* 83:137-140, 1991.
27. Coppa GF, et al: Management of penetrating wounds of the back and flank, *Surg Gynecol Obstet* 159:514-518, 1984.
28. Henao F, Jimenez H, Tawil H: Penetrating wounds of the back and flank: analysis of 77 cases, *South Med J* 80:21-25, 1987.
29. Phillips T, et al: Use of the contrast-enhanced CT enema in the management of penetrating trauma to the flank and back, *J Trauma* 26:593-601, 1986.
30. Vanderzee J, Christenberry P, Jurkovich GJ: Penetrating trauma to the back and flank: a reassessment of mandatory celiotomy, *Am Surg* 53:220-222, 1987.
31. Grossman MD, et al: Determining anatomic injury with computed tomography in selected torso gunshot wounds, *J Trauma* 45:446-456,1998.
32. Patel VG, Walker ML: The role of "one-shot" intravenous pyelogram in evaluation of penetrating abdominal trauma, *Amer Surg* 63:350-353,1997.

33. Mattox KL: Approached to trauma involving the major vessels of the thorax, *Surg Clin North Am* 69:77-91, 1989.
34. Kirsh MM, et al: *Blunt chest trauma,* Boston, 1977, Little Brown.
35. Pigman EC: Pulmonary and pleural injuries. In Harwood-Nuss AL, et al (editors): *The clinical practice of emergency medicine,* ed 2, Philadelphia, 1996, Lippincott-Raven.
36. Collins JC, Levine G, Waxman K: Occult traumatic pneumothorax: immediate tube thoracostomy versus expectant management, *Am Surg* 58:743-746, 1992.
37. Evans JT, et al: Meta-analysis of antibiotics in tube thoracostomy, *Amer Surg* 61:215-219,1995.
38. Nichols RL, et al: Preventive antibiotic usage in traumatic thoracic injuries requiring closed tube thoracostomy, *Chest* 106: 1493-1498,1994.
39. Vukich DJ, Markovchick V: Chest trauma: thoracic trauma. In Rosen P, et al (editors): *Emergency medicine: concepts and clinical practice,* ed 4, 1998, St Louis, Mosby.
40. Ma OJ, Mateer JR: Trauma ultrasound examination versus chest radiography in the detection of hemothorax, *Ann Emerg Med* 29:312-315,1997.
41. Singh G, Arya N, Safaya R, et al: Role of ultrasonography in blunt abdominal trauma, *Injury* 28:667-670,1997.
42. Kaplan AJ, Norcross ED, Crawford FA, et al: Predictors of mortality in penetrating cardiac injury, *Am Surg* 59:338, 1993.
43. Brown J, Grover FL: Trauma to the heart, *Chest Surg Clin North Am* 7:325-341, 1997.
44. Ivatury RR, Rohman M: The injured heart, *Surg Clin North Am* 69:93-110, 1989.
45. Shockey LW: Blunt cardiac injuries. In Harwood-Nuss AL, et al (editors): *The clinical practice of emergency medicine,* ed 2, Philadelphia, 1996, Lippincott-Raven.
46. Sakles JC, et al: Effect of immediate fluid resuscitation on the rate, volume, and duration of pulmonary vascular hemorrhage in a sheep model of penetrating thoracic trauma, *Ann Emerg Med* 29:392-399, 1997.
47. Lee RB: Traumatic injury of the cervicothoracic trachea and major bronchi, *Chest Surg Clin North Am* 7:285-304, 1997.
48. Markovchick VJ, Edney J: Bony thorax and diaphragm injuries. In Harwood-Nuss AL, et al (editors): *The clinical practice of emergency medicine,* ed 2, Philadelphia, 1996, Lippincott-Raven.
49. Boulanger BR, Mirvis SE, Rodriguez A: Magnetic resonance imaging in traumatic diaphragmatic rupture: case reports, *J Trauma* 32:89-93, 1992.
50. May HL, editor: *Emergency medicine,* ed 2, Boston, 1992, Little, Brown.
51. Mattox KL, Allen MK: Emergency department treatment of chest injuries, *Emerg Med Clin North Am* 2:783-797, 1984.

19 Blunt Abdominal Trauma

PETER C. FERRERA

Teaching Case

A 20-year-old man involved in a head-on motor vehicle crash (MVC) complained of trouble breathing and right thigh pain. His Glasgow Coma Scale (GCS) was 15, and he denied abdominal pain or tenderness. Examination showed an abrasion across his chest, a right femur deformity, and no abdominal tenderness. A chest radiograph demonstrated a left pulmonary laceration. After approximately 1 hour, he began coughing up blood. He was intubated and a diagnostic peritoneal lavage (DPL) returned 10 cc gross blood. Laparotomy demonstrated lacerations of his liver, spleen, and kidney. He exsanguinated in the operating suite.

The multiply-injured victim of blunt trauma is at high risk for intraabdominal injury (IAI), and damage to abdominal viscera is responsible for at least 10% of all trauma deaths. Missed abdominal injury remains a major cause of preventable trauma deaths. Occasionally, abdominal injuries are initially occult, but ultimately require emergent laparotomy.[1,2] If the injury is not quickly recognized, mortality ranges from 15% to 58%.[3]

HISTORY

Historical information provides important clues to abdominal trauma; prominent among these factors is mechanism of injury. Bicyclists and pedestrians struck by cars, victims of motor vehicle and motorcycle crashes, and those who fall greater than one story are at greatest risk for blunt abdominal trauma.[4] The use of a lap belt without a shoulder harness predisposes to hollow viscus injury. "Spearing-type" injuries occur when a significant force is concentrated over a small area. Examples include a fall onto a bicycle handlebar, a football helmet or foot contacting the anterior abdomen, or a kick by a horse. A spearing injury to the epigastrium is associated with duodenal hematomas, pancreatic trauma, or small bowel injury, each of which can present with a relatively benign examination during the first several hours after trauma.

PHYSICAL EXAMINATION

Patients with significant IAI may have a benign examination on presentation to the emergency department (ED). Conversely, some patients with significant abdominal tenderness have no visceral injury. The initial physical examination in blunt abdominal trauma is only 65% accurate.[5,6] Serial examinations are often more important than the initial finding. Several factors predict an unreliable physical examination, including the presence of drugs, alcohol, head trauma, and other causes of altered mental status.[2] Additional confounding factors include sensory abnormalities from spinal cord injury or preexisting neurologic disorders, mental retardation, or psychiatric disorders.

Although most alert patients with IAI will have abdominal tenderness,[7,8] a small proportion have a falsely negative abdominal examination secondary to associated extraabdominal injuries. These injuries may "distract" the patient's attention away from the pain of an IAI.[4,8-11] One recent study[8] defined *distracting injuries* as injuries that may obscure intraabdominal pathology in awake and alert adult victims of blunt trauma. Seven percent of these patients without abdominal pain or tenderness had IAI. All patients had extraabdominal injuries, including extremity fractures, blunt chest trauma (including rib fractures, pneumothoraces, pulmonary contusions, chest wall contusion, clavicle fracture, and pulmonary laceration), and pelvic fracture.

The physical examination begins with inspection. Physicians often (and incorrectly) believe that abdominal distension is due to hemoperitoneum. Even 2 liters of blood in the peritoneal cavity will not produce a significant increase in girth.[12] The distended abdomen is usually secondary to an ileus or, rarely, a pneumoperitoneum. Conversely, a flat abdomen can hide liters of blood within its enigmatic confines.

Look for abdominal bruising. Ecchymosis in the distribution of a lap belt should trigger further investigations for bowel injury. Occasionally the emergency physician (EP) will see ecchymosis at the umbilicus (**Cullen's sign**) or the flanks (**Grey Turner's sign**). However, these stigmata of retroperitoneal bleeding usually take hours to develop.

Palpate the lower chest for rib fractures, since they presage hepatic or splenic injury. Splenic injury occurs in up to 20% of patients with left lower fractures, and hepatic injury in 10% of patients with right-sided fractures.[13] Palpate each quadrant of the abdomen separately and evaluate for tenderness and peritoneal signs. Evaluate the pelvis for stability, and palpate the lumbar spine for tenderness. **Kehr's sign** is pain in the shoulder secondary to irritation of the diaphragm and is often present in patients with splenic trauma. A rectal examination will determine the presence of an abnormal prostate, lack of rectal tone, and heme-positive stools. A "high-riding" (bulging outward towards the examining finger) or boggy prostate suggests urethral disruption and the need for a urethrogram before Foley catheterization. (See Chapter 50 for a full discussion regarding the digital rectal examination in trauma.)

DIAGNOSTIC TESTING

Hemodynamically stable patients with nontender (or only mildly tender) abdomens, a clear sensorium, and no significant distracting injuries may require only serial examinations. However, many trauma patients present with an altered sensorium, equivocal abdominal examinations, or history of hypotension, and thus require further investigation. Patients with combined head and abdominal injuries require objective testing of the abdomen, either computed tomography (CT), diagnostic peritoneal lavage (DPL), or ultrasound (US), since normal vital signs do not rule out serious IAI in the comatose patient (Fig. 19-1).[12]

Extensive testing may harm, as well as help. Certain patients need immediate laparotomy. The patient with a rigid abdomen who presents in frank shock may require only a chest radiograph and a type and crossmatch before laparotomy, provided no other likely sources of blood loss exist.

Plain Radiographs

A **chest radiograph (CXR)** is perhaps the most important plain film in the patient with blunt trauma. The CXR determines the presence of obvious intrathoracic and diaphragmatic injuries. Patients with diaphragmatic ruptures on CXR need no further diagnostic evaluation of the abdomen in the ED and should proceed for laparotomy as soon as possible. An anteroposterior (AP) view of the pelvis is indicated if there is tenderness, instability, or an altered sensorium. Plain films of the abdomen are seldom helpful in blunt trauma and should not be routine.

Laboratory Studies

Laboratory tests also play a limited role in the diagnosis of IAI. Although an abnormal test helps confirm the suspicion of visceral injury, a normal test never rules it out. The initial hemoglobin or hematocrit only provides a baseline for serial measurements. Preinjury levels, rate of blood loss, the amount of intravenous fluids given, and fluid shifts into and out of the intravascular space all influence the initial hematocrit.[1] However, a hemoglobin of less than 8 g/dl on arrival usually indicates serious hemorrhage and also demonstrates the patient's marginal anatomic reserve.[14] Patients with a high likelihood of IAI may benefit from a type and screen, or if hypotensive, a full crossmatch. Although many trauma centers measure amylase as part of the "trauma package," no data support this practice. Serum amylase determinations are neither sensitive nor specific for pancreatic injury.[15,16]

One frequently overlooked test in the patient with blunt abdominal trauma involves the acid-base status. Metabolic acidosis in the presence of blunt trauma implies shock. The base deficit, serum lactate, and even serum bicarbonate all provide information regarding anaerobic metabolism. Lactate in particular is a more sensitive indicator of shock than either blood pressure or even sophisticated invasive monitoring.[17,18] Although a normal base deficit does not rule out IAI, a deficit more negative than –6 alerts the EP to the possibility of occult IAI.

The most consistent sign of serious renal injury is *gross* hematuria. All patients with gross hematuria require investigation of the genitourinary system, either before laparotomy in the stable patient, or after or during laparotomy for the patient with intractable shock. For the stable patient, if the urine is clear yellow, significant renal injury is unlikely. A dipstick or microscopic evaluation is indicated in all children and in those adults with shock or severe abdominal/flank trauma.[19]

Several studies suggest that patients with hepatic

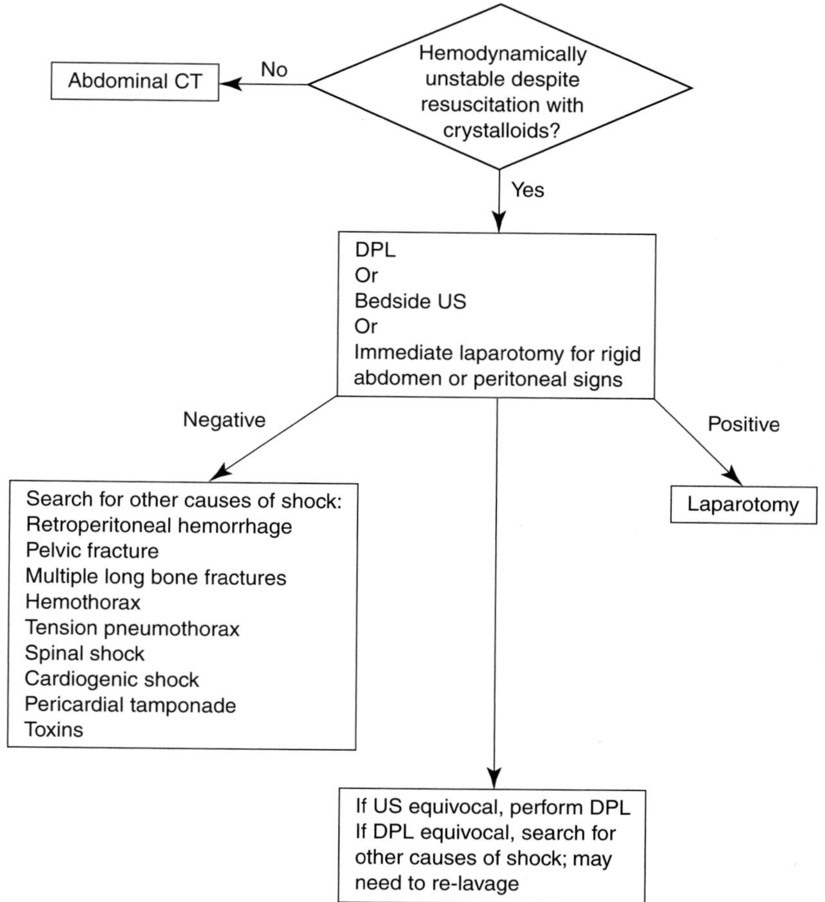

Fig. 19-1 Algorithm for evaluation of suspected abdominal injuries.

injury have elevated liver function tests (LFTs). These reports are small and unconvincing. Normal LFTs should not dissuade the EP from further evaluation of the traumatized abdomen.[20,21]

Objective Testing—Diagnostic Peritoneal Lavage, Computed Tomography, and Ultrasound

Because of the limitations of physical examination, many patients at risk for IAI require an objective test, such as DPL, CT, or US. The choice between an objective test (or the choice of *which* objective test) and serial examinations depends on many factors. The EP must consider patient factors such as the mechanism of injury, hemodynamic and neurologic stability, results of plain films and other bedside tests, and the degree of injury suggested by the physical examination. Factors relating to the ED setting include the number of patients in the department, hospital resources (both in terms of equipment and personnel), and consultant availability. Serial abdominal examinations are not feasible in patients who are undergoing general anesthesia for repair of other injuries. Patients who clearly need transfer to a trauma center based on their initial examination may benefit more from early transfer than extensive testing.

DIAGNOSTIC PERITONEAL LAVAGE

Diagnostic peritoneal lavage revolutionized the management of multiple trauma. Before DPL, nearly 20% of patients with abdominal trauma died secondary to an unrecognized abdominal injury.[22] Since the first report by Root et al,[23] many studies have confirmed its exquisite sensitivity. An analysis of multiple studies containing over 10,000 patients demonstrates DPL to be 97.3% accurate, with 1.4% false-positive and 1.3% false-negative results.[6] The complication rate is lower than 1%.

Although CT and US investigations are important

and noninvasive procedures, the performance of a DPL by skilled EPs, as well as surgeons, still has a role in blunt trauma. Hemodynamically unstable patients are never appropriate candidates for CT scanning. The only absolute contraindication to the performance of a DPL is obvious need for laparotomy (i.e., evisceration or peritoneal signs). The various techniques for the performance of a DPL and the interpretation of the lavage fluid results are discussed in Chapter 51. Hemodynamically unstable patients who have a positive peritoneal aspirate should proceed for laparotomy.

DPL has a high sensitivity, specificity, and negative predictive value.[24-27] However, DPL offers no information about the status of retroperitoneal organs, nor does it allow for the determination of which organ has been injured.[28] Although DPL may overlook small bowel injuries,[29] many authorities consider it more accurate than CT for this indication.[30] DPL is relatively "blind" to injuries of the diaphragm and bladder since they result in minimal bleeding.[31,32]

DPL has been criticized as being overly sensitive in the detection of IAI. Nonbleeding liver or spleen lacerations resulting in positive DPLs often result in nontherapeutic laparotomies. DPL is therefore best reserved for hemodynamically unstable patients to determine the need for emergent operation.

Overall, DPL remains a highly sensitive test for the hypotensive, multiply-injured blunt trauma patient, especially in centers that do not have immediate bedside US. The advantages of DPL over CT are rapidity and relative inexpensiveness, as well as having the patient in sight at all times.

ABDOMINAL COMPUTED TOMOGRAPHY

During the late 1970s, the introduction of **computed tomography** began the second great evolution in trauma management. Unlike DPL, CT approximates the amount of intraperitoneal blood and grades organ injury. Patients with injuries to the head, neck, and chest also benefit from this newer technology.

Indications for abdominal CT are similar to those for DPL, with one central caveat—*the patient who undergoes abdominal CT must be hemodynamically stable.* Hemodynamically unstable patients require DPL, bedside US, or immediate laparotomy.[33] Emergency physicians must strictly adhere to the imperatives of patient selection. DPL or US may be better suited to an agitated or intoxicated subject who might require sedation or even chemical paralysis to obtain an adequate CT scan. The CT suite must have adequate monitoring and resuscitative capabilities. Finally, the scanner should be a third- or fourth-generation device and located close to, or preferably within, the ED.[34]

The standard trauma scan begins at the dome of the diaphragm and continues down to the symphysis pubis. If the pelvis is not included, free fluid or blood that accumulates in this area will be missed.[35] Although most protocols require both intravenous (IV) and oral contrast for trauma CTs, routine oral contrast may not be necessary.[36,37]

Accuracy of CT is extremely reader-dependent.[38] Of note, the literature demonstrates a marked disparity between initial CT reading and subsequent review by an experienced tomographer. To use CT effectively, an expert tomographer must interpret the films.

The greatest risk of CT is the decompensation of a hemodynamically unstable patient outside of a resuscitation area. When deciding whether CT is appropriate for a seriously injured patient, consider the time the patient will spend outside of the safety of the ED. Modern spiral scanners require only 3 to 5 minutes for data acquisition. However, other factors such as patient preparation and transport times add considerable delays. The interval between the ED order and the CT interpretation may be hours.[39]

Where DPL is more sensitive than specific, CT is more specific than sensitive. The radiologist may underestimate or overlook hemoperitoneum. Pancreatic trauma is often misdiagnosed with both false-positive and false-negative results,[40,41] and scans routinely miss hollow viscus injuries.[41-43] In one review, CT missed 13 injuries in 92 patients, one of which contributed to the death of the individual.[44] Some experience with CT in detecting bowel injuries has been poor,[38,39,45,46] but other studies demonstrate a higher sensitivity.[47-49]

Prospective Comparative Trials of Diagnostic Peritoneal Lavage Versus Computed Tomography. Since 1985 nine prospective trials have directly compared DPL with CT in blunt abdominal trauma.[26,34,45,50-55] Most studies have found CT more specific but less sensitive than DPL. In general, DPL may lead to more unnecessary laparotomies than CT, but CT results in more missed injuries and therapeutic delays.[34,45,53] In most studies, DPL better predicts the need for operation. Over the years, a combination of advanced technology and growing experience in interpretation has increased the sensitivity of CT.

Of all the prospective studies directly comparing CT with DPL, only one found CT more sensitive and specific than DPL.[51] In a meta-analysis of all the prospective studies comparing CT with DPL, lavage had a sensitivity of 98% and a specificity of 92%, with an accuracy of 93%. Conversely, CT only had a sensitivity of 60%, a specificity of 98%, and an accuracy of 87%.[56] However, this statistic includes results of early trials, which employed first-generation CT scanners. These scanners provided less detail than modern devices. If only studies from the 1990s are considered, CT has a sensitivity of 88%.[56]

ULTRASOUND

The use of ED **ultrasound** is on the rise in the United States. However, in much of the industrialized world, US has been the standard for trauma evaluation for years.[50,57-62] Ultrasound is noninvasive, involves no radiation, and causes little patient discomfort. Serial examinations are easy to perform and inexpensive, and can provide early evidence of delayed bleeding.[63,64]

The indications for US mirror those for CT and DPL. The advantages include ease of use, portability, rapid results, noninvasiveness, lack of complications, and ability to repeat examinations as often as necessary. As with DPL, US is excellent for the unstable patient. Like DPL, it best screens for hemoperitoneum and is less capable of grading organ injury. The examination is noninvasive and can be safely performed at the bedside of any trauma patient.

The sensitivity, specificity, and accuracy of trauma US evaluations in experienced hands closely approximate that of DPL and CT.[50,57,61,65-72] Although some experts may discern actual organ injury, the EP should approach the examination with a single question in mind: "Is there free fluid in the abdomen?" The concept of the **FAST (Focused Abdominal Sonography in Trauma)** examination champions this notion.

The greatest advantage is the minimal time required to detect hemoperitoneum. On average, abdominal US can provide diagnostic information within 5 minutes.[33,57,66,69] In many patients, the EP can detect the presence or absence of hemoperitoneum in less than 3 minutes,[57] and a survey of Morison's pouch takes less than 1 minute.[73] Ultrasound may be particularly well suited for mass-casualty events. During the 1988 Armenian earthquake, physicians used US to screen thousands of patients for IAI. The studies took approximately 4 minutes each, with 1% false-negative and no false-positive results.[74]

Assessment of hemoperitoneum is the primary goal of trauma US, and time taken to localize and grade organ injuries may be ill-spent.[57] All US techniques emphasize imaging the abdominal recesses (i.e., those dependent parts of the abdomen where free blood collects). Although evaluation of Morison's pouch provides the highest yield, additional sonographic windows add to the sensitivity.[73] The most studied approach is the four-view technique that images Morison's pouch (hepato-renal) (Fig. 19-2), Douglas' pouch (recto-pelvic), left upper quadrant (to view spleen), and epigastric (to view pericardium).[57,61,63] Additional sonographic windows may include the right and left pericolic gutters.

The unstable patient with a positive US requires laparotomy, whereas stable patients with an equivocal examination should have their study repeated, ideally

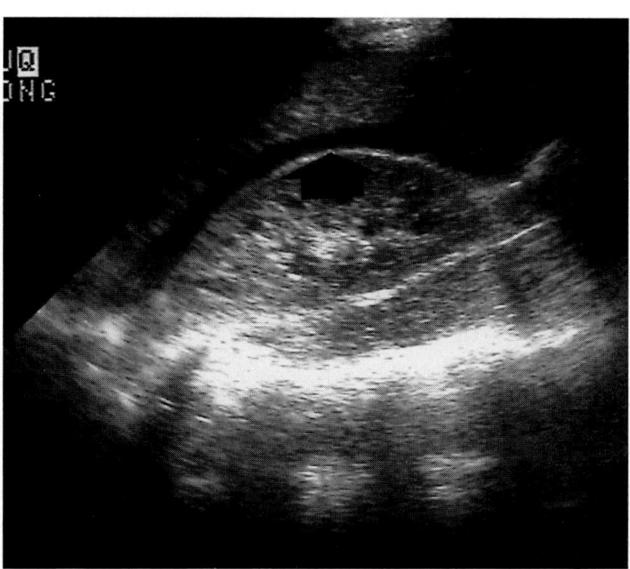

Fig. 19-2 Ultrasound image demonstrating fluid in Morison's pouch *(arrowhead).*

within the hour. Alternatively, the EP can employ CT for further evaluation if the patient is stable.

Although US is an excellent study, it has several shortcomings.[50,57,60,75] The uncooperative, agitated patient is difficult to scan. The presence of subcutaneous air or ileus distorts the ultrasonic images.[50,57,60,63] Images are coarsened or vague in the extremely obese patient and in those with large amounts of bowel gas.[50,57,63] In patients with prior abdominal surgery, adhesions may trap intraperitoneal blood, limiting distribution of free blood. Subcapsular hemorrhages of solid organs may be missed, since they do not produce significant free fluid. Like CT, US is insensitive for bowel injury. Finally, retroperitoneal structures are not well visualized. For these reasons, perform further diagnostic studies when the suspicion for IAI is high despite a negative US.[50,71,72,76] Not withstanding these limitations, ED US has improved emergency care and may soon supplant DPL in the initial evaluation of the unstable patient with blunt abdominal trauma.

Who Should Perform Ultrasound? The battle as to who will perform US in this country's EDs has begun. Most researchers agree that experience is necessary for accurate interpretation, and studies demonstrate a learning curve for accuracy. However, years of US experience improve specificity but not sensitivity. In one study, novice ultrasonographers demonstrated 100% sensitivity for IAI, compared with 92% sensitivity for those with more than 3 years of experience. However, as an individual's experience grew, specificity rose from 94% to 98%.[66]

Because of the time-sensitive nature of trauma care, many experts believe that EPs and surgeons should perform the initial ultrasound examinations.[77] Only 2 hours of physician training—1-hour theory, 1-hour practical—is necessary to detect hemoperitoneum more than 90% of the time.[76] Among EPs with only 10 hours of instruction, sensitivity was 90%, specificity 99%, and accuracy 99% in victims of blunt abdominal trauma.[69]

DIAGNOSTIC PERITONEAL LAVAGE, ULTRASOUND, AND COMPUTED TOMOGRAPHY AS COMPLEMENTARY STUDIES

DPL, CT, and US are not mutually exclusive, and in some patients the tests may be complementary. In some institutions, as a result of cost and logistical considerations, DPL or US is used as a screening examination for all patients with suspected blunt IAI, even if they are hemodynamically stable. Patients who are hemodynamically stable and have a positive DPL or US may benefit from subsequent CT.[78] In patients with an equivocal CT, a subsequent DPL may aid in decision making.[45] As experience with ED US grows, it may become the first study of choice in alert, hemodynamically stable patients with suspected IAI.

Ancillary Studies

LAPAROSCOPY

Laparoscopy has been used in hopes of decreasing the rate of nontherapeutic laparotomies.[79,80] Although laparoscopy can directly visualize organs, it offers little advantage over DPL in the initial evaluation of blunt abdominal trauma.[81] Its greatest utility may be in the hemodynamically stable patient with a hemoperitoneum diagnosed by DPL or ultrasound.[82]

OTHER STUDIES

A variety of other tests are occasionally useful in the evaluation of blunt abdominal trauma. **Endoscopic retrograde cholangiopancreatography (ERCP)** is indicated when the surgeon suspects a pancreatic duct injury. The consultant should order this study after the patient is hospitalized. **Nuclear medicine studies** (liver-spleen scans) popular in the 1970s have been replaced by CT. Lack of availability, high cost, and prolonged scanning times render **magnetic resonance imaging (MRI)** ineffectual in the acute setting. Although the surgical consultant may order an MRI to evaluate for diaphragmatic injury, the study is usually performed as an inpatient procedure. **Contrast duodenography** demonstrates duodenal hematomas and may be valuable in the patient with persistent, unexplained vomiting after a blow to the upper abdomen.

PRIORITIES IN MANAGEMENT

Patients sustaining blunt trauma typically have multisystem injuries. They face death from multiple causes, including severe intracranial, intraabdominal, intrathoracic, or pelvic hemorrhages. The pace of ED evaluation and treatment depends on the patient's hemodynamic and neurologic stability.

Although the issues regarding fluid resuscitation remain controversial (see Chapter 8), hypotensive victims of blunt abdominal trauma usually receive crystalloids, and if necessary blood, in an attempt to restore normotension. Definitive therapy for known or suspected active intraperitoneal hemorrhage or hollow viscus perforation is laparotomy.

Concomitant Thoracic Aortic and Intraabdominal Injuries

The majority of patients with traumatic aortic injuries (TAIs) have serious extrathoracic injuries.[83-86] If the CXR in a hypotensive patient suggests a TAI, recognize that undiagnosed IAIs may pose the most urgent threat to life.[83]

If the initial CXR is suggestive of a TAI, further evaluation of the thoracic aorta is needed.[86] Although an aortogram has been considered the gold standard, **helical computed tomography** scanning in the stable patient is an excellent alternative study.[87,88] Helical CT scanning is particularly valuable in the hemodynamically stable patient with multisystem injury who will need CT scans of other body regions. In the unstable patient, **transesophageal echocardiography (TEE)** is particularly useful and may be performed at the bedside or in the operating suite during laparotomy. Several studies attest to the high accuracy of TEE.[89,90]

There are several diagnostic options available to evaluate the abdomen in the hemodynamically stable patient (Fig. 19-3). A bedside US can rapidly detect large amounts of free intraabdominal fluid and may be available in major trauma centers. A DPL may also be performed in the trauma bay and should take minutes in experienced hands. Alternatively, a helical CT scan can rapidly evaluate the patient's abdomen and pelvis in less than 10 minutes and can image the thoracic aorta as well.

Kirsh et al[91] advocate immediate repair of aortic injuries, with thoracotomy preceding all other operative interventions with the exception of epidural hemorrhage or massive intraabdominal bleeding. These authors found 12 patients with concomitant intraabdominal and thoracic aortic injuries, 6 who underwent laparotomy before thoracotomy and 6 patients who had thoracotomy preceding laparotomy. Five of

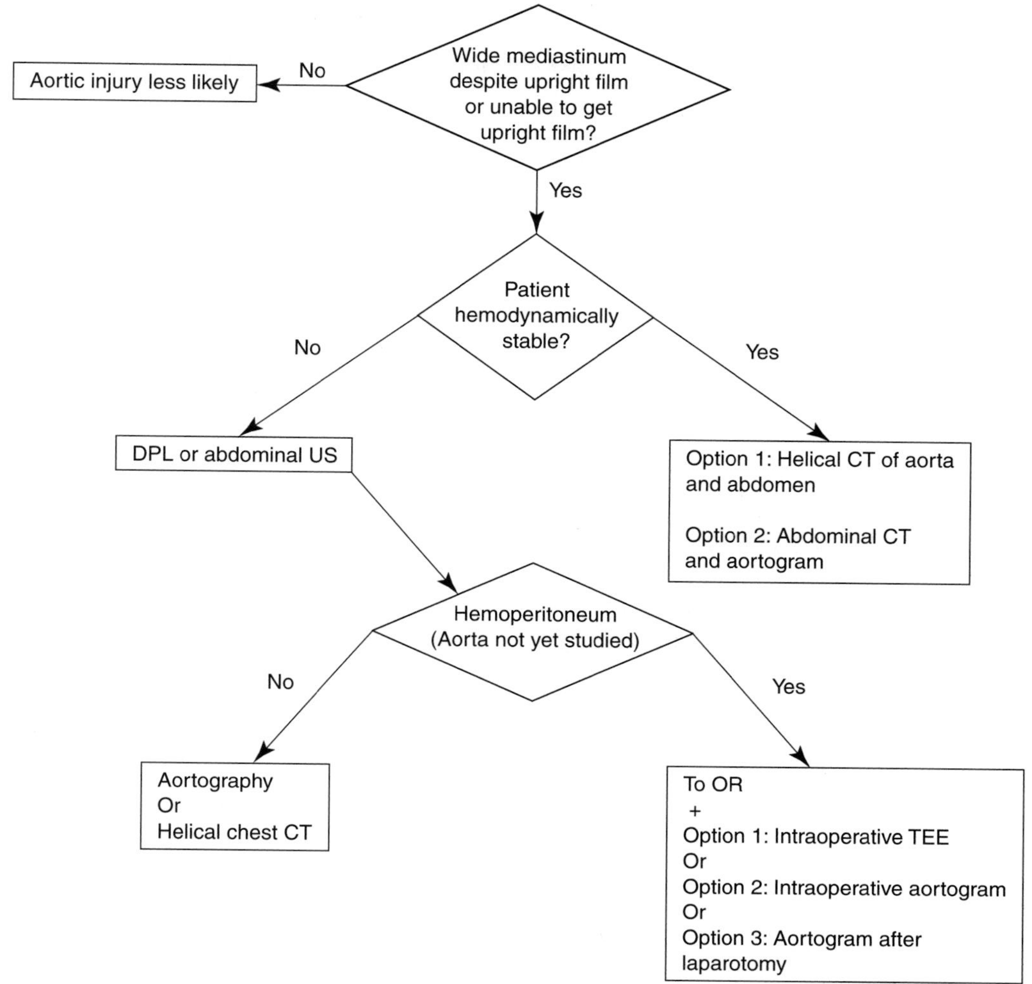

Fig. 19-3 Algorithm for patient with a wide mediastinum and suspected abdominal injury.

the six patients with laparotomy preceding thoracotomy died as a result of free rupture of the aortic injury, whereas all six patients who underwent aortic repair before laparotomy survived.

Conversely, Lee et al[83] have argued that IAIs should take precedence over TAI, and therefore these patients should be taken for laparotomy if any of the abdominal evaluations is suggestive of intraabdominal hemorrhage. After operation, the patient may then proceed for aortography, or in some centers, an on-table TEE can be performed. Similarly, Borman et al[92] advocate laparotomy before thoracotomy in patients with concomitant aortic and intraabdominal injuries. In addition to controlling hemorrhage, laparotomy will also identify and eliminate spillage of enteric contents, which may serve as a source for aortic graft contamination.

Richardson et al[84] believe that in the face of a DPL negative by gross inspection but positive by cell count, aortography may precede laparotomy; if the aortogram is positive in these cases, thoracotomy may precede laparotomy. Hunt et al[85] found no statistically significant difference in mortality whether laparotomy preceded thoracotomy or whether thoracotomy preceded laparotomy; however, there were only three instances where thoracotomy was performed first, compared with 32 patients undergoing laparotomy before thoracotomy.

In hemodynamically unstable or labile patients with suspected TAI, it is imperative to exclude intraabdominal hemorrhage immediately.[84,92,93] Patients with obvious peritoneal signs should proceed immediately to the operating suite for laparotomy to control hemorrhage. In equivocal situations, abdominal US or DPL may be performed rapidly to exclude intraabdominal hemorrhage. If the US or DPL is grossly positive, the patient should be rapidly transported to the operating suite for laparotomy before definitive evaluation of the aorta. An intraoperative TEE is a diagnostic option and may be carried out simultaneously with laparotomy. If the patient with a negative abdominal evaluation and suspected TAI remains hemodynamically unstable, then thoracotomy may need to be performed even without the performance of an aortogram.

Concomitant Intracranial and Intraabdominal Injuries

In contradistinction to patients sustaining TAI, it is unusual for blunt trauma patients with operable IAIs to have concomitant operable intracranial mass lesions (e.g., epidural or subdural hemorrhages).[94,95] Nonetheless, the patient with altered level of consciousness following blunt trauma should be suspected of having both intracranial and intraabdominal injuries until proven otherwise, regardless of hemodynamic stability (Fig. 19-4).[12]

With regards to mechanism of injury, Gutman et al[96] found that patients sustaining MVCs are much more likely to sustain a torso injury than an intracranial mass lesion. Conversely, patients sustaining falls were more likely to have an intracranial mass lesion, especially if they were 70 years of age or older. In addition, these authors concluded that unstable patients are also more likely to have a significant torso injury.

Thomason et al[95] prospectively evaluated the need for emergent craniotomy versus emergent laparotomy in hypotensive victims of blunt trauma and found that there is an 8.5-fold need for laparotomy over craniotomy. On the other hand, 33% of patients requiring craniotomy had an IAI requiring laparotomy. Similarly, Wisner et al[94] reviewed the need for craniotomy and laparotomy among blunt trauma victims and found that only 3 of 800 patients had both an operable intracranial lesion and IAI. These authors found that the only independent predictors of operable intracra-

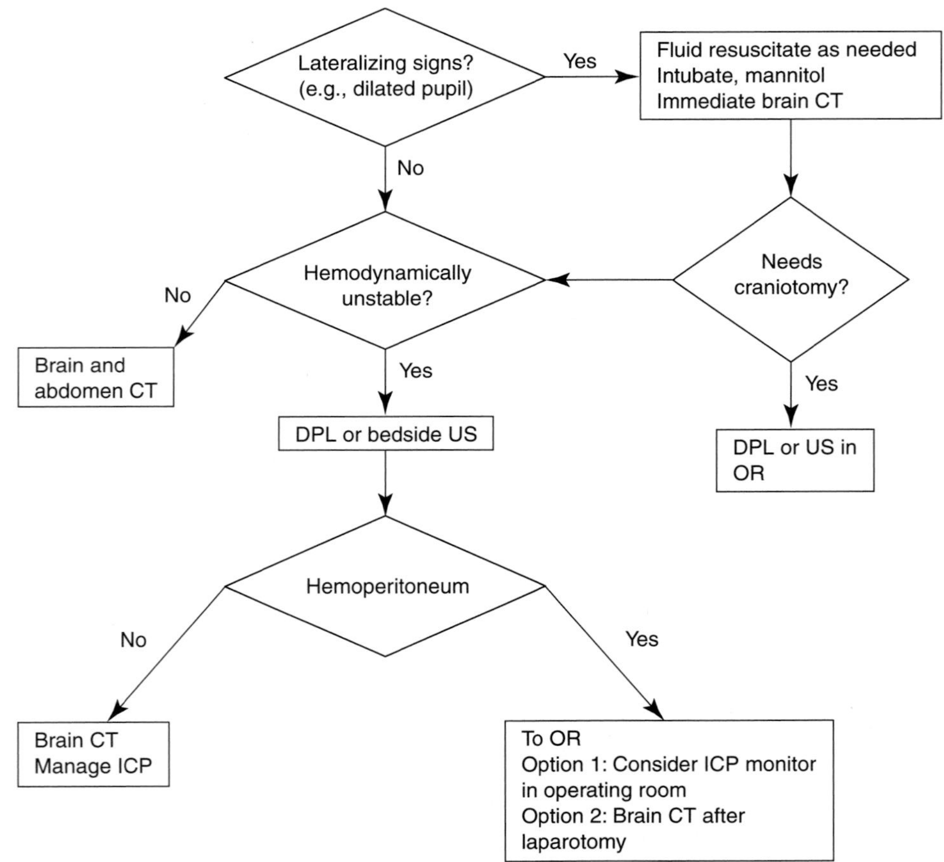

Fig. 19-4 Algorithm for patient with head injury and suspected abdominal injury.

nial lesions were field intubation and lateralizing findings, although none of the 3 patients with both operable intracranial and intraabdominal injuries had lateralizing findings.

PATIENTS WITH LATERALIZING FINDINGS

Patients with suspected severe intracranial injuries who have lateralizing findings (fixed unilateral pupil, unilateral hemiplegia) should first undergo brain CT scanning before laparotomy, even in the presence of a positive DPL, since herniation may be eminent.[94] In the neurologically unstable patient with a positive brain CT scan, abdominal CT scanning may be deferred in favor of emergent craniotomy, if the CT scan would consume valuable time. Such a patient may undergo DPL or US in the operating suite.

PATIENTS WITHOUT LATERALIZING FINDINGS

When there are no lateralizing findings of intracranial mass lesions, unstable patients with IAIs should first undergo laparotomy to prevent ongoing hemorrhage. Hypotension is one of the most dangerous insults suffered by the injured brain.[96] In cases where there is the need for emergent laparotomy, an intraoperative intracranial pressure monitor may be placed by a neurosurgeon simultaneously with the laparotomy.[94,95] Alternatively, emergent brain CT scanning may be performed immediately following laparotomy.

SPECIFIC ORGAN INJURIES

Splenic Injury

Teaching Case

A 43-year-old woman was involved in a motor vehicle crash. She complained of bilateral lower extremity, right elbow, and facial pain. Her abdomen was soft and nontender. Radiographs revealed multiple extremity fractures. Computed tomography of both her brain and abdomen were normal. She remained hemodynamically stable throughout her emergency department course and was taken to the operating suite for repair of her orthopedic injuries.

On the following day, she complained of abdominal pain and her hematocrit fell. A bedside DPL was positive for gross blood. At laparotomy, she was found to have a splenic rupture. ■

The spleen is the most commonly injured intraabdominal organ in patients with abdominal trauma.[97] Depending on the institution, the majority of these injuries may be secondary to either blunt or penetrating trauma. The spleen's fixed position under the left lower rib cage makes it prone to laceration from accompanying chest trauma. Patients presenting with left upper quadrant pain and tenderness have a splenic injury until proven otherwise. Up to 60% of patients with splenic injury may present with Kehr's sign, characterized by referred pain in the left shoulder caused by blood irritating the diaphragm.

Once felt to be a nonessential organ, the spleen's role in various immune functions emphasizes the need for its preservation when possible. Asplenic patients are at increased risk of infection, especially by gram-positive encapsulated organisms.[98,99]

Emergency Department Evaluation

Although a variety of diagnostic studies can identify IAI, CT scanning best demonstrates splenic trauma (Fig. 19-5). In addition to demonstrating obvious splenic contusions or lacerations, the IV contrast-enhanced scan may show a **contrast blush**, which is a hyperdense, well-circumscribed pooling of contrast media within the splenic parenchyma (Fig. 19-6).[100] The contrast blush helps predict which patients will fail nonoperative management.[100]

Ultrasonography is a rapid and noninvasive means to evaluate IAI, including splenic trauma. When US is used to evaluate the spleen, as opposed to screening for hemoperitoneum, order a formal radiographic study and do not rely on the ED FAST technique. Lesions vary from anechoic to hyperechoic when compared with normal splenic tissue.[101] One concern regarding the use of US in the diagnosis of splenic injury is the possibility of a missed hematoma. False-negative studies in the early posttraumatic period have been attributed to the initial isoechogenicity of the injury and inadequate studies limited by the patient's tenderness.[101]

Classification

Several classification systems exist for the evaluation of splenic injury (Boxes 19-1 to 19-4).[97,102-104] Although some predictions can be made on which patients require operative management, no one classification system is foolproof in determining which patients go on to splenic rupture, as is evident in the teaching case (see Controversies section).

Emergency Department Management

Once the diagnosis of splenic injury is made, the patient requires admission. **Splenectomy** was considered the procedure of choice for splenic injury for most of the twentieth century. However, after nu-

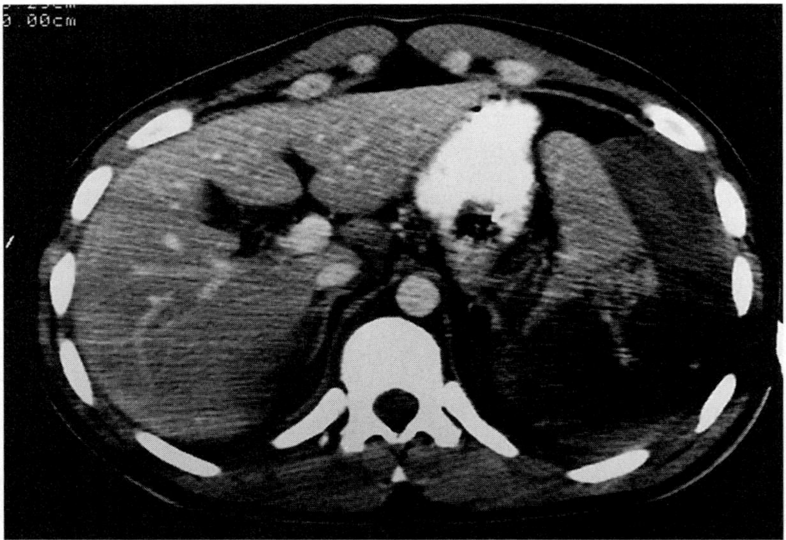

Fig. 19-5 Splenic laceration.

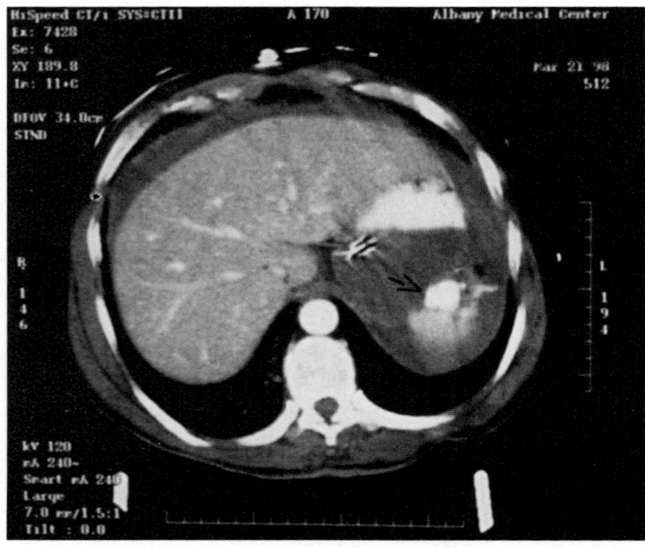

Fig. 19-6 Contrast blush within splenic laceration *(arrow).*

merous reports of the success of splenic salvage techniques in children and the concern of the risk for **overwhelming postsplenectomy infections** (**OPSI**), nonoperative management or attempts at splenic conservation (i.e., splenorrhaphy, angiographic embolization, or application of hemostatic agents) following blunt injury to the spleen are now the standard of care in selected groups of patients.[98,105-113]

The ultimate management decision relies on the clinical status of the patient more than the findings of diagnostic studies. Patients with higher injury severity scores (ISS) have sustained more serious trauma than patients with lower ISS and are more likely to require operative management of their splenic injuries.[97,110,114] Smith et al[112] have recently shown that patients over the age of 55 years usually fail nonsurgical management. Impaired level of consciousness resulting from intracranial trauma or intoxication, or the presence of associated intraabdominal or extraabdominal injuries, is also thought by some authors to preclude nonoperative management because of the unreliability of the sequential physical examinations.[107,112] However, pediatric and adolescent patients with splenic trauma sustaining additional injuries, including intracerebral trauma, have been successfully managed nonoperatively.[114] Patients with decreasing hematocrits despite blood transfusions, persistent hypotension, or worsening abdominal pain while in the ED or on the ward are considered to have failed nonoperative intervention and require laparotomy.[107,112,114]

Select patients with splenic injuries are candidates for transcatheter arterial embolization. Hemodynamically stable patients with (1) angiographic findings of extravasation of IV contrast, or (2) arterial disruption or major arteriovenous fistula are considered appropriate for embolization.[115,116]

Pediatric Considerations

Several explanations exist for the greater success of conservative management in children compared with adults. First, the size ratio of the splenic capsule to the parenchyma is greater in children and contributes to hemostasis.[107,117] Second, the more elastic ribs of children are less likely to fracture and puncture the spleen

BOX 19-1

Grading of Splenic Injuries Based on Findings at Autopsy, Laparotomy, or Radiologic Study

GRADE	INJURY
I	Subcapsular hematoma <10% surface area or nonbleeding capsular tear <1 cm deep
II	Capsular tear with active bleed; subcapsular hematoma 10% to 50% surface area; parenchymal hematoma <2 cm wide
III	Subcapsular hematoma >50% surface area or ruptured subcapsular hematoma; intraparenchymal hematoma >2 cm wide; deep parenchymal laceration >3 cm, not extending into hilar vessels
IV	Parenchymal laceration with extension into hilar vessels or actively bleeding ruptured intraparenchymal hematoma
V	Fragmented or devascularized spleen

Adapted from Moore EE et al: *J Trauma* 29:1664-1666, 1989.

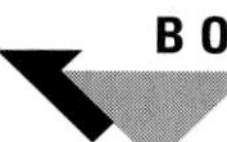

BOX 19-2

Grading of Splenic Injuries Based on Computed Tomography Findings

GRADE	FINDINGS
I	Capsular avulsion, superficial laceration or subcapsular hematoma <1 cm
II	Parenchymal laceration 1 to 3 cm in depth, subcapsular hematoma <3 cm
III	Parenchymal laceration >3 cm in depth, subcapsular hematoma >3 cm
IV	Fragmented or devascularized spleen

Adapted from Mirvis SE, Whitley NO, Gens DR: *Radiology* 171: 33-39, 1989.

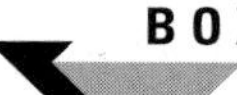

BOX 19-3

Grading of Splenic Injuries Based on Computed Tomography Findings with the Addition of Other Intraabdominal or Extraabdominal Injuries

CLASS	INJURY
I	Subcapsular hematoma or localized capsule tear
II	Capsular or parenchymal tears not extending into hilum
III	Parenchymal tears extending into hilar vessels
IV	Shattered spleen or pedicle disruption

A) No concomitant intraabdominal injuries
B) Concomitant intraabdominal injuries (B_1, solid viscus; B_2, hollow viscus)
C) Concomitant extraabdominal injury

Adapted from Buntain WL, Gould HR, Maull KI: *J Trauma* 31: 974-977, 1991.

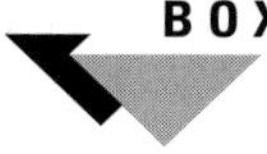

BOX 19-4

Grading of the Degree of Splenic Injury with the Amount of Hemoperitoneum

SITE	SCORE
Parenchyma	0 = Intact
	1 = Laceration
	2 = Fracture
	3 = Fragmented
Capsule	0 = Intact
	1 = Perisplenic fluid
Hemoperitoneum	0 = None
	1 = Any intraperitoneal fluid except perisplenic fluid
Pelvic fluid	0 = None
	1 = Any intraperitoneal pelvic fluid

Adapted from Resciniti A, et al: *J Trauma* 28:828-831, 1988.

as in adult patients.[108,113] Third, blunt abdominal injury is more likely to create splenic tears that run parallel to the splenic vessels; these tears tend not to bleed as much as if an object such as a knife or a fractured rib penetrated the spleen.[108,113] Fourth, local hemostasis is better achieved in children, since their vessels are better able to contract in the absence of atherosclerosis and vascular degenerative disease.[117] As a person ages, the spleen loses elastic tissue and is prone to brisk hemorrhage.

Complications

Complications following nonoperative management include **delayed splenic rupture** of an expanding subcapsular hemorrhage or pseudoaneurysm and the potential for missed associated IAIs.[118-121] Delayed rupture may occur days to weeks after an initially normal CT scan.[118-120] There is a distinction between delayed rupture (normal initial CT) and delayed *recognition* of rupture (no initial CT or misread CT).

Splenosis

An interesting side note concerning blunt splenic injury is the spontaneous autotransplantation of splenic tissue, a condition called **splenosis**. Most commonly found in the peritoneal cavity, nodules of splenic tissue have also been reported in the thoracic cavity following trauma to both the left hemidiaphragm and the spleen.[122] Splenosis is usually asymptomatic, but the appearance of splenic nodules on a chest radiograph may be mistaken for neoplasms.[122] The splenic nodules are not within the lung substance itself, but rather form within the pleura or interlobar fissures.[122] These ectopic splenic nodules have been reported to have splenic activity and may account for the low incidence of OPSI following splenectomy after trauma.[123]

Long-Term Disposition

Recent studies have shown that low-grade splenic injuries in children managed nonoperatively will demonstrate healing on CT scan within 4 months' time, usually within 6 weeks.[111,124,125] Grade III injuries may require up to 6 months to heal, and grade IV lesions require almost 1 year to show resolution on CT.[124] Although some authors advocate routine follow-up CT scans,[110] their value has been criticized because it is unknown whether residual parenchymal lesions are at risk for hemorrhage, and also because patients who remain clinically stable do not appear to benefit from a repeated scan.[126,127]

A current recommendation as to when resumption of contact sports or strenuous activity can occur is when a follow-up CT scan shows no residual lesions.[98] Pranikoff et al[111] have recommended that patients maintain a low activity level for 3 months postinjury if no follow-up CT scan is obtained. However, if patients with grade I or II injuries have a CT scan performed at 6 weeks and resolution is seen, they may resume normal activities.[111]

Controversies

Several authors have attempted to correlate the CT findings of splenic injury with operative findings, need for laparotomy, or feasibility of nonoperative management.[97,103,104,128,129] Others have disputed claims that CT scanning is reliable in predicting which patients will require laparotomy.[103,106,129,130] CT scans have been criticized for both overgrading and undergrading the actual damage to the spleen noted at laparotomy.[97,129,130] CT grading and intraoperative discrepancies may be due to the difficulty in assessing perisplenic fluid or when peritoneal lavage has been performed before scanning.[128,130]

Although some authors have stated that splenectomy is indicated for type IV or V splenic injuries,[97,131] others have noted resolution of these high-grade injuries without operative intervention.[130] Conversely, low-grade injuries have occasionally required late operative intervention after delayed rupture.[130]

HEPATIC INJURY

Teaching Case

A 48-year-old man was the unrestrained driver of a car that struck a brick wall. Physical examination showed lower chest and upper abdominal tenderness, the remainder of the examination being normal. The initial ED vital signs included a pulse of 60 beats/min and a blood pressure of 130/80 mmHg. Initial hematocrit was 28%. Abdominal CT showed a laceration of the left lobe of the liver and decreased flow to his right kidney. Renal angiography revealed an intimal flap at the level of the renal artery. The patient was taken to the operating room where he underwent an exploratory laparotomy. Operation revealed a grade IV liver laceration and a left perirenal aortic contusion. A partial hepatectomy of the left lobe was performed. ■

The liver is the second most commonly injured intraabdominal organ in blunt abdominal trauma.[132,133] Alert patients usually present with pain in the right upper quadrant, with occasional referred pain to the right shoulder.[134] However, injuries to the bare area of the liver (i.e., the posterior segment of the right hepatic lobe not covered by peritoneal reflections) may result in minimal or no abdominal pain or tenderness.[133] Physical examination in alert patients usually reveals abdominal tenderness, and a significant number of patients present with hemodynamic instability.[134]

Emergency Department Evaluation

In most patients, CT scanning is the preferred diagnostic measure. It can quantify injury and identify associated intraabdominal and retroperitoneal trauma.[135,136] Although US remains a rapid, noninva-

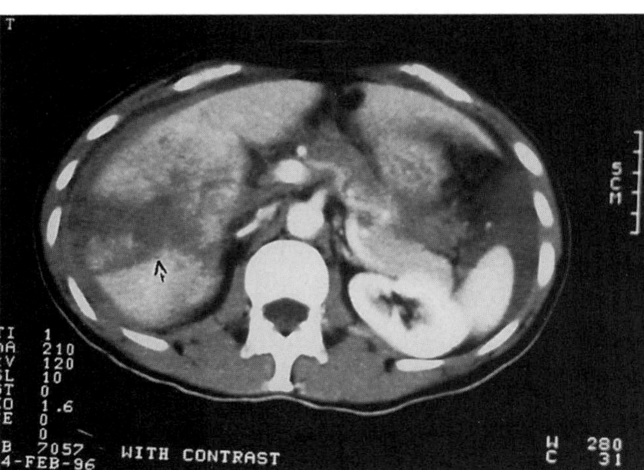

Fig. 19-7 Hepatic laceration *(arrow).*

sive, and inexpensive means of identifying hepatic trauma, it has several shortcomings compared with CT scanning. Ultrasonography in the setting of acute hepatic trauma cannot visualize the superior aspect of the hepatic parenchyma.[135] In addition, ribs, overlying bowel gas, and lack of inspiratory effort by the patient may decrease the accuracy.[135]

On CT scans, hepatic lacerations are hypodense and may be linear, round, or branching defects (Fig. 19-7).[136-138] Subcapsular hematomas are lenticular hypodense lesions adjacent to the capsule associated with indentation of the subjacent parenchyma.[136-138] On occasion, blood tracking around the liver may be the only indication of injury.[138] Artifacts from adjacent ribs, external tubes, or an air-contrast level in the stomach can lead to false-positive diagnoses.[136,138] False-negative diagnoses occur in the setting of a fatty liver as a result of its low attenuation, or when hepatic lacerations simulate biliary or vascular structures.[134,138]

Classification

The currently used classification system of hepatic injuries was described by Moore et al[102] and is based on the most accurate determination at autopsy, laparotomy, or radiologic study (Box 19-5). Mirvis et al[139] discuss a classification scheme based on CT findings in Box 19-6.

Although CT can accurately detect the presence of intrahepatic hematomas, operative findings often poorly correlate with CT estimation of hepatic lacerations.[140,141] In one study only 16% of patients had CT findings in agreement with operative findings; CT both underestimated and overestimated injury.[140] Computed tomography is also limited in its ability to detect injuries near the falciform ligament.

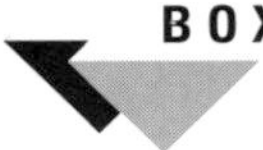

BOX 19-5
Grading Hepatic Injuries Based on Autopsy, Laparotomy, or Radiologic Study

GRADE	FINDINGS
I	Nonexpanding subcapsular hematoma, <10% surface area; nonbleeding capsular tear <1 cm deep
II	Nonexpanding subcapsular hematoma, 10% to 50% surface area; nonexpanding intraparenchymal hematoma, <2 cm wide; actively bleeding capsular laceration, 1 to 3 cm deep, <10 cm long
III	Expanding or >50% surface area subcapsular hematoma; ruptured subcapsular hematoma; intraparenchymal hematoma >2 cm or expanding; laceration >3 cm deep
IV	Ruptured intraparenchymal hematoma; parenchymal laceration involving 25% to 50% of lobe
V	Parenchymal laceration >50% of lobe; juxtahepatic venous injuries
VI	Hepatic avulsion

Adapted from Moore EE, et al: *J Trauma* 29:1664-1666, 1989.

Emergency Department Management

All patients with hepatic injuries require admission. Before the early 1980s, operation was routine.[142,143] Treatment consisted of suturing, vessel ligation, debridement, or partial resection, depending on the severity of the injury.[144-146] However, as many as 70% of patients taken for laparotomy had no active hepatic bleeding.[147-150] With the advent of improved radiographic techniques, principally abdominal CT, today's trend is towards nonoperative management for select pediatric and adult patients.*

Although some authors favor nonoperative management only for low-grade injuries,[141,154] even major hepatic injuries (grades III to V) have been successfully treated without laparotomy.[139,142,150,155] However, most grade V injuries are prone to hemodynamic instability and need operative intervention.[142] For nonoperative management to be successful, patients must remain hemodynamically stable after initial resuscitation, have no other indications for laparotomy, and require no more than two hepatic-related transfusions.[142,152,154]

*References 108, 109, 132, 134, 139, 141, 142, 148-155.

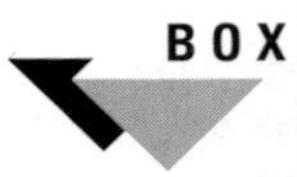

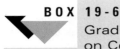

BOX 19-6

Grading Hepatic Injuries Based on Computed Tomography Findings

GRADE	CT FINDINGS
1	Capsular avulsion, lacerations <1 cm in depth, subcapsular hematoma <1 cm thick, or periportal tracking only
2	Lacerations 1 to 3 cm in depth, central/subcapsular hematomas 1 to 3 cm thick
3	Lacerations >3 cm in depth, central/subcapsular hematomas >3 cm thick
4	Massive central/subcapsular hematoma, lobar maceration, or devascularization
5	Bilobar maceration or devascularization

Adapted from Mirvis SE, et al: *Radiology* 171:27-32, 1989.

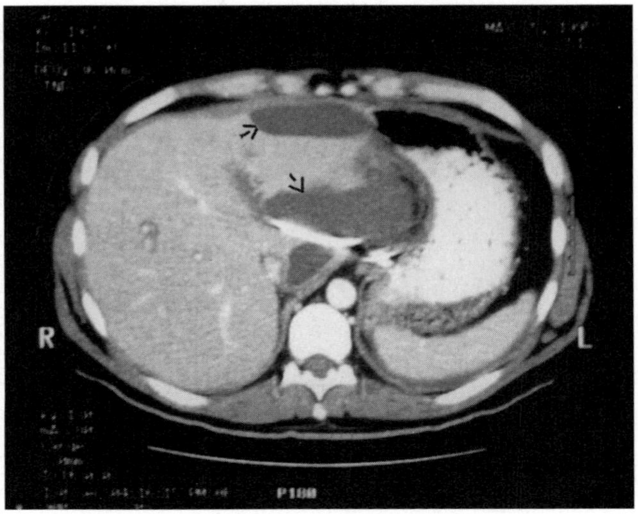

Fig. 19-8 Bilomas *(arrows).*

Hemodynamic instability during a trial of nonoperative management mandates laparotomy.[154] However, patients with falling hematocrits and CT scan evidence of ongoing bleeding are candidates for selective angiography and embolization if they are hemodynamically stable.[154,156] Patients who fail angiographic embolization require laparotomy.[154]

Complications

Bile peritonitis from intraperitoneal bile leaks, bilomas (Fig. 19-8), hemobilia, delayed hemorrhage, late intrahepatic bile duct stenosis, and subhepatic or subphrenic abscesses complicate hepatic injuries.* Hepatic dysfunction may occur in the face of enlarging biliary collections, and patients may develop hypoalbuminemia, anasarca, coagulopathies, jaundice, and ascites.[157] Some authors believe that mortality relates more to concomitant injuries rather than the hepatic trauma.[143,151]

Long-Term Disposition

Patients with subsequent CT scans demonstrating resolving hemoperitoneum and stable hepatic injuries may be discharged after in-hospital observation provided they have no other injuries requiring hospitalization.[141] Simple lacerations or subcapsular hematomas usually resolve within 2 to 4 months, whereas larger injuries may require 6 months to heal.[160] Patients may resume full activity when CT or US shows near-complete resolution, usually between 3 and 6 months postinjury.[154]

*References 142-144, 153, 154, 157-159.

GALLBLADDER INJURY

Teaching Case

A 46-year-old man fell 30 feet from a tree. His abdomen was firm and only mildly tender in the epigastrium. An abdominal CT scan showed pericholecystic and perihepatic fluid. He was taken to the operating suite for a diagnostic laparoscopy, which revealed an isolated perforation of the gallbladder. A cholecystectomy was performed, and he made a good recovery. ■

Compared with other intraabdominal organs, injury to the gallbladder (GB) is rare.[161,162] The protection from blunt trauma afforded to the GB is due to its small size, recessed location within the liver, and the surrounding omentum and rib cage.[162-166] Most authors report a high incidence of concomitant IAIs, with isolated GB injuries being a rare occurrence.[162,164-167]

Clinical Presentation

When laparotomy is not performed, a delay of up to several weeks may occur before the diagnosis of perforation is made.[162] Lack of symptoms in the early postinjury period is attributed to the lack of peritoneal signs in the presence of uninfected bile or if there is

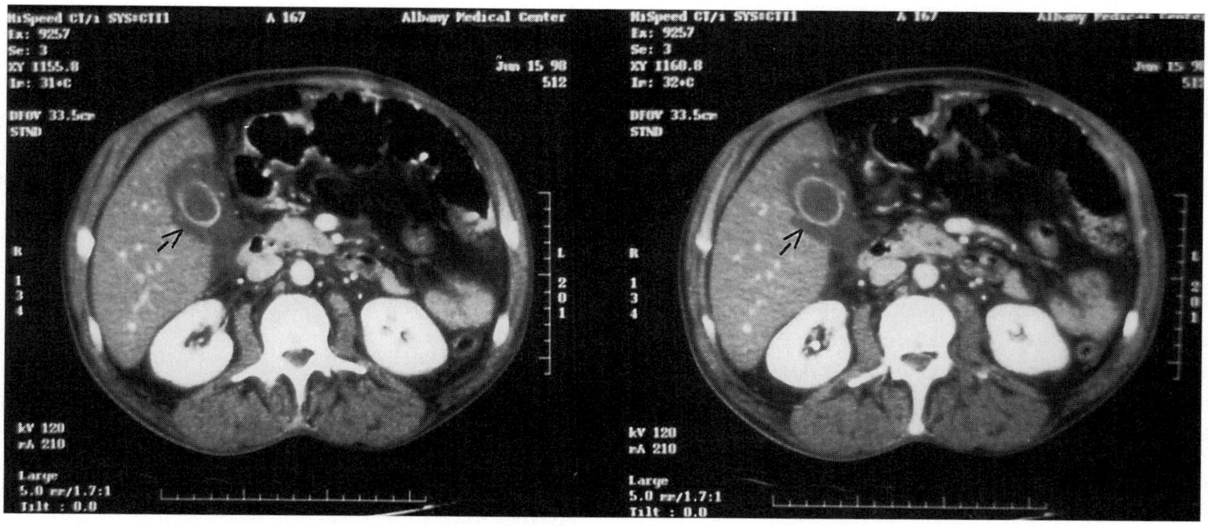

Fig. 19-9 Gallbladder avulsion *(arrows)*.

encapsulation of the bile within the peritoneal cavity by the surrounding omentum.[161,162,168-171] Bile in the peritoneal cavity causes fluid egress from the extracellular fluid compartment, leading to a hypovolemic state in the early postinjury period.[165,168,172] Early on patients may only complain of right upper-quadrant or nonlocalized abdominal pain or of referred pain to the right shoulder, but the physical examination may only show mild abdominal tenderness.[163,167] In the ensuing days or weeks following the injury, the patient may complain of increasing abdominal pain, nausea, and vomiting and become jaundiced or have acholic stools.[161,167] Jaundice results from absorption of bile pigments from the peritoneal cavity.[168,170]

Emergency Department Evaluation

Ultrasound may suggest the diagnosis by showing a contracted GB with a surrounding fluid collection in the subhepatic space, and hemobilia is detected by the presence of an intraluminal echogenic mass.[173-175] Abdominal CT scanning may show a blood collection within the gallbladder fundus or a fluid collection in the gallbladder fossa (Fig. 19-9).[169,174]

Emergency Department Management

Management options are related to the extent of injury. Nonoperative treatment may be carried out in selected cases of nonperforating injuries.[162] When the organ is severely injured or completely avulsed, or when the cystic artery is lacerated, cholecystectomy is recommended.[162,164] The long-term prognosis is excellent provided the injury is recognized and treated and there are no other associated injuries.[162,165,168]

PANCREATIC INJURY

Teaching Case

A 15-year-old boy flipped over his bicycle, his abdomen striking the handlebars before he landed. He had mild abdominal tenderness and vomited several times. An abdominal CT scan did not show any internal injuries. His initial amylase was normal, and he was discharged. Three days after injury his abdominal pain increased and he returned to the ED. A repeat abdominal CT scan showed a fracture of the body of the pancreas. The amylase level was now markedly elevated. He went to the operating suite for repair of a pancreatic injury. ■

Introduction and Pathophysiology

A concentrated force applied at the anterior abdomen, such as occurs with a forceful kick to the epigastrium or a fall onto a bicycle handlebar, may compress the pancreas against the spine. Isolated pancreatic injuries occur relatively infrequently. The proximity of the pancreas to the aorta, portal vein, inferior vena cava, renal veins, left kidney, liver, duodenum, and spleen account for the significant morbidity and mortality associated with injury to this region.[176,177] Most deaths from trauma to the pancreas occur within 48 hours after injury, often secondary to hemorrhage from the surrounding large vessels.[177,178] Deaths related exclusively to the pancreatic injury itself are rare.[178]

Clinical Presentation

Some patients remain asymptomatic for weeks following the initial injury.[176,178] The retroperitoneal location of the pancreas combined with decreased secretion and inactivity of pancreatic enzymes following injury may account for the paucity of early physical signs.[176,178] Some patients may complain of epigastric pain out of proportion to tenderness.[178] Patients with a remote history of trauma (days to weeks prior) may not recognize the connection between previous trauma and current symptoms.

Emergency Department Evaluation

Diagnosing isolated pancreatic injuries can be challenging. Measurement of serum amylase in the ED is not useful.[179-181] As many as one third to three quarters of patients with proven pancreatic injury initially have normal serum amylase levels.[178,179,181] Conversely, only a minority of patients with hyperamylasemia have pancreatic injury.[178] Confounding this issue, hyperamylasemia occurs with isolated intracranial hemorrhage.[182] Increased pancreatic amylase fractions may occur in the setting of preexisting pancreatitis or renal failure.[183] Although serum amylase levels obtained greater than 3 hours after admission may be more useful than initial values,[184] the EP should not routinely order a serum amylase in patients with blunt abdominal trauma.

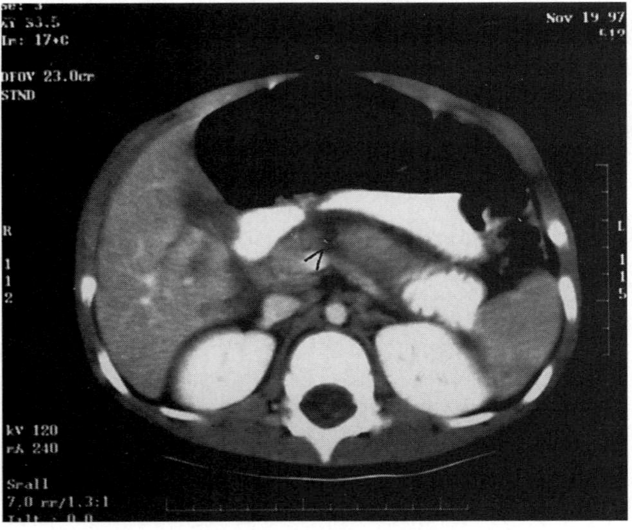

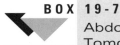

Fig. 19-10 Pancreatic fracture *(arrowhead)*.

Abdominal CT is widely used in the initial diagnosis of intraabdominal and retroperitoneal injuries in hemodynamically stable patients (Fig. 19-10). Diagnosis of pancreatic injuries on CT is not always evident, especially in children, where there is little surrounding retroperitoneal fat.[136,185] In cases where the fracture line is not evident, CT findings suggestive of pancreatic injury include edema of the peripancreatic fat, thickened left anterior perirenal (Gerota's) fascia, edema surrounding the superior mesenteric artery, fluid between the splenic vein and pancreas, and the presence of a pseudocyst (Box 19-7) (Fig. 19-11).[138,186,187] Potential causes of missed CT diagnoses include failure to recognize injury, hematoma masking the fracture line, and close approximation of the fracture ends.[186] False-positive diagnoses have been attributable to streak artifacts from objects such as nasogastric tubes, normal folding of the pancreas, and the juxtaposition of unopacified jejunum and the pancreas, simulating a fracture.[136,138,186]

The FAST examination by the EP is unlikely to reveal pancreatic trauma. However, formal US performed by a radiologist may play a role in diagnosis (Fig. 19-12). Ultrasound scanning can demonstrate pancreatic pseudocysts, as well as parenchymal and ductal fractures.[188]

In acute trauma, overlying ileus is likely to obscure pancreatic anatomy. Overall, US is a second-line test for pancreatic injury. Endoscopic retrograde cholangiopancreatography may demonstrate the injury in suspicious cases where all other imaging modalities have failed.

Emergency Department Management

The detailed operative management of pancreatic injuries is beyond the scope of this text, but a few comments on post ED interventions are helpful. Treatment

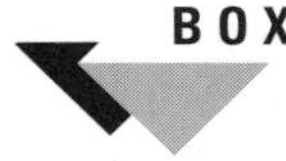

BOX 19-7
Abdominal Computed Tomography Findings Suggestive of Pancreatic Injury

Edema of peripancreatic fat
Thickened left perirenal fascia
Edema surrounding superior mesenteric artery
Fluid between splenic vein and pancreas
Presence of pseudocyst

plans are based on the classification of the injury found at operation (Box 19-8).

In the past, type I injuries generally required external drainage, whereas types II through IV required some form of resection, possibly with complete removal of the duodenum and diversion of the remaining pancreatic stump into the jejunum following more severe injuries.[178,189-191] More recent studies, especially involving children, have shown that a nonsurgical approach is often possible with grade I and II injuries.[192,193] Morbidity following pancreatic injury has decreased significantly with the use of intraoperative pancreatography for evaluation of the proximal pancreatic duct.[178] Postoperative enteral nutrition is important in the rehabilitative process.[189,190]

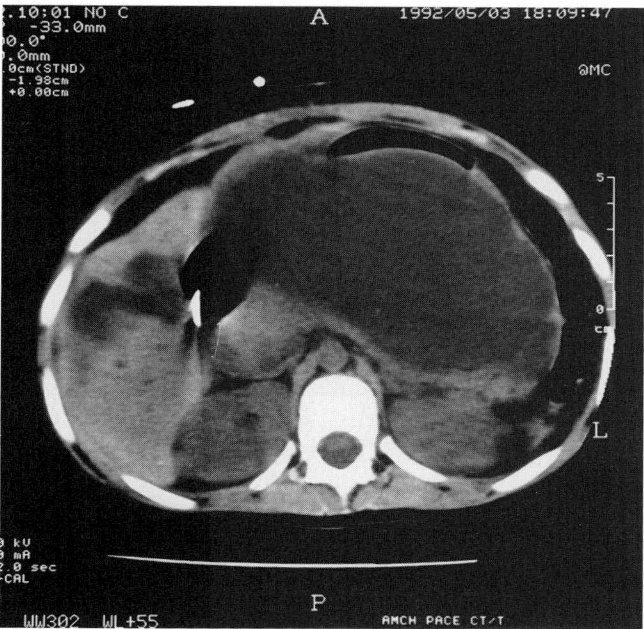

Fig. 19-11 Computed tomography illustrating pseudocyst.

Complications

As many as one third of patients experience complications from pancreatic injury.[178] Pancreatic fistulae, abscesses, pseudocysts, and pancreatitis are commonly reported sequelae; most result from injury to the pancreatic duct.[178,187,194,195] Postoperative hemorrhage re-

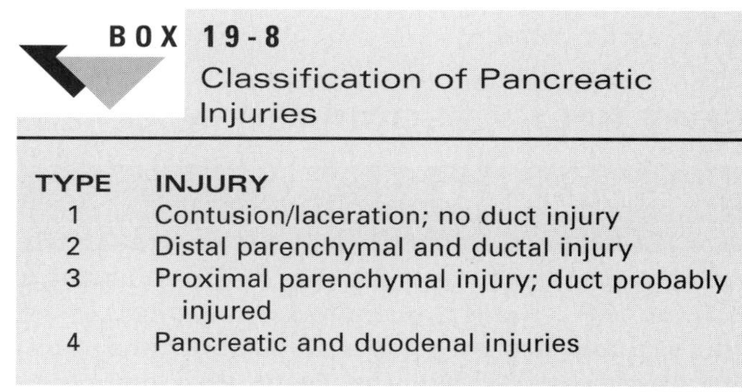

BOX 19-8
Classification of Pancreatic Injuries

TYPE	INJURY
1	Contusion/laceration; no duct injury
2	Distal parenchymal and ductal injury
3	Proximal parenchymal injury; duct probably injured
4	Pancreatic and duodenal injuries

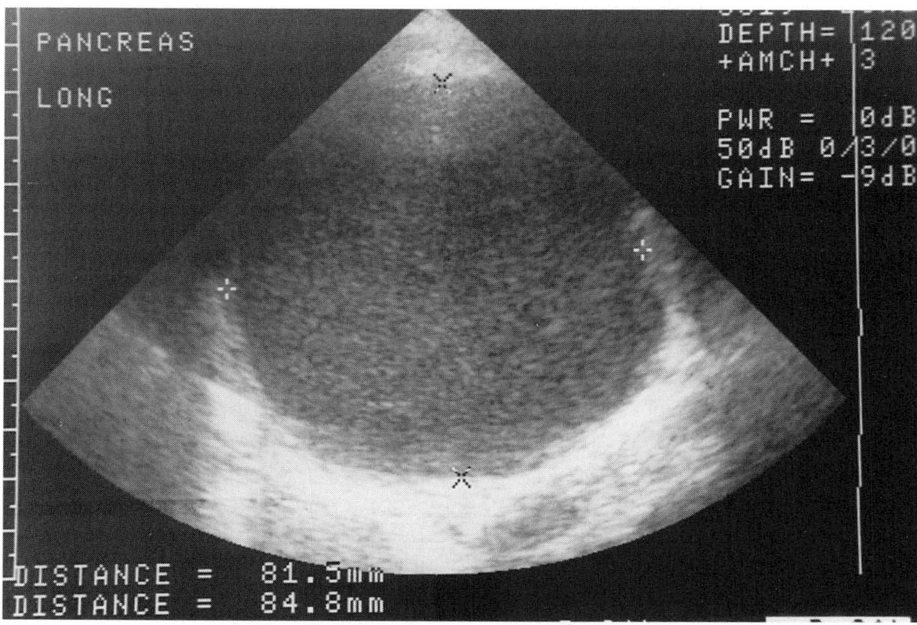

Fig. 19-12 Ultrasound of pseudocyst.

sults if leaking pancreatic enzymes erode into surrounding vessels.[178,191] Pseudocysts, which are fluid collections without a true epithelial lining, arise weeks to months after injury. Depending on the location of the ductal injury, pseudocysts may require aspiration, external drainage, or surgical resection, but nonoperative management has also been successful in selected cases.[189,195-197]

Diabetes mellitus is rare following pancreatic injury, since up to 80% to 90% destruction of the gland is required for endocrine dysfunction.[178,191] Provided that the pancreatic duct has access to the small intestine, impairment of exocrine functions (i.e., digestion and absorption of food products) is unusual.[178]

Disposition

All patients with proven pancreatic injuries, or those with high suspicion of occult injury despite normal imaging studies, require admission for observation and IV fluid therapy.

SEAT BELT–ASSOCIATED INJURIES

Teaching Case

An 11-year-old girl was brought to the ED following a two-car MVC. She was restrained by a lap belt in the rear seat and had no complaints of abdominal pain. She was released without diagnostic tests, but on discharge began to vomit. A more detailed physical examination showed a midabdominal ecchymosis overlooked on initial examination. An abdominal CT scan demonstrated free fluid without evidence of organ injury. She was admitted for observation, developed progressive abdominal tenderness, and was taken to the operating suite. At laparotomy, she had complete transection of her small bowel. ■

Over the past four decades, the routine use of seat belts has saved many lives. However, seat belts, lap belts in particular, are linked to certain types of injury. These injuries include Chance fractures of the lumbar spine, mesenteric or seromuscular avulsions and intestinal perforations, and abdominal wall avulsions and hernias. Dissections of the descending aorta and iliac artery are less common. The classic "*seat-belt sign*" consists of abdominal bruising over the lap belt distribution (Fig. 19-13). A patient with a seat belt sign requires diagnostic studies and repeated clinical examinations.[198] IAI may occur in as many as 64% of patients with the seat belt sign.[199] Patients with an abdominal seat belt sign have a nearly 8-fold increase in intraabdominal trauma (23% versus 3%) compared with patients without this finding.[200]

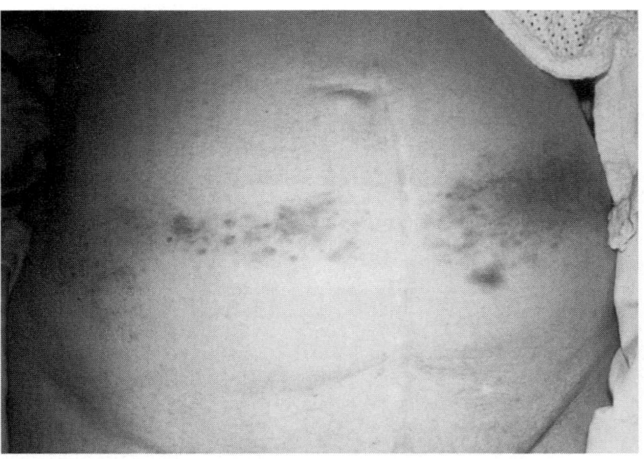

Fig. 19-13 Photograph of seat belt abrasion.

Children are at particularly increased risk of injury from the use of lap belts, since these restraints were designed for adults.[201] Lap belts tend to be positioned over the midabdomen in children, since their iliac spines are not fully developed and also because they usually do not sit upright.[201-204] The thin abdominal wall and narrow anteroposterior diameter of children afford little protection from the lap belt during deceleration of the motor vehicle.[198,202] Finally, since the center of gravity is higher in a child, there are increased deceleration forces if the upper torso is unrestrained.[202,203]

Chance Fractures

In 1948, Chance[205] commented on an uncommon fracture of the spine caused by extreme flexion that disrupted the posterior elements. These injuries did not compress the vertebral bodies or dislocate the apophyseal joints. Twenty years later, Smith and Kaufer[206] referred to these injuries as **Chance fractures** and noted their strong association with lap belts. Many authors have since commented on this correlation.[201,207-210]

The majority of Chance fractures occur between the first and third lumbar vertebrae, whereas most thoracolumbar compression fractures occur at the twelfth thoracic or first lumbar vertebra.[206,209] The mechanism of injury is thought to involve both hyperflexion of the body around the lap belt and distraction of the vertebrae during sudden deceleration.[206] These fractures rarely cause neurologic deficits unless shearing or rotatory forces displace the vertebral bodies.[206] Children, however, have a higher incidence of paraplegia associated with Chance fractures, attributed to

BOX 19-9
Types of Chance Fractures

TYPE	DESCRIPTION
I	Fracture through spinous process, laminae, apophyseal joints, pedicles, and transverse processes extending into vertebral body
II	Identical to type I, but spares spinous process
III	Posterior elements and vertebral body on one side are involved

their relatively higher center of gravity and increased degree of body distraction from the lumbar spine.[211] Three types of fracture patterns have been described (Box 19-9).

Although the fracture may not be readily apparent on quick inspection of the radiograph, there are several clues to its presence. In the anteroposterior view, the posterior elements may be so disrupted that they no longer are projected over the vertebral body, the so-called "*empty vertebrae sign*" (Fig. 19-14).[209] In addition, discontinuity of the oval-shaped pedicles or the tear-shaped spinous process in the AP view reveals the fracture.[209] The lateral radiograph should confirm disruption of posterior element disruption (Fig. 19-15).

Patients are usually treated by conservative measures (i.e., bed rest or body cast for 6 to 8 weeks) but surgical fixation may be required when the posterior ligaments and facet joints are disrupted.[208] The prognosis for healing and functional recovery is good provided that adequate reduction is achieved.[208]

INTESTINAL PERFORATIONS AND MESENTERIC AVULSIONS

Intraabdominal hollow viscus injury is another major injury pattern associated with the use of lap belts. Gastrointestinal perforations, particularly of the small bowel, are common.[212-216] Seromuscular tears without intestinal perforation and avulsions of the mesentery are also found in patients sustaining lap belt injuries.[212,213,216,217] Either a sudden rise in intraluminal pressure or shear of the mesentery at points of attachment may cause gastrointestinal injuries.[212,213]

Delayed intestinal obstruction may occur when mesenteric tears are not diagnosed on initial presentation.[218] Furthermore, patients with Chance fractures are at increased risk of intestinal injuries.[202,203] Children are especially prone to the constellation of lap-

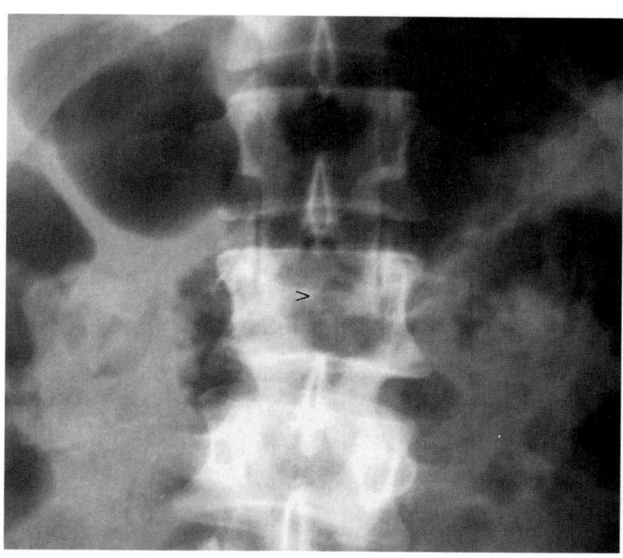

Fig. 19-14 Anteroposterior view of "empty vertebrae sign" associated with L2 Chance fracture *(arrowhead).*

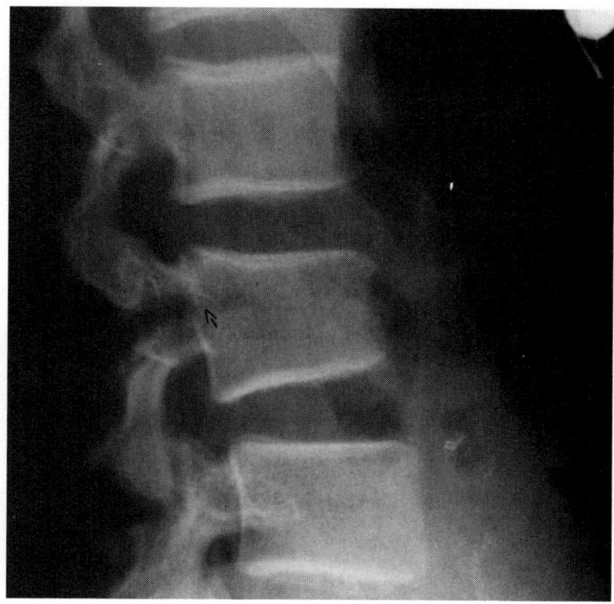

Fig. 19-15 Lateral view of L2 Chance fracture *(arrow).*

belt ecchymosis, Chance fracture, and hollow viscus injury. The presence of any two of these findings should prompt a search for the third part of the triad.

Delayed diagnosis of intestinal perforation is common, and the injury may not be recognized for up to a week.[46,213] More commonly, however, the injury will be apparent within 12 to 24 hours. Physicians often attribute distension, vomiting, and decreased bowel sounds to ileus resulting from associated injuries, such as retroperitoneal hematoma or lumbar spine fracture.[213] The initial physical examination may be benign.[204]

Some series report that CT of the abdomen is of limited use in the diagnosis of intestinal perforation, unless free intraperitoneal air is present (Fig. 19-16).[46,198,204,217] However, suggestive findings include unexplained peritoneal fluid collections (Fig. 19-17), bowel wall thickening, and focal bowel hematomas.[46,201] The presence of extravasated intravenous contrast material outside the lumen of the bowel suggests a torn mesenteric vessel.[219] If the CT is negative, serial physical examinations can detect intestinal perforation without dangerous delays in laparotomy, provided the patient is not head injured.[220]

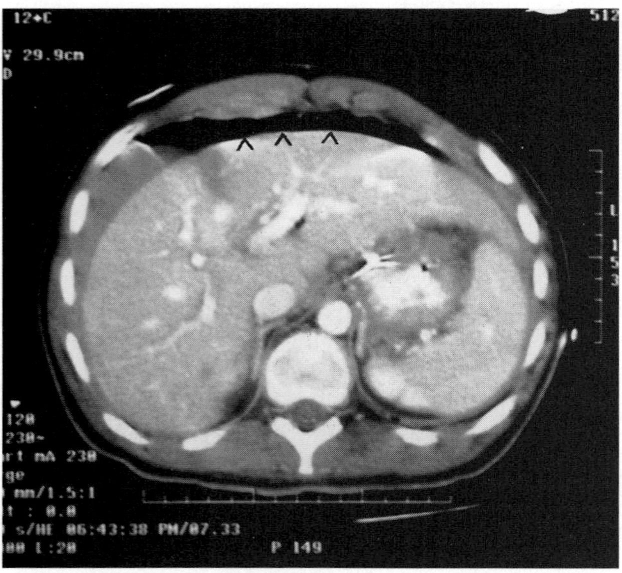

Fig. 19-16 Computed tomography shows free intraperitoneal air *(arrowheads).*

In cases where CT or physical examination is equivocal, DPL can provide important information.[198] Although the utility of the white blood cell (WBC) count in the lavage fluid is controversial, an elevated count in the presence of a positive seat belt sign is an important clue to hollow viscus injury. If the DPL is positive and the suspicion for bowel injury is high, laparotomy is indicated. The injured segment of bowel often needs to be resected and reanastomosed.[217] Seromuscular tears not involving more than two thirds of the circumference of the bowel may be repaired primarily without resection.[217]

Abdominal Wall Disruption and Delayed Ventral Hernia

Abdominal wall disruption is an uncommon injury that is strongly associated with the use of lap belts (Fig. 19-18).[212,215,216,221-223] However, cases have occurred that did not involve the use of seat belts or even involve MVCs.[224,225] The same mechanism that leads to pancreatic injury can disrupt the abdominal wall, as with "handle-bar hernias" in cyclists who crash their bikes.[226] The subcutaneous fat and overlying abdominal musculature are disrupted, and pa-

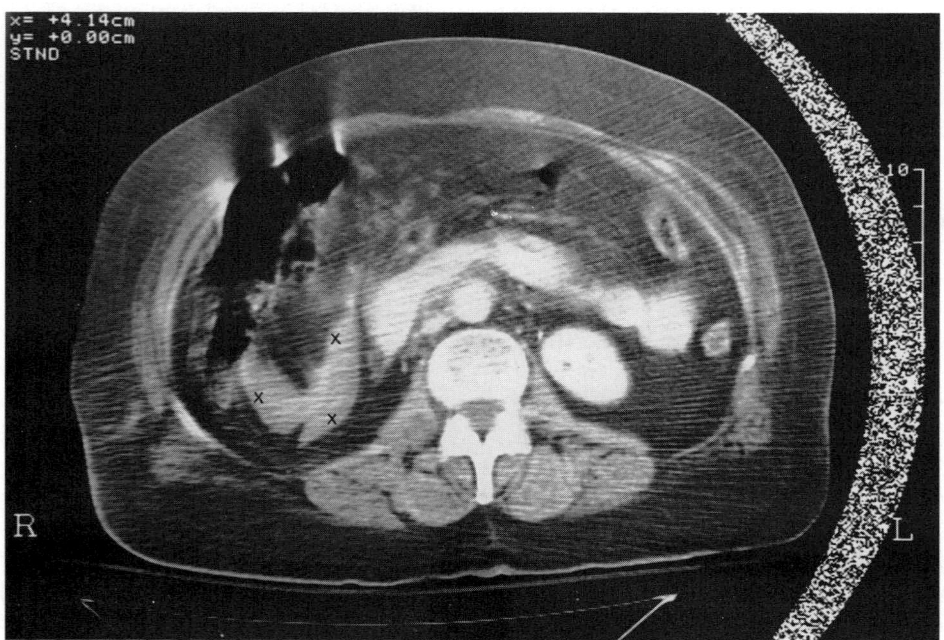

Fig. 19-17 Peritoneal fluid collection *(x)* in patient with mesenteric avulsions.

tients may present with a tender mass or muscular defect, usually located in the anterior midline between the rectus muscles.[221,222,227] Rarely, the defect lies in the lumbar region.[223] Loops of bowel may fill the hernia defect.[221-223] Disruption of the abdominal wall usually does not occur above the umbilicus, possibly because of the strength of the posterior rectus sheath above the arcuate line.[227]

The appearance of ventral hernias may be significantly delayed. Hurwitt and Silver[228] reported the appearance of a left upper quadrant hernia 7 months after the initial accident in which the victim was restrained by a lap belt. Delayed ventral hernias may either be asymptomatic or have associated pain.[228]

CT may help to distinguish a rectus sheath hematoma (Fig. 19-19) from a muscular disruption.[227]

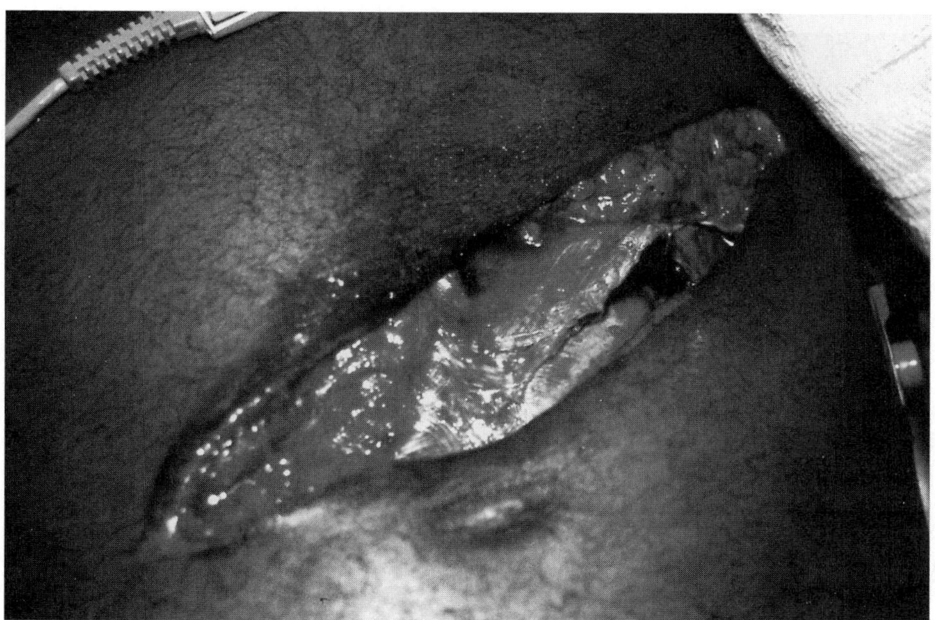

Fig. 19-18 Photograph of abdominal wall avulsion caused by a seat belt.

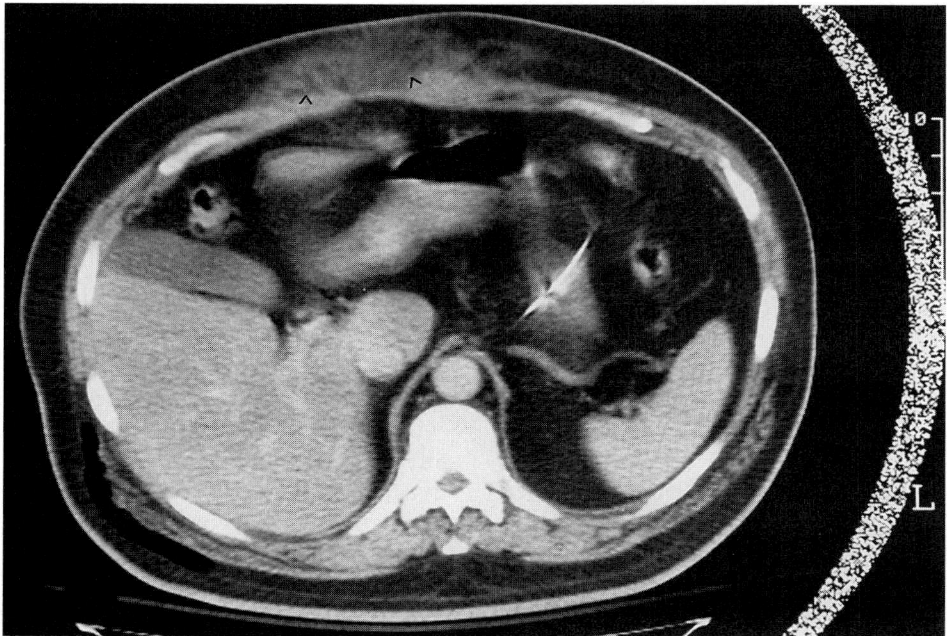

Fig. 19-19 Computed tomography of rectus sheath hematoma *(arrowheads)*.

CT also helps to delineate the anatomy of the muscle layers and presence of bowel contents within the defect.[223]

When the diagnosis of abdominal wall disruption is made, laparotomy is indicated to delineate the extent of the defect, as well as to detect associated IAIs.[227] Initial repair of the hernia is usually not feasible because of extensive muscle damage.[221] Late hernia repair can be postponed for months and is indicated for symptomatic disability.[227]

Abdominal Aortic Dissections and Aneurysm

Dissection of the abdominal aortic intima and traumatic abdominal aortic aneurysm are other injuries reported in association with seat belts.[229-231] Abdominal aortic injuries are much less common than thoracic aortic injuries because of the protection afforded by the retroperitoneum and the vertebral column.[229,232] Atherosclerosis increases the likelihood traumatic dissection.[229,232,233] Cases of isolated thrombosis or contusion of the iliac arteries without aortic involvement occur in patients with other lap-belt injuries.[234] The dissection often travels caudally into the iliac arteries.[235]

Patients may present with cold lower extremities, diminished peripheral pulses, and decreased sensation.[231,235] However, distal pulses may be palpable since the pulse wave is transmitted through clot.[230,234] Listen for abdominal bruits, which may be heard in some patients.[229] In some cases, diagnosis of the aortic injury is delayed for weeks, as occlusion may not occur immediately.[229] In the hemodynamically stable patient, aortography may delineate the aortic injury in cases where peripheral pulses are decreased.[234]

Rupture and exsanguination, occlusion with resultant ischemia and possibly subsequent gangrene can complicate unrepaired aortic aneurysms.[229] Thromboendarterectomy is required for cases associated with advanced atherosclerosis.[230] Repair without the use of grafts is preferred in the setting of bowel perforation because of the risk of contamination.[229,230] However, synthetic grafting is necessary is cases of severe damage to the aorta.[229,230]

HOLLOW VISCUS INJURIES

Teaching Cases

Case 1: A 16-year-old woman was a passenger in a high-speed MVC. She arrived in the ED complaining of right lower chest and right-sided abdominal pain. Her abdomen was diffusely tender. A chest radiograph revealed fractures of the right ninth and tenth ribs. An abdominal CT scan demonstrated a large amount of free intraperitoneal air and fluid. She was taken urgently to the operating suite for an exploratory laparotomy. Her duodenum was transected just distal to the pylorus and was repaired. She was ultimately discharged home tolerating a full diet.

Case 2: A 3-year-old girl pulled a television set onto herself from a height of 3 feet. She complained of upper abdominal pain and vomited once before arrival in the ED. Her examination revealed tenderness in the midepigastrium and left upper quadrant and a periumbilical ecchymosis. Radiographs of the chest and pelvis were negative and an abdominal CT scan was normal. The patient was not tolerating a liquid diet and was admitted for observation. The next morning the patient developed a low-grade fever and her abdominal pain and tenderness increased. She exhibited abdominal guarding and would not ambulate. She was taken to the operating suite for an exploratory laparotomy, where a jejunal perforation was found and repaired. Her postoperative course was uncomplicated. ■

Blunt trauma may cause numerous injuries to the hollow viscera including duodenal hematomas, bowel perforations, and mesenteric injuries. Hollow viscus perforations soil the peritoneal cavity and patients may ultimately develop intraabdominal sepsis. Mesenteric avulsions may result in necrotic bowel.

Specific Injury Patterns

STOMACH PERFORATIONS

Isolated gastric perforations as a result of blunt trauma are rare.[236-238] Gastric injuries are rare due to protection by the overlying ribs, lack of fixation, thick walls, and its usually empty state.[236,237] The stomach becomes more susceptible to injury after eating, since the stomach assumes a lower position in the abdomen.[238,239]

Patients with rupture of the stomach usually present with abdominal pain and distention, and may eventually develop peritonitis.[237,238] If the perforation occurs near the esophageal hiatus, air tracking into the mediastinum may produce subcutaneous emphysema.[237] Blood loss from gastric perforations is usually minimal, but hemorrhage occurs from coincident injuries such as splenic lacerations.[237] Diaphragmatic injury may also accompany gastric trauma.

Since the stomach normally has a low bacterial count, peritonitis from gastric perforations is unlikely. However, after eating a meal gastric bacterial flora increases, as the pH of the stomach becomes more neutral. Therefore peritoneal contamination by gastric perforations is more likely to occur in patients who have recently ingested a meal.[240] Morbidity of gastric perforations is usually due to associated intraabdominal injuries and includes intraabdominal abscess, multisystem organ failure, and thoracic empyema if the diaphragm is also injured.[240]

DUODENAL HEMATOMA AND DUODENAL PERFORATION

Duodenal injuries are more often seen in children and in those who suffer a concentrated force over the epigastrium, such as a handlebar injury or other "spearing-type" mechanism. Sports-related activities appear to be responsible for most cases.[241] Although these mechanisms often produce isolated duodenal hematomas without concomitant injuries, pancreatic trauma may also occur.[239,241] Consider child abuse in children with unexplained duodenal trauma.[242,243] Duodenal hematomas are rarely life threatening, and perforation is infrequent.[241,244] Hemophilia, von Willebrand's disease, and idiopathic thrombocytopenic purpura all predispose to hematoma formation.[241,245]

Patients with duodenal hematomas may have relatively benign ED presentations. They may complain of upper abdominal pain and vomiting, the emesis occasionally being frankly bloody.[241,244,246] In the ensuing 12 to 24 hours, the patient usually develops intractable vomiting. However, it may require several days for symptoms or signs to arise.[239,242,247]

Patients sustaining duodenal perforations following blunt epigastric trauma may have significant delay in diagnosis caused by a relative lack of definitive peritoneal signs.[247] Concomitant IAIs are frequently seen in patients with duodenal perforations and are often responsible for the associated morbidity and mortality.[247,248]

SMALL BOWEL PERFORATIONS AND MESENTERIC AVULSIONS

Although perforations and devascularizations of the intestines are the third most common injuries in the setting of blunt trauma,[30] the majority of small bowel injuries result from penetrating trauma.[249] Small bowel injuries tend to occur much more frequently in adults than in children.[250,251] In the setting of blunt trauma, these injuries result mainly from MVCs; falls, assaults, and bicycling are less common mechanisms.[30,249,252] The use of lap belts correlates with bowel perforations and mesenteric tears.

The physical examination of patients with small intestinal injuries may be deceptively minimal shortly after the injury.[49,251,253] The abdomen may only be slightly tender, and bowel sounds are often present. Patients usually complain of pain, and although vomiting, distention, and decreased bowel sounds suggest the diagnosis, they are often absent on presentation.[254] Ultimately, peritoneal signs will arise in all patients, but may take several hours or days to occur.[49,251-253] Concomitant IAIs are usually present.

Several different patterns of bowel injury result from blunt trauma.[230] First, blunt forces can transect or perforate the bowel wall, usually between the ligament of Treitz and the ileocecal valve.[30] Second, trauma can contuse the seromuscular layer, with a predilection for the colon.[30] Finally, the injury can avulse the mesentery from the bowel or lacerate the mesenteric vessels, resulting in bowel ischemia. An individual patient may experience combinations of devascularizations and perforations.[252]

COLONIC PERFORATIONS AND APPENDICEAL INJURIES

Colonic injuries resulting from blunt force are less common than small bowel injuries. Their scarcity may be secondary to the lack of redundancy of the colon, preventing the formation of closed loops that are prone to perforation by increased intraluminal pressure.[30]

Traumatic appendicitis caused by blunt and penetrating trauma is exceptionally rare.[255-257] Isolated blunt appendiceal injuries present similarly to spontaneous cases of appendicitis.[255,256] A proposed mechanism of isolated appendiceal injury after blunt trauma is that the mesoappendix is avulsed during sudden deceleration, leading to ischemia and necrosis of the distal appendix.[256]

Emergency Department Evaluation

DUODENAL HEMATOMAS

Although plain radiography is rarely helpful for the diagnosis of duodenal hematomas, upper gastrointestinal contrast studies are of great value in delineating the injury (Fig. 19-20). Instillation of oral barium or Gastografin reveals thickened mucosal folds in the proximal duodenum. Distally, the contrast will demonstrate a sharply marginated intramural mass widening the lumen.[246] The valvulae conniventes overlying the intramural mass often take on a "*coiled spring*" appearance, a finding pathognomonic for duodenal hematoma.[246] Abdominal CT may also demonstrate the injury (Fig. 19-21).

HOLLOW VISCUS PERFORATIONS

Plain films are occasionally helpful in suspicious cases, since *pneumoperitoneum* occurs in 25% to 50% of patients with hollow viscus perforation.[250,258,259] Miller and Nelson[260] showed experimentally that as little as 1 cc of air injected within the peritoneal cavity could be visualized under the right hemidiaphragm. A caveat, however, lies with proper patient positioning, since they demonstrated that a minimum of 10 minutes in the left lateral decubitus position, followed

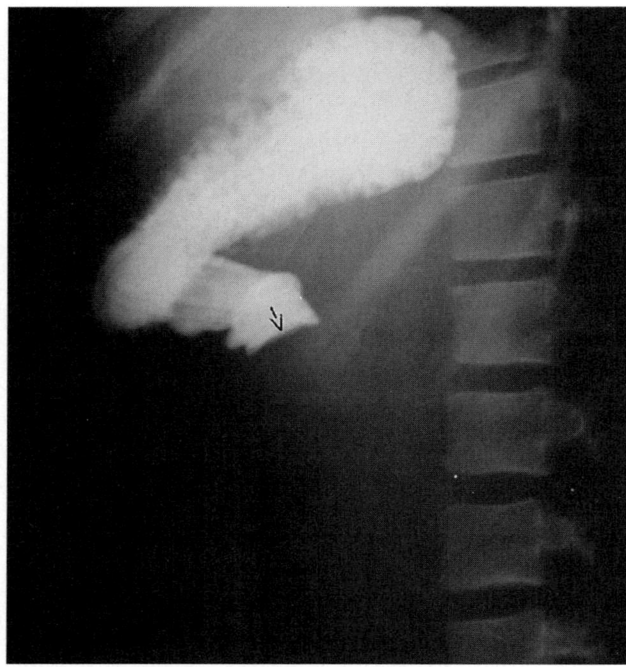

Fig. 19-20 Upper gastrointestinal study showing duodenal hematoma *(arrow)*.

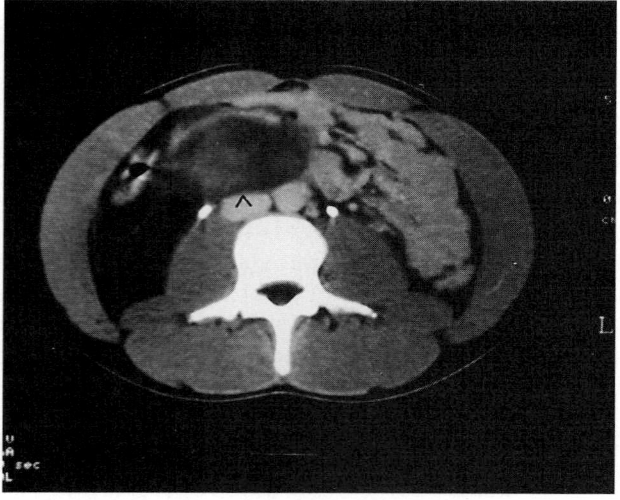

Fig. 19-21 Computed tomography of duodenal hematoma *(arrowhead)*.

by 10 minutes in the erect position, is required to show the free subdiaphragmatic air. However, in the traumatized patient with the potential for an unstable spine these maneuvers may not be readily performed. Perforations may be missed on plain abdominal radiographs as a result of a variety of causes (Box 19-10).[260] Occasionally, pneumoperitoneum may result from thoracic or female genital tract injuries, or following placement of thoracostomy tubes.[258,261-263]

Diagnostic peritoneal lavage is an inexpensive and rapid test for hollow viscus injury. The aspiration of enteric contents confirms the diagnosis. An elevated WBC count in the DPL fluid may be the only indicator of bowel injury.[264] Because the inflammatory response to leaked enteric contents often takes more than 3 hours, a DPL performed soon after injury may miss the diagnosis of bowel disruption.[264]

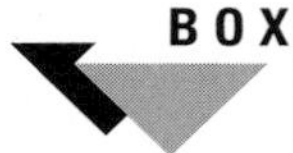

BOX 19-10
Causes of False-Negative Abdominal Radiographs for Intestinal Perforations

1. Adhesions that obliterate the right hemidiaphragm
2. Sealing off of the perforation by intraluminal fluid, food, peritoneum, or omentum
3. Absence of gas at the perforated site
4. Gas trapping within recesses or between bowel loops

CT scans are useful in the evaluation of hollow viscus injury. CT scanning for abdominal trauma must include the pelvis, since leaked enteric contents may manifest as free pelvic fluid. CT may demonstrate the rare duodenal perforation, since DPL may not detect blood cells with injury to this retroperitoneal organ.[239]

CT can reveal free air that has collected in the anterior abdomen in the supine trauma patient. However, as with pneumoperitoneum seen on plain radiographs, thoracic trauma, intraperitoneal bladder rupture, and antecedent DPL may all be responsible for this finding.[48] In addition, radiologists may be fooled by a condition known as **pseudopneumoperitoneum**. In this situation, extraperitoneal air, loculated by musculofascial septa, has an apparent intraperitoneal location.[263]

In the absence of free air or extravasation of oral contrast from the bowel, the diagnosis of hollow viscus or mesenteric injury is suggested by several CT findings (Box 19-11). A streaky density within the mesentery surrounded by a thickened bowel wall suggests hollow viscus rupture.[265] This density may represent bleeding and inflammatory cell infiltration within the mesentery and is not seen in patients without bowel rupture.[265] Nonspecific but helpful findings include free peritoneal fluid, bowel wall or mesenteric thickening, and ileus.[47-49,254,266] CT is valuable in demonstrating an intramural blood collection in cases of duodenal hematomas and can often distinguish perforations of the duodenum from hematomas.[241,267]

Some authorities criticize CT for its lack of sensitivity for intestinal injuries. Accurate interpretation requires a skilled radiologist and proper technique (e.g., lack of patient movement).[249,252] However, as experi-

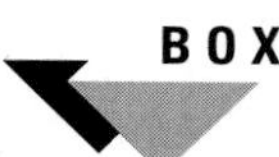

BOX 19-11

Nonspecific CT Findings Suggestive of Hollow Viscus Injury

1. Streaky density within the mesentery surrounded by a thickened bowel wall
2. Free peritoneal fluid
3. Bowel wall or mesenteric thickening
4. Ileus

ence with abdominal CT scanning grows, the sensitivity and specificity of CT for blunt intestinal and mesenteric injuries approaches 90% in some centers.[49,254]

The most important intervention for patients without definitive findings on diagnostic testing is repeated abdominal examination in the early postinjury period.[49] During this time, patients with hollow viscus injuries develop peritonitis. Patients with rigid abdomens, vomiting, and peritoneal signs require either laparoscopy or laparotomy to rule out intestinal injury.

Emergency Department Management

DUODENAL HEMATOMAS

The management of duodenal hematomas has evolved over the years, primarily because of better diagnostic modalities. Nonoperative management, consisting of nasogastric tube decompression, repeated physical examinations, and parenteral hyperalimentation, is currently the preferred treatment.[241,244,245,268] Oral feeding begins once obstruction resolves, usually within 7 to 10 days.[241] When damage to the duodenum is extensive or is accompanied by perforation, or if obstruction lasts longer than 14 days, surgical repair becomes necessary.[241,268] Patients undergoing bypass procedures such as gastroenterostomy for duodenal hematomas are at risk for bowel obstructions.[241]

HOLLOW VISCUS PERFORATIONS

Patients with hollow viscus perforations evident by DPL or CT require immediate laparotomy. Give antibiotics appropriate for bowel flora as soon as the diagnosis is made. Antibiotic coverage should include enteric aerobic bacteria such as *Escherichia coli*, enterococci, and *Klebsiella*, as well as anaerobic organisms such as *Clostridia* and *Bacteroides fragilis*.[269,270] Intravenous ampicillin/sulbactam (3 grams), cefotetan (2 grams), or a combination of ampicillin, clindamycin, and gentamicin is commonly used. The *preoperative* administration of antibiotics significantly decreases the risk of intraabdominal infection compared with patients who receive intraoperative or postoperative antibiotics.[271,272] Duration of antibiotic therapy for longer than 1 day does not appear to confer any advantage in preventing infection.[269,270]

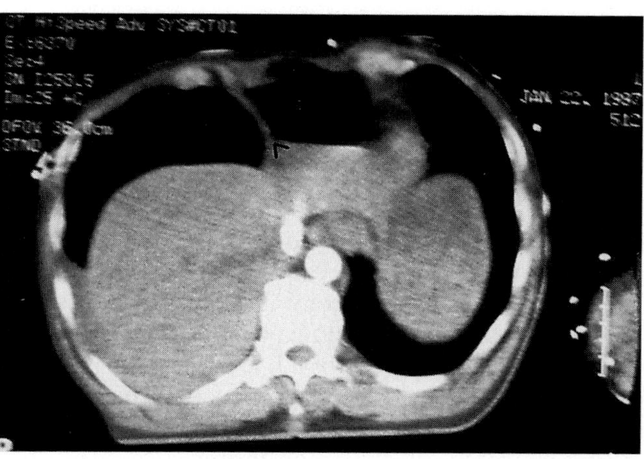

Fig. 19-22 Computed tomography of tension pneumoperitoneum; arrowhead points to falciform ligament.

Complications

The mortality of intestinal injuries is usually low if surgical repair is not delayed for more than 10 to 24 hours. Mortality from blunt intestinal injury ranges from 2% to 30% and is closely related to the severity of associated injuries.[30,249,251] Complications include intraabdominal abscess, wound dehiscence, wound infection, short bowel syndrome, intestinal obstruction, and fasciitis.[30,249,251,252] Abdominal septic complications such as intraabdominal abscess and peritonitis occur in up to as many as 35% of patients with colonic perforations.[273,274]

TENSION PNEUMOPERITONEUM

An unusual complication of bowel perforations is the development of **tension pneumoperitoneum (TP),** defined as the accumulation of air under pressure beneath the diaphragm. In addition to gastrointestinal perforation, TP may also occur with pneumothorax and as a complication of positive pressure ventilation.[275-277] Patients present with abdominal distention, circulatory collapse, and dyspnea.[275] Increased intraabdominal pressure restricts the diaphragm, severely limiting tidal volume, and downward displacement of the liver compromises venous return to the heart.[277] Abdominal CT shows posterior compression of the liver by the accumulated air (Fig. 19-22).[277] Treatment is by urgent decompression of the peritoneal cavity with a chest tube.[275]

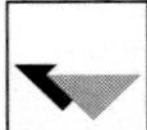

PEARLS & PITFALLS

- The presence of a distracting injury may cause the EP, patient, or both to overlook a serious abdominal injury.
- A spearing injury to the epigastrium is associated with duodenal hematomas, pancreatic trauma, or small bowel injury.
- Patients with combined head and abdominal injuries require objective testing of the abdomen, either CT, DPL, or US.
- Lactate is a more sensitive indicator of shock than blood pressure or even sophisticated invasive monitoring.
- DPL and US are rapid, accurate, and safe. They are the preferred initial studies in hemodynamically unstable patients.
- The only absolute contraindication to DPL is the need for emergency laparotomy.
- Hemodynamic stability is the major limitation for CT in trauma—unstable patients are not appropriate candidates.
- When the suspicion for IAI is high despite a negative US, perform further diagnostic studies.
- In hemodynamically unstable patients with suspected TAI, exclude intraabdominal hemorrhage immediately.

Splenic Injury

- The spleen is the most frequently injured intraabdominal organ.
- Left lower rib fractures are frequently associated with splenic injury.
- Pain in the left shoulder is often seen with splenic injuries (Kehr's sign).
- CT scanning is the most accurate means of preoperative diagnosis.
- The ultimate management relies more on the clinical status of the patient than on diagnostic studies.
- Management has shifted to nonoperative care or towards splenic salvage in blunt injuries.
- Splenectomy is indicated for hemodynamic instability or increased transfusion requirements.
- Delayed rupture may occur with nonoperative management.
- Physical activity is usually limited for at least 3 months after injury.

Hepatic Injury

- The liver is the second most commonly injured intraabdominal organ.
- Injuries to the bare area may not be clinically evident.
- CT scanning is the diagnostic method of choice in stable patients.
- Operative findings correlate poorly with CT estimation.
- The trend is towards nonoperative management in stable patients.
- Complications include bile peritonitis, bilomas, hemobilia, delayed hemorrhage, late biliary duct stenosis, and subhepatic/subphrenic abscesses.
- Full activity may resume when CT shows complete resolution.

Gallbladder Injury

- Blunt injuries to the gallbladder are rare.
- High incidence of concomitant intraabdominal injuries.
- Diagnosis infrequently made before laparotomy.
- Early clinical findings often nonspecific or minimal.
- Management depends on the severity of injury and physiologic condition of the patient.
- The prognosis is excellent if the injury is recognized and there are no other serious injuries.

Pancreatic Injury

- Diagnosis of pancreatic trauma is often difficult. Suspect the diagnosis if patients suffer a concentrated blow to the epigastrium.
- Amylase is not a reliable indicator of pancreatic trauma.
- CT findings of peripancreatic edema, thickening of Gerota's fascia, fluid between the splenic vein and pancreas, and pseudocyst are clues to diagnosis.
- Mortality is primarily due to injury of surrounding viscera and vascular structures.
- Complications include fistulae, abscesses, pseudocyst, and postoperative hemorrhage.

Seat Belt–Associated Injuries

- Seat belt associated injuries include Chance fractures of the lumbar spine, mesenteric or seromuscular avulsions, intestinal perforations, and abdominal wall avulsions or hernia.
- Properly expose patients. Abdominal wall abrasions are markers for serious intraabdominal pathology and should be vigorously investigated.

- Patients with abdominal bruising following an MVC are considered to have a seat belt associated injury until diagnostic studies prove otherwise.
- Serial abdominal examinations, CT, and DPL are all reasonable approaches to the diagnosis of hollow viscus injury associated with a seat belt sign.
- Children are at increased risk of injury as a result of lap belt use, since these restraints were devised for adults.

Hollow Viscus Injuries

- Consider the mechanism of injury. "Spearing-type" injuries to the epigastrium produce duodenal hematomas, small bowel perforations, and mesenteric injuries.
- Perforations of the stomach, duodenum, and colon are much more common with penetrating injuries than with blunt injuries.
- Physical examination and diagnostic study findings may be nonspecific and minimal in the immediate postinjury period in the presence of hollow viscus injuries.
- Concomitant solid organ intraabdominal injuries are often associated with significant morbidity and mortality in the setting of hollow viscus injuries.
- Pneumoperitoneum on plain film radiography or located by CT usually indicates hollow viscus perforation, but in rare instances may arise from extraabdominal injuries.
- The inflammatory response to leaked enteric contents takes at least 3 hours to become evident, and the initial DPL white blood cell count may be normal.
- Repeated abdominal examination in the early postinjury period is the most important diagnostic tool for hollow viscus injuries.
- Broad-spectrum antibiotics should be administered preoperatively to patients with suspected hollow viscus perforations.
- Mortality of intestinal injuries can be minimized if surgical repair is not delayed greater than 10 to 24 hours.

REFERENCES

1. McAnena OJ, Moore EE, Marx JA: Initial evaluation of the patient with blunt abdominal trauma, *Surg Clin North Am* 70: 495-515, 1990.
2. Davis JJ, Cohn I Jr, Nance FC: Diagnosis and management of blunt abdominal trauma, *Ann Surg* 183:672-678, 1976.
3. Bivins BA, Sachatello CR: Diagnostic exploratory celiotomy: an outdated concept in blunt abdominal trauma, *South Med J* 72:969-970, 1979.
4. Colucciello SA: Blunt abdominal trauma, *Emerg Med Clin North Am* 11:107-123, 1993.
5. Olsen WR, Hildreth DH: Abdominal paracentesis and peritoneal lavage in blunt abdominal trauma, *J Trauma* 11:824-829, 1971.
6. Powell DC, Bivins BA, Bell RM: Diagnostic peritoneal lavage, *Surg Gynecol Obstet* 155:257-264, 1982.
7. Kleinert HE, Romero J: Blunt abdominal trauma: review of cases admitted to a general hospital over a 10 year period, *J Trauma* 1:226-240, 1961.
8. Ferrera PC, et al: Injuries distracting from intraabdominal injuries after blunt trauma, *Am J Emerg Med* 16:145-149, 1998.
9. Mackersie RC, et al: Intra-abdominal injury following blunt trauma, *Arch Surg* 124:809-813, 1989.
10. Sorkey AJ, et al: The complimentary roles of diagnostic peritoneal lavage and computed tomography in the evaluation of blunt abdominal trauma, *Surgery* 106:794-801, 1989.
11. Menick F, Kim MC: Blunt abdominal trauma, *NY State J Med* 70:1897-1902, 1970.
12. Prall JA, et al: Early definitive abdominal evaluation in the triage of unconscious normotensive blunt trauma patients, *J Trauma* 37:792-797, 1994.
13. Hill AC, Schecter WP, Trunkey DD: Abdominal trauma and indications for laparotomy. In Mattox KL, Moore EE, Feliciano DV (editors): *Trauma*, Norwalk, CT, 1988, Appleton & Lange.
14. Knottenbelt JD: Low initial hemoglobin levels in trauma patients: an important indicator for ongoing hemorrhage, *J Trauma* 31:1396-1399, 1991.
15. Buechter KJ, et al: The use of serum amylase and lipase in evaluating and managing blunt abdominal trauma, *Am Surg* 56:204-208, 1990.
16. Mure AJ, et al: Serum amylase determination and blunt abdominal trauma, *Am Surg* 57:210-213, 1991.
17. Davis JW, Shackford SR, Holbrook TL: Base deficit as a sensitive indicator of compensated shock and tissue oxygen utilization, *Surg Gynecol Obstet* 173:473-476, 1991.
18. Davis JW, et al: Base deficit as an indicator of significant abdominal injury, *Ann Emerg Med* 20:842-844, 1991.
19. Knudson MM, et al: Hematuria as a predictor of abdominal injury after blunt trauma, *Am J Surg* 164:482-485, 1992.
20. Hennes HM, et al: Elevated liver transaminase levels in children with blunt abdominal trauma: a predictor of liver injury, *Pediatrics* 86:87-90, 1990.
21. Sahdev P, et al: Evaluation of liver function tests in screening for intra-abdominal injuries, *Ann Emerg Med* 20:838-841, 1991.
22. Perry JF: A five-year survey of 152 acute abdominal injuries, *J Trauma* 5:53, 1965.
23. Root HD, et al: Diagnostic peritoneal lavage, *Surgery* 57:633-637, 1965.
24. Henneman PL, et al: Diagnostic peritoneal lavage: accuracy in predicting necessary laparotomy following blunt and penetrating trauma, *J Trauma* 30:1345-1355, 1990.
25. Fischer RP, et al: Diagnostic peritoneal lavage: fourteen years and 2,586 patients later, *Am J Surg* 136:701-704, 1978.
26. Davis RA, et al: The use of computerized axial tomography versus peritoneal lavage in the evaluation of blunt abdominal trauma: a prospective study, *Surgery* 98:845-848, 1985.
27. Davis JW, et al: Complications in evaluating abdominal trauma: diagnostic peritoneal lavage versus computerized axial tomography, *J Trauma* 30:1506-1509, 1990.
28. Gomez GA, et al: Diagnostic peritoneal lavage in the management of blunt abdominal trauma: a reassessment, *J Trauma* 27:1-5, 1987.

29. Engrav LH, et al: Diagnostic peritoneal lavage in blunt abdominal trauma, *J Trauma* 15:854-857, 1976.
30. Dauterive AH, Flancbaum L, Cox EF: Blunt intestinal trauma: a modern-day review, *Ann Surg* 201:198-203, 1985.
31. Freeman T, Fischer RP: The inadequacy of peritoneal lavage in diagnosing acute diaphragmatic rupture, *J Trauma* 16:538-542, 1976.
32. Tibbs PA, et al: Diagnosis of acute abdominal injuries in patients with spinal shock: value of diagnostic peritoneal lavage, *J Trauma* 20:55-57, 1980.
33. Feliciano DV: Diagnostic modalities in abdominal trauma: peritoneal lavage, ultrasonography, computed tomography scanning, and arteriography, *Surg Clin North Am* 71:241-256, 1991.
34. Meyer DM, et al: Evaluation of computed tomography and diagnostic peritoneal lavage in blunt abdominal trauma, *J Trauma* 29:1168-1170, 1989.
35. Bresler MJ: Computed tomography of the abdomen, *Ann Emerg Med* 15:280-285, 1986.
36. Kinnunen J, et al: Emergency CT in blunt abdominal trauma of multiple injury patients, *Acta Radiol* 35:319-322, 1994.
37. Clancy TV, et al: Oral contrast is not necessary in the evaluation of blunt abdominal trauma by computed tomography, *Am J Surg* 166:680-684, 1993.
38. Peitzman AB, et al: Prospective study of computed tomography in initial management of blunt abdominal trauma, *J Trauma* 26:585-591, 1986.
39. Kearney PA Jr, et al: Computed tomography and diagnostic peritoneal lavage in blunt abdominal trauma: Their combined role, *Arch Surg* 124:344-347, 1989.
40. Federle MP, Jeffrey RB Jr: Hemoperitoneum studied by computed tomography, *Radiology* 148:187-192, 1983.
41. Cook DE, et al: Upper abdominal trauma: pitfalls in CT diagnosis, *Radiology* 159:65-69, 1986.
42. Sherck JP, McCort JJ, Oakes DD: Computed tomography in thoracoabdominal trauma, *J Trauma* 24:1015-1021, 1984.
43. Sherck JP, Oakes DD: Computed tomography in the management of thoracic, abdominal and pelvic trauma, *Int Surg* 4:505, 1985.
44. Padhani AR, et al: Computed tomography in blunt abdominal trauma: an analysis of clinical management and radiological findings, *Clin Radiol* 46:304-310, 1992.
45. Meredith JW, et al: Computed tomography and diagnostic peritoneal lavage: complementary roles in blunt trauma, *Am Surg* 58:44-48, 1992.
46. Sherck JP, Oakes DD: Intestinal injuries missed by computed tomography, *J Trauma* 30:1-5, 1990.
47. Rizzo MJ, Federle MP, Griffiths BG: Bowel and mesenteric injury following blunt abdominal trauma: Evaluation with CT, *Radiology* 173:143-148, 1989.
48. Bulas DI, Taylor GA, Eichelberger MR: The value of CT in detecting bowel perforation in children after blunt abdominal trauma, *AJR* 153:561-564, 1989.
49. Sherck J, et al: The accuracy of computed tomography in the diagnosis of blunt small-bowel perforation, *Am J Surg* 168:670-675, 1994.
50. Liu M, Lee CH, P'eng FK: Prospective comparison of diagnostic peritoneal lavage, computed tomographic scanning, and ultrasonography for the diagnosis of blunt abdominal trauma, *J Trauma* 35:267-270, 1993.
51. Goldstein AS, et al: The diagnostic superiority of computerized tomography, *J Trauma* 25:938-944, 1985.
52. Fabian TC, et al: A prospective study of 91 patients undergoing both computed tomography and peritoneal lavage following blunt abdominal trauma, *J Trauma* 26:602-608, 1986.
53. Frame SB, et al: Computed tomography versus diagnostic peritoneal lavage: usefulness in immediate diagnosis of blunt abdominal trauma, *Ann Emerg Med* 18:513-516, 1989.
54. Marx JA, et al: Limitations of computed tomography in the evaluation of acute abdominal trauma: a prospective comparison with diagnostic peritoneal lavage, *J Trauma* 25:933-937, 1985.
55. Pagliarello G, et al: Abdominopelvic computerized tomography and open peritoneal lavage in patients with blunt abdominal trauma: a prospective study, *Can J Surg* 30:10-13, 1987.
56. Catre MG: Diagnostic peritoneal lavage versus abdominal computed tomography in blunt abdominal trauma: a review of prospective studies, *Can J Surg* 38:117-122, 1995.
57. Hoffmann R, et al: Blunt abdominal trauma in cases of multiple trauma evaluated by ultrasonography: a prospective analysis of 291 patients, *J Trauma* 32:452-458, 1992.
58. Lucciarini P, et al: Ultrasonography in the initial evaluation and follow-up of blunt abdominal injury, *Surgery* 114:506-512, 1993.
59. Gruessner R, et al: Sonography versus peritoneal lavage in blunt abdominal trauma, *J Trauma* 29:242-244, 1989.
60. Kimura A, Otsuka T: Emergency center ultrasonography in the evaluation of hemoperitoneum: a prospective study, *J Trauma* 31:20-23, 1991.
61. Rothlin MA, et al: Ultrasound in blunt abdominal and thoracic trauma, *J Trauma* 34:488-495, 1993.
62. Bode PJ, et al: Abdominal ultrasound as a reliable indicator for conclusive laparotomy in blunt abdominal trauma, *J Trauma* 34:27-31, 1993.
63. Rozycki GS, et al: Prospective evaluation of surgeons' use of ultrasound in the evaluation of trauma patients, *J Trauma* 34:516-526, 1993.
64. Glaser K, et al: Ultrasonography in the management of blunt abdominal and thoracic trauma, *Arch Surg* 129:743-747, 1994.
65. Goletti O, et al: The role of ultrasonography in blunt abdominal trauma: results in 250 consecutive cases, *J Trauma* 36:178-181, 1994.
66. Forster R, et al. Ultrasonography in blunt abdominal trauma: influence of the investigators' experience, *J Trauma* 34:264-269, 1992.
67. McKenney M, et al: Can ultrasound replace diagnostic peritoneal lavage in the assessment of blunt abdominal trauma? *J Trauma* 37:439-441, 1994.
68. Boulanger BR, et al: A prospective study of emergent abdominal sonography after blunt trauma, *J Trauma* 39:325-330, 1995.
69. Ma OJ, et al: Prospective analysis of a rapid trauma ultrasound examination performed by emergency physicians, *J Trauma* 38:879-885, 1995.
70. Boulanger BR, et al: Emergent abdominal sonography as a screening test in a new diagnostic algorithm for blunt trauma, *J Trauma* 40:867-874, 1996.
71. Healey MA, et al: A prospective evaluation of abdominal ultrasound in blunt trauma: is it useful? *J Trauma* 40:875-883, 1996.
72. Akgur FM, et al: Prospective study investigating routine usage of ultrasonography as the initial diagnostic modality for the evaluation of children sustaining blunt abdominal trauma, *J Trauma* 42:626-628, 1997.
73. Jehle D, Guarino J, Karamanoukian H: Emergency department ultrasound in the evaluation of blunt abdominal trauma, *Am J Emerg Med* 11:342-346, 1993.
74. Sarkisian AE, et al: Sonographic screening of mass casualties for abdominal and renal injuries following the 1988 Armenian earthquake, *J Trauma* 31:247-250, 1991.

75. Pearl WS, Todd KH: Ultrasonography for the initial evaluation of blunt abdominal trauma: a review of prospective trials, *Ann Emerg Med* 27:353-361, 1996.
76. Tso P, et al: Sonography in blunt abdominal trauma: a preliminary progress report, *J Trauma* 33:39-43, 1992.
77. Drost TF, et al: Diagnostic peritoneal lavage: limited indications due to evolving concepts in trauma care, *Am Surg* 57:126-128, 1991.
78. Baron BJ, et al: Nonoperative management of blunt abdominal trauma: the role of sequential diagnostic peritoneal lavage, computed tomography, and angiography, *Ann Emerg Med* 22: 1556-1562, 1993.
79. Brandt CP, Priebe PP, Jacobs DG: Potential of laparoscopy to reduce non-therapeutic trauma laparotomies, *Am Surg* 60:416-420, 1994.
80. Townsend MC, et al: Diagnostic laparoscopy as an adjunct to selective conservative management of solid organ injuries after blunt abdominal trauma, *J Trauma* 35:647-651, 1993.
81. Salvino CK, et al: The role of diagnostic laparoscopy in the management of trauma patients: a preliminary assessment, *J Trauma* 34:506-513, 1993.
82. Larson GM: Laparoscopy for abdominal emergencies, *Scand J Gastroenterol* 208:62-66, 1995.
83. Lee RB, Stahlman GC, Sharp KW: Treatment priorities in patients with traumatic rupture of the thoracic aorta, *Am Surg* 58:37-43, 1992.
84. Richardson JD, Wilson ME, Miller FB: The widened mediastinum: diagnostic and therapeutic priorities, *Ann Surg* 211:731-736, 1990.
85. Hunt JP, et al: Thoracic aorta injuries: management and outcome of 144 patients, *J Trauma* 40:547-555, 1996.
86. Turney SZ, et al: Traumatic rupture of the aorta: a five-year experience, *J Thorac Cardiovasc Surg* 72:727-732, 1976.
87. Gavant ML, et al: Blunt traumatic aortic rupture: detection with helical CT of the chest, *Radiology* 197:125-133, 1995.
88. Fabian TC, et al: Prospective study of blunt aortic injury: helical CT is diagnostic and antihypertensive therapy reduces rupture, *Ann Surg* 227:666-676, 1998.
89. Chirillo F, et al: Usefulness of transthoracic and transesophageal echocardiography in recognition and management of cardiovascular injuries after blunt chest trauma, *Heart* 75:301-306, 1996.
90. Vignon P, et al: Role of transesophageal echocardiography in the diagnosis and management of traumatic aortic disruption, *Circulation* 92:2959-2968, 1995.
91. Kirsh MM, et al: The treatment of acute traumatic rupture of the aorta: a 10-year experience, *Ann Surg* 184:308-316, 1976.
92. Borman KR, Aurbakken CM, Weigelt JA: Treatment priorities in combined blunt abdominal and aortic trauma, *Am J Surg* 144:728-731, 1982.
93. Hanschen S, Snow NJ, Richardson JD: Thoracic aortic rupture in patients with multisystem injuries, *South Med J* 75:653-656, 1982.
94. Wisner DH, Victor NS, Holcroft JW: Priorities in the management of multiple trauma: intracranial versus intra-abdominal injury, *J Trauma* 35:271-276, 1993.
95. Thomason M, et al: Head CT scanning versus urgent exploration in the hypotensive blunt trauma patient, *J Trauma* 34:40-44, 1993.
96. Gutman MB, et al: Relative incidence of intracranial mass lesions and severe torso injury after accidental injury: implications for triage and management, *J Trauma* 31:974-977, 1991.
97. Buntain WL, Gould HR, Maull KI: Predictability of splenic salvage by computed tomography, *J Trauma* 28:24-31, 1988.
98. Lucas CE: Splenic trauma: Choice of management, *Ann Surg* 213:98-112, 1991.
99. Zarrabi MH, Rosner F: Serious infections in adults following splenectomy for trauma, *Arch Intern Med* 144:1421-1424, 1984.
100. Schurr MJ, et al: Management of blunt splenic trauma: computed tomographic contrast blush predicts failure of nonoperative management, *J Trauma* 39:507-512, 1995.
101. Siniluoto TMJ, et al: Ultrasonography in traumatic splenic rupture, *Clin Radiol* 46:391-396, 1992.
102. Moore EE, et al: Organ injury scaling: spleen, liver, and kidney, *J Trauma* 29:1664-1666, 1989.
103. Mirvis SE, Whitley NO, Gens DR: Blunt splenic trauma in adults: CT-based classification and correlation with prognosis and treatment, *Radiology* 171:33-39, 1989.
104. Resciniti A, et al: Nonoperative treatment of adult splenic trauma: development of a computed tomographic scoring system that detects appropriate candidates for expectant management, *J Trauma* 28:828-831, 1988.
105. Longo WE, et al: Nonoperative management of adult blunt splenic trauma: criteria for successful outcome, *Ann Surg* 210: 626-629, 1989.
106. Elmore JR, et al: Selective nonoperative management of blunt splenic trauma in adults, *Arch Surg* 124:581-586, 1989.
107. Cogbill TH, et al: Nonoperative management of blunt splenic trauma: a multicenter experience, *J Trauma* 29:1312-1317, 1989.
108. Delius RE, Frankel W, Coran AG: A comparison between operative and nonoperative management of blunt injuries to the liver and spleen in adult and pediatric patients, *Surgery* 106: 788-793, 1989.
109. Haller JA Jr, et al: Nonoperative management of solid organ injuries in children: is it safe? *Ann Surg* 219:625-628, 1994.
110. Jalovec LM, Boe BS, Wyffels PL: The advantages of early operation with splenorrhaphy versus nonoperative management for the blunt splenic trauma patient, *Am Surg* 59:698-705, 1993.
111. Pranikoff T, et al: Resolution of splenic injury after nonoperative management, *J Pediatr Surg* 29:1366-1369, 1994.
112. Smith JS Jr, Wengrovitz MA, DeLong BS: Prospective validation of criteria, including age, for safe, nonsurgical management of the ruptured spleen, *J Trauma* 33:363-369, 1992.
113. Upadhyaya P, Simpson JS: Splenic trauma in children, Surg Gynecol Obstet 126:781-790, 1968.
114. Coburn MC, Pfeifer J, DeLuca FG: Nonoperative management of splenic and hepatic trauma in the multiply injured pediatric and adolescent patient, Arch Surg 130:332-338, 1995.
115. Hagiwara A, et al: Nonsurgical management of patients with blunt splenic injury: efficacy of transcatheter arterial embolization, *AJR* 167:159-166, 1996.
116. Sclafani SJ, et al: Nonoperative salvage of computed tomography-diagnosed splenic injuries: utilization of angiography for triage and embolization for hemostasis, *J Trauma* 39: 818-825, 1995.
117. Lynch JM, et al: Is early discharge following isolated splenic injury in the hemodynamically stable child possible? *J Pediatr Surg* 28:1403-1407, 1993.
118. Farhat GA, Abdu RA, Vanek VW: Delayed splenic rupture: Real or imaginary? *Am Surg* 58:340-345, 1992.
119. Kluger Y, et al: Delayed rupture of the spleen: myths, facts, and their importance: case reports and literature review, *J Trauma* 36:568-571, 1994.
120. Pappas D, Mirvis SE, Crepps JT: Splenic trauma: false-negative CT diagnosis in cases of delayed rupture, *AJR* 149:727-728, 1987.
121. Hiraide A, et al: Delayed rupture of the spleen caused by an intrasplenic pseudoaneurysm following blunt trauma: case report, *J Trauma* 36:743-744, 1994.
122. Normand JP, et al: Thoracic splenosis after blunt trauma: frequency and imaging findings, *AJR* 161:739-741, 1993.

123. Pearson HA, et al: The born-again spleen: return of splenic function after splenectomy for trauma, *N Engl J Med* 298:1389-1392, 1978.
124. Benya EC, et al: Splenic injury from blunt abdominal trauma in children: follow-up evaluation with CT, *Radiology* 195:685-688, 1995.
125. Do HM, Cronan JJ: CT appearance of splenic injuries managed nonoperatively, *AJR* 157:757-760, 1991.
126. Federle MP: Splenic trauma: is follow-up CT of value? *Radiology* 194:23-24, 1995.
127. Lawson DE, et al: Splenic trauma: Value of follow-up CT, *Radiology* 194:97-100, 1995.
128. Scatamacchia SA, et al: Splenic trauma in adults: impact of CT grading on management, *Radiology* 171:725-729, 1989.
129. Sutyak JP, et al: Computed tomography is inaccurate in estimating the severity of adult splenic injury, *J Trauma* 39:514-518, 1995.
130. Becker CD, et al: Blunt splenic trauma in adults: can CT findings be used to determine the need for surgery? *AJR* 162:343-347, 1994.
131. Pachter HL, et al: Experience with selective operative and nonoperative treatment of splenic injuries in 193 patients, *Ann Surg* 211:583-589, 1990.
132. Giacomantonio M, Filler RM, Rich RH: Blunt hepatic trauma in children: experience with operative and nonoperative management, *J Pediatr Surg* 19:519-522, 1984.
133. Patten RM, et al: Traumatic laceration of the liver limited to the bare area: CT findings in 25 patients, *AJR* 160:1019-1022, 1993.
134. Richie JP, Fonkalsrud EW: Subcapsular hematoma of the liver: nonoperative management, *Arch Surg* 104:781-784, 1972.
135. Vock P, Tschaeppeler H: Blunt liver trauma in children: the role of computed tomography in diagnosis and treatment, *J Pediatr Surg* 21:413-418, 1986.
136. Raptopoulos V: Abdominal trauma: emphasis on computed tomography, *Radiol Clin North Am* 32:969-987, 1994.
137. Moon KL Jr, Federle MP: Computed tomography in hepatic trauma, *AJR* 141:309-314, 1983.
138. Roberts JL, et al: CT in abdominal and pelvic trauma, *Radiographics* 13:735-752, 1993.
139. Mirvis SE, et al: Blunt hepatic trauma in adults: CT-based classification and correlation with prognosis and treatment, *Radiology* 171:27-32, 1989.
140. Croce MA, et al: AAST organ injury scale: correlation of CT-graded liver injuries and operative findings, *J Trauma* 31:806-812, 1991.
141. Durham RM, et al: Management of blunt hepatic injuries, *Am J Surg* 164:477-481, 1992.
142. Boone DC, et al: Evolution of management of major hepatic trauma: Identification of patterns of injury, *J Trauma* 39:344-350, 1995.
143. Defore WW Jr, et al: Management of 1,590 consecutive cases of liver trauma, *Arch Surg* 111:493-497, 1976.
144. Carmona RH, Lim RC Jr, Clark GC: Morbidity and mortality in hepatic trauma: a 5 year study, *Am J Surg* 144:88-93, 1982.
145. Cogbill TH, et al: Severe hepatic trauma: a multi-center experience with 1,335 liver injuries, *J Trauma* 28:1433-1438, 1988.
146. Fabian TC, et al: Factors affecting morbidity following hepatic trauma: a prospective analysis of 482 injuries, *Ann Surg* 213: 540-548, 1991.
147. Davis JJ, Cohn I Jr, Nance FC: Diagnosis and management of blunt abdominal trauma, *Ann Surg* 183:672-678, 1976.
148. Hiatt JR, et al: Nonoperative management of major blunt liver injury with hemoperitoneum, *Arch Surg* 125:101-103, 1990.
149. Hollands MJ, Little JM: Non-operative management of blunt liver injuries, *Br J Surg* 78: 968-972, 1991.
150. Meredith JW, et al: Nonoperative management of blunt hepatic trauma: the exception or the rule? *J Trauma* 36:529-534, 1994.
151. Coburn MC, Pfeifer J, DeLuca FG. Nonoperative management of splenic and hepatic trauma in the multiply injured pediatric and adolescent patient, *Arch Surg* 130:332-338, 1995.
152. Federico JA, et al: Blunt hepatic trauma: nonoperative management in adults, *Arch Surg* 125:905-909, 1990.
153. Foley WD, et al: Treatment of blunt hepatic injuries: role of CT, *Radiology* 164:635-638, 1987.
154. Pachter HL, Hofstetter SR: The current status of nonoperative management of adult blunt hepatic injuries, *Am J Surg* 169:442-454, 1995.
155. Sherman HF, et al: Nonoperative management of blunt hepatic injuries: safe at any grade? *J Trauma* 37:616-621, 1994.
156. Hagiwara A, et al: Nonsurgical management of patients with blunt hepatic injury: efficacy of transcatheter arterial embolization, *AJR* 169:1151-1156, 1997.
157. Bynoe RP, et al: Complications of nonoperative management of blunt hepatic injuries, *J Trauma* 32:308-314, 1992.
158. Gates JD: Delayed hemorrhage with free rupture complicating the nonsurgical management of blunt hepatic trauma: a case report and review of the literature, *J Trauma* 36:572-575, 1994.
159. Halme L, et al: Late biliary stenosis after conservative management of traumatic liver rupture: case report, *J Trauma* 36:740-742, 1994.
160. Karp MP, et al: The nonoperative management of pediatric hepatic trauma, *J Pediatr Surg* 18:512-518, 1983.
161. Breen PC: Rupture of the gallbladder after blunt abdominal trauma, *South Med J* 68:658-660, 1975.
162. Sharma O: Blunt gallbladder injuries: presentation of twenty-two cases with review of the literature, *J Trauma* 39:576-580, 1995.
163. Greenwald G, Stine RJ, Larson RE: Perforation of the gall bladder following blunt abdominal trauma, *Ann Emerg Med* 16:452-454, 1987.
164. McNabney WK, Rudek R, Pemberton LB: The significance of gallbladder trauma, *J Emerg Med* 8:277-280, 1990.
165. Penn I: Injuries to the gall-bladder, *Br J Surg* 49:636-641, 1962.
166. Soderstrom CA, et al: Gallbladder injuries resulting from blunt abdominal trauma: an experience and review, *Ann Surg* 193:60-66, 1981.
167. Laffey DA, Hay DJ: Isolated perforation of the gall bladder following blunt abdominal trauma, *Postgrad Med J* 55:212-214, 1979
168. Delgado RR, Mullen JT, Ehrlich FE: Transection of the gallbladder as a sequela to blunt abdominal trauma, *VA Med* 104:233-236, 1977.
169. Jeffrey RB Jr, et al: Computed tomography of blunt trauma to the gallbladder, *J Comput Assist Tomogr* 10:756-758, 1986.
170. Spigos DG, et al: Diagnosis of traumatic rupture of the gallbladder, *Am J Surg* 141:731-735, 1981.
171. Weiner I, Watson LC, Wolma FJ: Perforation of the gallbladder due to blunt abdominal trauma, *Arch Surg* 117:805-807, 1982.
172. Davis WC, German JD: Traumatic rupture of the gallbladder without a penetrating wound of the abdominal wall, *Am J Surg* 99:103-105, 1960.
173. Gottesman L, et al:Diagnosis of isolated perforation of the gallbladder following blunt trauma using sonography and CT scan, *J Trauma* 24:280-281, 1984.
174. Kambayashi M, et al: Hemobilia due to gallbladder contusion following blunt trauma—sonography and CT scanning for early detection: case report, *J Trauma* 34:440-442, 1993.
175. Kauzlaric D, Barmeir E: Sonography of intraluminal gallbladder hematoma, *J Clin Ultrasound* 13:291-294, 1985.

176. Horst HM, Bivins BA: Pancreatic transection: a concept of evolving injury, *Arch Surg* 124:1093-1095, 1989.
177. Stone HH, et al: Experiences in the management of pancreatic trauma, *J Trauma* 21:257-261, 1981.
178. Jurkovich GJ, Carrico CJ: Pancreatic trauma, *Surg Clin North Am* 70:575-593, 1990.
179. Olsen WR: The serum amylase in blunt abdominal trauma, *J Trauma* 13:200-204, 1973.
180. Moretz JA III, et al: Significance of serum amylase level in evaluating pancreatic trauma, *Am J Surg* 130:739-741, 1975.
181. White PH, Benfield JR: Amylase in the management of pancreatic trauma, *Arch Surg* 105:158-162, 1972.
182. Bouwman DL. Altshuler J, Weaver DW: Hyperamylasemia: a result of intracranial bleeding, *Surgery* 94:318-322, 1983.
183. Bouwman DL, Weaver DW, Walt AJ: Serum amylase and its isoenzymes: a clarification of their implications in trauma, *J Trauma* 24:573-577, 1984.
184. Takishima T, et al: Serum amylase level on admission in the diagnosis of blunt injury to the pancreas: Its significance and limitations, *Ann Surg* 226:70-76, 1997.
185. Sivit CJ, et al: Blunt pancreatic trauma in children: CT diagnosis, *AJR* 158:1097-1100, 1992.
186. Dodds WJ, et al: Traumatic fracture of the pancreas: CT characteristics, *J Comput Assist Tomogr* 14:375-378, 1990.
187. Lane MJ, et al: CT diagnosis of blunt pancreatic trauma: Importance of detecting fluid between the pancreas and the splenic vein, *AJR* 163:833-835, 1994.
188. Gothi R, Bose NC, Kumar N: Case report: ultrasound demonstration of traumatic fracture of the pancreas with pancreatic duct disruption, *Clin Radiol* 47:434-435, 1993.
189. Mansour MA, et al: Conservative management of combined pancreaticoduodenal injuries, *Am J Surg* 158:531-535, 1989.
190. Wynn M, et al: Management of pancreatic and duodenal trauma, *Am J Surg* 150:327-332, 1985.
191. Wilson RH, Moorehead RJ: Current management of trauma to the pancreas, *Br J Surg* 78:1196-1202, 1991.
192. Keller MS, Stafford PW, Vane DW: Conservative management of pancreatic trauma in children, *J Trauma* 42:1097-1100, 1997.
193. Arkovitz MS, Johnson N, Garcia VF: Pancreatic trauma in children: mechanisms of injury, *J Trauma* 42:49-53, 1997.
194. Carr ND, et al: Late complications of pancreatic trauma, *Br J Surg* 76:1244-1246, 1989.
195. Lewis G, et al: Traumatic pancreatic pseudocysts, *Br J Surg* 80:89-93, 1993.
196. Grace PA, Williamson RC: Modern management of pancreatic pseudocysts, *Br J Surg* 80:573-581, 1993.
197. Vitas GJ, Sarr MG: Selected management of pancreatic pseudocysts: operative versus expectant management, *Surgery* 111:123-130, 1992.
198. Newman KD, et al: The lap belt complex: intestinal and lumbar spine injury in children, *J Trauma* 30:1133-1138, 1990.
199. Chandler CF, Lane JS, Waxman KS: Seatbelt sign following blunt trauma is associated with increased incidence of abdominal injury, *Am Surg* 63:885-888, 1997.
200. Velmahos GC, Tatevossian R, Demetriades D: The "seat belt mark" sign: a call for increased vigilance among physicians treating victims of motor vehicle accidents, *Am Surg* 65:181-185, 1999.
201. Sivit CJ, et al: Safety-belt injuries in children with lap-belt ecchymosis: CT findings in 61 patients, *AJR* 157:111-114, 1991.
202. Reid AB, Letts RM, Black GB: Pediatric Chance fractures: association with intra-abdominal injuries and seatbelt use, *J Trauma* 30:384-391, 1990.
203. Anderson PA, et al: The epidemiology of seatbelt-associated injuries, *J Trauma* 31:60-67, 1991.
204. Tso EL, Beaver BL, Haller JA Jr: Abdominal injuries in restrained pediatric passengers, *J Pediatr Surg* 28:915-919, 1993.
205. Chance GQ: Note on a type of flexion fracture of the spine, *Br J Radiol* 21:452-453, 1948.
206. Smith WS, Kaufer H: Patterns and mechanisms of lumbar injuries associated with lap seat belts, *J Bone Joint Surg* 51-A:239-254, 1969.
207. Williams JS, Kirkpatrick JR: The nature of seat belt injuries, *J Trauma* 11:207-218, 1971.
208. Gumley G, Taylor TK, Ryan MD: Distraction fractures of the lumbar spine, *J Bone Joint Surg* 64-B:520-525, 1982.
209. Rogers LF: The roentgenographic appearance of transverse or Chance fractures of the spine: the seat belt fracture, *AJR* 111: 844-849, 1971.
210. Gertzbein SD, Court-Brown CM: Flexion-distraction injuries of the lumbar spine: mechanisms of injury and classification, *Clin Orthop Rel Res* 227:52-60, 1988.
211. Rumball K, Jarvis J: Seat-belt injuries of the spine in young children, *J Bone Joint Surg* 74-B:571-574, 1992.
212. Appleby JP, Nagy AG: Abdominal injuries associated with the use of seatbelts, *Am J Surg* 157:457-458, 1989.
213. Sube J, Ziperman HH, McIver WJ: Seat belt trauma to the abdomen, *Am J Surg* 113:346-350, 1967.
214. Rutledge R, et al: The spectrum of abdominal injuries associated with the use of seat belts, *J Trauma* 31:820-826, 1991.
215. Grace DM, Fenton JA, Duncanson ME: Devastating lap-belt injury: a plea for effective rear-seat restraints, *Can Med Assoc J* 151:331-333, 1994.
216. Doersch KB, Dozier WE: The seat belt syndrome: the seat belt sign, intestinal and mesenteric injuries, *Am J Surg* 116:831-833, 1968.
217. Asbun HJ, et al: Intra-abdominal seatbelt injury, *J Trauma* 1990; 30:189-193
218. Shalaby-Rana E, et al: Intestinal stricture due to lap-belt injury, *AJR* 158:63-64, 1992.
219. Campbell RS, Zammit-Maempel I: Case report: mesenteric arterial rupture following blunt abdominal trauma: demonstration by computed tomography, *Br J Radiol* 67:205-206, 1994.
220. Bensard DD, et al: Small bowel injury in children after blunt abdominal trauma: is diagnostic delay important? *J Trauma* 41:476-483, 1996.
221. Payne DD, et al: Seat belt abdominal wall muscular avulsion, *J Trauma* 13:262-267, 1973.
222. Damschen DD, et al: Acute traumatic abdominal hernia: case reports, *J Trauma* 36:273-276, 1994.
223. Esposito TJ, Fedorak I: Traumatic lumbar hernia: case report and literature review, *J Trauma* 37:123-126, 1994.
224. Malangoni MA, Condon RE: Traumatic abdominal wall hernia, *J Trauma* 23:356-357, 1983.
225. Dubois PM, Freeman JB: Traumatic abdominal wall hernia, *J Trauma 21*:72-74, 1981.
226. Colucciello SA, Plotka M: Abdominal trauma, *Phys Sportsmed* 21:33-40, 1993.
227. Brenneman FD, Boulanger BR, Antonyshyn O: Surgical management of abdominal wall disruption after blunt trauma, *J Trauma* 39:539-544, 1995.
228. Hurwitt ES, Silver CE: Seat-belt hernia: a ventral hernia following an automobile crash, *JAMA* 194:829-831, 1965.
229. Matolo NM, Danto LA, Wolfman EF Jr: Traumatic aneurysm of the abdominal aorta. Report of two cases and review of the literature, *Arch Surg* 108:867-869, 1974.
230. Thal ER, Perry MO, Crighton J: Traumatic abdominal aortic occlusion, *South Med J* 64:653-656, 1971.
231. Dajee H, Richardson IW, Iype MO: Seat belt aorta: acute dissection and thrombosis of the abdominal aorta, *Surgery* 85:263-267, 1979.

232. Borja AR, Lansing AM: Thrombosis of the abdominal aorta caused by blunt trauma, *J Trauma* 10:499-501, 1970.
233. Hewitt RL, Grablowsky OM: Acute traumatic dissecting aneurysm of the abdominal aorta, *Ann Surg* 171:160-162, 1970.
234. Nitecki S, et al: Seatbelt injury to the common iliac artery: Report of two cases and review of the literature, *J Trauma* 33: 935-938, 1992.
235. Tomatis LA, Doornbos FA, Beard JA: Circumferential intimal tear of aorta with complete occlusion due to blunt trauma, *J Trauma* 8:1096-1101, 1968.
236. Bussey HJ, McGehee RN, Tyson KR: Isolated gastric rupture due to blunt trauma, *J Trauma* 15:190-191, 1975.
237. Yajko RD, Seydel F, Trimble C: Rupture of the stomach from blunt abdominal trauma, *J Trauma* 15:177-183, 1975.
238. Brunsting LA, Morton JH: Gastric rupture from blunt abdominal trauma, *J Trauma* 27:887-890, 1987.
239. Grosfeld JL, et al: Gastrointestinal injuries in childhood: analysis of 53 patients, *J Pediatr Surg* 24:580-583, 1989.
240. Durham RM, Olson S, Weigelt JA: Penetrating injuries to the stomach, *Surg Gynecol Obstet* 172:298-302, 1991.
241. Jewett TC Jr, et al: Intramural hematoma of the duodenum, *Arch Surg* 123:54-58, 1988.
242. Kleinman PK, Brill PW, Winchester P: Resolving duodenal-jejunal hematoma in abused children, *Radiology* 160:747-750, 1986.
243. Cooper A, et al: Major blunt abdominal trauma due to child abuse, *J Trauma* 28:1483-1486, 1988.
244. Winthrop AL, Wesson DE, Filler RM: Traumatic duodenal hematoma in the pediatric patient, *J Pediatr* 21:757-760, 1986.
245. Touloukian RJ: Protocol for the nonoperative treatment of obstructing intramural duodenal hematoma during childhood, *Am J Surg* 145:330-334, 1983.
246. Felson B, Levin EJ: Intramural hematoma of the duodenum: a diagnostic roentgen sign, *Radiology* 63:823-829, 1954.
247. Levison MA, et al: Duodenal trauma: experience of a trauma center, *J Trauma* 24:475-480, 1984.
248. Kelly G, et al: The continuing challenge of duodenal injuries, *J Trauma* 18:160-164, 1978.
249. Guarino J, Hassett JM Jr, Luchette FA: Small bowel injuries: mechanisms, patterns, and outcome, *J Trauma* 39:1076-1080, 1995.
250. Chatterjee H, Jagdish S: Intestinal injuries in childhood: analysis of 32 cases, *J Pediatr Surg* 27:583-585, 1992.
251. Brown RA, et al: Gastrointestinal tract perforation in children due to blunt abdominal trauma, *Br J Surg* 79:522-524, 1992.
252. Wisner DH, Chun Y, Blaisdell FW: Blunt intestinal injury: keys to diagnosis and management, *Arch Surg* 125:1319-1323, 1990.
253. Winton TL, et al: Delayed intestinal perforation after nonpenetrating abdominal trauma, *Can J Surg* 28:437-439, 1985.
254. Donohue JH, et al: Computed tomography in the diagnosis of blunt intestinal and mesenteric injuries, *J Trauma* 27:11-17, 1987.
255. Burgess CM: Traumatic appendicitis, *JAMA* 111:699-700, 1938.
256. Geer DA, Armanini G, Guernsey JM: Trauma to the appendix: a report of two cases, *Arch Surg* 110:446-447, 1975.
257. Simstein NL, Mattox KL: Penetrating injuries of the appendix, *Am J Surg* 134:415, 1977.
258. Roh JJ, et al: Value of pneumoperitoneum in the diagnosis of visceral perforation, *Am J Surg* 146:830-833, 1983.
259. Kovacs GZ, et al: Hollow viscus rupture due to blunt trauma, *Surg Gynecol Obstet* 163:552-554, 1986.
260. Miller RE, Nelson SW: The roentgenologic demonstration of tiny amounts of free intraperitoneal gas: experimental and clinical studies, *AJR* 112:574-585, 1971.
261. Gantt CB Jr, Daniel WW, Hallenback GA: Nonsurgical pneumoperitoneum, *Am J Surg* 134:411-414, 1977.
262. Madura MJ, Craig RM, Shields TW: Unusual causes of spontaneous pneumoperitoneum, *Surg Gynecol Obstet* 154:417-420, 1982.
263. Hamilton P, et al: Significance of intra-abdominal extraluminal air detected by CT scan in blunt abdominal trauma, *J Trauma* 39:331-333, 1995.
264. Root HD, Keizer PJ, Perry JF Jr: The clinical and experimental aspects of peritoneal response to injury, *Arch Surg* 95:531-536, 1967.
265. Hagiwara A, et al: Early diagnosis of small intestine rupture from blunt abdominal trauma using computed tomography: significance of the streaky density within the mesentery, *J Trauma* 38:630-633, 1995.
266. Hara H, Babyn PS, Bourgeois D: Significance of bowel wall enhancement on CT following blunt abdominal trauma in childhood, *J Comput Assist Tomogr* 16:94-98, 1992.
267. Kunin JR, et al: Duodenal injuries caused by blunt abdominal trauma: value of CT in differentiating perforation from hematoma, *AJR* 160:1221-1223, 1993.
268. Czyrko C, et al: Blunt abdominal trauma resulting in intestinal obstruction: When to operate? *J Trauma* 30:1567-1571, 1990.
269. Fabian TC, et al: Duration of antibiotic therapy for penetrating abdominal trauma: a prospective trial, *Surgery* 112:788-795, 1992.
270. Dellinger EP: Antibiotic prophylaxis in trauma: penetrating abdominal injuries and open fractures, *Rev Infect Dis* 13(Suppl):S847-857, 1991.
271. Fabian TC: Prevention of infections following penetrating abdominal trauma, *Am J Surg* 165 (suppl 2-A):14S-19S, 1993.
272. Fullen WD, Hunt J, Altemeier WA: Prophylactic antibiotics in penetrating wounds of the abdomen, *J Trauma* 12:282-288, 1972.
273. Stewart RM, et al: Is resection with primary anastomosis following destructive colon wounds always safe? *Am J Surg* 168: 316-319, 1994.
274. Thompson JS, Moore EE, Moore JB: Comparison of penetrating injuries of the right and left colon, *Ann Surg* 193:414-418, 1981.
275. Higgins JR, Halpin DM, Midgley AK: Tension pneumoperitoneum: a surgical emergency, *Br J Hosp Med* 39:160-161, 1988.
276. Ogle JW, Klofas E: Tension pneumoperitoneum after blunt trauma, *J Trauma* 41:909-911, 1996.
277. Winer-Muram HT, Rumbak MJ, Bain RS Jr: Tension pneumoperitoneum as a complication of barotrauma, *Crit Care Med* 21:941-943, 1993.

20 Penetrating Abdominal Trauma

PETER C. FERRERA

Teaching Case

A 30-year-old man was grinding metal, when an 8-inch copper spike impaled his left chest. The entry site was just medial to the nipple at the fifth intercostal space. He had the good sense not to pull out the spike. He was quickly taken to the operating suite, where he was found to have perforations of his stomach, spleen, left hemidiaphragm, and left ventricle. After surgery he made an uneventful recovery. ■

EPIDEMIOLOGY

The incidence of violent crimes continues to rise,[1] and young males account for the overwhelming majority of victims.[2,3] Gunshot wounds most often injure the small and large bowel, followed by the liver and abdominal vasculature, whereas stab wounds are most likely to penetrate the liver and small bowel.[1,2] Gunshot wounds routinely violate the peritoneum, whereas many stab wounds to the abdomen never reach the viscera.[4]

The unwary emergency physician (EP) may overlook the abdominal implications of penetrating chest trauma. During exhalation, the diaphragm rises to the fourth intercostal space anteriorly and the scapular tip posteriorly. Patients with stab wounds below the level of the nipples or tip of the scapula are at risk of intraabdominal injury (IAI). Gunshot wounds can traverse several body regions before stopping in the abdomen.

When vascular structures are uninjured, survival is likely following stab wounds and even most gunshot wounds.[2] However, patients who are profoundly hypotensive (systolic blood pressure <60 mmHg) or require emergency thoracotomy usually do poorly and die as a result of either massive hemorrhage or transfusion-related coagulopathies.[2]

PREHOSPITAL MANAGEMENT

The unstable victim of penetrating abdominal trauma needs surgery, and time to operation can determine outcome. Unfortunately, there is often significant delay in treating the patient, since law enforcement agents must first "secure the scene." The "scoop-and-run" dogma should rule for victims of penetrating trauma; paramedics must manage the airway and attempt other procedures only while en route to the emergency department (ED).[1,3]

Most studies demonstrate no benefit to the pneumatic antishock garment (PASG) or military antishock trousers (MAST) in penetrating torso trauma.[3,5-8] In fact, the application of MAST to patients with penetrating torso injuries may decrease survival.[7] Possible reasons for the poor outcomes include increased scene time, augmented afterload, and accelerated hemorrhage from increased blood pressure and subsequent clot disruption.[7]

EMERGENCY DEPARTMENT EVALUATION AND MANAGEMENT

Paramedics should alert the ED with details of the patient's condition well before hospital arrival, allowing for activation of the trauma team and preparation of the operating suite. When patients arrive in the ED resuscitation suite, the priorities include large-bore venous access, cardiac monitoring, and assessment for concomitant pneumothoraces or cardiac injury. Although massive volume resuscitation remains controversial, and may theoretically worsen outcomes in penetrating trauma, most centers continue the practice of giving crystalloid and blood to the hypotensive patient (see Chapter 8). If large-volume resuscitation is employed, a fluid warmer will mitigate hypothermia and associated coagulopathies. If the patient is impaled, leave the offending object in place, since ED removal may result in uncontrolled hemorrhage. *Protruding objects are best removed in the operating suite.*[3,9]

Initial Diagnostic Studies

If the patient's condition permits, obtain an upright chest radiograph to exclude intrathoracic injuries.[3] Free subdiaphragmatic air implies peritoneal penetration, not necessarily visceral perforation. In stab wounds, this isolated finding does not mandate laparotomy.[3] However, subdiaphragmatic air must prompt further investigation for intraperitoneal injury. In the unstable patient, a supine chest film is acceptable. The role of a "one-shot" intravenous pyelogram (IVP) is discussed in the following section.

Laboratory Studies

Perhaps the most important laboratory study in the patient with penetrating abdominal trauma is a crossmatch for blood. However, the moribund patient may require emergency uncrossmatched blood. A bedside test for hemoglobin or hematocrit establishes a baseline. Many patients in hemorrhagic shock may have normal levels on ED presentation, since they have not had time to equilibrate across the intravascular and extravascular spaces. A visual examination of the urine should detect gross hematuria, which suggests renal injury.

Management

Give preoperative intravenous antibiotics to patients with a high likelihood of bowel penetration; generally a cephalosporin or semisynthetic penicillin combined with an antianaerobic agent is sufficient.[1,10] Administer tetanus toxoid as indicated.

Patients who become pulseless while in the ED or shortly before arrival may be candidates for ED thoracotomy and aortic cross clamping.[1] However, the greatest chance of survival for ED thoracotomy occurs in patients with penetrating mediastinal trauma. Survival for pulseless victims of penetrating abdominal trauma is dismal. In rare circumstances, ED thoracotomy may prevent further hemorrhage until definitive control of intraabdominal hemorrhage is obtained.[11]

Patients with hemodynamic instability, signs of peritoneal irritation, bowel evisceration, or gastrointestinal (GI) bleeding need immediate laparotomy.[1,12,13] Patients who have omental evisceration without bowel protrusion and who are otherwise hemodynamically stable do not necessarily require laparotomy.[3,14,15]

STAB WOUNDS

Several diagnostic options can determine the severity of the abdominal wound in hemodynamically stable patients. Stab wounds penetrate the peritoneum in two thirds of cases, and only 50% to 75% of these have significant visceral or vascular injury. For this reason, not every patient with a stab wound to the abdomen requires laparotomy. It has been reported that routine laparotomy is frequently nontherapeutic.[1,3,15,16] In addition, false-negative laparotomies prolong hospital stay and increase overall morbidity.[17,18] Selective management of abdominal stab wounds is possible with the use of local wound exploration (LWE), diagnostic peritoneal lavage (DPL), laparoscopy, and observation using serial examinations (Fig. 20-1).

Local Wound Exploration

Local wound exploration requires adequate local anesthesia, good lighting, and an assistant to retract the wound edges. Do not explore wounds of the lower chest since this maneuver may cause intrathoracic hemorrhage or iatrogenic pneumothorax.[3] The exception to this rule would be slash wounds that are particularly amenable to LWE and are unlikely to cause an iatrogenic injury to the patient. Generally the EP should prepare the wound with a povidone-iodine solution, place a sterile field, and then extend the wound in both directions. The wound should be explored tissue layer by tissue layer, extending the wound in depth and not simply in length. It is necessary to reach the absolute bottom of the implement tract. If the wound is *clearly* superficial to the peritoneum, close the incision after copious irrigation. If the wound is contaminated, pack it and leave it open.[1] It is then safe to discharge the patient if there are no other injuries requiring further evaluation, treatment, or admission.[3,15,16]

In many cases, the ultimate depth of the wound is not clear. These injuries and wounds that penetrate the abdominal fascia may violate the peritoneum and injure viscera. When peritoneal violation is evident or uncertain, DPL or laparoscopy is usually indicated. However, some centers use serial abdominal examinations in place of these studies. Furthermore, some centers use serial abdominal examination in lieu of LWE as well.

Finally, LWE should only be entertained in those patients who present with a stab wound and are coop-

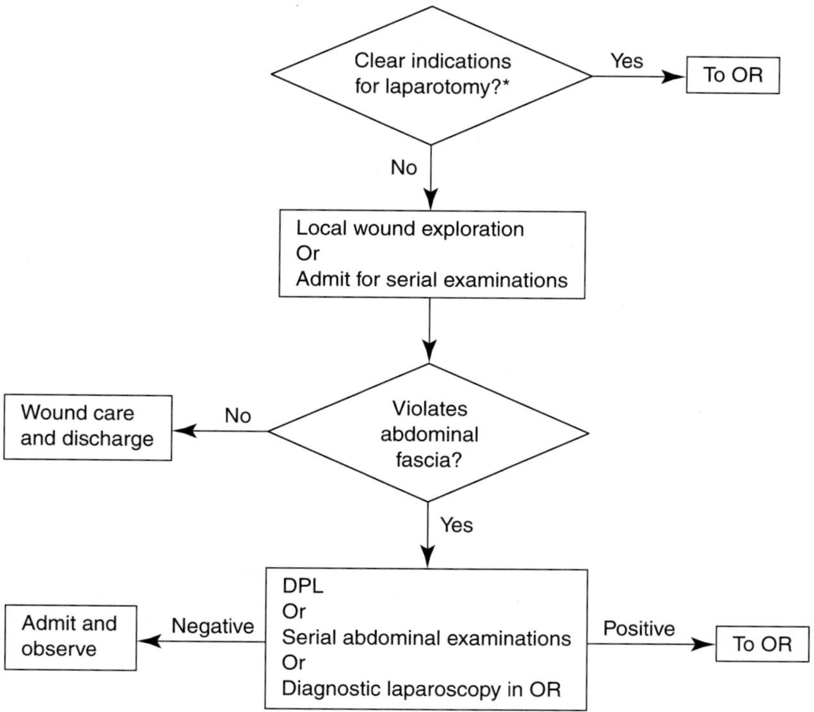

Fig. 20-1 Management of abdominal stab wounds.

erative, hemodynamically stable, and have no other indication for urgent laparotomy.

Diagnostic Peritoneal Lavage

Diagnostic peritoneal lavage is helpful in the management of penetrating low thoracic wounds, as well as patients with abdominal stab wounds.[19-21] It is particularly useful in patients with evidence of peritoneal penetration. Patients with negative DPLs seldom require subsequent laparotomy, and the EP should avoid the long- and short-term morbidities associated with an unnecessary operation.[19] On the other hand, for those patients that the EP cannot determine whether or not there has been peritoneal penetration, the DPL is an extremely sensitive indicator of intraabdominal injury.

One of the major controversies surrounding DPL in penetrating trauma is the definition of a positive test. Although ≥100,000/mm^3 red blood cells (RBCs) is considered positive for blunt abdominal injuries, significant intraperitoneal injury may exist after penetrating injuries despite a lavage RBC count <50,000/mm^3.[3,19] To increase specificity for anterior abdominal stab wounds, a RBC count between 20,000 and 100,000/mm^3 is considered indeterminate and should prompt further investigation or observation.[9] Stab wounds of the lower chest often injure the diaphragm, which tends not to bleed.[3] The RBC count cutoff in patients with either lower chest stab wounds or abdominal gunshot wounds is considered to be positive at ≥5000/mm^3.[3,9,16,20] Lavage white blood cell (WBC) counts are unreliable indicators of intraperitoneal injury.[9] Admit all patients with penetrating abdominal trauma and negative DPLs for 24-hour observation. This approach may limit the number of missed injuries, especially hollow viscus perforations.[15,16,21,22]

Diagnostic Laparoscopy

Laparoscopy is used to determine peritoneal violation in cases of penetrating abdominal, flank, and back injuries or whenever the possibility of injury to the diaphragm is entertained.[23-29] It is only indicated in hemodynamically stable patients, since those with indications for laparotomy need formal operative exploration. Laparoscopy accurately detects hemoperitoneum, solid organ injuries, diaphragmatic injuries, and retroperitoneal hematomas.[25,26] Patients without peritoneal penetration are spared an operation. The cost of laparoscopy is lower than the cost of laparotomy.[30] The major drawback with laparoscopy is a low sensitivity in detecting hollow viscus injuries.[25-27] Unlike DPL, it is very operator dependent; a novice laparoscopist can miss serious injury.

Serial Physical Examinations

Although some authors feel that asymptomatic victims of abdominal stab injuries should undergo DPL,[2] others believe that clinical criteria using serial examinations is the optimal approach.[13,14,22,31] In several trials, those patients who were initially observed, and later developed peritoneal signs, suffered no greater morbidity than the immediate laparotomy group.[13,32,33]

The use of serial examinations, while at first glance appearing cost-effective, has several drawbacks. It requires experienced personnel to perform round-the-clock examinations (usually every 2 hours)—a resource unavailable at most community hospitals. In addition, the presence of intoxicants, other "distracting" extraabdominal injuries, or head trauma undermines the reliability of the physical examination.[9] The risk of missed diaphragmatic injuries must always be considered in any patient undergoing serial examinations.

Abdominal Computed Tomography

Unlike DPL, abdominal computed tomography (ACT) can detect retroperitoneal injuries, and may demonstrate intraperitoneal or retroperitoneal air and fluid.[34] For this reason, some authors recommend ACT scanning for patients with stab wounds of the abdomen, back, and flank. Candidates must be hemodynamically stable and have no evidence of peritoneal signs. However, there are important limitations to CT scans in penetrating abdominal trauma. In particular, ACT cannot exclude bowel and diaphragmatic lacerations.[34]

GUNSHOT WOUNDS

Many authors believe in mandatory laparotomy for all abdominal gunshot wounds.[22,35] They cite the fact that 90% of such patients have an intraabdominal injury that requires surgery. Others reverse these same statistics and argue that low-velocity gunshot wounds may be managed based on clinical criteria, since 10% have negative laparotomies.[32,33,36] These authors advocate a policy of observation in patients without an obvious need for laparotomy.

However, the overwhelming majority of patients with abdominal gunshot wounds have an intraabdominal lesion necessitating an operation. Although some centers have successfully used nonoperative management of gunshot wounds to the right upper quadrant in selected patients,[37] this approach remains for the most part experimental. As regards abdominal gunshot wounds, it is best to follow the old surgical dictum that "it is better to look and see, than to wait and see."

For wounds with uncertain trajectories (i.e., tangential wounds), some centers use DPL, diagnostic laparoscopy,[38] or even computed tomography scanning to determine peritoneal penetration. If DPL is employed, lowering the RBC count increases sensitivity. A few studies document that CT scanning accurately determines if a bullet penetrates the abdominal cavity.[39,40] CT scanning for gunshot wounds to the abdomen is *not* indicated for patients with clear signs of peritoneal penetration, including those with shock, peritoneal signs, GI bleeding, or obvious intracavitary trajectory. Emergency physicians and surgeons should use CT *only* to determine if there is peritoneal penetration, and not employ this test to make other operative decisions. If there is intracavitary violation, most patients require laparotomy.

LUMBAR AND FLANK WOUNDS

Patients with penetrating injuries to the flank and lumbar back pose a diagnostic challenge. Victims of penetrating flank and back wounds are at significantly less risk for intraabdominal injuries than those with anterior abdominal injuries.[1,22,41-43] As such, a more selective approach is warranted in such patients without obvious indications for laparotomy. Close observation or contrast-enhanced ACT scanning combined with serial abdominal examinations is reasonable.[12,22,41,42,44]

Renal injuries occur in 6% to 8% of patients with penetrating abdominal, lumbar back, and flank wounds.[45,46] These injuries may lead to little or no hematuria.[3,45,47,48] Hemodynamic stability determines the radiographic evaluation of the urinary tract. Some authors suggest complete radiographic examination for all patients with penetrating flank or abdominal trauma.[47,48] In some centers, a **"one-shot" intravenous pyelogram (IVP)** is standard before laparotomy to ascertain the presence of two functioning kidneys in case nephrectomy is required.[3,45,46] Opponents of one-shot IVPs argue the studies are suboptimal, often yield false information, and delay definitive care.[49,50] False-positive studies may occur as a result of renal hypoperfusion,[50] and many individuals with abnormal IVPs have no renal injuries on exploration. In addition, less than 1% of patients have only one functioning kidney.[49,50] Some authors recommend a one-shot IVP be limited to patients with a flank wound and gross hematuria.[51]

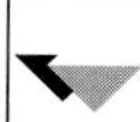

PEARLS & PITFALLS

- ◆ Avoid the use of PASG in prehospital care of penetrating torso trauma.
- ◆ Stab wounds penetrate the peritoneum in two thirds of cases, and only half of these patients have a significant visceral or vascular injury.
- ◆ Patients with shock, impalement, or blood on NG or rectal examination, or those with peritoneal signs need emergent laparotomy.
- ◆ Selective management of abdominal stab wounds includes local wound exploration, diagnostic peritoneal lavage, laparoscopy, and observation using serial examinations.
- ◆ The major controversy surrounding DPL in penetrating trauma is the definition of a positive test. A red blood cell count between 20,000 to 100,000/mm^3 is indeterminate and requires further investigation.
- ◆ ≥5000 RBCs/mm^3 is considered positive for lower chest stab wounds or abdominal gunshot wounds.
- ◆ If the trajectory of a gunshot wound clearly crosses the peritoneum, the patient requires a laparotomy.
- ◆ Patients with flank, back, and tangential gunshot wounds may benefit from a contrast CT of the abdomen to determine *peritoneal violation*. If the missile penetrates the abdominal cavity, nearly all patients will require laparotomy.

REFERENCES

1. Feliciano DV, Rozycki GS: The management of penetrating abdominal trauma, *Adv Surg* 28:1-39, 1995.
2. Feliciano DV, et al: Abdominal gunshot wounds: an urban trauma center's experience with 300 consecutive patients, *Ann Surg* 208:362-367, 1988.
3. Henneman PL: Penetrating abdominal trauma, *Emerg Med Clin North Am* 7:647-666, 1989.
4. Lacqua MJ, Sahdev P: Effective management of penetrating abdominal trauma, *Hosp Prac* 28:31-32, 34-38, 1993.
5. Mattox KL, et al: Prospective randomized evaluation of antishock MAST in post-traumatic hypotension, *J Trauma* 26:779-784, 1986.
6. Mattox KL: (Letter) *J Trauma* 27:1095, 1987.
7. Mattox KL, et al: Prospective MAST study in 911 patients, *J Trauma* 29:1104-1111, 1989.
8. Chang FC, et al: PASG: Does it help in the management of traumatic shock? *J Trauma* 39:453-456, 1995.
9. Marx JA: Penetrating abdominal trauma, *Emerg Med Clin North Am* 11:125-135, 1993.
10. Nichols RL, Smith JW: Risk of infection, infecting flora and treatment considerations in penetrating abdominal trauma, *Surg Gynecol Obstet* 177(suppl):50-54, 1993.
11. Mazzorana V, et al: Limited utility of emergency department thoracotomy, *Am Surg* 60:516-520, 1994.
12. Burns RK, Sariol HS, Ross SE: Penetrating posterior abdominal trauma, *Injury* 25:429-431, 1994.
13. de Lacy AM, et al: Management of penetrating abdominal stab wounds, *Br J Surg* 75:231-233, 1988.
14. Kent AL, et al: Ten year review of thoracic and abdominal penetrating trauma management, *Aust N Z J Surg* 63:772-779, 1993.
15. Thompson JS, et al: The evolution of abdominal stab wound management, *J Trauma* 20:478-483, 1980.
16. Moore EE, Marx JA: Penetrating abdominal wounds: rationale for exploratory laparotomy, *JAMA* 253:2705-2708, 1985.
17. Renz BM, Feliciano DV: Unnecessary laparotomies for trauma: a prospective study of morbidity, *J Trauma* 38:350-356, 1995.
18. Renz BM, Feliciano DV: The length of hospital stay after an unnecessary laparotomy for trauma: a prospective study, *J Trauma* 40:187-190, 1996.
19. Danne PD, Piasio M, Champion HR: Early management of abdominal trauma: the role of diagnostic peritoneal lavage, *Aust N Z J Surg* 58:879-887, 1988.
20. Henneman PL, et al: Diagnostic peritoneal lavage: accuracy in predicting necessary laparotomy following blunt and penetrating trauma, *J Trauma* 30:1345-1355, 1990.
21. Merlotti GJ, et al: Peritoneal lavage in penetrating thoraco-abdominal trauma, *J Trauma* 28:17-21, 1988.
22. McCarthy MC, et al: Prediction of injury caused by penetrating wounds to the abdomen, flank, and back, *Arch Surg* 126:962-966, 1991.
23. Berci G, Sackier JM, Paz-Partlow M: Emergency laparoscopy, *Am J Surg* 161:332-335, 1991.
24. Fernando HC, et al: Triage by laparoscopy in patients with penetrating abdominal trauma, *Br J Surg* 81:384-385, 1994.
25. Ivatury RR, Simon RJ, Stahl WM: A critical evaluation of laparoscopy in penetrating abdominal trauma, *J Trauma* 34:822-827, 1993.
26. Livingston DH, et al: The role of laparoscopy in abdominal trauma, *J Trauma* 33:471-475, 1992.
27. Smith RS, et al: Therapeutic laparoscopy in trauma, *Am J Surg* 170:632-636, 1995.
28. Sosa JL, et al: Laparoscopy in abdominal gunshot wounds, *Surg Laparosc Endosc* 3:417-419, 1993.
29. Zantut LF, et al: Diagnostic and therapeutic laparoscopy for penetrating abdominal trauma: a multicenter experience, *J Trauma* 42:825-829, 1997.
30. Marks JM, Youngelman DF, Berk T: Cost analysis of diagnostic laparoscopy vs laparotomy in the evaluation of penetrating abdominal trauma, *Surg Endosc* 11:272-276, 1997.
31. Zubowski R, et al: Selective conservatism in abdominal stab wounds: the efficacy of serial physical examination, *J Trauma* 28:1665-1668, 1988.
32. Demetriades D, et al: Gunshot wound of the abdomen: role of selective conservative management, *Br J Surg* 78:220-222, 1991.
33. Shaftan GW: Indications for operation in abdominal trauma, *Am J Surg* 99:657-664, 1960.
34. Rehm CG, Sherman R, Hinz TW: The role of CT scan in evaluation for laparotomy in patients with stab wounds of the abdomen, *J Trauma* 29:446-450, 1989.

35. Thal ER, May RA, Beesinger D: Peritoneal lavage: its unreliability in gunshot wounds of the lower chest and abdomen, *Arch Surg* 115:430-433, 1980.
36. Muckart DJ, Abdool-Carrim AT, King B: Selective conservative management of abdominal gunshot wounds: a prospective study, *Br J Surg* 77:652-655, 1990.
37. Chmielewski GW, et al: Nonoperative management of gunshot wounds of the abdomen, *Am Surg* 61:665-668, 1995.
38. Sosa JL, et al: Laparoscopic evaluation of tangential abdominal gunshot wounds, *Arch Surg* 127:109-110, 1992.
39. Carrillo EH, et al: The role of computed tomography in selective management of gunshot wounds to the abdomen and flank, *J Trauma* 45:1005-1009, 1998.
40. Grossman MD, et al: Determining anatomic injury with computed tomography in selected torso gunshot wounds, *J Trauma* 45:446-456, 1998.
41. Easter DW, Shackford SR, Mattrey RF: A prospective, randomized comparison of computed tomography with conventional diagnostic methods in the evaluation of penetrating injuries to the back and flank, *Arch Surg* 126:1115-1119, 1991.
42. Hauser CJ, et al: Triple-contrast computed tomography in the evaluation of penetrating posterior abdominal injuries, *Arch Surg* 122:1112-1115, 1987.
43. Boyle EM, et al: Diagnosis of injuries after stab wounds to the back and flank, *J Trauma* 42:260-265, 1997.
44. Whalen G, Angorn IB, Robbs JV: The selective management of penetrating wounds of the back, *J Trauma* 29:509-511, 1989.
45. Scott R Jr., Carlton CE Jr., Goldman M: Penetrating injuries of the kidney: an analysis of 181 patients, *J Urol* 101:247-253, 1969.
46. Carroll PR, McAninch JW: Staging of renal trauma, *Urol Clin North Am* 16:193-201, 1989.
47. Mee SL, McAninch JW: Indications for radiographic assessment in suspected renal trauma, *Urol Clin North Am* 16:187-192, 1989.
48. Mee SL, et al: Radiographic assessment of renal trauma: a 10-year prospective study of patient selection, *J Urol* 141:1095-1098, 1989.
49. Patel VG, Walker ML: The role of "one-shot" intravenous pyelogram in evaluation of penetrating abdominal trauma, *Am Surg* 63:350-353, 1997.
50. Stevenson J, Battistella FD: The 'one-shot' intravenous pyelogram: is it indicated in unstable trauma patients before celiotomy? *J Trauma* 36:828-833, 1994.
51. Nagy KK, et al: Routine preoperative "one-shot" intravenous pyelography is not indicated in all patients with penetrating abdominal trauma, *J Am Coll Surg* 185:530-533, 1997.

Genitourinary Tract and Renovascular Trauma

21

MICHAEL A. GIBBS AND ROBERT SCHNEIDER

Teaching Case

A 72-year-old man fell on the ice. He presented to the emergency department (ED) the following day complaining of abdominal pain and inability to urinate. His abdomen was diffusely tender. Urinalysis showed gross hematuria. An abdominal computed tomography (CT) scan showed a possible splenic laceration and moderate intraperitoneal fluid. He was admitted for observation.

The following day his pain increased. A repeat CT scan showed a small amount of free air anterior to the liver. He was taken to the operating suite with a presumptive diagnosis of bowel perforation. No bowel or splenic lacerations were found, but he did have a 3 cm intraperitoneal (IP) bladder rupture. His bladder was subsequently repaired. ■

Genitourinary (GU) injury occurs in 10% to 15% of patients sustaining major trauma.[1] Because these injuries can be clinically subtle, they are frequently overlooked during the initial patient evaluation, often leading to significant morbidity. Although the management of other life-threatening injuries takes precedence, early diagnosis of urologic insult is essential to avoid potentially serious complications. It is important for the emergency physician (EP) to recognize the signs of urologic trauma and to develop a rationale, repetitive approach to the diagnosis, staging, and management of these injuries.

A GENERAL DIAGNOSTIC APPROACH

The evaluation of the GU tract should be individualized, depending on several factors. The first is the *clinical status of the patient.* In the hemodynamically unstable patient with other indications for emergent laparotomy, the presence of gross hematuria should be noted. No further radiologic studies should be obtained in the ED, since these evaluations waste precious time. The integrity of the kidneys, ureters, and bladder can be assessed intraoperatively. In stable patients, diagnostic imaging can proceed in a systematic fashion.

The second is the *presence, absence, and degree of hematuria.* The presence of gross hematuria is an important sign of urologic injury and should prompt a diligent and targeted evaluation. *Gross hematuria* is broadly defined as urine any color other than clear or yellow. When gross hematuria is absent, urologic injury is less likely. The presence of *microscopic hematuria,* defined as greater than 5 red blood cells (RBCs)/hpf, should be interpreted in the context of the injury. Microscopic hematuria associated with hypotension (BP <90 mmHg) is an indication for further work-up.

The third is the *mechanism of injury* (i.e., blunt or penetrating). The evaluation of the urologic injury in *blunt trauma* is based on hemodynamics and whether or not hematuria is present, and if so to what degree. In general, diagnostic imaging is indicated in all blunt trauma patients with (1) microscopic hematuria and shock (BP <90 mmHg) or (2) gross hematuria. *Penetrating injury* of the urinary system is often clinically subtle and may exist even when hematuria is absent. For this reason, evaluation should be considered in all patients with penetrating wounds "in proximity" to the urinary tract (e.g., back, abdomen, flank, or groin), regardless of the presence, degree, or absence of hematuria.

The fourth is the *suspected anatomic site of injury.* For diagnostic and staging purposes, the urologic system is divided into the *upper tract* (ureters and kidneys) and *lower tract* (external genitalia, urethra, and bladder). Specific radiologic studies are required for imaging of the upper and lower tract. Equally important, tests must be performed in the correct sequence. As a general rule, urologic injuries should always be assessed in a retrograde fashion. Lower tract injury should be excluded before evaluation of the upper tract.

When lower tract injury is suspected (e.g., pelvic fracture and hematuria), the urethra should be evaluated before the bladder. When upper tract injury is suspected (e.g., rapid deceleration; direct blow to the back, flank, abdomen; penetrating torso injury), a targeted radiologic evaluation of the ureters and kidneys is appropriate. When injuries to both the upper and the lower tract may coexist, first evaluate the urethra and bladder, then the ureters and kidneys. This approach is effective and reduces the risk of iatrogenic complications and spurious information.

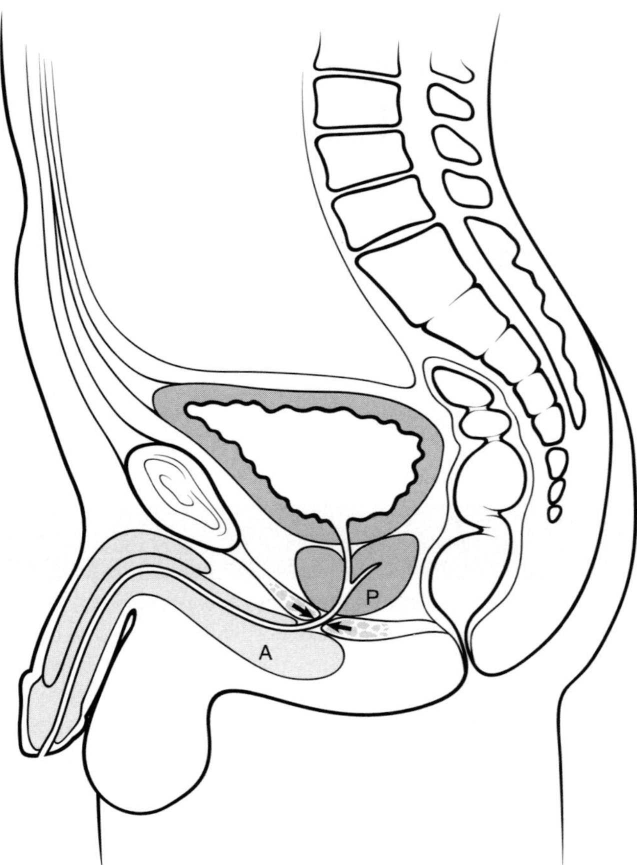

Fig. 21-1 Normal anatomy of the male urethra. The urogenital diaphragm *(arrow)* divides the urethra into anterior and posterior segments.

THE ASSESSMENT OF HEMATURIA

Hematuria is the most important sign of urologic injury. All patients suffering blunt multisystem trauma and those with penetrating "proximity" injuries should have a urine sample examined. A urinary catheter should be inserted after completion of the secondary survey, provided there are no signs of urethral injury (i.e., blood at the urethral meatus, gross hematuria, and perineal or scrotal hematoma). Catheterization allows for timely collection of a urine sample and can also be used to accurately monitor urine output and the patient's response to resuscitation. Because hematuria is often transient and may clear after voiding or following aggressive resuscitation with crystalloid, it is critical that the first portion of the catheterization specimen be collected.[2,3]

Testing for hematuria begins at the bedside with simple inspection of the urine for gross hematuria. Many different substances, including myoglobin, foods (e.g., beets, berries, food colorings), and medications (e.g., phenazopyridine, rifampin, alphamethyldopa, phenolphthalein-containing laxatives, metronidazole), may cause a red or brown discoloration of the urine. The observation of gross hematuria should always be confirmed by dipstick analysis. Commercially available dipsticks detect the presence of RBCs with a high degree of accuracy, although they are not quantitatively precise.[4,5] It should be remembered that both free hemoglobin and myoglobin will yield a false-positive dipstick result in the absence of microscopic RBCs. Therefore a positive dipstick should also be confirmed by microscopic urinalysis.

URETHRAL TRAUMA

Although urethral trauma is far less common than injury to the kidneys or bladder, it is potentially the most debilitating of all urologic injuries because of the high incidence of complications (e.g., strictures, impotence, incontinence). Early detection and appropriate management is imperative.[4]

For purposes of injury staging, the male urethra is anatomically divided into posterior and anterior segments by the urogenital diaphragm (Fig. 21-1). The *posterior urethra* is within and above the urogenital diaphragm and includes the prostatic and membranous urethra. The posterior urethra is firmly attached to the pubis by the puboprostatic ligaments. An injury to the posterior urethra should always be suspected in a patient with anterior pelvic ring trauma, particularly pubic rami fractures or symphyseal disruptions (Fig. 21-2). Between 5% and 25% of patients with pelvic fractures have an associated urethral injury. Conversely, a pelvic fracture is present in over 95% of patients with an injury to the posterior urethra.[4,5]

The *anterior urethra* is located below the urogenital diaphragm and includes the bulbous and penile urethra. The anterior urethra is surrounded by the corpus spongiosum, which is enveloped by Buck's fascia. In anterior urethral disruptions in which Buck's fascia is

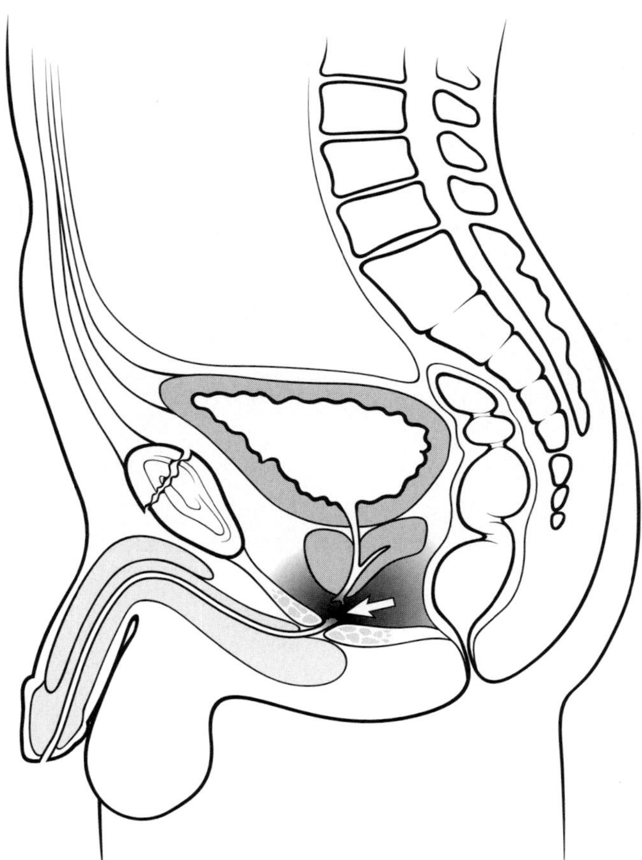

Fig. 21-2 Transection of the posterior urethra *(arrow)*. Disruption of the puboprostatic ligament and hematoma formation pushes the prostate upwards, resulting in a "high-riding" prostate on rectal examination.

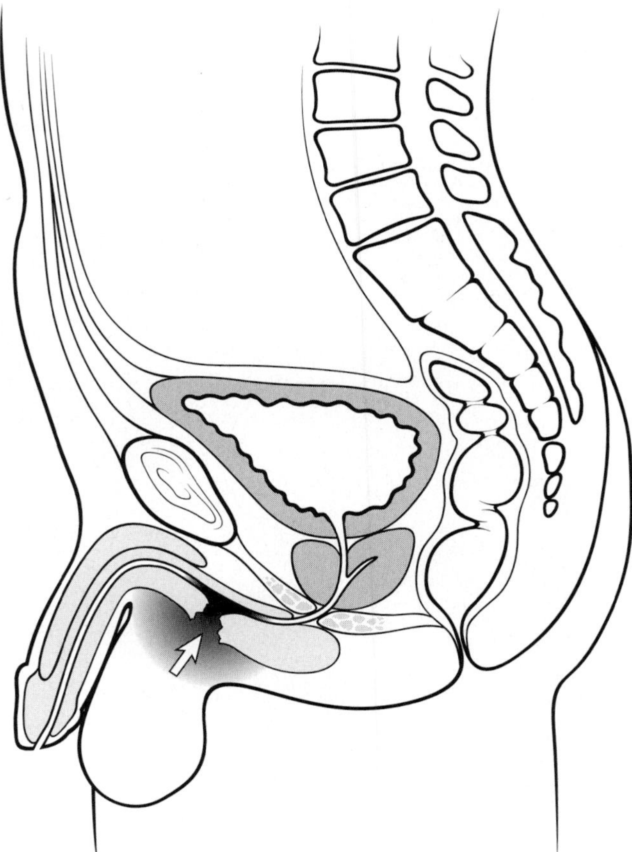

Fig. 21-3 Transection of the anterior urethra *(arrow)*. Extravasation of blood and urine is confined to the penis. The prostate remains in the normal position.

transected, extravasated urine dissects freely into the perineum, scrotum, and anterior abdominal wall (Fig. 21-3). If Buck's fascia remains intact, extravasation is confined to the penile shaft, resulting in fusiform swelling. Injuries to the anterior urethra are usually the result of a straddle injury or a direct blow to the perineum.

In contrast to the male urethra, the female urethra is not fixed to the pelvis. Increased mobility and a shorter length protect it somewhat from injury. Urethral trauma in the female patient is exceedingly rare, with only occasional case reports in literature.[6,7] Lacerations of the labia and vagina may be associated with urethral injury.

Diagnosis

The patient with a urethral injury typically complains of perineal pain, dysuria, or the inability to void. Micturition may cause swelling of the penis and perineum. Blood at the urethral meatus (Fig. 21-4) is the hallmark of urethral trauma, although this finding

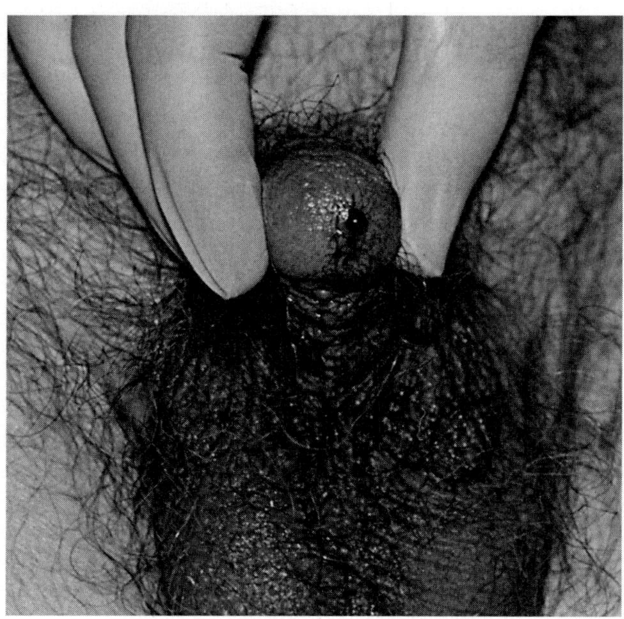

Fig. 21-4 Blood at the urethral meatus.

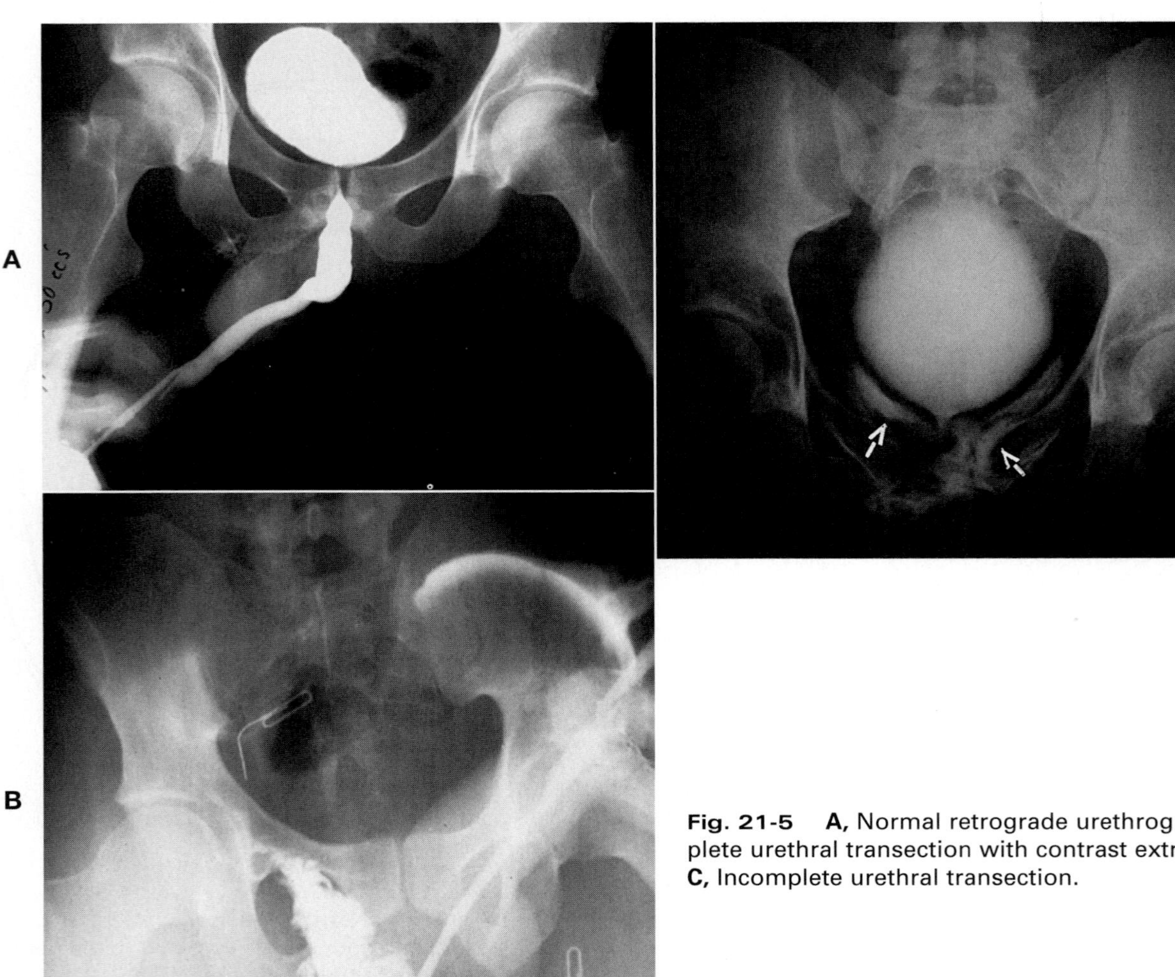

Fig. 21-5 **A,** Normal retrograde urethrogram. **B,** Complete urethral transection with contrast extravasation. **C,** Incomplete urethral transection.

is not present in all cases.[4,8] Although perineal discoloration and swelling may be present, it is usually a late finding. On rectal examination the prostate may not be palpable if the puboprostatic ligaments are transected, the so-called "high-riding prostate." This finding may be misleading because the consistency of a tense pelvic hematoma sometimes mimics prostatic tissue.

In patients with a suspected urethral injury, urinary catheterization is contraindicated, because it increases the incidence of infection, stricture formation, and conversion of a partial urethral transection into a complete one. Once signs and symptoms suggest urethral injury, the diagnosis is confirmed by retrograde urethrography. Urethrography is mandatory in any trauma patient with blood at the urethral meatus. The study is also recommended in patients with major anterior pelvic ring fractures in whom placement of a urinary catheter is met with resistance. Urethrography is quick, accurate, and carries virtually no risk. The retrograde urethrogram is performed as follows: (1) the tip of an irrigating syringe filled with contrast is seated tightly in the urethral meatus, (2) the penis is gently stretched and angled 45° from the midline, and (3) 50 to 60 ml of water-soluble contrast diluted to a 10% solution is slowly injected as an anteroposterior (AP) radiograph is taken.[4]

A normal urethrogram shows smooth flow of contrast into the bladder (Fig. 21-5). When the urethra is transected, contrast extravasates. In the presence of extravasation, contrast in the bladder denotes a partial injury. If the bladder does not fill, a complete transection has occurred. Since urethrography cannot be performed in the female patient, the diagnosis is

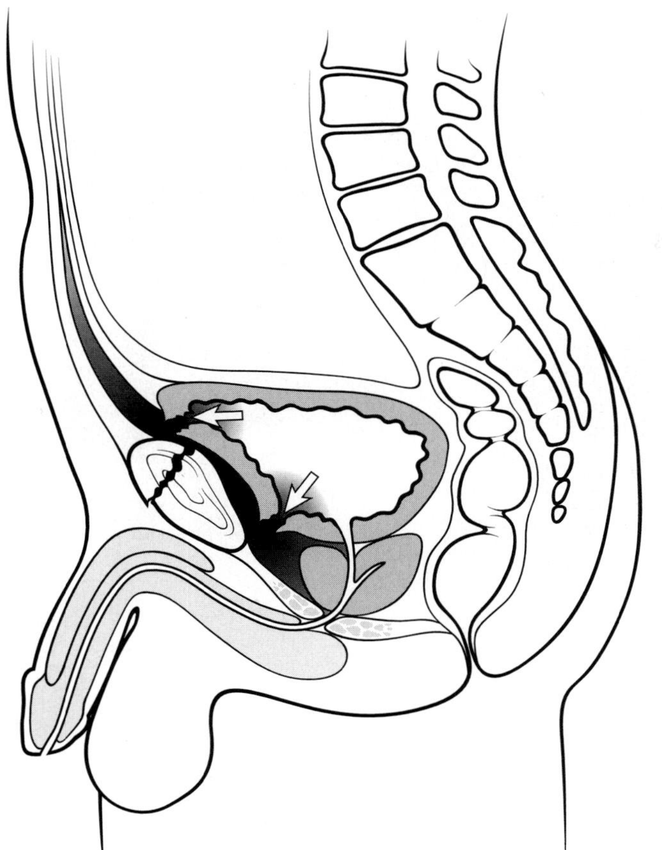

Fig. 21-6 Extraperitoneal bladder rupture.

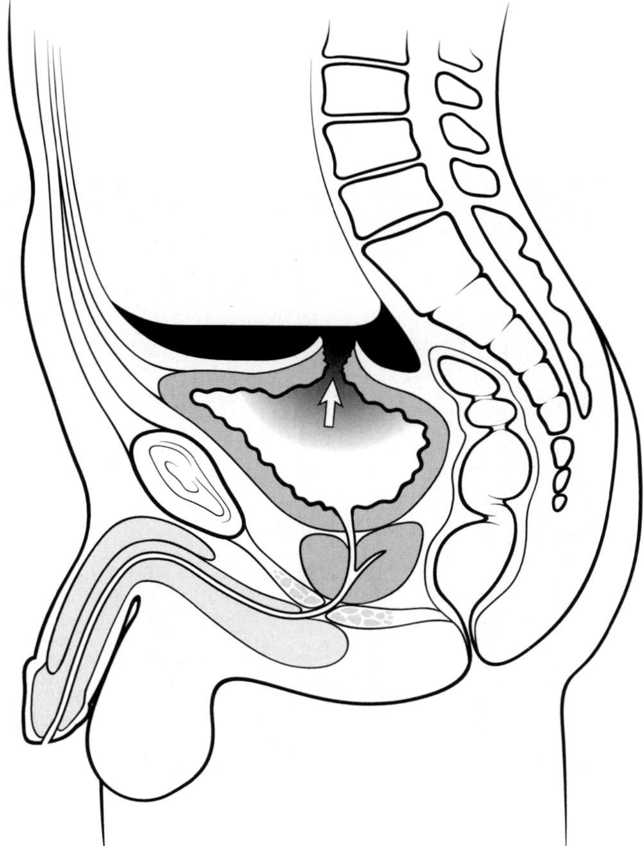

Fig. 21-7 Intraperitoneal bladder rupture.

made clinically if blood is present at the urethral meatus or if a gentle attempt at catheterization is met with resistance.

BLADDER TRAUMA

Bladder injuries are usually the result of motor vehicle crashes (MVCs) or crush injuries to the pelvis. Between 70% and 95% of patients with bladder injuries have associated pelvic fractures. Conversely, between 4% and 8% of patients with pelvic fractures have an associated bladder injury. The fracture types most often associated with bladder injury include pubic arch fractures, symphyseal fractures, and displaced two-part pelvic fractures. A blow to the lower abdomen (as might be seen with a steering wheel or seat-belt injury) may also cause bladder injury without an associated fracture.[9-14]

Bladder injury can be classified into three categories: (1) partial-thickness bladder wall contusions; (2) extraperitoneal (EP) rupture, involving a laceration below the pelvic peritoneum (Fig. 21-6) and; (3) intraperitoneal (IP) rupture, which violates the pelvic peritoneum and communicates with the peritoneal cavity (Fig. 21-7).

Diagnosis

The patient with a bladder injury usually complains of lower abdominal pain. Physical examination may reveal bruising and tenderness of the lower abdomen. Pelvic instability may be noted. Hematuria is always present, although it does not correlate with the degree of injury. A patient with a simple contusion may display gross hematuria, whereas an IP rupture may be associated with only microscopic hematuria.[9]

The diagnosis of bladder injury is made by retrograde cystography. If a urethral injury is suspected, the cystogram should be done *after* a retrograde urethrogram. Retrograde cystography is performed as follows: (1) a Foley catheter is gently inserted and contrast is instilled under gravity. Most authors recommend that 300 to 400 cc of water-soluble contrast material be used to ensure complete distension.[15-17] Since the natural elasticity of the detrusor muscle

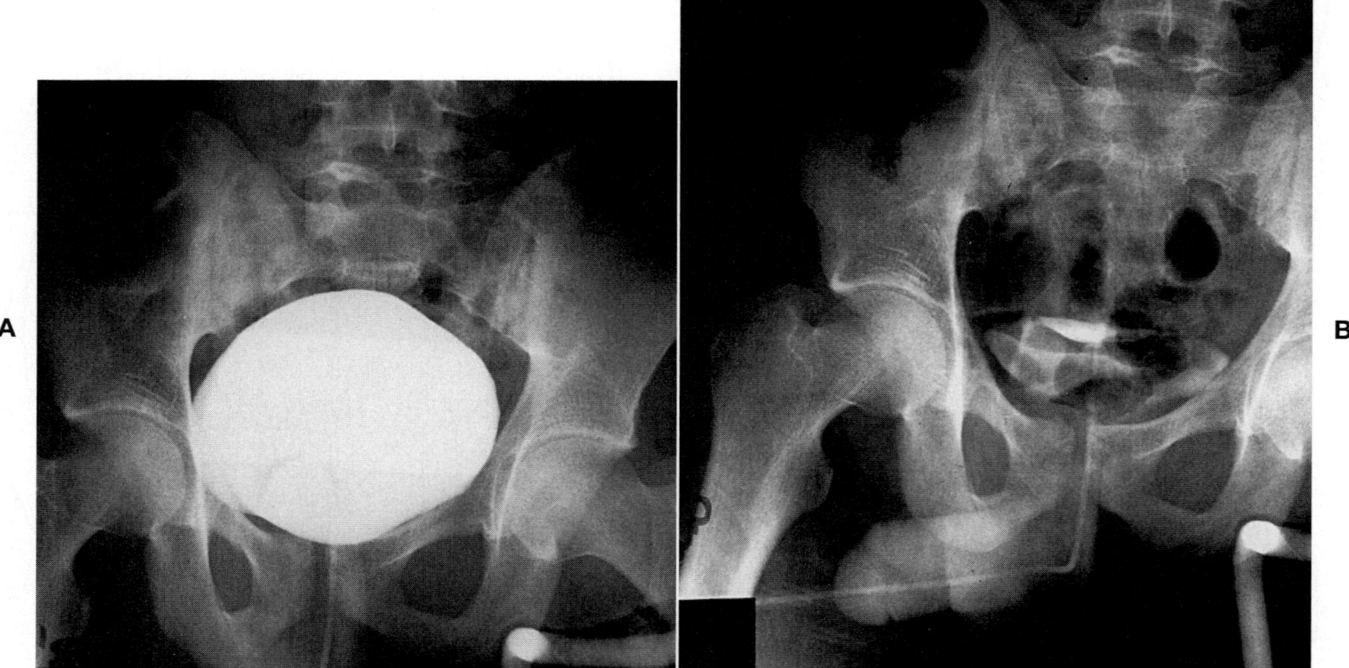

Fig. 21-8 **A,** Normal retrograde cystogram (anteroposterior view). **B,** Normal retrograde cystogram (post-void view)

tends to approximate the edges of a bladder wall tear, contrast may not extravasate if the bladder is inadequately distended. (2) The Foley catheter is then clamped, and an AP radiograph is taken (Fig. 21-8, *A*). (3) Next, the bladder is drained and a second AP postdrainage radiograph is performed (Fig. 21-8, *B*). This "post-void" view is important to demonstrate extravasated contrast material situated posteriorly, which be may obscured on the initial film. Although an intravenous pyelogram (IVP) can be used to assess the upper urinary tract, this anterograde study is inadequate to exclude an injury to the bladder.[18] In addition, several studies have shown that the routine abdominopelvic CT is not a reliable method for evaluating bladder injuries.[19,20] When accurate imaging of the bladder is desired in patients undergoing abdominal CT scanning, first instill contrast retrograde via a Foley catheter to distend the bladder, clamp the catheter, and then perform the CT scan.

When evaluating the cystogram, first look at the shape and position of the contrast-filled bladder. Patients with large pelvic hematomas may demonstrate an intact bladder that is compressed to assume a tear-drop appearance or deviated to one side of the pelvic cavity (Fig. 21-9). Next, look for contrast extravasation. In patients with EP rupture, extravasated contrast is confined to the pelvis (Fig. 21-10), whereas those with IP rupture demonstrate intraperitoneal contrast (Fig. 21-11) (e.g., layering of contrast in the dependent portion of the peritoneal cavity, in the paracolic gutters, between adjacent loops of bowel, or adjacent to the liver and spleen). Always scrutinize the post-void view for contrast that may have been obscured by the contrast-filled bladder on the initial radiograph. Patients with IP ruptures need to go to the operating suite for exploratory laparotomy.

URETERAL TRAUMA

Ureteral injuries are rare and account for less than 1% of all urologic injuries. There is a predilection towards children, with only about one third of cases involving adults. The right side is involved 3 times more often than the left side. Ureteral injuries almost always result from penetrating trauma,[21-24] although there are rare case reports of avulsion of the ureter at either the ureteropelvic or ureterovesical junction following blunt trauma with rapid deceleration.[25-27] Re-

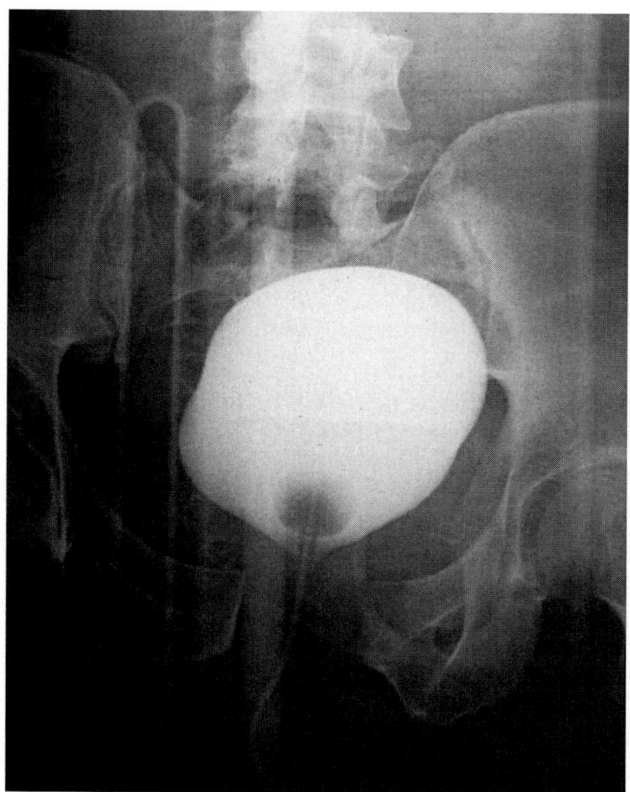

Fig. 21-9 Intact bladder deviated by a pelvic hematoma.

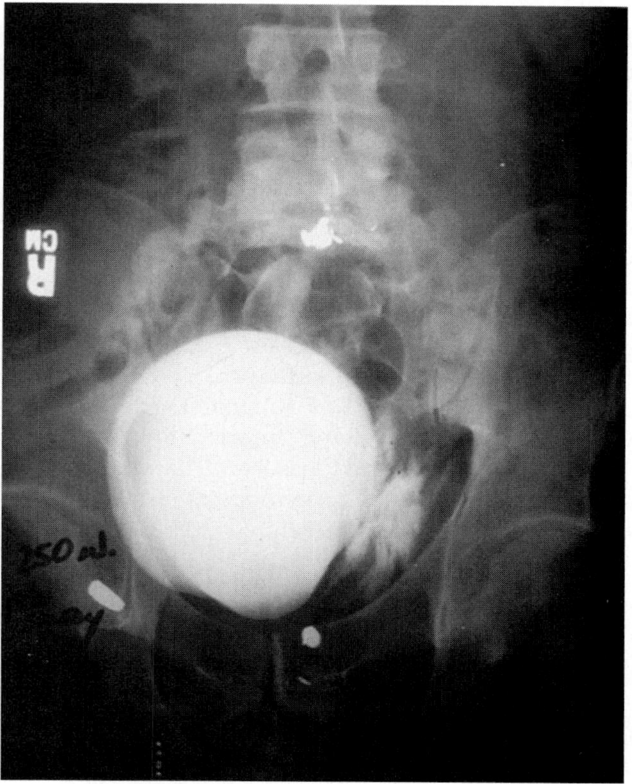

Fig. 21-10 Extraperitoneal bladder rupture.

gardless of the mechanism, more than 90% of ureteral injuries are associated with other intraabdominal injuries.

Diagnosis

Transection of the ureter does not cause any specific signs or symptoms, and this injury cannot be diagnosed or excluded clinically. For this reason, the diagnosis is often delayed. Although hematuria is present in 80% to 90% of cases, it is usually microscopic. Symptoms typically do not develop until extravasated urine produces local inflammation, or there is obstruction to urine flow from the ipsilateral kidney. Complications of unrecognized ureter injury include urinoma or abscess formation, strictures, hydronephrosis, pyelonephritis, loss of renal function, and ileus formation secondary to irritation from urine.[21]

Intravenous pyelography remains the technique of choice for the detection of ureteral injury, with a sensitivity of over 90%.[21] Although the sensitivity of CT scanning has never been tested in a prospective fashion, there is the potential to miss a ureteral injury between consecutive cross-sectional images. It is also important to recognize that because of the speed of helical CT imaging, extravasation of contrast from the damaged ureter may not be seen on the initial (nephrogram phase) images. Obtaining delayed images of the kidneys at 5 to 8 minutes makes misdiagnosis less likely.[28]

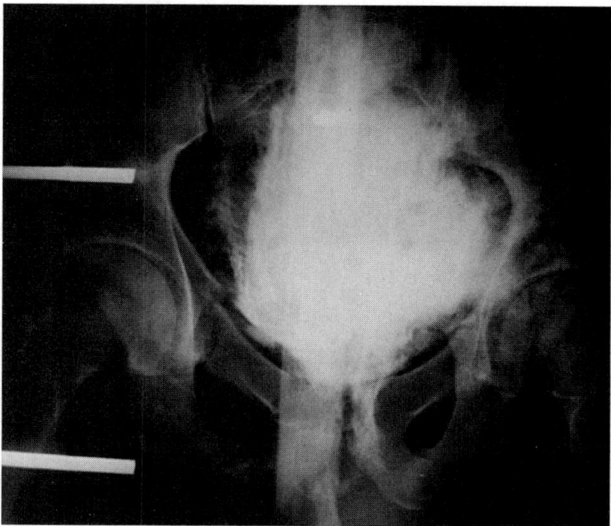

Fig. 21-11 Intraperitoneal bladder rupture.

RENAL TRAUMA

Renal injury can result from either penetrating or blunt trauma. In most case series, 5% to 10% of renal injuries are a consequence of penetrating trauma (stab or gunshot wound), whereas 90% to 95% are due to blunt trauma (MVCs, falls, or direct blows). These injuries are classified (Fig. 21-12) as Class 1 (contusions or subcapsular hematomas), Class 2 (superficial cortical lacerations not involving the medulla or collecting system), Class 3 (deep lacerations extending into the medulla and/or collecting system), Class 4 (renal vascular pedicle injuries), or Class 5 (completely shattered and devascularized kidneys).

Between 85% and 90% of all renal injuries are Class 1 and 2 and are considered "minor." Five percent to 10% of renal injuries are Class 3 and 4 and are considered "major."[1,3] Fig. 21-13 demonstrates a minor and major renal injury, respectively.

Diagnosis

Patients with renal injury usually complain of abdominal, flank, or back pain. Physical examination may reveal tenderness, rigidity, or ecchymosis of the involved area. A palpable abdominal or flank mass, representing an expanding retroperitoneal hematoma, is seen in rare cases. Decreased bowel sounds may be noted in the patient with a secondary ileus. Almost all patients with renal injury demonstrate either microscopic or gross hematuria. However, the degree of hematuria does not correlate with the degree of injury.

Adult Patients with Microscopic Hematuria and Blunt Trauma

The management of renal injury has evolved over the last two decades. Most early studies recommended that all patients with blunt abdominal

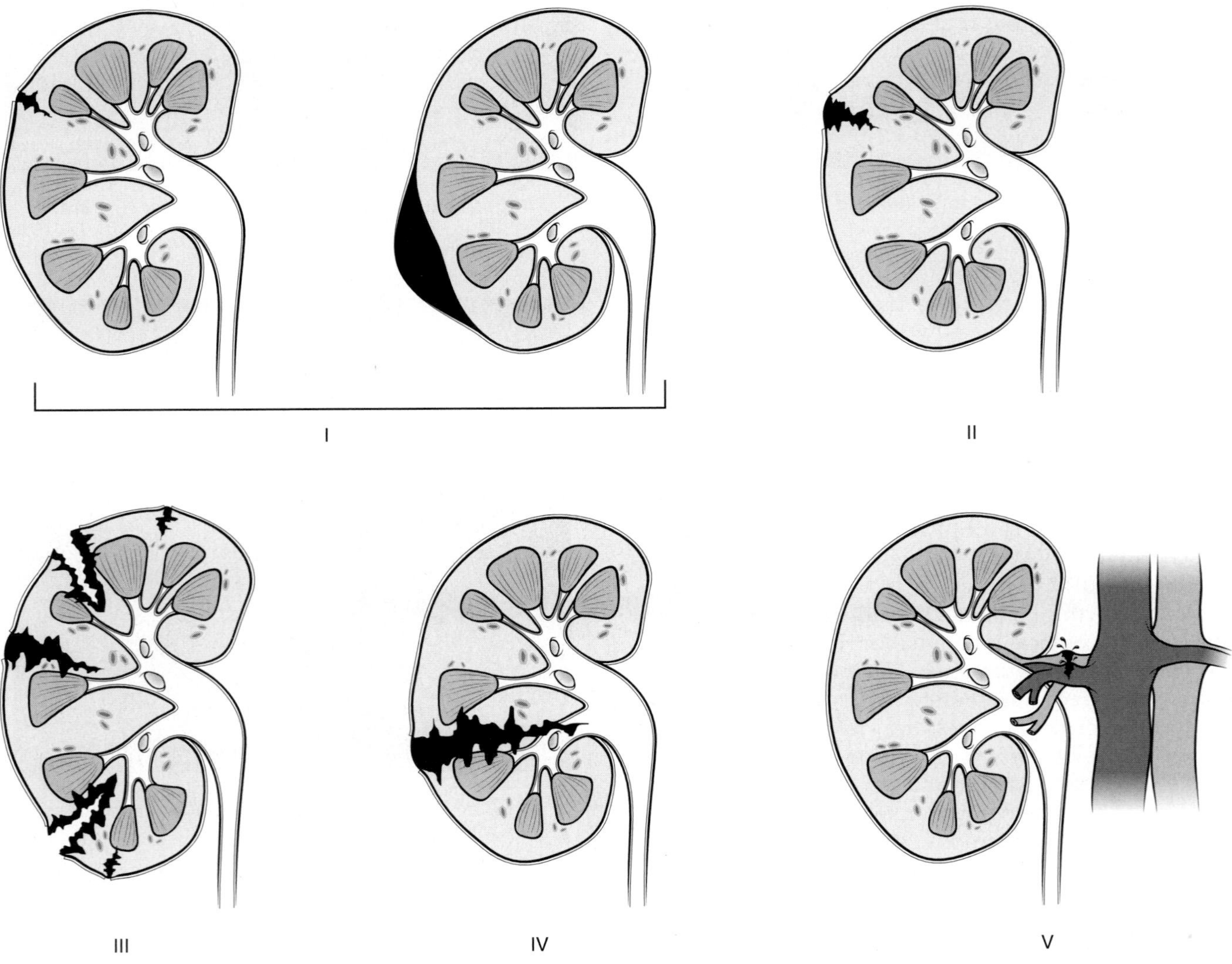

Fig. 21-12 Staging of renal injury.

trauma and any degree of hematuria undergo immediate radiologic evaluation.[29,30] This approach, while expensive and time-consuming, was defended on the basis of a small number of patients with major renal injuries presenting with microscopic hematuria. There is now a growing body of literature that supports a more selective approach. Pooled data from several independent studies have shown that in hemodynamically stable (BP >90 mmHg) blunt trauma patients with microscopic hematuria (>5 RBCs/hpf), the risk of major renal injury is exceedingly low (approximately 0.05%).[3,31-38] The vast majority of these patients have no demonstrable injury, or minor renal contusions that can be managed nonoperatively. Diagnostic studies can be safely withheld in this situation. Depending on the individual patient, a brief period of observation with repeat physical examination and a follow-up urinalysis may be indicated.[3] This approach to testing offers significant cost savings, since stable patients with microscopic hematuria represent 80% to 90% of all cases. This approach also decreases the potential morbidity associated with intravenous contrast and may expedite the evaluation and management of other injuries.

Children with Microscopic Hematuria

The management of children with traumatic hematuria has also evolved in the past two decades. Traditionally, teaching emphasized the need for renal imaging in all pediatric blunt trauma victims with any degree of hematuria. This recommendation was based on two assumptions: (1) hypotension is not a reliable indicator of significant renal injuries in children, and (2) the pediatric kidney is more vulnerable to injury because of its proportionally larger size and limited thoracic and perinephric fat protection.[39] This approach has recently been challenged by newer data demonstrating that the majority of renal injuries in children, like in adults, are minor and heal uneventfully with nonoperative management.[40] A meta-analysis of reported series of children with suspected renal injuries after blunt trauma in which the degree of hematuria was quantified (n=728) demonstrated that only 2% of patients with <50 RBC/hpf had significant renal injuries.[41-48] The incidence of significant renal injuries in patients with >50 RBC/hpf increases to 8%. Gross hematuria is associated with major renal injury in 32% of patients. In addition, all children with significant renal injuries were victims of severe multisystem trauma and would have undergone renal imaging during the evaluation for suspected abdominal trauma.

Gross Hematuria

All patients with blunt trauma and gross hematuria, regardless of age, require imaging of the GU tract. In the case of a pelvic fracture, evaluate the lower tract first.

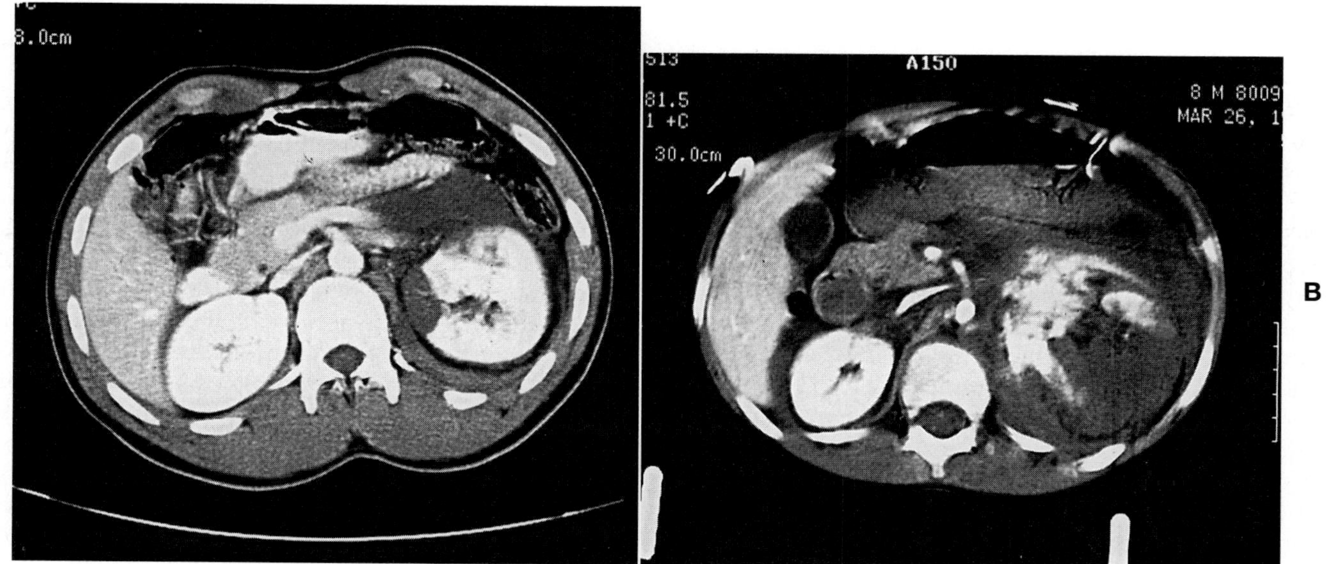

Fig. 21-13 **A,** "Minor" renal injury. **B,** "Major" renal injury.

IMAGING STUDIES

Current indications for radiologic assessment of suspected renal injury include:

1. Penetrating trauma in proximity to the GU tract with or without hematuria
2. Blunt trauma associated with hypotension and any degree of hematuria (many of these patients proceed directly to laparotomy)
3. Blunt trauma and gross hematuria
4. Pediatric blunt trauma with >50 RBCs/hpf

Plain-Film Radiography

Abdominal radiographs should not be ordered to evaluate renal injury. Although several findings are associated with renal injury, these findings are neither sensitive nor specific. Plain-film findings include: (1) fractures of the lower ribs or transverse processes; (2) loss of the renal outline or psoas shadow; (3) scoliosis, concave to the side of injury; and (4) focal ileus over the renal shadow.

Computed Tomography

Contrast-enhanced CT has replaced IVP as the diagnostic modality of choice for the diagnosis of renal injury.[49-54] Computed tomography offers two important advantages: (1) the severity of renal injury can be more precisely defined, and (2) associated intraabdominal injuries can also be detected. Associated injuries are present in 80% of patients with penetrating renal injuries and 20% of patients with blunt renal injuries.[1,51] Patients who demonstrate active extravasation of intravenous (IV) contrast should proceed to angiography.

Intravenous Pyelography

Although CT has replaced IVP in most centers as the diagnostic modality of choice for stable patients with suspected renal injury, the "one-shot" IVP may be useful in certain situations. In patients being resuscitated for immediate laparotomy, the IVP can provide critical information. This test is performed by rapidly injecting water-soluble intravenous contrast (2 cc/kg) via a central or peripheral intravenous line and obtaining a single 10-minute post-injection abdominal radiograph. The IVP film can verify the presence, or absence, of two functioning kidneys, and can demonstrate major parenchymal disruption or urinary extravasation.[1,50] Keep in mind that the IVP should be done in the operating suite whenever possible to reduce potential delays. In addition, it should be recognized that the IVP is not a perfect test and is associated with a significant number of false-negative and false-positive results.[55]

RENOVASCULAR INJURIES

Injuries to the renal artery and vein are extremely uncommon, seen in <3% of all patients with renal injuries.[56] Left-sided injuries outnumber right-sided injuries in blunt trauma, probably because the left renal artery is shorter and at a more acute angle than the artery on the right.[56,57] Rarely, bilateral renal artery injury has been reported.[58,59] The most common injury is thrombosis of the renal artery, which is produced by an intimal tear and dissection. Lacerations or avulsions of the renal pedicle may also occur in more severe injuries and usually require urgent exploration for hemorrhage control.[60] Associated injuries are the rule, and up to 85% of patients require laparotomy for other intraabdominal injuries.[56,57]

Hematuria may be lacking in about one third of patients with major renovascular trauma.[56] Since almost all patients have other indications for evaluation of intraabdominal injuries, CT scanning is probably the first study that detects these injuries in stable patients. The CT scan findings supporting renal arterial injury include lack of contrast enhancement (Fig. 21-14), nonopacification of the renal calyces, abrupt cessation of an enhancing renal artery, and the "cortical rim sign."[57,61] The latter finding represents minimal flow to the cortex from collateral vessels. Renal vein injury is suggested by displacement of the renal hilum and parenchyma by a central or large hematoma.[57]

The management of unilateral renal artery thrombosis has been controversial.[60] Since there is often a delay to definitive diagnosis and arrival to the operating suite, many hours of warm ischemia time result.[56] As such, revascularizations are usually met with nonpreservation of renal function.[56,57,62] All attempts must be made for renal salvage in patients with bilateral renal artery occlusion or in patients with a solitary kidney.[57,62] Some authors feel that if the CT scan demonstrates this injury, confirmatory angiography (Fig. 21-15) only delays the patient's chances for renal salvage.[61] Endovascular stent placement may be attempted for intimal tears of the renal artery.[63] Venous injuries have a better prognosis than arterial injuries and are usually managed by primary repair or ligation.[56,57]

The development of late hypertension after renal artery thrombosis may be seen in 50% of patients.[56] Nephrectomy may be required for blood pressure control in patients with severe hypertension.[62]

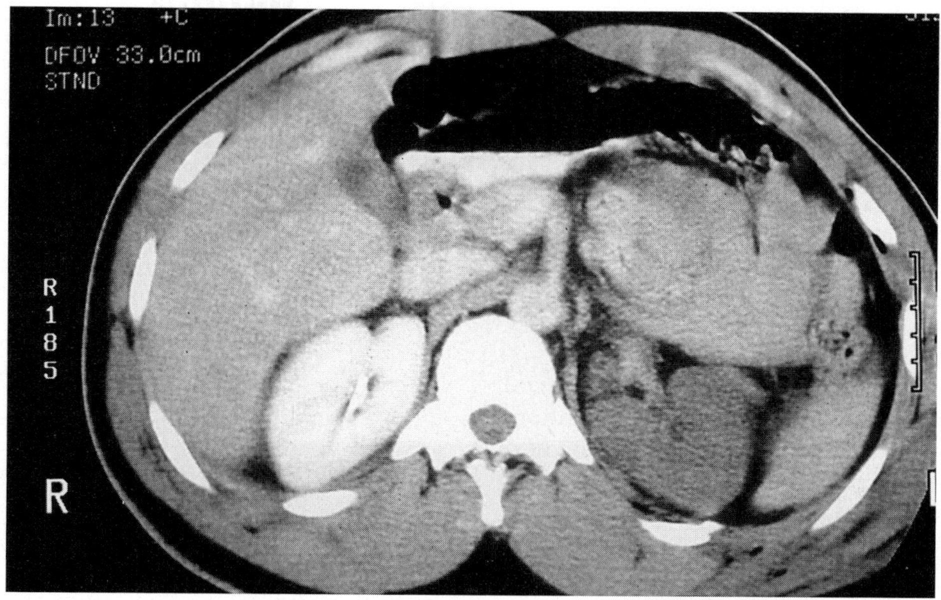

Fig. 21-14 Avascular left kidney in a patient with a renovascular injury.

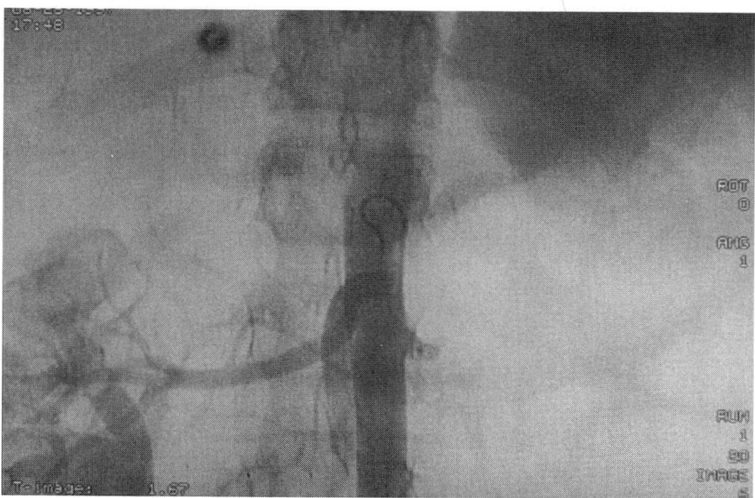

Fig. 21-15 Arteriogram shows occlusion of left renal artery.

Renal artery pseudoaneurysm has been reported mainly following penetrating injuries. However, blunt trauma has also been rarely reported as a cause for these lesions.[64,65] Pseudoaneurysms may be evident as large, enhancing collections within the kidney on CT scanning.[64] The danger in not treating these injuries is the risk of delayed rupture and death and renal loss.[64] Embolization with coils is a viable treatment option for these lesions.[64,65] Surgery may also result in renal salvage.[65]

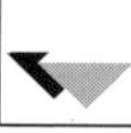

PEARLS & PITFALLS

- Examine the *initial* urine output to determine need for further studies.
- Timing of studies depends on patient stability. The hemodynamically unstable patient may require urgent operation.
- Always evaluate the GU tract in a *retrograde* fashion.

- Consider urethral injury in the patient with anterior pelvic ring fractures.
- When performing retrograde cystography, ensure that the bladder is adequately distended with contrast, and always obtain a post-void film.
- The indications for renal imaging in blunt trauma include (1) gross hematuria and (2) microscopic hematuria with shock.
- Children with >50 RBCs/hpf in their urine need abdominal CT scanning to rule out significant renal injury.
- Use of the "one-shot" IVP is controversial and rarely provides valuable information. It should not delay a needed operation and can be done in the operating suite.

REFERENCES

1. Schneider RE: Genitourinary trauma, *Emerg Med Clin North Am* 11:137-145, 1993.
2. Chandhoke PS, MaAninch JW: Detection and significance of microscopic hematuria in patients with blunt renal trauma, *J Urol* 140:16, 1988.
3. Daum GS, et al: Dipstick evaluation of hematuria in abdominal trauma, *Am J Clin Pathol* 89:538, 1988.
4. McAninch JW: Traumatic injuries to the urethra, *J Trauma* 21: 291-297, 1981.
5. Pontes JE, Pierce JM Jr: Anterior urethral injuries: four years of experience at the Detroit General Hospital, *J Urol* 120:563-564, 1978.
6. Carter CT, Schafer N: Incidence of urethral disruption in females with traumatic pelvic fractures, *Am J Emerg Med* 11:218-220, 1993.
7. Diekmann-Guiroy B, Young DH: Female urethral injury secondary to blunt pelvic trauma, *Ann Emerg Med* 20:1376-1378, 1991.
8. Devine PC, Devine CJ: Posterior urethral injuries associated with pelvic fractures, *Urology* 20:467-470, 1982.
9. Brosman SA, Paul JG: Trauma of the bladder, *Surg Gynecol Obstet* 143:605-608, 1976.
10. Cass AS: Bladder trauma in the multiple injured patient, *J Urol* 115:667-669, 1976.
11. Corriere JN Jr, Sandler CM: Management of the ruptured bladder: seven years of experience with 111 cases, *J Trauma* 26:830-833, 1986.
12. Cass AS: Diagnostic studies in bladder rupture: indications and techniques, *Urol Clin North Am* 16:267-273, 1989.
13. Clark SS, Prudencio RF: Lower urinary tract injuries associated with pelvic fractures: diagnosis and management, *Surg Clin North Am* 52:183-201, 1972.
14. Tile M: Pelvic fractures: operative versus nonoperative treatment, *Orthop Clin North Am* 11:423-464, 1980.
15. Carroll PR, McAninch JW: Major bladder trauma: the accuracy of cystography, *J Urol* 130:887-888, 1983.
16. Cass AS, Ireland GW: Bladder trauma associated with pelvic fractures in severely injured patients, *J Trauma* 13:205-212, 1973.
17. Lieberman AH, et al: Negative cystography with bladder rupture: presentation of 2 cases and review of the literature, *J Urol* 123:428-430, 1980.
18. Schiff M, Glickman MG, Herter GE: Radiologic procedures for the evaluation of urinary tract trauma. In Roberts JR, Hedges JR (editors): *Clinical procedures in emergency medicine*, Philadelphia, 1991, Saunders.
19. Mee SL, McAnich JW, Federle MP: Computerized tomography in bladder rupture: diagnostic limitations, *J Urol* 137:207-209, 1987.
20. Rehm CG, et al: Blunt traumatic bladder rupture: the role of retrograde cystogram, *Ann Emerg Med* 20:845-847, 1991.
21. Guerriero WG: Ureteral injury, *Urol Clin North Am* 16:237-248, 1989.
22. Holden S, et al: Gunshot wounds of the ureter: a 15-year review of 63 consecutive cases, *J Urol* 116:562-564, 1976.
23. Walker JA: Injuries of the ureter due to external violence, *J Urol* 102:410-413, 1969.
24. Presti JC, Carroll PR, McAninch JW: Ureteral and renal pelvic injuries from external trauma: diagnosis and management, *J Trauma* 29:370-374, 1989.
25. Boston VE, Smith BT: Bilateral pelvi-ureteric avulsion following closed trauma, *Br J Urol* 47:149-151, 1975.
26. Diokno AC: Avulsion of the proximal ureter secondary to blunt trauma, *J Urol* 111:412-414, 1974.
27. Rao CR: Ureteral avulsion secondary to blunt abdominal injury, *J Urol* 110:188-190, 1973.
28. Mulligan JM, et al: Ureteropelvic junction disruption secondary to blunt trauma: excretory phase imaging (delayed films) should help prevent a missed diagnosis, *J Urol* 159:67-70, 1998.
29. Bright TC, White K, Peters PC: Significance of hematuria after trauma, *J Urol* 120:455-456, 1978.
30. Cass AS, et al: Clinical indications for radiographic evaluation of blunt renal trauma, *J Urol* 136:370-371, 1986.
31. Eastham JA, Wilson TG, Ahlering TE: Radiographic assessment of blunt renal trauma, *J Trauma* 31:1527-1528, 1991.
32. Guice K, et al: Hematuria after blunt trauma: when is pyelogram useful? *J Trauma* 23:305-311, 1983.
33. Hardeman SW, et al: Blunt urinary tract trauma: identifying those patients who require radiological diagnostic studies, *J Urol* 138:99-101, 1987.
34. Klein S, et al: Hematuria following blunt abdominal trauma: the utility of intravenous pyelography, *Arch Surg* 123:1173-1177, 1988.
35. Mee SL, et al: Radiographic assessment of renal trauma: a 10-year prospective study of patient selection, *J Urol* 141:1095-1098, 1989.
36. Nicolaisen GS, et al: Renal trauma: Re-evaluation of the indications for radiographic assessment, *J Urol* 133:183-187, 1985.
37. Peterson NE, Schulze KA: Selective diagnostic uroradiography for trauma, *J Urol* 137:449-451, 1987.
38. Thomason RB, et al: Microscopic hematuria after blunt trauma: is pyelogram necessary? *Am Surg* 55:145-150, 1989.
39. Miller RC, et al: The incidental discovery of occult abdominal tumors in children following blunt abdominal trauma, *J Trauma* 6:99-106.
40. Smith EM, Elder JS, Spirnak JP: Major blunt renal trauma in the pediatric population: is a nonoperative approach indicated? *J Urol* 149:546-548, 1993.
41. Morey AF, Bruce JE, McAninch JW: Efficacy of radiographic imaging in pediatric blunt renal trauma, *J Urol* 156:2014-2018, 1996.
42. Stein JP, et al: Blunt renal trauma in the pediatric population: indications for radiographic evaluation, *Urology* 44:406-410, 1994.
43. Hashmi A, Klassen T: Correlation between urinalysis and intravenous pyelography in pediatric abdominal trauma, *J Emerg Med* 13:255-258, 1995.
44. Middlebrook PF, Schillinger JF: Hematuria and intravenous pyelography in pediatric blunt renal trauma, *Can J Surg* 36:59-62, 1993.

45. Lieu TA, et al: Hematuria and clinical findings as indications for intravenous pyelography in pediatric blunt renal trauma, *Pediatrics* 82:216-222, 1988.
46. Fleisher G: Prospective evaluation of selective criteria for imaging among children with suspected blunt renal trauma, *Pediatr Emerg Care* 5:8-11, 1989.
47. Cass AS: Blunt renal trauma in children, *J Trauma* 23:123-127, 1983.
48. Bass DH, Semple PL, Cywes S: Investigation and management of blunt renal injuries in children: a review of 11 years' experience, *J Pediatr Surg* 26:196-200, 1991.
49. Bretan PN Jr., et al: Computerized tomographic staging of renal trauma: 85 consecutive cases, *J Urol* 136:561-565, 1986.
50. Cass AS, Vieira J: Comparison of IVP and CT findings in patients with suspected severe renal injury, *Urology* 29:484-487, 1987.
51. Lang EK: Intra-abdominal and retroperitoneal organ injuries diagnosed on dynamic computed tomograms obtained for assessment of renal trauma, *J Trauma* 30:1161-1168, 1990.
52. McAninch JW, Federle MP: Evaluation of renal injuries with computerized tomography, *J Urol* 128:456-460, 1982.
53. Sandler CM, Toombs BD: Computed tomographic evaluation of blunt renal injuries, *Radiology* 141:461-466, 1981.
54. Federle MP, et al: The role of computed tomography in renal trauma, *Radiology* 141:455-460, 1981.
55. Stevenson J, Battistella FD: The "one-shot" intravenous pyelogram: is it indicated in unstable trauma patients before celiotomy? *J Trauma* 36:828-833, 1994.
56. Cass AS: Renovascular injuries from external trauma: diagnosis, treatment, and outcome, *Urol Clin North Am* 16:213-220, 1989.
57. Carroll PR, et al: Renovascular trauma: risk assessment, surgical management, and outcome, *J Trauma* 30:547-552, 1990.
58. Frassinelli P, et al: Bilateral renal artery thrombosis secondary to blunt trauma: case report and review of the literature, *J Trauma* 42:330-332, 1997.
59. Klink BK, et al: Traumatic bilateral renal artery thrombosis diagnosed by computed tomography with successful revascularization: case report, *J Trauma* 32:259-262, 1992.
60. Dinchman KH, Spirnak JP: Traumatic renal artery thrombosis: evaluation and treatment, *Semin Urol* 13:90-93, 1995.
61. Smith SD, Gardner MJ, Rowe MI: Renal artery occlusion in pediatric blunt abdominal trauma: decreasing the delay from injury to treatment, *J Trauma* 35:861-864, 1993.
62. Haas CA, et al: Traumatic renal artery occlusion: a 15-year review, *J Trauma* 45:557-561, 1998.
63. Goodman DN, Saibil EA, Kodama RT: Traumatic intimal tear of the renal artery treated by insertion of a Palmaz stent, *Cardiovasc Intervent Radiol* 21:69-72, 1998.
64. Swana HS, et al: Renal artery pseudoaneurysm after blunt abdominal trauma: case report and literature review, *J Trauma* 40:459-461, 1996.
65. Jebara VA, et al: Renal artery pseudoaneurysm after blunt abdominal trauma, *J Vasc Surg* 27:362-365, 1998.

22 Pelvic Ring Fractures

MICHAEL A. GIBBS AND MICHAEL J. BOSSE

Fractures that disrupt the pelvic ring are a common and often life-threatening consequence of major trauma. These injuries pose a unique challenge to the emergency physician (EP), and are frequently complicated by injuries to the genitourinary (GU) tract, pelvic vessels, abdominal viscera, chest, and central nervous system. Because of the high risk of associated injury and hemorrhage, the emergency department (ED) management of pelvic trauma requires a sound understanding of the biomechanics of injury, clinical presentation, and essentials of early resuscitation. A reasoned diagnostic and therapeutic plan, and the involvement of a multidisciplinary team is pivotal in the initial care of these complex injuries.

Approximately 60% of pelvic ring injuries are the result of vehicular trauma. Motorcycle crashes and pedestrians struck by cars contribute an additional 9% and 12% of cases, respectively. Falls from a height cause another 10%, and direct pelvic crush injuries make up the balance.[1,2] Pelvic fractures are the third most common cause of death in motor vehicle crashes (MVCs), ranking behind traumatic brain injury and blunt aortic disruption. The overall mortality associated with pelvic trauma remains approximately 10%.[3-6]

ANATOMIC CONSIDERATIONS

The pelvic ring is made up of three bones, the sacrum and two innominates. Each innominate is formed by the fusion of three separate centers of ossification, the ilium, the ischium, and the pubis. They meet at the triradiate cartilage, which fuses by 16 years of age. The posterior pelvis transmits the major weight bearing forces across the sacroiliac joint into the lower extremities. Its integrity is critical for pelvic ring stability. The posterior pelvic ring is strengthened by several ligaments: the anterior and posterior sacroiliac ligaments, sacrospinous ligament, and sacrotuberous ligament (Fig. 22-1). Anteriorly the pubic symphysis acts as a strut, preventing collapse of the pelvis. Disruption of the symphysis alone does not lead to instability, provided that the posterior ligamentous structures remain intact.

It is impossible to divorce pelvic ring trauma from injury to adjacent soft tissues, which may be clinically far more serious that the primary bony insult. Vascular injury of the internal and external iliac vessels and their branches is particularly likely following disruption of the posterior pelvis. The ureters, bladder, and urethra are in close proximity, and are vulnerable to injury in pelvic trauma. The lumbosacral plexus and its nerve roots that pass through and exit the sacrum are also susceptible.

CLASSIFICATION

When forces are applied to the pelvic ring, it breaks or dislocates in reproducible patterns that correlate with these force vectors.[7] An understanding of these forces help the clinician predict specific injury patterns during the early phase of patient evaluation and treatment. Several different classification systems have been developed for pelvic ring injuries. A common objective is assessment of pelvic instability based on the admission anteroposterior (AP) radiograph. The nature and degree of pelvic instability can predict the risk of hemorrhage and associated injury. The most widely accepted classification system is based on the mechanism of injury and direction of the causative force vector. This concept was originally developed by Pennal et al,[8] and several modifications of this system have since been published.[9-11] Using this approach, the EP can identify patients at risk for hemodynamic deterioration, formulate a comprehensive diagnostic plan, and communicate effectively with

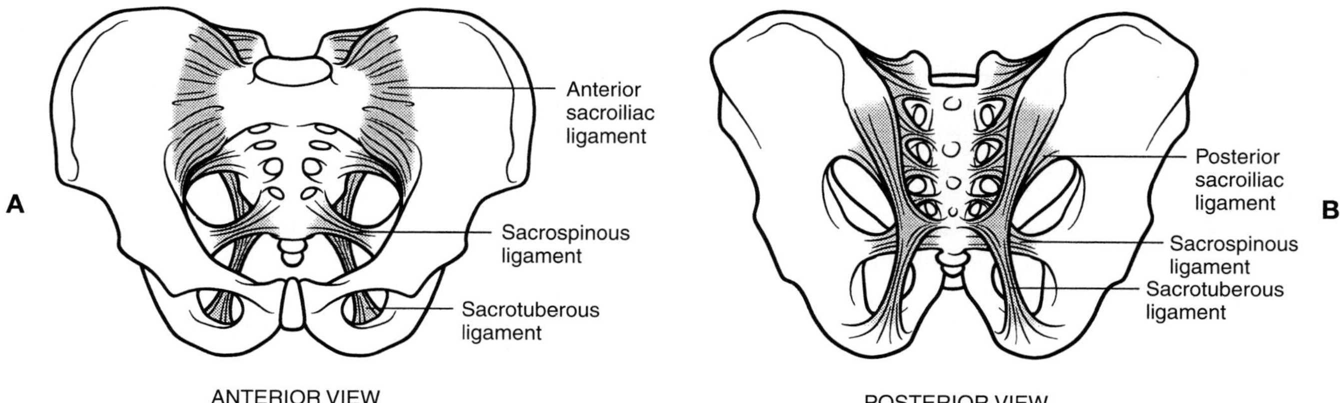

Fig. 22-1 Ligamentous support of the bony pelvis, anterior **(A)** and posterior **(B)** views. The posterior pelvic ring is stabilized by several strong ligaments. Disruption in this region implies major energy transfer and the potential for significant multisystem injury.

the consulting traumatologist and orthopedic surgeon during the early phase of patient resuscitation.

There are three types of force that may produce pelvic fractures: *lateral compression, anteroposterior compression,* and *vertical shear.* "Complex patterns" describe injuries that are the result of more than one force vector, although in most cases a dominant vector is usually identified. History obtained from the patient and prehospital care providers is helpful in predicting injury patterns.

Lateral Compression

Lateral compression fractures are the most common injury, accounting for roughly half of all pelvic ring injuries. As the name suggests, the force is delivered to the pelvis from the side. These injuries most commonly occur in "T-bone" MVCs or when a pedestrian is struck from the side. Lateral compression injuries are associated with a high incidence of traumatic brain injury, which is usually the primary cause of morbidity and mortality.

Anteroposterior Compression

Anteroposterior compression fractures account for 20% to 30% of pelvic ring fractures. Force is delivered in an anteroposterior, and less commonly in a posterior-anterior, direction. AP compression may occur following a head-on MVC, or when a pedestrian is struck head-on by an oncoming vehicle. Patients with AP compression injuries have a high incidence of thoracic, abdominal, and pelvic vascular injuries. Morbidity and mortality are the result of the combined effect of pelvic bleeding and other visceral injuries.

Vertical Shear

Vertical shear injuries are rare. They occur when a vertically oriented force is delivered to the pelvis via the extended femurs. Vertical sheer usually is the result of a fall from a height, or following a head-on MVC in which the occupant has the leg fully extended. Alternatively, a downward force delivered to the pelvis via the spine, as may occur when a heavy object falls on the back or shoulders, may produce a vertical shear injury. Patients with vertical shear fractures have a similar injury pattern to patients with lateral compression injuries.

ASSOCIATED INJURIES

Because of the magnitude of force required to disrupt the pelvic ring, associated trauma is common. Associated injuries include injuries of adjacent viscera, as well as organs distant to the pelvis. In one series of 348 patients with pelvic fractures, only 32 patients (9%) had injury isolated to the pelvic ring.[12] Pelvic fracture survivors sustain an average of 1.89 injuries in addition to their fracture, whereas nonsurvivors sustain 2.95 additional injuries.[13] A review of over 1000 pelvic fractures found associated neurologic injury in 27%, thoracic injury in 26%, and abdominal injury in 14%.[14] The fracture pattern on the admission pelvic radiograph may predict the severity of associated injuries. Dalal et al[1] reviewed a series of patients with pelvic fractures in an attempt to define the relationship between the causative force vector and associated injuries. The authors noted that AP compression fractures were associated with severe injuries to the torso, whereas lateral compression fractures were associated with traumatic brain injury. A pelvic fracture in a patient suffering blunt trauma should not be viewed as a "broken bone," but rather as a red flag for life-threatening multisystem injury.

Pelvic fractures are associated with aortic injury, increasing the risk of blunt aortic disruption two- to five-fold compared with the overall trauma population.[15] Aortic injury is especially likely in patients with AP compression fractures, being eight times more frequent than in the overall blunt trauma population.[16]

The incidence of urologic complications associated with pelvic fractures is reported to be as high as 25%.[17,18] In 200 consecutive patients with pelvic fractures, researchers found bladder injuries in 9%, urethral injuries in 13.5%, and combined injuries in 1%.[19] The posterior urethra is firmly attached to the pubis by the puboprostatic ligament, making it prone to injury following anterior pelvic ring fractures. Between 5% and 25% of patients with pelvic fractures have an associated urethral injury. Conversely, a pelvic fracture is present in over 95% of patients with an injury to the posterior urethra.[20,21] Bladder injury is usually the result of perforation by fracture spicules. Between 4% and 8% of patients with pelvic fractures have an associated bladder injury, and 70% to 95% of patients with bladder injuries have concomitant pelvic fractures.[22-24] The fracture types most often associated with bladder injury include pubic ramus fractures, and the likelihood of bladder injury increases when multiple rami are fractured. Symphyseal diastasis and displaced two-part pelvic fractures also endanger the bladder.

Injuries of the vagina are a rare complication of pelvic fracture. Niemi et al[25] reviewed 114 females with pelvic fractures and found vaginal lacerations in only 4 patients (3.5%). Most result from penetration of a bone fragment through the vaginal wall. Shearing forces caused by pubic diastasis, or displacement of disrupted fracture segments, may also cause soft tissue injury and vaginal tears. Vaginal lacerations are often associated with urologic or rectal trauma, and the presence of one of these injuries should prompt a search for the others.[26,27] Pelvic fractures associated with vaginal or rectal lacerations are considered open, and prophylactic antibiotics (e.g., first-generation cephalosporin and aminoglycoside) should be administered. Early detection and repair of these injuries avoids potentially serious sequelae, including pelvic abscesses, vaginal-visceral fistulas, strictures, dyspareunia, osteomyelitis, and chronic pelvic pain.[28]

For anatomic reasons, pelvic injury about the sacroiliac joint and sciatic notch imperils the lumbosacral plexus. The sciatic nerve and its roots (L4, L5, and S1-3) are close to this area, and recent series estimate the overall incidence of neurologic injury complicating pelvic fractures to be 10% to 21%.[29-31] Unstable pelvic ring fractures with posterior disruption carry the considerably higher risk of 40% to 50%.[32-34] Clinically, most neurologic injuries involve the L5 or S1 nerve root.[34] Such patients may present with distal motor weakness (impaired dorsiflexion and/or plantarflexion of the great toe), numbness on the dorsal and lateral aspect of the foot, and a diminished Achilles tendon reflex.

OPEN PELVIC FRACTURES

Open pelvic fractures are invariably associated with severe injuries of the pelvic visceral, and in the past 30% to 50% of these patients died.[35,36] Brisk pelvic hemorrhage and associated torso and intracranial injury contribute to a high mortality. In survivors of the early resuscitation phase, heavy contamination of perineal wounds resulting from damage of the rectum and GU tract causes localized abscesses, sepsis, and multisystem organ failure.

A structured multidisciplinary approach to these devastating injuries, involving (1) aggressive hemodynamic stabilization, (2) internal pelvic ring stabilization, (3) primary repair of rectal injuries with diverting colostomy, and (4) primary repair of genitourinary injury and urinary diversion with a suprapubic catheter, has improved outcome and reduced mortality to under 10%.[37,38]

ASSESSMENT

Physical Examination

During the initial assessment of all patients suffering significant multisystem trauma the clinical imperative is to rapidly identify injuries posing a threat to life. The patient should be immediately exposed and a thorough primary and secondary survey completed. Airway management, hemodynamic stabilization, and the maintenance of adequate tissue perfusion are the priorities of initial care. Hypotension in the patient suspected of having a pelvic fracture is a critical finding, and a rapid and diligent search for the source of hypotension should be instituted at once. Once the airway is secure and hemodynamic stabilization initiated, the clinician can then perform a careful examination of the pelvis.

The goals of the examination of the pelvis are to (1) estimate the likelihood of fracture (and thus the need for radiography) based on clinical grounds, (2) assess the degree of pelvic ring stability, and (3) identify injuries of the adjacent viscera. Lower abdominal tenderness is common to all pelvic fractures, but does not reliably differentiate pelvic from intraabdominal injury. Systematically inspect and palpate the

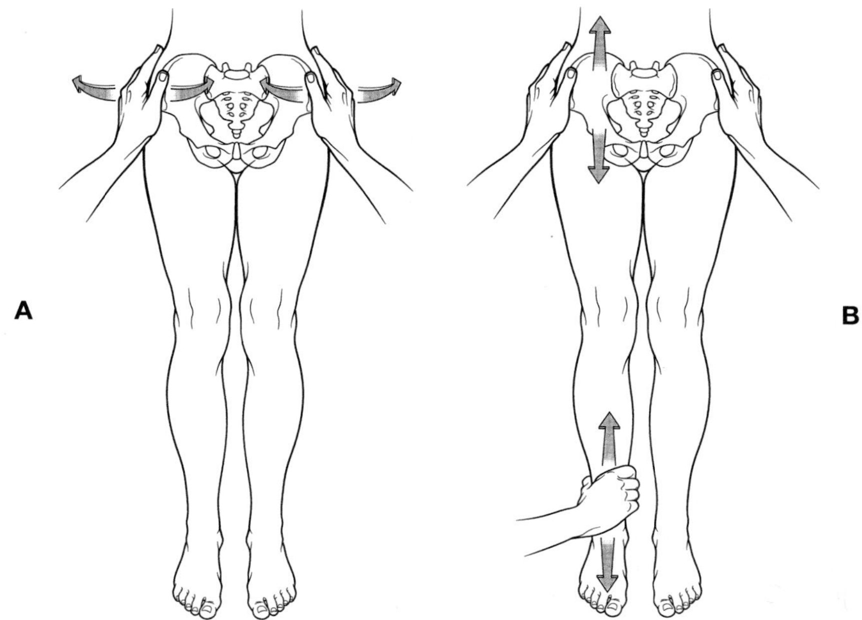

Fig. 22-2 Maneuvers to assess pelvic instability in the horizontal **(A)** and vertical **(B)** planes should be performed during the secondary survey. Since repeated pelvic movement may disrupt a stable pelvic hematoma, these maneuvers should be done once by an experienced examiner.

front and back of the pelvic ring to detect abrasions, contusions, lacerations, or crepitance. Look for tenderness or palpable instability with active hip flexion, direct downward pressure on the pubic bone, compression on the iliac wings, distractive pressure on the iliac crest, and vertical distraction of the extremities (Fig. 22-2). In one study the inability to actively flex the hip was the maneuver most reliably predictive of a pelvic fracture, with a sensitivity of 90% and a specificity of 95%.[39] The best examination is the first examination, and in the hemodynamically unstable patient, repeated overzealous pelvic manipulation is discouraged, since this maneuver may disrupt a pelvic hematoma and cause further bleeding.

The genitalia and perineum should be examined for signs of urologic injury (e.g., blood at the urethral meatus, penile or scrotal hematoma, abnormal prostate examination). A scrotal hematoma is a particularly important sign and may herald brisk pelvic bleeding. In patients with blood at the urethral meatus, perineal hematoma, or a high-riding prostate, perform a urethrogram *before* the insertion of a Foley catheter to avoid worsening of an incomplete urethral tear. A urethrogram should also be considered in patients with significant pelvic instability caused by anterior ring disruption. Once a urethral injury has been excluded, a retrograde cystogram should be performed in all patients with gross hematuria to rule out a bladder injury. A careful bimanual and speculum examination is mandatory in all female patients suffering pelvic trauma. Inspect perineal lacerations to identify associated intravaginal mucosal tears. Bleeding is the hallmark of vaginal trauma, although ongoing hemorrhage may not be grossly apparent because of vaginal muscle spasm. Hematuria, vaginal urine or stool, difficulty urinating, or difficulty passing a Foley catheter should also raise suspicion of a vaginal injury. Despite the need to consider associated injuries in pelvic fractures, always consider the priorities: vaginal, urethral, and bladder injuries never pose an immediate threat to life. Do not waste time in the hemodynamically unstable patient evaluating the genitourinary system when urgent laparotomy or pelvic vascular embolization is needed.

Perform a neurologic examination of the lower extremity, with particular attention to the L5 and S1 nerve roots to detect associated injury of the lumbosacral plexus. The L5 nerve root should be tested by assessing dorsiflexion of the great toe against resistance and sensation on the dorsum of the foot. Test the S1 nerve root by evaluating plantar flexion of the great toe against resistance, sensation on the lateral aspect of the foot, and the Achilles tendon reflex. Sphincter tone and perianal sensation should also be documented.

Pelvic Radiography

During the initial resuscitation of the patient suffering blunt trauma, the radiographic identification of a pelvic fracture has several important implications, which include the following:

- Reflects a major force-vector and risk for serious multisystem injury
- Rapidly identifies a potential site of life-threatening hemorrhage
- Provides clues to the likelihood of pelvic soft tissue and vascular injuries
- May alter the method and/or sequence of diagnostic testing
- Helps the clinician develop and prioritize management plan

INDICATIONS FOR PELVIC RADIOGRAPHY

Traditional teaching recommends routine pelvic radiography in all patients suffering significant blunt trauma.[40] Although this approach is effective at excluding injury, it comes at the expense of a large number of negative radiographs. Pelvic radiography should be routine in the severely injured blunt trauma patient who is either hemodynamically unstable or obtunded, or who has clinical evidence of abdominopelvic injury. Conversely, data suggest that a thorough physical examination can be used to identify the patient at low risk for pelvic fracture who can be managed safely without radiography; such patients include those without clinical signs and symptoms of pelvic injury. Civil et al[41] prospectively evaluated 265 patients suffering blunt multisystem trauma. There were 26 pelvic fractures (10%), none occurring in the awake, alert, and asymptomatic group. Another group studied 717 blunt trauma patients, and found no pelvic fractures in 125 patients who were hemodynamically stable, alert, and without pelvic pain or tenderness, gross hematuria, or presence of a femur fracture.[42] In a prospective study of 608 blunt trauma patients the negative predictive value of a negative physical examination was 99%.[43] In another study of 810 alert, asymptomatic blunt trauma patients only three (0.4%) had pelvic fractures, all of which were minor and did not affect the clinical course.[44] Selective use of pelvic radiography has obvious financial implications, reduces unnecessary exposure to radiation, and avoids potential delays in evaluation and treatment.

RADIOGRAPHIC PROJECTIONS

Anteroposterior View. The AP radiograph is obtained with the patient supine, and the beam directed perpendicular to the midpelvis and radiographic plate (Fig. 22-3). It should include the iliac crests, fifth lumbar vertebrae, each hip joint, and the proximal portion of each femur. The anatomic landmarks visible on the AP radiograph include the pubic symphysis, superior and inferior rami, anterior-superior and

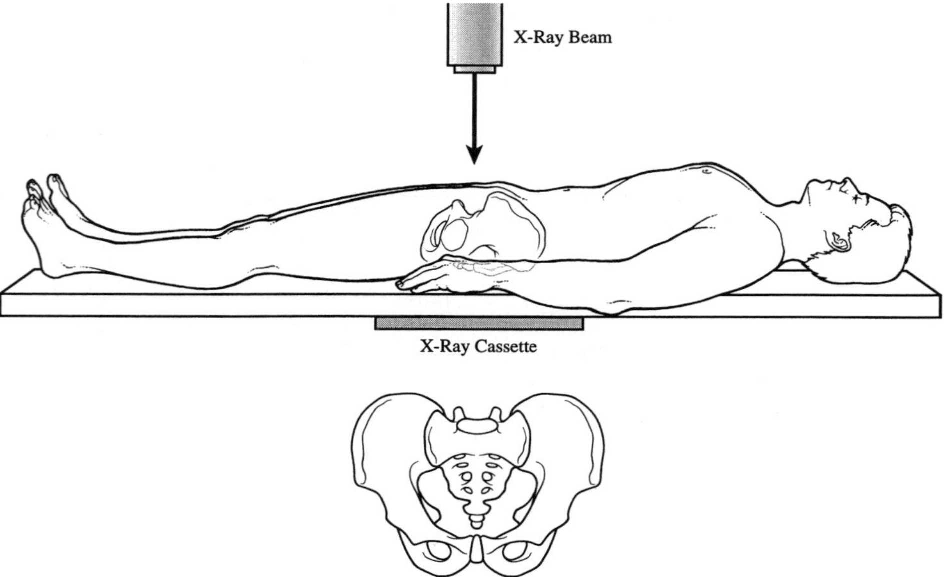

Fig. 22-3 The anteroposterior (AP) view of the pelvis. This view will demonstrate the majority of injuries, and it should be obtained early in the resuscitation. The AP view is 45° to 60° oblique to the pelvic brim. Radiographs at right angles to each other (inlet and outlet views) provide a more accurate assessment of ring disruption and pelvic displacement.

anterior-inferior iliac spines, sacroiliac joints, sacral ala, sacral foramen, and L5 transverse processes. Examine the anterior ring for pubic rami fractures, symphysis disruption, or combined lesions. Posterior pathology can present as iliac wing fractures, sacral fractures, or sacroiliac fracture dislocations.

The AP radiograph identifies most pelvic fractures and in most cases is sufficient to guide early management.[9,46] However, it is important to remember that in the supine position the pelvis lies 45° to 60° oblique to the long axis of the skeleton, making the AP radiograph an oblique view to the pelvic brim. Radiographs at right angles to each other (inlet and outlet views) provide a more accurate picture of pelvic displacement. Once hemodynamic stabilization is underway, the AP view can be supplemented by these views as needed. In the unstable patient do not delay or interrupt resuscitative efforts to obtain these additional views, especially when there is an indication for immediate laparotomy, pelvic angiography, or interfacility transport.

Inlet View. The inlet view is obtained with the patient supine, and the beam directed from the head to the midpelvis at an angle of approximately 35° to 40° from vertical (Fig. 22-4). This projection is perpendicular to the pelvic brim and affords a view of the entire pelvic ring. It provides excellent visualization of the sacral promontory, sacroiliac joint, ala and body of the sacrum, iliopectineal line, and the geometry of the pubic symphysis and ischial spines. The inlet view shows anterior and posterior displacement in the plane of the pelvis better than any other projection and is useful to assess displacement of the sacroiliac joint and iliac wings

Outlet View. The outlet view is obtained with the patient supine, and the beam directed cephalad from the foot to the symphysis at an angle of approximately 35° to 40° from vertical (Fig. 22-5). This view provides the best view of superior migration of the anterior hemipelvis, as might be seen in a vertical shear injury. It provides a true AP view of the sacral body and foramina and is useful to define fractures in this region. The inferior pubic ramus is also brought into full view.

RADIOGRAPH INTERPRETATION

Pelvic fractures are classified according to the mechanism of injury and predominant force vector. Each of these fracture types has characteristic radiologic features that can usually be identified on the AP radiograph.

Lateral Compression Fracture. Laterally directed compressive forces cause inward movement of the ipsilateral hemipelvis, hinging on the sacroiliac joint (Figs. 22-6 to 22-8). Since forces are primarily compressive, ligamentous injury may be minimal. Types LC-I through LC-III injuries describe progressive disruption of the posterior pelvic ring and resultant in-

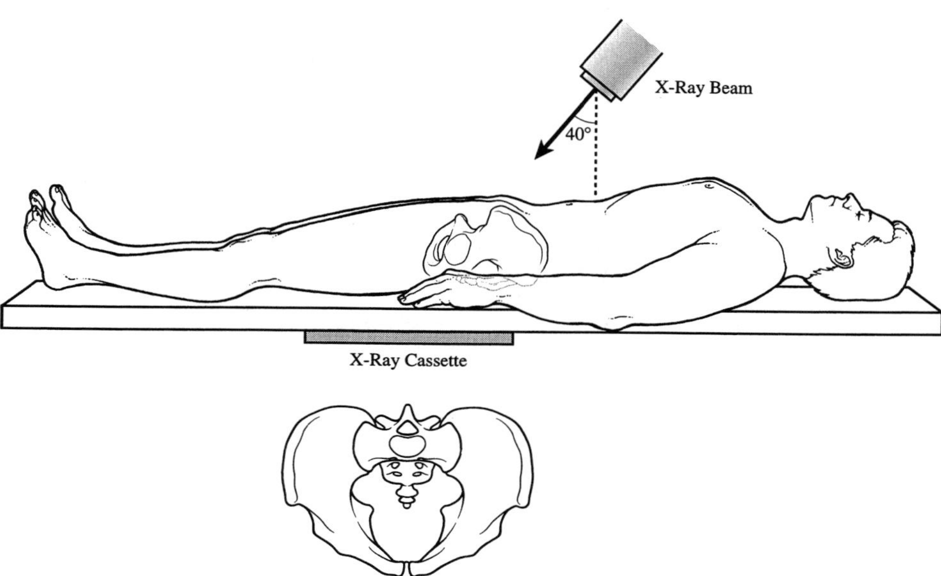

Fig. 22-4 Inlet view of the pelvis. This projection is perpendicular to the pelvic brim and provides the best view of the entire pelvic ring. The inlet view demonstrates anterior and posterior displacement in the plane of the pelvis better than any other projection.

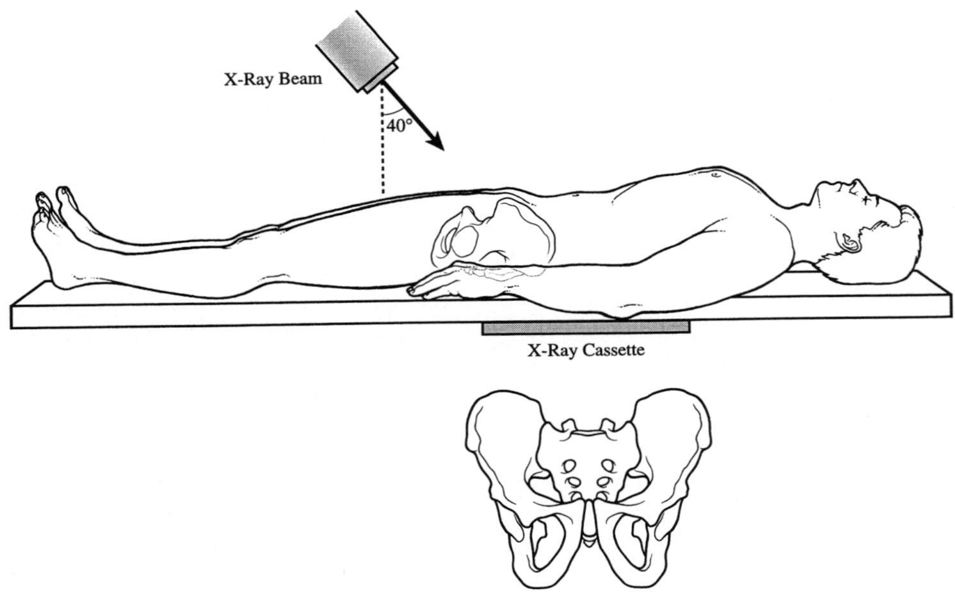

Fig. 22-5 Outlet view of the pelvis. This projection provides excellent visualization of the anterior pelvic ring and sacral body. The outlet view provides the most accurate assessment of vertical instability.

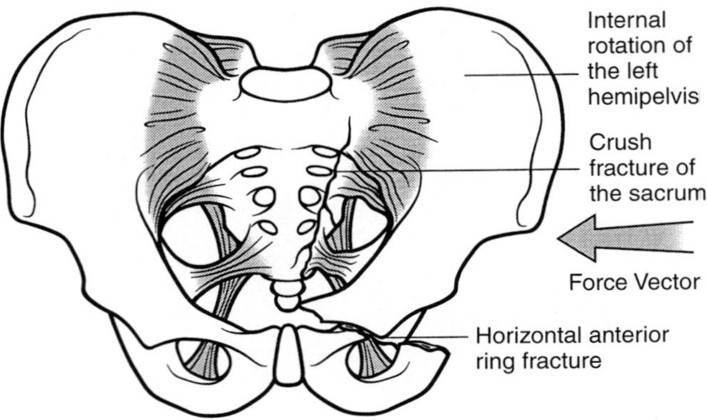

Fig. 22-6 Lateral compression injury. The characteristics of this injury pattern include (1) internal rotation of the affected hemipelvis, (2) an ipsilateral crush fracture of the sacrum, and (3) a distinctive *horizontal* anterior ring fracture.

stability, with increasing potential for hemorrhage and associated injury. Essential radiographic features of lateral compression fractures include the following:

1. Distinctive *horizontal* pubic rami fractures. These fractures are visible 80% of time on the AP view, 86% of time on the inlet view, and 100% of the time when these two views are used in combination. This feature alone is highly suggestive of lateral compression injury.
2. Crush fractures of the sacrum (88% of cases). These fractures may be subtle, visible only as a disruption of the arcuate lines. When combined with number 1, this feature is diagnostic of a lateral compression fracture.
3. Fractures of the acetabulum, quadrilateral plate, or central hip dislocations may also be seen.
4. Sacroiliac joint diastasis, in combination with the first three items, is also strongly suggestive of a lateral compression injury.

Anteroposterior Compression Fracture. A force vector delivered to the anterior elements of the pelvis causes rupture of the symphyseal ligament and diastasis of the anterior pelvic ring (Figs. 22-9 and 22-10). Cadaver studies have demonstrated that the posterior ligaments will tolerate up to 2.5 cm of diastasis. Beyond this point, progressive widening of the symphysis results in disruption of the anterior and then posterior sacroiliac joint, as well as the sacrospinous and sacrotuberous ligaments. Type I through type III injuries describe this progression. These injuries are referred to as "open book" pelvic fractures. Typically, radiographs demonstrate the following:

1. Vertically oriented pubic rami fractures, symphyseal diastasis, or both. Diastasis of greater than 2.5 cm reflects posterior ligament disruption (although the reverse does not always hold true).
2. A variable degree of sacroiliac joint disruption and instability.
3. Acetabular fractures may be seen in up to 52% of patients.

Vertical Shear Fractures. Vertical shear fractures result from a severe vertical force delivered over

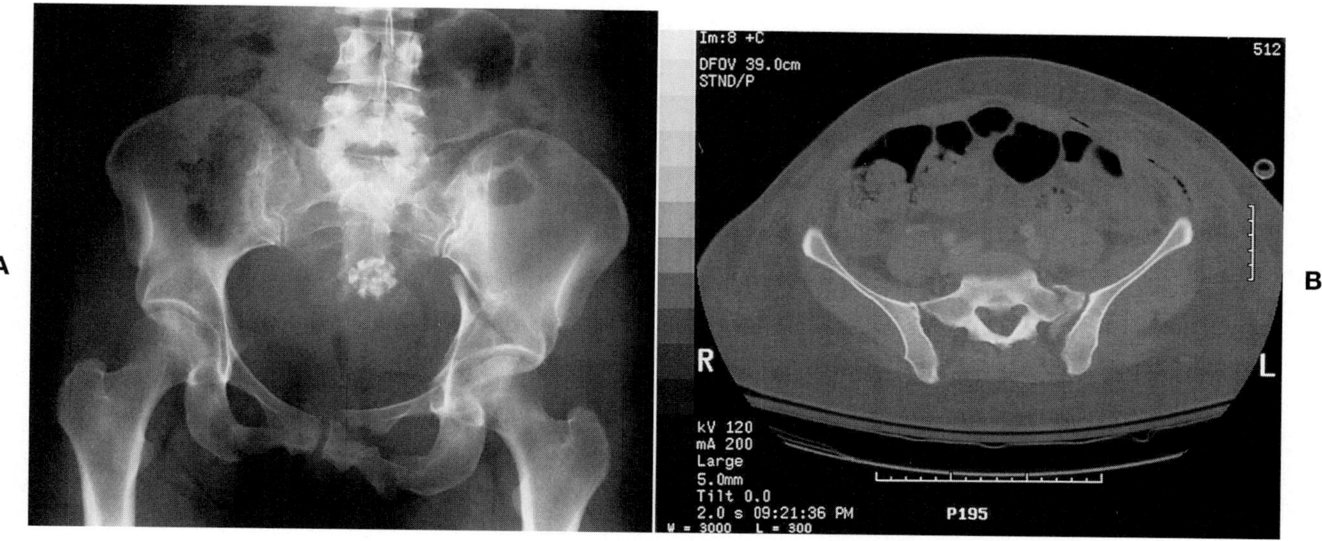

Fig. 22-7 Lateral compression injury. **A,** Anteroposterior projection demonstrating the characteristic horizontal anterior ring fracture *(arrow)* and ipsilateral sacral crush fracture. **B,** The sacral fracture is well visualized on the pelvic CT.

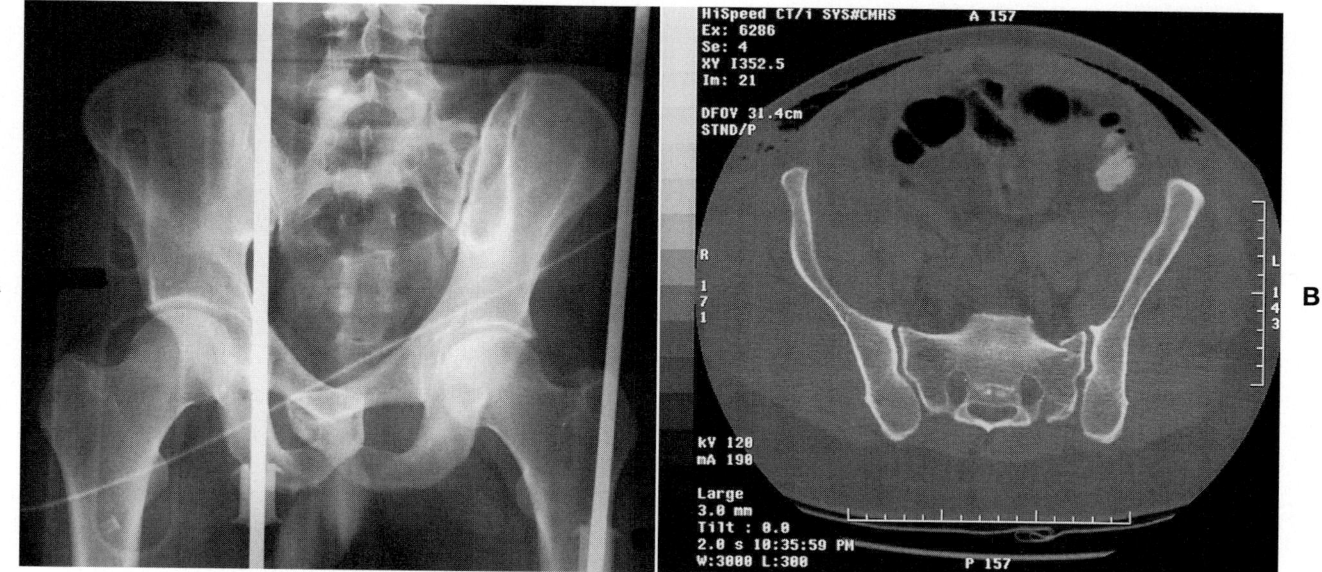

Fig. 22-8 Lateral compression injury. **A,** Anteroposterior projection demonstrating inward rotation of the left hemipelvis causing overlap of the anterior pelvic ring ("locked symphysis"). **B,** Computed tomography of the pelvis demonstrating the characteristic sacral crush fracture.

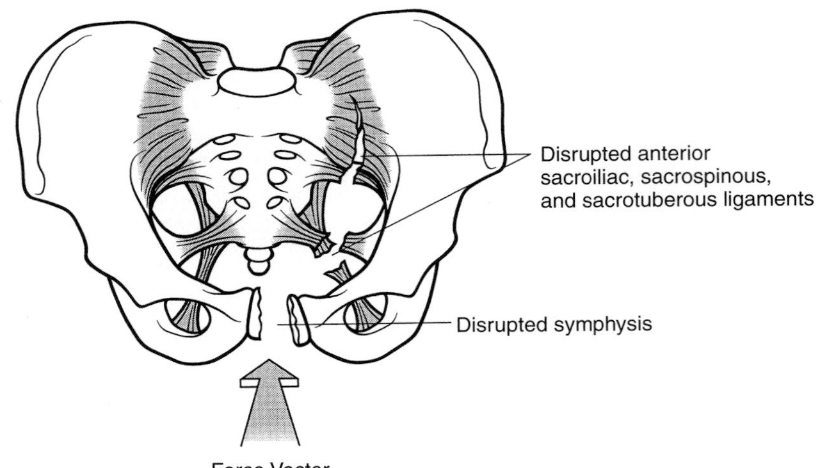

Fig. 22-9 Anteroposterior compression injury. The characteristics of this injury pattern include (1) severe posterior disruption manifest as either complete sacroiliac joint disruption, a vertical sacral fracture, or medial iliac wing fracture, and (2) symphyseal disruption or vertical pubic rami fractures.

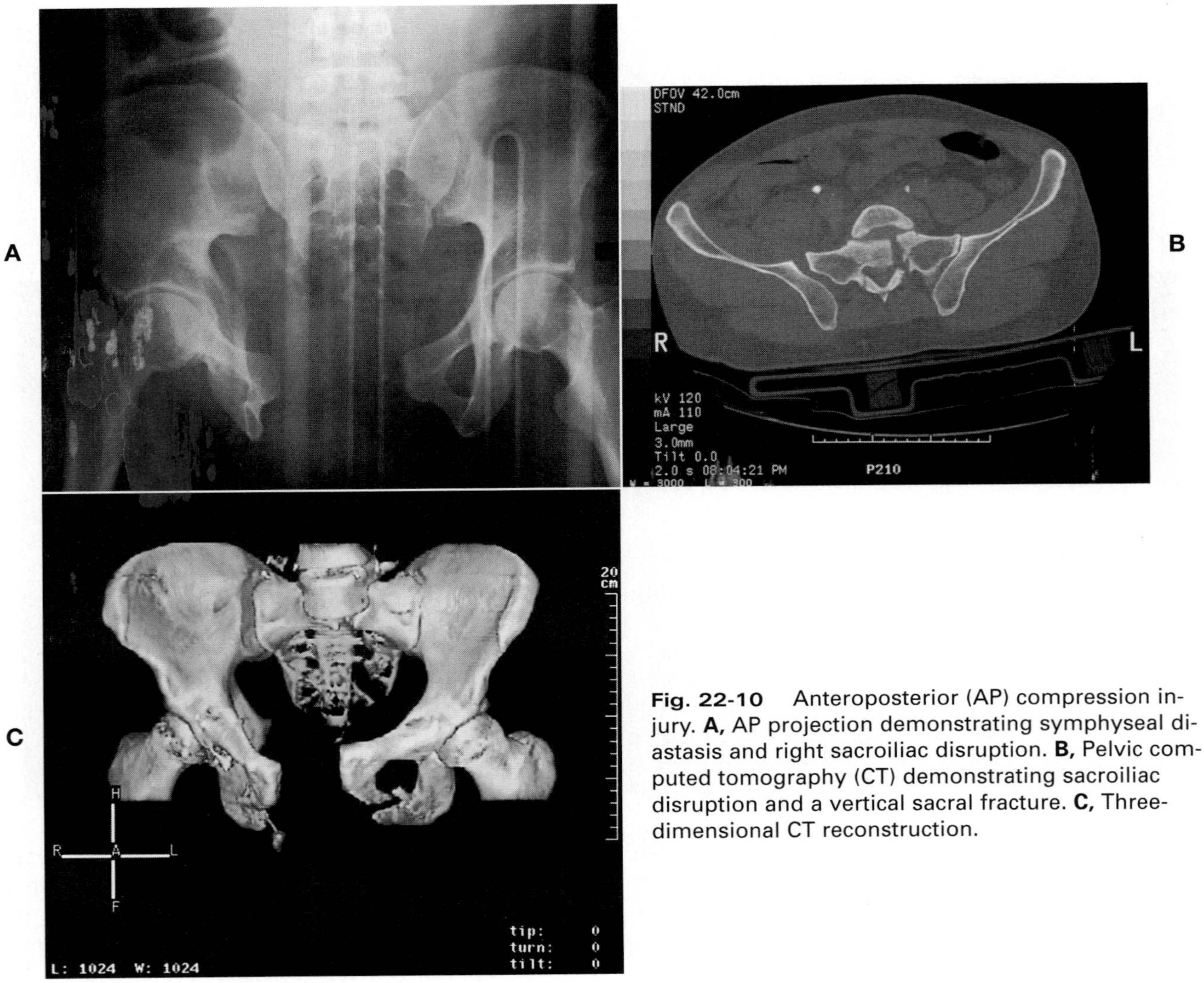

A

B

C

Fig. 22-10 Anteroposterior (AP) compression injury. **A,** AP projection demonstrating symphyseal diastasis and right sacroiliac disruption. **B,** Pelvic computed tomography (CT) demonstrating sacroiliac disruption and a vertical sacral fracture. **C,** Three-dimensional CT reconstruction.

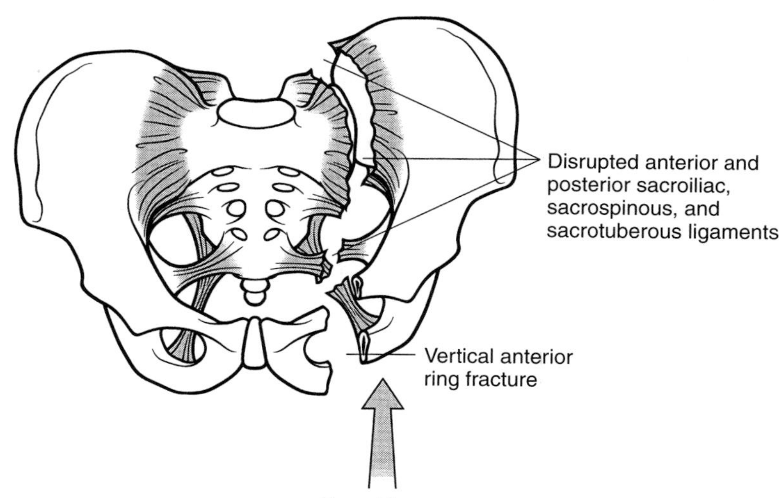

Fig. 22-11 Vertical shear injury. Characteristics of this injury pattern include (1) severe posterior disruption manifest as either complete sacroiliac joint disruption, a vertical sacral fracture, or medial iliac wing fracture; (2) vertical displacement of the hemipelvis; and (3) associated symphyseal disruption or vertical pubic rami fractures.

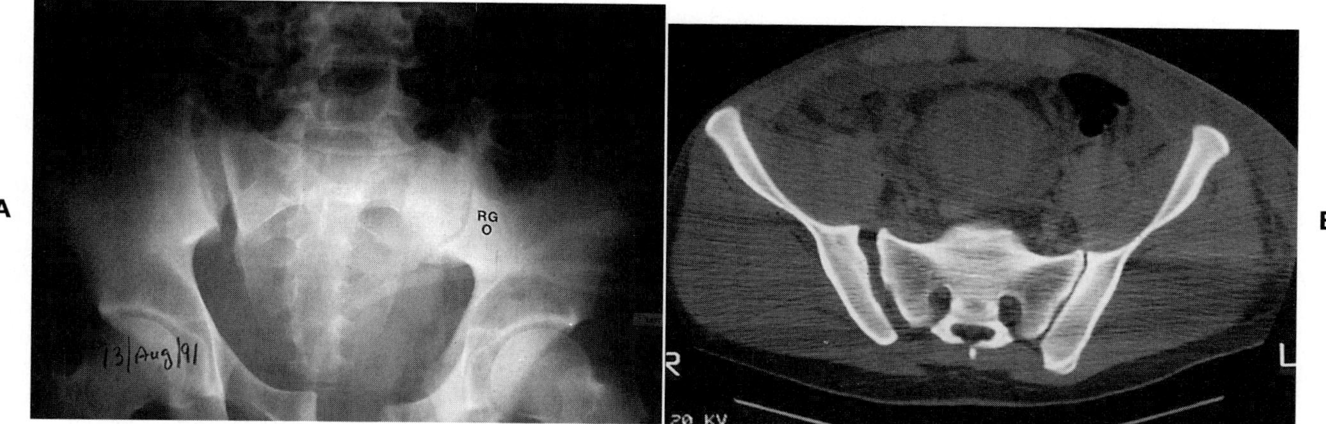

Fig. 22-12 Vertical shear injury. **A,** Anteroposterior projection demonstrating right sacroiliac joint disruption and vertical migration of the right hemipelvis. **B,** Pelvic computed tomography demonstrating right sacroiliac joint disruption.

one or both sides of the pelvis lateral to the midline (Figs. 22-11 and 22-12). These injuries are associated with disruption of both the anterior and posterior ring. Asymmetry of the hip joints in the vertical plain is a useful clue of vertical migration of one hemipelvis relative to the other. The outlet view is the best projection to assess superior displacement of fracture fragments. Radiographs will show the following:

1. Severe posterior disruption, manifest as either complete sacroiliac joint disruption, a vertical sacral fracture, or a medial iliac wing fracture.
2. Associated symphyseal disruption or pubic rami fractures.

Acetabular Fractures. Acetabular fractures are not considered pelvic ring injuries, although they may occur in combination with pelvic ring disruption. Acetabular fractures are often radiographically subtle, and can be easily missed on the AP film. In the stable patient with a known or suspected acetabular fracture, the AP radiograph should be supplemented by the Judet oblique views.[47] Although these plain radiographs are sufficient for fracture classification, they are usually followed by CT. Computed tomography images provide superior fracture definition, delineate the presence and extent of intraarticular fracture fragments, and give important preoperative information to the orthopedic surgeon.[48,49]

Early Detection of Intraperitoneal Hemorrhage

During the resuscitation of the hemodynamically unstable patient with pelvic trauma, it is critical to rapidly identify the predominant site of hemorrhage. Should pelvic bleeding pose the primary life-threat, angiography and skeletal stabilization is indicated. Conversely, if clinical instability is primarily the result of intraabdominal hemorrhage, laparotomy should be performed first. Taking a patient down the wrong branch of the algorithm can have devastating consequences: either uncontrolled pelvic hemorrhage in the operating suite or intraabdominal exsanguination in the angiography suite. Using diagnostic peritoneal lavage or ultrasonography, the EP can make an appropriate decision at the bedside (Fig. 22-13).

The objective of diagnostic peritoneal lavage (DPL) in this situation is to detect *life-threatening* abdominal hemorrhage, and *not* just the presence of intraperitoneal blood. The results of the DPL cell count can be misleading in patients with pelvic fractures and are not immediately relevant.[46,50] Instead, the DPL *aspirate* should be used to guide decision making. The aspiration of 5 to 10 cc of gross blood following the introduction of the catheter is considered "positive" and indicative of life-threatening abdominal hemorrhage. A positive peritoneal aspirate mandates immediate laparotomy, whereas a negative aspirate should be followed by pelvic angiography and vascular embolization. Moreno et al[5] studied the DPL results in 72 unstable patients with pelvic fractures. The DPL was negative in 22 patients and positive in 51 patients. Of note, 84% of patients with a positive DPL *aspirate* had active intraperitoneal hemorrhage at laparotomy, whereas all 19 patients with only a positive *cell count* had minor intraabdominal bleeding. In another study of 83 patients with pelvic fractures the DPL was negative in 37 patients and positive in 46. Once again, a negative DPL *aspirate* accurately excluded significant intraperitoneal hemorrhage in 100% of cases.[51] The open supraumbilical technique is preferred in patients with pelvic fractures.[52-54] Open DPL avoids the risk of blindly entering an anterior abdominal wall hematoma dissecting cephalad from the pelvis, and obtaining a false-positive aspirate. However, when this technique is used, it may be difficult to aspirate pelvic fluid because of the increased distance from the pelvic cavity, and the catheter must be fully advanced.

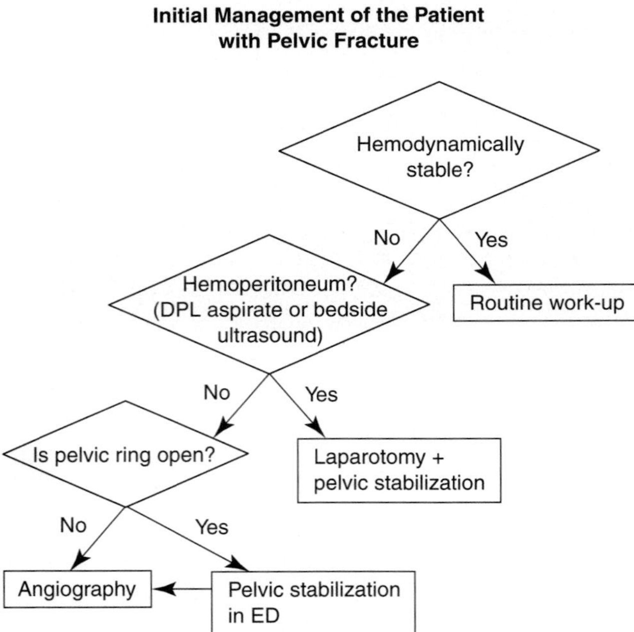

Fig. 22-13 Algorithm for the rapid bedside evaluation of the unstable pelvic fracture patient. It is critical to immediately identify the primary source of life-threatening hemorrhage. A diagnostic peritoneal *aspirate* or bedside ultrasound is used to evaluate for hemoperitoneum. When either study is positive, immediate laparotomy is indicated. If these studies are negative, stabilize the pelvis in the emergency department (e.g., pneumatic antishock garment, sheet wrapped around the pelvis) if the pelvic ring is open. This maneuver should be followed by pelvic angiography for vascular embolization.

Bedside ultrasonography (US) is rapidly becoming an important diagnostic tool in the ED evaluation of the trauma patient. A growing body of literature demonstrates the accuracy of US in the rapid bedside detection of hemoperitoneum.[55-59] In experienced hands, it can be performed within minutes during the secondary survey. When US demonstrates significant hemoperitoneum in the unstable patient with a pelvic fracture, immediate laparotomy is indicated.

MANAGEMENT

ABCs

Patients with pelvic fractures have the potential to deteriorate rapidly. For this reason, aggressive hemodynamic stabilization and vigilant monitoring of the patient's airway is essential. Stabilization is especially important before long trips to the radiology suite and certainly before interfacility transport. Should intubation be required, rapid sequence intubation (RSI) is the preferred technique for endotracheal intubation in the trauma patient.[60,61] It should be remembered that sedatives, which are an integral component of the RSI sequence, may cause or worsen hypotension in the volume-depleted patient. Agents with a favorable hemodynamic profile (e.g., etomidate, ketamine) are preferred over those more likely to worsen cardiovascular instability (e.g., barbiturates, benzodiazepines).[60-65]

A common pitfall in the initial management of the patient with significant pelvic injury is the failure to *anticipate* hypotension and initiate early aggressive resuscitation. In the setting of major blunt trauma, a pelvic fracture is an ominous finding and should immediately heighten the concern of the treating clinician. Adequate IV access with at least two large-bore IV catheters and careful monitoring is absolutely essential. Bedside determination of hemoglobin should be done at once, and blood should be sent for a complete blood count and crossmatch for type-specific blood. The serum lactate[66,67] and base deficit[68,69] may also provide an assessment of tissue perfusion and the adequacy of resuscitation. In the unstable patient, vigorous resuscitation with warmed crystalloid and early transfusion is essential. Because critically injured patients are at high risk for hypothermia, the core temperature should be monitored and measures taken to keep the patient warm.

Pelvic Stabilization

In patients with displaced pelvic ring fractures venous and arterial injury can be significant. Injuries that increase pelvic volume (i.e., AP compression and vertical shear injuries) create a potential space for unabated hemorrhage. Rubash et al[70] described a normal pelvic volume of 1.5 liters. This volume increased to 3 and 6 liters with diastasis of the pubic symphysis of 3 and 6 cm respectively. Pelvic stabilization provides benefit by reducing pelvic volume, stabilizing displaced fracture segments, and providing a tamponade effect on venous bleeding. Stabilization can be accomplished by several simple measures in the ED before the application of an external fixator or definitive operative repair. Internally rotating the lower extremities and wrapping a sheet tightly around the pelvis will close the pelvic ring to some degree in patients with anterior disruption. A pneumatic antishock garment (PASG) or vacuum splint will help maintain reduction, limit pelvic motion, and tamponade venous bleeding.[71,72] The use of PASG is especially well suited for the prehospital setting and for interfacility transport. When patients are brought to altitude during helicopter transport, the PASG must be monitored for expansion and deflated as needed.[73] Because prolonged use of the PASG has been reported to cause lower extremity compartment syndrome, this device should be considered a temporizing measure.[74,75] Several vacuum-splints, which envelope the patient and compress the pelvis, are also available. However, clinical experience with these devices in pelvic fracture patients is very limited.

Although its use has not been validated by prospective randomized trials, many clinical series advocate the early application of an external fixator in the unstable patient. External fixation reduces pelvic volume, provides a tamponade effect on venous bleeding, and decreases osseous bleeding by immobilizing and approximating the bones. Moreno et al[5] demonstrated that external pelvic fixation in the unstable patient decreased the average blood product requirement from 7.4 to 3.7 units. Others have noted a similar decrease on transfusion requirements following early pelvic stabilization.[76] Riemer et al[77] described a decrease in mortality from 41% to 21% in patients with pelvic fracture who were admitted with a systolic blood pressure of <100 mmHg after early external fixation. The pelvic C-clamp provides an alternative to standard external fixation, and can be rapidly applied in the ED.[78,79] Application of the C-clamp can be associated with serious iatrogenic complications, and we recommend that this device only be used by an experienced orthopedic surgeon. In addition to external fixation, skeletal traction should be applied to the ipsilateral lower extremity to control migration of the hemipelvis in patients with posterior instability.

Therapeutic Angiography

Venous bleeding is responsible for the majority of pelvic bleeding following blunt injury. Decreasing pelvic volume and stabilizing fracture segments will arrest venous bleeding in the vast majority of cases. However, injury of major pelvic arteries results in brisk hemorrhage resistant to pelvic stabilization alone. Arterial injury is uncommon in vertical compression injury, but can be found in up to 20% of patients with AP compression and lateral shear injuries.[80,81] In a series of 63 patients referred for angiography, Kam et al[82] found 123 arterial injuries in 49 patients. The superior gluteal, internal pudendal, obturator, and lateral sacral arteries were the most commonly injured vessels. Continued hemodynamic instability despite fracture stabilization is an indication for immediate pelvic angiography, after hemoperitoneum is ruled out by diagnostic peritoneal aspiration or by ultrasound. When arterial injury is present, vascular embolization is effective in 86% to 100% of cases, and improves outcome.[83,84] Because the time to embolization impacts survival, the angiography team should be mobilized as soon as possible.

Disposition and Transfer Issues

Patients with complex pelvic fractures benefit from the resources of regional trauma centers. A multidisciplinary team is essential in the care of these patients, and the rapid availability of an operating suite and/or angiography suite saves lives. Because patients may deteriorate swiftly, rapid transport to a trauma center or other hospital capable of handling such injuries is essential. The most common, and most lethal, errors in the early management of these patients are the failure to recognize and treat shock, and prevent delays in transfer. Preparation of the pelvic fracture patient for interfacility transport should include (1) appropriate clinical stabilization, (2) temporary stabilization of fractures that open the pelvic ring (e.g., PASG, vacuum splint, or a sheet wrapped tightly around the pelvis), (3) communication with the accepting clinical care team, and (4) transfer of appropriate medical documents.

A small minority of patients with pelvic fractures can be managed as outpatients. An example of this situation might be a patient with an isolated pubic ramus fracture who does not have evidence of additional injury after a thorough evaluation. The mechanism of injury and age of the patient should also be factored into the decision to send the patient home. When this option is chosen, consultation with an orthopedic surgeon, careful discharge instructions, and timely follow-up are absolutely essential.

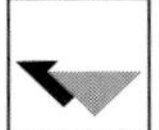

PEARLS & PITFALLS

- ◆ Recognize that pelvic trauma can be a cause of life-threatening hemorrhage.
- ◆ Aggressively resuscitate the patient and closely monitor his or her airway.
- ◆ Rapidly detect or exclude hemoperitoneum at the bedside using DPL or ultrasonography.
- ◆ Consider and evaluate for associated visceral injury (torso, genitourinary, neurologic).
- ◆ Temporarily immobilize fractures that open the pelvic ring (e.g., PASG, wrapped sheet).
- ◆ Initiate timely transfer to a level I trauma center.
- ◆ Failure to recognize shock and delays in transfer are important causes of preventable morbidity and mortality.

REFERENCES

1. Dalal SA, Burgess AR: Pelvic fracture in multiple trauma: classification by mechanism is key to pattern of organ injury, resuscitative requirements, and outcome, *J Trauma* 29:981:1988.
2. Melton LJ III, et al: Epidemiologic features of pelvic fractures, *Clin Orthop* 155:43, 1981.
3. Rothenberger DA, et al: The mortality associated with pelvic fractures, *Surgery* 84:356, 1978.
4. Gilliland MD, et al: Factors affecting mortality in pelvic fractures, *J Trauma* 22:691, 1982.
5. Moreno C, et al: Hemorrhage associated with major pelvic fractures: a multidisciplinary challenge, *J Trauma* 26:987, 1986.
6. McMurtry R, et al: Pelvic disruption in the polytraumatized patient: a management protocol, *Clin Orthop* 151:22, 1980.
7. Bucholz RW: Pathomechanics of pelvic ring disruptions, *Adv Orthop Surg* 10:167, 1987.
8. Pennal GF, et al: Pelvic disruption: assessment and classification, *Clin Orthop Rel Res* 151:12, 1980.
9. Young JWR, Burgess AR, Brumback RJ: Lateral compression fractures of the pelvis: the importance of plain radiography in the diagnosis and surgical management, *Skelet Radiol* 15:102, 1986.
10. Young JWR, et al: Pelvic fractures: value of plain radiography in the early assessment and management, *Radiology* 160:445, 1986.
11. Bucholz R: The pathological anatomy of malgaigne fracture dislocations of the pelvis, *J Bone Joint Surg* 63A:500, 1981.
12. Poole GV, Ward EF: Causes of mortality in patients with pelvic fractures, *Orthopedics* 17:691, 1994.
13. Fox MA, et al: Pelvic fractures: an analysis of factors affecting pre-hospital triage and patient outcome, *South Med J* 83:785, 1990.
14. Eastridge BJ, Burgess AR: Pedestrian pelvic fractures: 5-year experience of a major urban trauma center, *J Trauma* 42:695, 1977.
15. Ochsner MG: Pelvic fracture as an indicator of aortic rupture, *J Trauma* 29: 1376, 1989.
16. Ochsner MG Jr, et al: Associated aortic rupture-pelvic fracture: an alert for orthopedic and general surgeons, *J Trauma* 33:429, 1993.
17. Antoci JP, Schiff M Jr: Bladder and urethral injuries in patients with pelvic fractures, *J Urol* 128:25, 1982.
18. Fallon B, Wendt JC, Hawtrey CE: Urologic injury and assessment in patients with fractured pelvis, *J Urol* 131:712, 1984.
19. Palmer JK, Benson GS, Corriere JN: Diagnosis and initial management of urologic injuries associated with 200 consecutive pelvic fractures, *J Urol* 130:712, 1983.
20. McAninch JW: Traumatic injuries to the urethra, *J Trauma* 21: 291, 1981.
21. Pontes JE, Pierce JM: Anterior urethral injuries: four years of experience at the Detroit General Hospital, *J Urol* 120:563, 1978.
22. Clark SS, Pruencio RF: Lower urinary tract injuries associated with pelvic fractures: diagnosis and management, *Surg Clin North Am* 52:183, 1972.
23. Carroll PR, McAninch JW: Major bladder trauma: the accuracy of cystography, *J Urol* 130:887, 1983.
24. Cass AS, Ireland GW: Bladder trauma associated with pelvic fractures in severely injured patients, *J Trauma* 13:205, 1973.
25. Niemi TA, Norton: Vaginal injuries in patients with pelvic fractures, *J Trauma* 25:547, 1985.
26. Bredael JJ, et al: Traumatic rupture of the female urethra, *J Urol* 122:560, 1979.
27. Parkhurst JD, et al: Traumatic avulsion of the lower urinary tract in the female child, *J Urol* 126:265, 1981.
28. Siegel RS: Vesico-vaginal fistula and osteomyelitis, *J Bone Joint Surg* 53-A:583, 1971.
29. Majeed SA: Neurologic deficits in major pelvic injuries, *Clin Orthop* 282:222, 1992.
30. Reilly MC, Zinar DM, Matta JM: Neurologic injuries in pelvic ring fractures, *Clin Orthop* 329:28, 1996.
31. Huittinen VM: Lumbosacral nerve injury in fracture of the pelvis: a postmortem radiographic and pathoanatomy study, *Acta Chir Scand* 429(suppl):3, 1972.
32. Hyuttinen VM, Slatis P: Nerve injury in double vertical pelvic fractures, *Acta Chir Scand* 138:571, 1972.

33. Denis F, Davis S, Comfort T: Sacral fractures: an important problem. Retrospective analysis of 236 cases, *Clin Orthop* 227:67, 1988.
34. Helfet D, et al: Intraoperative somatosensory evoke potential monitoring during acute pelvic fracture surgery, *J Orthop Trauma* 9:28, 1995.
35. Birolini D, et al: Open pelvicoperineal trauma, *J Trauma* 30:492, 1990.
36. Davidson SB, et al: Pelvic fractures associated with open perineal wounds: a survivable injury, *J Trauma* 35:36, 1993.
37. Leenen LPH, et al: Internal fixation of open unstable pelvic fractures, *J Trauma* 35: 220, 1993.
38. Faringer PD, et al: Selective fecal diversion in complex open pelvic fractures from blunt trauma, *Arch Surg* 129:958, 1994.
39. Ham SJ, van Walsum AD, Vierhout PA: Predictive value of the hip flexion test for fractures of the pelvis, *Injury* 27:543, 1996.
40. American College of Surgeons, Committee on Trauma: *Advanced Trauma Life Support. ATLS Instructor Manual,* Chicago, 1988, ACS.
41. Civil ID, et al: Routine pelvic radiography in severe blunt trauma: is it necessary? *Ann Emerg Med* 17:488, 1988.
42. Koury HI, Peschiera JL, Welling RE: Selective use of pelvic roentgenograms in blunt trauma patients, *J Trauma* 34:236, 1993.
43. Yugueros P, et al: Unnecessary use of pelvic X-ray in blunt trauma, *J Trauma* 39:722, 1995.
44. Salvino CK, et al: Routine pelvic X-ray in awake blunt trauma patients: a sensible policy? *J Trauma* 33:413-416, 1992.
45. Mostafivi HR, Tornetta III P: Radiologic evaluation of the pelvis, *Clin Orthop* 329:6, 1996.
46. Hubbard SG, et al. Diagnostic errors with peritoneal lavage in patients with pelvic fractures, *Arch Surg* 114:844, 1979.
47. Hunter JC, Brandser EA, Tran KA: Pelvic and acetabular trauma, *Radiol Clin North Am* 35:559, 1997.
48. Brandser EA, El-Khoury GY, Marsh JL: Acetabular fractures: a systematic approach to classification, *Emerg Radiol* 2:18, 1995.
49. Mayo K: Fractures of the acetabulum, *Orthop Clin North Am* 18:43, 1987.
50. Gilliland MD, et al: Fractures affecting mortality in pelvic fractures, *J Trauma* 22:691, 1982.
51. Evers BM, Cryer HM, Miller FB: Pelvic fracture hemorrhage: priorities in management, *Arch Surg* 124:422, 1989.
52. Flint LM, et al: Definitive control of bleeding from severe pelvic fractures, *Ann Surg* 189:709, 1979.
53. Cochran W, Sobat WS: Open versus closed diagnostic peritoneal lavage: a multiphasic prospective randomized comparison, *Ann Surg* 200:24, 1984.
54. Rothenberger D, et al: The mortality associated with pelvic fractures, *Surgery* 84:356, 1978.
55. Kimura A, Otsuka T: Emergency center ultrasonography in the evaluation of hemoperitoneum: a prospective study, *J Trauma* 31:20, 1991.
56. Rozycki GS, et al: Prospective evaluation of surgeons' use of ultrasound in the evaluation of trauma patients, *J Trauma* 34: 516, 1993.
57. Bode PJ, et al: Abdominal ultrasound as a reliable indicator for conclusive laparotomy in blunt abdominal trauma, *J Trauma* 34: 27, 1993.
58. Ma OJ, et al: Evaluation of hemoperitoneum: using a single vs multiple view ultrasonographic examination, *Acad Emerg Med* 2:581, 1995.
59. Jehle D: Bedside ultrasonographic evaluation of hemoperitoneum: The time has come, *Acad Emerg Med* 2:575, 1995.
60. Walls RM: Airway management, *Emerg Med Clin North Am* 11: 53, 1993.
61. Walls RM: Rapid sequence intubation in head trauma, *Ann Emerg Med* 22:1008, 1993.
62. Bergen JM, Smith DC: A review of etomidate for rapid sequence intubation in the emergency department, *J Emerg Med* 15:221, 1997.
63. Ebert TJ, et al: Sympathetic responses to induction of anesthesia in humans with propofol or etomidate, *Anesthesiology* 76:725, 1992.
64. Gauss A, Heinrich H, Wilder-Smith OH: Echocardiographic assessment of the hemodynamic effects of propofol: a comparison with etomidate and thiopentone, *Anaesthesia* 46:99, 1991.
65. Batjer HH: Cerebral protective effects of etomidate: experimental and clinical aspects, *Cerebrovasc Brain Metab Rev* 5:17, 1993.
66. Abramson D, Scalea TM, Hitchcock R, et al: Lactate clearance and survival following injury, *J Trauma* 36:584, 1993.
67. Mizock BA, Falk JL: Lactic acidosis in critical illness, *Crit Care Med* 20:80, 1992.
68. Davis JW, et al: Base deficit as a guide to volume resuscitation, *J Trauma* 28:1464, 1988.
69. Davis JW, et al: Base deficit as an indicator of significant abdominal injury, *Ann Emerg Med* 20:842, 1991.
70. Rubash HE, Mears DC: External and internal fixation of the pelvis. In *AAOS Intsr Course Lect,* St Louis, 1983, Mosby.
71. Brown JJ, et al: Vascular injuries associated with pelvic fractures, *Am Surg* 50:150, 1984.
72. Clarke G, Mardel S: Use of MAST to control massive bleeding from pelvic injuries, *Injury* 24:628, 1993.
73. Sanders AB, Meislin HW: Effect of altitude change on MAST suit pressure, *Ann Emerg Med* 12:140, 1983.
74. Aprahamian C, et al: MAST-associated compartment syndrome (MACS): a review, *J Trauma* 29:549, 1989.
75. Kunkel JM: Thigh and leg compartment syndrome in the absence of lower extremity trauma following MAST application, *Am J Emerg Med* 5:118, 1987.
76. Edwards CC, et al: Results treating 50 unstable pelvic injuries using primary external fixation, *Orthop Trans* 9:434, 1985.
77. Riemer BL, et al: Acute mortality associated with injuries of the pelvic ring: the role of early patient mobilization and external fixation, *J Trauma* 35:671, 1993.
78. Ganz R, et al: The antishock pelvic clamp, *Clin Orthop* 267:71, 1991.
79. Buckle R, Browner BD, Morandi M: Emergency reduction for pelvic ring disruptions and control of associated hemorrhage using the pelvic stabilizer, *Tech Orthop* 9:258, 1994.
80. Burgess AR, et al: Pelvic ring disruptions: effective classification system and treatment protocols, *J Trauma* 30:785, 1990.
81. O'Neill PA, et al: Angiographic findings in pelvic fractures, *Clin Orthop* 329:60, 1996.
82. Kam J, Jackson H, Ben-Menachem Y: Vascular injuries associated with blunt pelvic trauma, *Radiol Clin North Am* 19:171, 1981.
83. Mucha P Jr., Farnell MB: Analysis of pelvic fracture management, *J Trauma* 24:376, 1984.
84. Agolini SF, Shah K, Jaffe J: Arterial embolization is a rapid and effective technique for controlling pelvic fracture hemorrhage, *J Trauma* 43:395, 1997.

Shoulder Trauma

23

MOHAMUD R. DAYA

The shoulder joint is a unique and complex articulation unit. It has the largest range of motion of any appendicular skeletal joint in the body and can be moved through a space that exceeds a hemisphere.[1] Unfortunately this wide range of motion also predisposes the joint to instability and injury. Shoulder injuries are frequently encountered in the emergency department (ED), and a recent study in Malmo, Sweden, documented an incidence of 219 per 100,000.[2] The most frequent injuries encountered in this study were fractures of the proximal humerus (53%), fractures of the clavicle (29%), and primary dislocations of the glenohumeral joint (11%). In general, children are vulnerable to the same injuries as adults. However, the presence of the epiphysis changes the pattern of injuries, since the strength of the joint capsule and its ligaments is two to five times greater than that of the epiphyseal plate.[3] Therefore an injury that produces a sprain or dislocation in an adult often causes a fracture through the hypertrophic zone of the growth plate in a child. This chapter focuses on the fractures and dislocations affecting the shoulder girdle complex, which consists of three bones (clavicle, humerus, and scapula), three joints (acromioclavicular, glenohumeral, sternoclavicular), and one articulation (scapulothoracic).

ASSESSMENT

History and Physical Examination

A thorough history and physical examination along with a radiologic evaluation are the keys to a precise diagnosis. Clinical evaluation begins with a thorough and well-directed history. The timing of the injury and its exact mechanism should be noted. Document the precise location of any pain and the presence of any systemic complaints. The history should also include the nature and results of any treatment before ED evaluation.

It is essential that the patient be disrobed so that both shoulders can be examined simultaneously. Any obvious deformity, ecchymosis, laceration, or hematoma should be noted. Begin palpation of the shoulder at the sternoclavicular (SC) joint and move laterally along the clavicle to the acromioclavicular (AC) joint. Palpation of the scapula, glenohumeral joint, and humerus completes the process. Any point tenderness, crepitus, swelling, or deformity should be noted. If possible, the active and passive range of motion should be tested in all patients. The degrees of abduction, forward flexion, extension, and internal and external rotation should be recorded and, where necessary, compared with the findings of the unaffected extremity. A thorough neurovascular examination should be performed and the results documented in all cases, before and following all manipulations.

Several simple maneuvers can detect rotator cuff tears. For example, the drop arm test is performed by elevating the arms over the head to each side (hyperabduction). Ask the patient to slowly lower them to his or her side. If the injured arm drops suddenly at around 90 degrees, the supraspinatus muscle is torn. In another test of the rotator cuff, the patient holds his or her arms extended in front at 90 degrees, with the thumbs pointing downward. A patient with a torn cuff will have weakness at the shoulder and be unable to resist downward pressure on the forearm.[1]

Radiology

Who deserves a shoulder x-ray? The issue is not completely clear, but it appears that few shoulder films contribute to management decisions. In one study, deformity on shoulder examination was the strongest predictor of an informative x-ray. No patients without a deformity or precipitating fall had a film that affected management. This decision rule may overlook patients with pathologic fractures and those with significant soft-tissue injuries—either fat or muscle—around the shoulder.[4]

The radiologic examination completes the clinical evaluation of the shoulder. Radiologic examination of any bone or joint in the appendicular skeleton requires a minimum of two views at right angles to one another. Standard anteroposterior (AP) views in internal and external rotation are considered unacceptable, since they project the shoulder in a single (frontal) plane.[5] At least one orthogonal projection must be included to complete the radiologic examination. Acceptable views include the axillary lateral, transscapular lateral, and apical oblique.[5-10] For traumatic injuries, Szalay and Rockwood[11] recommend a three-view series of radiographs consisting of a true AP (45° lateral), transscapular lateral, and axillary lateral. The true AP view is preferred over the standard AP projections since it projects the glenohumeral joint en face without any bony overlap.[11]

The preferred orthogonal view to date has been the axillary lateral (axillary view), which projects the glenohumeral joint in a cephalocaudal plane. This view is particularly useful in defining the relationship of the humeral head with the glenoid fossa and in identifying lesions of the coracoid process, humeral head, and glenoid rim.[6,12,13] Unfortunately, the axillary lateral is often difficult and painful in the setting of trauma, which has led to the popularity of the transscapular lateral or Y-view. The transscapular view is particularly useful in identifying anterior and posterior glenohumeral dislocations. Unfortunately, fine bony details are difficult to appreciate with this view. The apical oblique view (obtained by placing the injured shoulder in a 45° oblique position and angling the central ray 45° caudad) provides a unique coronal picture of the glenohumeral joint.[8,9] The view can be obtained easily and painlessly and studies have suggested that it is more sensitive than the transscapular view for detecting bone and joint abnormalities in the injured shoulder.[7,8]

The strict radiologic definition of the shoulder joint is restricted to the proximal humerus, distal clavicle, and scapula.[12] Additional views are necessary to complete the evaluation of the clavicle, humerus, and scapula. These views are reviewed in the appropriate sections. Lastly, developmental changes (acromial or coracoid apophysis) must not be mistaken for fractures in pediatric patients. These epiphyses, which appear at infancy, close at skeletal maturity (18 to 21 years of age).

SHOULDER COMPLEX DISLOCATIONS

Sternoclavicular Dislocations

Teaching Case

A 39-year-old male patient presents to the ED complaining of left-sided neck and shoulder pain 12 hours after a motor vehicle crash. He has an obvious seatbelt mark across his chest and his head is tilted to the left. There is tenderness to palpation over the medial end of the left clavicle. Range of motion testing in all directions is limited by pain and the neurovascular examination is intact. His radiographs are reported as normal and the patient is discharged with his arm in a sling.

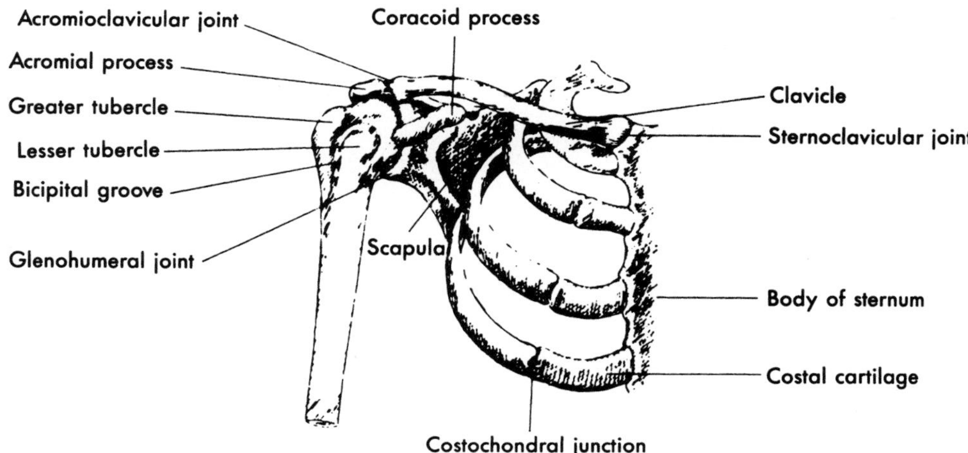

Fig. 23-1 Ligaments and the interarticular disk of the sternoclavicular joint. (Redrawn from DePalma AF: *Surgery of the shoulder,* ed 3, Philadelphia, 1983, JB Lippincott. In Rosen P, et al [editors]: *Emergency medicine: concepts and clinical practice,* ed 4, St Louis, 1998, Mosby.)

The sternoclavicular (SC) joint (Fig. 23-1) is the only true articulation point between the upper extremity and the axial skeleton. The articular surface of the sternal end of the clavicle fits poorly with the clavicular notch on the manubrium sterni and the stability of the joint is largely dependent on associated ligaments. These ligaments include the anterior and posterior SC ligaments, as well as the interclavicular and costoclavicular (CC) ligaments.[14] The latter opposes the pull of the sternocleidomastoid muscle and is considered the most important of the stabilizing ligaments.[15] The SC joint participates in all movements of the upper extremity and is the most moved joint in the body.[16] Immediately posterior to the joint lies the superior mediastinum with its vital structures.

EPIDEMIOLOGY

The SC joint is the least frequently dislocated major joint in the body. Significant forces are required to disrupt the strong ligamentous stabilizers of this joint. The SC joint can dislocate in an anterior or posterior direction but the former is much more common (9-to-1 ratio).[16]

PATHOPHYSIOLOGY

The usual mechanism of injury (Fig. 23-2) of an anterior dislocation involves an anterolateral force to the shoulder accompanied by backward rolling. Posterior dislocations (Fig. 23-2) can result from a direct blow to the medical clavicle or from a posterolateral force to the shoulder followed by inward rolling.[16] Posterior dislocations can be associated with life-threatening injuries within the superior mediastinum.

CLASSIFICATION

Injuries to the SC joint can be divided into three types.[17] Grade I injury is a mild sprain secondary to stretching of the SC and CC ligaments. A grade II injury is associated with subluxation of the joint (anterior or posterior) secondary to rupture of the SC ligaments. The CC ligament remains intact. Complete rupture of the CC and SC ligaments results in a grade III injury (dislocation). It is important to note that under the age of 25, grade III injuries actually represent Salter type I injuries since the medial epiphysis of the clavicle is still open.[18]

EMERGENCY DEPARTMENT PRESENTATION

Patients present with the injured extremity foreshortened and supported against the trunk by the opposite arm. There is pain with any movement of the upper extremity or lateral compression of the shoulders. The SC joint is usually swollen and tender to palpation. With an anterior dislocation, the displaced medial end of the clavicle may be palpable. Posterior dislocations are associated with more severe pain and the neck is frequently flexed towards the injured side.[17] The clavicular notch of the sternum may be palpable on the affected side, and there may be complaints of hoarseness, dysphagia, dyspnea and weakness, or paresthesias in the upper extremities. These patients should be examined thoroughly to identify any injuries to superior mediastinal or intrathoracic structures and, where necessary, obtain appropriate consultation.

DIAGNOSTIC STUDIES

Although the diagnosis of SC dislocations can often be made clinically, radiographic confirmation is re-

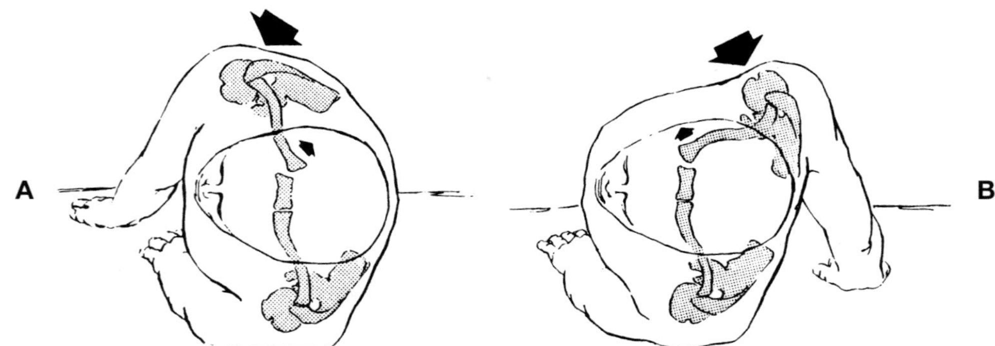

Fig. 23-2 Mechanism of injury causing sternoclavicular joint dislocations. **A,** When the patient is lying on the ground, and a compression force is applied to the posterior lateral aspect of the shoulder, the medial end of the clavicle is displaced posteriorly. **B,** When the lateral compression force is directed from the anterior position, the medial end of the clavicle is dislocated anteriorly. (From Neer CS, Rockwood CA: Fractures and dislocations of the shoulder. In Rockwood CA, Green DP [editors]: *Fractures in adults,* ed 2, Philadelphia, 1984, JB Lippincott.)

quired in most cases. Standard anteroposterior, oblique views, and special views (40° cephalic tilt) can be difficult to interpret because of overlapping rib, sternum, and vertebral shadows.[14] Overreliance on plain-film radiography can result in a failure to diagnose these injuries. These dislocations and any associated superior mediastinal injuries are best visualized by computed tomography (Fig. 23-3) scans.[14]

EMERGENCY DEPARTMENT MANAGEMENT AND DISPOSITION

Treatment of grade I and grade II injuries includes immobilization (simple sling or clavicular splint), adequate analgesia, and appropriate follow-up. Clavicular (figure-of-eight) splints (Fig. 23-4) are often preferred since they tend to maintain the clavicle in a more normal anatomic position.

Anterior dislocations may be reduced in the ED following appropriate consultation and intravenous (IV) analgesia (Fig. 23-5). A rolled sheet is placed between the shoulders in the supine position. Traction is applied to the arm in an extended and abducted position. If reduction does not occur, an assistant can add

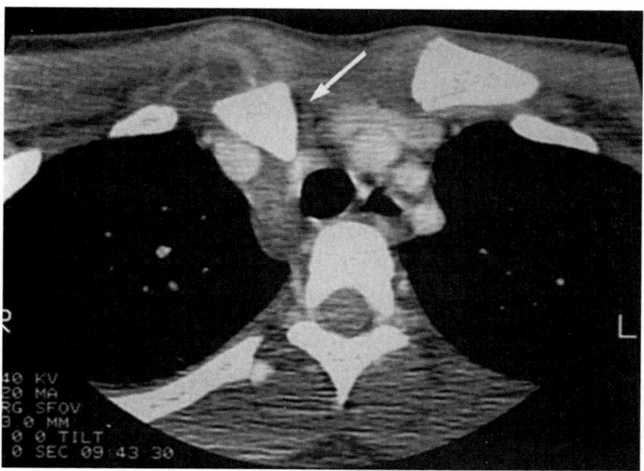

Fig. 23-3 CT scan showing posterior dislocation of the right sternoclavicular *(arrow)* joint with compression of the superior mediastinum. (Courtesy of Donald Sauser, MD.)

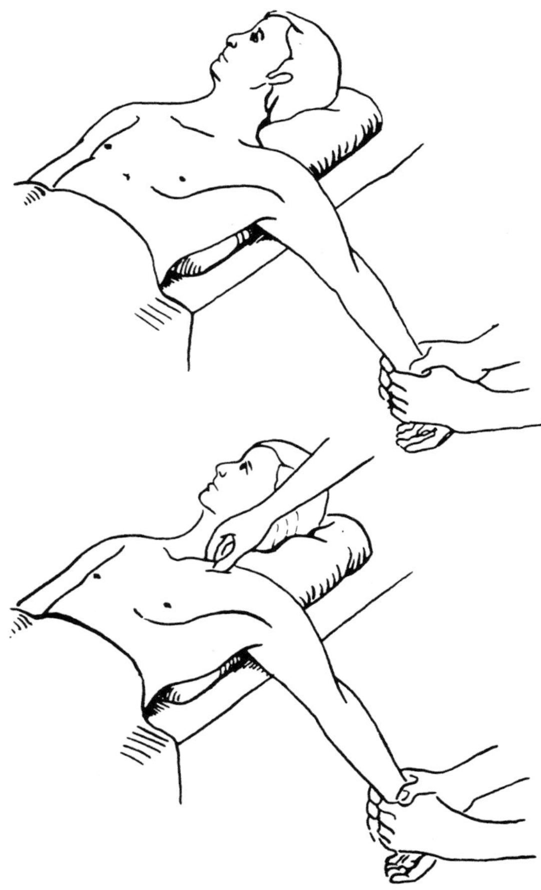

Fig. 23-5 Reduction of dislocated sternoclavicular joint. (From Simon RR, et al: *Emergency orthopedics: the extremities,* ed 2, Norwalk, Conn, 1987, Appleton & Lange.)

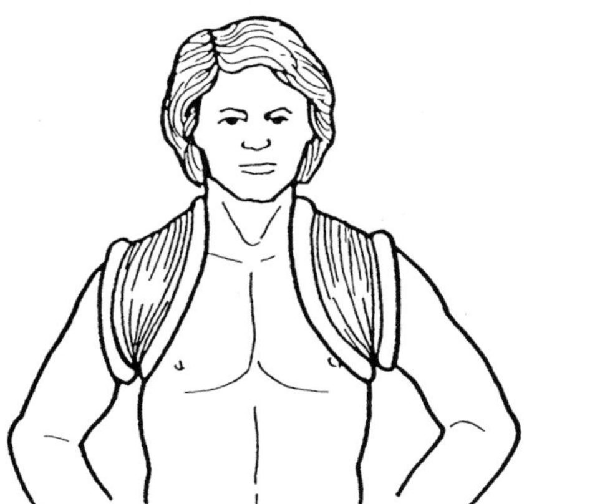

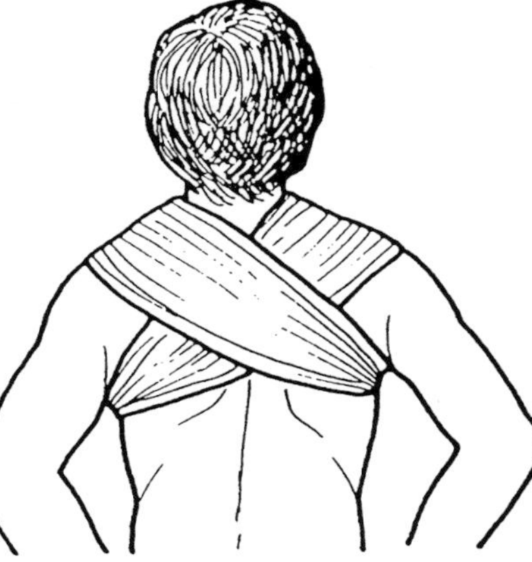

Fig. 23-4 Clavicular or figure-of-eight splint. (From Daya M: Shoulder. In Rosen P, et al [editors]: *Emergency medicine: concepts and clinical practice,* ed 4, St Louis, 1998, Mosby.)

inward pressure on the medial end of the clavicle. Stable reduction should be maintained in a clavicular splint and referred for orthopedic follow-up.[16,17] Unfortunately, the majority of reductions are invariably unstable. Since the deformity is primarily cosmetic and not functional, open reduction and internal fixation is not recommended.

Posterior dislocations are true orthopedic emergencies and should be reduced expeditiously.[17] At least one authority suggests posterior dislocations should be attempted in the operating suite under general anesthesia with a cardiopulmonary bypass team and a vascular surgeon on standby in case of massive hemorrhage.[19] Patients are placed supine with a rolled towel between their shoulders and traction is applied as previously described. The medial end of the clavicle is then grasped either manually or with a sterile towel clip and pulled outward. If diagnosed early, most posterior dislocations can be reduced in a closed fashion and stabilized with a clavicular splint.

COMPLICATIONS

Up to 25% of posterior SC joint dislocations may be complicated by injuries to intrathoracic and superior mediastinal structures.[20] Since the great vessels (i.e., the aorta and its branches, jugular vein, and superior vena cava) lie immediately posterior to the SC joint, vascular damage is a serious potential complication.[21] Injury to the trachea, esophagus, and recurrent laryngeal nerve is also possible. Pneumothorax should also be ruled out. These associated injuries can be life threatening and should be addressed immediately.[21]

Acromioclavicular Joint Dislocations

Teaching Case

A 20-year-old male complains of severe left shoulder pain after being tackled to the ground during a football match. He landed directly on the point of his shoulder. The left arm is held close to the body and the lateral end of the clavicle is prominent. ■

The AC joint connects the lateral end of the clavicle with the medial aspect of the acromion process (Fig. 23-6). Like other joints within the shoulder girdle complex, the stability of the AC joint is largely dependent on its associated ligaments and muscles. These structures include the relatively weak anterior, posterior, superior, and inferior AC ligaments, as well as the clavicular and acromial attachments of the deltoid and trapezius muscles.[16] The most important stabilizer of the joint is the powerful CC ligament, which is composed of two parts. The trapezoid ligament arises from the shaft of coracoid process and runs superiorly

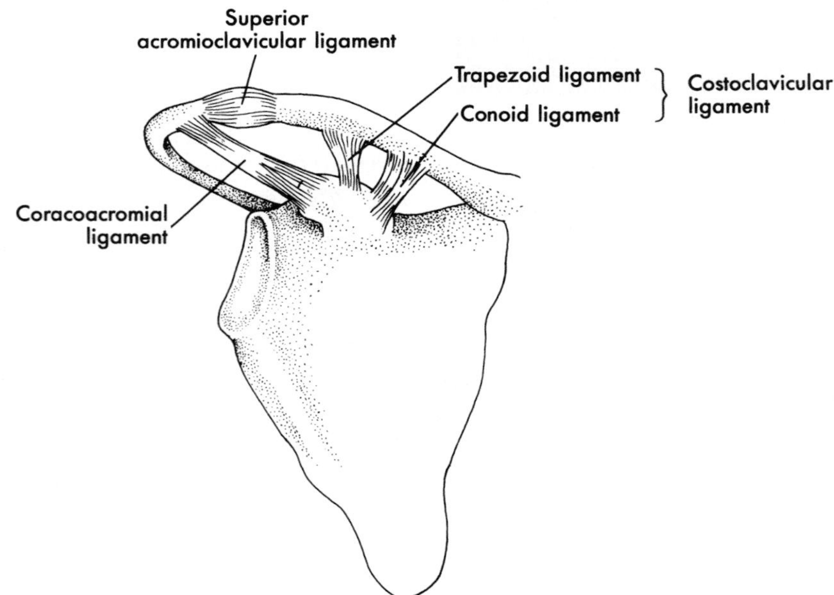

Fig. 23-6 Ligaments of the acromioclavicular joint. (Redrawn from DePalma AF: *Surgery of the shoulder,* ed 3, Philadelphia, 1983, JB Lippincott. In Rosen P, et al [editors]: *Emergency medicine: concepts and clinical practice,* ed 4, St Louis, 1998, Mosby.)

to insert onto the inferior surface of the lateral clavicle.[22] The conoid ligament arises from the base of the coracoid process and inserts more medially on the inferior surface of the distal clavicle. The normal distance from the undersurface of the clavicle to the superior aspect of the coracoid process varies between 11 and 13 mm in the standing adult.[16] Although the AC joint itself has a very limited range of movement, it does allow for 40 to 50 degrees of clavicular rotation, which is essential for a full range of motion at the glenohumeral joint.

EPIDEMIOLOGY

Injuries of the AC joint occur primarily in males (incidence of 15 per 100,000) and account for 25% of the dislocations about the shoulder girdle.[2] AC joint injury is the number one injury sustained in bicycle accidents. Many injuries are the result of participation in contact sports such as football, rugby, ice hockey, and wrestling. A smaller percentage result from motor vehicle crashes and falls.[23]

PATHOPHYSIOLOGY

The most common mechanism of injury involves a fall or direct blow to the point of the shoulder with the arm adducted.[23] The resultant force drives the scapula downward and medially to produce the injury.[22] The weak AC ligaments rupture first. With increasing force, the CC ligament ruptures and the attachments of the deltoid and trapezius muscles are torn from the distal clavicle.[24] The joint can also be injured following a fall on the outstretched hand. In these circumstances, the resultant indirect force is transmitted to the AC ligaments only. The CC ligament is relaxed in this position and remains uninjured.[16]

CLASSIFICATION

The three-part Allman classification of these injuries (Fig. 23-7) is based on the degree of damage sustained by the AC and CC ligaments.[23] Grade I injuries are basically sprains of the AC ligaments and the radiograph appears normal. Grade II injuries are associated with disruption of the AC ligaments. The joint space is

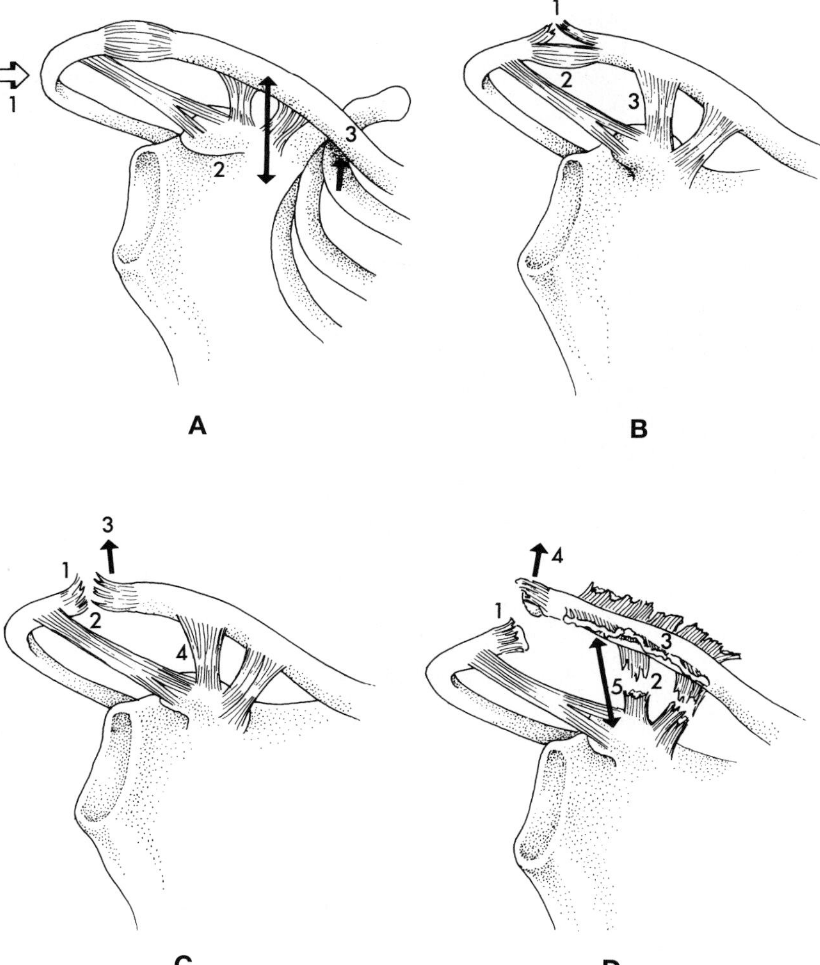

Fig. 23-7 Mechanism of injury and classification of acromioclavicular joint injuries. **A,** The direct force is applied to the point of the shoulder *(1);* the scapula and attached clavicle are forced downward and medially, the clavicle approaches the first rib *(2).* If the force continues, the first rib abuts the clavicle, producing a counterforce *(3).* Depending on the magnitude of the force, a grade I, II, or III sprain may occur. **B,** Grade 1 sprain. A few fibers of the acromioclavicular ligament stretch and a few tear *(1);* the acromioclavicular joint is stable *(2);* the coracoclavicular ligament is intact *(3).* **C,** Grade II sprain (subluxation). The capsule and the acromioclavicular ligament rupture *(1);* the joint is lax and unstable *(2);* the end of the clavicle rides upward, usually less than one half of the width of the end of the clavicle *(3);* the coracoclavicular ligament remains intact *(4);* the attachments of the trapezius and deltoid remain intact *(5).* **D,** Grade III sprain (dislocation). the capsule and acromioclavicular ligaments rupture *(1);* the coracoclavicular ligament ruptures *(2);* the insertions of the trapezius and deltoid tear away *(3);* the clavicle rides upward *(4);* the interval between the clavicle and the coracoid process is greatly increased *(5).* (From DePalma AF: *Surgery of the shoulder,* ed 3, Philadelphia, 1983, JB Lippincott.)

widened, and the clavicle displaces slightly upwards. There are minor tears in the attachments of the deltoid and trapezius, but the CC ligament remains intact. A grade III injury occurs when there is complete disruption of the AC ligaments, CC ligament, and muscle attachments. The joint space is widened and the CC distance is increased. The clavicle is displaced upward by the pull of the trapezius, and the shoulder is displaced downward by the effect of gravity.[22,24]

EMERGENCY DEPARTMENT PRESENTATION

It is important to examine the patient in the sitting or standing position because the supine position tends to mask any associated joint deformity.[22] Grade I injuries are associated with mild tenderness and swelling over the AC joint margin. There is no deformity and a full range of motion is usually possible, although painful. Grade II injuries produce moderate to severe pain. The distal end of the clavicle may lie slightly superior or posterior to the acromion. Patients with grade III injuries usually present with the arm adducted close to the body.[22] The shoulder hangs downwards, and the clavicle rides high, producing an obvious clinical deformity (Fig. 23-8).

DIAGNOSTIC STUDIES

The energy settings used for the standard radiographic trauma series over-penetrates the AC joint. Therefore order specific AC joint views, which use a third to two thirds less intensity.[22] The recommended views include an AP with a 15° cephalic tilt and an axillary lateral view.[16] The axillary lateral view is very useful for identifying associated fractures and posterior dislocation of the clavicle. Type I injuries have essentially normal radiographs. Type II injuries show slight widening of the joint and a slight upward or posterior displacement of the clavicle. The CC distance is normal. Type III injuries (Fig. 23-9) are characterized by more significant widening of the joint and an increased CC distance (normally 11 to 13 mm). A difference of >5 mm in this distance between the injured and uninjured side is diagnostic of a complete AC disruption.[16] Historically, stress views (using suspended weights) of the AC joint were recommended in an attempt to differentiate between type II and III

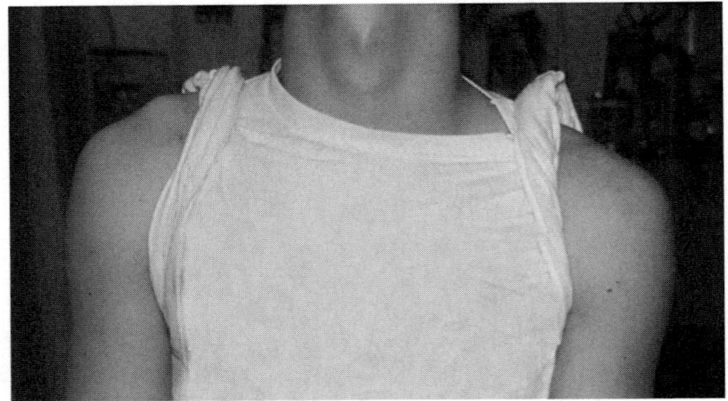

Fig. 23-8 Grade III acromioclavicular joint injury.

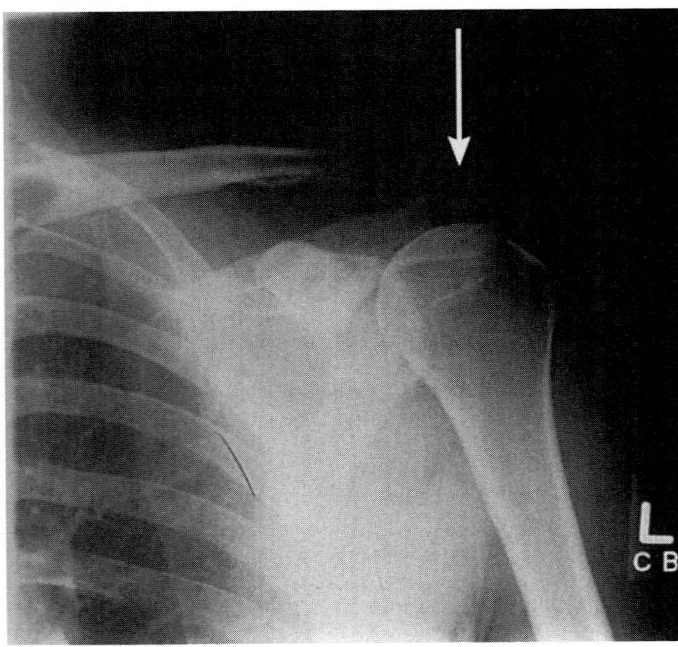

Fig. 23-9 Third degree sprain of the acromioclavicular joint. The coracoclavicular distance measures 18 mm *(arrow)*. (Courtesy of David Nelson, MD.)

injuries.[16] Weighted views have been shown to lack efficacy for this purpose and should be abandoned.[25]

EMERGENCY DEPARTMENT MANAGEMENT AND DISPOSITION

Grade I and grade II injuries should be immobilized in a sling for comfort and to protect against further injury, and patients should be referred for follow-up with their primary care physician.[26] Once pain has subsided (1 to 2 weeks), the patient can begin range-of-motion exercises. Grade III injuries are the subject of much controversy with regard to treatment (operative versus conservative).[24,27,28] Most studies have concluded that conservative (nonoperative) therapy provides equal or, in some cases, better results than surgical treatment. However, severe lesions (AC displacements of >20 mm) in younger individuals appear to have better outcomes in terms of residual pain, strength, and range of movement following early surgery.[27,28] Treatment of grade III injuries in the ED should consist of sling immobilization and prompt (<72 hours) orthopedic referral. The initial therapy in all cases should always include adequate analgesia.

COMPLICATIONS

The most common concurrent injuries are associated fractures of the clavicle and coracoid process. Pain that interferes with sleep and activities may persist in a small percentage of patients and necessitate lateral resection of the clavicle for relief. Osteoarthritis is a potential long-term complication of an acute injury to the AC joint.[26,27]

Glenohumeral Joint Dislocations

Teaching Case

A 20-year-old male and his older brother borrowed their father's high-performance ocean-racing boat. Attempting to water ski while barefoot, the younger brother grabbed the towrope and yelled to his sibling to "take off." When the 480-horsepower engine suddenly engaged, he sustained bilateral anterior dislocations of his shoulders. Only his lifejacket prevented his drowning. ■

The glenohumeral articulation is classified anatomically as a ball-and-socket type joint. Although the glenoid fossa is deepened by a rim of fibrocartilage (the glenoid labrum), it provides a bearing surface for only one half of the humeral head at any one time.[29] This absence of congruent surfaces makes the joint mechanically unstable but also permits a range of motion that is greater than that of any other joint in the body.[29] The stability of the joint is primarily dependent on associated muscles and ligaments. A loose and redundant fibrous capsule surrounds the joint's synovial membrane. Anteriorly, this capsule is thickened to form the superior, middle, and inferior glenohumeral ligaments. Superiorly, the acromial process and the coracoacromial ligament protect the capsule. The long head of the biceps muscle and the rotator cuff group of muscles further stabilize the superior and anterior parts of the joint. The neurovascular bundle runs anteriorly and the axillary nerve lies close to the inferior aspect of the joint. Movements of the glenohumeral joint include flexion, extension, abduction, adduction, internal rotation, external rotation, and circumduction.

The glenohumeral joint can dislocate anteriorly, posteriorly, inferiorly, or superiorly. Anterior dislocations account for 95% to 97% of all glenohumeral dislocations. Posterior dislocations account for the majority of the remainder, whereas inferior and superior dislocations are very rare.[11]

ANTERIOR SHOULDER DISLOCATIONS

Epidemiology. Anterior shoulder dislocations account for more then 50% of all major joint dislocations encountered in the ED. One Danish study reported an incidence of 17 per 100,000 with two distinct incidence peaks.[30] The first is in males aged 20 to 30 and the second in women aged 61 to 80.

Pathophysiology. Anterior dislocations can result from indirect or direct forces. The most common mechanism of injury consists of an indirect force transferred to the anterior capsule, from a combination of abduction, extension, and external rotation. In younger individuals, the injury is usually sustained during athletic activities.[31,32] A quarterback may have his arm "intercepted" in mid-pass, or the hapless water-skier may have the driver take off in full throttle. In older patients and in snow skiers, a fall onto the outstretched arm is the common cause of injury.[31] An increased abduction component will produce the subglenoid variety.[16] Rarely, a direct force applied to the posterolateral aspect of the shoulder can force the humeral head out of the glenoid fossa anteriorly.[32]

Classification. Anterior dislocations can be classified according to their etiology (traumatic or nontraumatic), frequency (primary or recurrent), and the anatomic position of the dislocated humeral head.[16,30] Following dislocation, the humeral head can assume a subcoracoid, subglenoid, subclavicular, or intrathoracic position (Fig. 23-10). The latter two types are extremely rare and the subcoracoid/subglenoid types account for 99% of all anterior dislocations.[16]

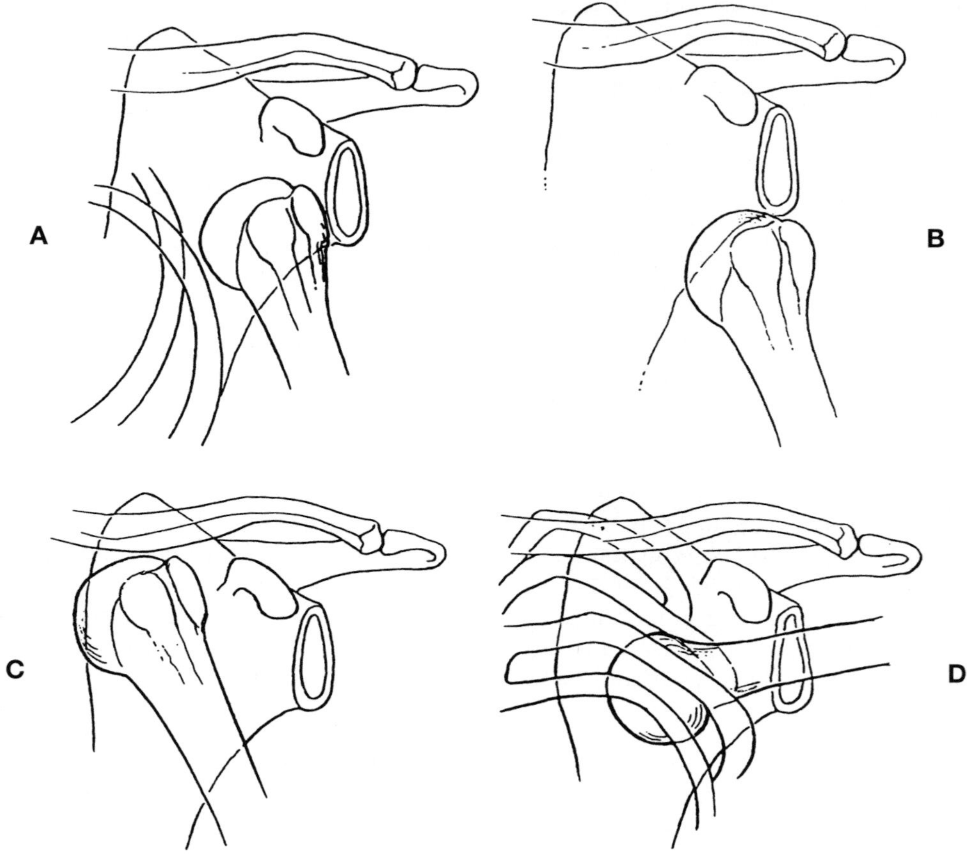

Fig. 23-10 Types of anterior shoulder dislocations. **A,** Subcoracoid; **B,** subglenoid; **C,** subclavicular; and **D,** intrathoracic. (From DePalma AF: *Surgery of the shoulder,* ed 3, Philadelphia, 1983, JB Lippincott.)

Emergency Department Presentation. The patient usually presents in severe pain with the dislocated arm held in slight abduction and external rotation by the opposite extremity. The lateral edge of the acromion process is prominent, and the shoulder often assumes a "squared off" appearance. The coracoid process is indistinct, and the anterior shoulder appears full. *The patient leans away from the injured side and cannot adduct or internally rotate the shoulder even slightly, without severe pain.*[32] A thorough neurovascular examination is essential to identify associated injuries of the axillary nerve, brachial plexus, radial nerve, or axillary artery. A pulse deficit mandates immediate reduction. Test for sensation over the deltoid muscle just below the lateral shoulder to determine sensory function of the axillary nerve. It is this nerve most often injured in anterior shoulder dislocations and may be associated with some deltoid weakness.

Diagnostic Studies. The trauma series of radiographs will confirm the clinical diagnosis and identify the resting position of the humeral head (Fig. 23-11). Associated fractures may be present in up to 50% of all cases,[33] although this number is lower in other series. The most common of these fractures is a compression fracture of the posterolateral aspect of the humeral head due to forceful impingement against the anterior rim of the glenoid fossa (Fig. 23-11). This defect in the humeral head, known as the Hill-Sachs deformity, is reported to be present in 11% to 50% of all anterior dislocations.[33] The actual incidence is probably higher since minor compression fractures are difficult to visualize on routine radiographs. A corresponding fracture of the anterior glenoid rim (Bankart's lesion) may also be present in some instances. Avulsion fractures of the greater tuberosity (more common in the elderly) may be detected in 10% to 15% of patients with anterior dislocations.[34]

Emergency Department Management and Disposition. Closed reduction of the dislocation should be accomplished expeditiously, since the incidence of complications increases with time.[34,35] Radiographic documentation of the type of dislocation and any associated fractures should be obtained before attempts at reduction in all cases. Reduction can be accomplished through the use of various techniques, most of

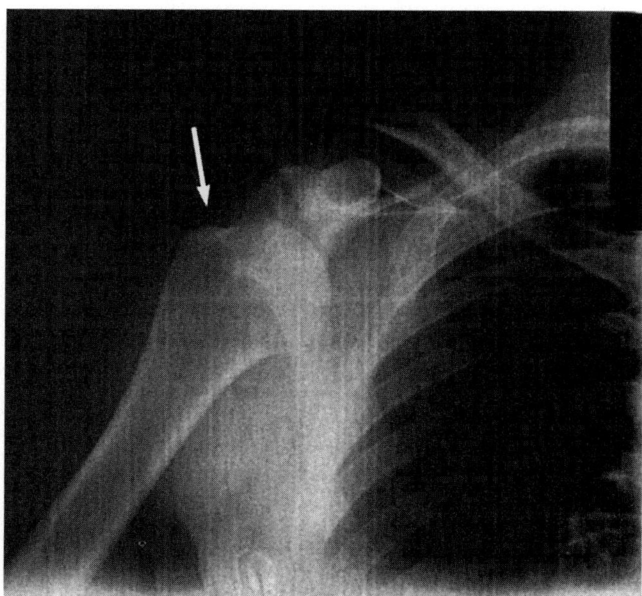

Fig. 23-11 Recurrent anterior subcoracoid dislocation with Hill-Sachs deformity of the humeral head *(arrow).* (From Daya M: Shoulder. In Rosen P, et al [editors]: *Emergency medicine: concepts and clinical practice,* ed 4, St Louis, 1998, Mosby.)

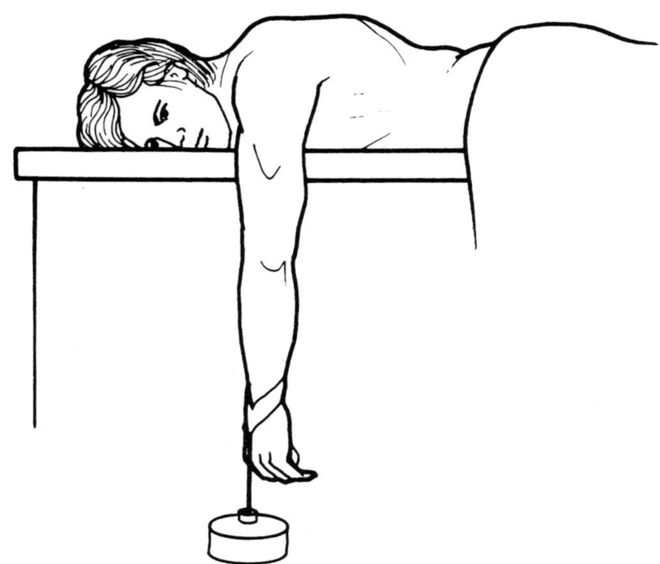

Fig. 23-12 Stimson technique for reducing anterior shoulder dislocations. (From Daya M: Shoulder. In Rosen P, et al [editors]: *Emergency medicine: concepts and clinical practice,* ed 4, St Louis, 1998, Mosby.)

which involve the use of traction, leverage, or scapular manipulation principles.[16,34]

Good muscle relaxation is the key to a successful reduction. Intravenous analgesics (opiates) and sedatives (benzodiazepines, methohexital) should be administered as needed before reduction. Reductions can sometimes be accomplished without the use of any analgesia, especially if the time from injury to reduction is short. Analgesia may also be provided by interscalene, supraclavicular, or suprascapular nerve blocks or by intraarticular injection of a local anesthetic agent.[20,36-39] In the latter, 20 ml of 1% lidocaine is injected into the lateral sulcus (2 cm inferior and directly lateral to the acromion) created by the absent humeral head using a 1.5-inch, 20-gauge needle.[38] This technique also allows for the aspiration of any associated hemarthrosis and is especially useful when IV sedation is contraindicated. Although conscious sedation has been popularized in recent years, the intraarticular technique appears to be very effective and has been associated with less cost and a shorter post-reduction length of stay in the ED.[38] The injection technique has the added advantage in a busy ED, since a nurse is not taken out of circulation to monitor a patient after conscious sedation. Key to this technique is allowing adequate time for the anesthetic response, usually 15 to 20 minutes.

Traction Methods. Gentle traction in various directions (forward flexion, abduction, overhead, lateral) is used to overcome the muscle spasm that holds the humeral head in its dislocated position.[34] Some authors prefer the Stimson or hanging weight technique (Fig. 23-12) as the initial method of reduction.[20] The patient is placed prone with the dislocated arm hanging over the edge of the examining table. A 10- or 15-lb weight attached to the wrist or lower forearm provides traction in forward flexion. Reduction usually occurs over 20 to 30 minutes.

Other clinicians prefer the traction-countertraction method (Fig. 23-13). Traction is applied along the abducted arm while an assistant using a folded sheet wrapped across the chest applies countertraction.

The forward elevation maneuver of Cooper and Milch is also simple and safe.[40] The arm is initially elevated 10° to 20° in forward flexion and slight abduction. Forward flexion is continued until the arm is directly overhead. Abduction is then increased and outward traction applied to complete the reduction.

The recently described Snowbird technique would appear to be an excellent technique since it is simple, quick, effective, requires little assistance, and can be executed without the use of analgesia in most cases.[41] In this technique the patient is seated in a chair and the affected arm is supported by the patient's unaffected extremity. A 3-foot loop of 4-inch cast stockinet is then placed around the proximal forearm of the involved extremity with the elbow at 90°. The patient is instructed to sit up (assist as needed) and the physician's foot is placed in the stockinet loop to provide firm downward traction. The physician's hands re-

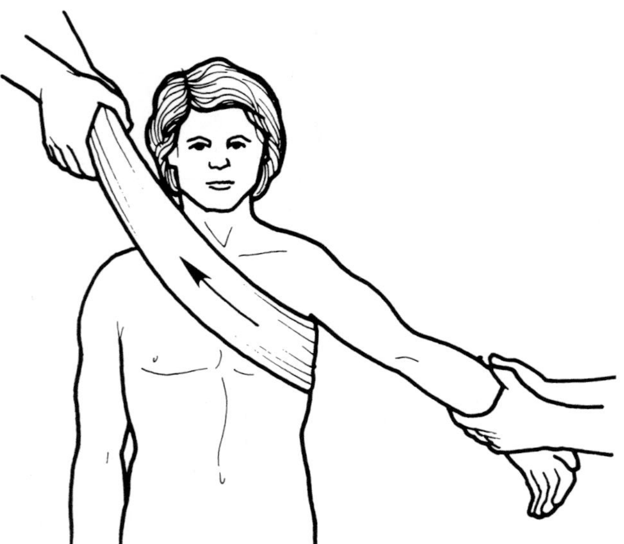

Fig. 23-13 Traction-countertraction technique for reducing anterior shoulder dislocations. (From Daya M: Shoulder. In Rosen P, et al [editors]: *Emergency medicine: concepts and clinical practice,* ed 4, St Louis, 1998, Mosby.)

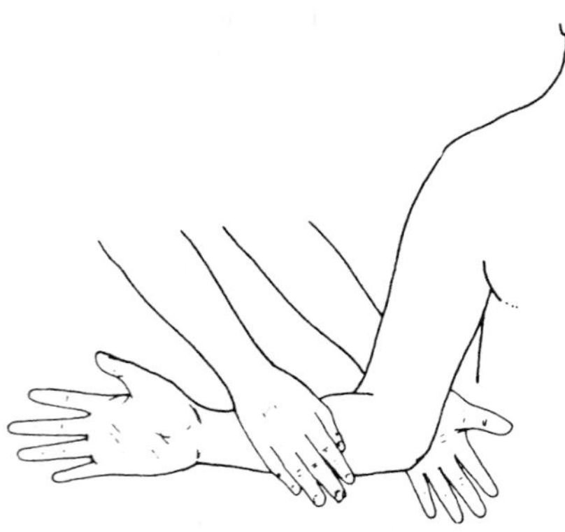

Fig. 23-14 External rotation technique for reducing anterior shoulder dislocations. The involved arm is slowly adducted to the patient's side and the elbow is flexed to 90 degrees. Gentle external rotation is then applied to the forearm to achieve reduction. (From Simon RR, et al: *Emergency othopedics: the extremities,* ed 2, Norwalk, Conn, 1987, Appleton & Lange.)

main free to apply any gentle external pressure or rotation as needed until the reduction has been obtained.[41]

Leverage Techniques. The most commonly recommended leverage technique is the external rotation method of Liedelmeyer.[42,43] With the patient in the supine position (or seated with the back firmly against the stretcher in an upright position), the involved arm is slowly and gently adducted to the side until it firmly abuts the chest. The elbow is flexed to 90° and

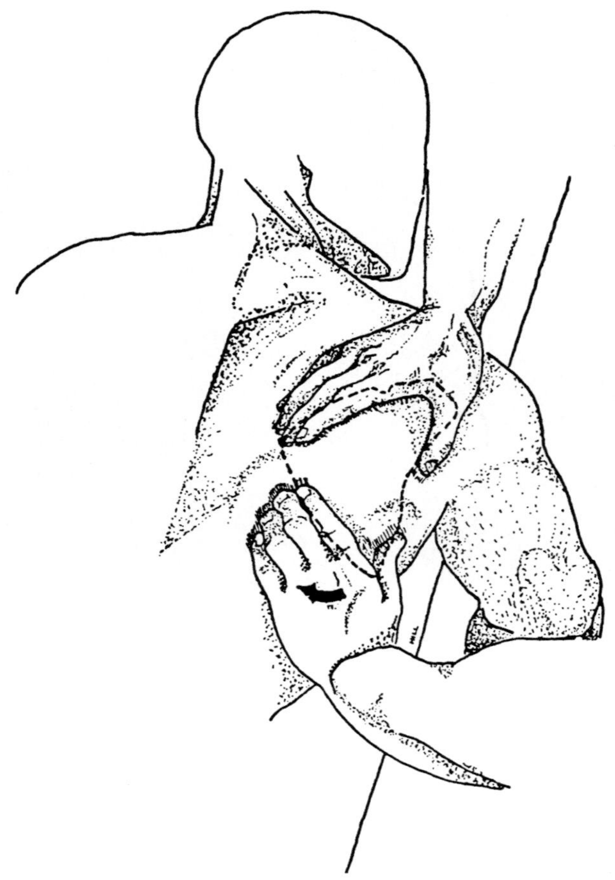

Fig. 23-15 Scapular manipulation technique for reducing anterior shoulder dislocations. (From Kothari RU, Dronen SC: *J Emerg Med* 8:625, 1990.)

slow, gentle external rotation is applied to the arm. It is essential to keep the patient's elbow against his or her chest wall, since it tends to drift outwards and decreases the success of the reduction (Fig. 23-14). The technique is simple and complications are rare.

Scapular Manipulation. Scapular manipulation accomplishes reduction by repositioning the glenoid fossa rather than the humeral head.[44,45] The patient is placed in the prone position with the affected arm hanging off the table as for the Stimson technique. After the application of downward traction (manual or hanging weights), the scapula is manipulated by rotating the inferior tip medially (Fig. 23-15) while simultaneously stabilizing the superior and medial edges with the opposite hand.[44] McNamara[45] has also described a seated modification of the scapular method, in which traction is applied in the forward horizontal position while the scapula is manipulated by an assistant. Scapular manipulation techniques can be difficult in obese or muscular individuals in whom it is often difficult to palpate and grasp the inferior tip of the scapula.

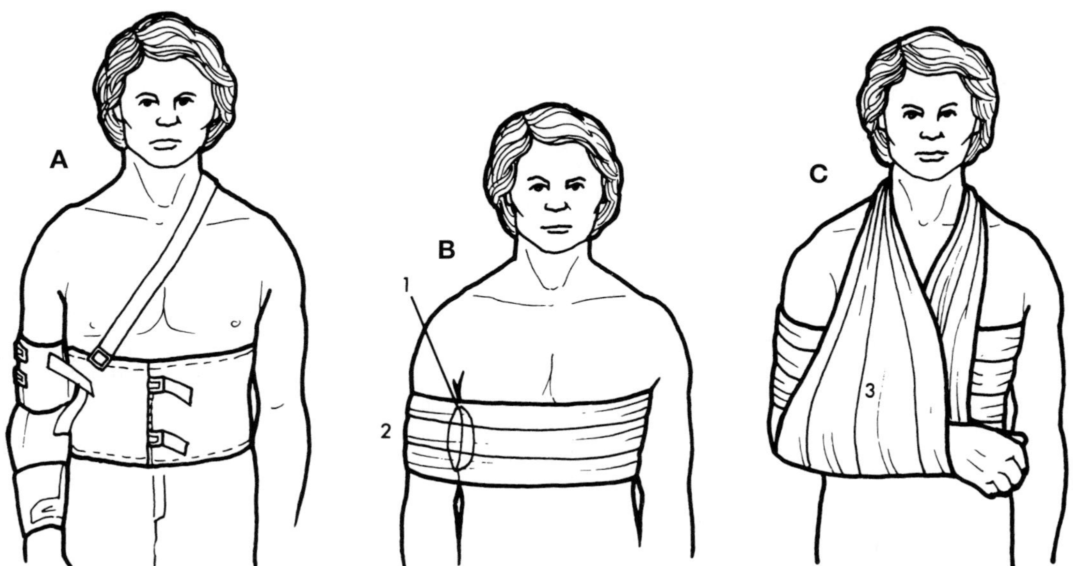

Fig. 23-16 Methods of shoulder immobilization. **A,** Commercial apparatus: **B,** application of swathe *(2)* with gauze padding *(1)* at point of skin contact; and **C,** application of sling *(3)* over swathe. (From Daya M: Shoulder. In Rosen P, et al [editors]: *Emergency medicine: concepts and clinical practice,* ed 4, St Louis, 1998, Mosby.)

The neurovascular examination must be repeated following any attempt at reduction. It is generally recommended that radiographs be repeated to confirm reduction and to identify any procedure-related fractures. Two small retrospective studies have questioned the need and cost-effectiveness of routine postreduction radiographs. Most reductions can usually be detected clinically (palpable clunk, decrease in pain, and improvement in range of motion) and in these studies, postreduction radiographs did not identify any clinically significant new fractures.[46,47] Larger prospective studies are required to confirm these findings and clarify the indications for postreduction radiographs.

Once reduced, the affected extremity may be immobilized using a sling-and-swathe bandage or a Velpeau sling made out of commercially available stockinet (Figs. 23-16 and 23-17). Patients should be discharged with adequate analgesia and appropriate follow-up. Primary dislocations and complicated cases (associated fracture, rotator cuff tear, axillary nerve injury, recurrent dislocation) should receive orthopedic follow-up. In uncomplicated cases, the shoulder is immobilized for 3 to 4 weeks in younger patients (<20 years) and 1 to 2 weeks in older (>40 years) individuals.[16] Early mobilization of the shoulder (pendular exercises) in the latter group reduces the risk of adhesive capsulitis ("frozen shoulder").

Complications. Complications include the aforementioned fractures and neurovascular injuries. The frequency of associated neurologic injuries ranges between 5% and 12%.[31] Most neurologic injuries (axillary nerve) are neuropraxic in nature and recover slowly over 3 to 12 months.[16,35] Rotator cuff tears may be present in 10% to 15% of cases.[33] Rotator cuff tears are more common in primary dislocations over the age of 40.[48] In this setting, failure to abduct the arm is often misdiagnosed as an axillary nerve injury. Most of these individuals require tendon and capsular repair to restore shoulder stability. Recurrence is also a common complication following anterior dislocation. Patients under the age of 30 have a reported recurrence rate of 79% to 100%.[30] Arthroscopic studies of first-time anterior dislocations in younger individuals have detected a high proportion of patients with detachment of the capsuloligamentous unit from the glenoid rim (Perthes-Bankart lesion). This injury is now believed to be the primary predisposing factor for recurrence and these studies have suggested the possible role for arthroscopic stabilization of first-time anterior dislocations in younger individuals.[49]

POSTERIOR SHOULDER DISLOCATIONS

Teaching Case

A heavy-set, middle-aged man presents to the ED complaining of right shoulder pain. He denies any trauma but admits to a history of alcohol intemper-

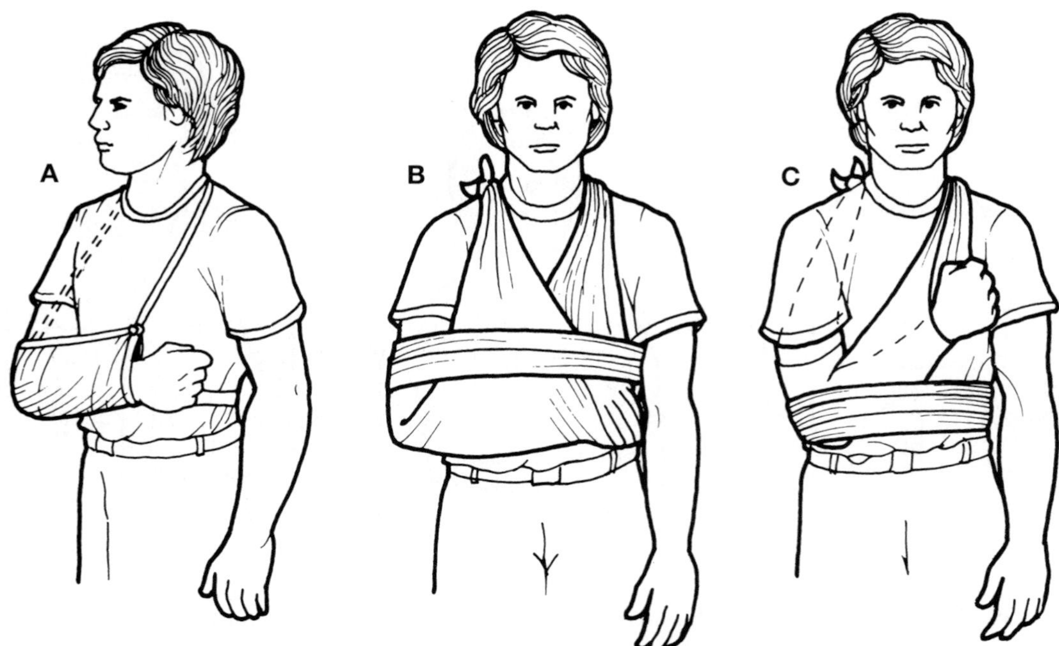

Fig. 23-17 Velpeau sling immobilization. **A,** Commercial version. **B** and **C,** Constructed using stockinette. (From Daya M: Shoulder. In Rosen P, et al [editors]: *Emergency medicine: concepts and clinical practice,* ed 4, St Louis, 1998, Mosby.)

ance, as well as epilepsy for which he takes carbamazepine. The affected extremity is held close to the chest and movement is severely restricted. There are no obvious external deformities and the neurovascular status is intact. A set of standard AP radiographs is obtained and read as normal. The patient is discharged and referred to his primary care physician with the presumptive diagnosis of a frozen shoulder.

■

Epidemiology. Posterior shoulder dislocations are rare and account for 2% to 4% of all glenohumeral dislocations.[50] Unfortunately, over 50% of posterior dislocations are missed on initial evaluation and many remain unrecognized ("locked dislocations") for weeks and months.[51]

Pathophysiology. Posterior dislocations can result from several distinct mechanisms of injury. Unilateral or bilateral posterior dislocations are often associated with seizures or electrical injuries.[50,52,53] An unconscious victim found on a golf course with a posterior shoulder dislocation is likely to be a victim of a lightning strike. In these instances, it is thought that the strong internal rotators (latissimus dorsi, pectoralis major, teres major, subscapularis) overpower the weak external rotators (infraspinatus, teres minor) to produce the injury.[51] A posterior dislocation can also occur during a motor vehicle crash or following a fall onto an outstretched hand with the arm held in flexion, adduction, and internal rotation. Rarely, a direct blow to the anterior aspect of the shoulder can produce this injury.

Classification. Posterior dislocations are classified into three types (subacromial, subglenoid, subspinous) based on the final resting position of the humeral head. The subacromial variety accounts for 98% of all posterior dislocations.[54]

Clinical Presentation. Early diagnosis is essential to prevent long-term functional and therapeutic complications. The initial examining physician misses the diagnosis with some regularity, in large part as a result of an over-reliance on radiologic findings and under-reliance on the clinical examination.[50,52] The patient typically presents in the "natural sling" position with the affected arm held across the chest in adduction and internal rotation. The patient is unable to externally rotate the arm. The injury is often painless and the normal round shoulder contour may be replaced by a flattened appearance ventrally.[51] The coracoid and acromion processes are prominent and easily palpated. The humeral head can often be palpated posteriorly beneath the acromion process. Abduction is limited and external rotation is completely blocked.

Diagnostic Studies. Standard AP radiographs can appear deceptively normal with posterior dislocations, especially if the diagnosis is not suspected clinically.[12] The frequent inability to diagnose posterior dislocation on the frontal film has led to the descrip-

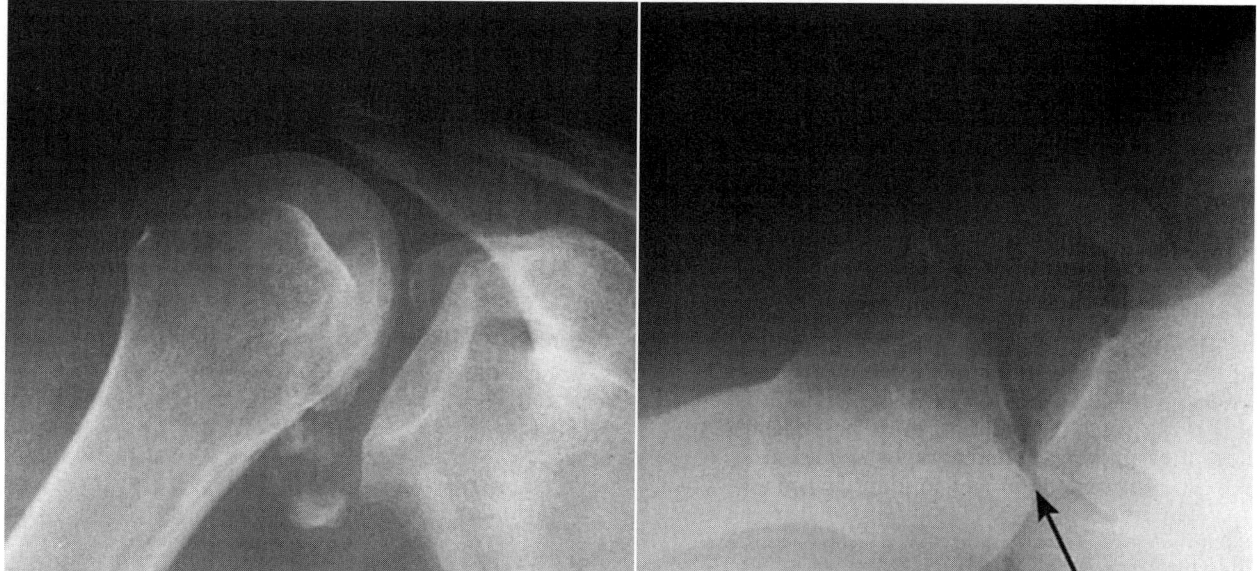

Fig. 23-18 Posterior shoulder dislocation. Note the widened joint space (rim sign), anteromedial impaction fracture of the humeral head, and curvilinear density parallel *(arrow)* to the articular surface (trough sign). (Courtesy of Donald Sauser, MD.)

tion of several radiologic findings to assist the clinician. Standard AP films show a loss of the normal half-moon elliptical overlap of the humeral head and glenoid fossa.[12,55] In addition, the distance ("rim sign") between the anterior glenoid rim and the articular surface of the humeral head is often increased.[12] The humeral head is typically profiled in internal rotation and can take on a "light bulb" or "drumstick" appearance (it may appear as a scoop of ice cream on a cone to the glucophile).[12,52] A true AP film shows abnormal overlap of the glenoid fossa with the humeral head.[55] Finally, an impaction fracture of the anteromedial humeral head (reverse Hill Sachs deformity) is often present (Fig. 23-18) and can produce a curvilinear density ("trough sign") on the frontal projection that parallels the articular cortex of the humeral head.[55] Despite these descriptions of characteristic findings on the frontal film, the best and most fail-safe method for establishing the diagnosis of a posterior dislocation is to obtain a good orthogonal view. The axillary lateral or the apical oblique views are especially valuable since they also demonstrate any associated fractures of the humeral head and posterior glenoid rim. Computed tomography may be of value in some instances but is rarely needed.[56]

Emergency Department Management and Disposition. Closed reduction of the acute dislocation can be attempted in the ED following IV analgesia and sedation. The technique of reduction incorporates axial traction in line with the humerus, gentle pressure on the posteriorly displaced head, and slow external rotation.[16] If this maneuver fails, reduction under general anesthesia is indicated. Cases that were missed initially and present as chronic or locked posterior dislocations should be referred promptly to the orthopedist for follow-up. Locked posterior dislocations usually require open reduction and internal fixation or hemiarthroplasty.[50,51]

Complications. Fractures of the glenoid rim, greater tuberosity, lesser tuberosity, and humeral head account for the majority of associated complications. In addition, the subscapularis muscle may be avulsed from its insertion site on the lesser tuberosity. Neurovascular injuries are rare because the anterior location of the neurovascular bundle protects it from direct injury. Recurrent dislocations occur in 30% of patients and can predispose the glenohumeral joint to degenerative changes.[16]

INFERIOR DISLOCATIONS (LUXATIO ERECTA)

Teaching Case

A 13-year-old girl developed sudden and severe left shoulder pain while attempting an overhead smash during a vigorous game of badminton. She is unable to lower her arm and immediately complains of numbness and tingling in her fingers. In the ED, the left arm was described as being abducted at the shoulder, flexed at the elbow, and pronated at the forearm with the hand resting on top of the head. ■

Epidemiology and Pathophysiology. Luxatio erecta is a rare type of glenohumeral dislocation in which the superior aspect of the humeral head is forced below the inferior rim of the glenoid fossa. It accounts for 0.5% of all shoulder dislocations and the mechanism of injury involves either direct or indirect forces.[57,58] Application of a direct axial load to an abducted shoulder can disrupt the weak inferior glenohumeral ligament and drive the humeral head downwards.[58] However, the majority of inferior dislocations are due to indirect forces that hyperabduct the affected extremity, resulting in impingement of the humeral head against the acromion process. Further levering of the humeral shaft against the acromion ruptures the capsule and dislocates the head inferiorly.

Emergency Department Presentation. These patients characteristically present with the arm locked overhead in 110° to 160° of abduction.[16] The elbow is usually flexed with the forearm resting on top of the head. The shoulder is fixed in this position and any attempts at movement results in significant pain. In thin individuals, the inferiorly displaced humeral head may be palpable along the lateral chest wall.

Diagnostic Studies. The radiographic features of luxatio erecta and subglenoid anterior dislocations are remarkably similar. However the dramatic clinical presentation of a patient with his or her upper arm held against the ear clearly distinguishes the luxatio from its mundane counterpart. Standard AP radiographs demonstrate the superior articular surface of the humerus to be inferior to the glenoid fossa. In addition, the humeral shaft characteristically lies parallel to the spine of the scapula (Fig. 23-19) on the AP view.[57] This feature is useful in distinguishing luxatio erecta from the subglenoid anterior dislocation since in the latter, the humeral shaft is perpendicular to the scapular spine. Associated fractures of the acromion, coracoid, clavicle, greater tuberosity, humeral head, and glenoid rim are common.

Emergency Management and Disposition. If possible, an orthopedic consultation should be obtained before attempts at reduction of this uncommon dislocation. Closed reduction can usually be accomplished in the ED using traction-countertraction ma-

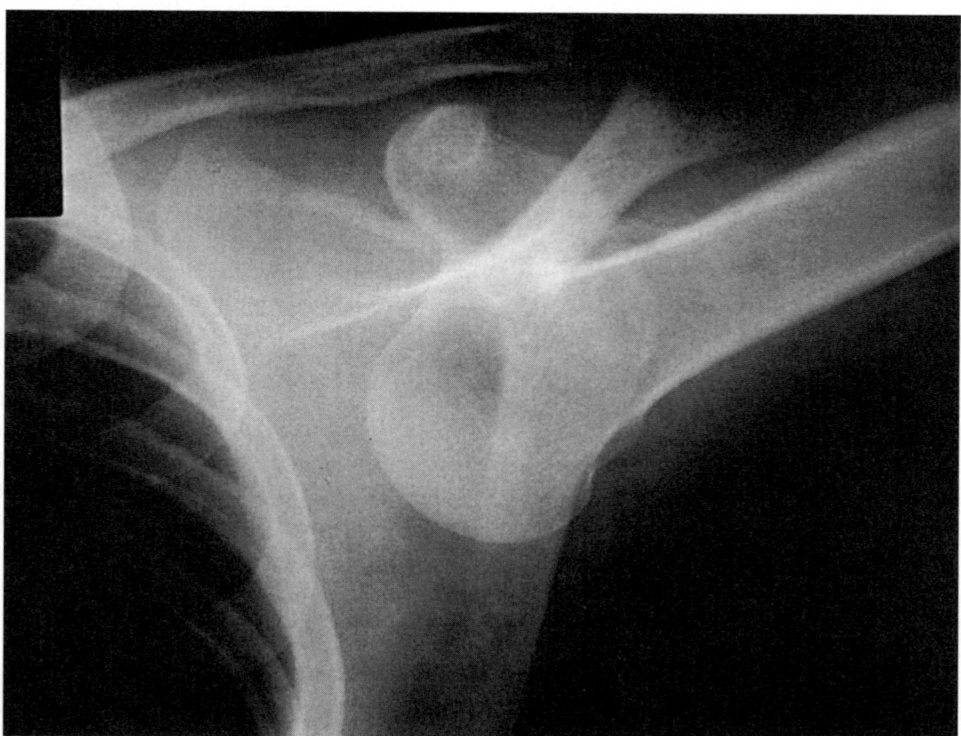

Fig. 23-19 Inferior shoulder dislocation. The humeral shaft lies parallel to the spine of the scapula. (From Daya M: Shoulder. In Rosen P, et al [editors]: *Emergency medicine: concepts and clinical practice,* ed 4, St Louis, 1998, Mosby.)

neuvers. Following IV analgesia and sedation, traction is applied in line with the humeral shaft while an assistant applies countertraction across the shoulder (Fig. 23-20). Gentle abduction usually reduces the dislocation and the arm is then brought down into an adducted position.[58] In rare instances, buttonholing of the capsule prevents closed reduction and necessitates an open reduction.

Complications. Trauma to brachial plexus is common and thrombosis of the axillary artery has also been reported with luxatio erecta.[16,59] Tears of the rotator cuff accompany most cases of luxatio erecta and may necessitate surgical repair.[57] Adhesive capsulitis is a common long-term complication of luxatio erecta.[58]

FRACTURES

Clavicle

EPIDEMIOLOGY

The clavicle is an S-shaped bone that acts as a strut to support the upper extremity. It is one of the most commonly fractured bones in the body. The recent Malmo study documented an incidence of 198 per 100,000 in the 0-to-14 year age group with clavicular fractures accounting for 87% of all shoulder injuries in this population.[2] In the same study, clavicular fractures accounted for 37% of all adult (age 15 to 64 years) shoulder injuries with an incidence of 46 per 100,000. Males predominated in both populations and the majority of injuries were related to sporting activities, falls, or traffic accidents.

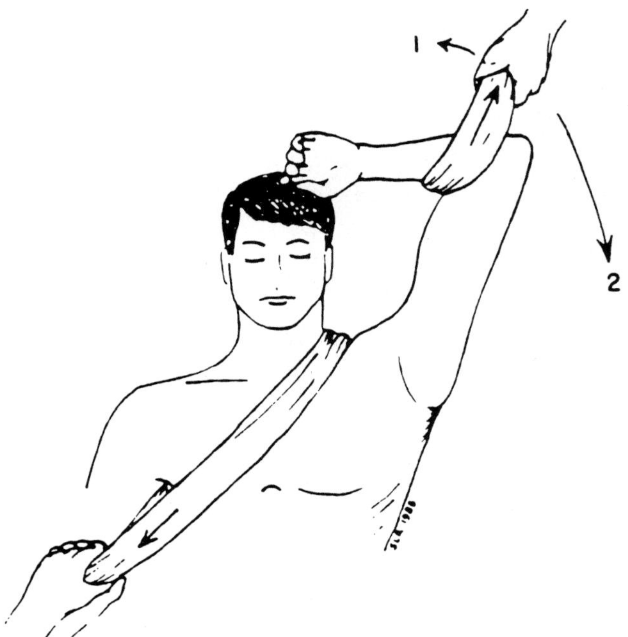

Fig. 23-20 Traction-countertraction method for reduction of luxatio erecta humeri. The initial maneuver *(1)* includes steady axial traction in line with humeral shaft position followed by gentle abduction, thereby reducing the glenohumeral dislocation. At this point *(2)* the arm is brought down to a position of adduction and internal rotation. (From Davids JR, Talbott RD: *Clin Orthop* 252:144, 1990.)

CLASSIFICATION

Clinically and mechanistically, clavicular fractures are classified into three main types.[60] Fractures of the proximal third result from a direct blow to the anterior chest and are uncommon (5%). Fractures of the middle third (Fig. 23-21) account for 80% of all injuries and are usually secondary to indirect forces, which when applied to the lateral aspect of the shoulder result in a shearing fracture of the clavicle proximal to the attachment of the coracoclavicular ligament.[16] Fractures of the distal third account for 15% of injuries and are a direct consequence of blows to the top of the shoulder. Fractures of the distal third are frequently overlooked and may be difficult to separate from AC dislocations. Distal-third fractures can be further classified into three subtypes.[16] Type I injuries (stable) are undisplaced fractures in which the coracoclavicular ligaments remain intact. Type II injuries (unstable) are associated with displacement and separation of the CC ligaments from the proximal fracture fragment. Type III injuries are intraarticular (Fig. 23-22).

EMERGENCY DEPARTMENT PRESENTATION

The patient most often presents with pain over the fracture site and the affected extremity held close to the body. With middle-third fractures, the shoulder is typically slumped downward, forward, and inward, as gravity and the pull of the pectoralis major and latissimus dorsi muscles act on the distal fragment.[61] The proximal fragment is frequently displaced upward by action of the sternocleidomastoid muscle. Crepitus and a palpable deformity may be present over the fracture site. Associated neurovascular injuries are rare. Children who fall and are not using their arm should be examined for clavicular fractures. Careful palpation of the clavicle should detect the injury.

DIAGNOSTIC STUDIES

Radiologic examination of the clavicle normally consists of a straight AP view and an AP view with the beam angled 45° cephalad.[12] The resulting radiographs are excellent for identifying middle-third fractures. CT scanning can visualize proximal-third fractures if the consultant believes further imaging

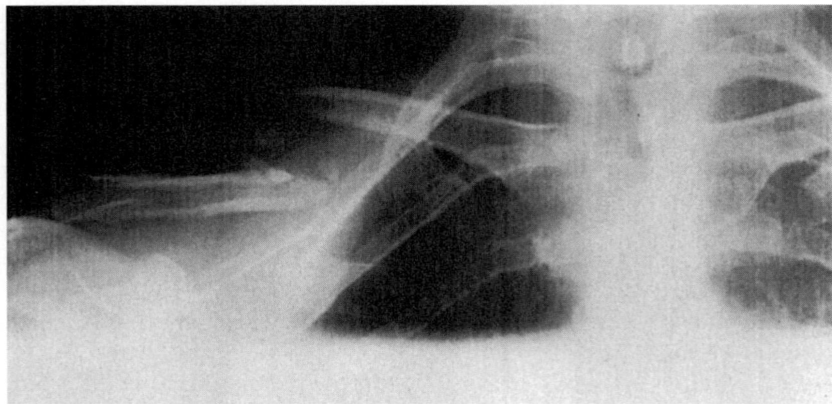

Fig. 23-21 Displaced midclavicular fracture. (From Daya M: Shoulder. In Rosen P, et al [editors]: *Emergency medicine: concepts and clinical practice,* ed 4, St Louis, 1998, Mosby.)

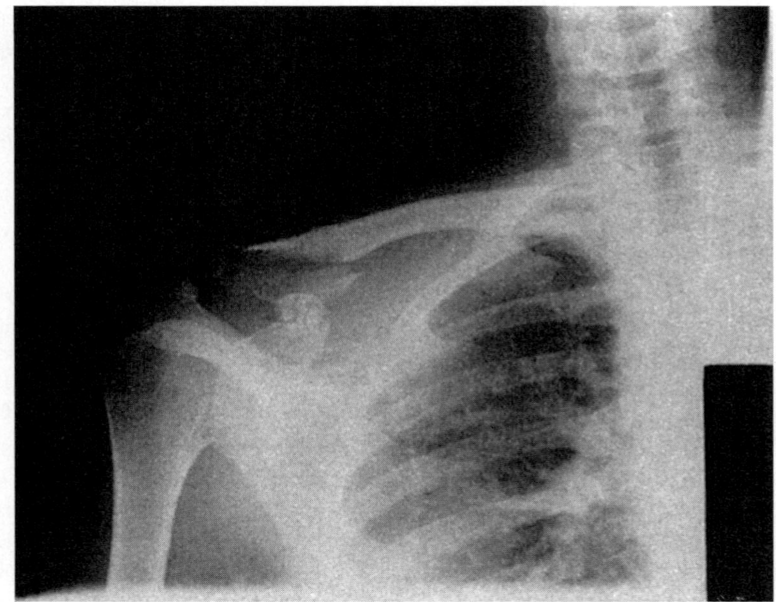

Fig. 23-22 Type III clavicle fracture. (From Daya M: Shoulder. In Rosen P, et al [editors]: *Emergency medicine: concepts and clinical practice,* ed 4, St Louis, 1998, Mosby.)

is necessary. Fractures of the distal-third are best visualized with the standard series of radiographs.[11,17]

EMERGENCY DEPARTMENT MANAGEMENT/ DISPOSITION

Principles of initial management include pain control, immobilization, and appropriate follow-up. Since malunion is generally associated with an acceptable functional and cosmetic outcome, treatment with a simple sling is the preferred treatment of clavicular fractures.[62] A sling and swathe or the Velpeau bandage may provide additional comfort for some patients during the first several days of treatment (Figs. 23-16 and 23-17). An older reduction technique was the clavicular (figure-of-eight) splint, which has generally fallen out of favor (Fig. 23-4). It is painful, is difficult to maintain, is often repeatedly tightened by the orthopedist and provides no benefit over a simple sling. Furthermore, patients treated with a figure-of-eight splint may develop skin irritation, as well as compression of the neurovascular bundle in the axilla.[61] Most fractures of the clavicle heal uneventfully.

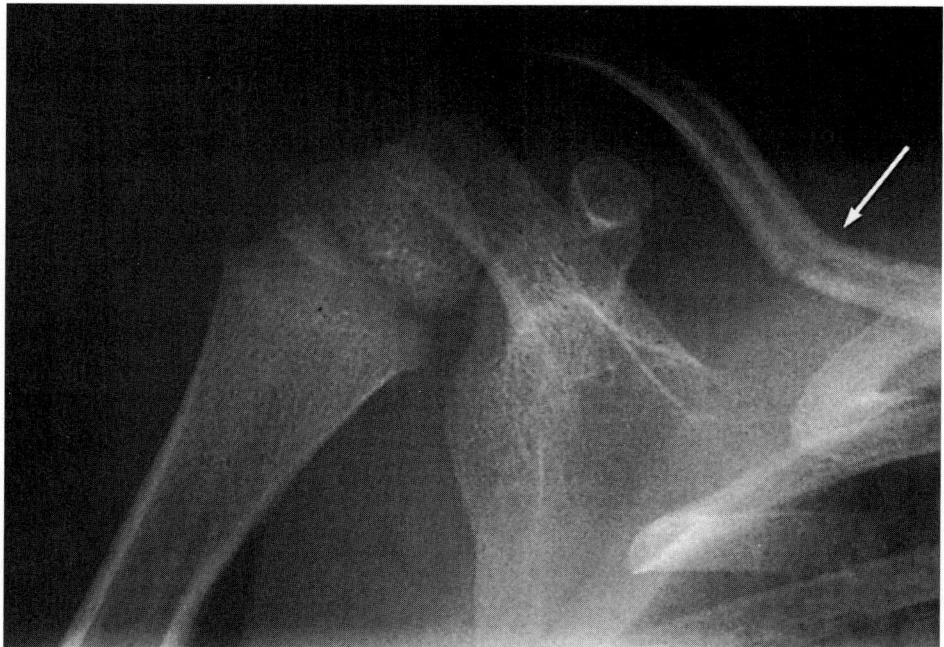

Fig. 23-23 Greenstick clavicle fracture. (From Daya M: Shoulder. In Rosen P, et al [editors]: *Emergency medicine: concepts and clinical practice,* ed 4, St Louis, 1998, Mosby.)

The sling should be worn until repeat radiographs demonstrate callus formation and healing across the fracture site. Younger children generally require shorter periods of immobilization (2 to 4 weeks) than adolescents and adults (4 to 8 weeks).[61] Vigorous competitive play should be avoided until the bone healing is solid.

More urgent orthopedic consultation (<72 hours) is required for type II distal fractures and immediate consultation should be sought for open fractures or fractures associated with neurovascular injuries or interposition of soft tissues. Type II distal fractures have a higher incidence of nonunion and usually require surgical repair.[16] Severely displaced middle-third (>20 mm of initial shortening) fractures in adults may also benefit from orthopedic referral since these have been noted to have a higher incidence of nonunion.[63]

Greenstick fractures of the midclavicle (Fig. 23-23) are common in the pediatric population. The majority of these fractures are undisplaced and heal uneventfully. The initial radiographs may appear normal despite suggestive clinical findings. In these instances, the arm should be immobilized in a simple sling and the radiographs repeated in 7 to 10 days if symptoms persist.

COMPLICATIONS

Complications are unusual with middle-third clavicle fractures. The old saying "the only time a broken clavicle does not heal is if the ends are in different rooms" is almost true. Complications of medial- and middle-third injuries resemble those associated with posterior sternoclavicular dislocations, and in rare instances may include injuries to the neurovascular bundle and the pleural dome. The impact forces associated with distal fractures can drive the clavicle inward resulting in associated rib fractures and other internal injuries. Articular surface injuries can lead to permanent pain because of subsequent arthritic changes.[16]

Scapula

The scapula is a flat, triangular bone that forms the posterior aspect of the shoulder girdle. The body of the scapula lies flat against the posterior thorax and widens laterally to form the glenoid fossa. The body of the scapula and its coracoid and acromial processes serves as attachment sites for many important muscles and ligaments. The most important aspect of scapular fractures is that it serves as a marker for significant injury to the chest, neck, and abdomen.

EPIDEMIOLOGY

Fractures of the scapula account for 1% of all fractures and less than 5% of all shoulder girdle injuries.[64] The incidence is 12 per 100,000 and the majority of these fractures occur in males between 30 and 40 years of age.[2,65]

PATHOPHYSIOLOGY

The scapula's thick muscle coat and ability to recoil along the chest wall protects it from injury. Most fractures are believed to be caused by direct trauma involving high energy transfer from sources such as high-speed vehicular accidents, falls from heights, or crush injuries.[64] Coracoid process fractures are frequently avulsive in nature and glenoid rim fractures are commonly encountered in association with anterior glenohumeral dislocations. An acromial process fracture is usually the result of a direct blow applied to the top of the shoulder. The most important clinical aspect of scapular fractures is the high incidence (75% to 98%) of associated injuries to the ipsilateral lung, chest wall, and shoulder girdle complex.[64,66,67] These injuries include fractures of the ribs, proximal humerus, and clavicle.[66] Associated lung injuries include pneumothorax, hemothorax, and pulmonary contusion, which may present in a delayed fashion 2 to 3 days following the initial injury.[68] More significant but less common are associated injuries of the brachial plexus and subclavian or axillary vessels.

CLASSIFICATION

Fractures of the scapula (Fig. 23-24) can be classified according to their anatomic location.[65, 69] Type I fractures involve the body and spine. Type II injuries involve the acromion or coracoid processes. Type III injuries involve the scapular neck and glenoid fossa (Fig. 23-25).

EMERGENCY DEPARTMENT PRESENTATION

The conscious patient presents with the shoulder adducted and the arm held close to the body. Any attempts at movement results in significant pain. There may be associated tenderness, crepitus, or hematoma over the fracture site. Hemorrhage into the rotator cuff associated with a scapula fracture can result in spasm and a temporary reflex inhibition of function.[60]

DIAGNOSTIC STUDIES

Fractures of the scapula are frequently overlooked as a result of the life-threatening nature of the associated pulmonary injuries.[70] The trauma series of shoulder radiographs identifies the majority of fractures, as will a careful examination of the scapula on the AP portable chest radiograph. The axillary lateral view is especially useful in evaluating fractures of the glenoid fossa and the acromion or coracoid processes.[65] The os acromiale (unfused acromial process epiphysis) is present in 3% of the population and should not be confused with a fracture of the acromion.[60] A comparison film can be useful since the abnormality is present bilaterally in 60% of cases.

EMERGENCY DEPARTMENT MANAGEMENT AND DISPOSITION

The majority of fractures of the body and spine, including those with severe comminution and displacement, do well with conservative therapy.[71] Initial therapy consists of analgesia and immobilization in a sling to support the ipsilateral upper extremity. Pen-

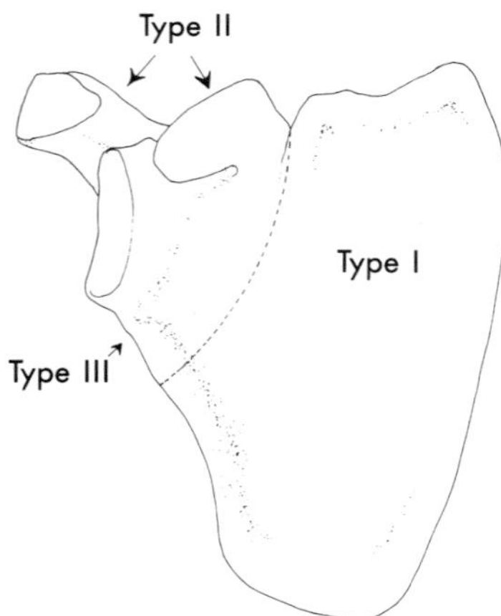

Fig. 23-24 Classification of scapular fractures. (Adapted from DeCloux MO, Minet P, Lemerle: *Lille Chir* 11:215, 1956. In Rosen P, et al [editors]: *Emergency medicine: concepts and clinical practice,* ed 4, St Louis, 1998, Mosby.)

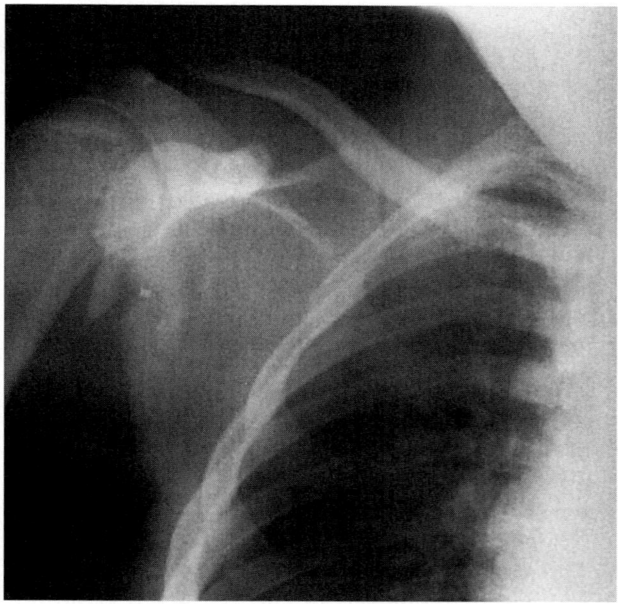

Fig. 23-25 Communuted type III scapular fracture. (Courtesy of David Nelson, MD.)

dular shoulder exercises (Fig. 23-26) should be initiated as soon as discomfort subsides to reduce the risk of adhesive capsulitis. In general, patients require a sling for 2 to 4 weeks.[64]

Undisplaced fractures of the acromion process also respond to conservative therapy. If the coracoclavicular ligaments remain intact, fractures of the coracoid process respond well to conservative therapy.[72] Severely displaced coracoid fractures with ruptured coracoclavicular ligaments may require open reduction and internal fixation.[72] Scapular neck and glenoid fossa fractures present the most difficult management issues. Although the majority of these injuries do well with conservative therapy, open reduction and internal fixation is recommended for severely displaced or angulated fractures.[64,71]

COMPLICATIONS

Associated injuries of the ipsilateral lung, chest wall, and shoulder girdle account for the majority of complications following fractures of the scapula. A shear type brachial plexus injury has been associated with fractures of the acromion process.[73] Neurovascular (brachial plexus, axillary artery) injuries have also been reported with fractures of the coracoid process.[16] Scapular neck, body, or spine fractures that extend into the suprascapular notch can injure the suprascapular nerve.[16] Delayed complications include adhesive capsulitis and rotator cuff dysfunction.[64]

When both the ipsilateral clavicle and scapular neck are fractured (Fig. 23-27), the scapular fracture becomes unstable, with the glenoid fragment pulled

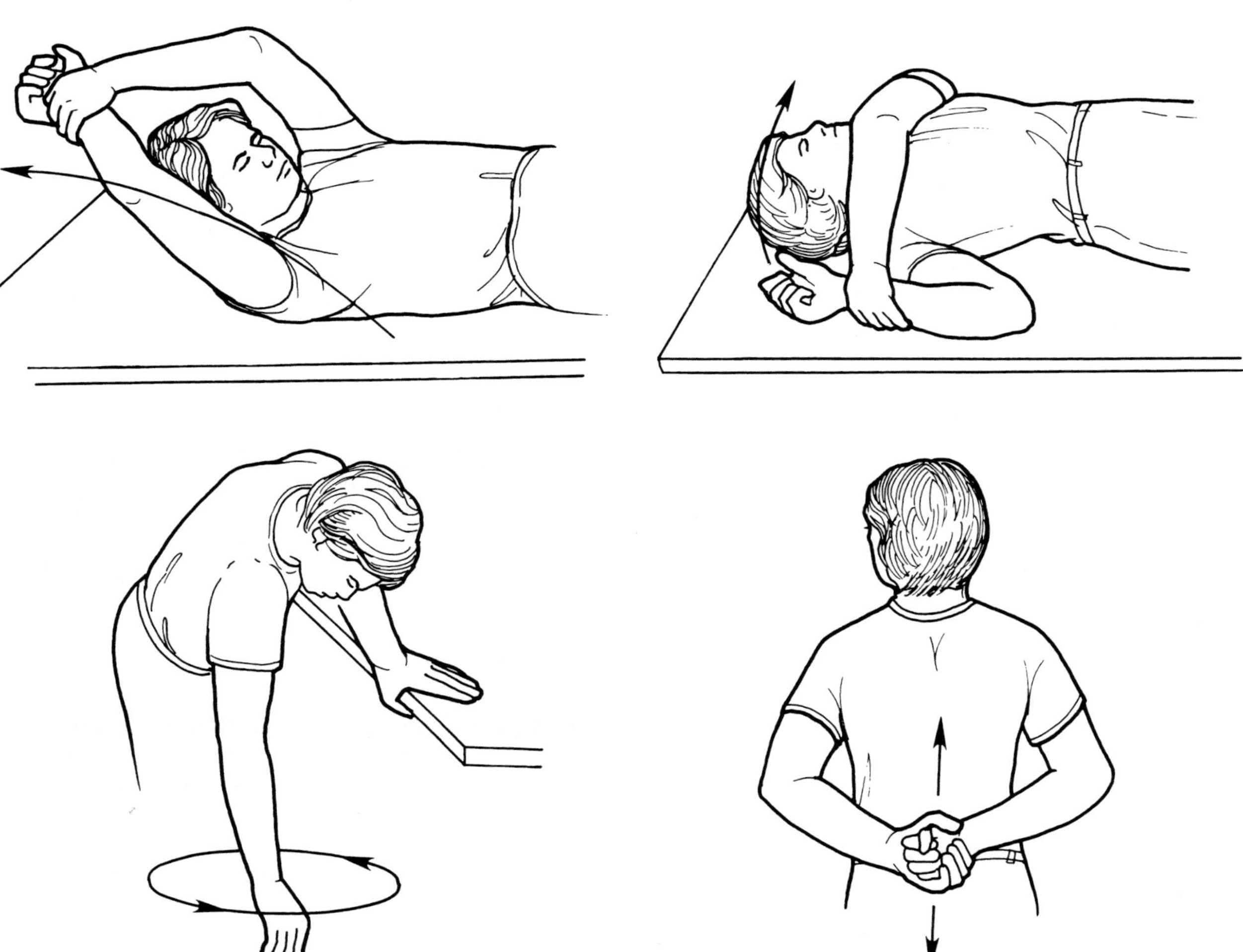

Fig. 23-26 Pendular shoulder exercises. (From Daya M: Shoulder. In Rosen P, et al [editors]: *Emergency medicine: concepts and clinical practice,* ed 4, St Louis, 1998, Mosby.)

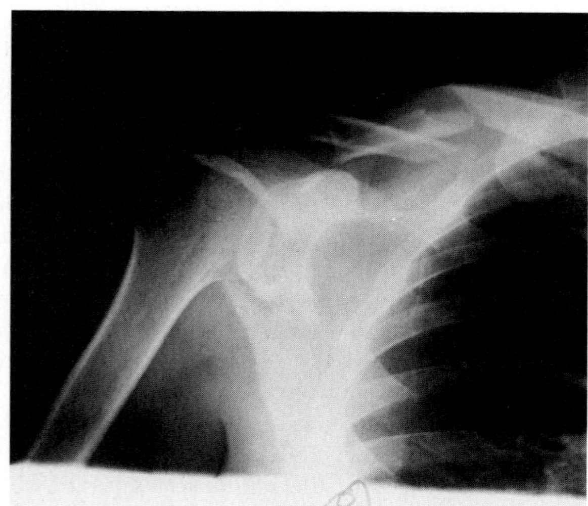

Fig. 23-27 Floating shoulder.

anteromedially and distally by the muscular attachments of the humerus and the weight of the arm.[74] This scenario is referred to as a "floating shoulder." Surgical intervention is required to attain good functional outcomes.[75,76]

Proximal Humerus

The proximal humerus provides for the attachment of a number of important muscle groups. These muscle groups include the rotator cuff group (supraspinatus, infraspinatus, teres minor, and subscapularis), which helps to stabilize the humeral head within the glenohumeral joint. Other muscle groups that insert onto the humerus are largely involved in movement about the glenohumeral joint. Displacements encountered with fractures of the humerus often reflect the pull of these attached muscle groups.[77]

EPIDEMIOLOGY

Fractures of the proximal humerus are common and account for 4% to 5% of all fractures.[78] Structural changes associated with aging (osteoporosis) weaken the proximal humerus, predisposing it to injury.[77] Nordqvist and Petersson[2] reported an incidence of 114 per 100,000 with a mean age of 67 and a female-to-male ratio of 3 to 1 in Malmo, Sweden.

PATHOPHYSIOLOGY

The classic mechanism of injury involves a fall onto an outstretched abducted arm. Concurrent pronation limits further abduction and levers the humerus against the acromial process. This mechanism produces a fracture or dislocation depending on the tensile strengths of the bone and surrounding ligaments.[77] Older patients are prone to fracture, whereas younger individuals are apt to dislocate.[16] The combined injury (fracture-dislocation) may be seen in middle-aged individuals. Proximal humerus fractures may also result from a direct blow to the lateral side of the arm or from an axial load transmitted through the elbow.[16] Patients with metastatic bone cancer or bone cysts may fracture through the weakened bone with minimal trauma. Patients with such pathologic fractures may have a deceptively mild mechanism of injury.

CLASSIFICATION

Fractures of the proximal humerus separate along old epiphyseal lines, producing four distinct segments consisting of the articular surface (anatomic neck), greater tuberosity, lesser tuberosity, and humeral shaft (surgical neck).[77] Neer[79] has developed a four-segment classification system (Fig. 23-28) for proximal humeral fractures based on the relationship of these four major segments. A segment is considered displaced if it is angled more than 45° or separated more than 1 cm from the neighboring segment. Since the classification system only considers displacement, the number of fracture lines is irrelevant. There are four major categories of fracture: minimal displacement (Fig. 23-29), two-part displacement (Fig. 23-30), three-part displacement, and four-part displacement. Anterior and posterior fracture-dislocations are included within the classification system. Impaction fractures of the humeral head are classified separately according to the percentage of articular surface involved. Head-splitting fractures are considered seperately.[79]

EMERGENCY DEPARTMENT PRESENTATION

The affected arm is held close to the body and all movements are restricted by pain. Tenderness, hematoma, ecchymosis, deformity, or crepitus may be present over the fracture site.

DIAGNOSTIC STUDIES

Orthogonal views of the humerus should be obtained in suspected cases. An axillary view of the glenohumeral joint can also be useful in clarifying the relationship of the humeral head and glenoid fossa in suspected fracture dislocations.[77]

EMERGENCY DEPARTMENT MANAGEMENT AND DISPOSITION

Minimally displaced fractures (Fig. 23-29) constitute 80% to 85% of all cases. There is no displacement or angulation and the fracture segments are held together by the capsule, periosteum, and surrounding muscles. Initial treatment consists of adequate analgesia and immobilization with a sling and swathe device. As soon as clinical union is achieved (head and shaft move together), functional exercises (Fig. 23-26)

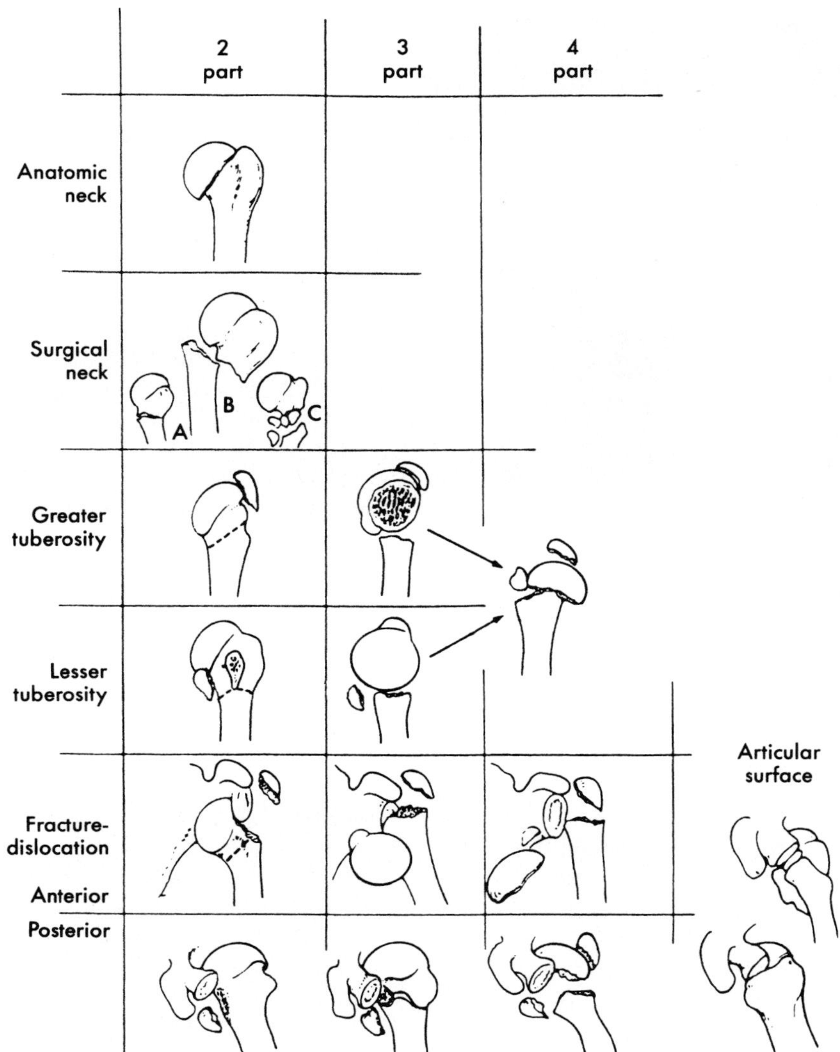

Fig. 23-28 Neer classification of proximal humerus fractures. (From Neer CS: *J Bone Joint Surg* 52A:1077, 1979.)

should be initiated. These exercises are especially important in the elderly. The emergency physician should warn the older patient that without daily range-of-motion exercises, they will develop adhesive capsulitis ("frozen shoulder"). Initial passive exercises are slowly replaced by more active and resistive exercises. Most undisplaced fractures heal over a period of 3 to 4 weeks.[77] The treatment of two-, three-, and four-part displaced fractures is beyond the scope of this discussion. An orthopedic surgeon should be consulted since many of these injuries require operative repair. Proximal humerus fracture-dislocation injuries should also be referred to the orthopedic surgeon since forceful attempted reductions of these injuries in the ED can lead to separation of previously undisplaced segments. Closed reduction under radiographic control and general anesthesia is preferred.[80]

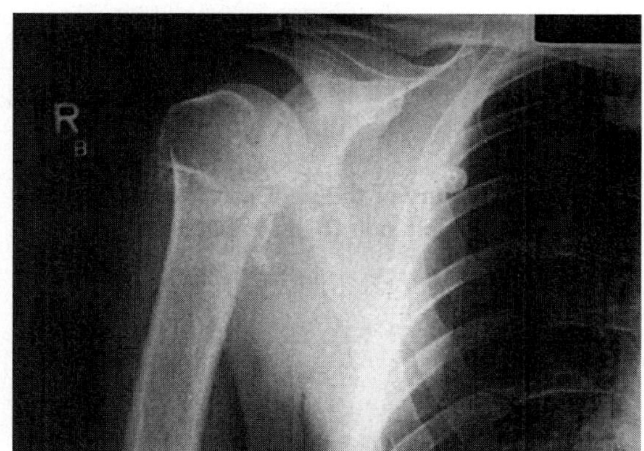

Fig. 23-29 Three-part minimally displaced proximal humerus fracture. (From Daya M: Shoulder. In Rosen P, et al [editors]: *Emergency medicine: concepts and clinical practice,* ed 4, St. Louis, 1998, Mosby.)

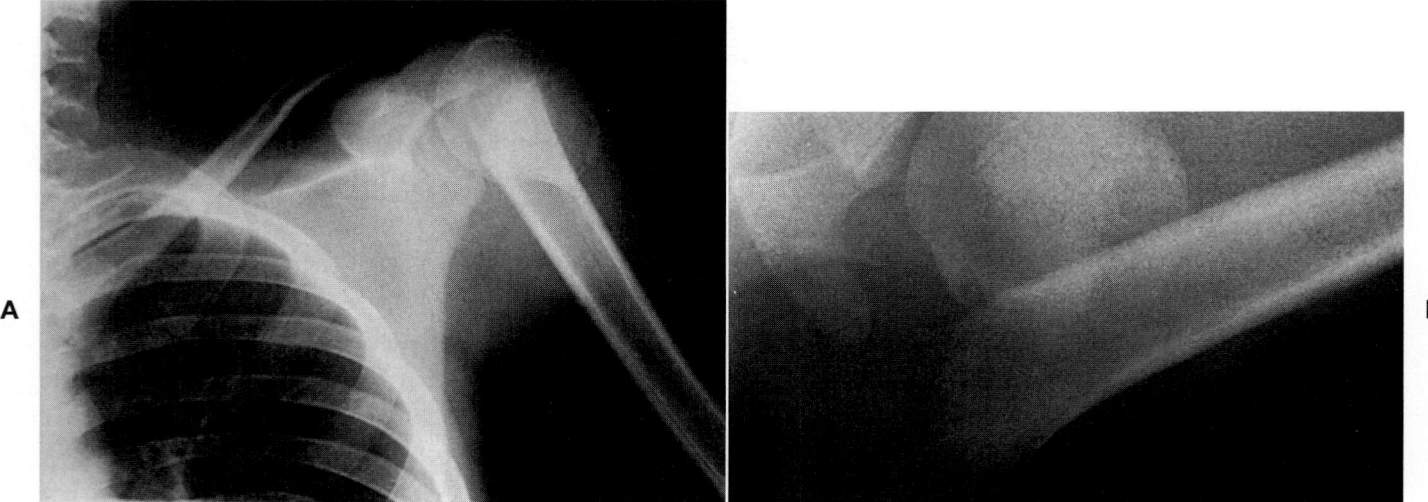

Fig. 23-30 Anteroposterior **(A)** and axillary **(B)** view of a two-part proximal humerus fracture. (Courtesy of David Nelson, MD.)

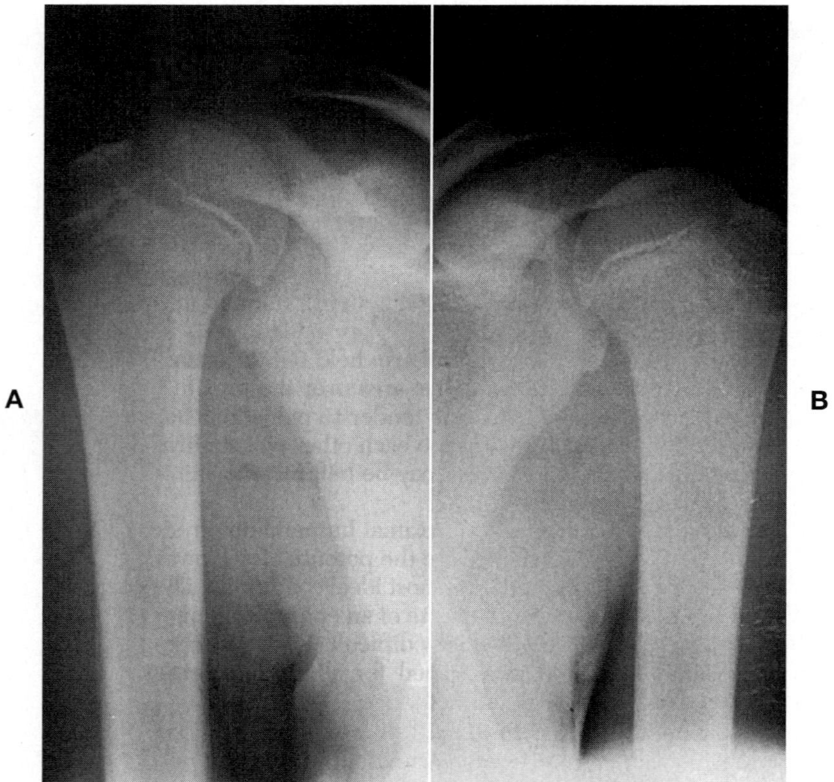

Fig. 23-31 Salter I fracture of proximal humeral epiphysis **(A).** Normal left side **(B)** is included for comparison. (From Daya M: Shoulder. In Rosen P, et al [editors]: *Emergency medicine: concepts and clinical practice,* ed 4, St Louis, 1998, Mosby.)

Impression fractures (a compression fracture characterized by a flattened humeral head) involving <20% of the articular surface are usually stable. With >20% involvement, the reduction is usually unstable and requires surgical repair.[77,79]

COMPLICATIONS

The most common complication of proximal humeral fractures is adhesive capsulitis ("frozen shoulder"), which can be prevented by the early initiation of a rehabilitation program. Two-part fractures of the articular surface and four-part fractures have a high incidence of avascular necrosis of the humeral head.[79] Repeated forceful attempts at reduction of fractures-dislocations can lead to subsequent heterotopic bone formation (myositis ossificans).[77] Neurovascular injuries (axillary nerve, brachial plexus, and axillary artery) may be encountered with displaced surgical neck fractures and fracture-dislocations.[78]

Proximal Humeral Epiphysis

EPIDEMIOLOGY

Fractures of the proximal humeral epiphysis are uncommon and account for 10% of shoulder fractures and 3% to 6% of all epiphyseal injuries in children.[81] The injury is usually seen in young males 11 to 17 years of age.[82]

PATHOPHYSIOLOGY/CLASSIFICATION

The most common mechanism of injury involves a fall onto the outstretched hand and the fracture typically occurs through the zone of hypertrophy in the epiphyseal plate. Injuries can be classified according to their location (Salter classification system), stability, and degree of displacement.[16]

EMERGENCY DEPARTMENT PRESENTATION

The patient presents with the injured arm held tightly against the body by the opposite hand. The area over the proximal humerus is usually swollen and extremely tender to palpation.

DIAGNOSTIC STUDIES

Radiographs obtained at 90° to each other confirm the diagnosis. Comparison views (Fig. 23-31) may be helpful especially with minimally displaced fractures.

EMERGENCY DEPARTMENT MANAGEMENT AND DISPOSITION

Fractures of the proximal humeral epiphysis should not be taken lightly since there is the potential for growth disturbance even under the most ideal of conditions. The very active healing process at the site of an epiphyseal injury makes delayed reduction extremely difficult. Orthopedic consultation should be obtained for all such injuries. Children under the age of 6 years usually have Salter I epiphyseal injuries (Fig. 23-31) and can be treated conservatively with sling and swathe immobilization and oral analgesics. Children over 6 years of age usually have a Salter II epiphyseal injury. Salter II injuries with greater than 20 degrees of angulation should be reduced under anesthesia.[81,82]

COMPLICATIONS

These injuries may be associated with damage to the neurovascular bundle, as well as growth plate disturbances and malunion.[16] Older patients with marked displacement or angulation are at higher risk for residual loss of mobility and dysmetria.[81]

SCAPULOTHORACIC DISSOCIATION

Scapulothoracic dissociation is a rare injury with a potentially devastating outcome.[83] The mechanism of injury involves a strong traction force applied to the upper extremity such as what might occur when a motorcyclist hangs onto the handlebars while the body is forced away during a high-speed crash.[84] Patients usually present with multisystem trauma and a characteristic triad of injuries, which include a chest wall hematoma, absent radial pulse (axillary or subclavian vessel injury), and complete brachial plexus palsy.[85] The chest radiograph demonstrates marked local soft tissue swelling in association with lateral displacement of the scapula.[84] Additional osseous injuries include acromioclavicular separation, displaced fractures of the clavicle, and dislocations of the sternoclavicular joint.[84] Outcome is generally poor with death in 10% of cases and a functionless extremity in survivors.[83,84]

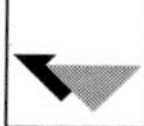

PEARLS & PITFALLS

Dislocation

- Obtain a true AP view of the shoulder as part of the trauma series.
- Always obtain orthogonal views (axillary lateral, apical oblique, or transscapular).
- Perform and document a thorough neurovascular examination before and after all manipulations.
- Suspect a grade III AC joint dislocation if the coracoclavicular distance is >11 to 13 mm or there is a difference of >5 mm in this distance between the injured and uninjured side.

- Suspect a sternoclavicular dislocation with tenderness over the medial clavicle, pain on any movement of the shoulder, and no obvious fracture of the clavicle.
- Obtain a CT scan to evaluate the mediastinal structures when investigating posterior dislocations of the SC joint.
- Good muscle relaxation, intraarticular anesthesia, or both are key to shoulder relocation.
- Include posterior dislocation in the differential diagnosis of any shoulder injury, especially if there is limited external rotation. An axillary or transscapular (Y-view) is helpful.
- Suspect a posterior dislocation in any individual who complains of shoulder pain or discomfort following a seizure.
- Suspect a scapular dissociation when you encounter the triad of chest wall hematoma, absent pulses, and a brachial plexus injury.

Fracture

- Refer severely displaced clavicle fractures for orthopedic follow-up.
- Examine the AP portable trauma chest radiograph closely for the presence of a scapular fracture.
- Remember to search for brachial plexus and vascular injuries, as well as ipsilateral lung trauma in patients with scapular fractures.
- Epiphyses in adolescents and young adults may mimic fracture lines.
- Order comparison films on a selective basis.
- Do not attempt reduction of two-part proximal humeral fracture dislocations in the ED.
- Request orthopedic consultation in all proximal humeral epiphysis fractures.

REFERENCES

1. Matsen FA III, Kirby RM: Office evaluation and management of shoulder pain, *Orthop Clin North Am* 13:453-475, 1982.
2. Nordqvist A, Petersson CJ: Incidence and cause of shoulder girdle injuries in an urban population, *J Shoulder Elbow Surg* 4:107-112, 1995.
3. Tibone JE: Shoulder problems of adolescents: how they differ from those of adults, *Clin Sports Med* 2:423, 1983.
4. Fraenkel L, Lavalley M, Felson D: The use of radiographs to evaluate shoulder pain in the ED, *Am J Emerg Med* 16:560-563,1998.
5. Neviaser RJ: Radiologic assessment of the shoulder. Plain and arthrographic, *Orthop Clin North Am* 18:343-349, 1987.
6. De Smet AA: Axillary projection in radiography of the nontraumatized shoulder, *Am J Roentgenol* 134:511-514, 1980.
7. De Smet AA: Anterior oblique projection in radiography of the traumatized shoulder, *Am J Roentgenol* 134:515-518, 1980.
8. Kornguth PJ, Salazar AM: The apical oblique view of the shoulder: its usefulness in acute trauma, *Am J Roentgenol* 149:113-116, 1987.
9. Brems-Dalgaard E, Davidsen E, Sloth C: Radiographic examination of the acute shoulder, *Eur J Radiol* 11:10-14, 1990.
10. Rubin SA, Gray RL, Green WR: The scapular "Y": a diagnostic aid in shoulder trauma, *Radiology* 110:725-726, 1974.
11. Szalay EA, Rockwood CA Jr: Injuries of the shoulder and arm, *Emerg Med Clin North Am* 2:279-294, 1984.
12. Harris JH, Harris WH: *The radiology of emergency medicine,* ed 2, Baltimore, 1981, Williams & Wilkins.
13. Flinn RM, et al: Optimal radiography of the acutely injured shoulder, *J Can Assoc Radiol* 34:128-132, 1983.
14. Destouet JM, et al: Computed tomography of the sternoclavicular joint and sternum, *Radiology* 138:123-128, 1981.
15. Salvatore JE: Sternoclavicular joint dislocation, *Clin Orthop Rel Res* 58:51-55, 1968.
16. Neer CS, Rockwood CA: Fracture and dislocations of the shoulder. In Rockwood CA, Green DP (editors): *Fractures in adults,* ed 2, Philadelphia, 1984, JB Lippincott.
17. Selesnick FH, et al: Retrosternal dislocation of the clavicle: report of four cases, *J Bone Joint Surg* 66-A:287-291, 1984.
18. Winter J, et al.: Retrosternal epiphyseal disruption of medial clavicle: case and review in children, *J Emerg Med* 7:9-13, 1989.
19. Kiroff GK, McClure DN, Skelley JW: Delayed diagnosis of posterior sternoclavicular joint dislocation, *Med J Aust* 164:242-243, 1996.
20. Simon RR, Koenigsknecht SJ, Stevens C: *Emergency orthopedics: the extremities,* ed 2, Norwalk, 1987, Appleton & Lange.
21. Cope R. Dislocations of the sternoclavicular joint, *Skel Radiol* 22:223-238, 1993.
22. Wickiewicz TL: Acromioclavicular and sternoclavicular joint injuries, *Clin Sports Med* 2:429, 1983
23. Allman FL Jr.: Fractures and ligamentous injuries of the clavicle and its articulation, *J Bone Joint Surg* 49-A:774-784, 1967.
24. Richards RR: Acromioclavicular joint injuries, *Instr Course Lect* 42:259-269, 1993.
25. Bossart PJ, et al: Lack of efficacy of 'weighted' radiographs in diagnosing acute acromioclavicular separation, *Ann Emerg Med* 17:20-24, 1988.
26. Neviaser JS: Injuries of the clavicle and its articulations, *Orthop Clin North Am* 11:233-237, 1980.
27. Larsen E, Bjerg-Nielsen A, Christensen P: Conservative or surgical treatment of acromioclavicular dislocation: a prospective, controlled, randomized study, *J Bone J Surg* 68-A:552-555, 1986.
28. Bannister GC, et al: The management of acute acromioclavicular dislocation: a randomised prospective controlled trial, *J Bone J Surg* 71-B:848-850, 1989.
29. Friedman SF: *Visual Anatomy III. Limbs and back,* ed 1, Hagerstown, 1981, Harper & Row.
30. Kroner K, Lind T, Jensen J: The epidemiology of shoulder dislocations, *Arch Orthop Trauma Surg* 108: 288-290, 1989.
31. Rowe CR: Acute and recurrent anterior dislocations of the shoulder, *Orthop Clin North Am* 11:253-270, 1980.
32. Aronen JG: Anterior shoulder dislocations in sports, *Sports Med* 3:224-234, 1986.
33. Tullos HS, Bennett JB, Braly WG: Acute shoulder dislocations: factors influencing diagnosis and treatment, *Instr Course Lect* 33:364-385, 1984.

34. Riebel GD, McCabe JB: Anterior shoulder dislocations: a review of reduction techniques, *Am J Emerg Med* 9:180-188, 1991.
35. Pasila M, Jaroma H, Kiviluoto O, et al: Early complications of primary shoulder dislocations, *Acta Orthop Scand* 49:260-263, 1978.
36. Underhill TJ, Wan A, Morrice M: Interscalene brachial plexus blocks in the management of shoulder dislocations, *Arch Emerg Med* 6:199-204, 1989.
37. Rollinson PD: Reduction of shoulder dislocations by the hanging method, *South Afr Med J* 73:106-107, 1988.
38. Matthews DE, Roberts T. Intraarticular lidocaine versus intravenous analgesia for reduction of acute anterior shoulder dislocations: a prospective randomized study, *Am J Sports Med* 23:54-58, 1995.
39. Gleeson AP, et al: Comparison of intra-articular lignocaine and a suprascapular nerve block for acute anterior shoulder dislocation, *Injury* 28:141-142, 1997.
40. Janecki CJ, Shahcheragh GH: The forward elevation maneuver for reduction of anterior dislocation of the shoulder, *Clin Orthop Rel Res* 164:177-180, 1982.
41. Westin CD, et al: Anterior shoulder dislocation: a simple and rapid method for reduction, *Am J Sports Med* 23:369-371, 1995.
42. Mirick MJ, Clinton JE, Ruiz E: External rotation method of shoulder dislocation reduction, *J Am Coll Emerg Phys* 8:528-531, 1979.
43. Danzl DF, et al: Closed reduction of anterior subcoracoid shoulder dislocation: evaluation of an external rotation method, *Orthop Rev* 15:311-315, 1986.
44. Kothari RU, Dronen SC: The scapular manipulation technique for the reduction of acute anterior shoulder dislocations, *J Emerg Med* 8:625-628, 1990.
45. McNamara RM: Reduction of anterior shoulder dislocations by scapular manipulation, *Ann Emerg Med* 22:1140-1144, 1993.
46. Harvey RA, Trabulsy ME, Roe L: Are postreduction anteroposterior and scapular Y views useful in anterior shoulder dislocations? *Am J Emerg Med* 10:149-151, 1992.
47. Hendey GW, Kinlaw K: Clinically significant abnormalities in postreduction radiographs after anterior shoulder dislocation, *Ann Emerg Med* 28:399-402, 1996.
48. Nevasier RJ, Nevasier TJ, Nevasier JS: Anterior dislocation of the shoulder and rotator cuff rupture, *Clin Orthop Rel Res* 291: 103-106, 1993.
49. Taylor DC, Arciero RA: Pathologic changes associated with shoulder dislocations: arthroscopic and physical examination findings in first-time traumatic anterior dislocations, *Am J Sports Med* 25:306-311, 1997.
50. McLaughlin HL: Posterior dislocation of the shoulder, *J Bone Joint Surg* 34-A:584-590, 1952.
51. Perrenoud A, Imhoff AB: Locked posterior dislocation of the shoulder, *Bull Hosp Joint Dis* 54:165-168, 1996.
52. Paton DF: Posterior dislocation of the shoulder: a diagnostic pitfall for physicians, *Practitioner* 223:111-112,1979.
53. May VR Jr.: Posterior dislocation of the shoulder: habitual, traumatic and obstetric, *Orthop Clin North Am* 11:271-285, 1980.
54. Heller KD, et al: Posterior dislocations of the shoulder: recommendations for a classification, *Arch Orthop Trauma Surg* 113: 228-231, 1994.
55. Cisternino SJ, et al: The trough line: a radiographic sign of posterior shoulder dislocation, *Am J Roentgenol* 130:951-954, 1978.
56. Wadlington VR, Hendrix RW, Rogers LF: Computed tomography of posterior fracture-dislocations of the shoulder: case reports, *J Trauma* 32:113-115, 1992.
57. Saxena K, Stavas J: Inferior glenohumeral dislocation, *Ann Emerg Med* 12:718-720, 1983.
58. Davids JR, Talbott RD: Luxatio erecta humeri, *Clin Orthop Rel Res* 252:144-149, 1990.
59. Rae PJ, Sylvester BS: Luxatio erecta: two cases without direct injury, *Injury* 19:361-362, 1988.
60. Newman AP: Fractures of the shoulder, *Top Emerg Med* 10:65, 1988.
61. Post M: Current concepts in the treatment of fractures of the clavicle, *Clin Orthop Rel Res* 245:89-101, 1989.
62. Andersen K, Jensen PO, Lauritzen J: Treatment of clavicular fractures: figure-of-eight bandage versus a simple sling, *Acta Orthop Scand* 58:71-74, 1987.
63. Hill JM, McGuire MH, Crosby LA: Closed treatment of displaced middle-third fracture of the clavicle gives poor results, *J Bone J Surg* 79-B:537-539, 1997.
64. Zuckerman JD, Koval KJ, Cuomo F: Fractures of the scapula, *Instr Course Lect* 42:271-281, 1993.
65. McGinnis M, Denton JR: Fractures of the scapula: a retrospective study of 40 fractured scapulae, *J Trauma* 29:1488-1493, 1989.
66. Ada JR, Miller ME: Scapular fractures: analysis of 113 cases, *Clin Orthop Rel Res* 269:174-180, 1991.
67. Thompson DA, et al: The significance of scapular fractures, *J Trauma* 25:974-977, 1985.
68. McLennan JG, Ungersma J: Pneumothorax complicating fracture of the scapula, *J Bone Joint Surg* 64-A:598-599, 1982.
69. DeCloux MP, et al: Omoplate, *Lille Chir* 11:215, 1956.
70. Harris RD, Harris JH Jr: The prevalence and significance of missed scapular fractures in blunt chest trauma, *Am J Roentgenol* 151:747-750, 1988.
71. Zdravkovic D, Damholt VV: Comminuted and severely displaced fractures of the scapula, *Acta Orthop Scand* 45:60-65, 1974.
72. Derosa GP, Kettlekamp DB: Fracture of the coracoid process of the scapula: case report, *J Bone Joint Surg* 59-A:696-697, 1977.
73. McGahan JP, Rab GT, Dublin A: Fractures of the scapula, *J Trauma* 20:880-883, 1980.
74. Herscovici D Jr, et al: The floating shoulder: ipsilateral clavicle and scapular neck fractures, *J Bone Joint Surg* 74-B:362-364, 1992.
75. Simpson NS, Jupiter JB: Complex fracture patterns of the upper extremity, *Clin Orthop Rel Res* 318:43-53, 1995.
76. Leung KS, Lam TP: Open reduction and internal fixation of ipsilateral fractures of the scapular neck and clavicle, *J Bone Joint Surg* 75-A:1015-1018, 1993.
77. Hawkins RJ, Angelo RL: Displaced proximal humeral fractures. Selecting treatment, avoiding pitfalls, *Orthop Clin North Am* 18: 421-431, 1987.
78. Kristiansen B, et al: Epidemiology of proximal humeral fractures, *Acta Orthop Scand* 58:75-77, 1987.
79. Neer CS II: Displaced proximal humeral fractures. Part 1. Classification and evaluation, *J Bone Joint Surg* 52-A:1077-1089, 1970.
80. Ferkel RD, Hedley AK, Eckardt JJ: Anterior fracture-dislocation of the shoulder: pitfalls in treatment, *J Trauma* 24:363-367, 1984.
81. Burgos-Flores J, et al: Fractures of the proximal humeral epiphysis, *Int Orthop* 17:16-19, 1993.
82. Williams DJ: The mechanisms producing fracture-separation of the proximal humeral epiphysis, *J Bone Joint Surg* 63-B:102-107, 1981.
83. Damschen DD, Cogbill TH, Seigel MJ. Scapulothoracic dissociation caused by blunt trauma, *J Trauma* 42:537-540, 1997.
84. Ebraheim NA, An HS, Jackson WT, et al: Scapulothoracic dissociation, *J Bone Joint Surg* 70-A:428-432, 1988.
85. Sampson LN, et al: The neurovascular outcome of scapulothoracic dissociation, *J Vasc Surg* 17:1083-1088, 1993.

24 Elbow and Forearm Injuries

ERIC W. OSSMAN

Of all the orthopedic injuries encountered by emergency physicians (EPs), injuries to the elbow and forearm are fairly common. Because of the functional importance of the elbow joint, the recognition and management of elbow injuries is paramount. This chapter reviews the types of injuries, the management decisions, and the disposition of patients to effect optimal treatment.

BIOMECHANICS

The elbow is a hinge joint, which functions primarily to flex and extend the forearm. The range of this joint is slightly greater than 180 degrees. Movement of the elbow rotates the olecranon of the ulna around the trochlea of the humerus. Flexion is limited by apposition of the anterior surfaces of the arm and forearm. Hyperextension causes the olecranon to impinge on the olecranon fossa of the humerus, preventing further movement.

The proximal and distal radioulnar joints allow the radius to rotate approximately 180 degrees about its axis. These articulations permit supination and pronation of the hand and forearm.

ANATOMY

The elbow and forearm are an anatomic unit composed of 3 bones, 3 major nerves, 3 major arteries, and 22 muscles. The elbow joint consists of three separate articulations: the proximal radioulnar joint, the humeroradial articulation, and the humeroulnar articulation.

Joint stability depends on the humeroulnar joint, which is completely enclosed in a fibrous capsule. The trochlea at the distal end of the humerus fits snugly into the U-shaped trochlear notch of the ulna. Thickened triangular bands along the medial and lateral aspects of the joint form the collateral ligaments. These ligaments provide the elbow with a great deal of stability against varus and valgus stress. Because the anterior and posterior aspects of the fibrous capsule are relatively thin, the cubital joint is susceptible to posterior and occasional anterior dislocations.

The capitellum articulates with the radial head at the humeroradial joint. This joint serves as a pivot for the radius to rotate about its long axis. The close application of the capitellum also prevents proximal migration of the radius. The annular ligament is a thick fibrous band attached to the ulna at the anterior and posterior margins of the radial notch. This ligament wraps around the radial head and maintains the relationship between the head of the radius and the radial notch of the ulna. The proximal articulation between the radius and ulna allows the radius to rotate about its long axis, but limits movement in other planes. The head of the ulna articulates at the ulnar notch with the distal end of the radius.

The interosseus membrane is a fibrous structure that spans the gap between the lateral aspect of the ulna and the medial aspect of the radius. In addition to approximating the radius and ulna, many of the deep muscles of the forearm attach to this structure.

Radiologic Anatomy

The lateral elbow film provides the most information regarding elbow fractures and dislocation. Many fractures are occult and do not demonstrate obvious lucencies. The presence of **fat pad** signs provides an important clue to injury. These lucencies occur with blood in the joint. Although the anterior fat pad ("sail sign") is occasionally a normal finding, a posterior fat pad is always pathologic.

Knowledge of normal alignment of the elbow also assists in radiographic interpretation. Two lines in particular are helpful. A line drawn down the anterior humerus should intersect the midcapitellum on the

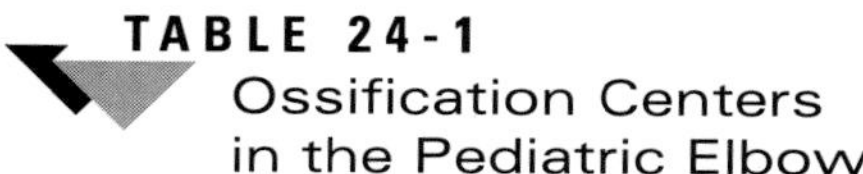

TABLE 24-1
Ossification Centers in the Pediatric Elbow

GROWTH CENTER	AGE OSSIFICATION CENTER APPEARS
Capitellum	2 years
Medial epicondylar apophysis	4 years
Trochlear epiphysis	8 years
Lateral epicondylar apophysis	10 years

AP radiograph, whereas a line through the center of the radius should bisect this same bone on the lateral radiograph. Using the border of another x-ray film held up as a straightedge against the lateral view is more accurate than an "eyeball" estimate of these relationships. On the lateral view, the overlapping condyles form a "figure-of-eight." A break in the continuity of this shape also suggests a fracture.

The numerous ossification centers in the pediatric elbow change with age (Table 24-1). Any standard radiologic text gives examples of the number and location of the ossification centers according to age, but on occasion, a comparison view of the normal elbow allows the distinction between a fracture and normal development.

INJURY PATTERNS

Distal Humerus Fractures

SUPRACONDYLAR FRACTURES

Mechanism of Injury. Forced hyperextension of the elbow joint produces most elbow dislocations and supracondylar fractures. In the adult, a *f*all *o*n an *o*utstretched *h*and (FOOSH) typically produces an elbow dislocation. In the pediatric population, this mechanism is more likely to lead to a supracondylar fracture, since the collateral ligaments surrounding the elbow joint are stronger than the distal humerus. Hyperextension drives the olecranon into the olecranon fossa on the posterior aspect of the humerus, breaking the bone.

Flexion-type injuries account for only a small percentage of supracondylar fractures. In a cadaveric model, flexion supracondylar fractures occur with a direct blow on the posterior aspect of the ulna with the elbow held in at least 110 degrees of flexion.[1] The mechanism is compatible with a fall or direct blow on a flexed elbow.

Fracture Classification. The classification of supracondylar fractures is relatively straightforward and based almost completely on the radiographic appearance of the elbow on the lateral view. The original three-stage system was described by Gartland in 1959 and has been in common use since. Classification of fractures based on the three-stage system demonstrates a high degree of intraobserver reliability (Table 24-2).

Supracondylar fractures are divided into the common extension type and relatively rare flexion type. The location of the distal fragment relative to the humeral shaft determines the fracture type (Fig. 24-1). On the lateral film, draw a line or hold a straightedge along the anterior border of the humeral shaft and determine the relative position of the distal fragment. In children, this line is compared with the position of the capitellum. This line drawn should transect the middle third of the capitellum. In an extension injury, the distal fracture fragment is displaced posteriorly and proximally. Subtle type I extension fractures can be very difficult to detect and careful attention to the anterior humeral line provides the diagnosis. The misplaced capitellum lies posterior to this line, or the line intersects the anterior third of the capitellum. A flexion type fracture displaces the distal fragment anteriorly.

Emergency Department Management. In any suspected supracondylar fracture, the EP should immediately assess the neurovascular status of the affected extremity. Because of their proximity to the supracondylar humerus, the brachial artery and radial nerve are at particular risk and require a focused examination to detect associated injury.

The management of type I extension and flexion supracondylar fractures is straightforward. Place the injured extremity in a padded posterior splint, with the elbow in 90 degrees of flexion and the forearm in the neutral position. Nonemergent orthopedic consultation is necessary for outpatient follow-up. Standard principles of ice, elevation, and analgesia apply.

Type II extension and flexion supracondylar fractures typically require orthopedic consultation for closed reduction in the emergency department (ED). It is unusual for these injuries to be associated with neurovascular injury, since the intact cortex prevents complete displacement of the fragments. The consultant may reduce and cast those fractures that are minimally displaced. Fractures with greater displacement typically require closed reduction and percutaneous pinning. The humerus-capitellar angle and Baumann's angle are better maintained with percutaneous pinning in the moderately displaced fracture.[3]

Type III supracondylar fractures always require emergent orthopedic consultation. Complications are frequent, and the most common problem is peripheral nerve injury. In one series, nerve injury occurred in nearly 10% of all type III fractures.[4] Although the most commonly injured nerve was the

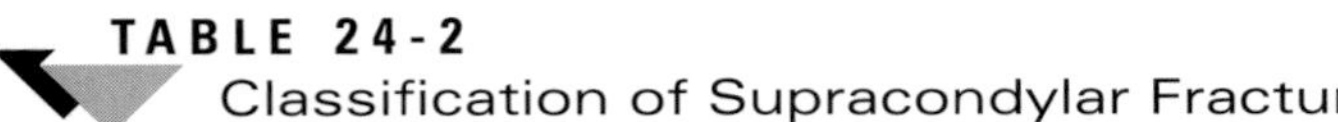

TABLE 24-2
Classification of Supracondylar Fractures

	TYPE I	TYPE II	TYPE III
Extension Supracondylar fracture	Distal fragment is minimally displaced posteriorly. The posterior cortex of humerus is intact.	Distal fragment is moderately displaced posteriorly. The posterior cortex of the humerus is intact.	Distal fragment is significantly displaced posteriorly. The posterior cortex of the humerus is disrupted.
Flexion Supracondylar fracture	Distal fragment is minimally displaced anteriorly. The anterior cortex of humerus is intact.	Distal fragment is moderately displaced anteriorly. The anterior cortex of the humerus is intact.	Distal fragment is significantly displaced anteriorly. The anterior cortex of the humerus is disrupted.

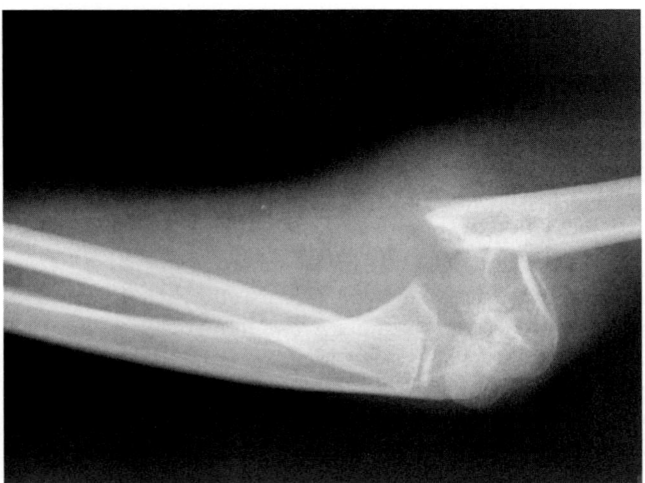

Fig. 24-1 Supracondylar humerus fracture.

anterior interosseus, injuries to the median, radial, and ulnar nerves also transpired. In the same series of 200 patients, physicians found 5 vascular injuries, 3 requiring operative intervention, and 1 requiring bypass.

The EP should attempt immediate reduction of a type III fracture only if vascular compromise is present. Reduction is most easily accomplished by applying axial traction to the forearm while manipulating the fragment in an anterior direction. Entrapment of the brachialis muscle may impede the emergent reduction of a type III fracture and is responsible for 90% of irreducible type III fractures.[5] The vast majority of type III fractures are treated by percutaneous pinning or open reduction and internal fixation, since instability makes closed reduction and casting impractical.

In addition to peripheral nerve injury, other complications of supracondylar fractures include **brachial artery entrapment**, **Volkmann's ischemic contracture**, and **cubitus varus**, the latter being a loss of the normally valgus carrying angle of the elbow. Volkmann's ischemic contracture results in permanent flexion of the fingers and is a consequence of a forearm compartment syndrome. Consider an acute compartment syndrome if the patient experiences pain in the forearm with passive extension of the fingers. Fasciotomy may be required to prevent this complication. A high index of suspicion and early measurements of compartment pressures are paramount in detecting this complication. Most compartment syndromes develop within the first 24 hours after the injury and, depending on the extent of the fracture and associated soft tissue injury, 12 to 24 hours of observation and repeated measurements may be the best strategy for the patient.

HUMERAL CONDYLAR FRACTURES

Mechanism of Injury. Isolated fractures of the humeral condyle are relatively rare in adults but, following supracondylar and radial neck fractures, are the third most common elbow fracture in children.[6] Lateral condylar fractures are caused by hyperextension combined with significant valgus stress. This mechanism results in an avulsion fracture of the lateral condyle. Hyperextension with varus stress results in the rare medial condylar fracture. In adults, these fractures are more likely a result of direct trauma to the respective condylar area.

The susceptibility of the pediatric elbow to lateral condylar fractures is in large part due to the differences in rates of ossification at the capitellar and trochlear epiphysis. The capitellar ossification center appears at about 12 months and begins to ossify at approximately 2 years of age. The trochlear ossification center does not appear until between 8 and 10 years of age.[7] Valgus stress on the hyperextended elbow produces a fracture that extends obliquely through the condyle into the weak space between the ossified capitellar epiphysis and the nonossified trochlear epiphysis.

TABLE 24-3
Adult Classification of Humeral Condylar Fractures

FRACTURE TYPE	DESCRIPTION	TREATMENT
Type I *Adult Lateral Epicondyle*	Stable Does not affect elbow joint integrity Trochlea remains intact, preserving stability of joint	Splint Posterior splint,* sling; orthopedic follow-up
Type II *Adult Lateral Epicondyle*	Lateral trochlear ridge disrupted, causing significant joint instability	Splint; orthopedic consultation for open reduction and internal fixation (ORIF)
Type I *Adult Medial Epicondyle*	Disruption of trochlea, lateral ridge remains intact Causes some joint instability	Splint Immediate orthopedic consultation for ORIF
Type II *Adult Medial Epicondyle*	Disruption of lateral trochlear ridge, significant joint instability	Splint Immediate orthopedic consultation for ORIF

*Note posterior splint with lateral molding, 90 degrees flexion at the elbow.

Fracture Classification. The pediatric classification is based on the integrity of the distal humeral epiphysis and the degree of distraction and rotation of the fracture fragment. In a stage I fracture, the distal humeral epiphysis remains intact, and there is minimal to no distraction of the fracture fragment. A stage II fracture is identified by the complete disruption of the distal humeral epiphysis with minimal to moderate displacement of the fracture fragment. Significant displacement and rotation of the fracture fragment is indicative of a stage III fracture.

The classification system is slightly different in adults because of the lack of cartilage in the adult distal humerus. Recall that the stability of the elbow joint in the adult is largely based on the humeroulnar articulation. Consequently, the classification in the adult is based on the integrity of the lateral trochlear ridge. In a type I lateral condylar fracture the trochlea remains intact, preserving the stability of the joint. A type II lateral condylar fracture occurs when the lateral trochlear ridge is disrupted, causing significant joint instability. The same principles apply to the classification of medial condylar fractures. A type I medial condylar fracture results in disruption of the trochlea, but the lateral ridge remains intact. A type II medial condylar fracture results in disruption of the lateral trochlear ridge and significant joint instability.

Emergency Department Management. The ED management of both adult and pediatric condylar fractures depends on the stability of the fracture based on the radiographic appearance (Tables 24-3 and 24-4).

A pediatric type I lateral condylar fracture is stable, since the integrity of the distal humeral epiphysis is maintained. More than 90% of these fractures with less than 2 mm of displacement heal with closed treatment in a long-arm cast or splint with the elbow flexed to 90 degrees.[8] Type II fractures with less than 2 mm of displacement are initially treated with a posterior splint with the elbow at 90 degrees of flexion, but must be followed very closely because of a propensity for later displacement.

Pediatric type III lateral condylar fractures demand immediate orthopedic consultation. These fractures require open reduction and internal fixation (ORIF). Patients who are operated on within 2 weeks of injury typically have good functional outcomes. If ORIF is delayed for more than 6 weeks or not attempted, significant complications may occur, including cubitus varus, cubitus valgus, nonunion, and osteonecrosis.[9]

In the adult patient, a type I lateral condylar fracture can typically be managed with a posterior splint and orthopedic follow-up. This fracture is stable and does not affect elbow joint integrity. A type II lateral condylar fracture disrupts the lateral trochlear ridge and causes joint instability. This fracture requires orthopedic consultation for ORIF.

A medial type I condylar fracture partially disrupts the trochlear ridge and causes some joint instability. Consequently, all medial type I condylar fractures require orthopedic consultation for ORIF. A type II medial condylar fracture results in significant joint instability and requires immediate ORIF.

HUMERAL INTERCONDYLAR FRACTURES

Mechanism of Injury. Intercondylar fractures are rare and occur mainly in the elderly. The typical mechanism of injury is a fall onto a flexed elbow or a

TABLE 24-4
Pediatric Classification of Humeral Condylar Fractures

FRACTURE TYPE	DESCRIPTION	TREATMENT
Type I *Pediatric Lateral Epicondyle*	Stable. Distal humeral epiphysis remains intact, minimal to no distraction of fracture fragment	Closed treatment in long-arm cast, splint,* or sling with elbow flexed (90% of these fractures with less than 2 mm of displacement) Follow-up in 5 days
Type II *Pediatric Lateral Epicondyle*	Complete disruption of distal humeral epiphysis, minimal to moderate displacement of fracture fragment	Splint. Elbow at 90 degrees of flexion Follow closely due to propensity for later displacement Orthopedic follow-up Possible open reduction and internal fixation (ORIF) (Fractures less than 2 mm of displacement)
Type III *Pediatric Lateral Epicondyle*	Significant displacement and rotation of fracture fragment	Splint. Immediate orthopedic consultation ORIF Patient operated on within 2 weeks of injury results in a good outcome Patient where ORIF delayed more than 6 weeks or not attempted results in significant complications (cubitus varus, cubitus valgus, nonunion, and osteonecrosis)

*Note posterior splint with lateral molding, 90 degrees flexion at the elbow.
(Based on the integrity of the distal humeral epiphysis, degree of distraction, and rotation of the fracture fragment.)

direct blow to the olecranon. This action can split the distal humerus via force applied through the trochlear notch.

Fracture Classification. By definition, all intercondylar fractures are intraarticular in nature. The distal fracture line typically splits the condyles, resulting in a T- or Y-shaped fracture. The most familiar classification system is based on the spatial and rotational relationship between the medial and lateral fracture fragments (Table 24-5).[10]

Emergency Department Management. Intercondylar fractures often present a management challenge. The elderly are typically osteopenic and often have concomitant medical problems. Initial ED management must ensure the distal neurovascular integrity. A flexion-type injury to the elbow can often result in a ulnar nerve injury. Typically, this injury manifests as a neuropraxia, but on occasion may become a permanent nerve injury.

Type I fractures require close orthopedic follow-up because of the potential for complications such as limitation in range of motion and persistent pain. Immobilize the affected arm with the elbow held at 90 degrees and the wrist slightly supinated. Immobilization is best accomplished using a posterior splint and sling.

Intercondylar fractures with any degree of separation or rotation require emergent orthopedic consultation for ORIF. The only exceptions are patients whose premorbid condition prohibits surgery. Early ORIF results in significantly better functional outcomes with less heterotopic bone formation than delayed or nonoperative treatment.[11] Approximately 25% of patients with such complex fractures have ulnar nerve injuries, emphasizing the importance of a thorough neurovascular examination.

Proximal Forearm Fractures

OLECRANON FRACTURES

Mechanism of Injury. Olecranon fractures typically result from a flexion-type elbow injury or from a direct blow over the olecranon. The triceps muscle inserts onto the posterior aspect of the olecranon and can exert significant strain.

Fracture Classification. Radiographic evaluation of olecranon fracture centers around determining whether the fracture is displaced (Fig. 24-2). A fracture

TABLE 24-5
Classification of Humeral Intercondylar Fractures

CLASSIFICATION	DESCRIPTION
Type I	Fracture line visible between medial and lateral condyles. No displacement.
Type II	Medial and lateral condyles are separated, but there is minimal rotation of the fracture fragments.
Type III	Medial and lateral condyles are separated, and there is significant rotational misalignment of the fracture fragments.
Type IV	Significant comminution, rotation, and displacement of the fracture fragments.

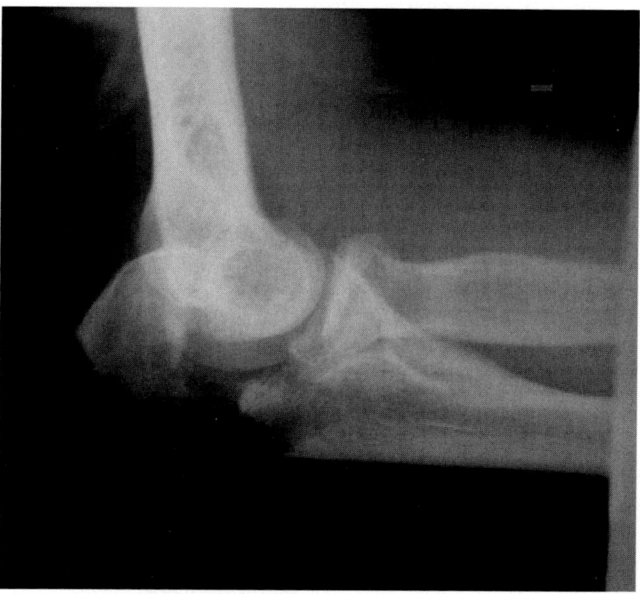

Fig. 24-2 Olecranon fracture.

that does not appear to be displaced in the lateral view with the elbow held at 90 degrees flexion may in fact displace with further movement of the joint. Thus, in seemingly nondisplaced fractures, it is prudent to obtain full flexion and extension lateral views of the olecranon.

The most useful system of classification for olecranon fractures is the Mayo system based on displacement, comminution, and joint stability (Table 24-6).[12] The initial evaluation requires that the EP evaluate the collateral ligaments of the elbow and the stability of the forearm in relation to the humerus. The lateral radiograph determines the degree of displacement and comminution of the fracture.

Emergency Department Management. Type I olecranon fractures are stable injuries. The lack of significant displacement indicates an intact triceps tendon aponeurosis. These injuries can best be managed with immobilization via a sling for 7 to 10 days and orthopedic follow-up. Range-of-motion exercises can typically begin within 2 weeks. On rare occasions, a type I fracture requires ORIF secondary to nonunion.

Type II olecranon fractures identified by greater than 3 mm of displacement require ORIF to obtain acceptable results. Orthopedic consultation for urgent follow-up (24 to 48 hours) is essential. Initial care should include immobilization of the extremity using a posterior splint in 45 degrees of flexion, analgesia, and elevation.

The critical component of ED management of the type III olecranon fracture is the assessment and reassessment of the distal neurovascular status. The unstable elbow implies a very significant mechanism with potential for neurovascular compromise. The ulnar nerve is most vulnerable in this type of injury. A type III injury necessitates orthopedic consultation for initial management and ultimately ORIF.

RADIAL HEAD FRACTURES

Mechanism of Injury. Radial head fractures are common in the adult population. The typical mechanism is a fall on an outstretched hand. This fracture commonly occurs in adults involved in bicycling accidents, in which they are pitched forward over the handlebars. This force drives the radial head into the capitellum, injuring the radial head and the articular surface of the capitellum. Because this mechanism also produces elbow dislocation and collateral ligament disruption, always test distal neurovascular integrity and joint stability.

Fracture Classification. In 1954 Mason[13] devised the most commonly used system of radial head fracture classification based on the radiographic appearance of the radial head (Table 24-7 and Fig. 24-3).

Type I radial head fractures are often missed because of their subtle radiographic appearance. The only clue may be the presence of a joint effusion on the lateral radiograph. The finding of a posterior effusion in the absence of an obvious fracture likely indicates a Mason type I radial head fracture.

The Mason classification system is limited because it does not account for associated injuries. Approximately 10% of radial head fractures are complicated by elbow dislocation.[14] Morrey[14] modified the system by subdividing fractures into simple or complex, based on the presence of an associated elbow disloca-

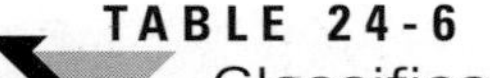

TABLE 24-6
Classification of Olecranon Fractures

MAYO CLASSIFICATION	FRAGMENT DISPLACEMENT	ELBOW JOINT STABILITY	COMMINUTION
Type IA	Undisplaced	Stable	Absent
Type IB	Undisplaced	Stable	Present
Type IIA	>3 mm displacement	Stable	Absent
Type IIB	>3 mm displacement	Stable	Present
Type IIIA	>3 mm displacement	Unstable	Absent
Type IIIB	>3 mm displacement	Unstable	Present

TABLE 24-7
Classification of Radial Head Fractures

MASON CLASSIFICATION	RADIAL HEAD DISPLACEMENT	COMMINUTION OF RADIAL HEAD
Type I	Nondisplaced	Absent
Type II	Greater than 2 mm displacement with involvement of more than 30% of the radial head	Absent
Type III	Greater than 2 mm displacement with involvement of more than 30% of the radial head	Present

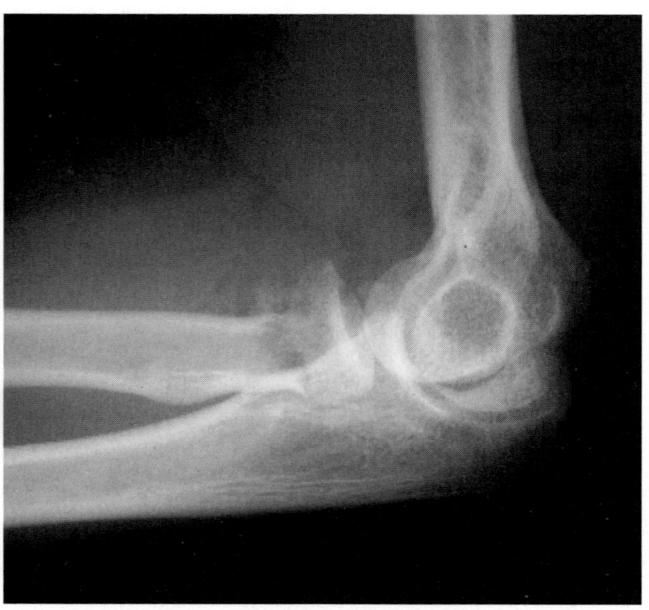

Fig. 24-3 Radial head fracture.

tion. This differentiation has important treatment implications and is essential to the orthopedic surgeon providing definitive care.

Emergency Department Management. Document the integrity of the medial and lateral collateral ligaments with stress testing. Any opening of the joint on a stress examination should be the impetus for a thorough distal neurovascular examination. Examine the radiocapitellar joint for the presence of a hemarthrosis, which presents as a squishy "fullness" in the triangle formed by the lateral condyle, olecranon, and radial head. Joint aspiration and instillation of a local anesthetic provides a great deal of relief and contributes to early mobilization. Immobilize the elbow with a sling and arrange early orthopedic follow-up. Limiting the period of immobilization and encouraging early range-of-motion exercises improves the functional outcome in Mason type I radial head fractures.

The treatment of Mason type II fractures is based on the range of motion of the elbow joint after application of a local anesthetic block at the radiocapitellar joint. The orthopedist can perform this test on an outpatient basis. Most patients can be managed nonoperatively if they can flex the elbow from 20 to 140 degrees after the anesthetic block.[15] If flexion is intact, the patient should be immobilized in a sling. The elbow is typically immobilized for 2 to 3 weeks before range-of-motion exercises begin. If the patient is unable to flex the elbow joint after the block, ORIF is indicated.

Mason type III fractures require orthopedic consultation for radial head excision within 48 hours of injury.[15] Immobilize the elbow via a posterior splint if surgery is to be delayed. Because nearly 10% of type

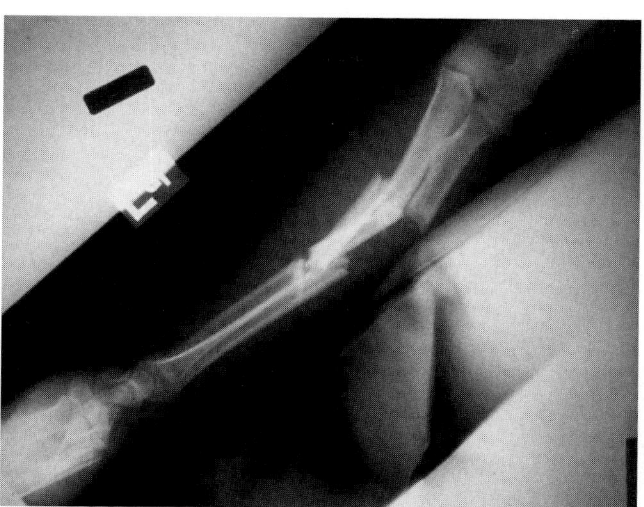

Fig. 24-4 Both bones forearm fracture.

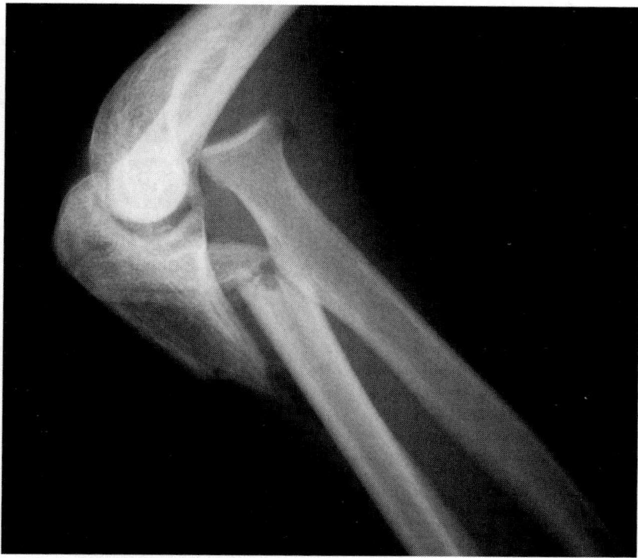

Fig. 24-5 Monteggia fracture.

III fractures are associated with dislocations of the elbow, carefully assess joint stability.

Radial head fractures are considered complex if associated with an elbow dislocation. All of these injuries require orthopedic consultation and immobilization in a posterior splint after reduction. The majority of type I injuries can be treated nonoperatively, but require close follow-up because of the possibility of joint instability.[16] Complex type II or III fractures require emergent consultation for ORIF or radial head excision.

FOREARM FRACTURES

Mechanism of Injury. The radius and ulna articulate at the proximal and distal radioulnar joints and the fibrous interosseous membrane holds the bones together. These articulations allow the radius and ulna to function as a united mechanical unit, and a fracture of one bone is usually associated with a fracture or dislocation of the other (Fig. 24-4). In one prospective series 114 out of 119 forearm fractures were both bone injuries.[17] Isolated fractures of the ulna or radius shaft are typically caused by a focal impact, such as a nightstick to the forearm. Thus, in the absence of a direct mechanism of injury, a diaphyseal fracture of the radius or ulna should prompt a careful search for an associated fracture or dislocation. Indirect mechanisms of injury typically result in a fracture-dislocation complex.

Fracture Classification. Identifying associated injuries is the most important aspect of forearm fracture classification. Carefully examine both the ulna and the radius for evidence of fracture or dislocation, and pay close attention to the articulations at the elbow and wrist. Radiographic evaluation of the forearm should generally include both the elbow and wrist, unless there is no suggestion of injury to these joints. Study the radiograph for angulation and displacement, as well as disruption of proximal and distal articulations. A forearm fracture is considered displaced if the radiograph reveals greater than 10 degrees of angulation or more than 50% displacement.[18]

Monteggia Fracture. The Monteggia fracture is a fracture of the ulnar shaft with an associated dislocation of the proximal radioulnar joint (Fig. 24-5). This injury is commonly overlooked because the obvious fracture to the ulna diverts attention from the subtle proximal radius dislocation. In a normal lateral elbow radiograph, the proximal radial line should bisect the capitellum, and deviation of this line suggests a proximal radius dislocation.

This system of fracture classification was first developed by Monteggia but later modified by Bado.[19] The subclassifications developed by Bado is based on the position of the dislocated radius and the angulation of the fractured ulna. The most common Monteggia fracture-dislocation is the Bado type I, representing 60% of Monteggia lesions (Table 24-8).

Galeazzi Fracture. The Galeazzi fracture is characterized by a fracture of the distal radius, usually at the junction of the distal and middle third, with an associated distal ulnar dislocation (Fig. 24-6). Galeazzi fractures in adults typically occur with hyperpronation of the outstretched forearm. Clinically, the ulnar styloid is very prominent and tender. On the lateral radiograph the distal ulna is usually displaced posteriorly with the fractured radius angulated anteriorly.

TABLE 24-8
Classification of Monteggia Fractures

MONTEGGIA LESION	FREQUENCY	PROXIMAL RADIUS DISLOCATION	ULNAR FRACTURE ANGULATION	PROXIMAL RADIUS FRACTURE
Bado type I	60%	Anterior	Anterior	Absent
Bado type II	15%	Posterior	Posterior	Absent
Bado type III	20%	Lateral or anterolateral	May be anterior, posterior, or lateral	Absent
Bado type IV	5%	Anterior	Anterior	Present

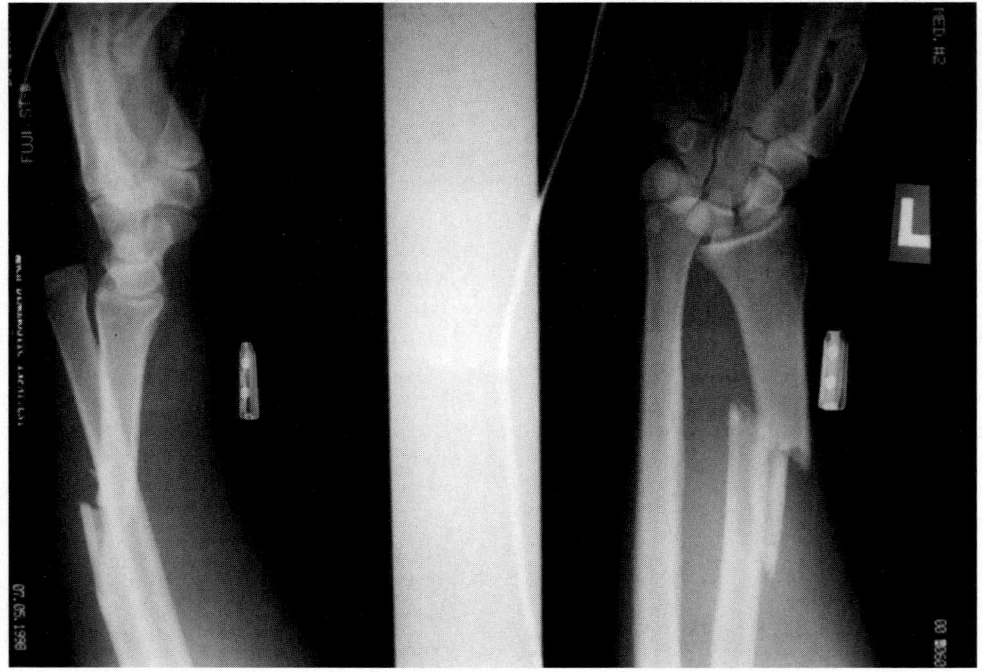

Fig. 24-6 Galeazzi fracture.

Emergency Department Management. The biomechanical linkage between the radius and ulna makes it nearly impossible to achieve adequate closed reduction in the majority of forearm fractures. The only exceptions to this rule are nondisplaced single bone fractures. Look for signs of developing compartment syndrome.

Isolated fractures of the ulna can be treated with closed reduction if there is minimal displacement and less than 10 degrees of angulation. Any single-bone fracture of the forearm that has greater than 10 degrees of angulation or more than 50% displacement requires orthopedic consultation for ORIF.

Both bone fractures and fracture-dislocations are inherently unstable and require emergent orthopedic consultation for ORIF. The most common complication of the Monteggia fracture is injury to the posterior interosseous branch of the radial nerve, which manifests as an inability to oppose the thumb with loss of finger extension.

Elbow Dislocations

Mechanism of Injury. The vast majority of elbow dislocations are posterior in nature and result from a fall onto an outstretched arm. Dislocations are rare in children because of the relative strength of the stabilizing ligaments. In the mineralized adult skeleton, the collateral ligaments typically give way, resulting in a posterior dislocation of the ulna onto the hu-

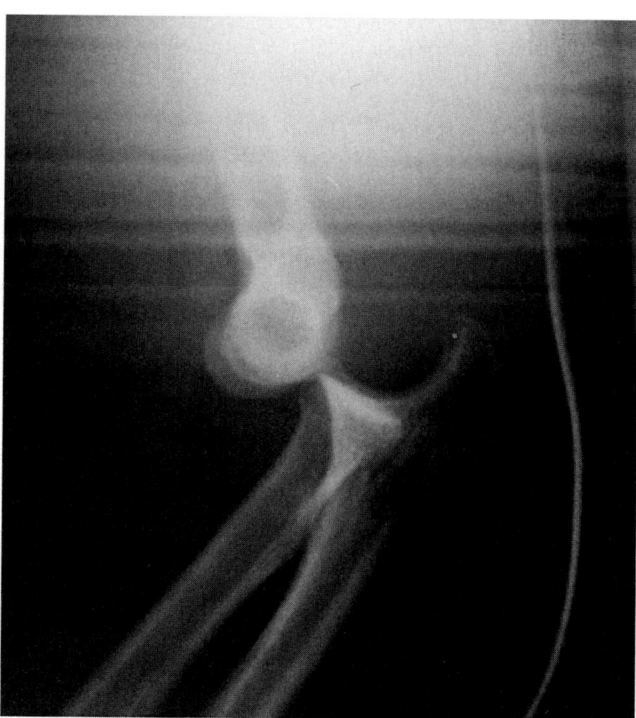

Fig. 24-7 Posterior elbow dislocation.

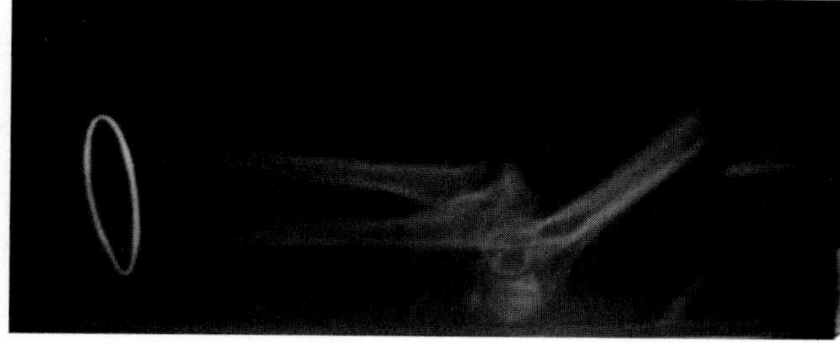

Fig. 24-8 Anterior elbow dislocation with associated humerus fracture.

merus. On very rare occasions, a direct blow to the posterior portion of the olecranon to a flexed arm results in an anterior dislocation.

Dislocation Classification. Elbow dislocations are classified according to the location of the displaced proximal ulna in relationship to the distal humerus (Figs. 24-7 and 24-8). Posterior and posterior-lateral dislocations are the most common. In most cases, the radius and ulna maintain their relationship because of the strength of the annular ligament of the radius and the proximal interosseous membrane. On occasion, a very severe mechanism of injury can produce an elbow dislocation with concomitant dislocation at the proximal radioulnar joint.

Emergency Department Management. The immediate assessment of the dislocated elbow should focus on the neurovascular status of the distal extremity. The findings of an open dislocation and no radial pulse strongly suggest the presence of a vascular injury.[20] In general, concomitant vascular injuries are rare, with only 84 reported cases since 1913.[21] Brachial artery injury is especially unusual in the presence of a closed posterior dislocation.[22] However, the location of the brachial artery in the antecubital fossa makes it susceptible to shear when the elbow dislocates anteriorly.

Nerve injuries are usually secondary to stretch injuries, and the vast majority resolve over time. The one exception to this rule is the pediatric dislocation with associated median nerve deficit. The high incidence of median nerve entrapment in this population makes surgical exploration and reduction optimal for this subgroup.[23]

Simple posterior dislocations are easily reduced by the EP. Anesthesia is best achieved with a parenteral sedative-hypnotic and opioid combination. An intraarticular injection of lidocaine often results in a significant diminution of pain and facilitates reduction. With the patient in the supine position, the clinician grabs the wrist and pulls along the axis of the forearm while an assistant applies counter-traction. Next, the clinician slowly flexes the elbow while maintaining traction, and thereby engaging the distal humerus into the trochlear notch. Alternatively, a single operator can reduce the elbow using his or her own arm as a fulcrum. Lateral or medial dislocations can be resolved with distraction in the opposite direction.

The EP should not reduce dislocations associated with fractures or concomitant radioulnar dislocations unless the distal vasculature is compromised. These injuries require emergent orthopedic consultation and management.

After successful reduction, reevaluate the neurovascular status of the distal extremity. Then immobilize the elbow with a posterior arm splint, with the joint in 90 degrees of flexion. Ensure orthopedic consultation for close follow-up. Most patients require strong outpatient pain medications.

Nursemaid's Elbow (Radial Head Subluxation). Subluxation of the radial head is a common injury in young children. It occurs when an adult or larger child attempts to lift the toddler by one arm. This traction can pull the radial head out from the annular ligament and the parents will state that the child will not use his or her arm. The injury can appear as a nerve palsy to the uninitiated, since the child holds the affected extremity limply at his or her side with the elbow in a partially flexed position.

If the history is classic, no films are necessary either

before or after reduction. The EP should place his or her thumb in over the radial head and fully supinate the child's forearm. Using the physician's thumb as a fulcrum, the child's elbow is hyperflexed over the thumb, then fully extended. A "click" felt over the radial head confirms reduction, and the child should begin to use his or her arm normally in 10 to 15 minutes.

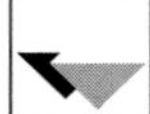

PEARLS & PITFALLS

- Supracondylar fractures are associated with peripheral nerve injuries and brachial artery entrapment; long-term complications include Volkmann's ischemic contracture and cubitus varus.
- Consider the possibility of a forearm compartment syndrome in children with supracondylar fractures.
- Radial head fractures are often missed because of their subtle radiographic appearance; the presence of a joint effusion on the lateral radiograph may be the only clue to diagnosis.
- The Monteggia fracture is a fracture of the ulnar shaft with an associated dislocation of the proximal radioulnar joint.
- The Galeazzi fracture is characterized by a fracture of the distal radius, usually at the junction of the distal and middle third, with an associated distal ulnar dislocation.
- Both bone fractures and fracture-dislocations are inherently unstable and require emergent orthopedic consultation for ORIF.
- Posterior elbow dislocations are much more common than anterior dislocations. Reduce simple dislocations after managing the pain, and immobilize the arm in a posterior splint and sling.

REFERENCES

1. Amis AA, Miller JH: The mechanisms of elbow fractures: an investigation using impact tests in vitro, *Injury* 26:163-168, 1995.
2. Barton KL, et al: Modified Gartland classification of supracondylar humerus fractures: an assessment of interobserver and intraobserver reliability, *Pediatrics* 100(abstract):478, 1997.
3. France J, Strong M: Deformity and function in supracondylar fractures of the humerus in children variously treated by closed reduction and splinting, traction, and percutaneous pinning, *J Pediatr Orthop* 12:494-498, 1992.
4. Dormans JP, Squillante R, Sharf H: Acute neurovascular complications with supracondylar humerus fractures in children, *J Hand Surg Am* 20:1-4, 1995.
5. Archibeck MJ, Scott SM, Peters CL: Brachialis muscle entrapment in displaced supracondylar humerus fractures: a technique of closed reduction and report of initial results, *J Pediatr Orthop* 17:298-302, 1997.
6. Landin LA, Danielsson LG: Elbow fractures in children: an epidemiological analysis of 589 cases, *Acta Orthop Scand* 57:309-312, 1986.
7. Harris JH, Harris WH, Novelline RA: Elbow. In Harris JH, Harris WH: *The radiology of emergency medicine,* Baltimore, 1993, Williams & Wilkins.
8. Bast SC, Hoffer MM, Aval S: Nonoperative treatment for minimally and nondisplaced lateral humeral condyle fractures in children, *J Pediatr Orthop* 18:448-450, 1998.
9. Dhillon KS, Sengupta S, Singh BJ: Delayed management of fracture of the lateral humeral condyle in children, *Acta Orthop Scand* 59:419-424, 1988.
10. Riseborough EJ, Radin EL: Intercondylar T fractures of the humerus in the adult: a comparison of operative and nonoperative treatment in twenty-nine cases, *J Bone Joint Surg* 51-A: 130-141, 1969.
11. Kundel K, et al: Intraarticular distal humerus fractures: factors affecting functional outcome, *Clin Orthop* 332:200-208, 1996.
12. Cabanela ME, Morrey BF: Fractures of the proximal ulna and olecranon. In Morrey BF (editor): *The elbow and its disorders,* ed 2, Philadelphia, 1993, Saunders.
13. Mason ML: Some observations on fractures of the head of the radius with a review of one hundred cases, *Br J Surg* 42:123-132, 1954.
14. Morrey BF: Fractures of the radial head. In Morrey BF (editor): *The elbow and its disorders,* ed 2, Philadelphia, 1993, Saunders.
15. Morrey BF: Current concepts in the treatment of fractures of the radial head, the olecranon, and the coronoid, *J Bone Joint Surg* 77-A:316-327, 1995.
16. Broberg MA, Morrey BF: Results of treatment of fracture-dislocations of the elbow, *Clin Orthop* 216:109-119, 1987.
17. Goldberg HD, et al: Double injuries of the forearm: a common occurrence, *Radiology* 185:223-227, 1992.
18. Anderson LD, Meyer FN: Fractures of the shafts of the radius and ulna. In Rockwood CA, Green DP, Bucholz RW (editors): *Fractures in adults,* ed 3, Philadelphia, 1991, JB Lippincott.
19. Bado JL: The Monteggia lesion, *Clin Orthop* 50:71-86, 1967.
20. Endean ED, et al: Recognition of arterial injury in elbow dislocation, *J Vasc Surg* 16:402-406, 1992.
21. Ferrera PC: Elbow dislocation complicated by brachial artery laceration, *Am J Emerg Med* 17:103-105, 1999.
22. Slowik GM, Fitzimmons M, Rayhack JM: Closed elbow dislocation and brachial artery damage, *J Orthop Trauma* 7:558-561, 1993.
23. Rao SB, Crawford AH: Median nerve entrapment after dislocation of the elbow in children: a report of 2 cases and review of literature, *Clin Orthop* 312:232-237, 1995.

Hand and Wrist Injuries

25

VINCENT P. VERDILE, PETER C. FERRERA, AND JAMES G. ADAMS

Teaching Case

A 40-year-old healthy woman slipped on her recently polished floor onto her outstretched left hand. In the process of falling, the vase she was carrying in her right hand smashed and lacerated the palmar aspect of her right hand. She presented to the emergency department (ED) for evaluation and treatment.

The left hand had no obvious deformity, but was tender in the anatomic snuffbox. The right hand had a palmar laceration with no active bleeding and a normal neuromuscular examination. Both hands were radiographed: the right hand to rule out a glass foreign body (FB) and the left wrist to rule out a fracture. Both radiographs were negative. The left hand was placed in a thumb spica splint for clinical evidence of a scaphoid fracture. After wound exploration, the right hand was closed with sutures. At a 2-week follow-up, a repeat radiograph of the left wrist showed a nondisplaced scaphoid fracture. ■

Although hand injuries may not at first appear to play a significant part in the overall toll injuries have on society and healthcare expenditures, some studies would suggest that an isolated hand injury might have grave personal and financial implications for the patient.[1-9] Studies have reported that hand-injured patients comprise 2% to 20% of the total ED patient volume.[4,10-13] The various mechanisms of injury, types of patients, and treatment approaches for hand-injured patients seen in the ED have also been described.[10-23]

ANATOMY

A standard nomenclature is generally used to describe the site of the injured region. The digits of the hand are usually referred to as thumb, index, middle, ring, and little fingers, rather than being numbered as 1 to 5. The side of the finger closest to the thumb is the **radial aspect**, whereas the side closest to the little finger is the **ulnar aspect**.

It is important to note that the close proximity of the tendons, nerves, and vascular supply to the surface of the skin adds to the potential complications associated with hand and wrist injuries. In addition, the grouping of the carpal bones with overlying and asymmetric articular surfaces makes radiographic interpretation of these fractures difficult at times.

Bones

The hand and wrist contain 27 bones: 14 phalanges, 5 metacarpals, and 8 carpal bones (Fig. 25-1). The eight small carpal bones in the region of the wrist are strongly united by ligaments and articulate with one another via synovial joints.

Muscles

The muscle supply to the hand is classified as extrinsic and intrinsic. **Extrinsic muscles** originate proximal to the wrist and serve either to flex or extend the hand and digits. The **extrinsic flexors** run along the volar forearm and are three layers deep. As the flexor tendons cross the wrist at the carpal canal, they are separated into three layers (Fig. 25-2). The **extrinsic extensors** run along the dorsal forearm. At the wrist there are six osseofibrous extensor compartments (Fig. 25-3).

The **intrinsic muscles** of the hand are those that arise distal to the wrist joint and insert within the hand. The intrinsics include the muscles of the thenar and hypothenar eminences, the abductor pollicis, the interossei, and the lumbricals.

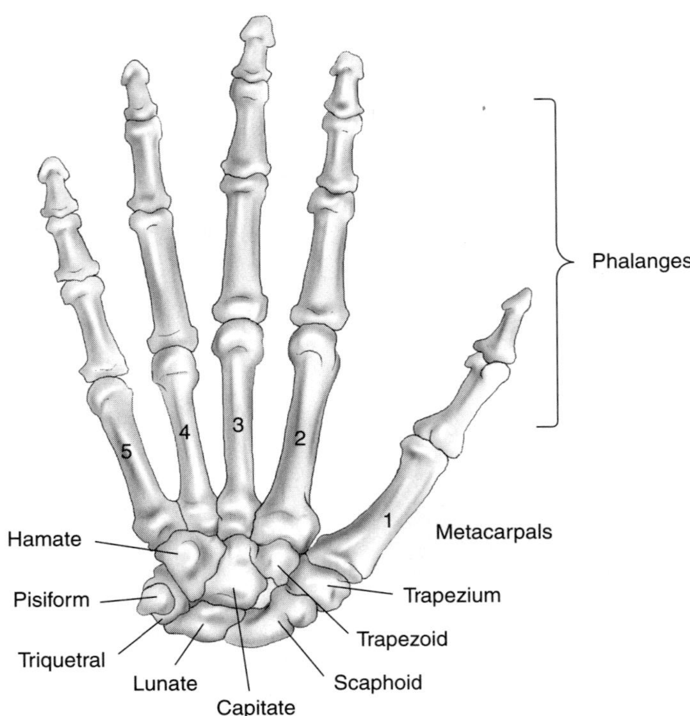

Fig. 25-1 Bones of the hand (volar aspect).

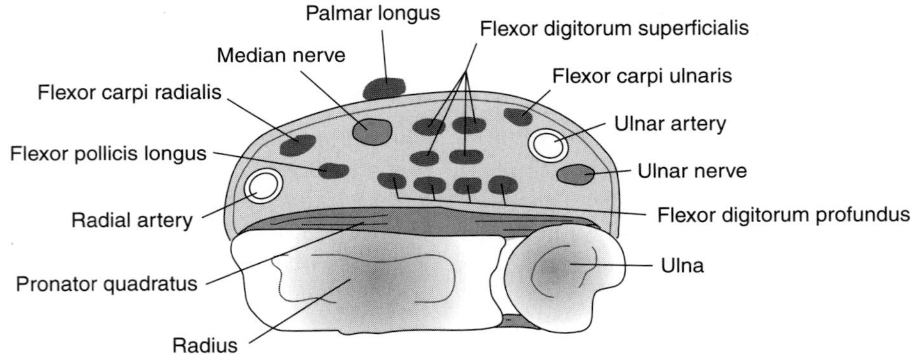

Fig. 25-2 Cross-section of flexor tendons at wrist proximal to flexor retinaculum.

Nerves

Three nerves provide motor and sensory innervation to the hand: the radial, ulnar, and median nerves. The **radial nerve** divides into the **posterior interosseous nerve** and **superficial radial nerve** in the forearm. The former branch provides motor function to the hand extensors, as well as sensation to the wrist. The latter branch provides sensation to the dorsal thumb and the proximal portions of the index finger, middle finger, and radial half of the ring finger (see Fig. 31-4).

The **ulnar nerve** gives motor branches to the flexor carpi ulnaris (FCU), the two ulnar flexor digitorum profundi (FDP) muscles in the forearm, and most of the intrinsic hand muscles. The ulnar nerve also supplies sensation to the little finger and ulnar half of the ring finger (see Fig. 31-4).

The branch of the **median nerve** within the forearm known as the **anterior interosseous nerve** provides motor function to the flexor pollicis longus (FPL), the pronator quadratus, and the radial half of the FDP muscles. Within the hand, the median nerve provides

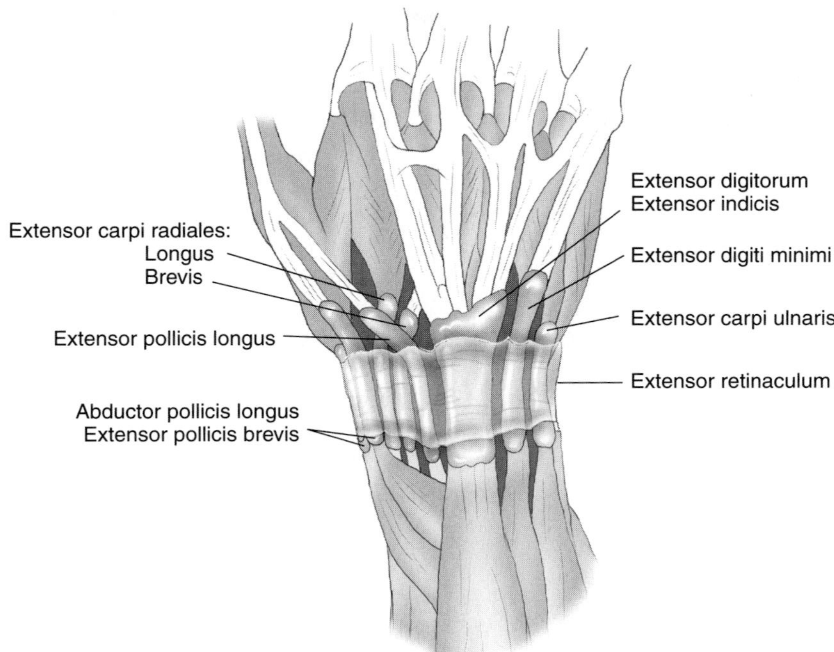

Fig. 25-3 Synovial sheaths encompassing the wrist extensors.

motor function to the thenar muscles. The median nerve also supplies sensation to the thumb and remaining portions of the hand not innervated by the radial and ulnar nerves (see Fig. 31-4).

Arteries

The **radial** and **ulnar arteries** provide blood to the hand. Extensive collateralization exists between the two vessels such that the hand can be perfused even if one of the vessels is damaged. The ulnar artery passes through Guyon's canal at the wrist, becoming the **superficial palmar arch**, which then spawns the digital arteries. This arch lies superficial to the nerves and tendons of the hand. The radial artery gives off superficial and deep branches at the wrist. The superficial branch provides blood to the thumb and ultimately forms an anastomosis with the ulnar artery's superficial arch. The deep branch forms the **deep palmar arch**, which lies deep to the flexor tendons. The deep palmar arch is the primary vasculature of the fingers.

APPROACH TO THE INJURED HAND

A multitude of pitfalls awaits the unwary EP who must deal with the injured hand and wrist. To avoid misstep, approach all patients with these injuries in a uniform manner. Although injuries may appear superficial, underlying soft tissue and bony structures may be damaged. General physical examination of every hand and wrist injury must include a general appearance, skin examination, neurovascular assessment, bone and joint evaluation, and musculotendinous evaluation (Box 25-1). The identification of injuries subjacent to the skin is important from both the standpoints of good patient outcome and risk management.[24-26]

History

A good history should include the circumstances surrounding the injury (e.g., fall onto outstretched hand versus direct crush), hand dominance, vocation, recreational activities, and prior injuries to the affected hand or wrist. In addition, patient co-morbidities and current medication usage may also complicate the injury. If a penetrating object was the offending agent, it is helpful to know its length, trajectory, and the position of the fingers or palm at the moment of contact. In penetrating injuries, determine what the offending object was made of (e.g., glass), which may show up on radiographs if embedded. In crushing injuries, determine whether an associated machine-induced thermal burn has also occurred. If there are amputated parts, ascertain what was done to protect and preserve them.

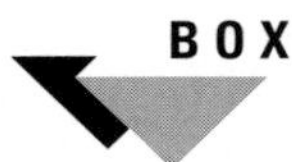

BOX 25-1
General Physical Examination

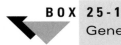

I. General appearance
  A. Active hemorrhage
  B. Amputation/avulsions
  C. Position at rest
II. Skin
  A. Integrity
  B. Moisture
  C. Swelling/edema
  D. Discoloration
  E. Inflammation
  F. Scars
III. Vascular
  A. Color/warmth
  B. Pulses
  C. Capillary refill
  D. Allen test
IV. Neurologic
  A. Motor function
    1. Ulnar nerve: finger abduction/adduction
    2. Radial nerve: wrist extension
    3. Median nerve: flexion of digits I, II, and III; thumb opposition
  B. Sensory function
    1. Ulnar nerve: tip of digit V
    2. Median nerve: tip of digit II
    3. Radial nerve: dorsal first web space
V. Bone and joint
  A. Deformity
  B. Local tenderness
  C. Pain with axial compression
  D. Joint range of motion
  E. Ligamentous stability: DIP, PIP, MCP joints
VI. Musculotendinous
  A. Function of each muscle-tendon group
  B. Strength against resistance
  C. Pain with motion

Physical Examination

GENERAL

The physical examination begins by noting the overall appearance of the hand and wrist to determine viability. Jewelry needs to be cut off so as not to compromise the distal blood flow to the fingers. Determine the possibility of an open fracture. Active bleeding needs to be controlled with direct pressure.

Look for rotational deformities of the digits, suggesting fractures or dislocations. Palpate each individual bone in the wrist and hand, noting tenderness. Tenderness in the **anatomic snuffbox** (i.e., the depression just distal to the radial styloid) is an important finding, especially in cases of occult scaphoid fractures. Tenderness in at the hook of the hamate is significant since it is the radial border of **Guyon's canal**, which contains the ulnar nerve and artery.

NEUROLOGIC

Determine the gross neurologic status of the affected hand. Sensation may be tested by two-point discrimination, position sense, or ability to detect vibrations. **Two-point discrimination** can be performed by using a bent paper clip. Normal two-point discrimination on the fingertips is 2 to 5 mm; anything greater represents an abnormal finding. A hand surgeon should be consulted if a nerve injury is present.[26-29]

Every hand examination should include motor testing. Three simple maneuvers are used to test motor function:

1. **Ulnar nerve.** Since the ulnar nerve innervates the first dorsal interossei, ask the patient to abduct his or her fingers (spread them apart against resistance).
2. **Median nerve.** Since the median nerve innervates the abductor pollicis brevis, have the patient lay his or her hand flat, palm up, and have the patient hold the thumb straight up from the palm (abduction) against resistance.
3. **Radial nerve.** The radial nerve supplies the motor function to wrist and finger extension via the extensor muscles of the forearm. Have the patient extend the wrist against gravity.

VASCULAR

Assess the vascular integrity of the hand and wrist by a variety of methods. Observe the color of the skin, measure capillary refill, palpate the radial and ulnar pulses, and note the skin temperature. These findings should then be compared with the noninjured side.

The **Allen test** determines the integrity of the radial and ulnar arteries and adequacy of collateral circulation. Have the patient raise the hand and clench the fist tightly several times. The examiner then firmly occludes both the ulnar and radial arteries. Initially release the radial artery and determine the length of time for the blanched hand to regain color. A normal test shows resumption of normal color within 3 seconds. Repeat the test by releasing the ulnar artery and testing its patency. The opposite hand serves as a control. A significant arterial injury in the hand or wrist endangers nearby neural structures, which often travel together in the wrist, hand, and digits.[1,20,26]

TENDONS

Careful assessment is necessary to diagnose a flexor tendon disruption and associated neurovascular injury. With a normal hand at rest, the fingers should fall into a cascade of flexion. The index finger is least flexed, while the fifth finger is the most flexed. If the finger has an abnormal position, especially if it appears to be less flexed than normal, a flexor tendon injury is likely. Complete disruption of the FDP tendon extends the distal interphalangeal (DIP) joint. A similar wound to the flexor digitorum superficialis (FDS) tendon results in partial extension of the proximal interphalangeal (PIP) joint.[30] A functional examination is important to confirm these findings.

Test the FDP and FDS separately. To test the FDP, have the patient flex the DIP joint. To test the FDS, isolate each finger. For instance, if you wish to test the FDS of the middle finger, hold all other fingers in extension while asking the patient to flex the PIP joint.

Patients may have a complete laceration of the FDS and still be able to flex the finger, because the FDP takes over as the primary flexor. Suspect flexor injuries if the patient complains of weakness, pain with flexion against resistance, or has an abnormal position of the hand at rest.[30] It is possible that testing a partially torn tendon against resistance may complete the tear.

Each extensor tendon should also be palpated individually. Tenderness implies strain or rupture of the tendon.

RANGE OF MOTION

Initially begin by testing active range of motion at the wrist. Normal wrist flexion is about 80 degrees, whereas normal wrist extension is about 70 degrees. Normal deviation of the wrist to the ulnar side is approximately 30 degrees, whereas normal deviation to the radial side is about 20 degrees.

To test for digit flexion and extension, have the patient make a fist and then extend the fingers. Note if the fingers move smoothly and evenly, or whether the patient has trouble moving any of the fingers.

To test for abduction and adduction, have the patient spread the fingers apart and then back together. Each finger should abduct about 20 degrees, and then adduct to abut the adjacent finger.

Flexion of the thumb across the palm tests for metacarpophalangeal and interphalangeal joint function. Thumb extension is tested by moving the thumb radially from the other fingers to a normal point of about 50 degrees. Normal opposition of the thumb is tested by touching the thumb to each fingertip pad.

Approach to Management

IMMOBILIZATION

As with any injury the ultimate goal is to restore function. Range of motion (ROM) must be preserved by immobilizing the injured area in a position of function; ROM exercises should be instituted as soon as possible. For example, the metacarpophalangeal (MCP) joints should be immobilized between 50 and 90 degrees of flexion. If these joints are not properly flexed, ligamentous shortening may ensue.

ANESTHESIA

Adequate anesthesia must be used. Always document the motor and sensory function of the hand and digits before placement of local anesthetic. Usually local infiltration or digital or intermetacarpal blocks suffice for finger injuries. Avoid placement of too much anesthetic during digital blocks to prevent compromise of the vasculature. Regional blocks are also helpful if the entire hand is involved. Epinephrine-containing anesthetics must be avoided to prevent necrosis of the fingers.

INFECTION CONTROL

Tetanus immunization must be ensured with open wounds. Grossly contaminated wounds, open fractures, and open joint lacerations require antibiotic coverage with agents such as cephalosporins.

SOFT TISSUE INJURIES

Soft tissue injuries of the hand or wrist are frequent in the ED. A fundamental knowledge of anatomy is essential to assess these injuries. Lacerations, punctures, and bite wounds disturb the integrity of the skin and may also injure underlying soft tissue or osseous structures.

Careful wound preparation minimizes infection or missed retained FB. After a wound is cleansed, anesthetized, and draped, an exploration identifies potential tendon injuries or retained FBs. Examining a wound through a full range of motion of the digit, hand, or wrist is essential to ensure that an injured tendon has not retracted from the area of the wound.

The use of a tourniquet provides a bloodless field and minimizes the risk of missing an injury. Although an automated pressure tourniquet is ideal, the emergency physician (EP) can fashion a simple tourniquet. Have the patient lie on the gurney with the arm held directly over head, that is, sticking straight out from the stretcher. Place a blood pressure cuff around the arm and encircle it twice with bandage tape. Inflate the cuff above systolic pressure. Be sure tourniquet time does not extend more than 20 minutes to avoid vascular compromise.

Evaluation of Foreign Bodies

Use diagnostic imaging when necessary to evaluate for FB. Imaging modalities may include plain films, computed tomography (CT), magnetic resonance imaging (MRI), or ultrasonography (US).[31-38] The choice of diagnostic imaging depends on the location, size and substance of the suspected FB. Plain films are good for glass and metals, whereas MRI and US are useful for nonradiopaque substances such as wood or plastic. Plain-film radiographs and US tend to be the most available to the EP and are reasonably good in detecting the presence of a retained FB. In addition, US and CT are useful for localizing and retrieving the foreign body.[34,37,38]

High-Pressure Injection Injuries

High-pressure injection injuries represent a special type of soft tissue injury. Initially, these injuries may appear innocuous and the patient may be minimally symptomatic. The patient may relate that the device was against the skin or remote from the finger. These devices can create serious injury even when they are inches away from the hand. The finger may demonstrate fusiform swelling, and hours later the digit becomes extremely painful, swollen, and pale. Vascular compromise may rapidly progress with ensuing tissue necrosis.[39,40] Initial management for the patient who presents shortly after injury involves splinting, hand elevation, ensuring tetanus immunization, analgesia, and coverage with broad-spectrum antibiotics. Avoid digital blocks because of the potential for further compromised blood flow. Urgent hand surgery consultation is warranted, since most cases require extensive surgical decompression and debridement.[39,40]

Bite Wounds

Patients may present to the ED with a bite wound from virtually any type of animal. Fortunately, the most common bite wounds encountered are from domestic dogs and cats. Dogs tend to have a starring impression type of injury that may create fractures, as well as soft tissue injuries. On the other hand, cat wounds tend to be puncture type wounds, which although seemingly innocuous often penetrate quite deeply into the soft tissues of the hand or wrist. These patients often present late because the initial injury appeared to be relatively trivial. Generally speaking, cat and dog bite wounds are particularly high risk for developing infectious complications. The hand, particularly over joints, can be very problematic.

Treatment consists of local wound care, ensuring tetanus immunization, immobilization, and empiric antibiotic treatment. The organisms most often encountered are *Streptococcus spp.*, *Staphylococcus aureus*, *Eikenella corrodens*, anaerobes, and, especially in cat bites, *Pasteurella multocida*. All of these organisms have reasonable sensitivity to amoxicillin/clavulanate (Augmentin). For the penicillin-allergic patient, a fluoroquinolone is a reasonable alternative.

Human bites tend to be fairly superficial in nature and have a relatively low incidence of infection. The most serious bite wound encountered is that which is sustained when a clenched fist strikes an opponent's tooth (“**clenched-fist injury**”), penetrating the extensor hood and joint capsule and possibly fracturing the metacarpal head. Inoculated bacteria can incubate within the closed space of the hand. Inspect the wound through a full range of motion, clean these wounds thoroughly, obtain radiographs to exclude fractures and FBs, and give antibiotic prophylaxis. Consult a hand specialist, since joint space injuries may require surgical debridement.

All bite wounds require close follow-up with a wound check in less then 24 hours and admission to the hospital in patients who have co-morbidities, which place them at higher risk for infection (e.g., diabetes mellitus, acquired immunodeficiency syndrome). Bite wounds that involve a tendon over a joint or disrupt a bone should also be considered for admission to the hospital. Lastly, patients who present with a delayed wound infection and have questionable reliability should also be admitted to the hospital. In general, puncture wounds are usually not sutured.

Burns

Although the management of burns is described elsewhere in this textbook, thermal injury to the hand and wrist comprises a special subset. Loss of function may be devastating. Admission to the hospital is required if there is significant partial- or full-thickness burns to one or both hands, or if the burns are circumferential. Vascular compromise may be heralded by paresthesias. **Digital escharotomy** is necessary in deep circumferential burns with evidence of vascular compromise.[41]

Tendon Injuries

Most tendon injuries to the hand or wrist are associated with lacerations or wounds, although crush injuries and sudden and significant stress can also result in tendon damage (Fig. 25-4). The tendons most at risk are those that are subjacent to the wound or laceration at the time of injury.

FLEXOR TENDON INJURIES

Flexor tendon injuries greater than 25% of the width of the tendon should be repaired exclusively by a hand surgeon. Primary repair is feasible if the wound is not contaminated. A delayed repair can occur up to 10 days after the injury if other injuries or illnesses

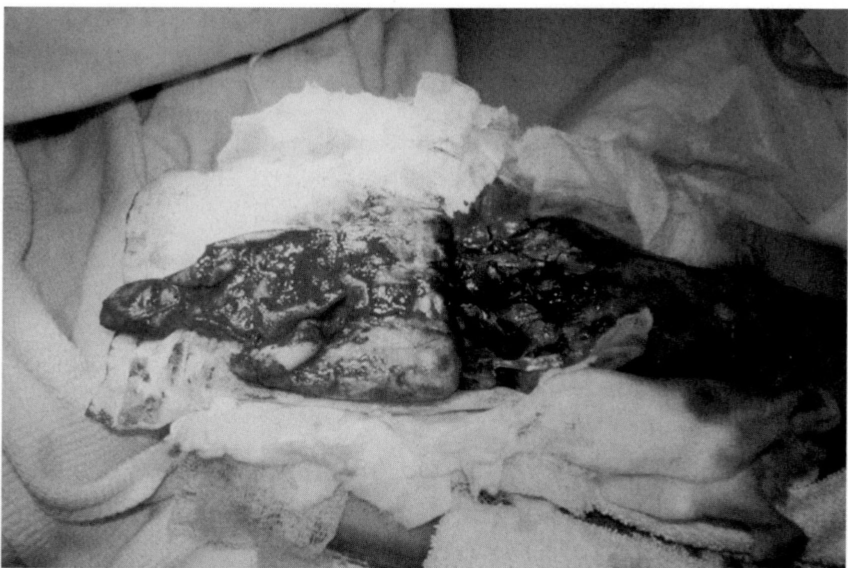

Fig. 25-4 Crush injury resulting in severe hand tendon damage.

prevent a primary repair. The role of the EP is to identify flexor tendon lacerations that involve more than 25% of the tendon substance.[27,30,42,43] Consult a hand surgeon if a flexor tendon laceration is identified. If the patient is not to have primary repair, the EP may close the wound, splint the digit, and refer for delayed repair.

EXTENSOR TENDON INJURIES

Although management of extensor tendons is generally felt to be easier than that for flexor tendons, there are several potential problems with these injuries. When an extensor tendon is severed at the wrist, the portion of the tendon within the forearm tends to retract several centimeters; therefore finding the proximal portion may be difficult. Lacerations over the interphalangeal joints are at risk for joint capsule violation because of the close apposition of the tendon with the joint. Full-thickness extensor tendon lacerations are best repaired in the operating suite by a hand surgeon.

Mallet Finger. A **mallet finger** (Fig. 25-5) is a unique tendon injury of the distal extensor apparatus. It often occurs after a direct blow to the tip of the finger, usually with a baseball. Mallet fingers may be associated with a fracture that is often a small avulsion where the extensor tendon attaches to the dorsal aspect of the distal phalanx. In the absence of a fracture, splint the DIP joint in slight hyperextension and refer to an orthopedic or hand specialist.[44,45] If the patient has a fracture to the distal phalanx, a splint is a temporary solution, but may ultimately require open reduction and internal fixation.

Boutonniere Deformity. When sudden forced flexion occurs at the PIP joint with the finger in extension, the lateral bands of the extensor mechanism may become displaced in a volar direction. This mechanism may cause rupture of the central slip of the extensor tendon. Contraction of the lumbrical muscles flexes the PIP joint, but since the lateral bands to the distal phalanx remain intact, the DIP joint remains in extension. There is usually a painful and swollen PIP joint and it is important to assess whether the patient can actively extend the PIP joint. Occasionally there is an associated avulsion fracture off the dorsal surface of the middle phalanx. Treatment is by splinting the PIP joint in full extension for at least 4 weeks. **The DIP joint should not be immobilized** so that the patient may actively perform flexion exercises while the rest of the finger is splinted. The patient should be referred to a hand surgeon on an outpatient basis.

Ulnar Collateral Ligament Injury (Gamekeeper's Thumb)

Injury to the **ulnar collateral ligament (UCL)** ("**gamekeeper's thumb**") was first described in Scottish gamekeepers. Repetitive twisting of the neck of hares ruptured the UCL. Today the most common cause of "gamekeeper's thumb" is skiing. This injury occurs when the thumb is dislocated radially and then it spontaneously relocates at the metacarpophalangeal joint. When the thumb moves radially, the UCL may rupture. Physical examination reveals swelling and tenderness over the ulnar border of the thumb MCP joint and a weak pinch. A stress test is key to the

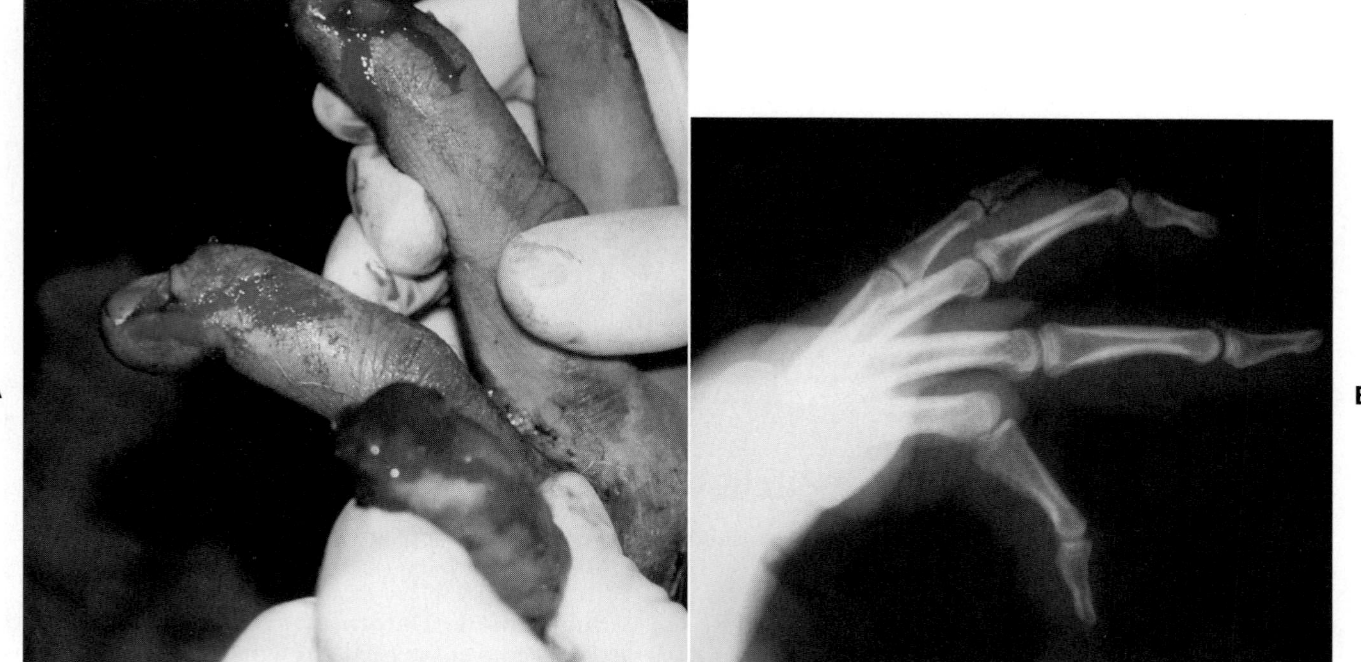

Fig. 25-5 **A** and **B**, Mallet finger.

diagnosis. Stress the UCL, both in full extension and then with the thumb IP joint in 30 degrees of flexion to avoid the stabilizing effect of the volar plate. If the patient has significant pain and guarding, a median and radial nerve block may be helpful. In the patient with a complete rupture, there is no end-point to radial abduction of the thumb. In questionable cases, use the other hand for comparison. Radiograph the joint before stressing it to rule out fracture or bony avulsion from the insertion of the UCL on the proximal phalanx. If a fracture is present, avoid stressing the ligament.

Partial ruptures of the UCL may be treated by a 3- to 4-week period of immobilization in a thumb spica cast. Patients with acute complete ruptures, or those who fail conservative therapy, require surgical repair. In the ED, patients with suspected rupture should be splinted with a thumb spica and referred to a hand surgeon.[46,47]

Nailbed Injuries

Nailbed injuries are also commonly seen in the ED. Severe injuries may result in nail deformities. Suspect a nailbed injury in the presence of a tuft fracture associated with a **subungual hematoma**, which is a collection of blood below the nail plate arising from the matrix below. Not all subungual hematomas are associated with nailbed lacerations. If the hematoma occupies less than 25% of the nail plate, the hematoma may simply be drained. The most common method of drainage in the ED is by use of a battery-operated microcautery, the hot tip of which quickly bores through the nail and allows for egress of blood. A superheated paperclip also works well if a cautery is not available. Larger hematomas require evaluation of the nailbed.

The nail must be removed and the nailbed repaired if a laceration is discovered. Using either a microspatula or small scissors, the nail may be easily separated from the underlying nailbed and eponychium. Lacerations are repaired with thin absorbable sutures.[48] The eponychium must not adhere to the proximal nailbed or adhesions may develop; the nail itself, petroleum gauze, or the aluminum foil from a suture package may be inserted between the eponychium and the nailbed.[48] The new nail will take several months to grow back. Until healing is complete, a sterile dressing is changed daily.

Fingertip Lacerations

Defects >1 cm^2 without exposed bone usually require skin grafts. Smaller wounds may heal by secondary

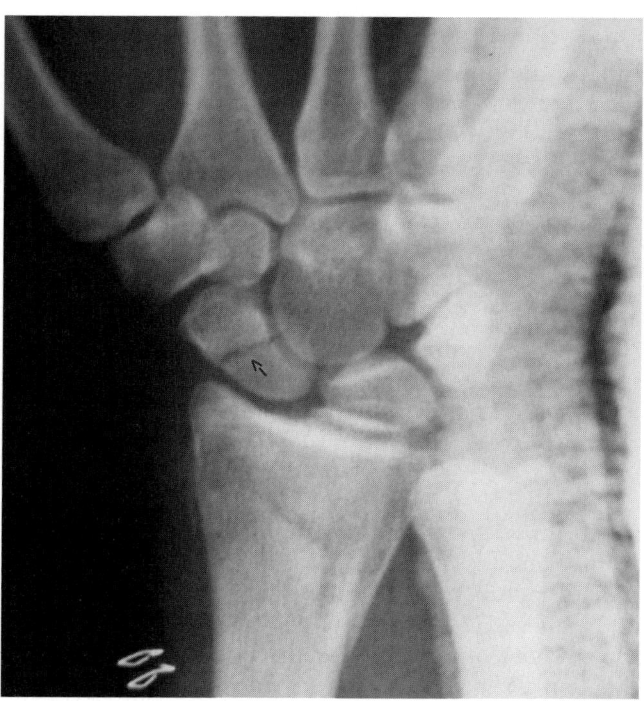

Fig. 25-6 Scaphoid fracture *(arrow).*

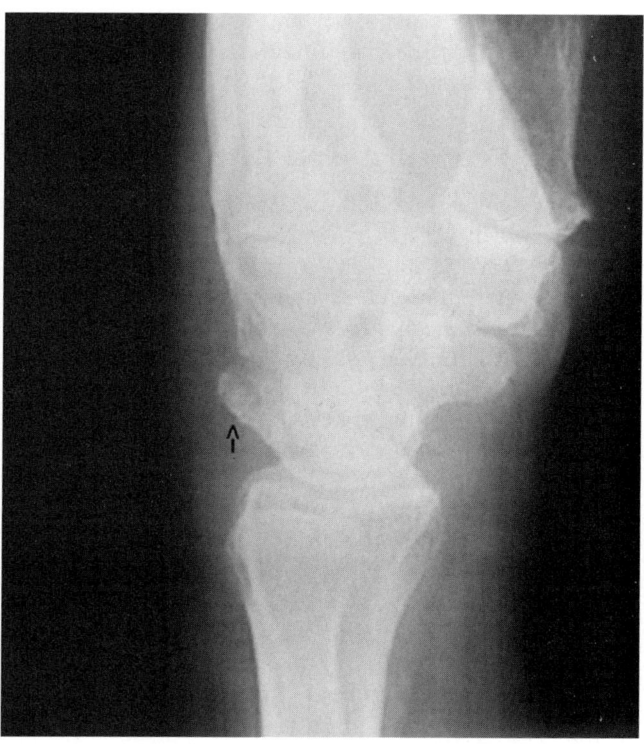

Fig. 25-7 Triquetral fracture *(arrow).*

intention. A hand surgeon may be required to construct flaps if bone is exposed.

FRACTURES AND DISLOCATIONS

Blunt injuries to the hand may be from direct blows, crush injuries, or include indirect forces such as twisting. Radiographic diagnosis of wrist fractures is complicated by the close proximity and overlap of the carpal bones. Wrist injuries are an important component of emergency practice and a systematic means of evaluating the wrist is essential. Common injuries are described in the following section.[49-51]

Scaphoid Fractures

The scaphoid is the most commonly fractured bone in the wrist. Unfortunately it is among the most challenging fracture to diagnose, and consequences of missed injury may be significant. The scaphoid is supplied by a single vessel that enters distally, resulting in a tenuous blood supply. **A missed scaphoid fracture may result in an avascular necrosis of the proximal fragment.**

A common mechanism of injury is falling onto an outstretched hand. The physical examination is fairly sensitive for scaphoid fracture. There are three prominent physical findings: (1) tenderness in the anatomic snuffbox (defined by the extensor pollicis longus on the dorsal border and the abductor pollicis longus on the volar border); (2) pain in the scaphoid with axial compression of the thumb;[49,52] and (3) pain with resisted pronation (i.e., shake the patient's hand and ask the patient to pronate his or her hand while exerting counter pressure).

Standard wrist films may demonstrate a scaphoid fracture (Fig. 25-6). A "scaphoid view," accentuates the cortex of the scaphoid. This film is taken with the wrist supinated and deviated towards the ulna. If the patient has tenderness in the anatomic snuffbox, consider the diagnosis of scaphoid fracture despite normal radiographs. Patients with clinical suspicion of scaphoid fracture should be immobilized in a thumb spica splint and have follow-up arranged. Repeat radiographs in 2 weeks may demonstrate the initially occult injury.

Triquetral Fractures

Triquetral fractures are evident on a lateral view radiograph of the wrist as a dorsal fleck of bone in the proximal wrist area (Fig. 25-7). Triquetral fractures are actually ligamentous avulsion fractures. The patient demonstrates tenderness in the dorsal proximal wrist with limited wrist motion. These fractures are managed initially with immobilization by splinting and complications are rare.

Lunate Fracture and Dislocation

The lunate is rarely fractured in isolation since it is fairly well protected by the radius. Similar to scaphoid fractures, the lunate is fractured as the patient falls onto an outstretched hand. The lunate can also dislocate with a hyperextension injury (Figs. 25-8 and 25-9). Patients may have **perilunate** or **lunate dislocation**. It is helpful to think of lunate and perilunate dislocations as different stages of the same injury rather than as separate entities.[53] These injuries are diagnosed on a "true lateral" wrist radiograph by drawing a line down along the center of the radius, through the midpoint of the distal radius, the lunate, and the capitate and looking for displacement.

In a **lunate dislocation**, the distal radius and the capitate remain partially aligned while the lunate is dislocated. In a **dorsal perilunate dislocation**, the radius and lunate align but the capitate appears misplaced dorsal to the lunate. A volar lunate dislocation may actually be the final stage of a dorsal perilunate dislocation, since the capitate spontaneously reduces by the forces of injury.[53] The **volar lunate/dorsal perilunate dislocation** is the most common injury pattern seen, with the dorsal **transscaphoid perilunate dislocation** being the next most common injury pattern. In the latter injury, the scaphoid is fractured and the distal pole is displaced dorsally with the capitate. It is exceptionally rare to see a **volar perilunate/dorsal lunate dislocation**, whereas the lunate dislocates dorsally and the capitate dislocates volarly.

The dorsal perilunate and volar lunate dislocations are managed identically since they represent different stages of the same injury. Anatomic restoration of the scaphoid lunate and capitate is essential.[52-55] Associated median nerve injury is common.[55]

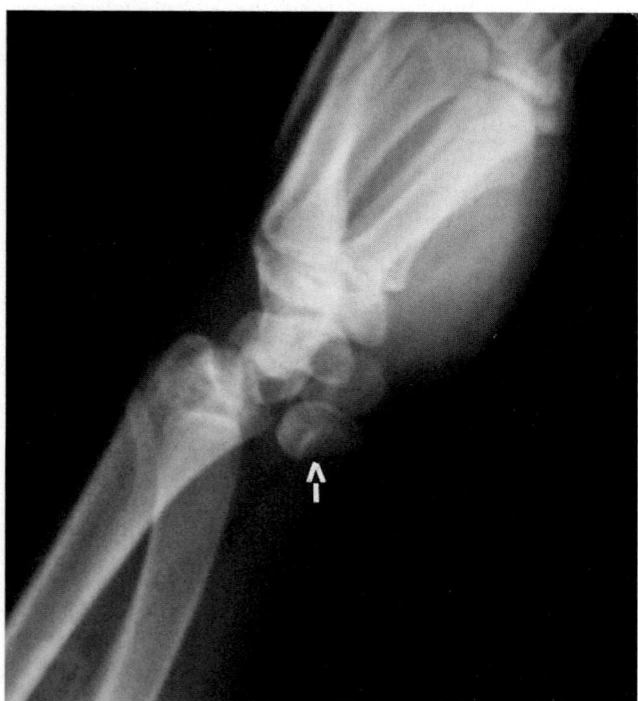

Fig. 25-8 Volar lunate dislocation *(arrow)*.

Other Carpal Fractures

Fractures of the other carpal bones (trapezium, pisiform, hamate, capitate, and trapezoid) are less common. Fracture of the hamate may occur in golfers and batters. The handle of the club may rest against the hamate, and when brisk contact is made with the ball or other animate/inanimate object, it can crack the hook of the hamate. A carpal tunnel view of the wrist may best demonstrate this injury. In general, point tenderness and diagnostic radiographs will guide management of carpal fractures other than lunate and scaphoid. Immobilize suspected fractures with a volar splint (i.e., a splint placed from the palm to the ventral surface of the forearm) and refer for follow-up. It is not essential to identify the specific fracture but rather to provide immobilization, pain control, and referral.

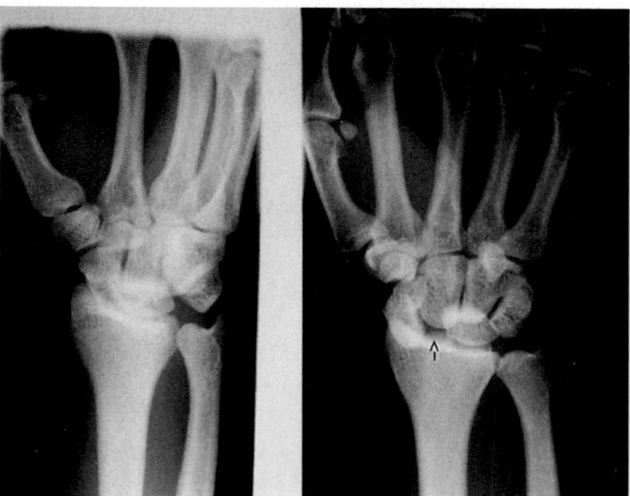

Fig. 25-9 Scapholunate widening *(arrow)* associated with perilunate dislocation.

Distal Radius/Ulna Fractures

These fractures are classified based on comminution, mechanisms of injury, displacement, and angulation. One of the most common fractures of the wrist is the **Colles' fracture**. This fracture of the distal radius occurs as a result of a fall onto an outstretched hand (Fig. 25-10). The lateral radiograph demonstrates dorsal angulation of the distal fracture fragment. A concomitant ulnar styloid fracture is frequently seen. Most Colles' fractures may be managed with ice, elevation, splinting, and pain medication. The orthopedic surgeon may perform a closed reduction and formal casting either in the ED or in the office. High-risk fractures include those that are open, neurovascularly compromised, or unstable. Unstable fractures have more than 30 degrees angulation with accompanying comminution or intraarticular involvement. These complex fractures should be evaluated promptly by the orthopedic surgeon.

A **Smith's fracture** represents the converse of the Colles' fracture. It is a distal radial fracture with a volar angulation of the distal fragment (Fig. 25-11). The Smith's fracture occurs from a blow or fall onto the dorsum of the hand. Evaluation and treatment of these fractures are comparable to Colles' fractures. Many patients may demonstrate a concomitant radial styloid fracture as the consequence of forces transmitted through the radial ligaments.

The **hematoma block** is a useful technique to provide analgesia in the ED. It is particularly well suited to patients with a Colles' fracture. Identify the site of the fracture by palpation and radiographs. Aspirate until blood is returned, then inject 10 cc of 1% or 2% plain lidocaine into the fracture site using a 21-gauge, 1.5 inch needle in a large syringe. Adequate analgesia is achieved within 15 minutes, allowing for reduction of the Colles' fracture. Supplemental opiates or hypnotics augment pain relief.

Phalangeal Fractures

Nondisplaced **shaft fractures** without rotational deformity may be splinted to the adjacent finger for 2 to 3 weeks. However, oblique fractures and fractures with rotational deformities are unstable and require operative fixation.

Distal phalangeal ("tuft") fractures are also frequently encountered in the ED. These fractures often have overlying subungual hematomas, as well as nailbed injuries. The subungual hematoma should be drained, and the nailbed evaluated for laceration.

Metacarpal Fractures

Nondisplaced fractures are usually treated by splinting in the ED, and a cast may be subsequently placed by an orthopedic or hand specialist. Unstable fractures (e.g., those that are obliquely oriented) require operative fixation.

BENNETT'S FRACTURE

A **Bennett's fracture** (Fig. 25-12) is an intraarticular fracture at the base of the thumb metacarpal, associated with a dislocation or subluxation of the carpometacarpal (CMC) joint. The ulnar portion of the metacarpal remains stable while the larger fragment subluxes dorsally when pulled by the adductor polli-

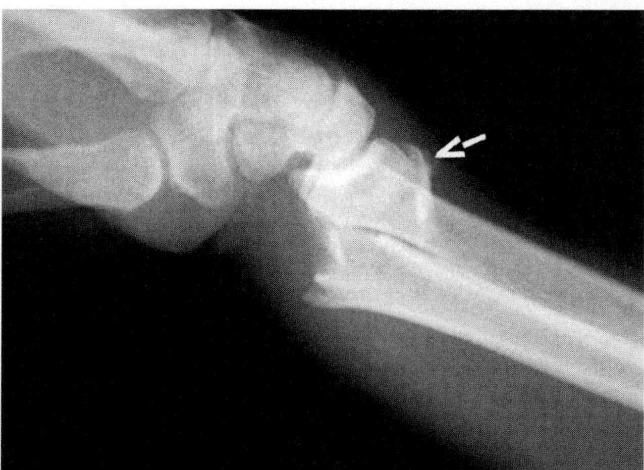

Fig. 25-10 Colles' fracture (*arrow* shows dorsal angulation of distal radius fragment).

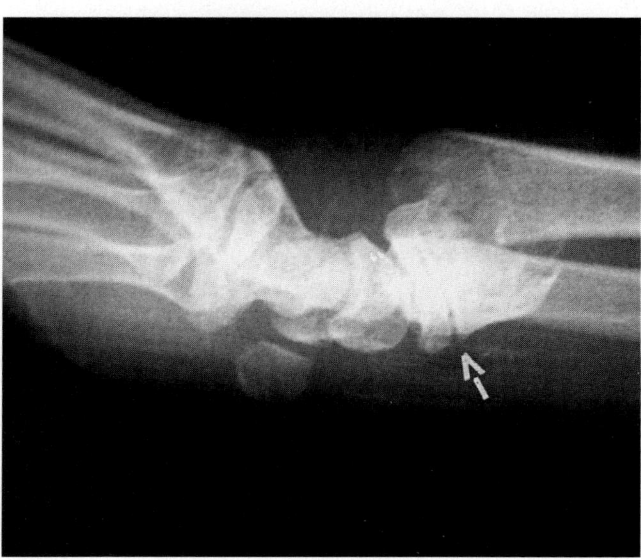

Fig. 25-11 Smith's fracture (*arrow* shows volar angulation of distal fragment).

cis longus and adductor pollicis. Anatomic reduction is essential to stabilize the CMC joint. In the ED, immobilize the patient in a thumb spica splint and refer to a hand surgeon. Definitive management may range from closed reduction to percutaneous pinning to open reduction and internal fixation.

ROLANDO FRACTURE

A **Rolando fracture** is a comminuted fracture of the base of the first metacarpal (Fig. 25-13). Plain radiographs may under-represent the severity of comminution. These fractures also require a thumb spica splint.

BOXER'S FRACTURE

This fracture of the distal little finger metacarpal usually occurs from pugilistics. The offending object is usually a chin, wall, or door. On examination, the distal aspect of the fifth metacarpal is tender and swollen. Radiographs confirm this fracture (Fig. 25-14). The EP must determine if the patient suffers a rotational deformity of the fifth digit. Have the patient place the hand palm up, and gently make a fist. All fingers should point in a cascade towards the patient's scaphoid bone. The plane of the fingernails should be uniform. When there is a rotational deformity, the fifth digit may overlap or underlap the fourth digit. Rotational deformities may require subsequent pinning. The ED management of this fracture includes an ulnar gutter splint, ice, elevation, and pain medication. The patient should be referred to an orthopedic or hand specialist.[1,51,56]

AMPUTATIONS

Advances in technology and procedures have led to increased success in reimplanting amputated digits and extremities. In academic health science centers where reimplantation procedures occur, the timely consultation with the reimplantation team is necessary. For the vast majority of EPs practicing outside of academic health science centers, preparing patients for a referral to a reimplantation center becomes paramount. Generally the wound should be cleaned with normal saline irrigation, wrapped in a sterile moist dressing, and splinted to protect further injury. Cold packs can be applied to the dressing to prevent warm ischemia. The amputated digit(s) or extremity is similarly prepared; after it is cleansed of major debris, it is wrapped in a sterile moist dressing and placed into a watertight container placed into a larger container containing ice.

The following amputation scenarios may require reimplantation: (1) multiple digits, (2) the thumb, (3) wrist and forearm, (4) sharp amputations with minimal to moderate avulsion proximal to the elbow, (5) single digits amputated between proximal inter-

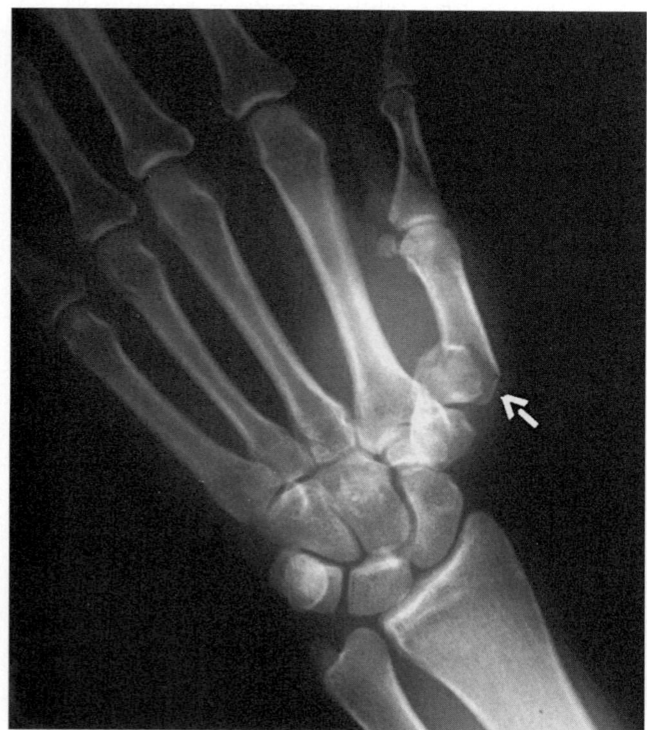

Fig. 25-12 Bennett's fracture *(arrow).*

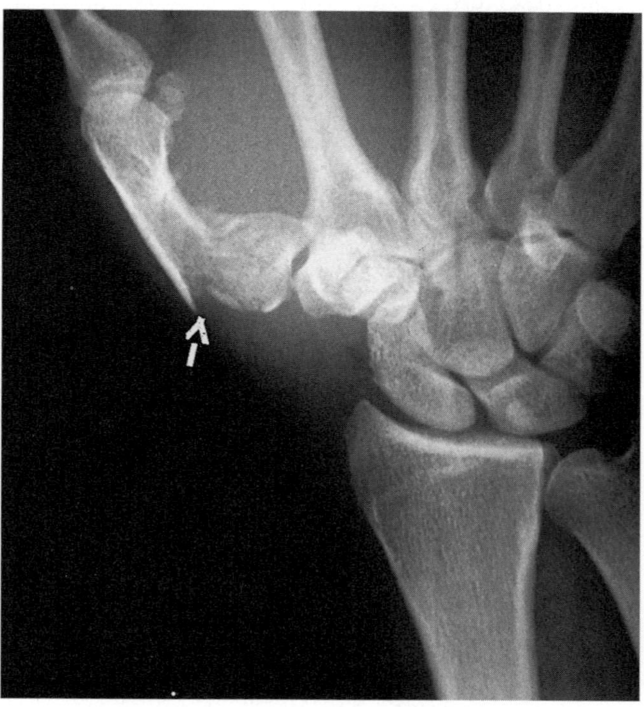

Fig. 25-13 Rolando fracture *(arrow).*

phalangeal joints and distal interphalyngal joints, and (6) all pediatric amputations.

Reimplantation is not appropriate in the following situations: (1) amputations in unstable patients with other life-threatening injuries, (2) multiple-level amputations (e.g., concomitant amputations of the mid-hand and fingers), (3) single-digit amputations proximal to the flexor digitorium superficialis insertion, (4) serious underlying disease such as peripheral vascular disease or complicated diabetes mellitus, and (5) extremes of age. With these stipulations in mind, the appropriate patients can be selected and referred for reimplantation (Box 25-2).[57,58]

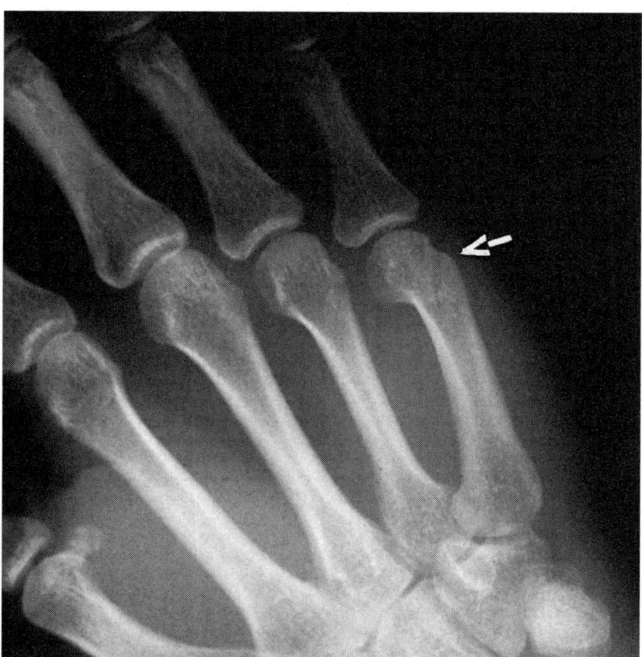

Fig. 25-14 Boxer's fracture *(arrow)*.

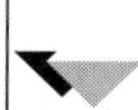

PEARLS & PITFALLS

- Examine hand lacerations through a full range of motion to ensure that a tendon has not been injured.
- Use a tourniquet when exploring hand wounds.
- Search for foreign bodies using plain-film radiographs, ultrasound, computed tomography, or magnetic resonance imaging.
- Consult a hand specialist after high-pressure injection injuries.
- Clenched fist bite wounds carry a high risk of infection.
- Assume that a scaphoid fracture exists in the presence of anatomic snuffbox tenderness, even if radiographs do not show a fracture.
- A lunate dislocation is the end stage of a perilunate dislocation.

REFERENCES

1. McGinnis JM, Foege WH: Actual causes of death in the United States, *JAMA* 270:2207-2212, 1993.
2. Runge JW: The cost of injury, *Emerg Med Clin North Am* 11:241-254, 1993.
3. Rice DP, et al: Cost of injury in the United States: a report to Congress. San Francisco, Institute for Health and Aging,

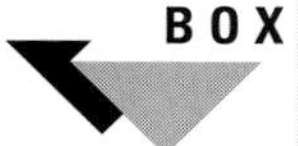

BOX 25-2
Indications and Contraindications for Replantation

INDICATIONS

Multiple digits

Thumb

Wrist and forearm

Sharp amputations with minimal-to-moderate

Avulsion proximal to the elbow

Single digits amputated between proximal interphalangeal joint and distal interphalangeal joint (distal to flexor digitorum superficialis insertion)

All pediatric amputations

CONTRAINDICATIONS

Amputations in unstable patients with other life-threatening injuries

Multiple-level amputations

Single-digit amputations proximal to the flexor digitorum superficialis insertion

Serious underlying disease such as vascular disease, complicated diabetes mellitus, congestive heart failure

Extremes of age

University of California, San Francisco, and Baltimore, Injury Prevention Center, The John Hopkins University, 1989.

4. Smith ME, Auchincloss JM, Ali MS: Causes and consequences of hand injuries, *J Hand Surg Br* 10:288-292, 1985.
5. Grunert BK, et al: Treatment of posttraumatic stress disorder after work-related hand trauma, *J Hand Surg Am* 15:511-515, 1990.
6. Grunert BK, et al: Sexual dysfunction following traumatic hand injury, *Ann Plast Surg* 21:46-48, 1988.
7. Cunningham LS, Kelsey JL: Epidemiology of musculoskeletal impairments and associated disability, *Am J Public Health* 74: 574-579, 1984.
8. Tanaka S, et al: The US prevalence of self-reported carpal tunnel syndrome: 1988 National Health Interview Survey data, *Am J Pubic Health* 84:1846-1848, 1994.
9. Broback LG, et al: Clinical and socio-economic aspects of hand injuries, *Acta Chir Scand* 144:455-461, 1978.
10. Burt CW: Injury-related visits to hospital emergency departments: United States, 1992, Advance Data, Center for Disease Control and Prevention 261:1-20, 1995.
11. Frazier WH, et al: Hand injuries: incidence and epidemiology in an emergency service, *JACEP* 7:265-268, 1978.
12. Clark DP, Scott RN, Anderson IW: Hand problems in an accident and emergency department, *J Hand Surg [Br]* 10:297-299, 1985.
13. Bhende MS, Dandrea LA, Davis HW: Hand injuries in children presenting to a pediatric emergency department, *Ann Emerg Med* 22:1519-1523, 1993.
14. Morbidity and Mortality Weekly Report. Snow-blower injuries-Colorado, New York, *MMWR* 32:77-78, 1983.
15. Bhairo NH, et al: Hand injuries in volleyball, *Int J Sports Med* 13:351-354, 1992.
16. Amadio PC: Epidemiology of hand and wrist injuries in sports, *Hand Clin* 6:379-381, 1990.
17. Johnson CF, Kaufman KL, Callendar C: The hand as a target organ in child abuse, *Clin Pediatr* 29:66-72, 1990.
18. Ross DJ, Smith ME, Angarita G: Hand injury in the accident and emergency service, *Arch Emerg Med* 2:155-160, 1985.
19. Redmon HA: Acute hand injuries: emergency room management, *J Fla Med Assoc* 76:633-636, 1989.
20. Altman RS, Harris GD, Knuth CJ: Initial management of hand injuries in the emergency patient, *Am J Emerg Med* 5:400-403, 1987.
21. St. Louis Emergency Physicians' Association Research Group: Evaluating acute hand injuries in the emergency department: a comparison of physicians with varying postgraduate training backgrounds, *Am J Emerg Med* 10:110-114, 1992.
22. Leaming DB, Walder DN, Braitwaite F: The treatment of hands: a survey of 10,668 patients treated in the hand clinic of the Royal Victoria Infirmary, Newcastle upon Tyne, *Br J Surg* 48: 247-270, 1960.
23. Edwards DH: The spectrum of hand injuries, *Hand* 7:46-50, 1975.
24. Billmire DA: Acute management of severe hand injuries, *Surg Clin North Am* 64:683-697, 1984.
25. Culver JE (editor): Injuries of the hand and wrist, *Clin Sport Med* 11:1-257, 1992.
26. Overton DT, Uehara DT: Evaluation of the injured hand, *Emerg Med Clin North Am* 11:585-600, 1993.
27. Corley FG Jr.: Examination and assessment of injuries and problems affecting the elbow, wrist, and hand, *Emerg Med Clin North Am* 2:295-312, 1984.
28. Carter PR: Injuries to the major nerve of the hand, *Emerg Med Clin North Am* 3:351-363, 1985.
29. Sloan EP: Nerve injuries in the hand, *Emerg Med Clin North Am* 11:651-670, 1993.
30. Hart RG, Kutz JE: Flexor tendon injuries of the hand, *Emerg Med Clin North Am* 11:621-636, 1993.
31. Lammers RL, Magill T: Detection and management of foreign bodies in soft tissue, *Emerg Med Clin North Am* 10:767-781, 1992.
32. Carneiro RS, Okunski WJ, Heffernen AH: Detection of a relatively radiolucent foreign body in the hand by xerography, *Plast Reconstr Surg* 59:862-863, 1977.
33. Kaplan PA, et al: Ultrasonography of post-traumatic soft-tissue lesions, *Radiol Clin North Am* 27:973-982, 1989.
34. Ginsburg MJ, Ellis GL, Flom LL: Detection of soft-tissue foreign bodies by plain radiography, xerography, computed tomography and ultrasonography, *Ann Emerg Med* 19:701-703, 1990.
35. Donaldson JS: Radiographic imaging of foreign bodies in the hand, *Hand Clin* 7:125-134, 1991.
36. Courter BJ: Radiographic screening for glass foreign bodies—what does a "negative" foreign body series really mean? *Ann Emerg Med* 19:997-1000, 1990.
37. Crawford R, Matheson AB: Clinical value of ultrasonography in the detection and removal of radiolucent foreign bodies, *Injury* 20:341-343, 1989.
38. Gilbert FJ, Campbell RS, Bayliss AP: The role of ultrasound in the detection of non-radiopaque foreign bodies, *Clin Radiol* 41: 109-112, 1990.
39. Pai C, Wei DC, Hou SP: High pressure injection injuries of the hand, *J Trauma* 31:110-112, 1991.
40. Lewis RC Jr: High-compression injection injuries to the hand, *Emerg Med Clin North* Am 3:373-381, 1985.
41. Drueck C III: Emergency department treatment of hand burns, *Emerg Med Clin North Am* 11:797-809, 1993.
42. Strickland JW: Flexor tendon surgery. Part I. Primary flexor-tendon repair, *J Hand Surg Br* 14:261-272, 1989.
43. Hart RG, Uehara DT, Kutz JE: Extensor tendon injuries of the hand, *Emerg Med Clin North Am* 11:637-649, 1993.
44. Katzman BM, et al: Immobilization of the mallet finger: effects on the extensor tendon, *J Hand Surg Br* 24:80-84, 1999.
45. Geyman JP, Fink K, Sullivan SD: Conservative versus surgical treatment of mallet finger: a pooled quantitative literature evaluation, *J Am Board Fam Pract* 11:382-390, 1998.
46. McCue FC III, Meister K: Common sports hand injuries: an overview of etiology, management and prevention, *Sports Med* 15:281-289, 1993.
47. Hossfeld GE, Uehara DT: Acute joint injuries of the hand, *Emerg Med Clin North Am* 11:781-796, 1993.
48. Stevenson TR: Fingertip and nailbed injuries, *Orthop Clin North Am* 23:149-159, 1992.
49. Chin HW, Visotsky J: Wrist fractures, *Emerg Med Clin North Am* 11:703-715, 1993.
50. O'Brien ET: Acute fractures and dislocations of the carpus, *Orthop Clin North Am* 15:237-258, 1984.
51. Watson FM Jr.: Fractures in the hand: metacarpals and phalanges, *Emerg Med Clin North Am* 3:293-310, 1985.
52. Culver JE: Sports-related fractures of the hand and wrist, *Clin Sports Med* 9:85-109, 1990.
53. Green DP, O'Brien ET: Classification and management of carpal dislocations, *Clin Orthop* 149:55-72, 1980.
54. Cooney WP, Dobyns JH, Linscheid RL: Fractures of the scaphoid: a rational approach to management, *Clin Orthop* 149:90-97, 1980.
55. Campbell RD Jr., Lance EM, Yeoh CB: Lunate and perilunar dislocations, *J Bone Joint Surg Br* 46:55-72, 1964.
56. McKerrell J, et al: Boxer's fractures: conservative or operative management? *J Trauma* 27:486-490, 1987.
57. Urbaniak JR, et al: The results of replantation after amputation of a single finger, *J Bone Joint Surg Am* 67:611-619, 1985.
58. Schlenker JD: Fingertip injuries and reimplantations, *Trauma Qtr* 1:38-45, 1985.

Proximal and Midshaft Femur Fractures and Hip Dislocations

26

JAMES E. GRUBER AND MICHAEL A. GIBBS

Teaching Case

A 30-year-old man was the victim of a motor vehicle crash (MVC). He had chest wall ecchymoses and a left lower extremity that was internally rotated, adducted, and shortened. He was admitted to the orthopedic surgeon on call. During surgery his blood pressure dropped and a stat hemoglobin demonstrated profound anemia. A diagnostic peritoneal lavage in the operating room was positive for gross blood.

Midshaft femur fractures indicate a severe mechanism of injury. Suspect associated trauma in such patients and recognize that a major distracting injury can obscure hemoperitoneum. ■

Fractures of the femur are frequently encountered in emergency practice. Patients with fractures of the proximal femur and midfemur can present to the emergency department (ED) in a variety of ways: from the 80-year-old ambulatory woman complaining of mild hip pain after a minor fall to the multiple-trauma victim in hemorrhagic shock after a high-speed motorcycle crash. Many principles of care for the orthopedic problems for these varying types of patients are similar and are reviewed here.

Patients with diaphyseal fractures of the femur have two primary threats to life: blood loss from other organ damage and hemorrhage from the femur fracture itself. Although a single break in the femur is unlikely to be immediately life threatening, the associated blood loss can endanger the patient with underlying medical disease or those with multiple-bleeding sites. Bilateral femur fractures, multiple fractures in the same extremity, or open fractures increase the risk of shock.

Severity may range from a minor avulsion of the lesser trochanter to the devastating open midshaft fracture. Although any midshaft femur fracture is serious, it reflects significant energy transfer to the patient and is frequently associated with other injuries. The pain of the fracture may obscure significant intraabdominal trauma. For this reason, a femur fracture must not distract the emergency physician (EP) from other, sometimes occult, threats to life.

Acute fractures of the proximal femur include hip fractures (encompassing femoral head, femoral neck, intertrochanteric, subtrochanteric, and isolated greater or lesser trochanteric fractures), as well as fractures of the femoral shaft. Stress fractures of the femoral neck, shaft, and subtrochanteric region can result from repeated application of submaximal forces. Additionally, in children, separation of the proximal femoral epiphysis can occur.

ANATOMY

The femur is the longest and strongest bone in the body. It is routinely subject to substantial forces from muscle contractions and weight transmission. In an anatomic position, the two femurs extend obliquely from the pelvis medially to the knee, bringing the legs closer to midline, where they can best support the body.[1]

The femoral head shape is ellipsoid and articulates with the acetabulum in a ball-and-socket joint at the hip. The femoral neck connects the femoral head with the shaft. The femoral neck resembles an oblique strut, between a horizontal beam (the pelvis) and a vertical beam (the shaft of the femur). The length, angle, and narrow circumference of the femoral neck facilitate range of motion at the hip, but also subject the neck to great shear forces, rendering it susceptible to fracture.[2]

The intertrochanteric line marks the junction of the femoral neck with the femoral shaft. The subtrochanteric region extends from the superior aspect of the lesser trochanter distally to the center of the isthmus of the femoral shaft.

Age and underlying disease affect bone physiology and anatomy. Age, sex, and gender predispose to injuries or pathologic conditions. Elderly women frequently suffer osteoporotic femoral neck fractures, associated with minor or no apparent trauma. Slipped capital femoral epiphysis (SCFE) is more frequent in boys than in girls and usually occurs between 10 and 15 years of age.

PREHOSPITAL CARE

Before moving the patient, prehospital care providers must assess the spine and, if indicated, provide immobilization. They should perform a brief neurovascular evaluation of the injured extremity and wrap open wounds with a sterile dressing. Direct pressure controls external hemorrhage. Prehospital care providers should immobilize the injured extremity before moving the patient. The leg is best supported in a position of comfort (usually flexed, abducted, and externally rotated at the hip) with a pillow placed under the thigh.[3] A Hare traction splint or similar device will reduce the fracture, limit thigh hemorrhage, and relieve pain. The two contraindications to this device include the presence of an open femur fracture and potential sciatic nerve injury. In patients with possible sciatic nerve injury, the splint may be placed to relieve pain without applying traction.

Ideally, medics should transport the patient with an isolated fracture of the proximal femur to a facility capable of handling this operative emergency. Transport to a level I or level II trauma center is advisable if (1) the patient is hypotensive, (2) there is evidence of neurovascular compromise of the injured extremity, or (3) there is suspicion of concomitant intraabdominal, pulmonary, cardiac, or neurologic injury.

EMERGENCY DEPARTMENT MANAGEMENT

History

The EP should obtain a detailed description of any antecedent trauma or other precipitating factor. In the elderly, a fall resulting in a broken hip may be the result of syncope. Recognition of syncope is fundamental in the evaluation of older adults, since this condition requires cardiac monitoring and medical consultation. Details of the mechanism of injury help predict the injury pattern. Minimal trauma resulting in a femur fracture may indicate a pathologic condition such as osteoporosis or metastatic disease. In children, a mechanism inconsistent with injury should prompt suspicion of nonaccidental trauma.

Pain from the lumbosacral spine, hip, or knee can be referred to the proximal thigh or midthigh; hence information about previous injuries or pathologic processes of these regions may be revealing. Systemic illnesses or known metabolic disorders should be noted, and current medications, as well as past steroid use, determined. Polypharmacy, particularly sedative use, is associated with falls and hip fractures in the elderly. Obtain the specifics of any previous neoplastic process, including chemotherapy or radiation therapy.

Physical Examination

Hemorrhagic shock can develop with an isolated femur fracture (particularly a femoral shaft fracture) since a liter or more of blood can be lost in the thigh. However, in the hypotensive trauma victim with an obvious extremity injury, consider thoracic, abdominal, pelvic, and retroperitoneal sources of blood loss. The presence of a midshaft femur fracture must prompt a diligent search for associated injury. Although the femur fracture is obvious, the hemoperitoneum is not.

After management of immediate life threats, evaluate the injured extremity. Because femoral nerve and arterial injuries are often associated with these fractures, a detailed neurovascular assessment is warranted. Vascular examination includes palpation of femoral, popliteal, dorsalis pedis, and posterior tibial pulses. Comparative Doppler signals between the injured and noninjured lower extremity sometimes yields useful information, particularly in penetrating trauma.[4] Neurologic examination includes an evaluation of light touch, vibratory, two-point discrimination, and pin-prick sensation, in addition to the motor examination. The EP must examine the hip and knee for associated trauma. If the leg has been splinted in the field, it is necessary to remove the splint to conduct an adequate examination.

Visual inspection of a painful proximal thigh or midthigh is important. Any lesions of the skin, discoloration, or disruption of integrity provide clues to injury. Observe the position of the leg, and check the leg for shortening or gross deformity. Palpating the skin, subcutaneous tissue, and musculotendinous units may elicit point tenderness, asymmetry, deformity, or warmth. Whenever possible, test active and passive range of motion and strength at both the hip and knee. If the patient is clinically stable and considered unlikely to have a fracture, weight-bearing may be attempted.

Laboratory Tests

Laboratory tests are usually indicated in patients with femur fractures. A measurement of metabolic acidosis, either lactate or base deficit, may detect occult shock in patients with relatively stable vital signs. Baseline hemoglobin identifies anemia and serial levels help monitor progressive blood loss. Consider obtaining a blood-type and screen for antibodies, or type and cross-match.[5] Indications for blood-typing include (1) signs of shock, (2) history of hypotension, (3) patients with multiple injuries, (4) need for operation, and (5) elevated lactate.

Radiology

Patients with midshaft femur fractures must be evaluated for major multisystem trauma. The pain associated with a femur broken at midshaft may render the physical examination of the abdomen unreliable. Some authorities would suggest routine computed tomography (CT) scanning of the abdomen for such patients, particularly if the patient will undergo urgent orthopedic surgery.[6,7]

If femur films can be obtained immediately, the splint should be left off until they are completed; otherwise the splint may obscure vital regions. It is essential to have both anteroposterior (AP) and lateral views. In proximal and midshaft fractures of the femur, make sure to radiograph the hip and knee to rule out associated fractures or dislocations. If a femoral fracture is suspected on clinical grounds, but is not seen with routine radiographs, magnetic resonance imaging (MRI) or CT scanning may be useful.[8-15] Following radiographic studies, reimmobilize the traumatized leg. Immediate operative repair is mandatory in the treatment of associated femoral artery injuries,[4,16-20] but in more subtle cases of potential vascular injury, ancillary studies such as contrast angiography, intraarterial digital subtraction angiography, or duplex ultrasonography may be indicated.[16,21-34] Venography is generally the most helpful study in the evaluation of potential femoral venous injuries.[30-32] Duplex ultrasonography is probably the most useful noninvasive test in assessing these injuries.[33,34]

True lateral and AP radiographs of the pelvis and femur are usually adequate for evaluating potential fractures of the proximal femur. However, radiologic abnormalities may be subtle, particularly with femoral neck fractures. Both the medial and lateral cortical margins of the femoral neck must be carefully examined for any irregularities suggestive of a fracture (Fig. 26-1). Occasionally, obtaining radiographs with the affected leg rotated internally or externally helps clarify the fracture line.

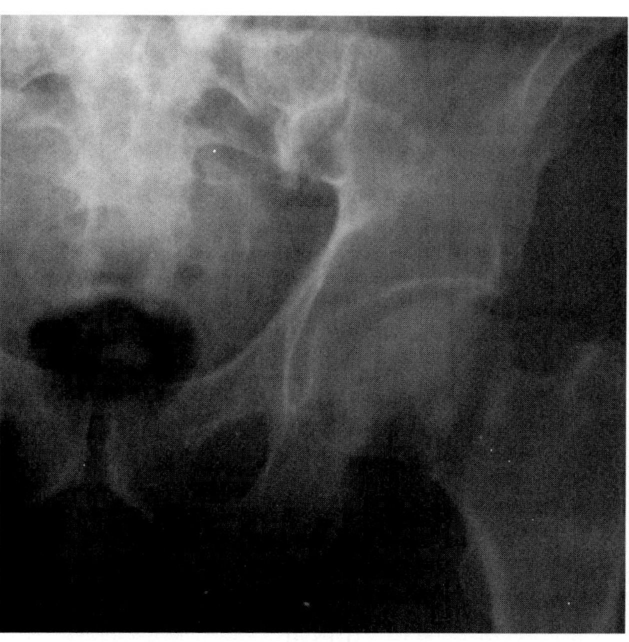

Fig. 26-1 Nondisplaced femoral neck fracture, showing disruption of cortical margins.

Several radiographic lines provide important clues to proximal femur fractures. Two of these lines are best seen on the AP pelvis film. The first is **Shenton's line.** This line runs up the medial femur and along the inferior border of the femoral neck and should continue smoothly into the inferior border of the superior pubic ramus (Fig. 26-2). In femoral neck fractures this line is disrupted, or is asymmetric compared with the opposite side. The other important line relates mostly to children and is termed **Klein's line** (Fig. 26-3). This line runs along the superior border of the femoral neck and intersects the femoral head. Discrepancies in Klein's line between the two hips occur with slipped capital femoral epiphyses.

Bone scintigraphy may be useful in a patient with a clinically suspected fracture that is not seen on a plain radiograph; however, this study is best left to the consultant. Within 24 hours of a fracture, about 80% of patients have an abnormal bone scan, and within 72 hours almost all patients have abnormal studies.[35,36] However, waiting 72 hours to diagnose a hip fracture involves prolonged bedrest and often mandates hospitalization. If a timely MRI study of a questionable hip fracture is feasible, a prolonged period of recumbency with the inherent associated costs can be avoided. If the MRI shows a fracture, the patient can

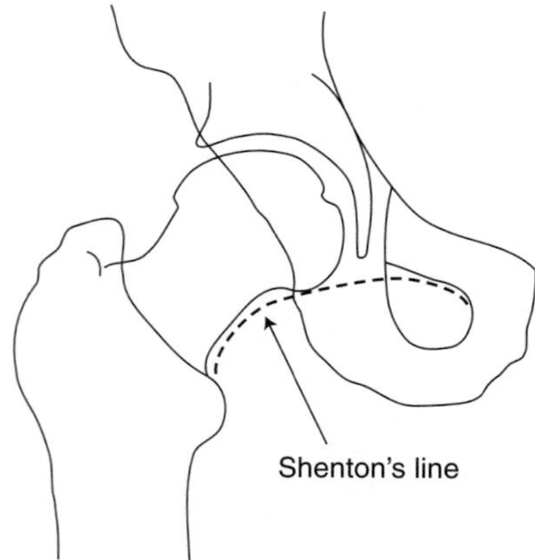

Fig. 26-2 Shenton's line.

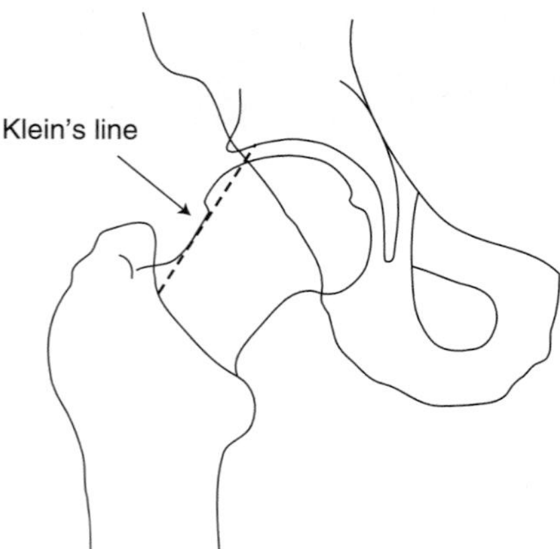

Fig. 26-3 Klein's line.

undergo early operative repair. With a negative MRI, the patient can be mobilized immediately.[9]

Emergency Department Interventions

If not already accomplished by prehospital providers, apply a traction splint in the ED after performing the extremity examination. Splints include the Hare and Sager traction devices. These devices decrease blood loss and pain associated by movement. Ensure distal pulses after application. It is helpful to mark the location of the dorsalis pedal pulse with a pen. These portable traction devices facilitate patient movement during other procedures, such as CT scanning of the abdomen.

Nearly all patients with femoral fractures are in significant pain, and analgesics should be given. Repeated small doses of an intravenous narcotic such as fentanyl or morphine provide safe, titratable relief. An alternative to parenteral analgesia is the femoral nerve block.[37] This block is particularly useful in multiple-trauma victims or in children and is performed after a detailed neurovascular examination of the lower extremity. The femoral nerve is approached lateral to the femoral artery at the inguinal crease. Five to 10 cc of a long-acting local anesthetic such as bupivacaine provides hours of relief. This block temporarily affects the motor and sensory function of the thigh, but does not change the neurologic examination in the leg below the knee.

Prophylactic antibiotics should be administered in the ED for the patient with an open fracture.[29,38,39] In a reasonably clean open fracture with a laceration of 1 cm or less, an intravenous bolus of 2 grams of a first generation cephalosporin is appropriate.[39] An antibiotic for gram-negative coverage should be added to the cephalosporin if the open fracture is associated with a laceration of greater than 1 cm, if there is extensive soft tissue injury, or if the wound appears contaminated. An intravenous loading dose of 2 mg/kg of an aminoglycoside such as gentamicin or tobramycin is effective, but once-a-day dosing using an initial load of 5 to 7 mg/kg is a safe and cost-effective alternative.[29,39] If the open fracture occurred in a highly contaminated environment, such as a farm, the addition of penicillin may prevent a Clostridial infection.[39] Prophylactic antibiotics are sometimes recommended for the patient who will undergo immediate internal fixation for closed fractures as well. The usual dose is 2 grams of a first-generation cephalosporin,[40] and can be given in the operating suite or the ED.

Disposition

Because midfemur fractures are associated with other serious injury, consultation with a general or trauma surgeon may be indicated. Although an orthopedic surgeon will address issues regarding fracture management, they may or may not be the admitting physician, depending on suspicion of other injuries.

Certain isolated fractures of the greater or lesser trochanter and selected stress fractures may be managed initially on an outpatient basis. To be considered for initial outpatient management, the patient must be reliable, have a good social situation, and not require ongoing parenteral analgesia for pain control. The patient must be able to use crutches and remain non–weight-bearing.

SPECIFIC INJURIES

Femoral Head Fractures

A fracture of the femoral head generally results from the shearing forces associated with a hip dislocation. With an anterior dislocation, the posterosuperior and

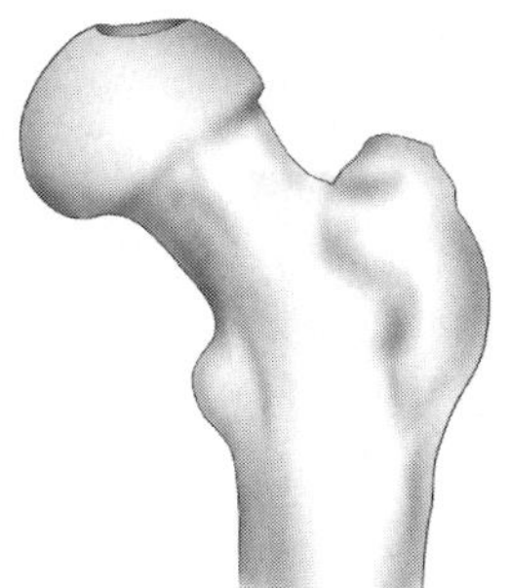

Fig. 26-4 Femoral head fracture.

lateral regions of the femoral head are usually affected (Fig. 26-4).[41] The reported incidence of an associated femoral head fracture in anterior hip dislocations ranges from 22% to 77%.[41-43] In a posterior dislocation, the posteroinferior and inferomedial aspect of the femoral head is most commonly injured. Between 10% and 16% of posterior hip dislocations have an associated fracture.[44-46] With severe impaction forces, comminuted fractures of the femoral head can occur in the absence of hip dislocation.

The femoral head is routinely subject to high mechanical stress; hence tremendous forces are necessary to fracture this region. Before the advent of high-speed travel, hip dislocations and femoral head fractures were quite rare.[47] Approximately 75% of these injuries result from MVCs.[48] Femoral head fractures predominate in young patients; an elderly patient with a similar mechanism of injury usually sustains a femoral neck fracture.[42,49,50]

The patient with a femoral head fracture generally has moderate to severe discomfort, with complete immobility at the hip joint. CT scanning or MRI of the hip may be useful when a femoral head fracture is suspected.[51]

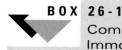

In addition to the complications seen with immobilizing injuries in elderly patients (Box 26-1), delayed complications that may develop following femoral head fracture or fracture-dislocation include posttraumatic arthritis, avascular necrosis (AVN) of the femoral head, and myositis ossificans.[42,43,48,52-55] The overall prognosis for a femoral head fracture is directly related to the severity of the initial trauma.[56,57]

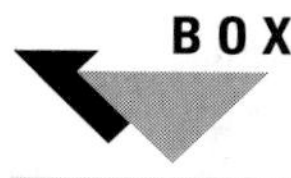

BOX 26-1

Complications of Immobilization in the Elderly[58,59]

Lower extremity thrombophlebitis
Pulmonary embolus
Pneumonia
Apathy, depression
Wound infections
Urinary tract infections
Decubitus ulcers
Congestive heart failure
Myocardial infarction
Cerebrovascular accidents
Gastrointestinal hemorrhage

Hip Dislocations

The hip joint is an extremely stable anatomic structure. The acetabulum and its labrum envelop the femoral head in any position of hip motion. The strong capsular complex, in association with powerful muscles, also protects it from dislocation.

Hip dislocations are classified as anterior, posterior, or central depending on the relationship of the dislocated femoral head to the acetabulum. **Posterior dislocations** account for between 80% and 90% of cases. **Anterior dislocations** are seen in 10% to 15% of patients. **Central dislocations**, which occur in 2% to 4% of cases, are often not true dislocations. Instead, the entire hip joint is forced through a comminuted fracture of the acetabulum.

The precarious blood supply to the femoral head jeopardizes the long-term outcome of a dislocation. During a dislocation, significant tension on surrounding vessels temporarily interrupts blood flow to the femoral head. **Avascular necrosis (AVN)** of the femoral head may develop in 1% to 17% of dislocations. The likelihood of AVN relates to both a delay in reduction and to the severity of the injury and the overall condition of the patient.

Traumatic hip dislocations occur primarily in patients suffering severe multisystem trauma, most often as a result of high-speed MVCs. The failure to use seat belts is a significant risk factor. In two large series, only 1% to 2% of patients with traumatic hip dislocation were restrained.[60]

Prehospital providers should support the involved extremity in the position of comfort, and document a brief neurovascular examination of both the injured and uninjured extremity. Splints minimize further movement and provide pain relief. If transport time is prolonged and pulses are absent, anatomic reduction is indicated. Reduction is contraindicated in the presence of a grossly contaminated wound or neuropraxia. Analgesics should be administered whenever possible.

All patients with suspected fractures or dislocations should be promptly transported to the nearest appropriate ED. If other significant trauma or hemodynamic compromise accompanies the injury to the hip, prehospital providers should proceed directly to a trauma center. Because of the forces involved, a hip dislocation is a "red flag" for multisystem trauma. These injuries are associated with other serious injuries in up to 95% of cases.[60,61]

Posterior dislocations are almost always the result of MVCs. The seated vehicle occupant typically has the hip adducted, flexed, and internally rotated at the time of impact. A direct blow of the knee against the dashboard transmits a force along the femoral shaft that dislocates the hip posteriorly. **Anterior dislocations** result from forceful extension, abduction, and external rotation of the femoral head. Anterior dislocations most often occur following an MVC when the occupant has the hip abducted and externally rotated at the time of impact. It may also result from a fall or sports injury, which forcefully hyperextends the hip.

In the course of the secondary survey, the lower extremities should be carefully examined and palpated for associated injury. Note the positioning, swelling, ecchymosis, and open wounds. Knee injuries, including fractures, ligamentous injuries, and dislocations are seen in up to 30% of cases of hip dislocation. Perform a complete neurovascular examination for both the injured and uninjured extremities. Sciatic nerve palsies, most commonly involving the peroneal nerve branch, are present in about 10% of patients with hip dislocations and such patients may demonstrate foot drop.[60] Document the strength and symmetry of pulses at the femoral artery and distal vessels. The femoral vessels are particularly prone to injury following an anterior dislocation.

The position of the injured extremity can provide valuable clues in the patient with a hip dislocation. The patient with a posterior dislocation typically holds the hip flexed, adducted, and internally rotated, with the knee of the affected extremity resting on the opposite thigh (Fig. 26-5). The extremity is usually shortened, and the greater trochanter and buttock may be unusually prominent. The patient with an anterior dislocation holds the hip in abduction, slight flexion, and external rotation (Fig. 26-6). It is important to remember that the physical findings described may be absent if an associated ipsilateral femoral shaft fracture is present, and the proximal hip injury can be easily missed.

Plain radiography identifies the majority of dislocations of the hip (Figs. 26-7 through 26-9). Radiologic investigation should begin with an AP radiograph of the pelvis on which both hips are seen. Position the hip with the maximum degree of internal rotation possible for the AP film. The AP view should include the entire pelvis and the proximal third of the femur to allow comparison of both hips.[62] The abnormal

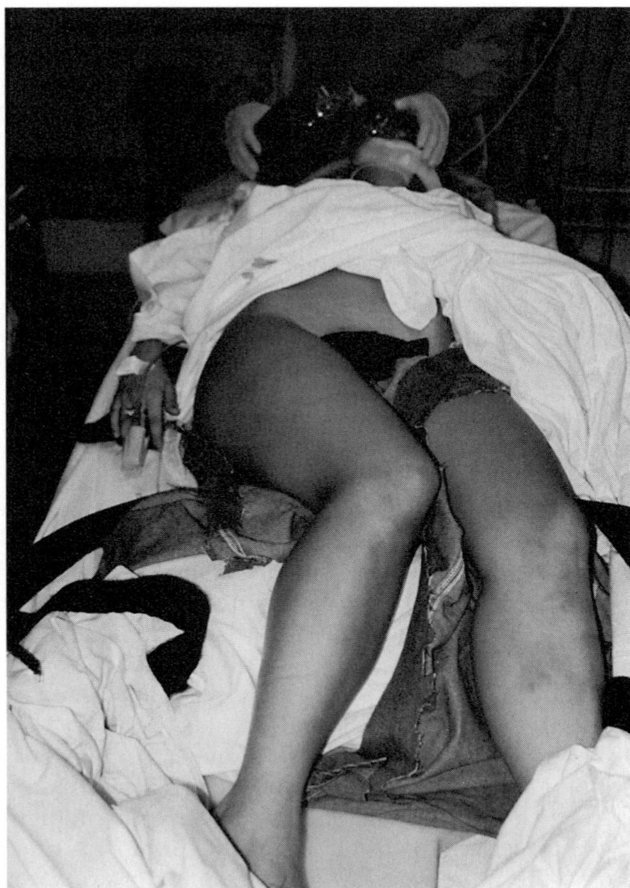

Fig. 26-5 Young woman with internal rotation, adduction, and shortening of right femur, consistent with her right posterior hip dislocation.

hip should be systematically compared with the normal one with regards to the joint space, contour of Shenton's line, and the lesser trochanter. Examine the trabecular pattern to identify disruptions and osteoporosis. The femoral head, femoral neck, and acetabulum should be carefully inspected for associated fractures. The lateral projection assists in identifying anterior and posterior dislocations, as well as femoral neck fractures.

All patients with hip dislocations should have adequate radiographic visualization of the acetabulum. If a fracture of the acetabulum is seen or suspected, it must be defined before closed reduction is attempted since intraarticular bone fragments may interfere with effective reduction. Oblique radiographs (Judet views) and CT scanning help visualize the acetabulum and precisely define the injury (Fig. 26-10).[63]

Hip dislocations are true orthopedic emergencies and reduction should be performed as soon as possible. The earlier the reduction within the context of the patient's overall condition the better the results

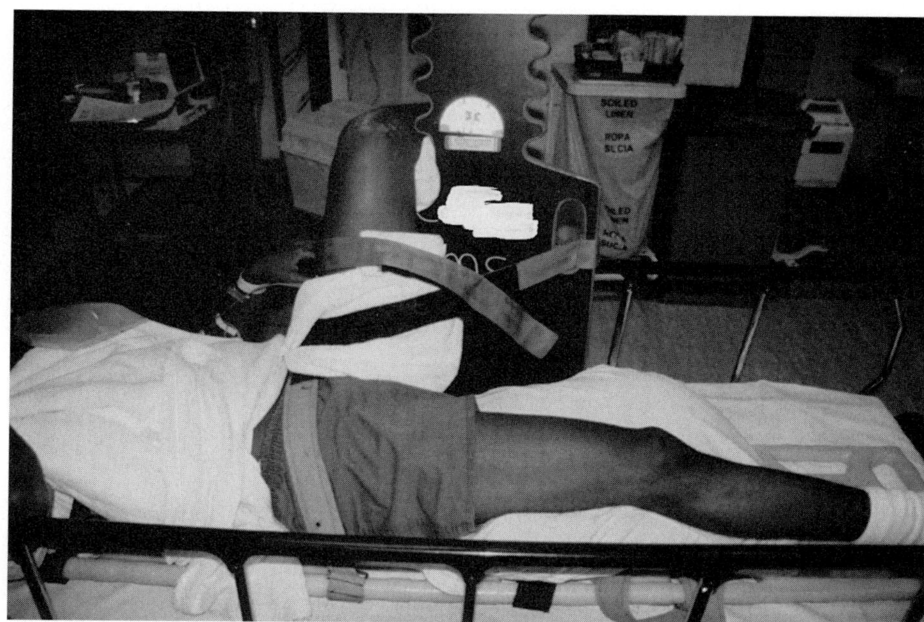

Fig. 26-6 Young man with hyperabduction of left femur, consistent with left anterior hip dislocation.

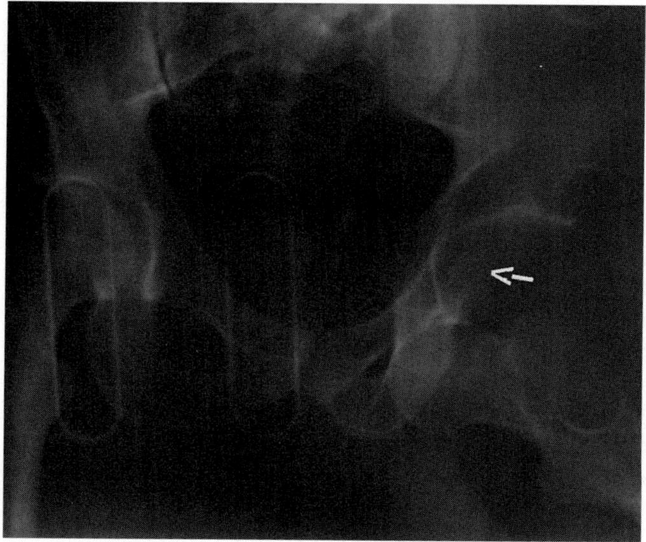

Fig. 26-7 Left anterior hip dislocation (arrow points to empty acetabulum).

should be. Delay in reduction is correlated with a higher incidence of AVN of the femoral head and posttraumatic arthritis.[64]

The timing and method of reduction is dependent on the overall condition of the patient, the type of dislocation, and the presence or absence of associated fractures. In cases of simple dislocations, closed reduction should be attempted first using intravenous sedatives. In the past, orthopedic surgeons have performed most reductions. However, if the orthopedist is not quickly available, the EP should reduce the dislocated hip. To achieve success, the patient must be adequately relaxed. Techniques of closed reduction are described in the following section.

POSTERIOR DISLOCATIONS

The **Stimson technique** is preferred for posterior dislocations by some authors.[65] This technique uses the weight of the limb and the force of gravity to reduce the dislocation, and is relatively atraumatic. Because it requires the patient to lie prone with the leg off the bed, it may not be feasible for the multiply-injured patient. It is performed as listed in the following:

1. The patient is placed prone with the leg hanging over the edge of the bed with the hip and knee flexed at 90 degrees
2. An assistant stabilizes the pelvis
3. The operator applies steady downward traction in line with the femur
4. The femoral head is gently externally rotated and the assistant pushes the greater trochanter towards the acetabulum
5. Once reduction is accomplished, the hip is brought to the extended position while traction is maintained

Since many patients have potential spinal injuries, reduction in the supine position is often performed (**Allis technique**). This technique is performed as follows:

1. The patient remains in the supine position and an assistant stabilizes the pelvis. (The assistant may simply lie across the patient's pelvis.)
2. With the knee slightly flexed, the operator applies steady traction in line with the deformity.

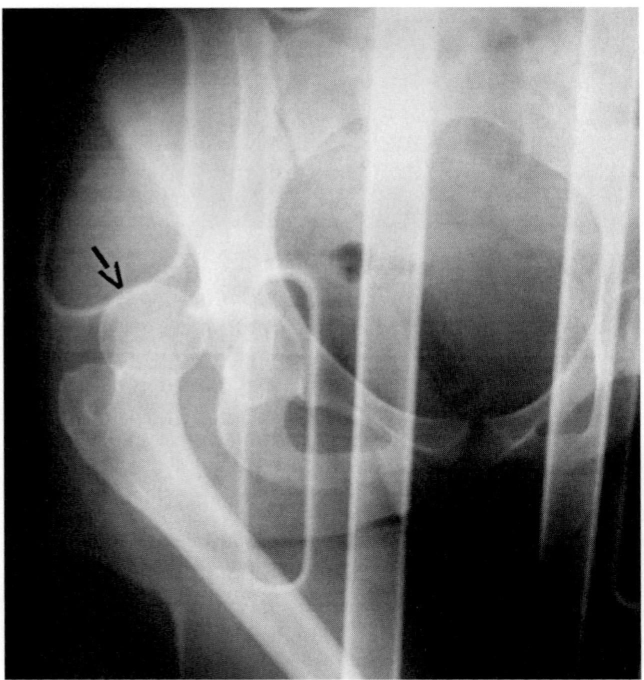

Fig. 26-8 Right posterior hip dislocation (*arrow* points to displaced femoral head).

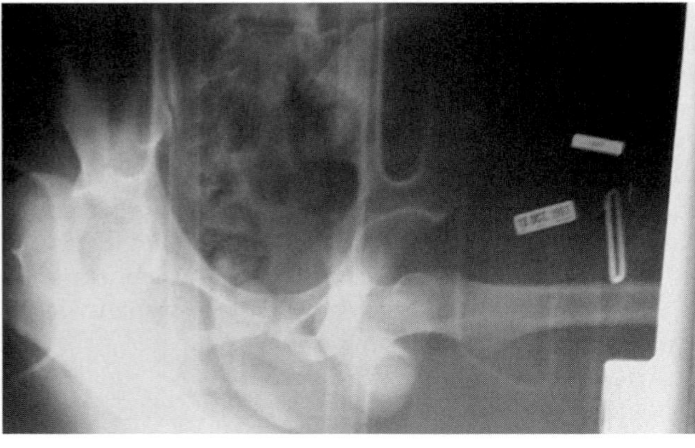

Fig. 26-9 Concomitant right posterior and left anterior hip dislocations.

3. The hip is slowly brought to 90 degrees of flexion, applying steady upward traction and gentle external rotation.
4. The assistant pushes the greater trochanter forward towards the acetabulum.
5. Once reduction is accomplished, the hip is brought to the extended position while traction is maintained.

Sometimes it helps the physician to stand on the patient's bed to accomplish this maneuver.

Following reduction, place a large abduction pillow between the patient's thighs to hold them widely apart to maintain reduction. The consultant may test

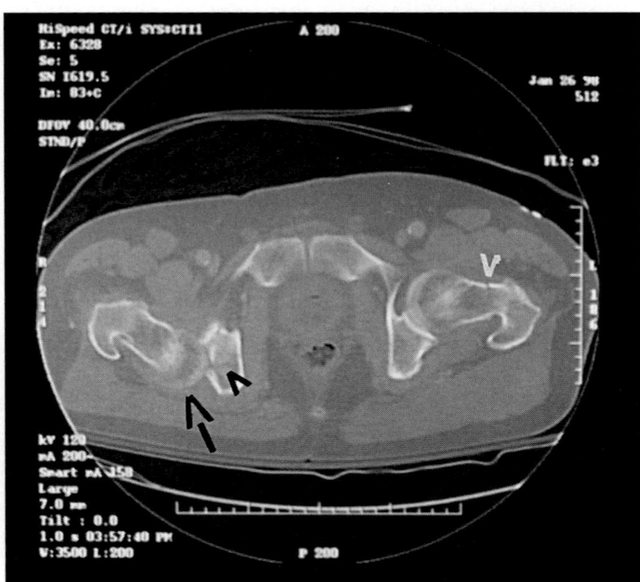

Fig. 26-10 CT scan shows right posterior hip dislocation *(black arrow),* right acetabular fracture *(black arrowhead),* and nondisplaced left femoral neck fracture *(white arrowhead).*

the hip for stability, gently placing it through a full range of motion to see if it will redislocate. Obtain an AP radiograph of the pelvis to verify the proper location of the femoral head in the acetabulum. The shaft of the femur should be in a neutral position. Examine Shenton's line and the profile of the lesser trochanter.

Occasionally a simple hip dislocation is irreducible because of incarceration of either a tendon, capsular structure, or an unrecognized osteochondral fracture fragment. In the case of an irreducible dislocation, closed reduction under general anesthesia or open reduction is often required.

In general, fracture-dislocations should be reduced using closed reduction under general anesthesia, or using open reduction. Attempted closed reduction of a fracture-dislocation by an EP is inappropriate, since the rate of complications and associated medicolegal risk is significant.

Dislocation after total hip arthroplasty is a common presentation to the ED. The reported incidence of postoperative dislocation ranges from less than 1% to almost 10%.[66] Although most dislocations occur within 30 days of surgery,[67] "late dislocations" have been reported up to 10 years after operation.[68] These dislocations can result from major trauma or from trivial events (e.g., rising from a seated position). Posterior dislocations account for 75% to 90% of cases.[66] Reduction techniques for prosthetic hip dislocations are identical to those described earlier. Consultation with an orthopedic surgeon is essential to develop a long-term treatment plan for the patient. Both nonoperative treatments (spica cast or knee immobilizer) and operative treatments have been used.

The forces required to dislocate a child's hip are often much less than in the adult patient. Seemingly minor trauma, such as tripping or suffering a minor fall, may dislocate the femoral head in the young child. In the school-age child, athletic injuries are the major cause of traumatic hip dislocation. In the teenage years, MVCs predominate as the cause.[69,70]

Femoral Neck Fractures

Fractures of the **femoral neck** are very common in the elderly, and quite rare in young patients with normal bone.[71,72] Age-related bone loss is perhaps the most important factor leading to femoral neck fractures.[73-75] As our population ages, the incidence of femoral neck fractures is expected to rise to greater levels.[74,76] The mean age of patients sustaining these fractures is 74 to 78 years, and women outnumber men by a 2:1 to 5:1 ratio.[77-79] Osteoporosis and sometimes osteomalacia or other bone defects are common.[80-86] Medications that affect bone density and strength, including corticosteroids, thyroxine, phenobarbital, phenytoin, and furosemide, increase the risk of femoral neck fractures.[78,87] Pathologic fractures, usually secondary to metastatic carcinoma, are also seen.[88]

The majority of femoral neck fractures are associated with trivial injuries, and most are secondary to primary skeletal pathologic conditions.[79] In one study, 60% of the patients with femoral neck fractures could give no history of injury.[78] Furthermore, a recent photoelastic stress analysis concluded that most hip fractures in osteoporotic individuals probably occur before the patient hits the ground.[89]

Garden has categorized femoral neck fractures into four types (Fig. 26-11), based on prereduction roentgenograms.[90-96] A **Garden I** fracture is an impacted (incomplete) fracture in which the trabeculae of the inferior femoral neck remain intact. In the **Garden II** fracture, the fracture extends completely across the femoral neck, but there is no displacement. A **Garden III** fracture is also complete, but with partial displacement. The **Garden IV** fracture is complete, with total displacement. With a Garden IV fracture there is no continuity between fracture fragments.

The signs and symptoms of a Garden I or II fracture may be minimal. These patients may complain of a slight pain in the groin or referred pain along the medial knee. Palpation of the anterior hip may reveal tenderness, induration, or swelling. Active or passive motion of the hip results in only minor discomfort, though pain increases with extremes of hip motion, particularly with flexion and internal rotation. The affected leg may be slightly shortened. Patients sustaining Garden I or II fractures are often ambulatory and walk with an antalgic gait (leaning to the side away from the injury) to minimize the pain associated with weight-bearing on the injured limb. The radiographic findings associated with a Garden I or II fracture may be subtle, requiring CT scanning, MRI, or bone scanning for detection.[7-13,35,36]

Displaced femoral neck fractures (i.e., Garden types III and IV) are more clinically apparent than incomplete, impacted, or nondisplaced fractures. Pain affects the entire hip region, and the patient will lie with the leg in external rotation and abduction. Slight shortening may be present, but the extreme deformity seen with hip dislocations or intertrochanteric fractures is rare. A displaced femoral neck fracture is unstable, and the patient cannot walk.

In impacted or incomplete fractures (Garden I) of the femoral neck, the bone fragments are in close apposition and do not shift during normal hip movement. The need for operative treatment remains controversial.[88,97-100] Nondisplaced Garden II fractures of the femoral neck are inherently unstable, and these fractures will likely become displaced unless they are internally fixated.

The morbidity and mortality of displaced femoral neck fractures, with or without comminution, is very high, but may be reduced by early surgery. In all displaced femoral neck fractures, the femoral head is at risk of AVN. Urgent treatment may reduce this complication.[101-103] If surgery is performed within the first 12 hours, the rate of AVN is reported to be about 25%. This rate rises to 30% with surgery between 13 and 24 hours, 40% between 25 and 48 hours, and 100% after 1 week.[104,105] The patient who cannot undergo surgery promptly should have the hip immobilized, with an effort made to decrease the external rotational deformity.

Intertrochanteric Fracture

The classic **intertrochanteric fracture** is extracapsular, occurring in a line between the greater and lesser trochanters. As the force of impact increases, the greater and lesser trochanters may avulse as separate fragments, yielding a four-part intertrochanteric fracture. The bone in the intertrochanteric region has an abundant blood supply and hence has an excellent potential for healing. Unfortunately, the healing process is often adversely affected by comminution of the bony fragments.

Intertrochanteric fractures are common, with an annual incidence in the United States of 98 per 100,000.[106] Reduction and internal fixation of an intertrochanteric fracture is the most frequently performed orthopedic operation.[107] Over 90% of these fractures result from falls, although they can also be seen with automobile and pedestrian accidents.[108] These fractures occur primarily in the elderly and osteoporosis or bone quality defects predispose to injury.[109-111]

The patient who sustains an intertrochanteric fracture is generally in significant pain and nonambulatory. However, the clinical presentation may be subtler in the elderly patient with impaired mentation who is normally not ambulatory.[112] The affected leg will be shortened and held in marked external rotation, sometimes up to as much as 90 degrees.[113] Swelling and ecchymosis of the hip may be seen. Attempts to move the hip are usually extremely painful and should be avoided.

A large number of classification systems for intertrochanteric fractures have been proposed[108,114-118]; however, none has gained widespread acceptance.[96] From a practical standpoint, it is best to simply define and describe these fractures based on their anatomic features.[96] The important aspects include: (1) the number of fracture fragments (two-part versus three-part versus four-part, etc.), (2) the extent of the fracture in terms of its boundaries proximally and distally,

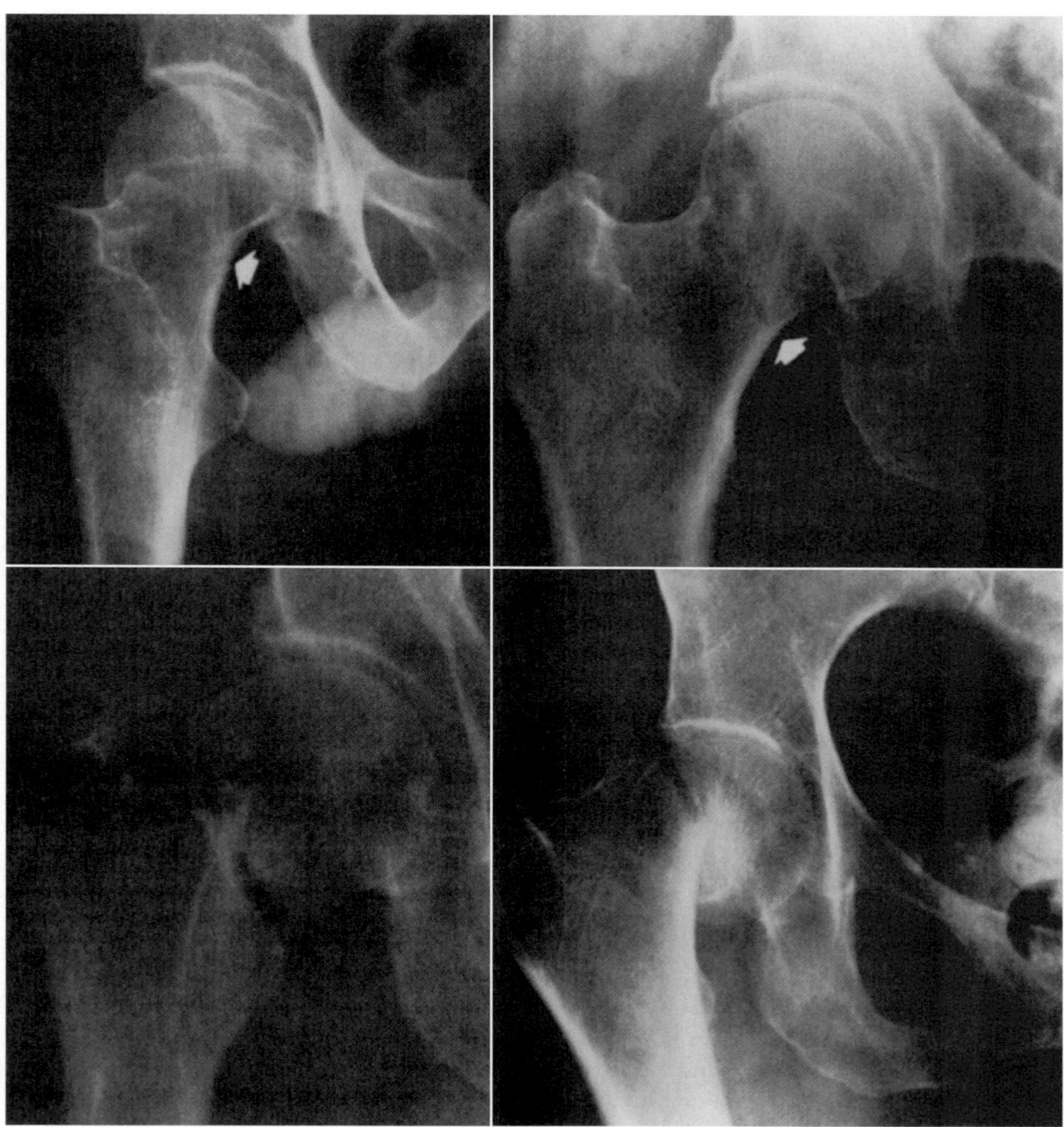

Fig. 26-11 Garden classification of femoral neck fractures. (From Rockwood CA, Green DP, Bucholz RW: *Fractures in adults,* ed 3, Philadelphia, 1991, JB Lippincott.)

(3) whether the fracture is open or closed, (4) whether the bone fragments are displaced or angulated, and (5) whether the greater or lesser trochanters are avulsed and displaced as separate fragments (Figs. 26-12 and 26-13).

The goal in managing an intertrochanteric fracture is to quickly restore the patient to preinjury level of function, generally through operative reduction and internal fixation.[65,119,120] The prognosis for patients sustaining intertrochanteric fractures varies with the patient population, the type of the fracture, and the treatment undertaken. Reported in-hospital mortality rates in different studies vary from 10% to 55%.[121-123]

Subtrochanteric Fracture

Subtrochanteric fractures account for 11% of all fractures of the proximal femur.[124] The mechanism of injury is usually direct trauma. Although young trauma victims may sustain this fracture, it is most commonly observed in elderly women.[125,126] Significant forces are usually needed to produce these fractures; how-

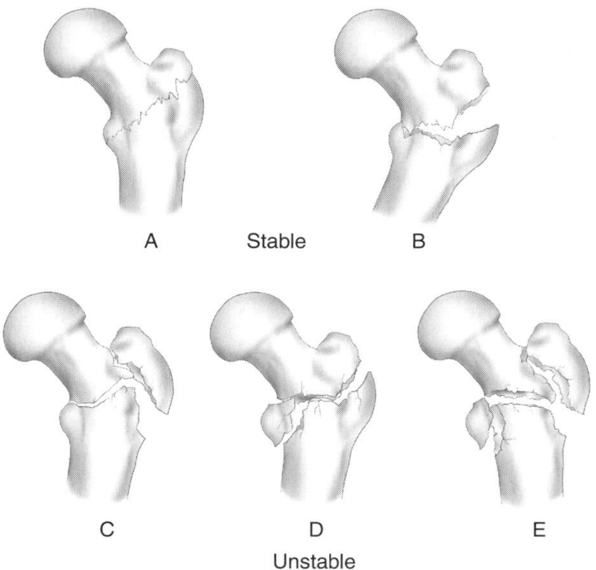

Fig. 26-12 Various types of intertrochanteric fractures. **A,** Nondisplaced, two-part fracture. **B,** Displaced, two-part fracture. **C,** Three-fragment fracture with detachment of greater trochanter. **D,** Three-fragment fracture with dislocation of lesser trochanter. **E,** Four-fragment fracture with detachment of both greater and lesser trochanter.

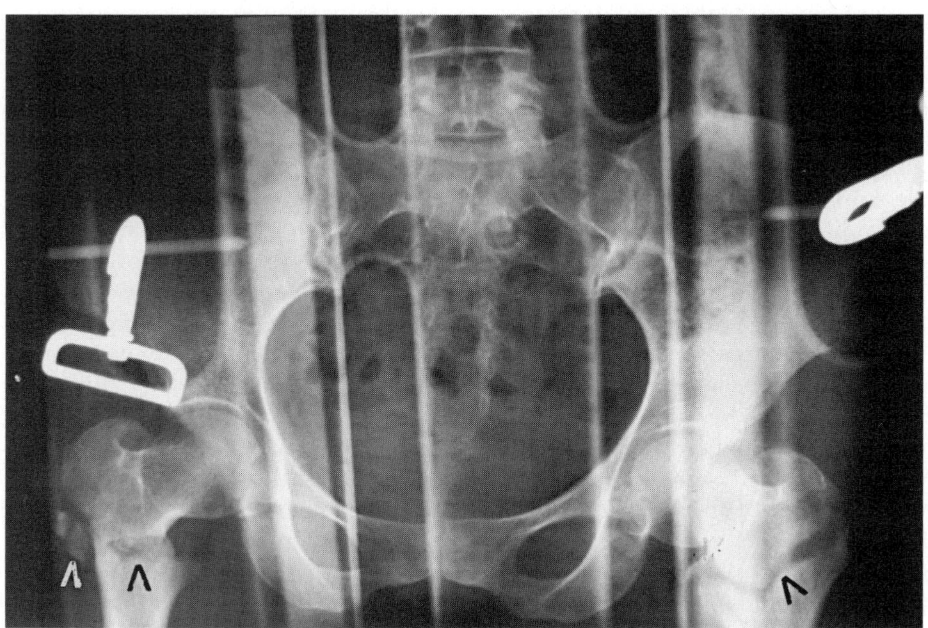

Fig. 26-13 Bilateral intertrochanteric fractures *(black arrowheads)* and avulsion of right greater trochanter *(white arrowhead).*

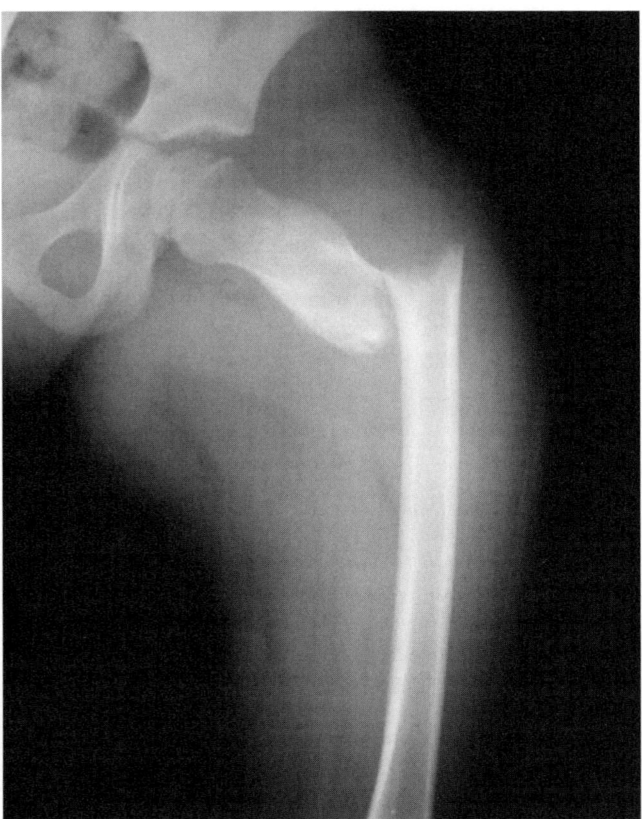

Fig. 26-14 Pathologic left subtrochanteric femur fracture (bone cyst).

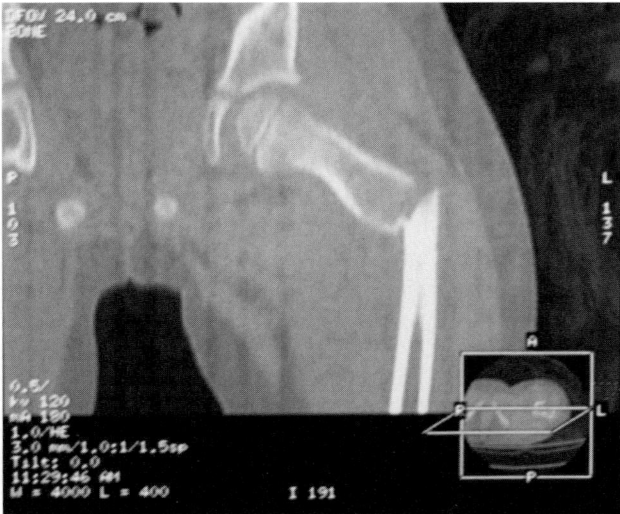

Fig. 26-15 CT scan of pathologic left subtrochanteric femur fracture (bone cyst).

ever, disorders affecting bone strength, such as Paget's disease, bone cysts, or renal osteodystrophy, may render this region susceptible to pathologic fractures (Figs. 26-14 and 26-15).[127] Subtrochanteric stress fractures occur in runners and military recruits.[128-130] The subtrochanteric femur is also a frequent site of skeletal metastases, with breast carcinoma being the most common primary tumor.

The patient with a subtrochanteric fracture presents in moderate to severe distress. Unbalanced muscles produce a characteristic flexion, abduction, and external rotation of the proximal fragment.[131] Also, the fracture site may be angulated, and the leg may be shortened.[132] The region of the greater trochanter protrudes outward, and the hip appears thick and swollen. The entire limb is in full external rotation, and slightly flexed at the knee. The patient keeps the leg still since it is very sensitive to any movement.[133] Ecchymosis is generally not present initially, but develops over the first few days.

Because of the extreme forces usually needed to produce subtrochanteric fractures, associated injuries are frequent, especially to the ipsilateral extremity. In one study, 30% of patients sustained other fractures, 4% suffered genitourinary trauma, 5% had intraabdominal injuries, and 6% neurologic injury.[134] Associated closed head injuries and chest trauma are common.[135]

Subtrochanteric fractures may be stable or unstable, depending on the displacement of the fragments and degree of comminution. A variety of classification systems for these fractures have been proposed,[114,115,135-139] but no system is widely accepted.[96] From a practical standpoint (as is the case with intertrochanteric fractures), it is best to describe these fractures on an anatomic basis. The relevant anatomic features of subtrochanteric fracture include (1) the location of the fracture (proximal versus distal), (2) the angle of the fracture (transverse, short-oblique, or long-oblique), (3) whether the fracture is open, and (4) whether the fracture is comminuted (Figs. 26-16 and 26-17). Transverse and short-oblique fractures tend to be found most commonly in younger patients sustaining injuries from severe trauma. Long-oblique fractures, seen predominantly in elderly patients, are usually the result of a low-velocity force with rotational stress, from slipping on ice or a loose rug. Comminution, whether associated with long- or short-oblique fractures, also tends to occur more often in the elderly and is commonly the result of high-velocity forces, usually applied directly to the trochanteric or subtrochanteric region.

Subtrochanteric fractures are the most difficult of all proximal femur fractures to treat, and the definitive management is a complex issue. The high stresses in this area make these fractures difficult to reduce and to maintain in reduction. Because the bone in the subtrochanteric region is predominantly cortical, healing is relatively slow, and numerous complications can develop.[126] The reported mortality rate from subtrochanteric fractures ranges from 12.2% to

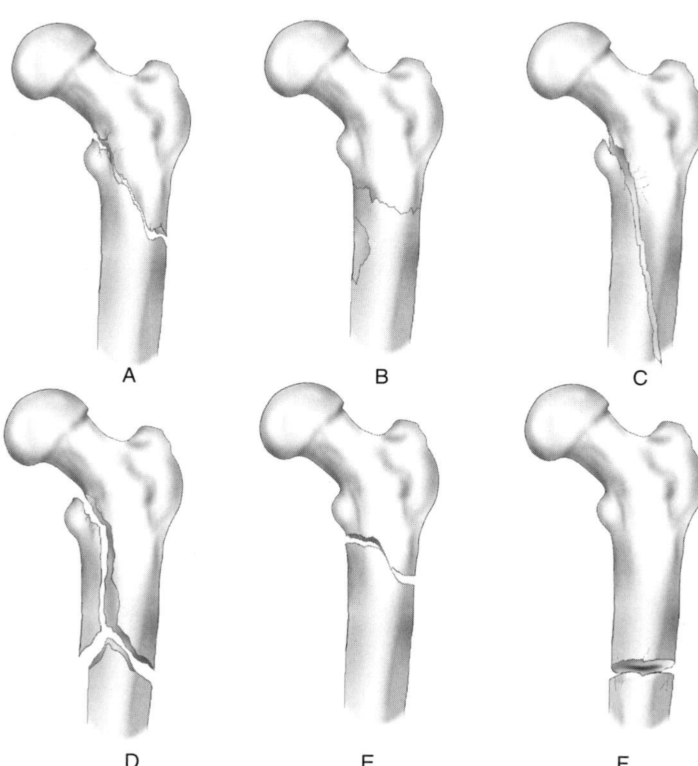

Fig. 26-16 Various types of subtrochanteric fractures. **A,** Short oblique fracture. **B,** Short oblique fracture with comminution. **C,** Long oblique fracture. **D,** Long oblique fracture with comminution. **E,** High transverse fracture. **F,** Low transverse fracture.

20.8%.[126,135] This relatively high degree of mortality reflects the severe force needed to produce these fractures, the common associated injuries, and the often advanced age of these patients. Operative repair with a variety of screws and plates or nails has been used in the management of these fractures in adults.[140]

Femoral Shaft (Diaphyseal) Fracture

Femoral shaft fractures (Fig. 26-18) are relatively common injuries. Most of these fractures result from blunt trauma, although penetrating trauma or torsional stress can also shatter the femur.[141] As a rule, these fractures are produced by high-energy forces, but they can also occur with only mild to moderate trauma in elderly patients with osteoporosis.[142,143] Sometimes, stress fractures of the femoral shaft can occur. The majority of femoral shaft fractures are transverse, although spiral and oblique fractures are also seen. Spiral fractures in young children should raise the specter of abuse. Comminuted or segmental fractures result from severe mechanism of injury.[144] Open fractures of the femoral shaft are not as frequent as closed fractures, and are usually associated with gunshot wounds.

A physical examination detects most femoral shaft fractures. The patient will have significant pain, tenderness, and swelling and will be unable to move either the hip or knee on the affected side. A diffusely

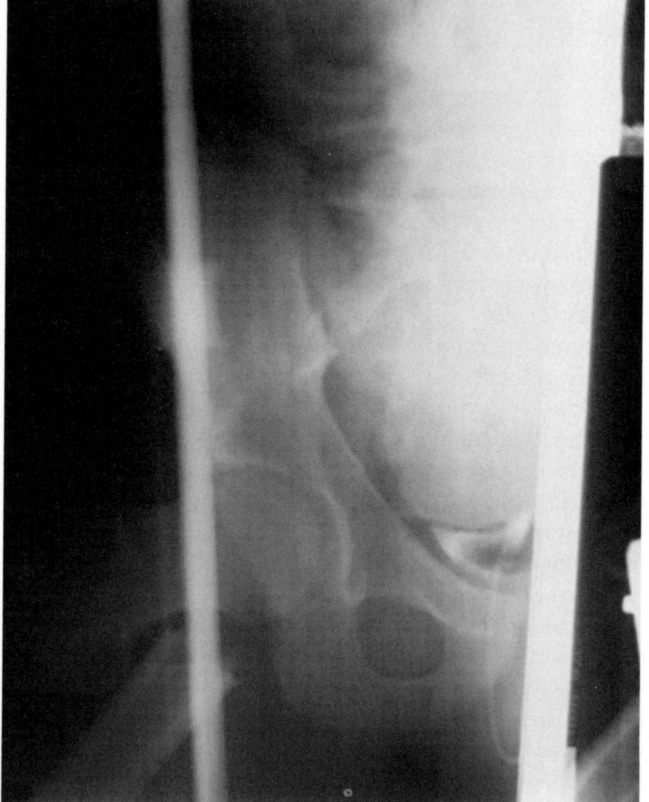

Fig. 26-17 High-transverse right subtrochanteric fracture.

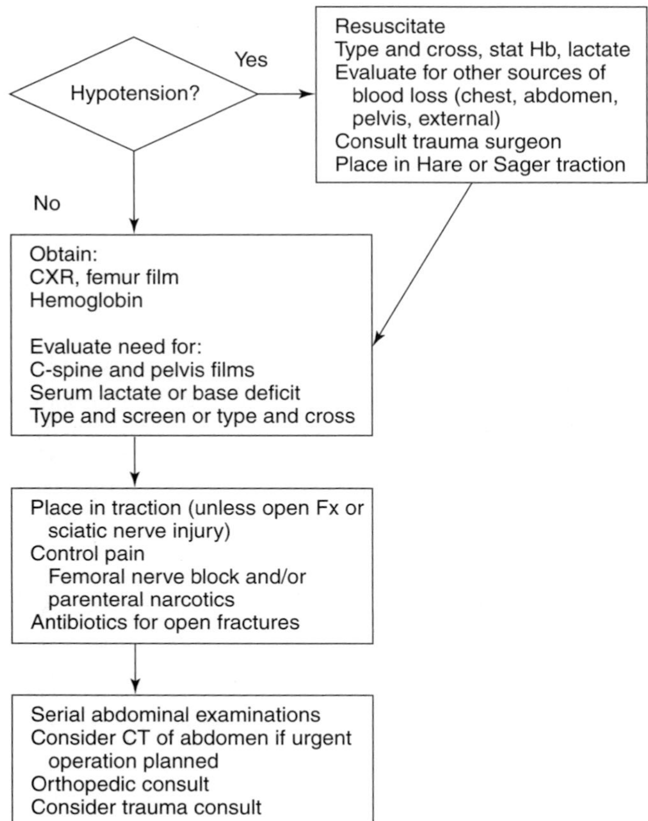

Fig. 26-18 Management of midshaft femur fractures.

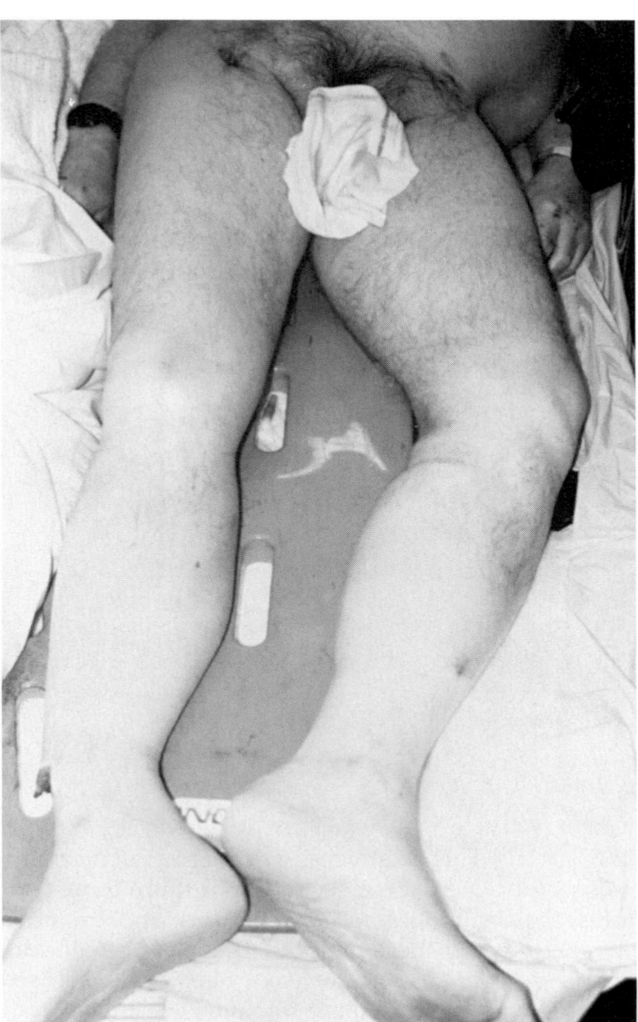

Fig. 26-19 Young man with external rotation, abduction, and shortening of the left femur, consistent with his midshaft fracture. Also note right tibia fracture.

expanding thigh indicates a large hemorrhage. Angulation of the thigh is pathognomonic (Fig. 26-19). The type of deformity depends on the location of the fracture. In a fracture of the proximal femoral shaft, the massive muscle attachments of the greater trochanter create an abduction deformity, whereas the iliopsoas causes a flexion-external rotation deformity of the proximal segment. With midshaft fractures, the thigh adductors produce a varus malformation. In both midshaft and distal shaft fractures, the gastrocnemius can flex the distal fragment.[145]

The initial evaluation of the patient sustaining acute femoral shaft fractures should include a careful survey to rule out associated trauma, especially to the head, neck, and torso. Hip and other lower extremity injuries are common, and include hip fractures or dislocations, femoral neck fractures, supracondylar femoral fractures, ligamentous injuries of the knee, and patellar fractures.[144,146,147] Plain radiographs usually are sufficient for defining these injuries (Fig. 26-20). Vascular compromise from arterial occlusion or disruption can occur (Fig. 26-21).[148-150] Nerve damage is rare because of the wide cushion of muscle between the bone and the nerve.[151]

If the patient arrives in the ED with the injured extremity immobilized in traction, it will be necessary to remove the traction to examine the hip and knee adequately. Analgesia should precede this maneuver, either parenterally or using a femoral nerve block after performance of the neurologic examination. Patients should be evaluated clinically for hip pain or tenderness. Range of motion at the hip is naturally limited by pain from the femoral shaft fracture. The knee should always be assessed for ligamentous instability, since these injuries can be easily missed. In one study, one third of patients with femoral shaft fractures had associated ligamentous damage of the knee.[147] A complete neurovascular examination of the lower extremity is also mandatory. The neurologic examination may be somewhat unreliable because the patient generally is in severe pain and unable to coop-

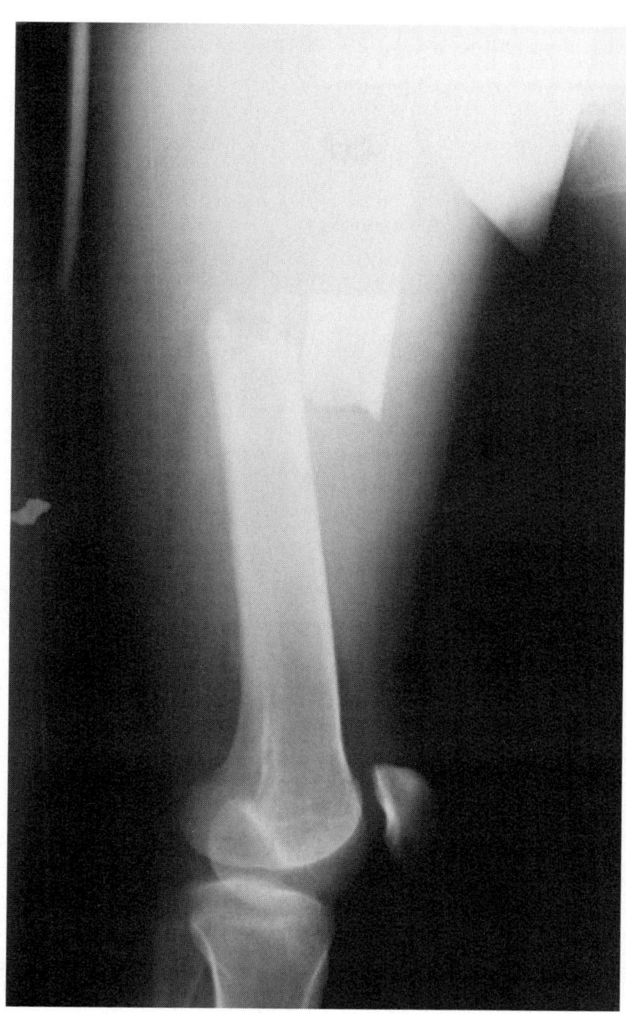

Fig. 26-20 Midshaft femur fracture with 100% displacement.

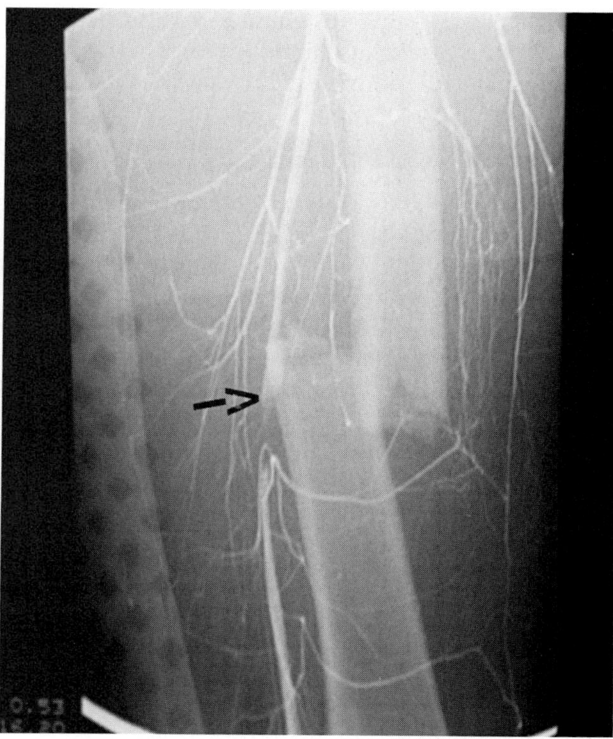

Fig. 26-21 Angiogram shows occlusion of left superficial femoral artery *(arrow)* associated with a femur fracture.

erate fully; however, an adequate vascular examination should be possible.

The vast majority of femoral shaft fractures heal quite well in time, regardless of the mode of treatment employed.[152] The ultimate goal is early return of strength and activity.[153,154] Treatment modalities include traction, cast bracing, external fixation, pins and plaster, or internal fixation. More severely comminuted fractures are more likely to be treated in a closed fashion, particularly if extensive soft-tissue damage is present.[151] However, with nonsegmental fractures internal fixation shortens both hospitalization and total disability time.[155,156]

Femoral shaft fractures have close to a 100% union rate.[157] However, a variety of complications can occur. The risks of prolonged immobilization in elderly patients are always of concern (see Box 26-1). The refracture rate may vary from 1% for those fractures treated by open method, to 6% for fractures treated by closed methods.[156] Nonunion is relatively uncommon, with an incidence of about 1%, but malunion or delayed union is not infrequent.[151,156] Even minor degrees of limb shortening or malalignment can lead to a limp and posttraumatic arthritis.[151] The incidence of osteomyelitis, a potentially disastrous complication, is significantly higher when open surgical repair is attempted. Although open fractures only occasionally become infected with conservative treatment,[158] open fractures treated with open fixation have an alarming infection rate of 14% to 21%.[159-161]

Isolated Greater Trochanter Fracture

An **isolated fracture of the greater trochanter** is a rare injury.[162,163] There are two types of these fractures. The most prevalent is an epiphyseal separation in which the entire greater trochanteric apophysis is avulsed from the femur.[162,164,165] This fracture occurs in children and adolescents between 7 and 17 years of age.[162] The mechanism of injury is generally a powerful muscle contraction of the lateral rotators of the hip joint, as might occur in a twisting fall.[163] The second type of isolated greater trochanter fracture is seen in adults. It is typically a comminuted fracture involving only part of the greater trochanter and usually results from a direct blow to this region. Most commonly, the avulsed fragments are displaced superiorly and posteriorly.[65]

The patient with an isolated greater trochanter fracture may be ambulatory. The greater trochanter is tender to palpation, and ecchymosis is common.[164] Pain and spasm may produce flexion of the hip.[163]

Several modes of treatment have been described for isolated greater trochanter fractures.[163] Usually the fracture can be treated as a soft-tissue injury, with protected weight-bearing until the patient is asymptomatic. Treatment generally necessitates several days of bed rest, followed by partial weight-bearing movements with crutches for 3 to 4 weeks.[65] In the young patient who has a noncomminuted fracture involving a large fragment with greater than 1 cm of separation of the avulsed fragment, open reduction and internal fixation may be indicated. Regardless of the type of treatment employed, the prognosis is good, and function following healing is generally excellent.[162-164]

Isolated Lesser Trochanter Fracture

An **isolated fracture of the lesser trochanter** generally occurs when a forceful contraction of the iliopsoas muscle avulses the lesser trochanter apophysis.[166,167] Usually, sudden or forceful hip flexion, often against resistance, produces this injury. The injury is most common in adolescent athletes, particularly dancers and gymnasts. Eighty-five percent of all cases occur in patients less than 20 years of age, with a peak incidence between 12 and 16 years.[166,168] When this injury is seen in adults over 25 years of age, it generally represents a pathologic fracture, secondary either to a metastatic neoplasm or severe osteoporosis.[169]

The patient who has sustained an isolated fracture of the lesser trochanter can usually walk. However, the femoral triangle is markedly tender, and hip flexion against resistance is painful. Iliopsoas insufficiency is common and the seated patient is unable to lift the foot of the affected leg from the floor (**Ludloff's sign**).[168]

The treatment of an isolated lesser trochanter avulsion fracture usually involves bed rest without a plaster cast and relatively early mobilization.[168] Most patients regain painless active hip flexion within 3 weeks. However, in cases of wide separation between the lesser trochanter and the femur, hospitalization for open reduction and internal fixation may be beneficial, especially if the patient is young and athletic.

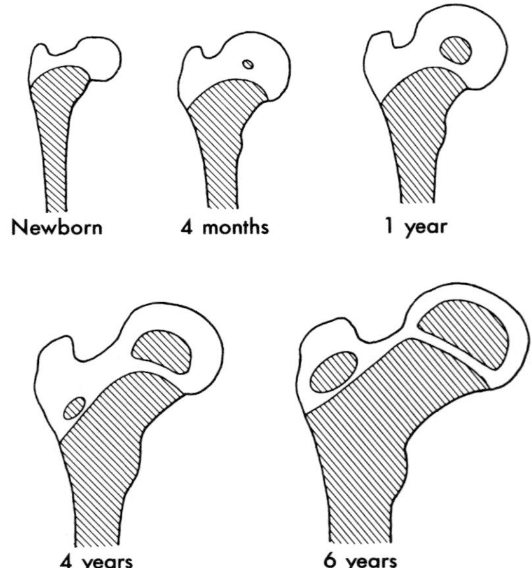

Fig. 26-22 Development of femoral head. (From Edgren W: *Acta Orthop Scand* 84[suppl]:24, 1965.)

SPECIAL CONSIDERATIONS IN THE CHILD WITH A PROXIMAL FEMUR OR HIP FRACTURE

In general, the presentation of children with proximal femur or hip fractures is similar to that of adults. However, several important differences are noteworthy. First, developmental anatomy must be considered in evaluating the young child with a possible proximal femoral injury (Fig. 26-22). Plain radiographs do not demonstrate an injury in a femoral head, neck, or trochanter that is still cartilaginous. Second, the incidence of hip fractures in children is extremely low compared with the incidence of hip fractures in adults with osteoporosis.[170] These fractures account for less than 1% of all pediatric fractures.[171] It usually takes a great deal of force to cause these fractures in children; therefore, the likelihood of associated injuries is much higher.[172-174] If a seemingly trivial injury has resulted in a hip fracture in a child, abuse-related injury or a pathologic fracture must be considered.[174-177] Third, fracture patterns and classification of hip fractures are different in children as compared with adults. Transepiphyseal separation can occur in children because of the weakness of the capital femoral epiphysis. Also, transcervical fractures in children are usually displaced, in contrast to the situation with adults, in whom impacted fractures often occur.

In children, fractures of the proximal femur have high complication rates,[174,175,178,179] in part as a result of the fact that the child's proximal femur must grow. The blood supply to the femoral head in children is more tenuous than in adults, and the rate of AVN for transcervical fractures in children has been reported to be as high as 43%.[172,180] Given these high complication rates, it is not surprising that there are various opinions about the best way to treat these fractures.[181] Early involvement of an orthopedist is essential for optimal care.

The prognosis for children with femoral shaft fractures is considerably better than it is for children with more proximal femur fractures. The vast majority of femoral shaft fractures heal well. Traditionally, infants and children under 10 years old have been managed by application of an early spica cast, unless there was more than 2 cm of overriding on a resting length radiograph. However, some authors now advocate internal fixation employing elastic intramedullary devices that avoid the physeal region. Internal fixation in these patients provides the advantages of early weight-bearing and reduced hospitalization time compared with conservative treatment.[182,183] External fixation is another treatment option that has been employed in these fractures, particularly in head-injured patients, since these children tend not to tolerate prolonged periods of traction.[183-185]

In children over 10 years of age, the potential for permanent leg shortening is greater, and an extensive period of traction (up to 6 weeks), followed by casting, is usually the preferred method of treatment.[186] The most common complication seen with this fracture is length malunion. Angular or rotational malunion can also occur if the fracture fragments are not properly aligned during healing. Nonunion is a rare complication that is seen almost exclusively in patients who have had open procedures, usually complicated by infection.[187]

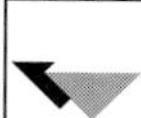

PEARLS & PITFALLS

- Consider the mechanism of injury. A hip fracture in the elderly patient may be a consequence of a malignant dysrhythmia producing syncope. A spiral fracture in a child may be the clue to child abuse.
- Beware the midshaft femur fracture! This fracture is a high-energy injury associated with multiple trauma. Liberalize criteria for abdominal CT scanning in such patients.
- Attempt reduction of a hip dislocation as soon as possible. However, reduction may need to be delayed if the patient has the potential for more serious injuries, for example, thoracic aortic injury.
- Control pain with parenteral narcotics or a femoral nerve block.
- Use radiographic lines. Shenton's line is useful to detect femoral neck fractures, whereas Klein's line helps detect slipped capital femoral epiphysis.
- Splint. Both the Hare traction splint and the Sager splint decrease bleeding and pain.
- Check the knee. In one study, one third of patients with femoral shaft fractures had associated ligamentous damage of the knee.[147]Disposition. Do not automatically admit all patients with a femur fracture to an orthopedist. A trauma surgeon is better suited to direct in-hospital care for the multiply-injured patient.

REFERENCES

1. Wadsworth CT: *Manual examination and treatment of the spine and extremities,* Baltimore, 1988, Williams & Wilkins.
2. Lockhart R, Hamilton GF, Fyfe FW: *Anatomy of the human body,* Philadelphia, 1959, JB Lippincott.
3. Needoff M, Radford P, Langstaff R: Preoperative traction for hip fractures in the elderly: a clinical trial, *Injury* 24:317-318, 1993.
4. Shaker IJ, et al: Special problems of vascular injuries in children, *J Trauma* 16:863-867, 1976.
5. Kurdy NM, Hokan R: A cross-matching policy for fractures of the proximal third of the femur, *Injury* 24:521-524, 1993.
6. Colucciello SA: Blunt abdominal trauma, *Emerg Med Clin North Am* 11:107-123, 1993.
7. Ferrera PC, et al: Injuries distracting from intraabdominal injuries after blunt trauma, *Am J Emerg Med* 16:145-150, 1998.
8. Weissman BN, Sledge CB: *Orthopedic radiology,* Philadelphia, 1986, Saunders.
9. Guanche CA, et al: The use of MRI in the diagnosis of occult hip fractures in the elderly: a preliminary review, *Orthopedics* 17:327-330, 1994.
10. Brake D: Imaging of femoral neck stress fracture, *Kans Med* 95:49, 1994.
11. Deutsch AL, Mink JH, Waxman AO: Occult fractures of the proximal femur: MR imaging, *Radiology* 170:113-116, 1989.
12. Sauser DO, et al: CT evaluation of hip trauma, *AJR* 135:269-274, 1980.
13. Lang P, et al: Imaging of the hip joint: computed tomography versus magnetic resonance imaging, *Clin Orthop Rel Res* 274:135-153, 1992.
14. Conway WF, Totty WG, McEnery KW: CT and MR imaging of the hip, *Radiology* 198:297-307, 1996.
15. Mitchell MJ, et al: Diagnostic imaging of lower extremity trauma, *Radiol Clin North Am* 27:909-928, 1989.
16. Saide R, et al: Management of peripheral vascular trauma, *Am Surg* 47:429-438, 1981.
17. Reynolds RR, et al: The surgical treatment of arterial injuries in the civilian population, *Ann Surg* 189:700-708, 1979.
18. Meagher DP, et al: Vascular trauma in infants and children, *J Trauma* 19:532-536, 1979.
19. Tilson MD, et al: Obturator canal bypass grafts for septic lesions of the femoral artery, *Arch Surg* 114:1031-1033, 1979.
20. Cargile JS, Hunt JL, Purdue GF: Acute trauma of the femoral artery and vein, *J Trauma* 32:364-370,1992.

21. Howard CA, et al: Intra-arterial digital subtraction arteriography in the evaluation of peripheral vascular trauma, *Ann Surg* 210:108-111, 1989.
22. David PC, Hoffman JC Jr: Work in progress. Intra-arterial digital subtraction angiography: evaluation in 150 patients, *Radiology* 148:9-15, 1983.
23. Norman D, et al: Intraarterial digital subtraction imaging cost considerations, *Radiology* 156:33-35, 1985.
24. Anderson RJ, et al: Reduced dependency on arteriography for penetrating extremity trauma: Influence of wound location and noninvasive vascular studies, *J Trauma* 30:1059-1063, 1990.
25. Berstein JM, et al: Pitfalls in the use of color-flow duplex ultrasound for screening of suspected arterial injuries in penetrated extremities, *J Trauma* 33:395-402, 1992.
26. Knudson MM, et al: The role of duplex ultrasound arterial imaging in patients with penetrating extremity trauma, *Arch Surg* 128:1033-1037, 1993.
27. Bynoe RP, et al: Noninvasive diagnosis of vascular trauma by duplex ultrasonography, *J Vasc Surg* 14:346-352, 1991.
28. Meissner M, Paun M, Johansen K: Duplex scanning for arterial trauma, *Am J Surg* 161:552-555, 1991.
29. Brien WW, et al: The management of gunshot wounds to the femur, *Orthop Clin North Am* 26:133-138, 1995.
30. Gerlock AJ Jr, Muhletaler CA: Venography of peripheral venous injuries, *Radiology* 133:77-80, 1979.
31. Gerlock AJ, Thal ER, Snyder WH III: Venography in penetrating injuries of the extremities, *AJR* 126:1023-1027, 1976.
32. Rich NM: Management of venous trauma, *Surg Clin North Am* 68:809-821, 1988.
33. Frykberg ER: Advances in the diagnosis and treatment of extremity vascular trauma, *Surg Clin North Am* 75:207-223, 1995.
34. Blumenthal J: Difficult venous injuries, *NY State J Med* 80:1689, 1980.
35. Matin P: The appearance of bone scans following fractures, including immediate and long-term studies, *J Nucl Med* 20: 1227-1231, 1979.
36. Fairclough J, et al: Bone scanning for suspected hip fractures, *J Bone Joint Surg* 69B:251-253, 1987.
37. Ronchi L, et al: Femoral nerve blockade in children using bupivacaine, *Anesthesiology* 70:622-624, 1989.
38. O'Meara PM: Management of open fractures, *Orthop Rev* 21: 1177-1185, 1992.
39. Gustilo RB, Merkow RL, Templeman D: The management of open fractures, *J Bone Joint Surg* 72A:299-304, 1990.
40. Burnett JW, et al: Prophylactic antibiotics in hip fractures: a double-blind, prospective study, *J Bone Joint Surg* 62A:457-462, 1980.
41. Dussault RG, et al: Femoral head defect following anterior hip dislocation, *Radiology* 135:627-629, 1980.
42. DeLee JC, Evans JA, Thomas J: Anterior dislocation of the hip and associated femoral-head fractures, *J Bone Joint Surg* 62A: 960-964, 1980.
43. Epstein HC: Traumatic dislocations of the hip, *Clin Orthop Rel Res* 92:116-142, 1973.
44. Roeder LF Jr, DeLee JC: Femoral head fractures associated with posterior hip dislocations, *Clin Orthop Rel Res* 147:121-130, 1980.
45. Epstein HC: Posterior fracture-dislocations of the hip: long term follow-up, *J Bone Joint Surg* 56A:1103-1127, 1974.
46. Ghormley RK, Sullivan R: Traumatic dislocation of the hip, *Am J Surg* 85:298-301, 1953.
47. Stimson LA: Five cases of dislocation of the hip, *NY Med J* 50:118-121, 1889.
48. Stewart MJ, Milford LW: Fracture-dislocation of the hip: an end result study, *J Bone Joint Surg* 36A:315-342, 1954.
49. Polesky RE, Polesky FA: Intrapelvic dislocation of the femoral head following anterior dislocation of the hip, *J Bone Joint Surg* 54A:1097-1098, 1972.
50. Pringle JH: Traumatic dislocation at the hip joint: an experimental study in the cadaver, *Glasgow Med J* 21:25, 1943.
51. Stein H: Computerized tomography for ascertaining osteocartilaginous intraarticular (slice) fractures of the femoral head, *Isr J Med Sci* 19:180-184, 1983.
52. Epstein HC: *Traumatic dislocation of the hip,* Baltimore, 1980, Williams & Wilkins.
53. Lutter LD: Post-traumatic hip redislocation, *J Bone Joint Surg* 55A:391-394, 1973.
54. Epstein HC: Posterior fracture-dislocations of the hip: comparison of open and closed methods of treatment in certain types, *J Bone Joint Surg* 43A:1079-1098, 1961.
55. Larson CB: Fracture-dislocations of the hip, *Clin Orthop Rel Res* 92:147-154, 1973.
56. Urist MR: Fracture-dislocation of the hip joint: the nature of the traumatic lesion, treatment, late complications and end results, *J Bone Joint Surg* 30A:699-727, 1948.
57. Urist MR: Injuries to the hip joint: traumatic dislocation incurred chiefly in jeep injuries in World War II, *Am J Surg* 74: 586-595, 1947.
58. Stevens J, Fardin R, Freeark RJ: Lower extremity thrombophlebitis in patients with femoral neck fractures: a venographic investigation and a review of the early and late significance of the findings, *J Trauma* 8:527-534, 1968.
59. Ecker ML, Joyce JJ, Kohl EJ: The treatment of trochanteric hip fractures using a compression screw, *J Bone Joint Surg* 57A:23-27, 1975.
60. Pietrafesa CA, Hoffman JR: Traumatic dislocation of the hip, *JAMA* 249:3342-3346, 1983.
61. Suraci AJ: Distribution and severity of injuries associated with hip dislocations secondary to motor vehicle accidents, *J Trauma* 26:458-460, 1986.
62. Sanville P, Nicholson DA, Driscoll PA: ABC of emergency radiology: the hip, *Br Med J* 308:524-529, 1994.
63. Hougaard K, Thomsen PB: Traumatic posterior fracture-dislocation of the hip with fracture of the femoral head or neck, or both, *J Bone Joint Surg* 70-A:233-239, 1988.
64. Dreinhofer KE, et al: Isolated traumatic dislocation of the hip: long-term results in 50 patients, *J Bone Joint Surg* 76-B:6-12, 1994.
65. DeLee JC: Fractures and dislocations of the hip. In Rockwood JC Jr, Green DP, Bucholz RW (editors): *Rockwood and Green's fractures in adults,* ed 3, vol 2, Philadelphia, 1991, JB Lippincott.
66. Morrey BF: Instability after total hip arthroplasty, *Orthop Clin North Am* 23:237-248, 1992.
67. Williams JF, Gottesman MJ, Mallory TH: Dislocation after total hip arthroplasty: treatment with an above-knee hip spica cast, *Clin Orthop* 171:53-58, 1982.
68. Coventry MB: Late dislocations in patients with Charnley total hip arthroplasty, *J Bone Joint Surg* 67-A:832-841, 1985.
69. McGoff JP, Ramoska EA: Traumatic hip dislocation in a child, *Ann Emerg Med* 16:108-110, 1987.
70. Offierski CM: Traumatic dislocation of the hip in children, *J Bone Joint Surg* 63-B:194-197, 1981.
71. Askin SR, Bryan RS: Femoral neck fractures in young adults, *Clin Orthop Rel Res* 114:259-264, 1976.
72. Protzman RR, Burkhalter WE: Femoral neck fractures in young adults, *J Bone Joint Surg* 58A:689-695, 1976.
73. Melton LJ, Riggs BL: Epidemiology of age-related fractures. In Avioli LV (editor): *The osteoporotic syndrome,* New York, 1983, Grune & Stratton.
74. Birge SJ: Osteoporosis and hip fracture, *Clin Geriatr Med* 9:69-86, 1993.

75. Cooper C: Femoral neck bone density and fracture risk, *Osteoporosis Int* 6(suppl 3):S24-S26, 1996.
76. Lewis AF: Fracture of the neck of the femur: changing incidence, *Br Med J Clin Res Ed* 283:1217-1220, 1981.
77. Lawton JO, Baker MR, Dickson RA: Femoral neck fractures-two populations, *Lancet* 2:70-72, 1983.
78. Muckle DS: Iatrogenic factors in femoral neck fractures, *Injury* 8:98-101, 1976.
79. Stott S, Gray DH: The incidence of femoral neck fractures in New Zealand, *NZ Med J* 91:6-9, 1980.
80. Knowelden J, Buhr AJ, Dunbar O: Incidence of fractures in persons over 35 years of age. Report to MRC Working Party on fractures in the elderly, *Br J Prev Soc Med* 18:130, 1964.
81. Bidner S, Finnegan M: Femoral fractures in Paget's disease, *J Orthop Trauma* 3:317-322, 1989.
82. Stevenson JC, Whitehead MI: Postmenopausal osteoporosis, *Br Med J Clin Res Ed* 285:585-588, 1982.
83. Merkow RL, Lane JM: Paget's disease of bone, *Orthop Clin North Am* 21:171-189, 1990.
84. Ralis ZA: Bone quality defect: a more significant factor than osteopenia in patients with fracture of the femoral neck, *J Bone Joint Surg* 65B: 365, 1983.
85. Stevens J, et al: The incidence of osteoporosis in patients with femoral neck fractures, *J Bone Joint Surg* 44B:520-527, 1962.
86. Chalmers J, Irvine GB: Fractures of the femoral neck in elderly patients with hyperparathyroidism, *Clin Orthop Rel Res* 229: 125-130, 1988.
87. Muckle DS, Miscony Z: Fractures of the femoral neck in the "young" elderly, *Injury* 12:41-44, 1980.
88. Bingold AC: The science of pinning the neck of the femur, *Ann Roy Coll Surg Engl* 59:463-469, 1977.
89. Cotton DW, et al: Are hip fractures caused by falling and breaking or breaking and falling? Photoelastic stress analysis, *Forensic Sci Int* 65:105-112, 1994.
90. Garden RS: Stability and union in subcapital fractures of the femur, *J Bone Joint Surg* 46B:630-647, 1964.
91. Garden RS: Malreduction and avascular necrosis in subcapital fractures of the femur, *J Bone Joint Surg* 53B:183-197, 1971.
92. Garden RS: The structure and function of the proximal end of the femur, *J Bone Joint Surg* 43B:576-589, 1961.
93. Garden RS: Low-angle fixation in fractures of the femoral neck, *J Bone Joint Surg* 43B:647-663, 1961.
94. Garden RS: Scientific thinking and clinical research, *Pro Mine Med Off Assoc* 47:47-52, 1967.
95. Garden RS: Reduction and fixation of subcapital fractures of the femur, *Orthop Clin North Am* 5:683-712, 1974.
96. De Boeck H: Classification of hip fractures, *Acta Orthoped Belg* 60(suppl 1):106-109, 1994.
97. Linton P: On the different types of intracapsular fractures of the femoral neck, *Acta Chir Scand* 86 (suppl), 1944.
98. Crawford HB: Experience with the non-operative treatment of impacted fractures of the neck of the femur, *J Bone Joint Surg* 47A:830-831, 1965.
99. Banks HH: Factors influencing the results in fractures of the femoral neck, *J Bone Joint Surg* 44A:931-964, 1962.
100. Fielding JW, Wilson HJ Jr, Zickel RE: A continuing end-result study of intracapsular fracture of the neck of the femur, *J Bone Joint Surg* 44A:965-972, 1962.
101. Zuckerman JD: Hip fracture, *N Engl J Med* 334:1519-1525, 1996.
102. Bredahl C, Nyholm B, Hindsholm KB: Mortality after hip fracture: results of operation within 12 h of admission, *Injury* 23:83-86, 1992.
103. Fox HJ, et al: Factors affecting the outcome after proximal femoral fractures, *Injury* 25:297-300,1994.
104. Massie WK: Treatment of femoral neck fractures emphasizing long term follow-up observations on aseptic necrosis, *Clin Orthop Rel Res* 92:16-62, 1973.
105. Massie WK: Extracapsular fractures of the hip treated by impaction using a sliding nail plate fixation, *Clin Orthop Rel Res* 22:180-201, 1962.
106. Lewinnek GE, et al: The significance and a comparative analysis of the epidemiology of hip fractures, *Clin Orthop Rel Res* 152:35-43, 1980.
107. Laskin RS, Gruber MA, Zimmerman AJ: Intertrochanteric fractures of the hip in the elderly. A retrospective analysis of 236 cases, *Clin Orthop Rel Res* 141:188-195, 1979.
108. Cleveland M, et al: A ten-year analysis of intertrochanteric fractures of the femur, *J Bone Joint Surg* 41A:1399-1408, 1959.
109. Aitken JM: Relevance of osteoporosis in women with fracture of the femoral neck, *Br Med J Clin Res Ed* 288:597-601, 1984.
110. Kannus P, et al: Epidemiology of hip fractures, *Bone* 18(suppl): 57S-63S, 1996.
111. Hayes WC, et al: Etiology and prevention of age-related hip fractures, *Bone* 18(suppl):77S-86S, 1996.
112. Lindberg EJ, Macias D, Gipe BT: Clinically occult presentation of comminuted intertrochanteric hip fractures, *Ann Emerg Med* 21:1511-1514, 1992.
113. Lowell JD: Fractures of the hip (concluded), *N Engl J Med* 274: 1480-1490, 1966.
114. Boyd HB, Griffin LL: Classification and treatment of trochanteric fractures, *Arch Surg* 58:853-863, 1949.
115. Evans EM: The treatment of trochanteric fractures of the femur, *J Bone Joint Surg* 31B:190-203, 1949.
116. Tronzo RG: *Surgery of the hip joint*, Philadelphia, 1973, Lea & Febiger.
117. Jensen JS: Classification of trochanteric fractures, *Acta Orthop Scand* 51:803-810, 1980.
118. Harrington KD, Johnston JO: The management of comminuted unstable intertrochanteric fractures, *J Bone Joint Surg* 55A:1367-1376, 1973.
119. Sisk DT: Fractures. In Edmonson AS, Crenshaw AH (editors): *Campbell's operative orthopaedics*, ed 7, St Louis, 1987, Mosby.
120. James ETR, Hunter GA: The treatment of intertrochanteric fractures: a review article, *Injury* 14:421-431, 1983.
121. Jensen JS: Trochanteric fractures: an epidemiological, clinical and biochemical study, *Acta Orthop Scand* 188(suppl):1-100, 1981.
122. Moore M Jr: Treatment of trochanteric femoral fractures with special reference to complications, *Am J Surg* 84:449-452, 1952.
123. Sherk HH, Crouse FR, Probst C: The treatment of hip fractures in institutionalized patients. A comparison of operative and nonoperative methods, *Orthop Clin North Am* 5:543-550, 1974.
124. Johnson LL, Lottes JO, Arnot JP: The utilization of the Holt nail for proximal femur fractures, *J Bone Joint Surg* 50A:67-78, 1968.
125. Cochran GV: Implantation of strain gages on bone in vivo, *J Biomech* 5:119-123, 1972.
126. Velasco RU, Comfort TH: Analysis of treatment problems in subtrochanteric fractures of the femur, *J Trauma* 18:513-523, 1978.
127. Chalmers J: Subtrochanteric fractures in osteomalacia, *J Bone Joint Surg* 52B:509-513, 1970.
128. Butler JE, Brown SL, McConnell BG: Subtrochanteric stress fractures in runners, *Am J Sports Med* 10:228-232, 1982.
129. Hallel T, Amit S, Segal D: Fatigue fractures of tibial and femoral shaft in soldiers, *Clin Orthop Rel Res* 118:35-43, 1976.
130. Morris J, Blickenstaff L: *Fatigue fractures, a clinical study*, Springfield, Ill, 1967, Charles C Thomas.
131. Froimson AI: Treatment of comminuted subtrochanteric fractures of the femur, *Surg Gynecol Obstet* 131:465-472, 1970.
132. Fielding JW: Subtrochanteric fractures, *Clin Orthop Rel Res* 92:86-99, 1973.
133. Leonidis S, Panagopoulos N: Surgical treatment of subtrochanteric fractures, *Injury* 6:70-76, 1974.

134. Zickel RE, Mouradian WH: Intramedullary fixation of pathological fractures and lesions of the subtrochanteric region of the femur, *J Bone Joint Surg* 58A:1061-1066, 1976.
135. Waddell JP: Subtrochanteric fractures of the femur: a review of 130 patients, *J Trauma* 19:582-592, 1979.
136. Fielding JW, Magliato HJ: Subtrochanteric fractures, *Surg Gynecol Obstet* 122:555-560, 1966.
137. Watson HK, Campbell RD, Wade PA: Classification, treatment, and complications of the adult subtrochanteric fracture, *J Trauma* 4:457-479, 1964.
138. Zickel RE: An intramedullary fixation device for the proximal part of the femur: nine years experience, *J Bone Joint Surg* 58A: 866-872, 1976.
139. Seinsheimer F III: Subtrochanteric fractures of the femur, *J Bone Joint Surg* 60A:300-306, 1978.
140. Parker MJ, et al: Subtrochanteric fractures of the femur, *Injury* 28:91-95, 1997.
141. Ryan JR, et al: Fractures of the femur secondary to low-velocity gunshot wounds, *J Trauma* 21:160-162, 1981.
142. Arneson TJ et al: Epidemiology of diaphyseal and distal femoral fractures in Rochester, Minnesota, 1965-1984, *Clin Orthop Rel Res* 234:188-194, 1988.
143. Hedlund R, Lindgren U: Epidemiology of diaphyseal femoral fracture, *Acta Othop Scand* 57:423-427, 1986.
144. Kulowski J: Fractures of the shaft of the femur resulting from automobile accidents, *J Int Coll Surg* 42:412-420, 1964.
145. Watson-Jones, R: *Fractures and joint injuries,* ed 4, vol 2, Baltimore, 1960, Williams & Wilkins.
146. Taylor MT, Banerjee B, Alpar EK: Injuries associated with a fractured shaft of the femur, *Injury* 25:185-187, 1994.
147. Walling AK, Seradge H, Spiegel PG: Injuries to the knee ligaments with fractures of the femur, *J Bone Joint Surg* 64A:1324-1327, 1982.
148. Flint LM, Richardson JD: Arterial injuries with lower extremity fracture, *Surgery* 93:5-8, 1983.
149. Kootstra G, et al: Femoral shaft fracture with injury of the superficial femoral artery in civilian accidents, *Surg Gynecol Obstet* 142:399-403, 1976.
150. Kluger Y, et al: Blunt vascular injury associated with closed mid-shaft fracture: a plea for concern, *J Trauma* 36:222-225, 1994.
151. Bucholz RW, Brumback RJ: Fractures of the shaft of the femur. In Rockwood JC Jr, Green DP, Bucholz RW (editors): *Rockwood and Green's fractures in adults,* ed 3, vol 2, Philadelphia, 1991, JB Lippincott.
152. Cave EF: *Fractures and other injuries,* Chicago, 1958, The Year Book Publishers.
153. Burkhalter WE: Experience with brace-cast for femoral fractures. Cast-bracing of fractures. A report of a workshop sponsored by the Committee on Prosthetics Research and Development, Division of Engineering, Washington, DC, 1971, National Research Council.
154. Moll JH: The cast-brace walking treatment of open and closed femoral fractures, *South Med J* 66:345-352, 1973.
155. Viljanto J, Paananen M: Return to work after femoral shaft fracture, *Ann Chir Gynaec Fenn* 62:30-35, 1973.
156. Carr CR, Wingo CH: Fractures of the femoral diaphysis: a retrospective study of the results and costs of treatment by intramedullary nailing and by traction and a spica cast, *J Bone Joint Surg* 1973; 55A:690-700, 1973.
157. Olerud S, Danckwardt-Lilliestrom G: Fracture healing in compression osteosynthesis in the dog, *J Bone Joint Surg* 50B:844-851, 1968.
158. Hicks JH: The relationship between metal and infection, *Proc R Soc Med* 50:842-844, 1957.
159. Wickstrom J, Corban MS, Vise GT Jr: Complications following intramedullary fixation of 324 fractured femurs, *Clin Orthop Rel Res* 60:103-113, 1968.
160. Dencker H: Shaft fractures of the femur: a comparative study of the results of various methods of treatment in 1003 cases, *Acta Chir Scand* 130:173-184, 1965.
161. Wickstrom J, Corban MS: Intramedullary fixation for fractures of the femoral shaft: a study of complications in 298 operations, *J Trauma* 7:551-583, 1967.
162. Armstrong GE: Isolated fracture of the great trochanter, *Ann Surg* 46:292, 1907.
163. Merlino AF, Nixon JE: Isolated fractures of the greater trochanter: report of twelve cases, *Int Surg* 52:117-124, 1969.
164. Milch H: Avulsion fracture of the great trochanter, *Arch Surg* 38:334-350, 1939.
165. Ratzan MC: Isolated fracture of the greater trochanter of the femur, *J Int Coll Surg* 29:359-363, 1958.
166. Eikenbary CF: Avulsion or fracture of the lesser trochanter, *J Orthop Surg* 3:464-468, 1921.
167. Milgram JE: Muscle ruptures and avulsions with particular reference to the lower extremities, *AAOS Instr Course Lect* 10: 233, 1953.
168. Poston HL: Traction fracture of the lesser trochanter of the femur, *Br J Surg* 9:256, 1921-1922.
169. Phillips CD, et al: Nontraumatic avulsion of the lesser trochanter: a pathognomonic sign of metastatic disease? *Skeletal Radiol* 17:106-110, 1988.
170. Kay SP, Hall JE: Fracture of the femoral neck in children and its complications, *Clin Orthop Rel Res* 80:53-71, 1971.
171. Ratliff AH: Fractures of the neck of the femur in children, *J Bone Joint Surg* 44B:528-542, 1962.
172. Canale ST, Bourland WL: Fracture of the neck and intertrochanteric region of the femur in children, *J Bone Joint Surg* 59A:431-443, 1977.
173. Swiontkowski MF, Winquist RA: Displaced hip fractures in children and adolescents, *J Trauma* 26:384-388, 1986.
174. Azouz EM, et al: Types and complications of femoral neck fractures in children, *Pediatr Radiol* 23:415-420, 1993.
175. Canale ST, King RE: Fractures of the hip. In Rockwood CA Jr, Wilkins KE, King RE (editors): *Fractures in children,* ed 3, vol 3, Philadelphia, 1991, JB Lippincott.
176. Rang M: *Children's fractures,* ed 2, Philadelphia, 1983, JB Lippincott.
177. Dalton HJ, et al: Undiagnosed abuse in children younger than 3 years with femoral fracture, *Am J Dis Child* 144:875-878, 1990.
178. Hughes LO, Beaty JH: Fractures of the head and neck of the femur in children, *J Bone Joint Surg* 76-A:283-292,1994.
179. McDonald GA: Pelvic disruptions in children, *Clin Orthop Rel Res* 151:130-134, 1980.
180. Ratliff AHC: Complications after fractures of the femoral neck in children and their treatment, *J Bone Joint Surg* 52B:175, 1970.
181. Levy J, Ward WT: Pediatric femur fractures: an overview of treatment, *Orthopedics* 16:183-190, 1993.
182. Parsch KD: Modern trends in internal fixation of femoral shaft fractures in children: a critical review, *J Pediatr Orthop* Part B 6:117-125, 1997.
183. Buckley SL: Current trends in the treatment of femoral shaft fractures in children and adolescents, *Clin Orthop Rel Res* 338: 60-73, 1997.
184. Cramer KE: The pediatric polytrauma patient, *Clin Orthop Rel Res* 318:125-135, 1995.
185. Porat S, et al: Femoral fracture treatment in head-injured children: use of external fixation, *J Trauma* 26:81-84, 1986.
186. Staheli LT: Fractures of the femoral shaft. In Rockwood CA Jr, Wilkins KE, King RE (editors): *Fractures in children,* ed 3, vol 3, Philadelphia, 1991, JB Lippincott.
187. Blount W: *Fractures in children,* Baltimore, 1955, Williams & Wilkins.

27 Knee Injuries

DANIEL M. ROBERTS

Teaching Case

A 42-year-old man arrives in the emergency department (ED) after a motor vehicle crash (MVC). He complains primarily of severe right knee pain. Examination reveals posterior displacement of the right knee. His femoral pulse is strong, but the dorsalis pedis and anterior tibial pulses are absent. Radiographs demonstrate a right acetabular fracture and a right posterior knee dislocation. After reduction, the distal pulses remain absent. The patient is taken to the operating suite by a vascular surgeon, where the popliteal artery is found to be torn. The artery is repaired by interposition of a saphenous vein graft and the patient makes an uneventful recovery.

In this case, arteriography is not necessary because the location of the arterial injury is known and arteriography would expose the patient to an unnecessary intravenous contrast load and delay operative repair. If his pulses were present but not as strong as on the contralateral side, an arteriogram would be indicated.

The knee is one of the most commonly injured joints, and the frequency of knee injuries is increasing, largely because of athletic injuries. Emergency physicians (EPs) in North American treat more than 1 million patients with acute knee injury each year.[1] In the United States, orthopedic surgeons operate on over 50,000 knee injuries annually.[2] Because of their frequency and potential for significant morbidity, the EP must become expert in acute knee injuries.

ANATOMY

The knee encompasses the patella, the distal femur, the tibia, the fibula, and associated soft tissues, including ligaments and tendons. Although the knee is primarily a hinge joint (flexion and extension), it may rotate slightly both laterally and medially. In full extension, no rotary motion is possible since the ligaments are taut. This tightening during extension is termed the *screwing home mechanism.*

HISTORY AND PHYSICAL EXAMINATION

The history must focus on the mechanism of injury and an account of prior knee injuries. The knee position at the time of injury provides important clues. A flexed knee dissipates force better than an extended knee. Note the time course of swelling. Because hip injuries may refer pain to the knee, examine the hip in all patients with knee complaints. Children with hip pathology are especially prone to misdiagnosis because of this phenomenon.

The examination is best begun with the patient supine. The physical examination includes inspecting the leg and knee for swelling, ecchymosis, effusions, and masses. Note the patellar location and size, thigh muscular development, erythema, evidence of local trauma, and leg length. Examine the knee for both range of motion and tenderness. Physicians will miss ruptures of the extensor mechanism unless they ask the patient to extend the knee against gravity.

Begin palpation in the nontender areas and move toward the tender areas last. This sequence promotes compliance with the examination. It is best to first examine the injured knee. Palpate for temperature (increased warmth), strength, sensation, and location/character of distal pulses.

Examine the patella with the knee in both flexion and extension. Balloting the patella is a sensitive means of detecting an effusion. The popliteal space may hide swelling or demonstrate a decreased pulse.[3]

Because of the potential for pain, stress the ligaments last. If there is a strong likelihood of fracture, obtain a radiograph before grappling the knee and displacing fragments. Always examine the uninjured knee first to gain the patient's confidence and determine the normal knee's motion limits. The first examination is often the most reliable since the patient is not guarding the knee. Compare the laxity encountered in an injured knee with that of the contralateral uninjured knee.

Perform **Lachman's test** first, since it produces less pain and joint motion. Position the knee in 15 to 20 degrees of flexion with the patient lying supine. Using one hand on the anterior aspect of the distal femur and the second hand behind the proximal tibia, try to displace the tibia forward on the femur. Lachman's test is positive for an anterior cruciate (ACL) injury if there is either >5 mm of anterior displacement of the tibia or a "soft, mushy" endpoint.[3] It performs well despite large knee effusions and hamstring sprains because the knee is not flexed to 90 degrees. Lachman's test can also identify partial ACL tears. It is highly specific for ACL injuries and, with adequate muscle relaxation, is a more sensitive test than the anterior drawer test.

Like the Lachman's test, the **anterior drawer (AD) test** also detects an ACL tear by attempting to displace the tibia forward on the femur. However, the AD test is done with the knee in 90 degrees of flexion (with the hip flexed to 45 degrees). Variants of the test place the leg in a variety of positions, including neutral, internal (posterolateral), and external (posteromedial) rotation. Although more than 6 mm of tibial displacement is considered positive for an ACL injury, there are significant false positives. The AD test is only 77% sensitive for complete ACL rupture.[4]

The **pivot shift test** is often discussed as an alternative diagnostic maneuver for possible ACL tears. However it is technically difficult, painful, and, because of associated pain and spasm, unreliable without anesthesia.

The **posterior drawer (PD) test** is done with the knee in 70 to 90 degrees of flexion, and is 90% sensitive and 99% specific for the diagnosis of a PCL injury.[5] The PD test is a reversal of the AD test. However, this time attempt to posteriorly displace the tibia from the femur. If the posterior displacement of the tibia is >5 mm, or if the endpoint is "soft,"[6] PCL injury is likely.

Another useful finding of a PCL injury is the "posterior sag sign." In this sign, the proximal tibia sags in relation to the femur when the hips and knees are both flexed to 90 degrees.[2,6] Evaluate the contour of the knees from the side.

Examine the Collateral Ligaments

The collateral ligaments must be tested in varus (pushing out on the medial side of the knee while pulling the leg medially) and valgus (pushing in on the lateral knee while pulling the leg laterally) stress. A frequent mistake involves positioning the leg only in extension during this test. During extension, the posterior capsule is taut. In this position, both varus and valgus pressure strain the posterior capsule and not the collaterals. Bend the knee 10 degrees to unload the posterior capsule, while the patient is supine. To stress the medial collateral, place one hand on the lateral aspect of the knee and grasp the foot and ankle with the other hand. Apply gentle abduction stress with slight external rotation of the foot and ankle. The slight external rotation tightens the MCL and detects laxity. If the knee is flexed to 30 degrees, the pressure will stress the ACL.

A varus stress is needed to evaluate the lateral collateral ligament.

Evaluate the Menisci

Several tests detect meniscal injury. The **McMurray's test** is done with the patient supine and the hip and knee flexed. Rotate the tibia and apply a valgus stress to the externally rotated foot. Pain may indicate a torn medial meniscal cartilage, especially if a pop or grind is felt along the lateral and/or medial joint lines when the leg is extended. Results are not definitive because rotation also stresses the collateral ligaments and may cause pain in an MCL or LCL sprain.[2] The lateral meniscus can be tested similarly with the foot internally rotated. The McMurray's test is not well tolerated if the patient is in pain or has limited movement of the knee because of spasm.

In the **Apley distribution (grinding) test** the patient is prone rather than supine. Flex the knee to a 90-degree angle and rotate it while under traction. Pain and popping in the knee indicate damage to the knee capsule or a tear in the posterior horn of the medial meniscus.

Payr's sign is increased pain with downward force of the knee while the patient is sitting with the legs crossed ("Indian style"). Payr's sign is associated with a medial meniscus posterior-horn injury.[2]

The **first Steinmann's sign** is pain in the anterolateral joint space noted with internal rotation of the flexed knee that signifies a lateral meniscus injury. Pain in the anteromedial joint space with external rotation of the flexed knee indicates a medial meniscus injury.[4]

The **"squat test"** can also detect meniscal injury. Have the patient squat several times with his or her feet alternately internally and externally rotated. Pain is usually localized to either the medial or the lateral joint line based on the location of the meniscal injury.[7]

If the patient is ambulatory, observe his or her gait.

RADIOGRAPHIC EXAMINATION

Routine radiographic views of the knee consist of the anteroposterior (AP), lateral, and oblique views (internally and externally rotated knee). The external and internal oblique projections accentuate the femoral condyles and tibial tuberosities not visible on standard AP and lateral films. In addition, the oblique views better define the patella. Some authors suggest a "tunnel" (notch) view to evaluate loose bodies in the joint space.[8] If a patellar injury is suspected, obtain an axial (tangential, "skyline," "sunrise," Hughston) view. This view is taken with the patient supine or prone and the knee flexed to 45 degrees. In children with an intact physis, comparison views of the uninjured knee are sometimes helpful.

Radiographs detect bony injury, as well as joint effusions. An effusion distends the joint capsule and displaces the quadriceps femoris muscle, suprapatellar tendon, and patella anteriorly. This finding appears radiographically as a soft tissue density within the suprapatellar bursa and an anterior convexity of the quadriceps tendon.[8]

Emergency physicians may be ordering too many knee films. Nearly all patients with knee injuries seen in U.S. emergency departments undergo radiography.[9] However, 90% of these films are negative. Three recent studies have looked at clinical decision rules for obtaining knee radiographs. These rules can significantly decrease unnecessary films.

In the Ottawa Knee Rules, a knee radiograph is only indicated in patients with acute knee injuries and one or more of the following:

1. Blunt knee trauma in a patient >55 years old
2. Tenderness of the head of the fibula on palpation
3. Isolated tenderness of the patella
4. Inability to flex the knee to 90°
5. Inability to bear weight immediately and inability to take four steps in the ED

Exclusion criteria for the use of the Ottawa Knee Rules include the following:

1. Isolated skin injuries
2. Referred patients from another ED or clinic
3. Injury greater than 7 days old
4. Patient returning for reevaluation
5. Distracting injuries (multiple trauma)
6. Altered mental status
7. Age <18 years old
8. Pregnant patients
9. Paraplegia

The Ottawa Knee Rules are highly reliable.[1,10] In a study of 3907 consecutive adult patients, the rules detected all 59 fractures. They can reduce knee radiographs by 26% to 28%.[10] Avoiding a radiograph reduces ED length of stay by 33 minutes and lessens charges by $103. Failure to obtain radiographs did not decrease patient satisfaction. The Ottawa Knee Rules were not designed to assess ligamentous injuries.[10]

A second clinical decision rule in acute knee injuries is known as "Weber's Clinical Decision Rule." It is intended for isolated, nonpenetrating knee trauma less than 24 hours old. If the patient can walk without limping and sustained a twist injury without effusion, knee radiographs are not indicated. Patients are excluded if they have multiple trauma, mental impairment, a prosthesis, or known fractures elsewhere. The decision rule is still undergoing clinical evaluation, but the initial study population had 100% sensitivity with a potential reduction in knee radiographs by 29%. Patients with fractures tended to be older than 50 years of age.[11]

A final decision rule known as the "Pittsburgh Rule" also reduces unnecessary knee radiographs. A subsequent validation and comparison study found the Pittsburgh Rules for knee radiographs to be more specific than the Ottawa Knee Rules (60% to 80% versus 27% to 49%) and just as sensitive (99% versus 97%).[9] The Pittsburgh Rules include patients of any age and are based on the flow chart shown in Fig. 27-1. Exclusion criteria for the Pittsburgh Rules include the following:

1. Injury >6 days old
2. Isolated skin injuries (superficial abrasions or lacerations)
3. Prior history of knee fracture or surgery
4. Repeat visit for the same injury

In the comparative study the Pittsburgh Rules could have reduced radiographs by 52% with one missed fracture. In contrast, the Ottawa Knee Rules could have decreased knee radiographs by 23% with three missed fractures.[9] The Pittsburgh Rules for Knee

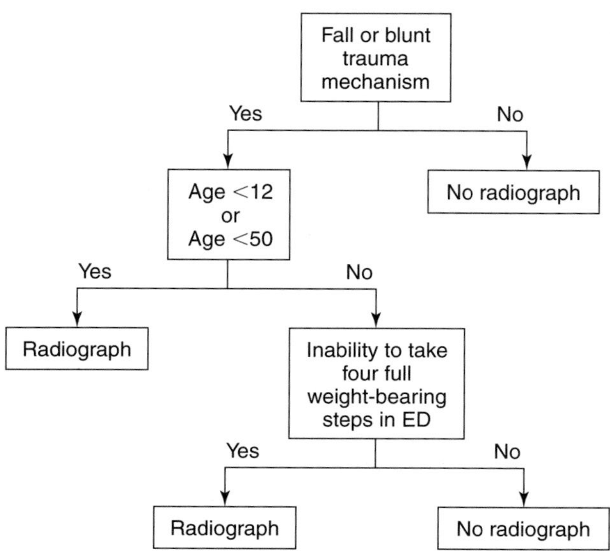

Fig. 27-1 Pittsburgh Rules for knee radiographs.

Radiographs may be more specific because patients must bear full weight (step on toe pads and the heel of each foot for 4 steps). The Ottawa Knee Rules require only foot transfer (including limping).

ARTHROCENTESIS

Swelling of the knee that occurs within minutes to a few hours of injury strongly suggests a hemarthrosis.[2] Delayed swelling (more than 4 hours after injury) is likely due to synovial irritation, and not hemarthrosis. If the knee capsule ruptures, fluid and blood extravasates into the surrounding soft tissue rather than distending the joint. This action explains why some severely injured knees may not swell.

Arthrocentesis of the knee serves both diagnostic and therapeutic purposes. After aspirating a hemarthrosis, squirt the blood into an emesis basin. Fat globules floating atop the blood indicate an osteochondral fracture, even despite negative radiographs. With the appropriate mechanism of injury, the presence of an acute hemarthrosis often indicates a tear of the anterior collateral ligament.

Aspiration may also relieve discomfort and improve knee function. A large effusion is painful and may block full extension of the knee. After aspiration, joint injection with morphine and/or bupivacaine provides significant pain relief.

The knee joint is the easiest joint in the body to tap and can be entered medially or laterally using sterile technique and an 18-gauge needle. Arthrocentesis of the knee is contraindicated in patients with known bleeding disorders, anticoagulant use, thrombocytopenia, or overlying cellulitis.[12]

The differential diagnosis of hemarthrosis with a negative radiograph includes the following:

1. Anterior cruciate ligament (ACL) injury (70% to 85%)[2,13]
2. Osteochondral fractures involving the cartilage and subchondral bone (including subtle tibial plateau fractures)
3. Medial collateral (tibial) ligament (MCL) injury
4. Posterior cruciate ligament (PCL) injury (usually only a small hemarthrosis, since the PCL is extra-synovial)
5. Peripheral meniscal tear (usually blood-tinged aspirate)

Penetrating Trauma

A deep laceration or penetrating injury near the knee must be evaluated for joint penetration (Fig. 27-2). After sterile preparation, inject dilute methylene blue into the knee joint; extravasation of the dye from the wound indicates violation of the joint. Because methylene blue stains the intraarticular structures, some orthopedists discourage its use, especially if the patient may need a subsequent arthroscopy. Instead of the dye, they advocate using a sterile saline solution.

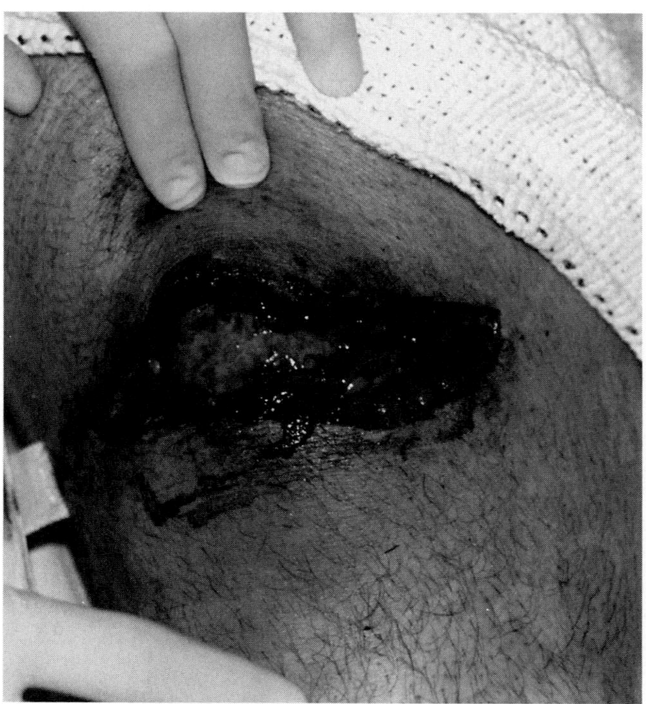

Fig. 27-2 Open right knee joint.

PAIN REDUCTION BY INTRAARTICULAR INJECTION

Both intraarticular morphine and bupivacaine help control severe knee pain. Although originally studied in postoperative patients, some EPs use intraarticular morphine in cases of acute knee trauma. In a postoperative knee trial, 5 mg of morphine injected directly into the knee significantly lowered pain scores and need for subsequent intravenous analgesics.[14] The analgesic effect can last for at least 24 hours. A second study found that a single 10 mg dose of intraarticular morphine was superior to 20 ml of intraarticular bupivacaine after knee arthroscopy.[15] Some authors believe that combining the intraarticular morphine with bupivacaine produces the best analgesic results.[16] However, the bupivacaine-morphine intraarticular mixture may be no more efficacious than either alone.[17]

PATELLAR FRACTURES

The patella is the largest sesamoid bone in the body and augments extension of the knee. Approximately

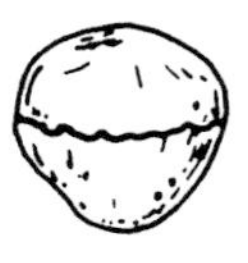
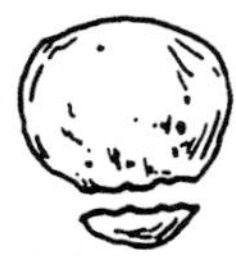
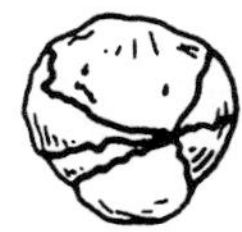
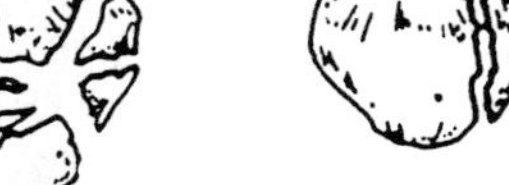
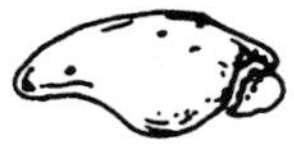

Fig. 27-3 Schematic of different types of patella fractures. (From Hohl M, Johnson EE, Wiss DA: Fractures of the knee. In Rockwood CA, Green DP, Bucholz RW [editors]: *Fractures in adults,* ed 3, Philadelphia, 1991, Lippencott.)

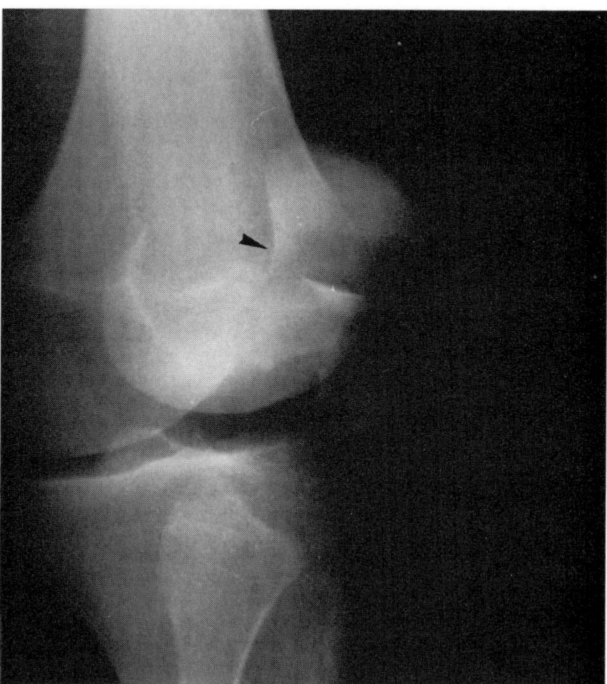

Fig. 27-4 Transverse patella fracture *(arrowhead).*

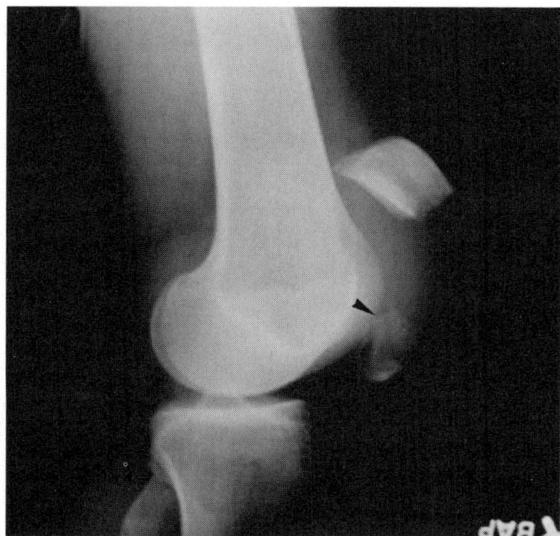

Fig. 27-5 Inferior pole patella fracture *(arrowhead).*

1% of all adult fractures involve the patella.[6] Fracture is rare in children since the patella is surrounded by thick cartilage. The majority of patellar fractures (up to 27% in one series) occur during an MVC when the flexed knee strikes the dashboard.[18]

Pathophysiology

The patella is usually fractured after a direct blow, such as a fall on a flexed knee. It can also be fractured after a forceful contraction of the quadriceps muscle. Types of patellar fractures (Fig. 27-3) include the following:

1. Transverse (Fig. 27-4)
2. Lower pole (Fig. 27-5)
3. Comminuted (stellate) (Fig. 27-6)
4. Vertical
5. Marginal

Transverse and comminuted (stellate) fractures of the patella are the most common and usually occur after a direct blow to the knee. Marginal fractures involve the medial and lateral borders of the patella and are relatively uncommon. Marginal fractures usually occur after a patellar dislocation or a direct blow to the edges of the patella. Patella fractures can be either displaced or nondisplaced. Displaced fractures are defined as >3 mm of bony separation and >2 mm of AP step-off. All fractures of the patella (except small avulsion, rim fractures) are intraarticular.

Clinical Presentation

The patient is usually unable to maintain the knee in active extension and may have a palpable defect or crepitus over the patella. There may be an associated knee effusion. Because most patellar fractures occur with the knee in flexion, look closely for other injuries, including knee dislocations, femur fractures, acetabular fractures, and hip dislocations.

Differential Diagnosis

Patellar fractures are often confused with a bipartite patella. In a bipartite patella, the two patellar ossifica-

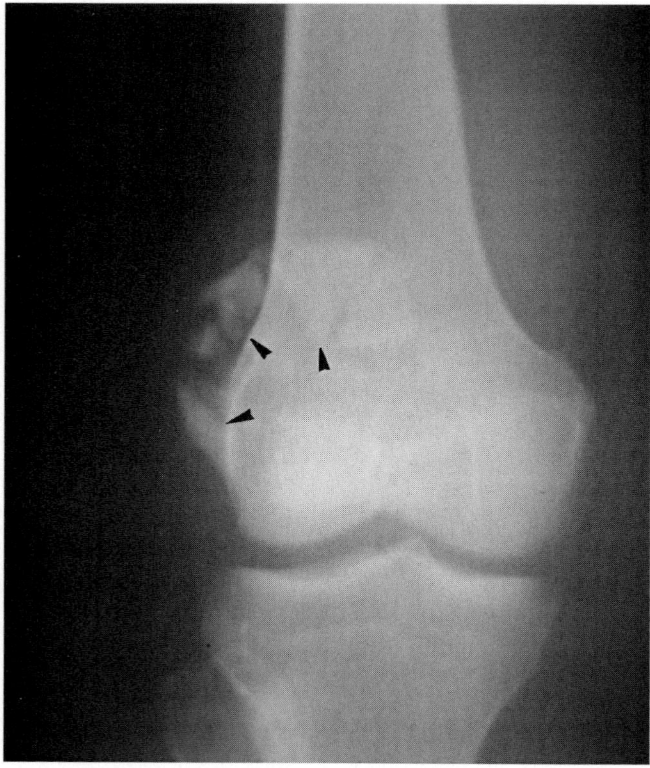

Fig. 27-6 Stellate patella fracture *(arrowheads).*

tion centers have not joined, leaving a smooth, sclerotic margin, usually on the superolateral aspect of the patella. Bipartite patellas are usually bilateral, so a comparison radiograph of the contralateral knee may be helpful. Most importantly, unlike a fractured patella, a bipartite patella is not significantly tender.

Physical Findings

Palpate the patella for pain and crepitus. Assess the medial and lateral patellofemoral grooves, the quadriceps and patellar tendons, and the tibial tuberosity for size, integrity, and pain.

Diagnostic Studies

The patella is best imaged with AP, lateral, and tangential ("sunrise") radiographs. The tangential view is useful for detecting intraarticular step-offs and for small vertical fractures. Tomograms and computed tomographic (CT) scans of the knee are unnecessary in isolated patellar fractures.

Treatment

Treat nondisplaced patellar fractures nonoperatively with a knee immobilizer and partial weight-bearing for 3 weeks.[6] Crutches can significantly relieve pain. Begin isometric quadriceps contractions early in the treatment.

Displaced fractures usually require an operation. Partial or total patellectomy is reserved for severely comminuted fractures.

PATELLAR DISLOCATIONS

Pathophysiology

A patellar dislocation is common in adolescent females. It occurs in association with an internal rotation of the leg, a direct blow to the outer aspect of the flexed knee, or a valgus stress applied to a flexed knee. The patella may also dislocate after a powerful contraction of the quadriceps in combination with sudden flexion and external rotation of the tibia on the femur. These injuries often occur while dancing or during sports. Patellar dislocations are more common in obese patients or those with flattening of the lateral femoral condyle. Other predisposing factors include patella alta ("high-riding patella"), excessive genu valgum ("knock knee"), elongated patella tendon, weak vastus medialis (quadriceps muscle), or excessive tibial torsion.[18] For anatomic reasons, the patella usually dislocates laterally. Up to 40% of acute patellar dislocations are associated with an osteochondral fracture often invisible on routine radiographs.[8] Months to years later, this osteochondral fracture becomes a loose body in the joint space, causing impaired motion, locking, or degenerative changes of the knee.

History

A patient with a patellar dislocation usually complains of a knee that "went out of place." Some report prior episodes, since 15% to 50% of patellar dislocations recur, especially in patients with anatomic predisposition.[6]

Physical Findings

A patient who has sustained a patellar dislocation, which has spontaneously reduced, complains of pain at the medial patella where the attachments have been torn. The patient also may have a positive **Patellar Apprehension Test** (**"Fairbank's Test"**). When positive, this test indicates instability of the patellofemoral joint. To perform the Patellar Apprehension Test, have the patient flex the knee to 30 degrees and, while supporting the foot with a relaxed quadriceps muscle, attempt to push the patella laterally. If excessive laxity exists (>1 cm), the patella is pushed up onto the lateral femoral condyle, producing the sensation of impend-

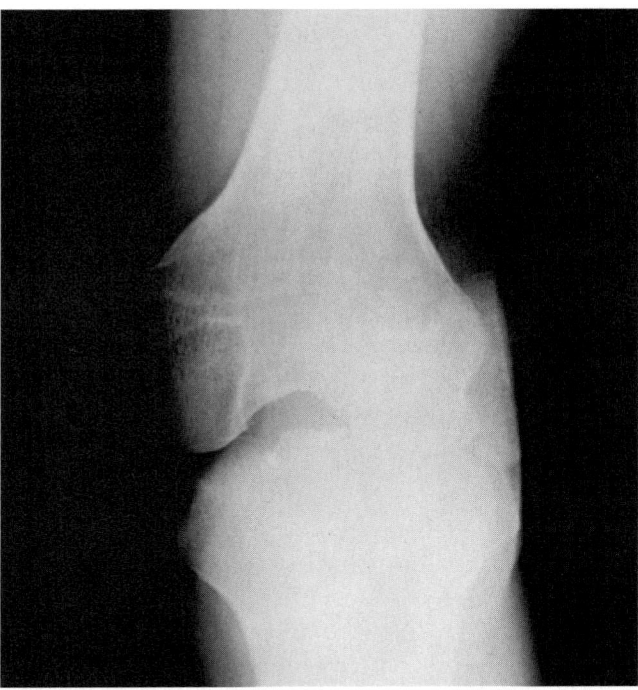

Fig. 27-7 Patella dislocation.

ing subluxation. The patient will involuntarily contract the quadriceps muscle and extend the knee, which pulls the patella medially. The patient may also grab the knee.

Up to 12% of all patients with patellar dislocations have a concomitant major ligamentous or meniscal injury.[6]

In an intracondylar dislocation, the edge of the patella locks between the femoral condyles. This condition results in a very prominent patella that sticks "straight up" from the knee.

The "lateral pressure syndrome" can develop after a patellar dislocation. This syndrome is an aching anterior knee joint pain with excessive use (especially when descending stairs) and after long periods of sitting ("movie-goers" knee).[18]

Diagnostic Studies

Radiographs include tangential, AP, and lateral views (Fig. 27-7). Postreduction radiographs may demonstrate a marginal or osteochondral fracture of the patella.

Treatment

Most patellar dislocations reduce spontaneously. If the patella is still dislocated on arrival in the ED, straighten the leg with the hip flexed to reduce tension on the quadriceps tendon and apply gentle pressure on the patella directed from lateral to medial. This maneuver may require procedural sedation. An intracondylar dislocation is difficult to reduce and often requires conscious sedation. Once the patient is sedated, straighten the knee and flex the hip by raising the leg toward the ceiling. This maneuver decreases the tension on the quadriceps muscle.

Once reduced, place the patient in a knee immobilizer in full extension for 3 to 7 weeks with progressive weight-bearing as tolerated. Some authors feel that prolonged periods of immobilization (up to 7 weeks) may slow recovery. Prolonged immobilization may have a deleterious effect on ligament strength and the joint cartilage, and may cause significant atrophy of the quadriceps muscle.[19]

Have the patient apply ice for the first 24 hours; a compressive dressing for the first 4 days may reduce postreduction effusion.[18] The patient should begin a quadriceps strength and stretching program once he or she can perform range-of-motion exercises without discomfort.[18] Even with rehabilitation, one third of patients with acute patellar dislocations develop patellar instability and other chronic problems.[19] Orthopedic referral is mandatory.

ANTERIOR KNEE DISLOCATIONS

Knee dislocations are true emergencies because of the associated vascular and neurologic injuries. Two thirds of all knee dislocations result from MVCs, with the remainder occurring during falls, sports, and industrial activities. The peak incidence of knee dislocations is in males (3:1) in their third decade of life. Knee dislocations are classified by the direction of tibial displacement with respect to the femur.[20] Although the knee can dislocate in any direction (Figs. 27-8 to 27-10), the majority are either anterior or posterior. In 50% to 60% of all cases, the knee dislocates anteriorly.

Pathophysiology

Anterior knee dislocations usually occur after a high-energy hyperextension injury (80%), although even a low-energy mechanism can disrupt the joint.[20] The knee hyperextends, tearing the posterior capsule and possibly the cruciates. As the hyperextension progresses, the popliteal artery is stressed or injured. The popliteal artery is tethered proximally at the adductor hiatus ("Hunter's canal") and distally by the immobile fibrous arch of the soleus muscle. These fixed points cause a traction tear and/or thrombosis after an anterior dislocation. The popliteal artery is the central vascular conduit for the lower leg since the knee has few collaterals that provide distal flow.

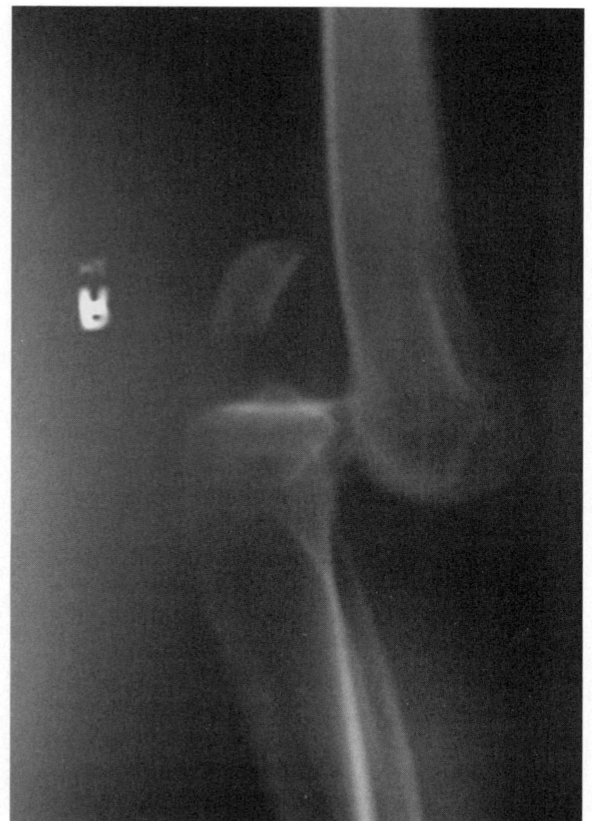

Fig. 27-8 Anterior knee dislocation.

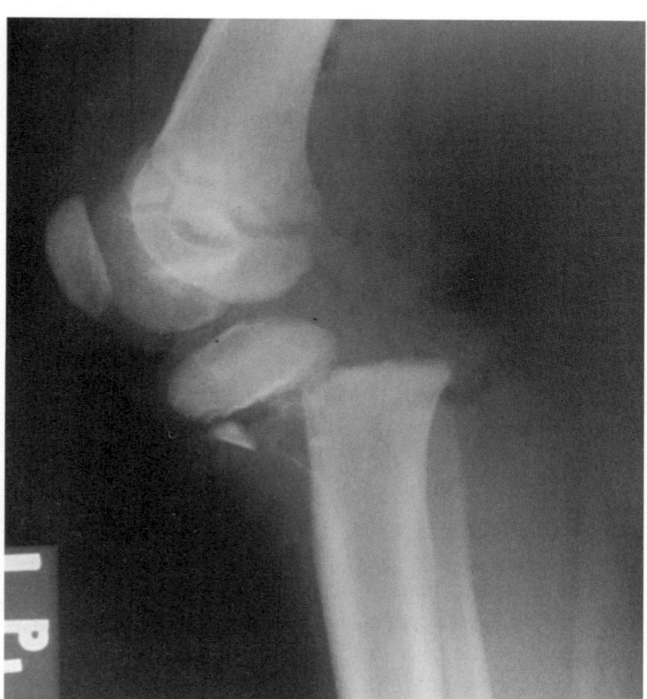

Fig. 27-9 Posterior knee dislocation.

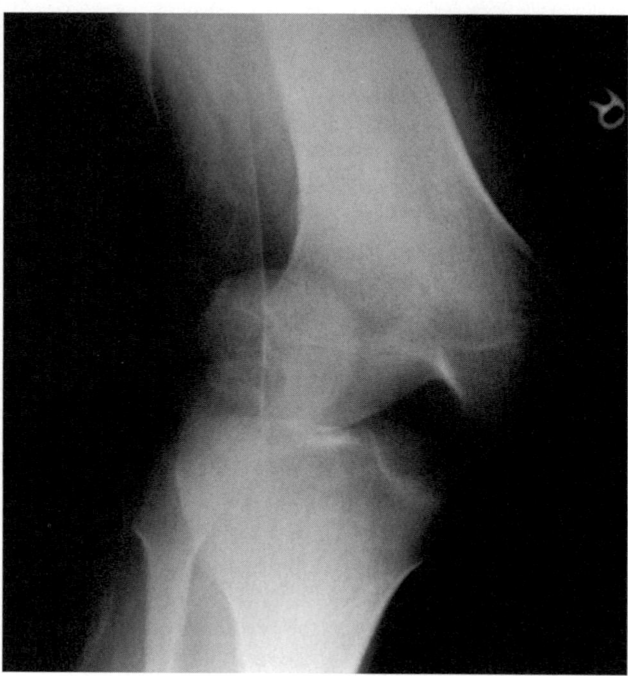

Fig. 27-10 Lateral knee dislocation.

Clinical Presentation

The dislocation is described in terms of the relationship of the tibia to the femur (distal to proximal) (Figs. 27-11 and 27-12), and is often associated with a fracture of the proximal tibia. Absence of gross deformity does not eliminate a dislocation, since many dislocations spontaneously reduce before arrival in the ED. Until proven otherwise, a grossly unstable knee after major trauma represents a reduced dislocation.

Anterior knee dislocations have a high incidence (5% to 40%) of associated vascular injuries, usually involving the popliteal artery. Of these, 20% to 50% result in amputation of the leg.[4,6]

The incidence of peroneal nerve injury after an anterior knee dislocation is reported at 14% to 40% of patients.[6] Peroneal nerve injury is permanent in 50% to 78% of cases.[6]

Physical Findings

The knee is often massively swollen, and stress of the ligaments reveals a completely flaccid joint. Evaluate the knee for valgus, varus, and hyperextension instability in 10 to 20 degrees of flexion. Consider a

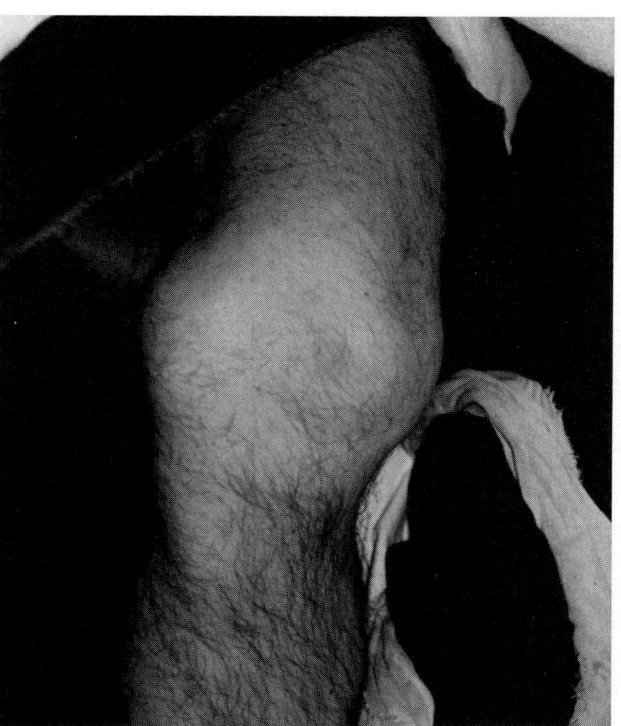

Fig. 27-11 Right lateral knee dislocation.

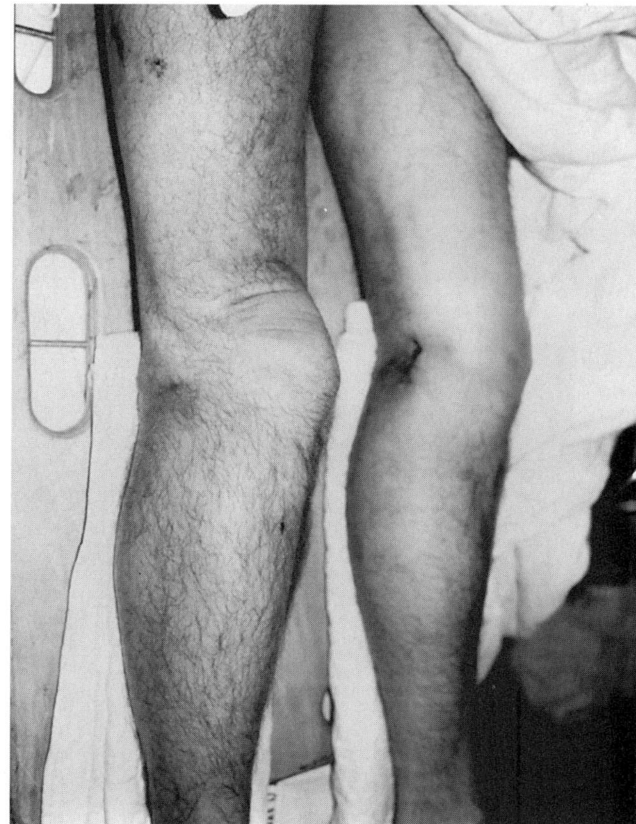

Fig. 27-12 Right anterior knee dislocation with overriding of tibia on femur.

grossly unstable knee as evidence for a knee dislocation until proven otherwise. Suspect neurovascular injuries. Markedly unstable knees require reconstructive surgery.

The vascular examination is paramount for the patient with a suspected knee dislocation. Are the pulses equal? Are blood pressures measured by Doppler in the arms identical to the pressures in the leg? The presence of distal pulses in the foot *does not* rule out an arterial injury. Ten percent of patients with injury to the popliteal artery have distal pulses.[20] An intimal tear can lead to delayed popliteal artery thrombosis.

Major vascular trauma is almost always associated with a popliteal nerve injury.[20] Check the peroneal nerve by determining sensation on the dorsal foot and by having the patient evert the foot. Plantar anesthesia and weak plantar flexion of the foot demonstrate injury to the tibial nerve. In one study, every patient with a tibial nerve injury had an ipsilateral peroneal nerve injury.

Early diagnosis of vascular trauma is essential. Irreversible muscle damage occurs 4 to 6 hours after injury, whereas irreversible nerve damage occurs after 12 hours.[6] If vascular repair is delayed for 8 hours from the time of injury, the amputation rate approaches 86%.[4]

Diagnostic Studies

Historically, an arteriogram (Fig. 27-13) was advocated for all anterior knee dislocations. Authorities suggested routine use of arteriography, even if pulses were normal. However, arteriograms are costly and invasive, and complications include anaphylaxis, femoral artery injury, and acute renal insufficiency.[21] Duplex Doppler ultrasound may supplant contrast studies.[20] Noninvasive Duplex Doppler studies correlate well with arteriography. The decision to perform an ultrasound versus an arteriogram is often based on the patient's ankle/brachial arterial index. A pressure ratio less than 0.8 should impel arteriography.[20]

There are good arguments against the need for arteriography if pulses are normal. Very few patients with normal distal pulses require arterial repair,[20] and those with minor or nonocclusive vascular injuries rarely need surgery.[21] Physical examination accurately identifies patients at risk for clinically significant arterial injury. Selective arteriography is based on serial

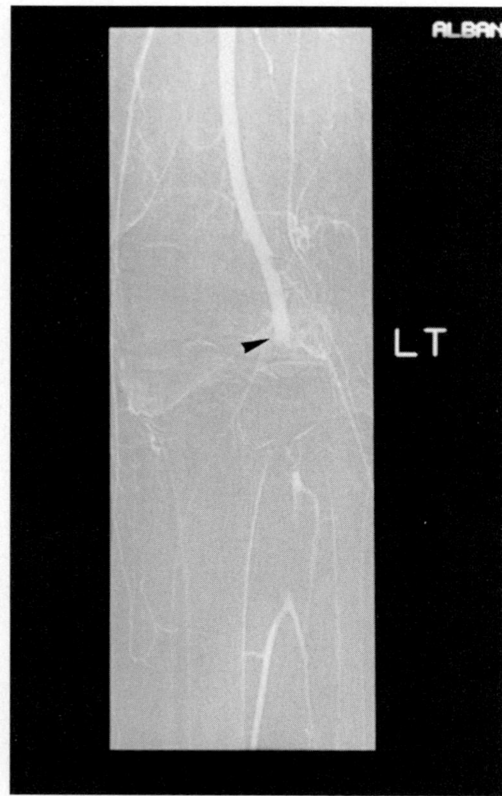

Fig. 27-13 Arteriogram showing disruption of left popliteal artery *(arrowhead).*

physical examinations during the first 24 to 48 hours.[21]

Arteriography should never delay surgical exploration in patients with obvious signs of arterial injury. Patients with a cool, cyanotic extremity should proceed directly to the operating suite for direct popliteal artery exploration. If necessary, the surgical team may order an intraoperative angiogram.[6]

Treatment

The goals of treatment include early reduction, immobilization, and emergency referral. Reduce the dislocated knee as soon as possible. Have an assistant apply longitudinal traction on the leg while the EP keeps one hand on the tibia and one on the femur. Lift the femur anteriorly and guide it back into position. Immobilize the knee with a posterior splint in 15 degrees of flexion to avoid tension on the popliteal artery,[18] and admit the patient for observation. If a popliteal artery injury is present, it must be repaired within 8 hours of injury. Depending on associated injuries, the surgeon may anticoagulate the patient for 7 or more days. Some surgeons apply an external fixator to the leg to protect the vascular repair.[22]

Historically, injuries to the popliteal intima uniformly prompted operation. Recently, some surgeons opt for nonoperative management and instead perform frequent serial examinations within the first 48 hours.[21]

Complications of an anterior knee dislocation include the following:

1. Progressive distal leg ischemia with amputation
2. Degenerative joint disease (arthritis)
3. Persistent joint instability
4. Compartment syndromes of the calf
5. Permanent motor and sensory deficits
6. Deep vein thrombosis

POSTERIOR KNEE DISLOCATIONS

Pathophysiology

Posterior dislocation of the tibia on the femur requires a much greater force than an anterior knee dislocation and accounts for up to 40% of knee dislocations.[4] A posterior knee dislocation occurs after a direct blow to the anterosuperior tibia with the knee flexed ("dashboard injury"). The posterior displacement of the tibia ruptures the posterior capsule and tears both cruciates.

Clinical Presentation and Diagnostic Studies

The clinical presentation resembles that of an anterior knee dislocation. Arterial injuries may be only slightly less common.[21] The diagnostic studies are as discussed for anterior knee dislocations.

Treatment

Reduce the knee as soon as possible by having an assistant stabilize the femur while the EP distracts and lifts the anterior tibia. After reduction, immobilize the knee in 15 degrees of flexion and treat as for anterior knee dislocation.[4]

TIBIAL SPINE FRACTURES

Pathophysiology

Isolated injuries to the tibial spine are uncommon, and occur when a force is directed against a flexed proximal tibia. Tibial spine fractures are more common in children than in adults.[18]

Clinical Presentation

A tibial spine fracture usually causes a painful, swollen knee, often with a hemarthrosis. The patient is unable to fully extend the knee and may have a positive Lachman's test. Tibial spine fractures are often

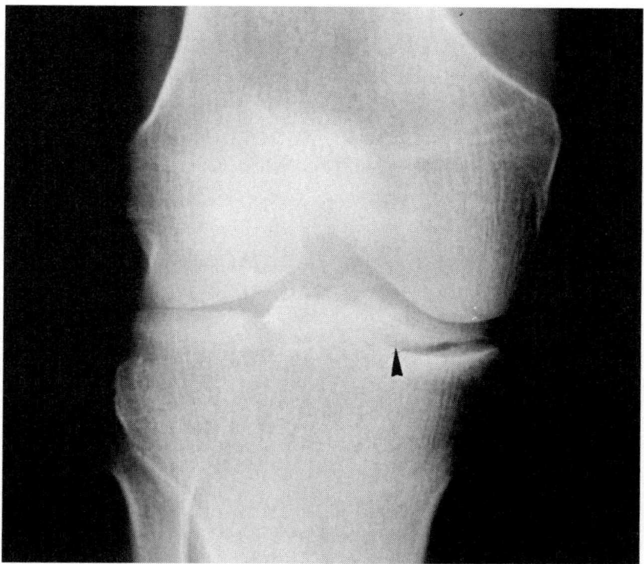

Fig. 27-14 Right tibial spine fracture.

associated with a tear of the medial collateral or anterior cruciate ligaments.

Diagnostic Studies

Radiographs occasionally demonstrate a subtle fracture line (Fig. 27-14). A "tunnel view" of the tibial notch may clarify the diagnosis, whereas a cross-table radiograph can show lipohemarthrosis. A CT scan reveals a tibial spine fracture clearly, but is not necessary for ED management.

Treatment

Treat minimally displaced fractures conservatively, and immobilize the knee in a flexed position to relax the ACL. Completely displaced tibial spine fractures require operation. Children with displaced medial tibial spine fractures generally need surgery.[18]

TIBIAL PLATEAU FRACTURES

Because of the sometimes subtle radiographic findings, tibial plateau fractures are frequently overlooked. They occur more commonly in the elderly, and are unusual in children. The injury usually results from falls or vehicular trauma, especially in pedestrians struck by cars.

Pathophysiology

Tibial plateau fractures usually occur after a valgus or varus force with axial compression ("bumper fracture").[18] Lateral fractures are most common. Displaced fractures may damage the peroneal nerve or anterior tibial artery. Depressed fractures, seen mostly in the elderly, usually occur in osteopenic bone after a low-energy valgus stress. In this injury, the lateral femoral condyle sinks into the lateral plateau.

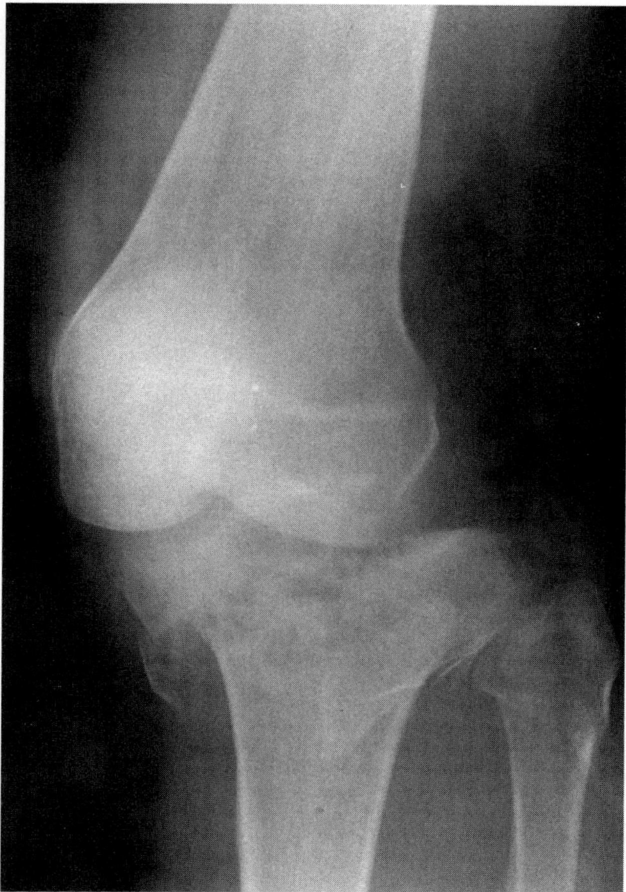

Fig. 27-15 Tibial plateau fracture.

Clinical Presentation

The patient with a tibial plateau fracture complains of painful swelling of the knee with decreased range of motion. Ligamentous instability, meniscal tears, or associated fractures are common. Tibial plateau fractures result in a major ligamentous injury in 7% to 16% of patients.[18] One study showed a 56% frequency of associated soft tissue injuries: 20% MCL, 20% menisci, 3% LCL, 3% peroneal nerve, and 10% ACL.[23] Hemarthrosis is common.

Diagnostic Studies

Radiographs may demonstrate a fracture (Fig. 27-15), but more likely exhibit an inconspicuous lipohemarthrosis on the cross-table lateral view. Oblique views

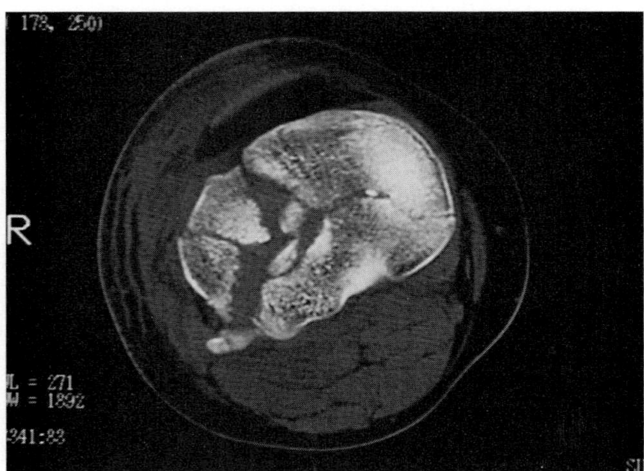

Fig. 27-16 Computed tomography scan of right tibial plateau fracture.

best illuminate nondisplaced fractures. If a tibial plateau fracture is likely, consider a five-view series: AP, lateral, two obliques, and 15° caudal plateau views.[6] Because the initial radiographs may be negative or inconclusive, reexamination in 10 to 14 days is often helpful in patients with significant pain or swelling.[18]

"Insufficiency fractures" of the tibial plateau may occur in elderly, osteoporotic patients with no history of significant trauma. These fractures resemble avascular necrosis or osteoarthritis on radiographs. Consultants may order nuclear medicine studies to clarify this diagnosis.[8]

Avulsion fractures of the lateral tibial plateau are invariably associated with an ACL rupture and can be seen on AP radiographs ("lateral capsular sign").[18]

A special type of tibial plateau injury is a Segond fracture. This small avulsion fracture occurs at the lateral edge of the tibial plateau and results from direct axial compression. A Segond fracture is associated with an ACL injury in up to 75% of patients.[24]

CT scanning and magnetic resonance imaging (MRI) often help the orthopedic surgeon evaluate for subtle tibial plateau or tibial spine fractures (Fig. 27-16). MRI may detect subtle abnormalities, as well as surrounding soft tissue injuries.[24]

Treatment

When describing a tibial plateau fracture to an orthopedic surgeon, it is important to relate three things:

1. How much of the plateau surface is involved
2. Whether the plateau is depressed
3. Whether the fragments are displaced

Ninety percent of patients with minimally or nondisplaced tibial plateau fractures do well with nonoperative treatment.[6] Immobilize the knee in a long-leg cast or knee immobilizer, and refer the patient to an orthopedic surgeon.[3] The patient is usually kept non–weight-bearing for up to 8 weeks, followed by toe-touch weight-bearing.[22] It is especially important to avoid unnecessary surgery in the elderly, osteopenic patient.

If the articular surface is significantly depressed, the patient will need an operation.

LIGAMENTOUS INJURIES

Anterior Cruciate Ligament

An estimated 90,000 acute ACL injuries occur in the United States each year, and the incidence has been increasing largely because of new athletic activities.[6] The ACL is taut in an extended knee, preventing rotatory motion. The ACL prevents excessive anterior movement of the tibia from the femur (hyperextension), excessive internal rotation of the tibia on the femur, and excessive lateral mobility of the knee in flexion and extension.

PATHOPHYSIOLOGY

Injuries to the ACL usually occur with sudden deceleration, hyperextension, and marked internal rotation of the tibia on the femur.

Ligamentous knee injuries in children are rare, and the pediatric patient usually fractures the epiphysis (Salter I). Children can also shatter the base of the intercondylar eminence or medial tubercle, which detaches the ACL from the proximal tibia. These children usually have a negative anterior drawer test.[8]

HISTORY

Important points include the following:

1. Mechanism of injury
2. Sudden onset of pain
3. Feeling or hearing a "pop"
4. Feeling knee "give out"
5. Inability to continue playing sport
6. Sudden swelling
7. Loss of knee motion
8. History of previous knee injury

Up to 50% of patients with acute knee injuries who report a "cracking" or "popping" sound have an ACL injury.[2] A complete ACL tear is immediately painful, then resolves, whereas the pain of a partial ACL tear may persist.

CLINICAL PRESENTATION

The ACL has a plentiful vascular supply, and a hemarthrosis usually develops within 2 hours of injury. Immediately after injury there is no effusion or spasm, and ACL injuries are easily identified. After a few hours, effusion and spasm complicate the diagnosis. One half to three quarters of patients with acute ACL tears have a meniscal tear, and 91% of patients with chronic ACL tears have torn menisci.[25]

PHYSICAL FINDINGS

Diagnose injury to the ACL by stressing the knee with the Lachman's and anterior drawer tests. Laxity is graded on a 1+, 2+, 3+ scale, as follows:

1+	3 to 5 mm of joint space opening
2+	6 to 10 mm of joint space opening
3+	>10 mm of joint space opening

DIAGNOSTIC STUDIES

Plain films cannot diagnose ligamentous injury. However, MRI is a valuable study for the orthopedist. MRI is 93% to 94% sensitive for ACL injury compared with 89% for a positive Lachman's test, and 78% for an AD test.[6,26] In the best of hands, the specificity is near 100% for all three tests.[6] MRI can also demonstrate a concomitant meniscal tear.

TREATMENT

The goals of treating an ACL injury are to reduce pain, swelling, and inflammation, and to restore the normal range of motion and strength as soon as possible. Have the patient reexamined in 1 to 2 days by an orthopedist after immobilization, apply ice and remain non–weight-bearing with use of crutches. Elevation and analgesics (nonsteroidal antiinflammatory drugs [NSAIDs]) provide additional relief. If a painful tense effusion is present, aspirate the knee and apply a compressive elastic wrap. Quadriceps and hamstring strengthening exercises are important for joint rehabilitation.

Complete ACL injuries in young, active adults usually require operation (especially athletic patients with a secondary ligament tear of the PCL or MCL). An associated meniscal injury will also drive surgical repair.[25] However, the optimal timing of repair is controversial.

Posterior Cruciate Ligament

The posterior cruciate ligament (PCL) is the primary static knee stabilizer that prevents knee rotation, as well as the primary restraint to posterior motion of the tibia.[5] The broader PCL is reportedly twice as strong as the ACL and is maximally taut in full knee flexion. PCL trauma comprises 7% to 23% of all knee ligament injuries. Only 4% of all PCL injuries occur in isolation.[6]

PATHOPHYSIOLOGY

Injury to the PCL usually results from a direct blow to the pretibial area when the knee is flexed (forcing the knee posteriorly). This "dashboard injury" often ruptures other ligaments or fractures the patella, femur, or acetabulum.[6] The PCL may also be torn with a fall onto a flexed knee with the foot in plantar flexion. PCL injuries are typically associated with severe trauma to the ACL and MCL. In one study, 83% of patients with a PCL injury suffered medial meniscal tears.[6]

HISTORY

The patient usually complains of pain and hears an audible pop, snap, or buckling sound at the time of injury. The knee may lock. As with an ACL tear, complete tears of the PCL are usually less painful than partial tears. The pain is increased when the patient descends stairs or during the push-off phase of running.

PHYSICAL FINDINGS

Test for the stability of the PCL with the posterior drawer and sag tests (see the previous discussion).

DIAGNOSTIC STUDIES

MRI is a useful adjunct to diagnose PCL injuries. MRI has a sensitivity of 99% for PCL injuries.[6] It is not a standard ED test, and is best left to the consultant.

TREATMENT

Place the patient with an injured PCL in a knee immobilizer. Have the patient use crutches, ice, and elevation, and arrange for orthopedic referral within a few days. The patient can usually begin isometric quadriceps exercises 1 to 2 weeks after the initial injury.

The surgical treatment of an isolated PCL injury depends on many factors, including the patient's usual level of activity.

Medial Collateral Ligament

The medial collateral ligament (MCL), also referred to as the tibial collateral ligament, is the most commonly injured ligament of the knee in adults and children. It is damaged during abduction, flexion, and internal rotation of the femur on the tibia. The MCL is a two-part structure that has 3 to 4 layers with a long superficial ligament overlying a deep capsular structure.

PATHOPHYSIOLOGY

The MCL limits rotation and abduction of the knee, and prevents valgus deformity of the knee in all stages of flexion. An isolated disruption of the MCL usually occurs after a direct blow to the lateral knee with the leg fixed.

CLINICAL PRESENTATION

MCL tears are often associated with a concomitant ACL injury (rotational with valgus injury as in an athlete making an abrupt pivot). Concomitant injuries to the cruciate ligaments and menisci are also frequent. Meniscal injuries occur in 13% of all MCL injuries.[6]

PHYSICAL FINDINGS

Diagnosis of the MCL tear involves valgus stress in flexion. Medial laxity of >10 mm without a firm endpoint suggests complete rupture of the MCL. Laxity <10 mm suggests the presence of an incomplete or partial tear.

TREATMENT

The treatment of an isolated MCL injury is nonoperative and consists of ice, elevation, and crutches. Immobilize the knee with a post-operative splint and the patient may weight-bear as tolerated. Begin range-of-motion exercises once the patient is pain free; full activity can usually be resumed in 3 to 9 weeks, depending on the tear's severity.[6]

Certain tears of the MCL are treated operatively, especially if the ACL or menisci are also injured. However, some studies have shown better results with nonsurgical treatment.[18]

Lateral Collateral Ligament

The lateral collateral ligament (LCL) is also known as the fibular collateral ligament. It is extracapsular and does not insert on the lateral meniscus. The LCL is the primary lateral knee stabilizer in all degrees of flexion and external rotation. It resists varus stress, and isolated injuries are uncommon. Three muscles reinforce the LCL: biceps femoris, popliteus, and iliotibial band.

PATHOPHYSIOLOGY

The LCL can be injured after an internal rotational (varus) stress with the knee in a dependent position. An isolated LCL injury results from a direct varus blow to the medial aspect of the knee with the leg fixed, as occurs with wrestlers.[6]

LCL injury is infrequent because the opposite leg protects the inner aspect of the knee. However, with injury, lateral instability of the knee is more disabling than medial instability.

PHYSICAL FINDINGS

Test for LCL injury by applying a varus force to the knee in extension and 30 degrees of flexion. Position the knee with the foot and leg first in a neutral position, apply the varus force, and repeat the maneuver with the leg first in internal rotation, then in external rotation. Lateral (varus) instability suggests damage to the LCL, or lateral capsule, as well as possible injury to the ACL and/or PCL, iliotibial band, or the popliteus/biceps femoris complex. Lateral laxity of >10 mm without a firm endpoint suggests complete LCL rupture. Varus laxity <10 mm is likely due to an incomplete or partial tear.

LCL tear is often associated with cruciate injury. The common peroneal nerve is also at risk.

TREATMENT

Usual treatment of an isolated LCL injury is nonoperative, consisting of a knee immobilizer, ice, and crutches with weight-bearing as tolerated. An isolated LCL injury generally does not lead to a disabling instability or loss of function. Operative treatment is reserved for LCL injuries associated with other major ligament damage.

MENISCAL KNEE INJURIES

The menisci are two crescent-shaped, fibrocartilaginous, avascular disks important in load-bearing and force transmission across the knee. The menisci are interposed between the condyles of the femur and tibia and are also known as the semilunar cartilages. The menisci are the "shock absorbers" of the knee. The periphery of each meniscus is attached to the femur and tibia by the joint capsule. The lateral meniscus is O-shaped and has only a single attachment, making it more mobile. However, the medial meniscus is C-shaped and relatively immobile, thus predisposing it to injury. The menisci move posteriorly with knee flexion and anteriorly with knee extension. The medial meniscus is injured twice as commonly as the lateral meniscus.[18]

Pathophysiology

The menisci are usually injured after a twisting motion to a flexed knee, and can cause the knee to lock in flexion. A displaced and torn meniscus produces a mechanical block leading to a "locked knee." Although this loss of full extension usually points to a mechanical factor such as a cartilage tear, ligament, or loose body, a large effusion is occasionally responsible.

These tears are usually longitudinal (bucket handle) and are displaced into the intercondylar notch. Nearly 80% of patients with medial meniscal tears have ACL injuries.[28]

History

Several historical questions aid the diagnosis of a meniscal injury. The probability of a meniscal injury increases if the patient experienced a rotational force at the time of injury. Unlike injuries to the MCL and LCL, the pain of a meniscal injury is worse with weight-bearing. The patient may have recurring episodes of instability, pain, catching, locking, audible snaps/pops, or a history of buckling. The patient often complains that he or she is unable to squat.

Physical Findings

The diagnostic triad of meniscal tears includes the following:

1. Joint line pain (Bragard's sign)
2. Swelling
3. Locking

Anteromedial joint line pain suggests a medial meniscal tear.[2] The locking occurs when the posterior segment of the meniscus jams between the articular surfaces, leaving the patient unable to fully extend the knee. Test the knee through extension and flexion, and evaluate range of motion. Normal range of motion is between 0 and 135 degrees. With a meniscal injury, range of motion is limited, especially in terminal phases of flexion and extension. The Apley grind and McMurray's tests, in conjunction with Payr's and Steinmann's signs, are all helpful in diagnosing meniscal injury.

Diagnostic Studies

Use radiographs of the knee (AP, lateral, tunnel, and tangential views) routinely to evaluate for other mechanical causes of a "locked knee," such as a dislocated patella or a loose calcific body (osteochondritis desiccans).

The consultant may perform a variety of tests for suspected meniscal injury. MRI is very helpful in making the diagnosis, and is performed on an outpatient basis.

Arthroscopy is valuable for diagnosing and treating meniscal tears, and may reveal other pathology such as a loose foreign body, chondral fracture, or torn ACL.

Treatment

Meniscal injury does not require urgent intervention unless the tear is displaced into the intercondylar notch, resulting in a "locked knee."[18] Reduce a locked knee within 24 hours of injury. Have the patient hang his or her legs off the edge of the bed with the knee in 90 degrees of flexion. Gravity will distract the tibia from the femur. Applying careful traction along the leg axis with mild rotation of the tibia should unlock the knee. Immobilize the knee, elevate it, and arrange for orthopedic follow-up in 2 to 4 days.

The use of arthroscopy has recently declined in favor because arthroscopic removal or resection of torn menisci increases the risk of future degenerative changes. Without the meniscus, the forces on the articular joint surface force double or triple. In many cases, excision of the meniscus leads to increased joint laxity.[18]

QUADRICEPS TENDON TEAR

The quadriceps tendon is the primary dynamic stabilizer of the knee. Four anterior quadriceps muscles (rectus femoris, vastus lateralis, vastus intermedius, and vastus medialis) join to form the quadriceps tendon. The quadriceps tendon envelops the patella in the retinaculum and inserts on the tibial tubercle as the patellar tendon. This mechanism is responsible for knee extension. Rupture of the quadriceps tendon is easily missed unless the physician tests for active extension. Patients can still walk with this injury and some have minimal or no pain on presentation.

Pathophysiology

The quadriceps tendon is injured during forced flexion of the knee with the quadriceps contracted, for example, stumbling while descending a staircase, a fall with the knee in flexion, or during springboard diving into a pool. Rupture can also occur during strenuous exercise when the knee is extended and the feet are fixed. Sudden indirect trauma, such as a basketball jump shot, can snap the quadriceps tendon. Several conditions predispose to rupture and include obesity, degenerative joint disease, gout, collagen vascular disorders, and fatty tendon degeneration. Metabolic disorders such as diabetes mellitus, chronic renal failure, and hypoparathyroidism also place the patient at risk. Repeated minor injury results in calcification and weakening of the quadriceps tendon.[18] The majority (88%) of quadriceps tendon ruptures occur in patients >40 years old, whereas 80% of the patellar ligament ruptures occur in patients <40 years old.[6]

History

A patient with an injury to the extensor mechanism complains of his or her knee giving way. The patient is unable to climb stairs without support, and the knee

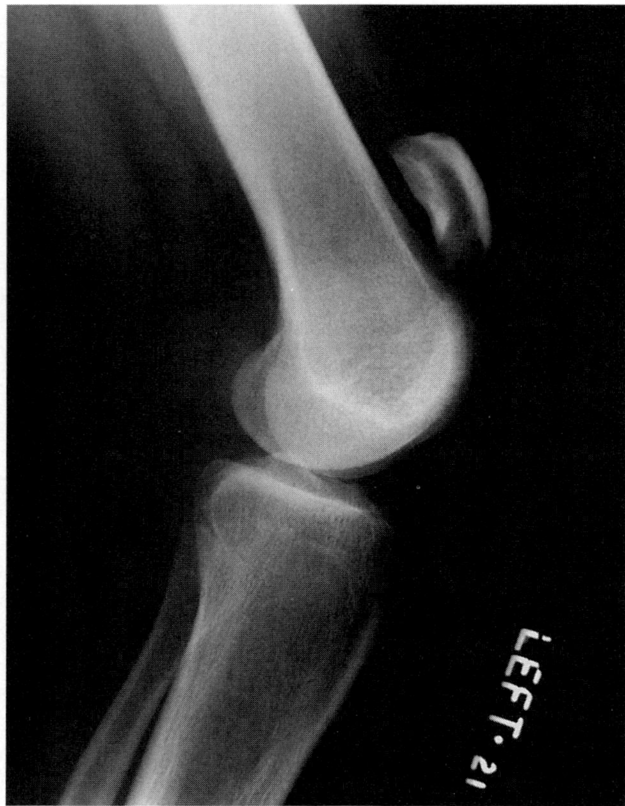

Fig. 27-17 Left patella tendon rupture (patella alta).

may collapse when the patient steps down (e.g., off a curb).[4]

Physical Findings

Patients with rupture of their extensor mechanism are able to walk with a peculiar forward-leaning gait. By the time they present to the ED, they may have minimal or no pain. The patient with a complete quadriceps tendon rupture cannot maintain the knee in active extension. A palpable defect lies above the patella, and the patient may have diffuse swelling around the knee. Patients with partial quadriceps tendon injuries have swelling superior to the patella and demonstrate weakness in extension. Suspect an extensor mechanism injury if the patient uses his or her hands to boost the injured leg up to the examining table.[2] If the physician moves the leg in full extension and lets go, the leg immediately drops.

Diagnostic Studies

Avulsion of the quadriceps tendon may result in fragments of bone anterior to the suprapatellar synovium (superior pole of patella) on radiographs. Radiographs may also show an effusion and/or patella alta ("high-riding" patella seen in Fig. 27-17). Many films may be normal or demonstrate only subtle findings.

Treatment

The application of a knee immobilizer for 4 to 6 weeks treats an incomplete quadriceps tendon injury (extension is weak but still possible). Early rehabilitation exercises prevent disuse atrophy during immobilization.[18,22] Complete tendon ruptures usually require surgical repair.

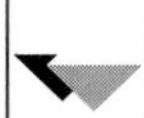

PEARLS & PITFALLS

- Injuries to the hip and acetabulum are commonly associated with severe knee trauma.
- The Pittsburgh and Ottawa knee rules are useful in determining the need for radiography.
- Assume penetrating wounds adjacent to the knee have violated the joint. Consider injection of sterile saline or methylene blue into the knee and observe for leakage from the wound.
- Aspiration of a hemarthrosis may decrease pain, whereas instillation of morphine or bupivacaine provides additional relief.
- Flex the knee when testing the collateral ligaments.
- Patients can walk despite a quadriceps rupture. Test for active extension against gravity.
- Knee dislocations are associated with injury to the popliteal artery. Such patients require serial vascular examinations, measurement of the ankle/arm index, and consultation.

REFERENCES

1. Stiell IG, et al: Prospective validation of a decision rule for the use of radiography in acute knee injuries, *JAMA* 275:611-615, 1996.
2. Sonzogni JJ Jr: Examining the injured knee, *Emerg Med* 28:76-86, 1996.
3. Tintinalli JE, Krome RL, Ruiz E, (editors): *Emergency medicine: a comprehensive study guide,* ed 3, New York, 1992, McGraw-Hill.
4. Simon RR, Koenigsknecht SJ: *Emergency orthopedics: the extremities,* ed 2, Norwalk, CT, 1987, Appleton & Lange.
5. Miller MD, Olszewski AD: Posterior cruciate ligament injuries: new treatment options, *Am J Knee Surg* 8:145-154, 1995.
6. Silski JM, ed: *Traumatic disorders of the knee,* New York, 1994, Springer-Verlag.
7. Crenshaw AH, (editor): *Campbell's operative orthopedics,* ed 8, St Louis, 1992, Mosby.

8. Harris JH, Harris WH, Novelline RA: *The radiology of emergency medicine,* ed 3, Baltimore, 1993, Williams & Wilkins.
9. Seaberg DC, et al: Multicenter comparison of two clinical decision rules for the use of radiography in acute, high-risk knee injuries, *Ann Emerg Med* 32:8-13, 1998.
10. Stiell IG, et al: Implementation of the Ottawa Knee Rule for the use of radiography in acute knee injuries, *JAMA* 278:2075-2079, 1997.
11. Graeme KA, Jackimczyk KC: The extremities and spine, *Emerg Med Clin North Am* 15:365-379, 1997.
12. Reinhardt RL: Emergency evaluation and management of the traumatic acute joint, *Crit Dec Emerg Med* 12:1-15, 1997.
13. Barkin RM, ed: *Pediatric emergency medicine: concepts and clinical practice,* ed 2, St Louis, 1997, Mosby.
14. Richardson MD, et al: The efficacy of intra-articular orphine for postoperative knee arthroscopy analgesia, *Arthroscopy* 13:584-589, 1997.
15. Cepeda MS, et al: Pain relief after knee arthroscopy: intra-articular morphine, intra-articular bupivacaine, or subcutaneous morphine, *Reg Anesth* 22:233-238, 1997.
16. Lundin O, et al: Analgesic effects of intra-articular morphine during and after knee arthroscopy: a comparison of two methods, *Arthroscopy* 14:192-196, 1998.
17. DeAndres J, et al: Intra-articular analgesia after arthroscopic knee surgery: comparison of three different regimens, *Eur J Anaesthesiol* 15:10-15, 1998.
18. Rosen P, et al: *Emergency medicine: concepts and clinical practice,* ed 3, St Louis, 1992, Mosby.
19. Garth WP Jr, Pomphrey M Jr, Merrill K: Functional treatment of patellar dislocation in an athletic population, *Am J Sports Med* 24:785-791, 1996.
20. Wascher DC, Dvirnak PC, DeCoster TA: Knee dislocation: Initial assessment and implications for treatment, *J Orthop Trauma* 11:525-529, 1997.
21. Treiman GS, et al: Examination of the patient with a knee dislocation, *Arch Surg* 127:1056-1063, 1992.
22. Perry CR, Elstrom JA, Pankovich AM, (editors): *Handbook of fractures,* New York, 1995, McGraw-Hill.
23. Bennett WF, Browner B: Tibial plateau fractures: a study of associated soft tissue injuries, *J Orthop Trauma* 8:183-188, 1994.
24. Holt MD, Williams LA, Dent CM: MRI in the management of tibial plateau fractures, *Injury* 26:595-599, 1995.
25. Shelbourne KD, et al: Correlation of joint line tenderness and meniscal lesions in patients with acute anterior cruciate ligament tears, *Am J Sports Med* 23:166-169, 1995.
26. O'Shea KJ, et al: The diagnostic accuracy of history, physical examination, and radiographs in the evaluation of traumatic knee disorders, *Am J Sports Med* 24:164-167, 1996.

28 Leg Injuries: Tibia and Fibula

E. PARKER HAYS, Jr.

Injuries to the lower leg are frequent, and fractures of the tibia and fibula are the most common long-bone fractures.[1,2] Typical mechanisms include pedestrians struck by cars, motor vehicle crashes (MVCs), falls, and sporting or skiing mishaps. Because it is covered only by thin skin through much of its length, the tibia is the most common open long-bone fracture.[3]

Emergency physicians (EPs) need to be familiar with fracture and dislocation patterns for accurate diagnosis and communication with consultants. We must stabilize, occasionally reduce, immobilize, and refer these injuries. Diagnosis and treatment must maintain function and avoid major complications, such as neurovascular compromise, and delayed-union or nonunion. In particular, the EP must remain alert to the subtleties of compartment syndrome, which is a common complication.

ANATOMY

General

The tibia bears the bulk of the body's weight (85% or more).[4] The smaller fibula stabilizes the tibia through its tibial-fibular articulations and the interosseous membrane. If intact, the fibula maintains leg length in tibial fractures. Familiarity with normal bony alignment, major vascular and neural structures, and compartments helps the EP assess and diagnose specific injuries.

Bones (Fig. 28-1)

The wide, slightly concave, articular surfaces on either side of the *tibial spine* constitute the *tibial plateaus* and are covered by synovium and the *medial* and *lateral menisci*. The patellar tendon attaches proximally on the anterior *tibial tuberosity*. The tibia narrows to a long shaft before widening distally to form the *plafond* (the "ceiling" of the ankle joint), and the *medial malleolus*. The posterior portion of the distal articular surface constitutes the *posterior malleolus*.

The fibula lies lateral and posterior to the tibia. It articulates proximally at the *superior* or *proximal tibia-fibula joint*, through its length by the fibrous *interosseous membrane*, and distally at the *inferior tibia-fibula joint* or *syndesmosis*.

Vessels

The *femoral artery* becomes the *popliteal artery* after traversing behind the knee. Here, at the *trifurcation*, it divides into the three vessels that supply the leg: the *anterior* and *posterior tibial arteries and the peroneal artery* (Fig. 28-1, *A*). The anterior tibial artery courses anteriorly over the top of the interosseous membrane and runs down the leg on the anterior surface of the membrane. Its integrity is evident clinically as the *dorsalis pedis pulse*. The posterior tibial artery continues behind the membrane to the medial ankle and is felt as the *posterior tibial pulse*. The peroneal artery courses down the posterior-lateral leg.

Nerves

Three nerves of clinical significance supply the leg and foot (Fig. 28-1, *B*, and Table 28-1). The *peroneal nerve* emerges from behind the fibular neck and divides into the *superficial peroneal* and *deep peroneal* nerves. The *tibial nerve* courses behind the tibia in the deep posterior compartment, whereas the *sural nerve* supplies the muscles that plantarflex the ankle (gastrocnemius, soleus) and provides sensation to the sole of the foot. The proximity of the peroneal nerves behind the fibular head makes injuries to these structures a concern (Fig. 28-1, *B*). Indeed, injury to the peroneal nerve is one of the most common neurologic deficits associated with leg fractures, and frequently results in foot drop.

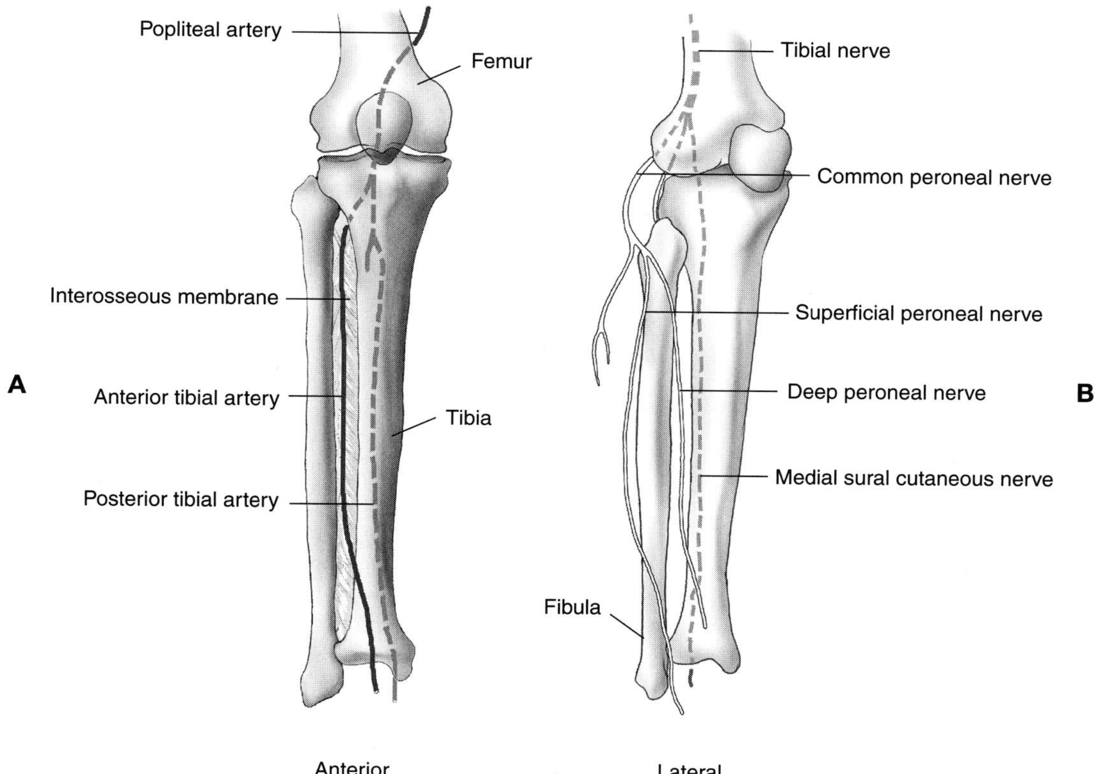

Fig. 28-1 Leg anatomy. **A,** The tibia and fibula are attached through their shafts by the interosseous membrane. The popliteal artery bifurcates into the anterior tibial artery and the posterior tibial artery. **B,** The peroneal nerve courses behind the fibular head and around the fibular neck, then branches into the (1) superficial peroneal nerve, and the (2) deep peroneal nerve. The (3) sural nerve runs in the posterior leg on its way to the heel. The tibial nerve (not shown) courses behind the tibia, running together with the posterior tibial artery.

TABLE 28-1
Nerves of the Leg and Foot

NERVE	*MOTOR*	*SENSORY*	*COMPARTMENT*
Superficial peroneal	Foot eversion	Lateral dorsal foot	Lateral
Deep peroneal	Foot dorsiflexion	First and second webspace	Anterior
Tibial	Plantarflexion of the toe (tibialis posterior, flexor digitorum longus)	Anterior sole of the foot	Deep posterior
Sural	Ankle plantarflexion (gastrocnemius, soleus)	Plantar aspect of the heel	Superficial posterior

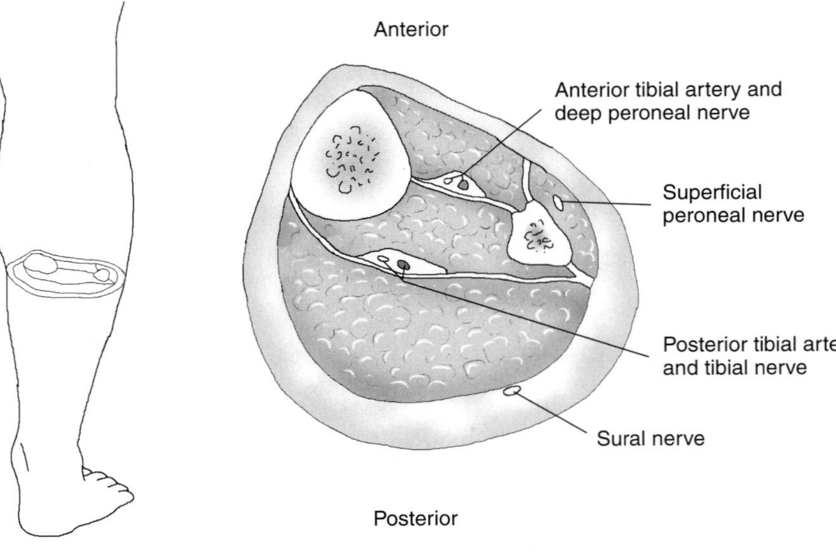

Fig. 28-2 The interosseous membrane runs between the tibia and fibula. The four compartments of the leg—anterior, lateral (peroneal), superficial posterior, and deep posterior—and their major neurovascular contents are shown.

Compartments

The upper third of the leg is divided into four compartments. Inelastic fibrous septae and bone separate these compartments. When pressure within a compartment rises, it can damage muscles and nerves confined within its space. The neurovascular structures in each compartment are depicted in Fig. 28-2.

SPECIFIC INJURY PATTERNS

Tibial Plateau Fractures

See Chapter 27 for additional discussion.

MECHANISM OF INJURY

Plateau fractures usually arise from a varus or valgus force, axial load, or forced hyperextension of the knee. Common scenarios include motor vehicle or motorcycle crashes, falls from a height, pedestrian struck by car, contact sports, and skiing mishaps. Fractures are often accompanied by ligamentous and meniscal injuries.[5] An intact collateral ligament on the side opposite the injurious force may act as a hinge. This hinge force may drive the femoral condyle down onto the meniscus and tibial plateau on the same side as the injuring force.[5] If the force continues and the opposite side of the joint widens, the "hinge" ligament may rupture. The weaker lateral plateau (approximately 70% of fractures) is much more commonly fractured than the medial plateau.[1,2]

CLINICAL PRESENTATION

Alert patients complain of knee pain and the great majority are nonambulatory. However, some patients can walk. *Therefore do not assume that ambulation precludes a tibial plateau fracture.* Effusion is common and associated skin and soft tissue injury is frequent, especially when the knee is injured from a direct blow (e.g., car bumper). The Ottawa Knee rules (see Chapter 27) are a good guide to determine the need for radiographs in patients with knee injuries.

DIAGNOSIS AND RADIOLOGY

Assess joint effusion by comparing the contralateral knee with the injured knee. Test for range of motion and compare with the contralateral knee. Decreased range of motion is common with effusions, especially limitation of flexion. Effusions appear on the lateral radiograph as a widening of the density between the quadriceps tendon and the femur; distention >5 mm suggests joint effusion.

Some fractures are radiographically subtle.[6] Oblique views may improve diagnostic sensitivity, especially if unexplained lucencies or slight deformities are seen on anteroposterior (AP) or lateral films (Fig. 28-3). The tibial plateau view involves angling the radiograph beam 10° to 15° caudad and "shoots" down on the joint. This view may demonstrate otherwise hidden fractures, and helps determine the degree of fracture depression (Fig. 28-4). The orthopedist may employ computed tomography (CT) to further define the extent of injuries.[7,8]

The three types of tibial plateau fractures[7] are represented schematically in Fig. 28-5.

EMERGENCY MANAGEMENT AND DISPOSITION

Carry out a careful assessment for associated injuries, evaluate distal sensory and motor function of the ankle and foot, and palpate the dorsalis pedis and posterior tibial pulses. Displaced fractures increase the risk

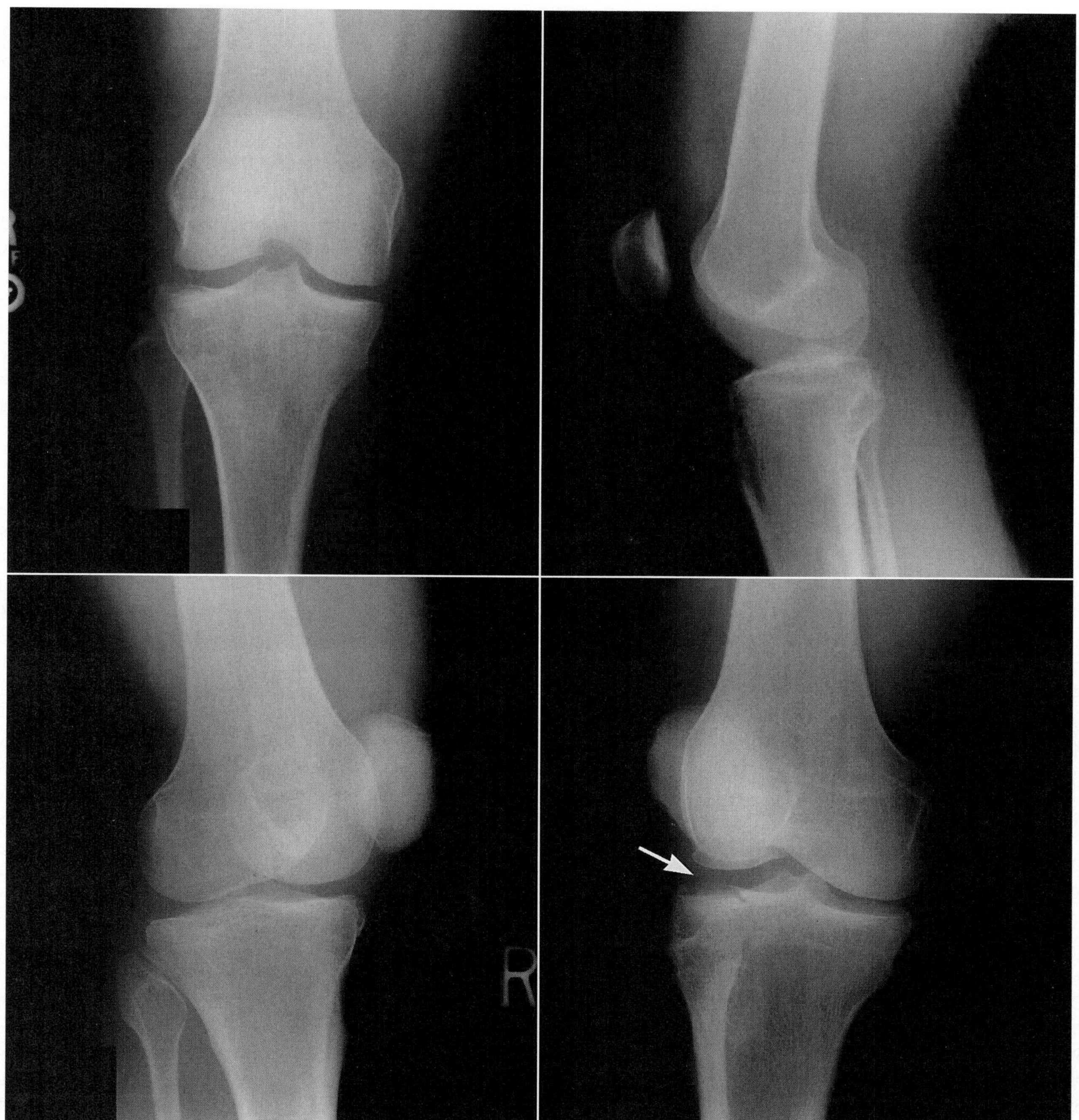

Fig. 28-3 Lateral tibial plateau fracture (local compression). This patient was sent back for oblique views when initial anteroposterior and lateral views did not show a fracture. The injury is only seen on one oblique view *(arrow)*. Tibial plateau views might help delineate the amount of depression.

for vascular injury.[3,9,10] Assess ligamentous stability since coexistent ligament rupture may necessitate operative repair.

Determine the amount of displacement or depression of the fracture fragments. Depression >3 to 8 mm may require surgery.[7,11] The acceptable range of displacement varies with the amount and location (anterior, medial, lateral) of articular surface involvement.

The emergency management of all plateau fractures involves immobilization and pain control. Displaced, depressed, high-energy, open, and comminuted or bicondylar fractures usually require sur-

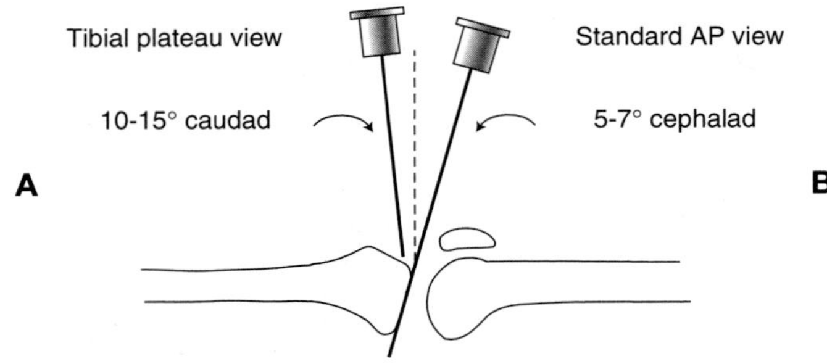

Fig. 28-4 Tibial plateau views. **A,** Standard anterior-posterior views of the knee are taken with the x-ray beam angled 5° to 7° cephalad. **B,** To visualize the tibial plateaus as flat surfaces, the x-ray beam is directed 10° to 15° caudad. With a tibial plateau fracture, the amount of fracture depression can then be more accurately measured.

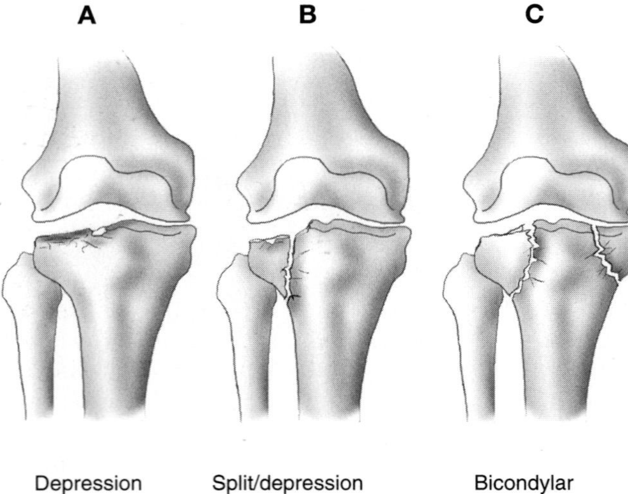

Fig. 28-5 Tibial plateau fracture types. For purposes of general treatment and surgical decision making, tibial plateau fractures can be described as one of three types. **A,** *Depression fractures,* where a part of the articular surface is compressed, but the lateral and medial cortices remain intact. **B,** *Split fractures* may also have a component of depression. The fracture extends through the cortex on the affected medial, lateral (shown), or posterior aspect of the tibia. **C,** *Bicondylar fractures* involve both medial and lateral cortices, are often comminuted, and may have depressed segment.

gery.[7,11,12] Prolonged non–weight-bearing is the rule, but early range of motion may encourage cartilaginous healing, avoid residual knee stiffness, and maintain functional range.[7,12] Nondisplaced depression or split fractures are sometimes managed without surgery.[7,11] Most patients managed nonoperatively are discharged with crutches, immobilization, and non–weight-bearing status. Early range of motion is employed to encourage cartilaginous healing and avoid residual knee stiffness.[7,12] Initial immobilization, elevation, non–weight-bearing, and close orthopedic follow-up may be appropriate after consultation.

Tibial Shaft Fractures

MECHANISM OF INJURY

The tibia's subcutaneous position predisposes it to direct violence. Common scenarios include the classic car bumper injury and industrial accidents. Direct trauma often results in transverse or comminuted fractures. Indirect violence or torsional mechanisms tend to produce oblique or spiral fractures; common examples include MVCs and skiing injury. Significant soft tissue injury may accompany these fractures, which are often open.[13]

CLINICAL PRESENTATION

As with any significant fracture, associated injuries may dominate the clinical picture. Patients with tibial shaft fractures are nonambulatory and complain of moderate to significant pain. In open fractures, soft-tissue injury ranges from protruding bone to pinpoint skin breaks. Indirect mechanisms (e.g., a skiing injury) may not have associated or distracting injuries. In indirect mechanisms, patients can usually locate the fracture site.

There are several mechanisms that produce unique tibial fractures. A "**toddler's**" fracture is an oblique or transverse fracture of the distal tibia that occurs when a small child catches his or her leg between furniture and then falls. When a ski stops suddenly from an obstruction, the skier may sustain a "**boot-top**" fracture. This transverse tibial fracture appears just above the top of the ski boot.

DIAGNOSIS AND RADIOLOGY (Fig. 28-6)

Radiographs should include the knee and ankle joints in addition to the leg. Determine if the fracture is open or closed and identify the fracture pattern (oblique/spiral, transverse, or comminuted). Note the presence or absence of an associated fibular fracture. Assess the feet for sensory and motor ability and for the presence of dorsalis pedis and posterior tibial pulses. Finally, determine the degree of soft tissue damage, any contamination of open wounds, and ligamentous injuries to the knee and ankle.

EMERGENCY MANAGEMENT AND DISPOSITION

Initial management of tibial shaft fractures consists of prompt immobilization in a radiolucent splint, local wound care, and analgesia. Definitive treatments include long-leg casting or open reduction and inter-

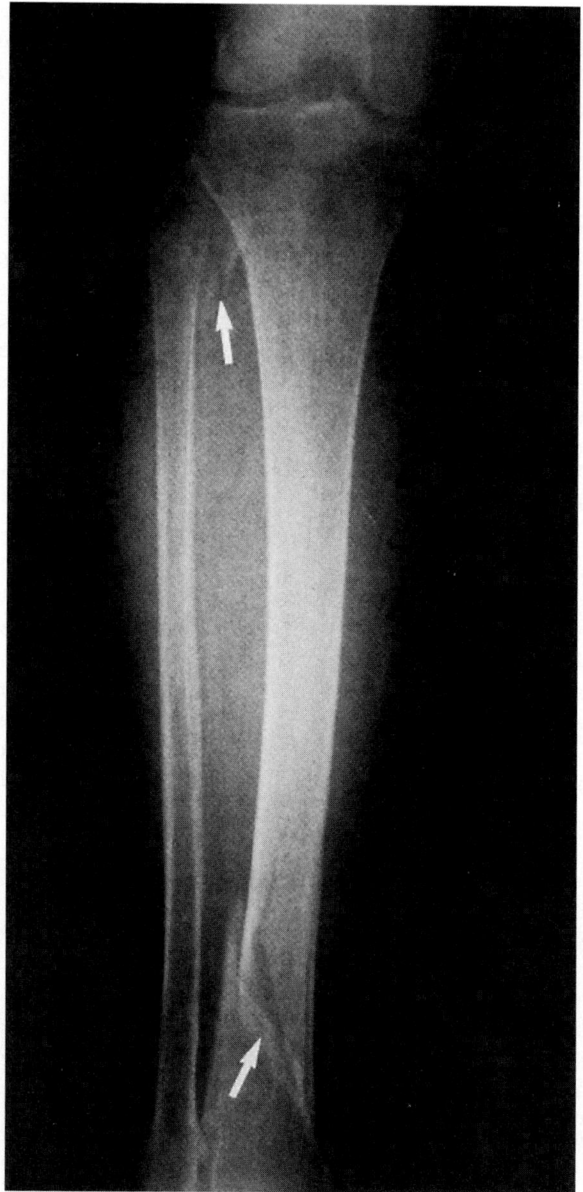

Fig. 28-6 Tibial shaft fracture. An oblique fracture of the distal tibial shaft is demonstrated. Note the accompanying fracture of the proximal fibula, also resulting from a twisting force. (From Jackimczyk KC, Goy W: Musculoskeletal trauma. In Rosen P, et al: *Diagnostic radiology in emergency medicine,* St Louis, 1992, Mosby.)

nal fixation (ORIF). External fixation may be used for open fractures. Major complications are infection, compartment syndrome, loss of leg length, and delayed-union or nonunion.

On occasion, EPs may manage certain low-risk fractures conservatively by immobilizing the patient in a long leg splint and arranging for close follow-up. Low-risk fractures include those that are closed, nondisplaced, have a low-energy mechanism, and no accompanying ligamentous or fibular injury. However, the greater majority of tibial fractures *must be admitted* for close observation. Compartment syndrome may occur in up to 20% of cases (see the following discussion).[2,14] Emergency department consultation with the orthopedic surgeon helps guide treatment.

TABLE 28-2
Classification Scheme for Open Tibial Fractures

TYPE	DESCRIPTION
Type I	Small skin laceration (<1 cm); minimal contamination and intact vascular supply
Type II	Moderate comminution, larger wound (>1 cm); minimal or moderate contamination and some crush component
Type IIIA	High-energy fracture, moderate contamination, extensive soft tissue injury
Type IIIB	Massive contamination, periosteal stripping, severe soft-tissue loss, requires flap for bony coverage
Type IIIC	Associated vascular injury that requires repair. Mechanisms include high-velocity gunshot wounds, close-range shotgun wounds, amputations, open fractures >8 hours old at presentation

Adapted from Gustilo RB, Anderson JT: *J Bone Joint Surg* 58A: 453, 1976 and Gustilo RB, Mendoza RM, Williams DN: *J Trauma* 24:742, 1984.

Open Fractures

An open fracture is a true orthopedic emergency. A classification system developed by Gustilo and Anderson[15,16] is commonly used to classify open fractures (Table 28-2). However, there are questions regarding interobserver reliability.[17]

TREATMENT

Promptly irrigate wounds, débride obvious contamination, dress with moist saline gauze, and immobilize the limb. Immediately administer parenteral broad-spectrum antibiotics (e.g., cefazolin 1g intravenous). In type II or type III injuries, add an aminoglycoside (e.g., gentamicin) to increase gram-negative coverage. For farm injuries or soil/fecal-contaminated wounds, add penicillin to cover *Clostridium* species.[18-21] Consult an orthopedic surgeon for emergent surgical débridement and fixation.

Fibular Shaft Fractures

MECHANISM OF INJURY

On occasion, patients may suffer isolated fibular fractures from a direct blow to the lateral leg.[1,3] However, most fibular fractures occur in conjunction with tibial injury. An intact fibula maintains leg length and stabilizes the leg through the interosseous membrane and the proximal and distal tibiofibular ligaments. However, with healing of the tibial fractures, the fibula can push the leg into varus deformity.[1]

CLINICAL PRESENTATION

Both bone fractures present similarly to tibial shaft fractures, but are associated with higher energy mechanisms. Patients with an isolated fibular fracture report a history of direct trauma and complain of lateral pain (Fig. 28-7). Because the fibula only bears 15% of weight,[4] the patient may be able to walk, and the injury may be mistaken for an "ankle sprain." In proximal fractures, the peroneal nerve is frequently injured due to its location just posterior to the fibular head and may result in foot drop or inability to evert the foot.

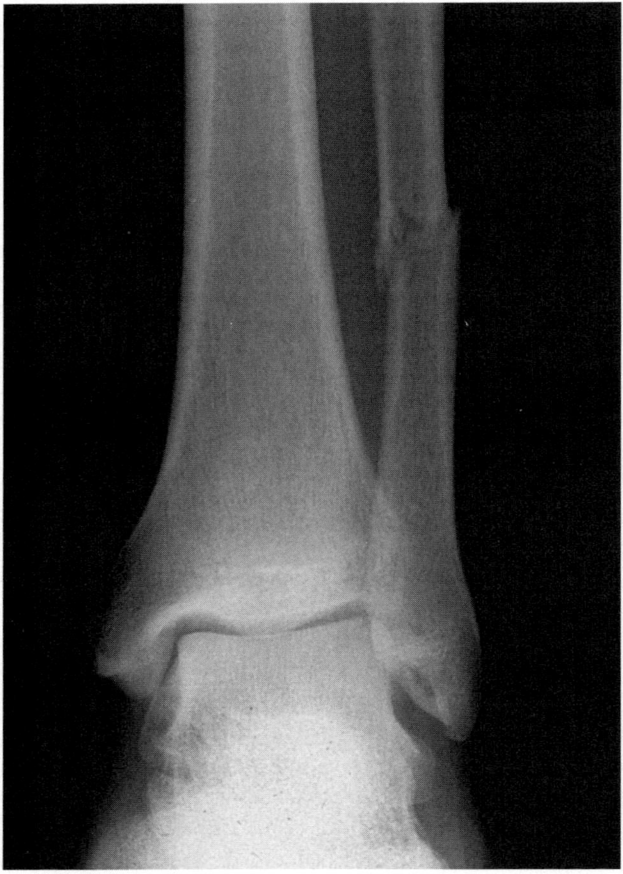

Fig. 28-7 Isolated fibular shaft fracture. This patient sustained a direct blow to the lateral leg to produce this transverse fracture. A fracture in this location should arouse suspicion of associated injury to knee ligaments or ankle injury.

DIAGNOSIS AND RADIOLOGY

Examine for soft tissue injury, neurovascular injury, and associated ligamentous instability; associated ligamentous injury is common for both proximal and distal fractures (Fig. 28-8). Obtain radiographs of the entire length of the fibula and examine for subtle, nondisplaced fractures or disruption of the normal tibiofibular articulation. A Maisonneuve or syndesmotic injury at the ankle is frequent.

EMERGENCY MANAGEMENT AND DISPOSITION

Manage open fractures with irrigation, intravenous antibiotics, saline dressings and urgent orthopedic evaluation. If the patient is ambulatory, treat closed fractures that are minimally displaced and have no significant associated injury with ice, analgesia, crutches as needed, and an elastic wrap. Alternatively, use a stirrup splint (for distal fractures) or a posterior/sugar-tong splint or short-leg cast in pa-

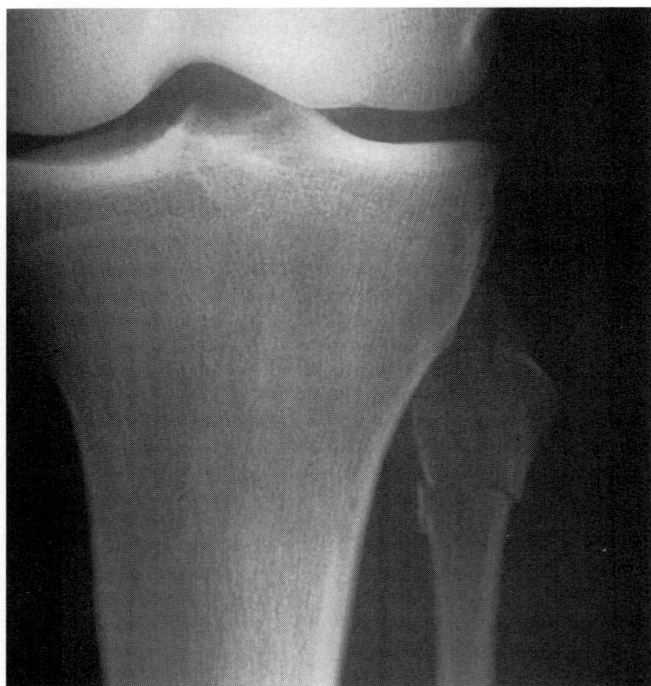

Fig. 28-8 Fibular neck fracture. A valgus force to the lateral knee area (a car bumper) caused this fibular neck fracture. This fracture should prompt suspicion for associated knee ligament injuries and peroneal nerve damage. This patient had ACL and medial collateral ligament injury.

tients with severe pain.[1-3] Consult an orthopedic surgeon before discharge from the ED.

Proximal Tibia-Fibula Dislocations

MECHANISM OF INJURY

The lateral collateral ligament (LCL) and the biceps femoris tendon oppose the anterior forces on the fibular head exerted by the peroneal muscles. If the knee is flexed, relaxing the LCL and biceps femoris, the fibular head may dislocate anteriorly and laterally (*anterolateral dislocation*). The classic mechanism occurs when a person falls from a height with the knee flexed beneath the femur.[2]

Damage to the anterior portion of the tibial-fibular joint capsule may allow the biceps femoris to pull the fibular head backward, resulting in a *posteromedial* dislocation. The LCL is commonly damaged as well. A common scenario for this injury is direct trauma from a car bumper. Superior dislocation of the joint may occur with associated tibial or ankle fractures. The common peroneal nerve or its branches are at risk in patients with all proximal fibular dislocations (see Fig. 28-1, *B*).

CLINICAL PRESENTATION

Patients complain of pain to the lateral knee, increased by movement of the knee or ankle. The fibular head is prominent in anterolateral dislocations and palpable in the lateral popliteal region in posteromedial dislocations.

DIAGNOSIS AND RADIOLOGY

In one series, this diagnosis was missed on initial presentation one third of the time.[22] The key to radiographic diagnosis lies in the knowledge of normal alignment. On a normal AP film, the fibular head should overlap the tibia by about one half of the fibular head width. In anterolateral dislocations, this overlap is lost and the fibula is displaced away from the tibia. In postero-medial dislocations, this overlap is increased.

On the normal lateral film, the fibula head should overlie the posterior portion of the tibia by about one half the fibular head's width. In anterolateral dislocations, this overlap is increased and the fibula may be tilted forward. In posteromedial dislocations, the fibular head may overlie the tibia only slightly or not at all.

EMERGENCY MANAGEMENT AND DISPOSITION

Carefully assess neurovascular integrity before and after any reduction attempts. With local or regional anesthesia or conscious sedation, reduce anterolateral dislocations by flexing the knee, dorsiflexing and inverting the foot, and applying direct posterior pressure to the fibular head.[2] If successful, place a knee immobilizer for 3 weeks, prohibit weight-bearing, and obtain orthopedic follow-up. Consult an orthopedic surgeon for posteromedial dislocations, which are usually treated surgically.[2] Superior dislocations commonly have associated fractures requiring urgent orthopedic consultation.

Compartment Syndrome

Development of a compartment syndrome is a frequent and, if unrecognized, a possibly devastating event. The EP must evaluate for this condition in every patient with a tibial fracture. Although this syndrome may be absent on initial presentation it may develop hours later in the ED or after discharge.

The most common site of all compartment syndromes is the lower leg, and is usually due to tibial fracture.[23,24] Bone and dense connective tissue or septae bind the four compartments of the lower leg (see Fig. 28-2). The relative nondistensibility of these closed compartments may offer no release of pressure if the structures within them increase in volume.

Compartment syndromes arise through the following mechanisms:

1. A fracture or other hemorrhage within a compartment.
2. Vascular injury leading to ischemia. Reperfusion injury results in muscle swelling, capillary leak, tissue edema, and a subsequent rise in compartment pressures.
3. Pressure within a compartment may also increase as a result of constrictive dressings or casts, full-thickness burns, and military antishock trousers (MAST) use.[25]

On a tissue level, an increase in compartment pressure may overcome venous pressure and interfere with capillary gradients. If tissue blood flow is inadequate, ischemic damage to muscles and nerves progresses, resulting in additional capillary leak and a spiral of increased compartment pressure. *Most patients with compartment syndrome have normal distal pulses.* Ischemia at the tissue level occurs well below diastolic pressure, and a normal pulse *in no way* rules out the diagnosis.

Compartment syndrome is easily overlooked in the ED. The time of onset for compartment syndrome may range from as short as 2 hours to 6 days after injury,[26] although most patients develop the clinical picture 15 to 30 hours after insult.[27] The earliest sign of compartment syndrome is pain.[2,3,23,27,28] Although it is easy to attribute the pain to the fracture or initial injury, patients usually have pain out of proportion to that expected for a given injury.

TABLE 28-3
Findings in Leg Compartment Syndromes

COMPARTMENT	SENSORY LOSS	WEAKNESS	THIS PASSIVE MOVEMENT. . .	CAUSES PAIN AT THE. . .
Anterior	First web space	Toe extension	Toe flexion	Shin
Deep posterior	Sole of foot	Toe flexion	Toe extension	Deep calf, Achilles
Lateral	Top of foot	Foot eversion	Foot inversion	Lateral leg
Superficial posterior	Lateral foot	Plantar flexion	Foot dorsiflexion	Calf

There are a number of physical findings associated with the compartment syndrome. The compartments may feel tight and palpation exacerbates the pain, often in areas remote to the fracture. When a muscle is stretched from its resting position, it elongates and increases in volume. *Pain with passive stretching of the muscle within the affected compartment is classic.*

The anterior compartment is the most common compartment involved. Passive plantar flexion of the toe stretches the toe extensors and produces pain at the shin. If the deep posterior compartment is involved, passive dorsiflexion of the toes results in deep calf pain.

Compression of nerves may result in decreased sensation early in the course of this syndrome.[2,23] In the anterior compartment syndrome, patients may demonstrate decreased sensation in the webspace between the first and second toes from compression of the deep peroneal nerve. Patients with the deep compartment syndrome may have numbness or hypesthesias over the sole, marking involvement of the posterior tibial nerve (Table 28-3).

Note that pulses are always intact early in the syndrome unless the initial injury directly interrupted the vasculature.[23,24] By the time pulses are absent in a compartment syndrome, structures within the compartment are irreversibly injured.[27]

DIAGNOSIS AND RADIOLOGY

If the EP suspects a compartment syndrome, immediate orthopedic consultation is mandatory. Compartment pressures may be measured with a needle/syringe/manometer setup or a commercial kit (Stryker I.C. monitor, Stryker Surgical, Kalamazoo, MI, Fig. 28-9). Normal compartment pressure should be <10 mmHg. Pressures in compartment syndrome typically are 40 to 60 mmHg or <30 mm below diastolic pressure.[27,29] Many authors suggest that fasciotomy is indicated in patients who demonstrate either of these findings. Patients with compartment pressures between 20 and 30 mmHg may be monitored and compartment pressures repeated in 1 to 2 hours.[2,24,25] Continuous compartment monitoring is possible by hooking a compartment pressure system to an arterial line monitor.

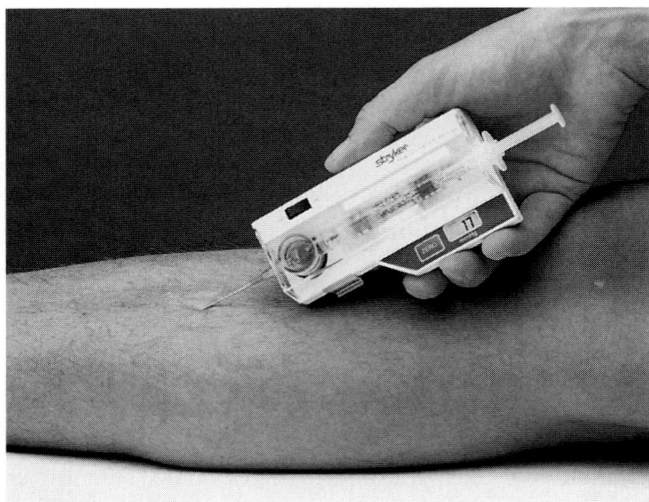

Fig. 28-9 Compartment pressure monitor. Compartment pressure can be measured using a commercial kit such as this, a manual set-up with intravenous tubing and a saline monitor, or by utilizing the pressure measurement ability on some overhead patient monitors.

The anterior, lateral (peroneal), and superficial posterior compartments are easily accessed for measurement. Pressures of the deep posterior compartment require introducing a needle posterior to the medial midshaft tibia and advancing until the needle tip is in the center of the leg.[2,25]

Correlating measured pressures with the clinical scenario is imperative (Table 28-4). False-positive measurements can occur if the needle is in tendon or fascia, whereas false-negatives are seen with air bubbles in the line, faulty equipment, or misplaced needles.

EMERGENCY MANAGEMENT AND DISPOSITION

Fasciotomy is the definitive treatment for compartment syndrome. Initial treatment involves removing compressive dressings or splitting casts. Elevate the

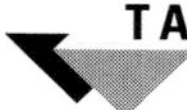

TABLE 28-4
Compartment Pressure Measurements and Actions

PRESSURE	ACTION*
<10 mmHg	Normal, observe
20 to 30 mmHg	Orthopedic consultation Observe closely and repeat pressures in 1 to 2 hours
>30 to 60 mmHg or within 30 mmHg of diastolic blood pressure	Immediate orthopedic consultation; fasciotomy

*Caveat: Correlate measured pressure with clinical findings since false readings can occur.

affected leg to the level of the heart. Patients require analgesia and continued monitoring. Emergent orthopedic consultation is essential.

Animal studies and retrospective human data indicate that the duration of elevated pressure determines outcome.* Relief of elevated pressure within 4 hours decreases residual deficit, whereas fasciotomy after 12 hours of symptoms usually results in poor outcome. An orthopedist should perform this procedure, certainly within 4 hours of symptoms and ideally as soon as the diagnosis is known. If the patient has a compartment syndrome, all four compartments are usually decompressed using a two-incision technique.[24,25,28] The orthopedist will open the anterior and lateral (peroneal) compartments with a linear vertical incision over the intercompartmental septum. This septum is located just anterior to the fibula; the incision will run the length of the compartment and through the outer fascia. The superficial peroneal nerve is in the lateral compartment and has a variable location.[28] A second linear vertical incision should be 2 cm posterior to the medial crest of the tibia and opens the posterior and the deep posterior compartments (Fig. 28-10).

*References 2, 3, 14, 23-28, 30-32.

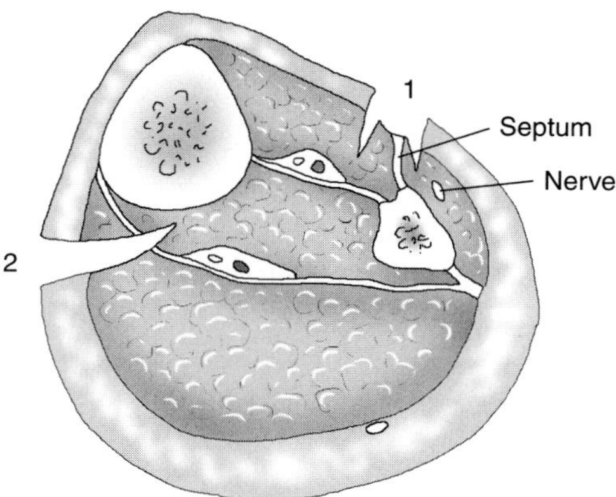

Fig. 28-10 Leg fasciotomy. To release all four compartments, a two-incision technique is used. (1) The anterior and lateral compartments are opened using an incision over the intermuscular septum and through the outer fascia of each. Avoid the superficial peroneal nerve. (2) The superficial posterior and deep posterior compartments are opened through a second incision.

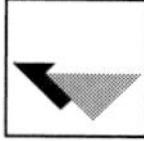

PEARLS & PITFALLS

- The tibia and fibula are the most common long-bone fractures. Tibial fractures are often open. Depressed and displaced tibial plateau fractures need surgery.
- Observe tibial shaft fractures for compartment syndrome.
- Beware of peroneal nerve injury with fibular head/neck fractures.
- Compartment syndrome has a variable time of onset, but may occur during the ED stay. Superficial compartments may feel tense, and patients may complain of pain remote from the fracture site.
- Patients with compartment syndromes often have normal distal pulses.
- Pain on passive range of motion is common with compartment syndrome.

REFERENCES

1. Alpert SW, et al: *Fractures and dislocations: a manual of orthopedic trauma,* New York, 1994, Lippincott-Raven.
2. Haller PR, Harris CR: The tibia and fibula. In Ruiz E, Cicero JJ (editors): *Emergency management of skeletal injuries,* St Louis, 1995, Mosby.
3. Rockwood CA, Green DP, Bucholz RW (editors): *Fractures in adults,* ed 3, vol 2, Philadelphia, 1991, JB Lippincott.
4. Takebe K, et al: Role of the fibula in weight-bearing, *Clin Orthop* 184:289-292, 1984.
5. Delamarter RB, Hohl M, Hopp E Jr: Ligament injuries associated with tibial plateau fractures, *Clin Orthop* 250:226-233, 1990.
6. Shearman CM, el-Khoury GY: Pitfalls in the radiologic evaluation of extremity trauma: Part II. The lower extremity, *Am Fam Physician* 57:1314-1322, 1998.
7. Dirschl DR, Dahners LE: Current treatment of tibial plateau fractures, *J South Orthop Assoc* 6:54-61, 1997.
8. Langer JE, Meyer SJ, Dalinka MK: Imaging of the knee, *Radiol Clin North Am* 28:975-990, 1990.

9. Cone JB: Vascular injury associated with fracture-dislocations of the lower extremity, *Clin Orthop* 243:30-35, 1989.
10. Gregory P, Sanders R: The management of severe fractures of the lower extremities, *Clin Orthop* 318:95-105, 1995.
11. Watson JT: High-energy fractures of the tibial plateau, *Orthop Clin North Am* 25:723-752, 1994.
12. Tscherne H, Lobenhoffer P: Tibial plateau fractures: management and expected results, *Clin Orthop* 292:87-100, 1993.
13. Johnson KD: Management of fractures of the femur, tibia, and upper extremity in the multiply injured patient, *Instr Course Lect* 39:565-576, 1990.
14. McQueen MM, Christie J, Court-Brown CM: Acute compartment syndrome in tibial diaphyseal fractures, *J Bone Joint Surg* 78B:95-98, 1996.
15. Gustilo RB, Anderson JT: Prevention of infection in the treatment of one thousand and twenty-five open fractures of long bones: retrospective and prospective analyses, *J Bone Joint Surg* 58A:453-458, 1976.
16. Gustilo RB, Mendoza RM, Williams DN: Problems in the management of type III (severe) open fractures: a new classification of type III open fractures, *J Trauma* 24:742-746, 1984.
17. Horn BD, Rettig ME: Interobserver reliability in the Gustilo and Anderson classification of open fractures, *J Orthop Trauma* 7:357-360, 1993.
18. Brumback RJ: Open tibial fractures: current orthopaedic management, *Instr Course Lect* 41:101-117, 1992.
19. O'Meara PM: Management of open fractures, *Orthop Rev* 21: 1117-1185, 1992.
20. Turen CH, DiStasio AJ: Treatment of grade IIIB and grade IIIC open tibial fractures, *Orthop Clin North Am* 25:561-571, 1994.
21. Wilkins J, Patzakis M: Choice and duration of antibiotics in open fractures, *Orthop Clin North Am* 22:433-437, 1991.
22. Ogden JA: Subluxation of the proximal tibiofibular joint, *Clin Orthop* 101:192-197, 1974.
23. Mabee JR: Compartment syndrome: a complication of acute extremity trauma, *J Emerg Med* 12:651-656, 1994.
24. van Essen GJ, McQueen MM: Compartment syndrome in the lower limb, *Hosp Med* 59:294-297, 1998.
25. Gulli B, Templeman D: Compartment syndrome of the lower extremity, *Orthop Clin North Am* 25:677-684, 1994.
26. Matsen FA III, Clawson DK: The deep posterior compartmental syndrome of the leg, *J Bone Joint Surg* 57A:34-39, 1975.
27. Roberts JR, Hedges JR (editors): *Clinical procedures in emergency medicine,* Philadelphia, 1998, Saunders.
28. Tornetta P 3rd, Templeman D: Compartment syndrome associated with tibial fracture, *Instr Course Lect* 46:303-308, 1997.
29. McQueen MM, Court-Brown CM: Compartment monitoring in tibial fractures: the pressure threshold for decompression, *J Bone Joint Surg* 78B:99-104, 1996.
30. Matsen FA 3rd: Compartmental syndromes, *Hosp Pract* 15:113-117, 1980.
31. Moore MN: Orthopedic pitfalls in emergency medicine, *South Med J* 81:371-378, 1988.
32. Styf J, Wiger P: Abnormally increased intramuscular pressure in human legs: comparison of two experimental models, *J Trauma* 45:133-139, 1998.

29 Ankle and Foot Injuries

E. PARKER HAYS, Jr.

ANKLE INJURIES

Injury to the ankle is a frequent emergency department (ED) complaint, and approximately 15% of these patients have clinically significant fractures.[1] Suboptimal management carries significant consequences: with each step the ankle bears the entire weight of the body; it is crucial to ambulation. Basic tenets of management include identifying specific injury, return to stable configuration, initial immobilization, and rapid return to function. Optimal emergency care may prevent long-term disability.

Anatomy

The ankle is a complex hinge joint, and allows movement along several directions. **Dorsiflexion** is extension of the ankle as the foot moves upward toward the shin. **Plantarflexion** is flexion of the ankle as the foot moves downward away from the shin. **Inversion** and **eversion** take place at the subtalar joint between the talus and calcaneus. **Internal** and **external rotation** occur at the subtalar joint as well.

The ankle **mortise**, comprised of the tibia, fibula, and talus, is held together by ligamentous structures and the joint capsule. Several tendons, including the Achilles, cross the joint tightly bound by retinacula. Neurovascular structures supplying the ankle and foot also cross the joint.

In general, the ankle joint is most stable in dorsiflexion, when the wider anterior portion of the talus is held between the malleoli. In plantarflexion (e.g., landing after a jump), the ankle is less stable because the narrower posterior portion of the talus is within the mortise and allows more laxity.[2-7]

The tibia's distal articular surface forms the **plafond** or **pilon** (French for "ceiling") of the ankle joint. Its medial extension, the **medial malleolus,** along with the terminal extension of the fibula, the **lateral malleolus,** provides bony reinforcement on each side of the talus. Supporting ligaments attach to the malleoli. The width of the joint space in neutral position is relatively uniform.

Laterally, three collateral ligaments fix the lateral malleolus to the foot.[8] The **anterior talofibular ligament (ATFL),** the **calcaneofibular ligament (CFL),** and the **posterior talofibular ligament (PTFL)** tend to sprain or rupture in this order (from front-to-back). Inversion injuries may avulse the distal fibula. The **deltoid ligament complex**[9] buttresses the medial ankle. This fan-shaped ligament is stronger than the lateral structures, but may be injured by eversion mechanisms or ankle dislocations (Fig. 29-1). The **anterior** (and **posterior**) **tibiofibular ligaments**, or **syndesmosis,** act with the **interosseous membrane** to maintain apposition of the tibia and fibula. Interruption of this membrane cripples the functional anatomy and usually requires surgery.

The nerves and arteries supplying the foot have already been discussed in Chapter 28.

Injury Patterns

ANKLE SPRAINS

Mechanism of Injury. The most common mechanism for ankle sprain is inversion, and results from sports, ambulatory trauma, motor vehicle crashes (MVCs), or falls. The lateral collateral ligaments are stretched and usually tear from front-to-back in varying degrees, typically affecting the ATFL, the CFL, and uncommonly the PTFL, in descending order of frequency (Fig. 29-2).[7,10]

Eversion or external rotation injuries may stretch or rupture portions of the deltoid ligament. This type of injury may be associated with damage to the tibiofibular ligaments or syndesmosis. Because the deltoid ligament may be stronger than bone, the medial malleolus can fracture before rupture of the deltoid.

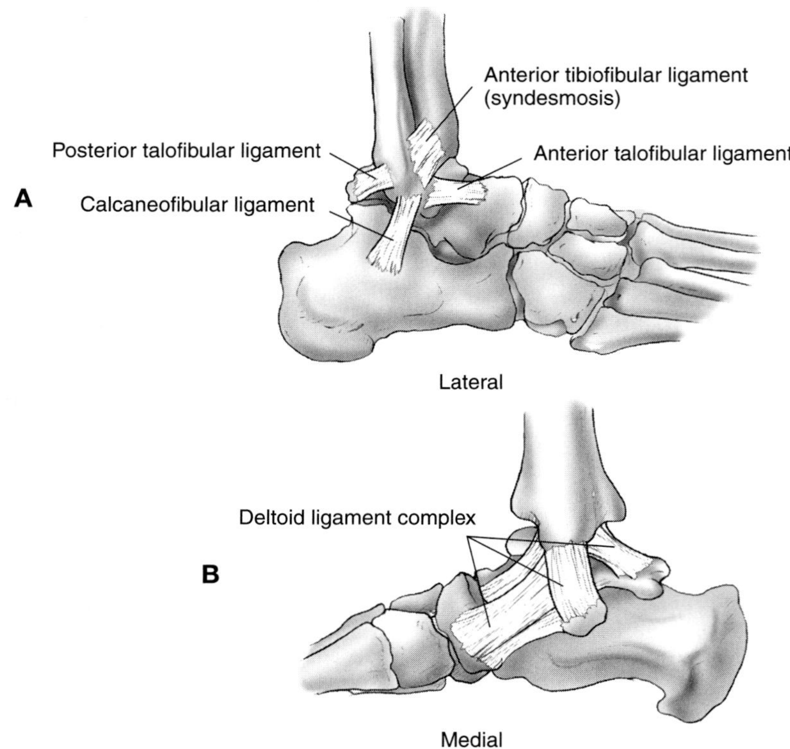

Fig. 29-1 Ligaments of the ankle. **A,** The lateral collateral ligaments consist of the anterior talofibular, calcaneofibular, and posterior talofibular ligament. **B,** The medial collateral ligament or deltoid ligament is a complex of navicular, talar, and calcaneal sections.

Many injuries involve a complex combination of forces. For example, inversion may be accompanied by external rotation, potentially injuring the lateral ligaments, as well as the medial structures and the syndesmosis.

Clinical Presentation. Patients typically complain of pain and swelling at the ankle and have decreased ability to ambulate. However, especially in stable sprains, patients may be able to walk or even continue sports immediately after injury. They seek care later when swelling and pain arise. In multiple-trauma patients with distracting injuries, the ankle may be an unrecognized or secondary complaint. However, the presence of swelling or instability on examination during the secondary survey should alert the emergency physician (EP).

Diagnosis and Radiology. Ask about the mechanism of injury and, in particular, inversion versus eversion forces. When inspecting the injured ankle, compare it with the opposite limb and look for swelling or ecchymosis. Pain with palpation of affected ligaments is a consistent sign. With inversion injuries, palpate the ATFL *last,* since the patient is likely to become less cooperative when tormented. Ask the patient to use one finger to point to the area of pain. Ask where the pain is worse, outside or inside (lateral or medial). If the medial malleolus is significantly painful, suspect a fracture or other serious injury.

Certain injuries to the foot and knee are associated with ankle sprains; palpate the proximal fibula just below the knee. A fracture of the proximal fibula in association with a syndesmotic rupture is known as a **Maisonneuve fracture.** Palpate the base of the fifth metatarsal to determine the presence of a **Dancer's** or **Jones fracture**. The integrity of the syndesmosis is an important consideration. Assess the syndesmosis by compressing the midportion of the tibia and fibula together (the "**squeeze test**") and look for referred pain to the ankle as the ligaments are stretched.[6,7,11] Achilles tendon rupture can also mimic ankle sprain; check its integrity with palpation and **Thompson's test.** To perform this test, have the patient lie prone on the stretcher and squeeze the midportion of the calf. If the Achilles tendon is intact, the foot will plantarflex.

To determine the stability of the ankle, use the **anterior drawer test**, by grasping the posterior calcaneus and attempting to move the foot forward on the leg.[7,12] The knee must be flexed and the muscles around the ankle relaxed. Look for a "dimpling" over the ATFL if significant swelling is absent, and com-

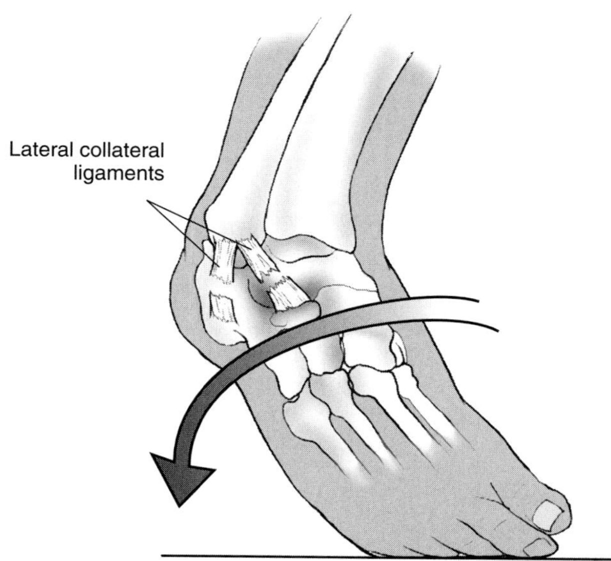

Fig. 29-2 Inversion ankle sprain. As the inverted foot "rolls," lateral ligaments tend to sprain or rupture from front-to-back, affecting the anterior talofibular ligament, calcaneofibular ligament, and posterior talofibular ligament.

pare the laxity in relation with the contralateral ankle (Box 29-1). Other stability tests are usually not practical in the ED because of pain.

Sprains are graded according to severity and degree of ligamentous disruption.[7,13,14] Partial stretching or tears are grade 1 or 2, characterized by mild-to-moderate swelling, ecchymosis, and functional impairment. Grade 3 sprains have complete ligament rupture and demonstrate marked swelling, ecchymosis, inability to bear weight, and instability on testing (Box 29-2).

Because ankle injury is so common, and because most radiographs are negative, researchers examined whether history and physical examination can determine the need for a radiograph. Traditionally 95% of ED patients with ankle injuries receive radiographs; however, 85% of these studies are negative.[15] A Canadian group developed and validated the Ottawa ankle rules (Box 29-3) to virtual 100% sensitivity in a variety of settings.[1,16-19] These rules have the potential to decrease costs for the emergency management of ankle injuries by $600,000 to over $3 million for every 100,000 patients.[20] The rules can decrease costs, waiting time, and unnecessary radiation exposure.

The Ottawa ankle rules highlight the value of an artful clinical evaluation. However, exercise caution in assessing a trauma patient with distracting injury, intoxication, or children with open epiphyseal plates. Such patients may require a lower threshold for obtaining radiographs and initiating treatment.

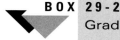

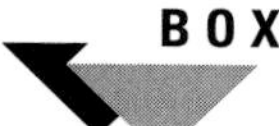

BOX 29-1 The Ankle Examination

INSPECTION
How did patient enter examination room, remove sock or shoe? Compare with opposite *exposed* ankle and foot
Note deformity, swelling, ecchymosis, previous scars, *and any* skin breaks

PALPATION
Start *away* from the probable site of injury
Assess the distal motor, sensory, and vascular function/pulses
Palpate the (proximal) fibular shaft, the base of the fifth metatarsal, the deltoid ligament
Palpate the posterior malleolar edges and tips

TESTS
Squeeze test
Anterior drawer test
Thompson's test

PALPATION
Palpate the lateral ligaments from back-to-front

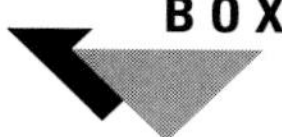

BOX 29-2 Grading Ankle Sprains

GRADE 1: STRETCHING OF LIGAMENT(S)
Minimal pain, swelling, ecchymosis, loss of functional ability; can bear weight

GRADE 2: PARTIAL TEAR OF LIGAMENT(S)
Increasing pain, swelling, ecchymosis, and loss of functional ability; usually difficulty with bearing weight

GRADE 3: COMPLETE TEAR OF LIGAMENT(S)
Severe pain, swelling, and ecchymosis, loss of functional ability; nearly always unable to bear weight; positive drawer sign

According to local protocol, triage nurses may apply these rules to order radiographs before physician evaluation—potentially saving both time and money. If the physician explains to the patient why a radiograph is unnecessary, patient satisfaction is the same in "no-films" compared with the irradiated group.

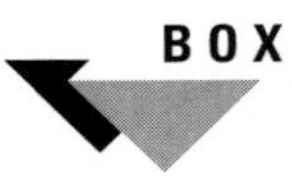

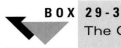

BOX 29-3
The Ottawa Ankle Rules

An ankle radiographic series is only required if there is pain in the ankle malleolar "zone" and any of these findings:

1. Bone tenderness at the posterior edge (distal 6 cm) or tip of the lateral malleolus

   or

2. Bone tenderness at the posterior edge (distal 6 cm) or tip of the medial malleolus

   or

3. Inability to bear weight both immediately and in ED (2 steps each leg)

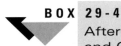

Emergency Management and Disposition. In grade 1 and 2 sprains, the physician should minimize inflammatory response, initially immobilize, and promote early mobilization and physical therapy to aid in healing and prevent functional instability.[7,13,21-29] Functional instability can occur in up to 40% of sprains and is characterized by persistent "giving way," subjective instability, or recurrent pain in a previously sprained ankle.[25] Correlated with more severe ankle sprains (especially those involving the syndesmotic and the calcaneofibular ligaments[10,25]), its incidence may be decreased with accurate initial assessment of severity, ligament protection, and an active physical therapy program.

Institute **RICE** (*r*est, *i*ce, *c*ompression, and *e*levation) **therapy** immediately after injury or as soon as possible to *prevent* subsequent swelling as much as to decrease existing edema. Treat pain and inflammation with a nonsteroidal antiinflammatory agent.[23]

Various immobilization or support devices are available, including over-the-counter appliances. Initially, elastic wraps provide compression, are inexpensive, and are readily available. They are appropriate for minor sprains (grade 1) without significant ligament involvement, since they provide little or no lateral support. Other devices such as air stirrup-splints restrict inversion/eversion but allow dorsiflexion/plantarflexion (a "functional brace").[30] These splints promote an earlier return to walking, daily activities, or work.[21,22,26,27] Choose appliances based on severity of ligamentous involvement and functional requirements, as well as expense and availability. On discharge, provide crutches for non–weight-bearing in the first 24 to 48 hours with instructions to advance as tolerated.

Detailed instructions for discharge and home physical therapy are crucial (Box 29-4). The concept of

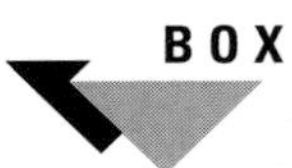

BOX 29-4
Aftercare for Grade 1 and Grade 2 Ankle Sprains

- *Initially,* RICE (*R*est by using crutches, *I*ce for 25 minutes at a time, *C*ompression with elastic wrap or air splint to prevent swelling, *E*levation of ankle above the level of the heart)
- *In first 48 hours or when pain allows,* begin range-of-motion exercises (drawing alphabet with toes)
- *When patient can bear standing weight comfortably,* begin strengthening exercises (dorsiflexing foot against a strap looped around chair leg, rolling a ball up wall with lateral foot) and gentle stretching of Achilles tendon
- *When range of motion is near-normal and pain allows,* begin proprioceptive exercises (one-leg standing, then with eyes closed)

Caveats: If pain and swelling increase, decrease intensity of therapy. Grade 2 sprains should be protected during therapy with a functional brace for 4 weeks.

functional management suggests that early return to protected range of motion prevents declines in strength and stability in an injured joint, and promotes edema resolution, increase in strength, and return in proprioceptive ability.[7,24,26,28,29] Instruct patients to follow up with their primary care doctor or orthopedist.

Patients with grade 3 sprains may require a plaster splint or cast and orthopedic referral. The air or gel stirrup devices may suffice for early follow-up. If protected with a functional brace for 3 to 6 months, most patients do well with early mobilization and physical therapy.[7,26,27,31] Although in the United States nonsurgical management is usually preferred, competitive athletes may be candidates for surgery.[7]

Even in the absence of fracture, patients with suspicion of syndesmotic injury as evidenced by localized pain, palpation tenderness, a positive squeeze test, or radiographic signs (Fig. 29-3) should be immobilized with a splint and provided prompt orthopedic referral.[32]

There is no universal agreement on splinting techniques. Ankle splints include the stirrup splint (in which the plaster straps go under the arch of the foot and up each side of the leg like a foot in a stirrup) and the posterior splint (where the strips go down the posterior leg, under the heel, and out the foot). A combination splint combines both splints on the same leg. For the unstable ankle, a stirrup or combination splint may provide greater support.

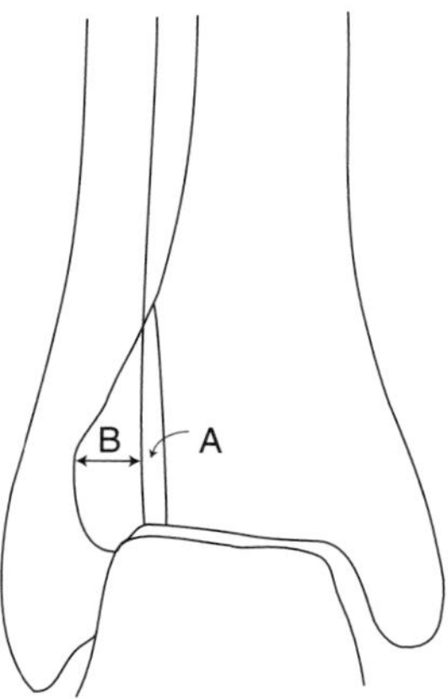

Fig. 29-3 Schematic showing syndesmotic injury. This patient has an isolated lateral malleolar fracture with normal syndesmotic relationships. Compare these measurements with Fig. 29-10.

ANKLE FRACTURES

Mechanism of Injury. Mechanisms similar to ankle sprains (inversion or eversion, rotation), axial loading, forced hyperdorsiflexion or hyperplantarflexion, may all result in fracture to the ankle. Inversion may cause the lateral ligaments to avulse fragments of bone from the lateral malleolus, whereas eversions may fracture either the lateral malleolus directly or avulse the medial malleolus. Falls with axial loading may transmit energy upward through the distal tibia resulting in a tibial pilon (plafond) fracture. Rotational forces may fracture the malleoli, disrupt the syndesmotic ligaments, or transmit up the fibula with a proximal spiral fracture.

The ankle has been compared with the ring structure of the pelvis,[33] where one break in the continuity of the joint tends to be associated with another injury in the circle.

Clinical Presentation. Pain, swelling, and inability to ambulate are nearly uniform findings. Attempts to ascertain the mechanism and position of the ankle at the time of injury may suggest specific fracture patterns.

Diagnosis and Radiology. A variety of classification systems describe ankle fractures.[3,26,34-36] Knowing the classification allows for excellent communication with the orthopedist and can determine the timing of follow-up or need for admission. The **Weber** system is most useful to describe distal fibular fractures.

The **Lauge-Hansen system** is based on pure injury patterns and accounts for the mechanism of force and the position of the ankle at injury. The Lauge-Hansen classification is still used by many orthopedists to assess for associated ligamentous injuries and to plan operative repair. However, its complexity and injury variations from the described patterns limit its use in the emergency evaluation.

The **Danis-Weber** (often just **Weber**, pronounced *va-ber*) classification is simpler and is based on the location of the fibular fracture in relation to the articular surface of the tibia. It carries implications for potential injury to the syndesmotic tibiofibular ligament:

- **Type A:** Fracture of the fibula below the level of the syndesmosis (at the plafond); an inversion (supination) avulsion fracture
- **Type B:** Oblique or spiral fracture of the fibula at or near the syndesmosis; external rotation force, causing disruption of the anterior tibiofibular (syndesmotic) ligament in 50% of cases
- **Type C:** Fibula fracture above the level of the syndesmosis with disruption of the syndesmotic ligament; often has medial malleolus fracture; includes Maisonneuve injury

A comparison of the Weber and Lauge-Hansen classification systems is depicted in Fig. 29-4. Regardless of the classification system used by orthopedists in a local area, the EP must be able to describe fracture components and mortise disruption to an orthopedic consultant to help guide subsequent therapy.[37,38]

Isolated Malleolar Fractures

Lateral Malleolar Fractures. **Single lateral malleolar fractures** may result from inversion stresses, avulsing the distal fibula through the pull of its collateral ligaments. Inversion stress injuries appear as transverse fractures, ranging from small chips to significantly displaced fragments. These fractures are usually seen at or below the top of the mortise on anteroposterior (AP) or radiographs corresponding to Weber A. An example of an unusually subtle Weber A fracture is seen in Fig. 29-5.

Oblique fibular fractures at the level of the syndesmosis (above the top of the mortise on radiograph) correspond to Weber B (Fig. 29-6). They may have associated transverse medial malleolar fractures, deltoid ligament rupture, and anterior syndesmotic disruption.

Weber A lateral malleolar fractures that are minimally displaced and do not have an associated medial fracture or mortise disruption do well. Treat such patients with a short-leg posterior splint, non–weight-bearing, RICE, and orthopedic follow-up within a week. Those patients with mortise widening or marked displacement require immobilization and orthopedic consultation. Assume that Weber B and C fractures may have syndesmotic injury. Immobilize and consult orthopedics.

Medial Malleolar Fractures. **Isolated medial malleolar fractures** are much less common than lateral fractures, usually occurring with bimalleolar or

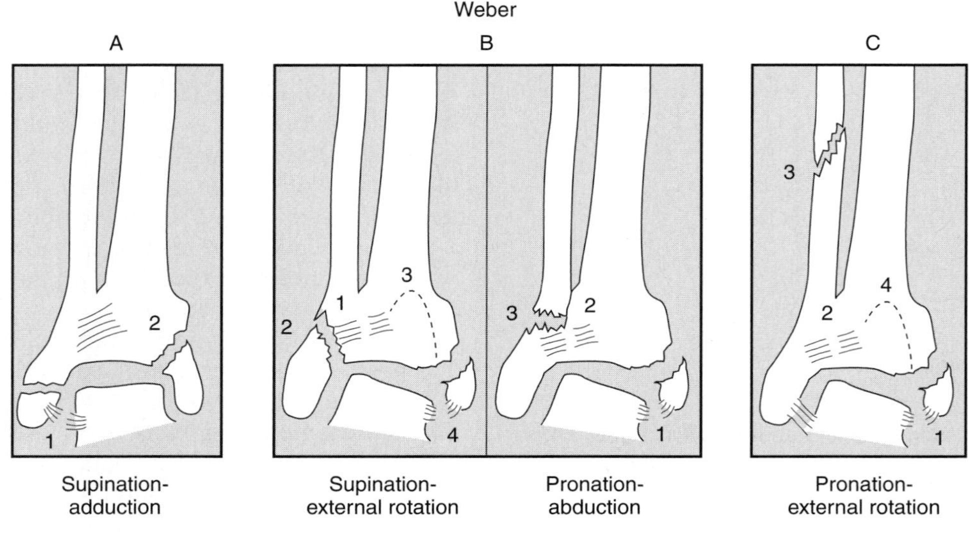

Fig. 29-4 Weber and Lauge-Hansen classifications. Weber types A, B, and C are determined by the location of the fibular fracture to the top of the mortise. Lauge-Hansen stages are indicated by the numbers and represent progression of injury severity.

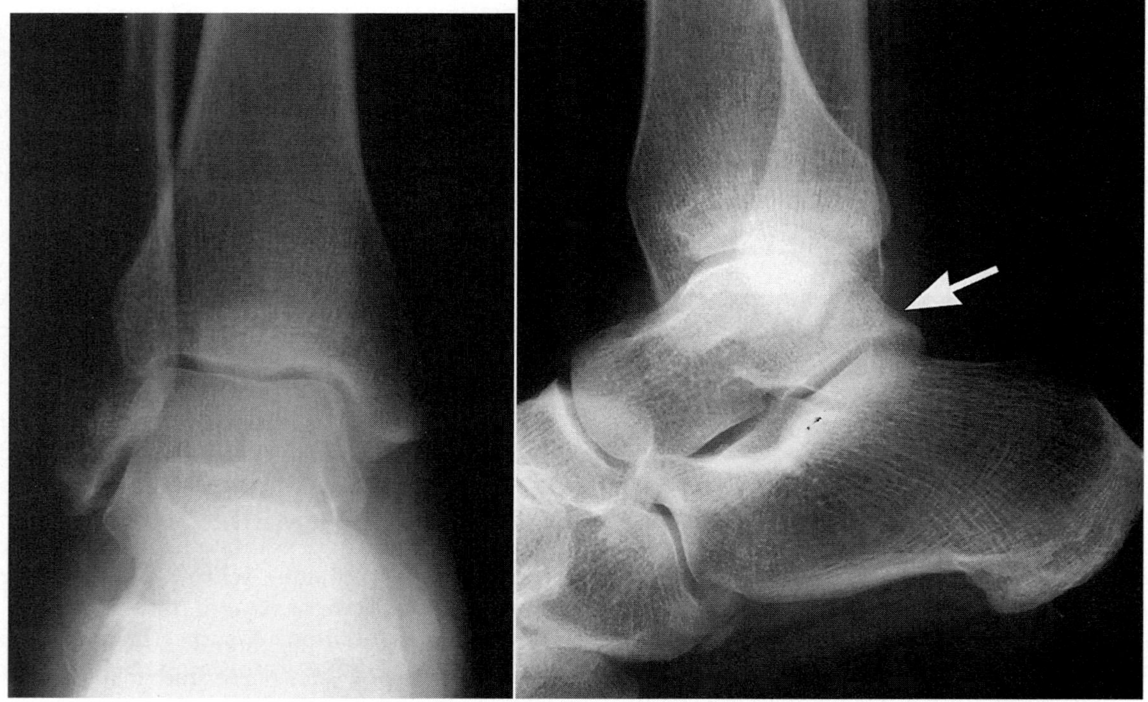

Fig. 29-5 Isolated lateral malleolus fracture. This subtle, minimally displaced fracture was only well visualized on the lateral projection. This fracture is a Weber A.

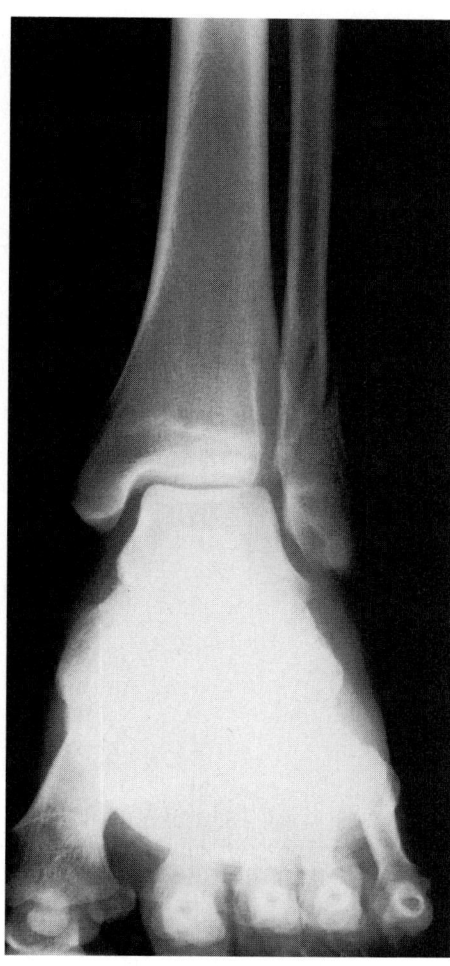

Fig. 29-6 Weber B ankle fracture. The fracture lines extend obliquely from the mortise. The medial joint line (between medial malleolus and talus) is somewhat widened. This patient had deltoid ligament rupture and was later treated with surgery.

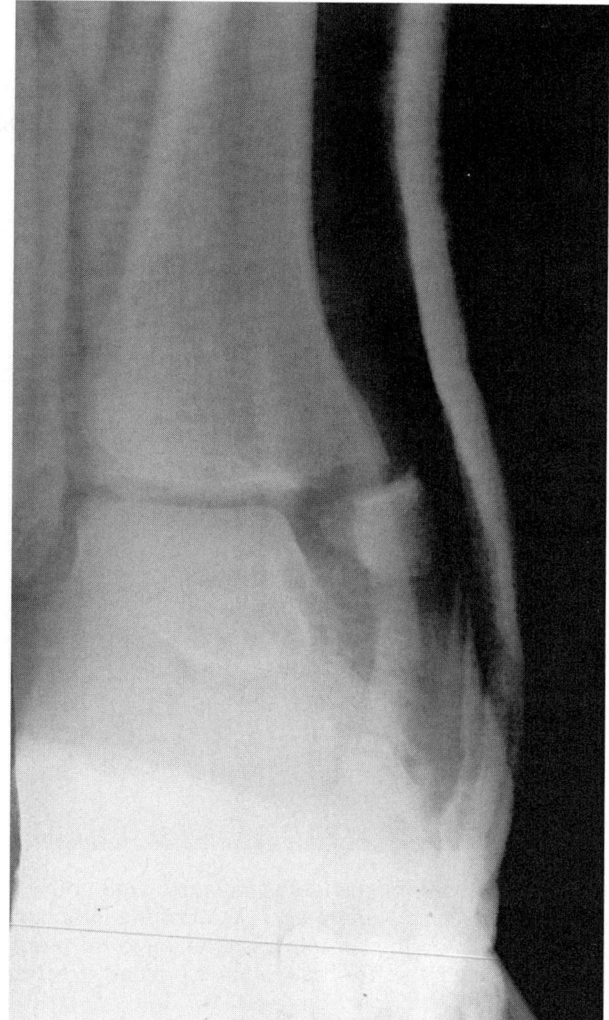

Fig. 29-7 Isolated medial malleolar fracture.

trimalleolar fracture patterns. Eversion mechanisms may result in an isolated transverse medial malleolar fracture, corresponding to Lauge-Hansen pronation-abduction stage I (Fig. 29-7). However, maintain a high degree of suspicion for syndesmotic injury (stage II) and fracture along the fibula (stage III).

Often the mortise is unstable and operative fixation is indicated; therefore prompt orthopedic consultation is warranted. If immediate follow-up is arranged, discharge with a bulky splint and non–weight-bearing.

Bimalleolar Fractures. Bimalleolar fractures consist of fracture to the lateral malleolus and either the medial or posterior malleolus.[39] Although frequently obvious on lateral projection, posterior malleolus fractures can be subtle, as seen in Fig. 29-8. Syndesmotic injury is common. It is important to communicate the degree of mortise disruption and fragment displacement to the orthopedist.

Because some bimalleolar fractures may represent spontaneously reduced dislocation, carefully assess neurovascular status. Immobilization in a bulky splint and padding and immediate orthopedic consultation are appropriate.

Trimalleolar Fractures. Trimalleolar fractures result from complex directional mechanisms and include fractures of the lateral, medial, and posterior malleoli. On occasion, these fractures involve dislocation or displacement of the talus relative to the tibia (Fig. 29-9). Treatment is essentially the same as for bimalleolar fractures.

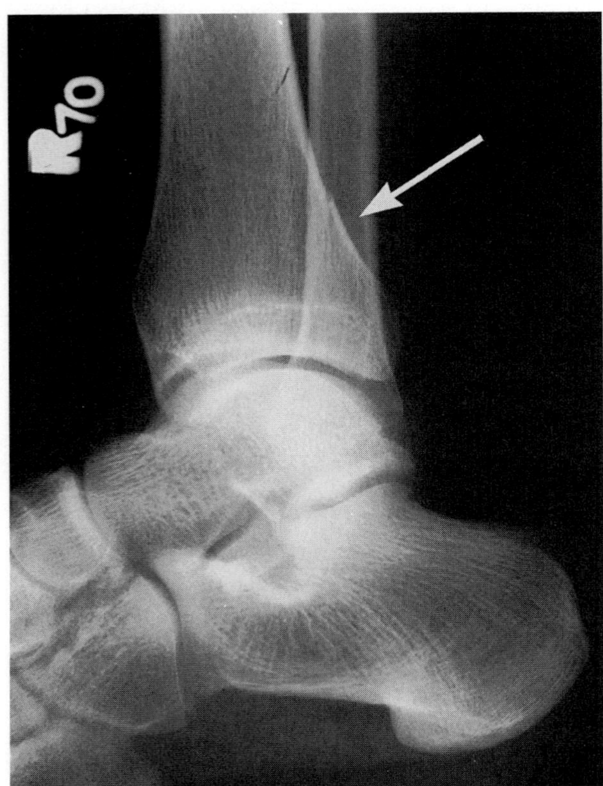

Fig. 29-8 Posterior malleolus fracture. This unusually subtle fracture was evident as a result of the interrupted cortical margin on the lateral view. The posterior process of the tibia (the posterior malleolus) is typically fractured with the lateral or medial malleoli.

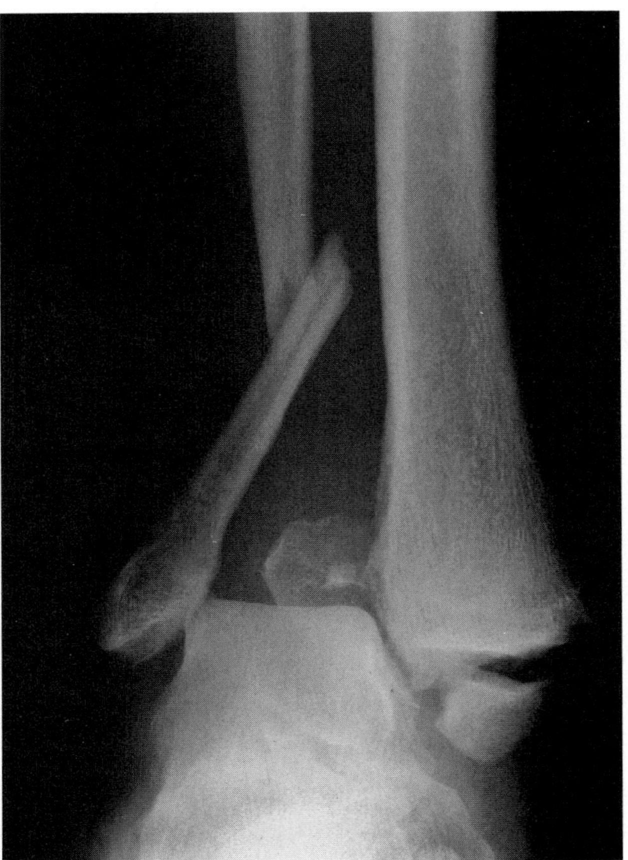

Fig. 29-9 Lateral ankle dislocation. The talus is dislocated laterally in conjunction with a trimalleolar fracture. In the initial view, note the posterior malleolus fragment just above the talus.

Maisonneuve Injury. This injury complex consists of a medial malleolar fracture or deltoid disruption, syndesmotic rupture, and a proximal oblique fibular fracture. The interosseous membrane may also tear. It results from external rotation of the inverted foot and is similar to bimalleolar fractures that might otherwise be a Weber B. However, the torque is transmitted up the fibula, fracturing it proximally. It can occur when a patient twists his or her ankle in a fall from a height. A Maisonneuve injury is a Weber C fracture (pronation-external rotation stage III). In Fig. 29-10, note that the deltoid ligament can rupture without fracture, and that the fracture of the fibular shaft runs from anterosuperior to posteroinferior.[2]

Always include palpation of the proximal fibula near the knee in patients with an ankle injury. After neurovascular assessment, perform reduction if indicated. Consultation for open reduction and fixation is the rule.

Plafond (Pilon) Fractures. In a violent axial load mechanism, the talus rams against the distal tibial plafond, resulting in complex oblique fracture lines (Fig. 29-11).[36,40] The synonyms for these injuries, **pilon** (French for "pile-driver") or **pylon** (Greek for supports of a doorway arch), reflect the injurious force through the roof of the mortise.[36] Sometimes the malleoli maintain their relative positions but the joint is unstable.

After neurovascular and soft-tissue assessment, place a bulky splint and padding and consult for surgical repair. Computed tomography (CT) may delineate fracture fragment location and guide surgery. This study is usually ordered by the orthopedist as he or she see fit.

Talar Dome Fractures (Osteochondritis Dessicans). The superior surface of the talus is covered with articular cartilage. This cartilage may tear with or without a fragment of underlying bone. The classic

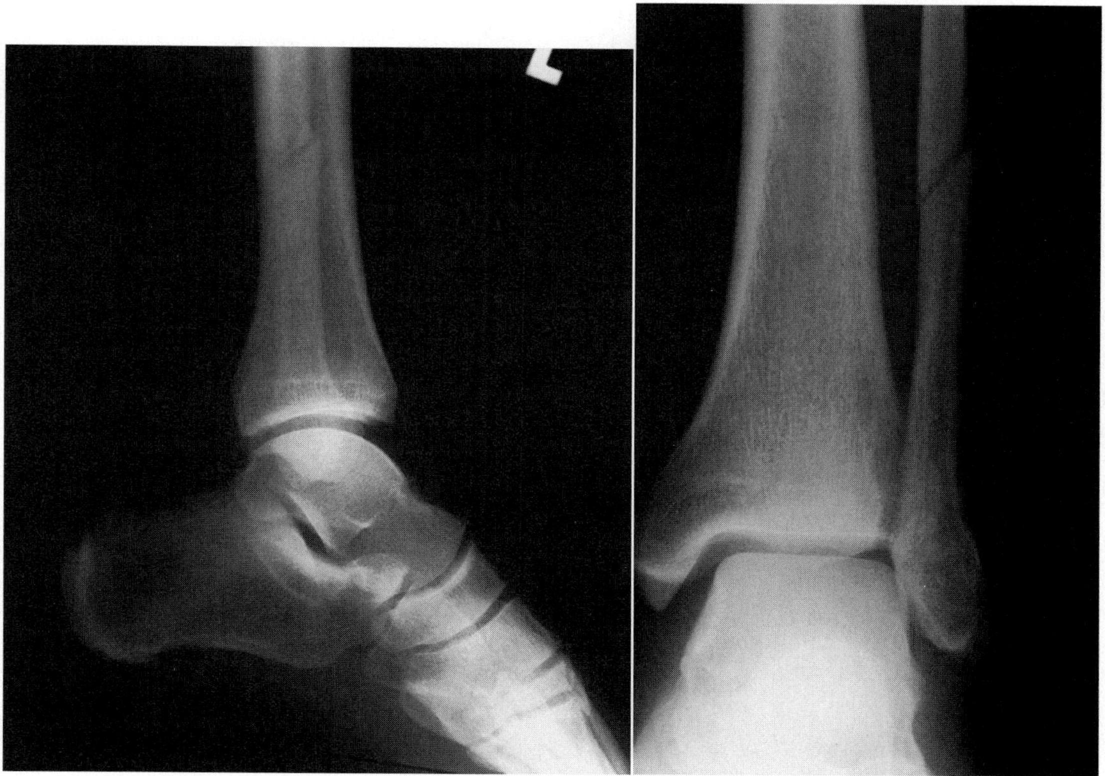

Fig. 29-10 Maisonneuve injury. Note the widened medial joint space, syndesmotic rupture (widened clear space and decreased tibiofibular overlap on anteroposterior view), and the oblique fracture of the proximal fibula. This fracture is a Weber C.

history is an ankle sprain that is not healing.[4,13,14,41] Patients may present with a hemarthrosis or delayed presentation until persistent pain or locking prompt evaluation.[41] The patient may have had a "negative" radiograph from a previous visit.

If carefully scrutinized, radiographs may reveal a subtle irregularity in the talus or densities within the joint space. CT scanning or magnetic resonance imaging (MRI) may be used nonemergently. Immobilize the ankle, prohibit weight-bearing, and provide orthopedic follow-up.

ANKLE DISLOCATIONS

Mechanism of Injury. The loss of articulation between the talus and the ankle mortise results from exaggerated mechanisms described for ankle sprains and fractures. Dislocations are virtually always accompanied by significant malleolar fracture and ligamentous disruption. For example, a posterior dislocation may result from axially loading and forcibly inverting a plantarflexed foot. Anterior dislocation may result from posterior forces on the tibia with a fixed foot, as in a motorcyclist's foot on the foot peg. Subtalar dislocations (foot dislocations) are described in the foot injury section that follows.

Clinical Presentation. Gross deformity with tenting of skin, swelling, and ecchymosis make the diagnosis obvious. However, spontaneously reduced dislocations must be considered in bimalleolar or trimalleolar fractures, especially those with neurovascular compromise.

Diagnosis and Radiology. Ankle dislocations are classified into three types with regards to the foot relative to the tibia: posterior, anterior, and lateral. Posterior dislocations are the most common. In addition to the posterior and lateral position of the talus, the anterior joint capsule and collateral ligaments are disrupted to varying degrees. Anterior dislocations are associated with bimalleolar fractures and collateral ligament disruption. Lateral dislocations, likewise, virtually always have associated lateral malleolus or bimalleolar fractures.

Emergency Management and Disposition. After assessment of the trauma patient for other significant injuries, give first priority to neurovascular status. Note time since injury, foot and toe color, temperature, sensation, capillary refill time, motor ability, and presence of palpable or Doppler dorsalis pedis and posterior tibial pulses. If significant compromise exists, reduce the dislocation promptly. Reduction may need to be accomplished even before radiographs are obtained if films are likely to significantly prolong ischemia time. However, if blood flow is not significantly compromised, get radiographs first to visualize fractures and look for intraarticular bony fragments. Obtain emergency orthopedic consultation either before or after ankle reduction. *However, the EP must reduce the ankle if there are any signs of vascular compromise.* Frequently reassess neurovascular status, especially after any reduction attempts.

Ankle dislocations are easy to reduce. In all the techniques, an assistant should stabilize the leg and apply countertraction when needed. Perform the reduction after adequate sedation and analgesia, with the hip and knee flexed to decrease tension on the gastrocnemius muscle and Achilles tendon.[42] Reduce posterior dislocations by holding the posterior heel with one hand, the dorsal foot with the other, and pulling the foot forward, as in removing a boot. Reduce anterior dislocations by plantarflexing the foot slightly and pushing the foot posteriorly. This maneuver may require initial traction to "unlock" the foot. Reduce lateral dislocations by applying traction and some medial pressure to the foot while an assistant applies countertraction. Again, reassess neurovascular status. Obtain postreduction radiographs and immobilize the ankle in a bulky splint and padding, anticipating surgical repair.

These injuries are frequently open (Fig. 29-12). Examine the skin very carefully for even minute wounds. An open injury requires intravenous (IV) antibiotics. Cefazolin 1 gm IV is appropriate for clean minor wounds, but add an aminoglycoside if the wound is >1 cm and has moderate contamination. If the injury occurred on a farm, add penicillin to cover for *Clostridium*.[37] Keep wounds clean and covered. Provide tetanus prophylaxis as indicated.

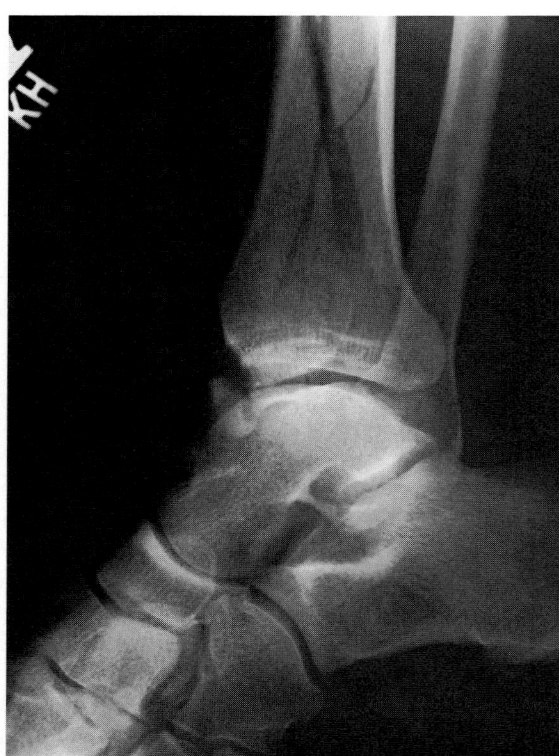

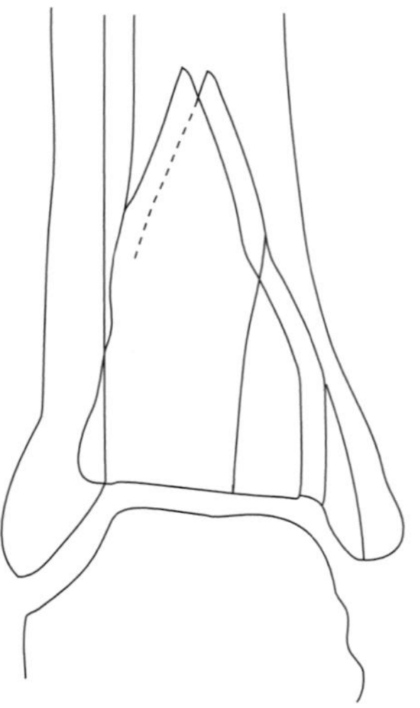

Fig. 29-11 Tibial plafond fracture. The talus acts as a ram, driving into the "ceiling" of the ankle joint, with resulting complex fracture lines.

FOOT INJURIES

The foot is a complex unit that absorbs shocks, is a base for ambulation, and transmits force to the ground. Its dependent peripheral location and relative lack of soft-tissue protection, together with the tremendous demands placed on it, make it susceptible to injury.[43] Foot injuries cause significant disability in multiply-injured trauma patients.[44]

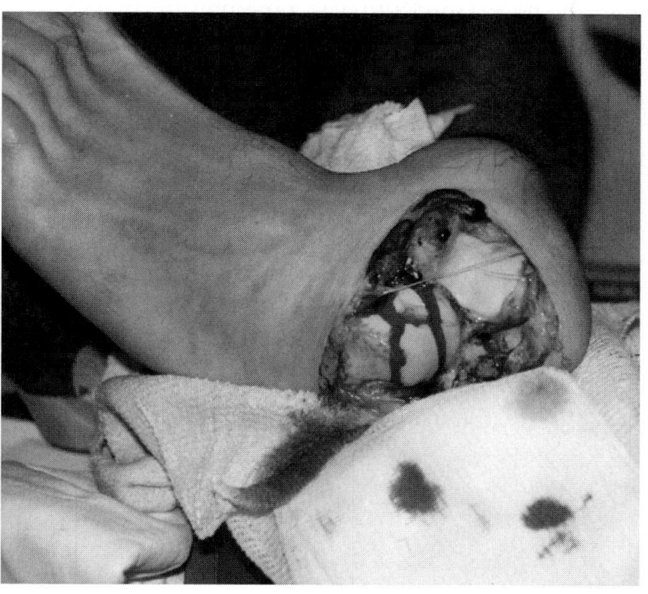

Fig. 29-12 Open tibiotalar dislocation.

Anatomy

The bony anatomy of the foot consists of 28 bones, and divides the foot into 3 parts: the hindfoot, the midfoot, and the forefoot (Fig. 29-13). The **hindfoot** contains the **talus** and the **calcaneus**. The calcaneus is the largest bone in the foot, with a thin cortical shell around trabecular bone. It projects posteriorly from the vertical axis of the leg, and functions as a shock absorber, making it susceptible to injury in falls. It articulates superiorly with the talus and anteriorly with the cuboid. Its blood supply is via ligamentous attachments to the talus. The largest of the calcaneotalar articulations is the **posterior facet**, which has important prognostic implications in calcaneal fractures.

The talus bears the entire weight of the body. It has a head, neck, and body. The body is trapezoidal in shape, being wider anteriorly, and fits between the malleoli on the distal tibia in the ankle mortise. It is almost entirely covered with articular cartilage. The talus sits on the anteromedial aspect of the calcaneus. The talar neck is relatively narrow on lateral view, and the lateral process protrudes into the recess of the calcaneus at the **crucial angle of Gissane**; this anatomy allows the talus to act as a "wedge," driving it into the calcaneus in axial load injuries.

Important vascular structures traverse the hindfoot. The **anterior tibial artery** progresses anterior to the talus and between the first and second toes, palpable over the midfoot as the **dorsalis pedis pulse**. The **posterior tibial artery** crosses from behind the medial malleolus (palpable as the **posterior tibial pulse**) over

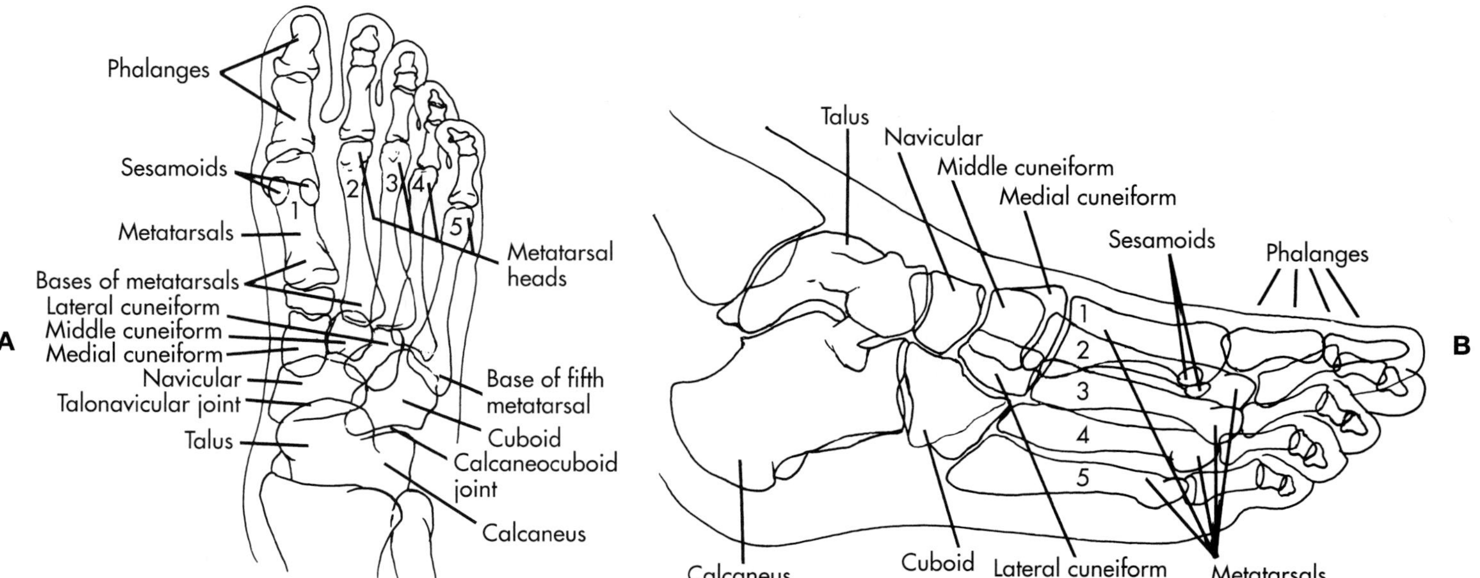

Fig. 29-13 Anatomic drawings of the foot. **A,** Anteroposterior projection. **B,** Medial oblique projection. (From Traughber PD: Imaging of the foot and ankle. In Coughlin MJ, Mann RA: *Surgery of the foot and ankle,* ed 7, St Louis, 1999, Mosby.)

the medial talus and calcaneus to form the plantar arteries supplying the sole.

The **flexor hallucis longus** tendon passes between the posterior tubercles of the talus and under the **sustentaculum tali** of the calcaneus. Fractures of these structures may cause pain if the patient moves the great toe.

Chopart's joint, collectively consisting of the talonavicular and calcaneocuboid articulations, is the boundary between the hindfoot and the midfoot.

The **midfoot** region of the foot contains the **navicular** medially, the **cuboid** laterally, and the three **cuneiforms** anterior to the navicular and medial to the cuboid. The middle or second cuneiform is recessed posteriorly, forming a notch in which sits the base of the second metatarsal. The navicular has some attachments of the **posterior tibial tendon**, which can cause avulsion fractures. The midfoot bones contribute to the arches of the foot. Their resultant prominence dorsally, along with the metatarsals, makes them prone to direct injurious blows from heavy objects.

The **forefoot** consists of the five **metatarsals**, the medial and lateral **sesamoids** at the distal first metatarsal, and the *phalanges*. The metatarsals are held to each other and the tarsals by ligamentous attachments, which when disrupted allows displacement in various directions. The proximal base of the fifth metatarsal is the insertion of the **peroneus brevis tendon**, which can cause an avulsion fracture with forcible inversion. Individual or neighboring metatarsals are particularly susceptible to falling object injuries, whereas the toes (phalanges) are prone to axial loads ("stubbing") or lateral displacement. The forefoot as a whole is susceptible to crush mechanisms, soft-tissue injury, and subsequent infection or other complications. The great toe is particularly important during the "push-off" phase of walking, and chronic pain or deformity after injury can be very debilitating.

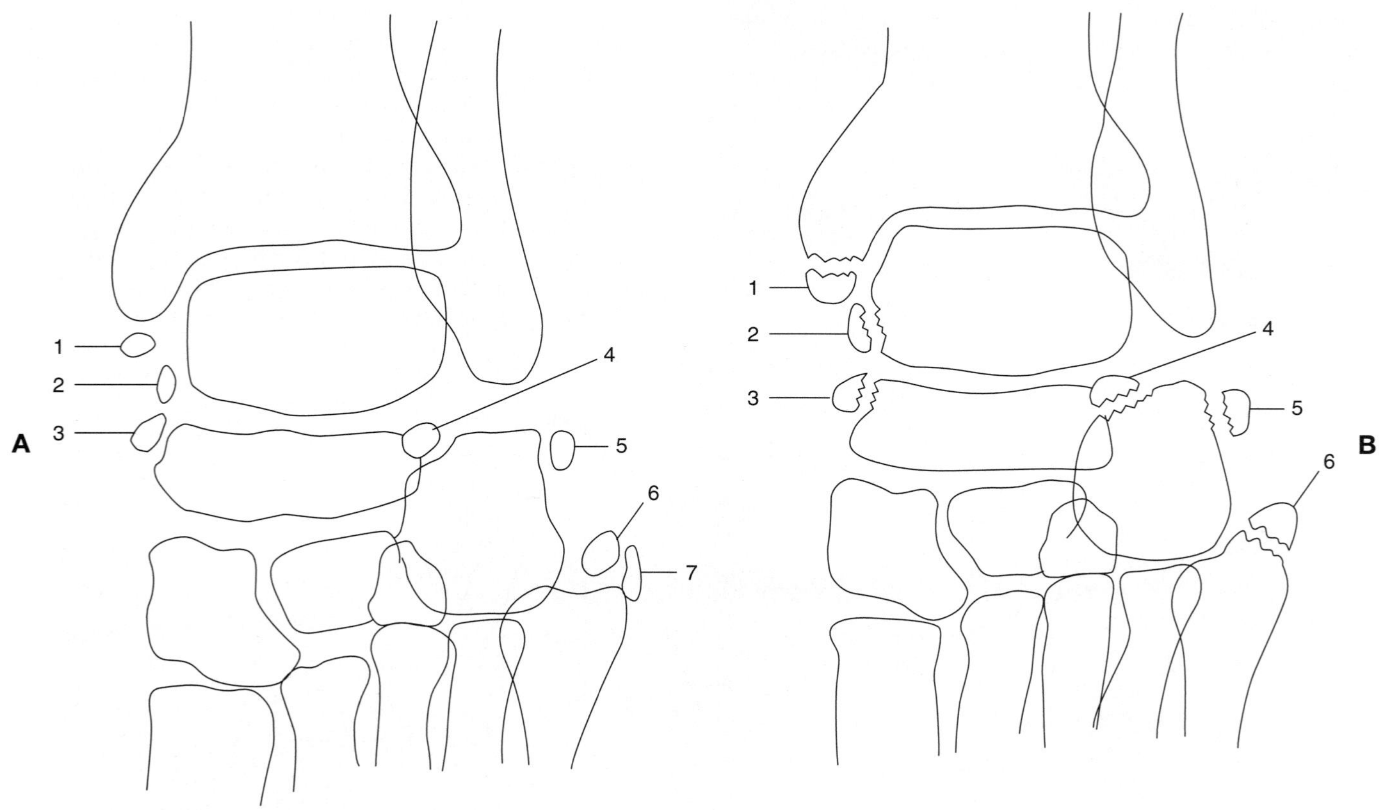

Fig. 29-14 Fractures versus accessory ossicles similarly located. **A,** Accessory ossicles. *1,* Os subtibiale; *2,* accessory talus; *3,* os tibiale externum; *4,* os cuboids secondarium; *5,* os peroneum; *6,* os vesalianum; *7,* apophysis of fifth metatarsal. **B,** Fractures. *1,* Tip of medial malleolus; *2,* medial border of talus; *3,* medial border of navicular; *4,* proximal medial tip of cuboid; *5,* proximal lateral border of cuboid; *6,* base of fifth metatarsal. (Adapted from Zatzkin HR: *Sem Roentgenol* 5:419, 1970.)

The articulation between the midfoot and the forefoot is called **Lisfranc's joint,** for the French military physician Jacques Lisfranc who first described amputation through this joint nearly a century ago.

Awareness of the various accessory bones of the foot (Fig. 29-14) is useful since these ossicles can be confused with acute fractures.[45] Accessory bones are typically round, oval, or triangular and have a smoother cortical margin than the jagged or irregular surfaces of fractures. The navicular is bipartite in some patients, and this variant can mimic a fracture on radiograph.

Injury Patterns

HINDFOOT INJURIES

Talus Fractures and Dislocations. A variety of mechanisms may result in chip fractures of the cortex, or fractures of the neck, body, or posterior process of the talus. Osteochondral (dome of the talus) injuries are covered in the preceding section. In general, the talus has a tenuous blood supply. This resultant high risk of nonunion warrants prompt orthopedic consultation for all but the most minor nondisplaced or cortical avulsion fractures.[46]

Cortical chip fractures are the most common talar fractures.[47] The anterior cortex can be avulsed in flexion or inversion injuries that stress the talonavicular ligament.[43,48] The dorsal talonavicular accessory bone may be confused with this fracture. The posterior process (specifically the lateral tubercle)[49] can be injured by excessive foot plantarflexion, where the posterior tibia compresses the process against the calcaneus. Patients may complain of pain at the fracture site if they wiggle their great toe. This fracture may be confused with the **os trigonum**, which represents the failure of the lateral tubercle to unite with the talar body during ossification (Fig. 29-15). Treat cortical chip fractures with immobilization in a rigid splint or cast and arrange orthopedic follow-up.

The **neck of the talus** may be injured by excessive dorsiflexion of the foot during which the anterior tibia contacts the talar neck.[50] The injury may be caused by falls or MVCs and was described in wartime airplane pilots whose feet rested on the rudder bar and were forcibly dorsiflexed in crashes ("aviator's astraga-

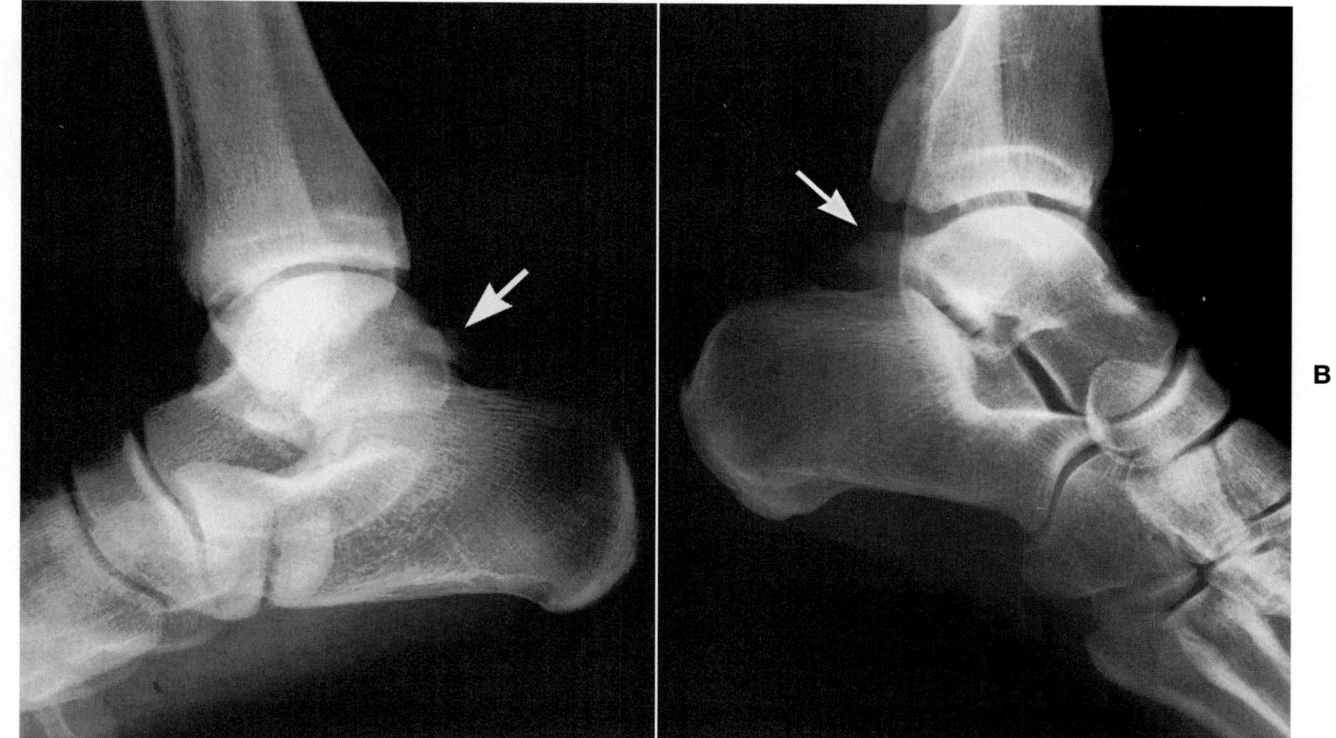

Fig. 29-15 Talus fracture versus os trigonum. A common accessory bone can be confused with injury. **A,** Os trigonum, with triangular shape and smooth margins. **B,** Nondisplaced posterior process fracture. Patient had pain with great toe movement. This injury was treated with casting and follow-up.

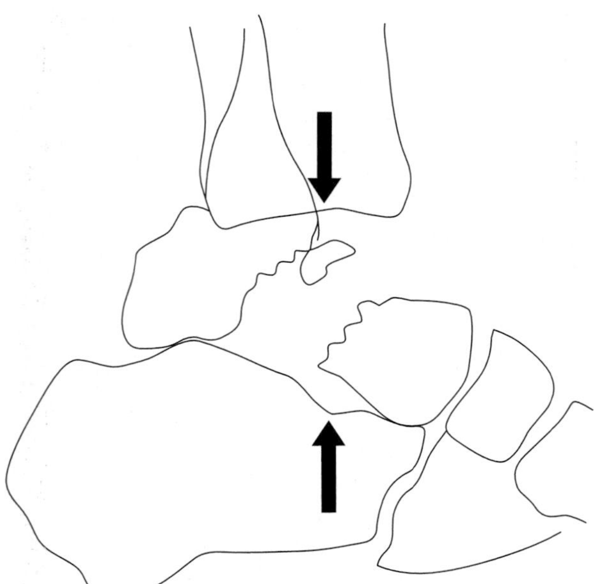

Fig. 29-16 Body of talus fracture. These fractures are caused by high-energy falls or axial-loading mechanisms.

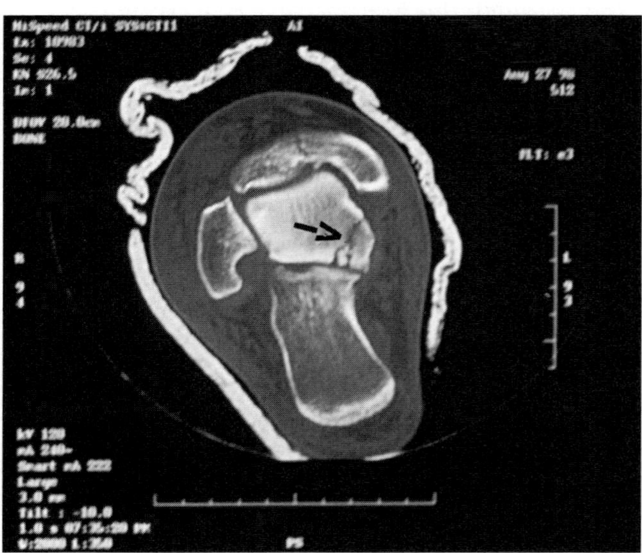

Fig. 29-17 Computed tomography scan of talus fracture.

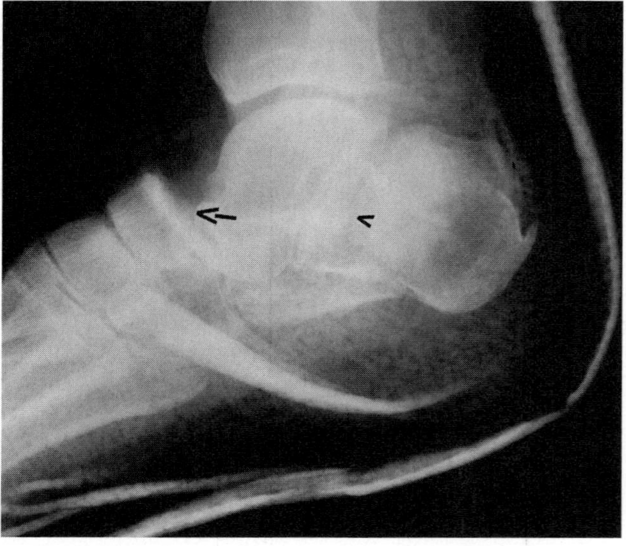

Fig. 29-18 Talonavicular dislocation. Arrow points to dislocation; arrowhead points to associated calcaneus fracture.

lus").[51] Three types have been described with different implications for their treatment.[43,52]

- **Type I:** Talar neck fracture with minimal displacement
- **Type II:** Talar neck fracture with subtalar dislocation or subluxation
- **Type III:** Talar neck fracture with dislocation of the body of the talus from the ankle joint

Treat type I fractures with non–weight-bearing and casting and refer for orthopedic evaluation. Type II and III injuries should be consulted emergently for closed or open reduction. The tenuous blood supply accounts for the high incidence of avascular necrosis.

Fractures of the **body of the talus** are typically caused by high-energy axial load mechanisms or falls (Fig. 29-16). In general, relatively subtle derangements or lucencies on plain films belie the damage and comminution evident on CT scanning (Fig. 29-17).[43] Nondisplaced fractures may initially be treated with a non–weight-bearing splint and urgent orthopedic follow-up. Displaced or comminuted fractures should be consulted for surgical consideration.

Subtalar dislocations involve the talonavicular and talocalcaneal joints after high-energy foot trauma (Figs. 29-18 to 29-20). Typically there is dramatic deformity.[43] The talus itself can dislocate medially or laterally, and should be promptly reduced because of skin compromise or vascular injury. The EP should reduce the foot in a way similar to the ankle dislocations described earlier. Concomitant talar neck fractures are common. Emergent orthopedic consultation is appropriate.

Calcaneus Fractures. The calcaneus is typically fractured by axial stresses such as a fall from height or in a MVC. A combination of shear and compressive forces may split it into pieces through the body.[47,53,54]

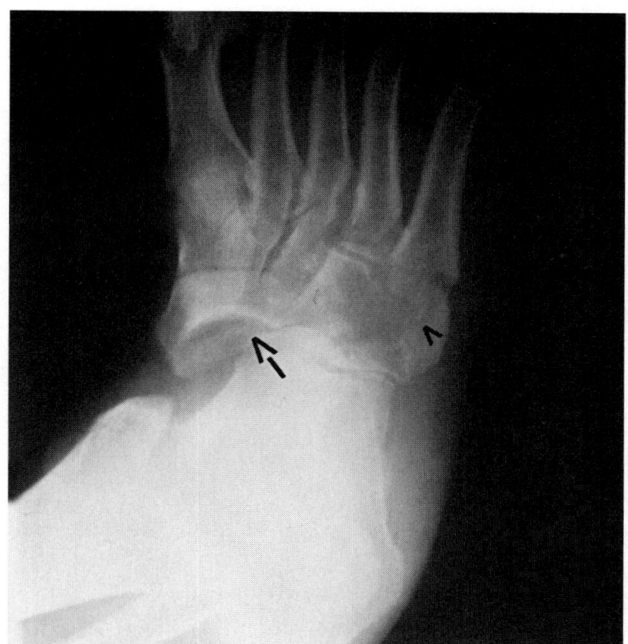

Fig. 29-19 Talonavicular dislocation. Arrow points to dislocation; arrowhead points to associated cuboid fracture.

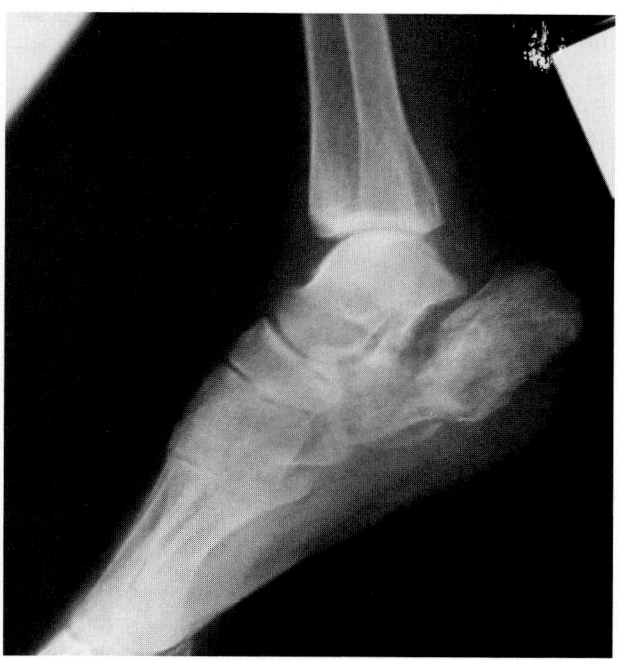

Fig. 29-20 Talocalcaneal dislocation.

Forcible dorsiflexion is another potential mechanism that results in fracture of the posterior tuberosity near the Achilles tendon insertion. In all patients with calcaneal fractures, consider typical associated injuries such as tibial plateau and lumbar fractures.

Clinically, patients complain of moderate to severe pain and swelling at the heel. There may be associated skin contusion, open wounds, or fracture blisters. A calcaneal fracture connotes significant injury force, and vigilance for associated injuries such as lumbar spine fractures is imperative.

Although the most commonly fractured tarsal bone,[47,52] calcaneal fractures can be difficult to diagnose, with 10% missed in the ED in one series.[55] Standard radiographs of the foot (AP, lateral, and oblique) should be supplemented with a Harris heel view (axial view of the calcaneus).[43,46,47] Study the radiograph for irregularities of the cortical shell and lucencies within the otherwise relatively homogeneous-looking trabecular bone. Because of the trabecular network, calcaneal fractures may appear as densities (crushed rays of bone) rather than the expected lucencies on the lateral view. The dome of the calcaneus may appear flat (i.e., abnormal Bohler's angle) (Fig. 29-21). The Harris view may demonstrate widening of the bone, sagittal fracture lines, or heel shortening.[46] Two angles on the lateral film, **Bohler's angle** (to assess the height of the posterior process, normally 20° to 40°),[47,54] and the **crucial angle of Gissane** (formed by cortical struts on the lateral calcaneus, normally about 135°) should be visualized (Fig. 29-22), especially in fractures of the body of the calcaneus.

Classification of calcaneus fractures is CT scan based, and centers around the fracture through the posterior facet articulation with the talus. The CT scan is often used for surgical decision making.[52,54,56,57] In general, fractures are categorized as extraarticular (25%) or intraarticular (75%) with regard to the subtalar joint.[47,53] Because the possibility of articular involvement cannot always be excluded by plain films, virtually all calcaneal fractures should be CT scanned at some point (Fig. 29-23).

Compartment syndrome of the foot can also follow calcaneal fracture and is characterized by severe pain, hypesthesias of the foot, and weakness.[58]

Extraarticular fractures involve the "beak" or posterior process of the calcaneus near the Achilles tendon insertion (forced dorsiflexion), the anterior processes of the calcaneus, or the sustentaculum tali (axial loading on inverted foot). The flexor hallucis longus tendon passes just adjacent to the sustentaculum tali, and passive movement of the great toe may cause referred pain to the medial calcaneus with sustentaculum tali fractures.[43,46,47] Initial treatment of extraarticular calcaneal fractures consists of elevation, bulky compressive (Jones) dressing, and analgesia. Weight-bearing is prohibited until orthopedic consultation has been obtained.

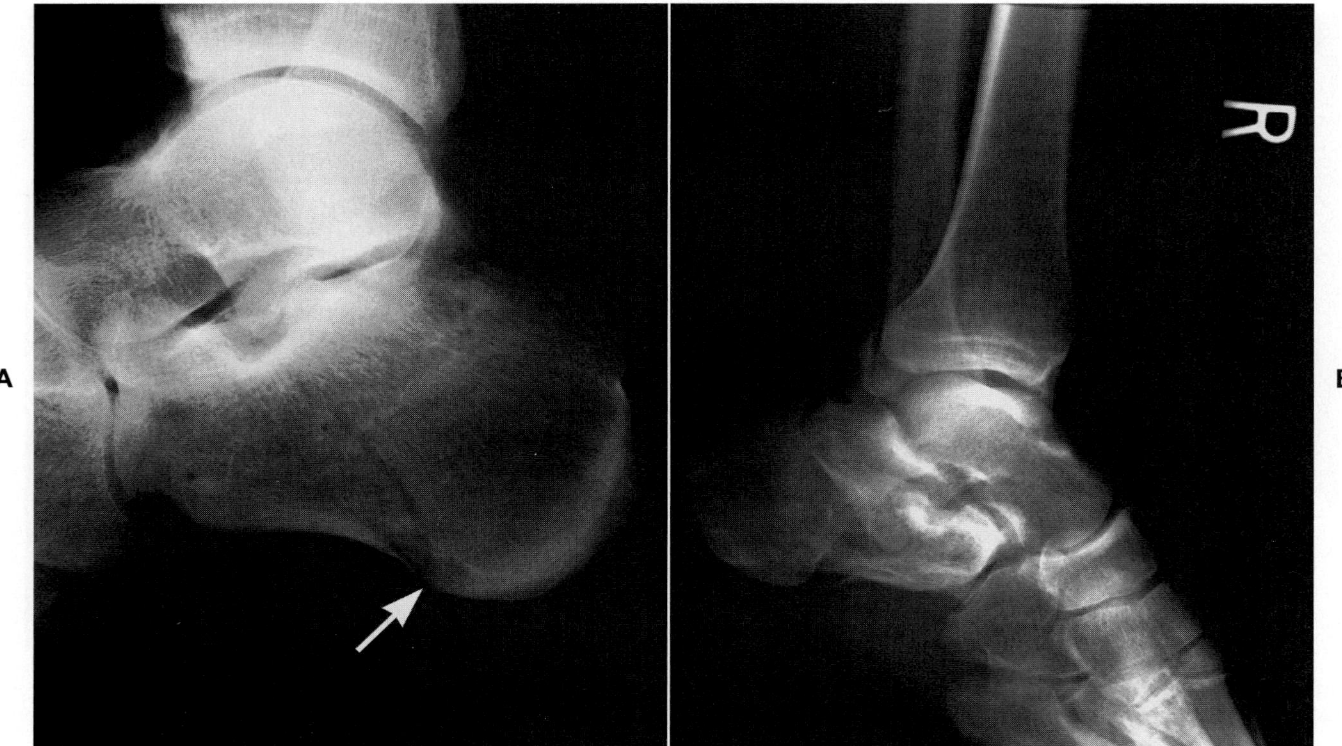

Fig. 29-21 Calcaneus fracture. Axial loads from falls or motor vehicle accidents may result in complex fractures of the heel bone. **A,** Relatively subtle fracture, notable by a small cortical defect and lucency through the trabecular bone. **B,** Complex comminuted intraarticular fracture.

Intraarticular fractures have a high risk for significant long-term debility. These injuries are typically caused by high-energy axial loading. The definitive treatment of intraarticular calcaneal fractures is the subject of controversy.[43,53,56] No single factor mandates a specific method of therapy. The best results are achieved by anatomic reduction of the posterior facet to achieve an effective talocalcaneal articulation and correct calcaneal width and heel height. Closed manipulations may be appropriate for some patients, although open reduction and fixation is also frequently used. Immediate orthopedic consultation is mandatory.

Chopart's Fracture-Dislocation. Injuries to the talonavicular or calcaneocuboid joints (Chopart's joints) are frequently misdiagnosed as ankle sprains.[59] The deformity may be obscured by marked swelling.[60] Prompt reduction is necessary for dislocations (Fig. 29-24).[60] Nondisplaced fractures are treated with short-leg casts for 6 weeks. Operative fixation may be required for severe injuries, and fusion with bone grafting is often necessary for extensive comminution.[60]

MIDFOOT INJURIES

Midfoot injuries may commonly involve multiple fractures or fracture-dislocations.[47]

Navicular Fractures. Eversion or inversion forces are associated with ***chip fractures*** off the dorsal anterior aspect (Fig. 29-25). This injury is the most common tarsal navicular fracture and is associated with lateral malleolar ligament injury.[47] Eversion mechanisms may cause **fractures of the navicular tuberosity** through avulsion of the posterior tibial tendon insertion. Forefoot abduction can also cause a concomitant compression fracture of the cuboid (**"nutcracker" fracture**) with an unstable midfoot.[61] Forced midfoot flexion or axial loading may result in **navicular body fractures.**[46,62] Treat nondisplaced or avulsion fractures with a rigid splint or short-leg walking cast. Nutcracker fractures are treated surgically.[61] Displaced body fractures likely require open reduction and internal fixation or arthrodesis.[59,62]

Cuboid Fractures. These unusual fractures may be easily missed. They are usually best seen on the oblique film,[46] and comparison views may be necessary.[47] Direct mechanism fractures are typically non-

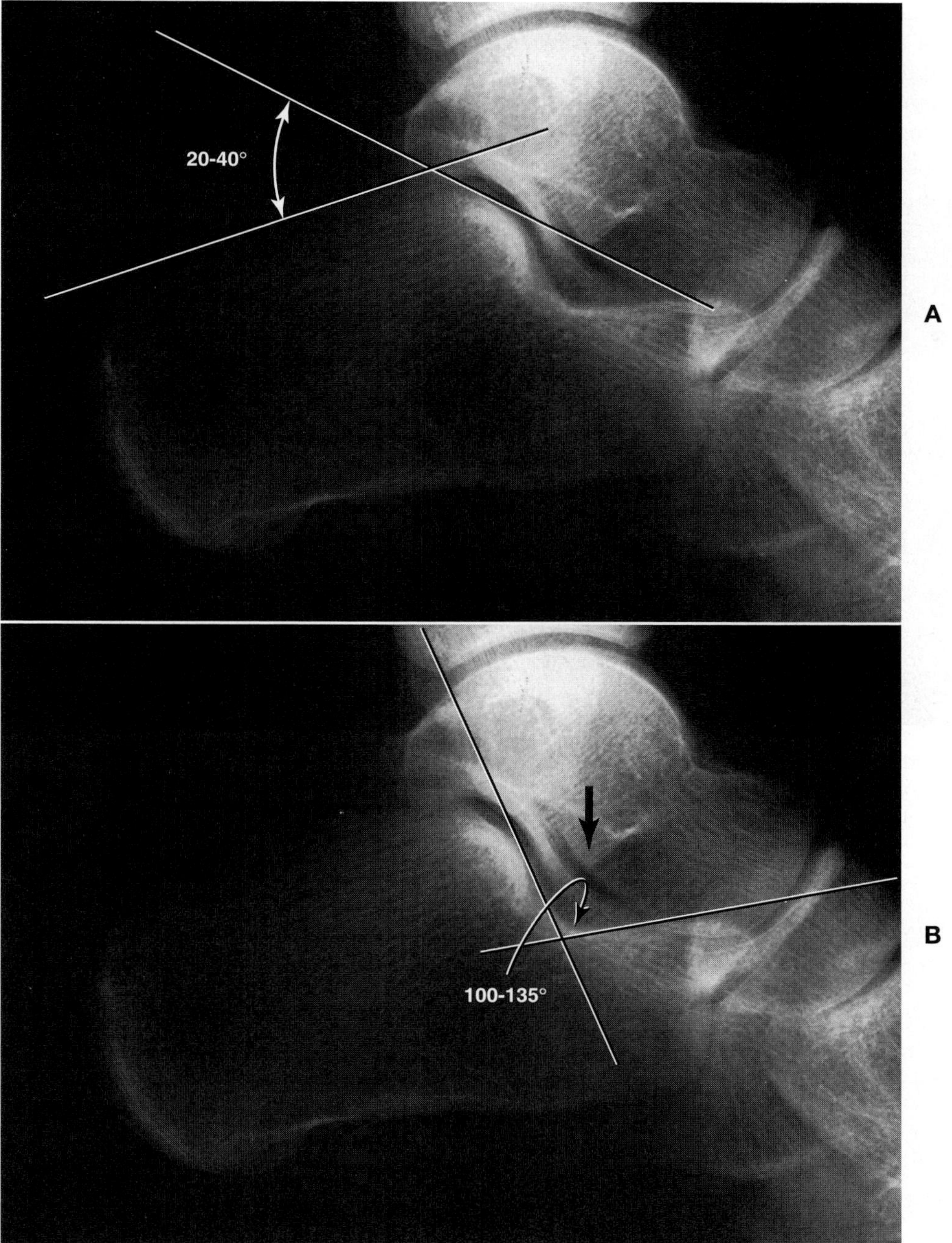

Fig. 29-22 Normal angles of the calcaneus. **A,** Böhler's angle is measured using the three "highest" points of the calcaneus. A flattened, widened, fractured calcaneus has a decreased angle. **B,** Crucial angle of Gissane. The talus may act as a wedge, driving through the calcaneus and decreasing this angle.

displaced (Fig. 29-26). Cuboid fractures are usually associated with other midfoot fractures or dislocations.[63,64] Treat with a non–weight-bearing short-leg cast and provide orthopedic follow-up. Fractures that are displaced, compacted (nutcracker), or associated with tarsometatarsal instability may require surgery.

Cuneiform Fractures. When fractured, the usual mechanism is a direct blow or crush, as in a heavy object dropped on the foot in an industrial accident. The best clues are clinical, with localized pain and swelling, because radiographs of this area are frequently difficult to interpret.[46] The navicular should articulate with each cuneiform equally on the AP view. Beware of associated Lisfranc injury with fractures of the distal cuneiforms or cuboid. If suspicious for fracture, immobilize in spite of negative radiographs and arrange follow-up. Treatment is with a short-leg walking cast unless associated fractures (e.g., Lisfranc joint injury) mandate urgent treatment by an orthopedist.

Lisfranc Injuries

Mechanism of Injury. Complex forces, usually high-energy, may result in injury to the metatarsal-tarsal (Lisfranc's) joint.[43,65,66] Direct crushing blows can displace the metatarsals in the direction of the force. More commonly, indirect or rotational mechanisms result in injury to the Lisfranc joint. Examples include falls from height, striking a fixed plantar-

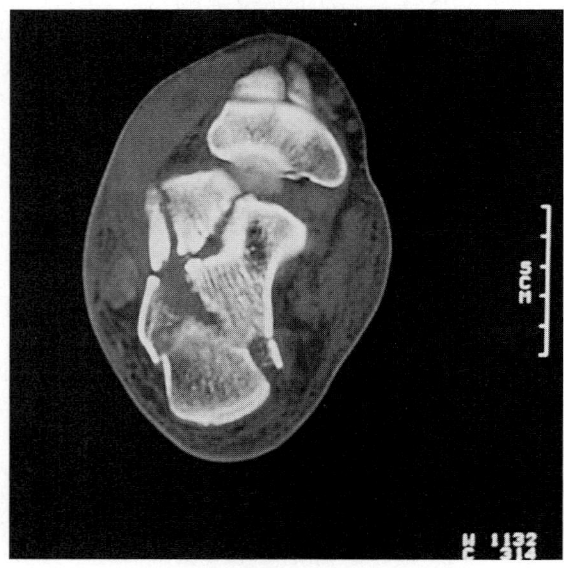

Fig. 29-23 Computed tomography scan of calcaneus fracture. In this view at least five separate fractures are seen.

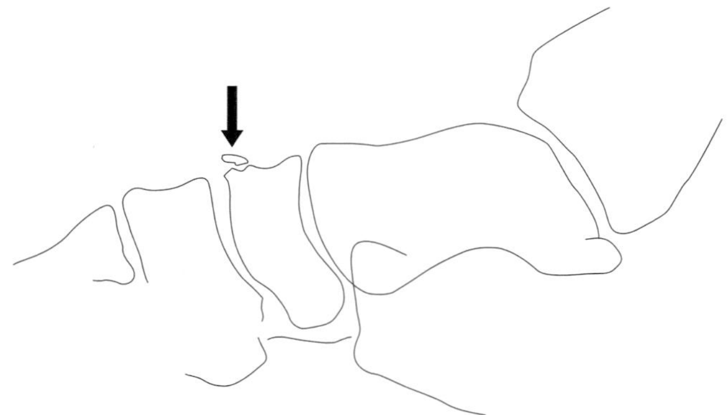

Fig. 29-25 Navicular chip fracture. Cortical chip fractures of the navicular are associated with twisting mechanisms.

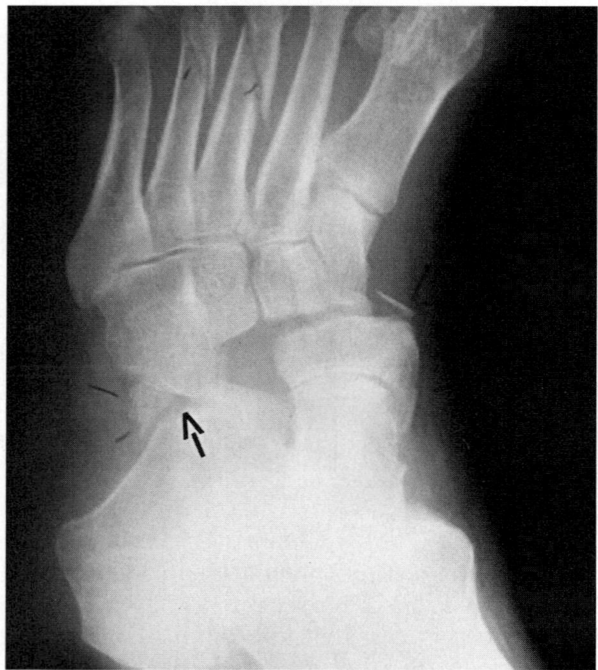

Fig. 29-24 Chopart's fracture-dislocation. Arrow points to fracture and dislocation at calcaneocuboid joint.

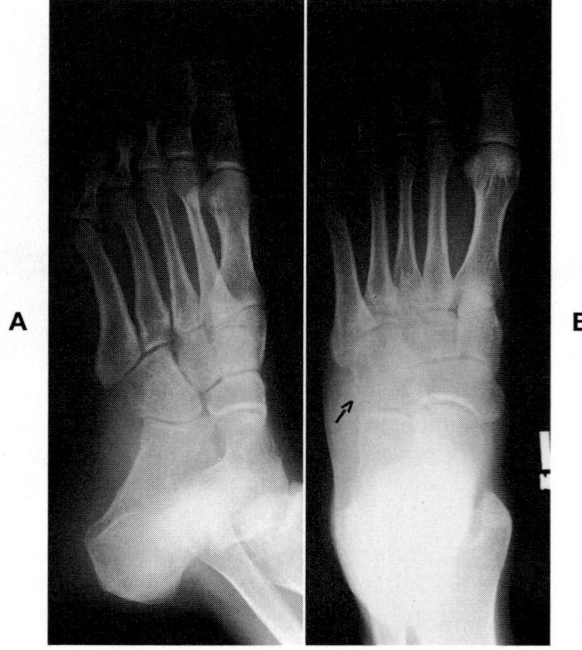

Fig. 29-26 Cuboid fracture. These fractures may be easily missed. **A,** Normal oblique view. **B,** Chip fracture of the lateral cuboid seen only on anteroposterior view.

flexed foot on the floorboard in a MVC, or even a misstep onto an uneven surface with axial force transmitted up the metatarsals, displacing them dorsally on the tarsals. Anatomically, recall that the second metatarsal sits in the second cuneiform in a notch created by the first and third cuneiforms, and is anchored medially to the first metatarsal and first cuneiform by transverse and oblique ligaments (Fig. 29-27). The third, fourth, and fifth metatarsals are prevented from lateral movement by transverse ligamentous attachments medially. Disruption of this medial anchoring allows the lateral displacement of the metatarsals in varying degrees. The injury may vary from ligamentous strain without apparent radiographic findings to fracture-dislocations with lateral shifting of all four lateral metatarsals relative to the midfoot (Fig. 29-28).

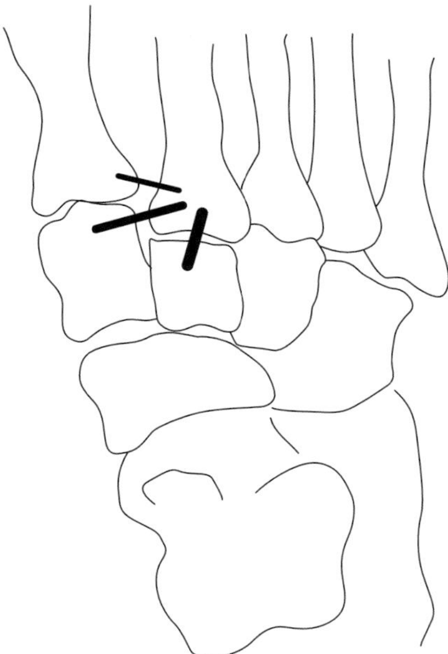

Fig. 29-27 Anatomy of Lisfranc's joint. The key ligamentous attachments anchoring the second metatarsal medially, demonstrated schematically.

Clinical Presentation. Patients commonly present with a characteristic history, midfoot pain, swelling, and decreased ability to bear weight. There may be a mid-foot ecchymosis on the plantar aspect.[67] Although some patients lack abnormalities on inspection, they indicate that the dorsal medial midfoot is the site of pain.

Diagnosis and Radiology. Lisfranc injuries are easy to miss and may be overlooked on initial presentation in up to 20% of cases.[53,64,68-70] Suspect this injury in any person complaining of midfoot pain, and palpate the joint from both the dorsal and plantar aspect. This deformity is seen best on the AP and oblique views of the foot. Fractures of the second metatarsal, cuboid, or navicular should increase suspicion. The most consistent radiographic finding is loss of the usual alignment between the medial borders of the second metatarsal and second cuneiform. *When looking at the radiographs, ascertain that the second metatarsal lines up with second cuneiform on the AP view,*

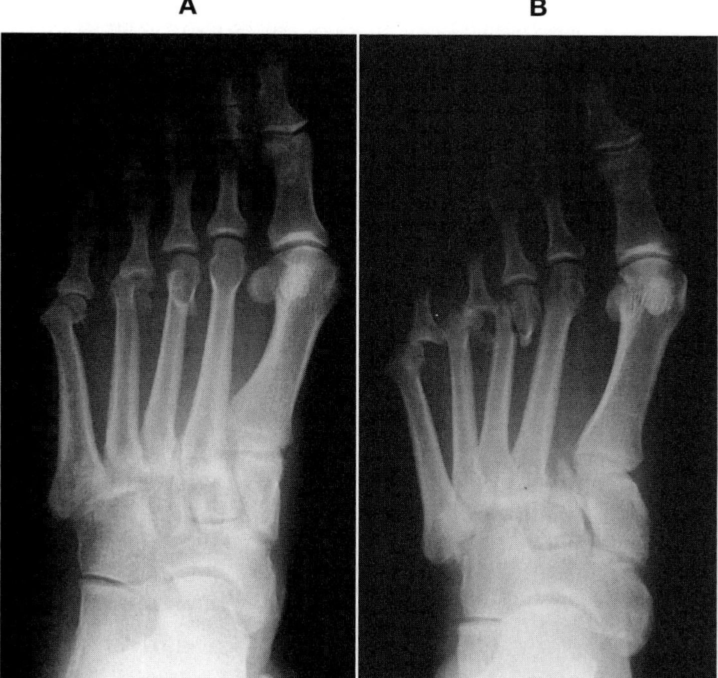

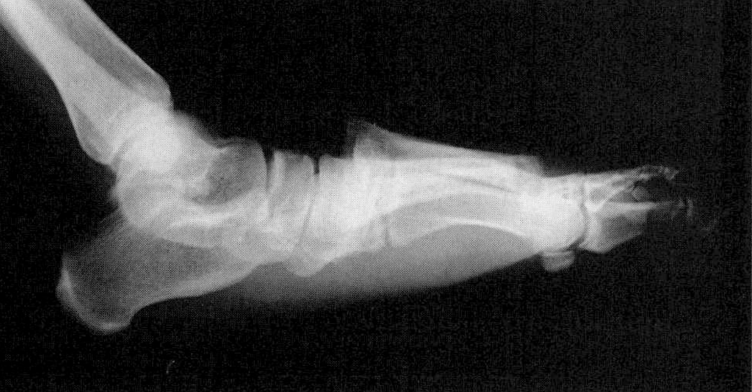

Fig. 29-28 Lisfranc fracture. **A,** In spite of the relatively normal alignment on the oblique view; **B,** the anteroposterior view shows misalignment and lateral shifting of the metatarsals. The pathognomonic fracture of the base of the second metatarsal is seen. **C,** The lateral view demonstrates dorsal displacement of the metatarsals. Multiple fracture-dislocations of the metatarsals and phalanges are present.

and that the cuneiforms are in line with the metatarsals on the lateral view. On the lateral view, metatarsals normally may be aligned with or slightly plantar to their respective tarsal, but should never be more dorsal (Box 29-5).

If initial radiographs are negative, consider weight-bearing comparison views (both AP and lateral projections). A misalignment may become apparent when the ruptured ligament(s) are stressed, particularly the second metatarsal/medial cuboid alignment on the AP view, or a dorsally displaced metatarsal on the lateral view.

BOX 29-5
Radiographic Findings and Lisfranc Injury

Normal alignments:
- Medial base of second metatarsal and medial border of second (medial) cuneiform
- Lateral base of third metatarsal and lateral border of third (lateral) cuneiform
- Medial base of fourth metatarsal and medial border of cuboid
- On lateral radiograph, a metatarsal should never be more dorsal than its respective tarsal

An avulsion fracture of the medial base of the second metatarsal or the lateral base of the first metatarsal is virtually pathognomonic.

Graeme KA, Jackimczyk KC: *Emerg Med Clin North Am* 15:365-379, 1997.

Emergency Management and Disposition. After assessing distal neurovascular status, immobilize patients with normal radiographic findings with a posterior splint, prohibit weight-bearing, and consult for immediate orthopedic follow-up. Consult orthopedic surgery for displaced fractures for reduction and casting. Open reduction and fixation is used if adequate reduction cannot be achieved or maintained, which is a common scenario as a result of soft-tissue interpositioning.[65]

FOREFOOT INJURIES

Metatarsal Injuries. The relatively long metatarsals are susceptible to injury from direct (often crushing) or indirect (often torsional) forces. Particular sections of bones may be involved because of partial protection from steel-toed footwear. Patients complain of pain, swelling, and inability to bear weight.

If examined promptly before significant swelling begins, patients may localize the pain and describe point tenderness. Pain may also be elicited with axial loading of the involved digit. Radiographs typically reveal transverse fractures after direct blows or oblique fractures after rotational mechanisms. Usually these injuries are seen well on the AP view, but the lateral film is important to assess dorsal or plantar angulation (Fig. 29-29).[53,59]

Because crushing mechanisms are frequently involved, closely assess the overlying skin and soft

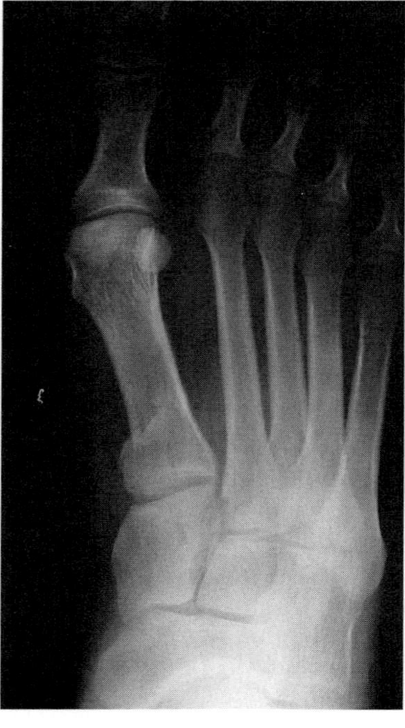

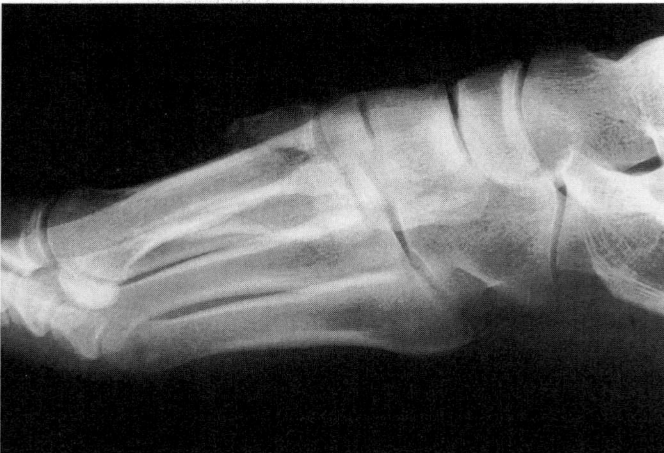

Fig. 29-29 Metatarsal fractures. These fractures are usually readily seen on the anteroposterior view, but the other views may demonstrate plantar angulation, which can result in painful callous formation. This severe fracture of the first metatarsal required operative repair.

tissue for devitalization or evidence of fracture communication. Significant tissue involvement or neurovascular compromise, even if underlying fractures are minimal, mandates consultation and admission.

Treat nondisplaced transverse fractures with a hard-soled shoe or short-leg walking cast for 2 to 4 weeks and orthopedic referral. Reduce significantly displaced or angulated fractures with Chinese finger trap traction, countertraction with weights on the tibia, and manual pressure opposite to the angulation.[47] Reduction is especially important for plantar-angulated fractures, which if allowed to heal may result in callous formation and chronic pain at the prominence in the sole. After reduction, place a short-leg cast and arrange prompt follow-up. Exercise caution with first metatarsal injuries and arrange orthopedic consultation as a result of the importance in the "push-off" phase of walking.[47] Irreducible fractures should be consulted in the ED.

Fifth Metatarsal Fractures. Acute traumatic injuries are usually one of two types, tuberosity avulsion fracture versus Jones fracture. Each has different prognoses and implications for treatment (Fig. 29-30). Inversion of the foot can avulse the proximal tip of the bone in varying degrees. This type of injury is called a **tuberosity avulsion fracture**. Confusion with an os versalianum accessory bone is possible (see Fig. 29-14). Tuberosity avulsion fractures typically heal well with symptomatic care.[47,57,59] A compressive dressing alone, a hard-soled shoe, or a posterior splint may be used based on the displacement, pain, and desire for rapid ambulation. Significantly displaced fractures are sometimes treated with open reduction and fixation, especially in performance athletes.[71]

Transverse fracture at the diaphyseal-metaphyseal junction within 1.5 cm of the tuberosity (**Jones fracture**) is consistent with the injury suffered by Sir Robert Jones "whilst dancing" and described by him in 1902.[72] This fracture has a greater tendency for nonunion than tuberosity avulsion fractures.[43,53,59,73] Place a short-leg cast, or combination splint, prohibit weight-bearing, and arrange prompt orthopedic follow-up.[53] Jones fractures are sometimes treated surgically, especially in active or athletic persons.[57,73]

Oblique distal shaft fractures are sometimes referred to as "**Dancer's fractures**," and are common in ballet dancers.[74] These injuries are usually treated nonoperatively with good results.

Phalanx Injuries. The phalanges of the toes are susceptible to fracture and dislocation from direct blows or "stubbing" mechanisms. Patients exhibit pain, swelling, and ecchymosis, and associated nail or

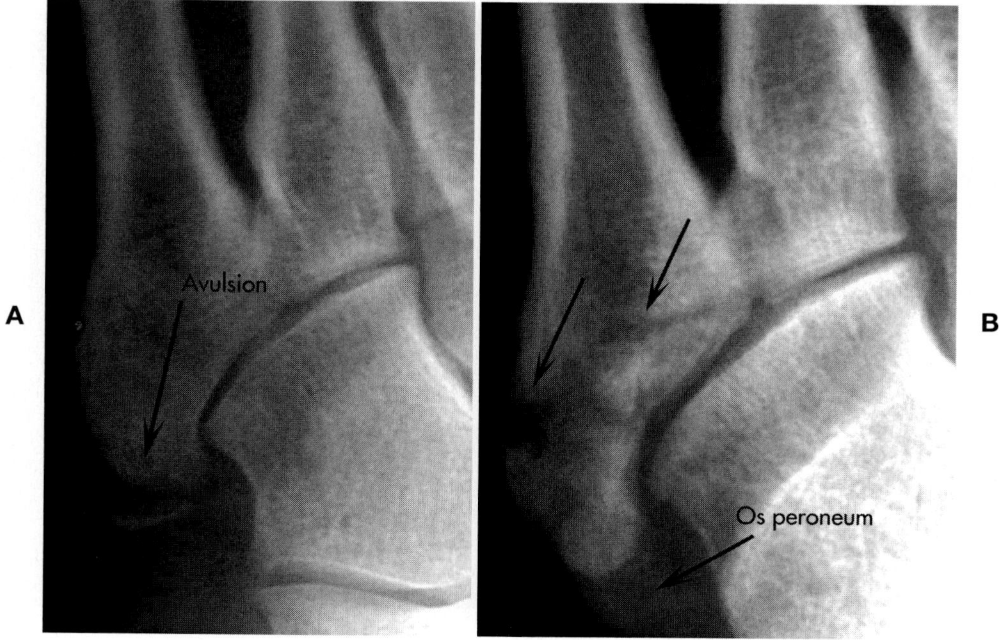

Fig. 29-30 Fifth metatarsal fracture types. Fractures near the base of the fifth metatarsal have different prognoses and implications for treatment. **A,** Tuberosity avulsion fracture. **B,** Jones' fracture, at the metaphyseal-diaphyseal junction. (From Sanders R: Fractures of the midfoot and forefoot. In Coughlin MJ, Mann RA: *Surgery of the foot and ankle,* ed 7, St Louis, 1999, Mosby.)

soft-tissue injuries may be present. Patients may need to remove nail polish to evaluate for subungual hematoma. Release subungual hematomas with nail trephination, either cautery or needle-drill technique.

Not all toe injuries require radiographic diagnosis, since toes 2 through 5 generally heal without problems. Straighten the toe and treat with buddy-taping. Intraarticular fractures of the great toe may require surgical alignment and pinning. For this reason, obtain radiographs for suspicious great toe injuries. Uncomplicated toe fractures can be treated with dynamic splinting or "buddy-taping" to an adjacent toe with interposed padding.[47,59] First toe injuries, displaced fractures (especially with plantar angulation), and dislocations should be reduced, immobilized, and prompt follow-up arranged, similar to the management of metatarsal injuries (Fig. 29-31).

Sesamoid Fractures. These unusual injuries are the result of a direct blow. The medial sesamoid is involved more frequently than the lateral.[47,48] Since the bones are encased in the flexor hallucis brevis tendon sheath (analogous to the patella), passive great toe movement exacerbates pain. The sesamoid may be bipartite in 34% of radiographs (Fig. 29-31, *B*),[48] but can be differentiated from fractures by the appearance of the cortical margins and wider distraction of frag-

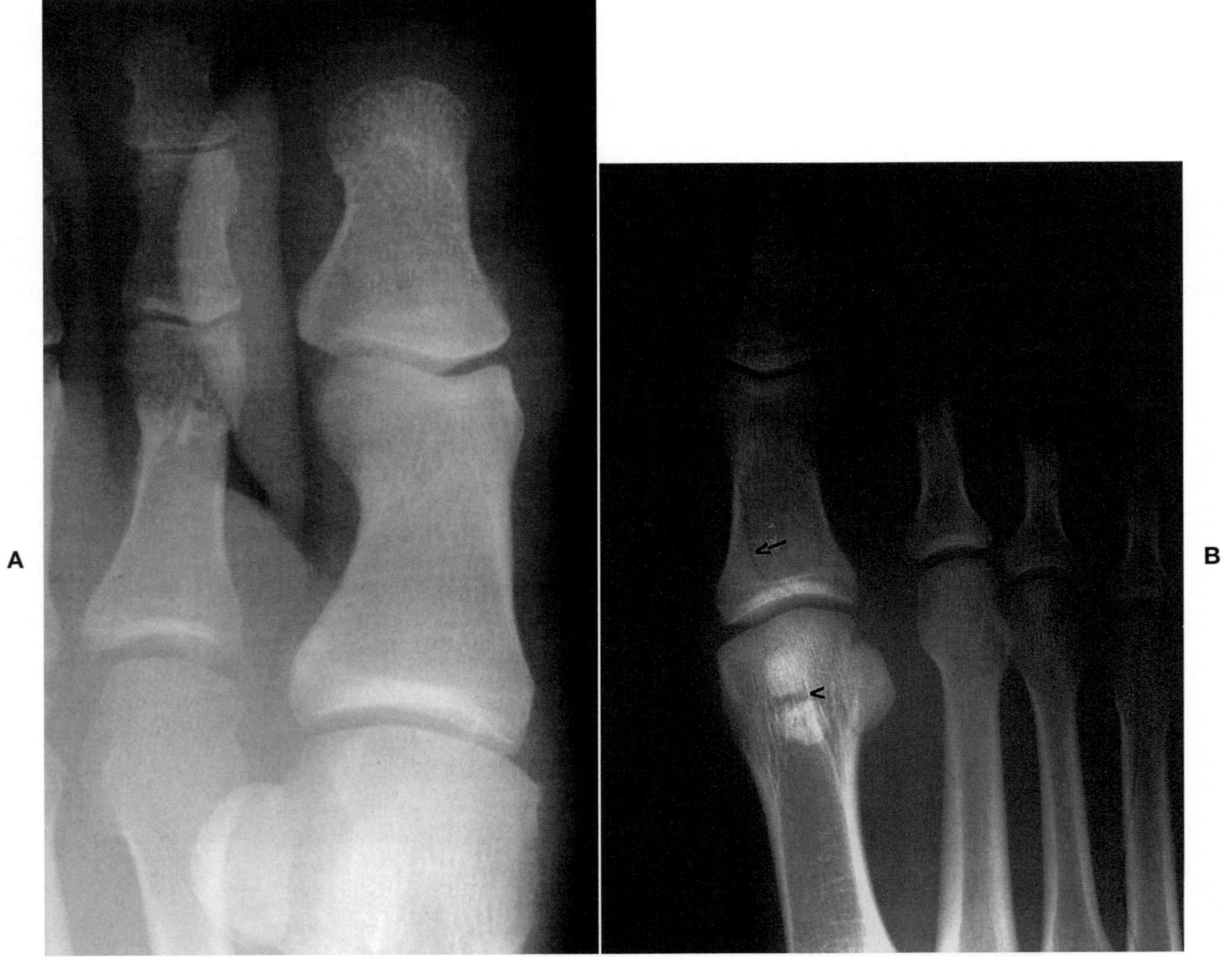

Fig. 29-31 Phalanx fractures. The toes are susceptible to crushing, torsional, and "stubbing" mechanisms. **A,** Transverse fracture of the second proximal phalanx. This fracture was treated with buddy tapping. **B,** Intraarticular nondisplaced proximal phalanx great toe fracture. This fracture was treated with a stiff-soled shoe and follow-up. Neither fracture had significant soft-tissue injury. A bipartite medial sesamoid was incidentally noted *(arrowhead).*

ments with fracture. These fractures are treated with brief immobilization and orthopedic follow-up.

PEARLS & PITFALLS

Ankle Injuries

- Injuries that mimic ankle sprain include Achilles tendon rupture, malleolar fractures, fifth metatarsal fracture, and talar dome injury.
- Use Ottawa ankle rules to determine need for a radiograph but use caution if the patient is intoxicated or has altered mental status, <18 years old, or has distracting injury. Explain to the patient why he or she does not need a radiograph.
- Always examine the foot and knee in patients with ankle injuries. Especially palpate the base of the fifth metatarsal, the navicular in the foot, and the fibular head at the knee.
- Reduce ankle dislocations promptly, especially if neurovascular compromise is present. Do not wait for an orthopedist.

Foot Injuries

- The talus has a tenuous blood supply, and fractures require early orthopedic follow-up. Quickly reduce subtalar fractures.
- The calcaneus is the most commonly fractured tarsal bone and fractures may be subtle. Obtain calcaneal views and look for flattening of the dome.
- Associated injuries are common with calcaneus fractures, such as other lower extremity and lumbar spine fractures.
- Cuboid and cuneiform injuries are easy to miss on radiographs.
- Beware of a spontaneously reduced Lisfranc injury with normal radiographs.
- Lisfranc fracture-dislocations may have a paucity of inspection findings, but the midfoot is painful. The radiographic finding most consistent with Lisfranc injury is loss of second metatarsal/second cuneiform alignment. Other findings include cuboid and cuneiform fractures.
- Straighten and buddy tape deformities of toes 2 through 5. Obtain films for suspected great toe fractures. Intraarticular fractures of the great toe may ultimately require surgery.

REFERENCES

1. Stiell IG, et al: Decision rules for the use of radiography in acute ankle injuries: refinement and prospective validation, *JAMA* 269:1127-1132, 1993.
2. Alpert SW, et al: *Fractures and dislocations: a manual of orthopedic trauma,* New York, 1994, Lippincott-Raven.
3. Danis R (editor): *Les fractures malléolaires. Théorie et pratique de l'osteosynthèse,* Paris, 1949, Masson et Cie.
4. Hamilton WC: Injuries of the ankle and foot, *Emerg Clin North Am* 2:361-389, 1984.
5. Herscovici D, Spiegel PG: Ankle fractures: when to manage, when to refer, *J Musculoskel Med* 14:79-91, 1997.
6. Hopkinson WJ, et al: Syndesmosis sprains of the ankle, *Foot Ankle* 10:325-330, 1990.
7. Trevino SG, Davis P, Hecht PJ: Management of acute and chronic lateral ligament injuries of the ankle, *Orthop Clin North Am* 25:1-16, 1994.
8. Milner CE, Soames RW: Anatomy of the collateral ligaments of the human ankle joint, *Foot Ankle Int* 19:757-760, 1998.
9. Milner CE, Soames RW: The medial collateral ligaments of the human ankle joint: anatomical variations, *Foot Ankle Int* 19:289-292, 1998.
10. Tochigi Y, et al: Acute inversion injury of the ankle: magnetic resonance imaging and clinical outcomes, *Foot Ankle Int* 19:730-734, 1998.
11. Teitz CC, Harrington RM: A biomechanical analysis of the squeeze test for sprains of the syndesmotic ligaments of the ankle, *Foot Ankle Int* 19:489-492, 1998.
12. Frost HM, Hanson CA: Technique for testing the drawer sign in the ankle, *Clin Orthop* 123:49-51, 1977.
13. Wexler RK: The injured ankle, *Am Fam Physician* 57:474-480, 1998.
14. Whitelaw GP, et al: The acutely painful ankle: differential diagnosis, *Hosp Med* 32:13-19, 1996.
15. Stiell I: Ottawa ankle rules, *Can Fam Physician* 42:478-480, 1996.
16. Lucchesi GM, et al: Sensitivity of the Ottawa rules, *Ann Emerg Med* 26:1-5, 1995.
17. Pigman EC, et al: Evaluation of the Ottawa clinical decision rules for the use of radiography in acute ankle and midfoot injuries in the emergency department: an independent site assessment, *Ann Emerg Med* 24:41-45, 1994.
18. Stiell IG, et al: A study to develop clinical decision rules for the use of radiography in acute ankle injuries, *Ann Emerg Med* 21:384-390, 1992.
19. Stiell IG, et al: Implementation of the Ottawa ankle rules, *JAMA* 271:827-832, 1994.
20. Anis AH, et al: Cost-effectiveness analysis of the Ottawa ankle rules, *Ann Emerg Med* 26:422-428, 1995.
21. Dettori JR, Basmania CJ: Early ankle mobilization. Part II: a one-year follow-up of acute, lateral ankle sprains (a randomized clinical trial), *Mil Med* 159:20-24, 1994.
22. Dettori JR, et al: Early ankle immobilization. Part I: the immediate effect on acute, lateral ankle sprains (a randomized clinical trial), *Mil Med* 159:15-20, 1994.
23. DuPont M, Beliveau P, Theriault G: The efficacy of antiinflammatory medication in the treatment of the acutely sprained ankle, *Am J Sports Med* 15:41-45, 1987.
24. Freeman MA, Dean MR, Hanham IW: The etiology and prevention of functional instability of the foot, *J Bone Joint Surg* 47-B:678-685, 1965.
25. Gerber JP, et al: Persistent disability associated with ankle sprains: a prospective examination of an athletic population, *Foot Ankle Int* 19:653-660, 1998.
26. Konradsen L, Holmer P, Sondergaard L: Early mobilizing treatment in grade III ankle ligament injuries, *Foot Ankle* 12:69-73, 1991.

27. Leanderson J, Wredmark T: Treatment of acute ankle sprain. Comparison of a semi-rigid ankle brace and compression bandage in 73 patients, *Acta Orthop Scand* 66:529-531, 1995.
28. Mascaro TB, Swanson LE: Rehabilitation of the foot and ankle, *Orthop Clin North Am* 25:147-160, 1994.
29. Smith RW, Reischl S: Treatment of ankle sprains in young athletes, *Am J Sports Med* 14:465-471, 1986.
30. Stover CN: Air stirrup management of ankle injuries in the athlete, *Am J Sports Med* 8:360-365, 1980.
31. Munk B, Holm-Christensen K, Lind T: Long-term outcome after ruptured lateral ankle ligaments. A prospective study of three different treatments in 79 patients with 11-year follow-up, *Acta Orthop Scand* 66:452-454, 1995.
32. Amendola A: Controversies in diagnosis and management of syndesmosis injuries of the ankle, *Foot Ankle* 13:44-50, 1992.
33. Neer CS II: Injuries of the ankle joint: evaluation, *Conn State Med J* 17:580-583, 1953.
34. Lauge-Hansen N: Fractures of the ankle. II. Combined experimental-surgical and experimental-roentgenologic investigations, *Arch Surg* 60:957-985, 1950.
35. Weber BG: *Die Verletzungen des oberen Sprunggelenkes,* ed 2, Bern, 1972, Verlag Hans Huber.
36. Daffner RH: Ankle trauma, *Radiol Clin North Am* 28:395-421, 1990.
37. O'Meara PM: Management of open fractures, *Orthop Rev* 21: 1177-1185, 1992.
38. Pettrone FA, et al: Quantitative criteria for prediction of the results after displaced fracture of the ankle, *J Bone Joint Surg* 65-A:66-77, 1983.
39. O'Keeffe D, et al: ABC of emergency radiology: the ankle, *BMJ* 308:331-336, 1994.
40. Karas EH, Weiner LS: Displaced pilon fractures: an update, *Orthop Clin North Am* 25:651-663, 1994.
41. Shea MP, Manoli A II: Osteochondral lesions of the talar dome, *Foot Ankle* 14: 48-55, 1993.
42. Roberts JR, Hedges JR (editors): *Clinical procedures in emergency medicine,* Philadelphia, 1991, Saunders.
43. Hamilton WC: Injuries of the ankle and foot, *Emerg Clin North Am* 2:361-389, 1984.
44. Turchin DC, et al: Do foot injuries significantly affect the functional outcome of multiply injured patients? *J Orthop Trauma* 13:1-4, 1999.
45. Keats TE: An atlas of roentgen variants that may simulate disease, ed 3, St Louis, 1984, Mosby.
46. Ling LJ: Foot and toes. In Ruiz E, Cicero JJ (editors): *Emergency management of skeletal injuries,* St Louis, 1995, Mosby.
47. Simon RR, Koenigsknecht: *Emergency orthopedics: the extremities,* Stanford, Conn, 1996, Appleton & Lange.
48. Connolly JF: Foot fractures. Catching the common troublemakers, *Emerg Med* 23:21-38, 1991.
49. Nadim Y, Tosic A, Ebraheim N: Open reduction and internal fixation of fracture of the posterior process of the talus: a case report and review of the literature, *Foot Ankle Int* 20:50-52, 1999.
50. Daniels TR, Smith JW: Talar neck fractures, *Foot Ankle* 14:225-234, 1993.
51. Anderson HG: *Medical and surgical aspects of aviation,* London, 1919, Oxford Medical.
52. Forrester DM, Kerr R: Trauma to the foot, *Radiol Clin North Am* 28:423-433, 1990.
53. Carr JB: Surgical treatment of the intra-articular calcaneus fracture, *Orthop Clin North Am* 25:665-675, 1994.
54. Lowery RB, Calhoun JH: Fractures of the calcaneus. Part I: anatomy, injury mechanism, and classification, *Foot Ankle Int* 17:230-235, 1996.
55. Freed HA, Shields NN: Most frequently overlooked radiographically apparent fractures in a teaching hospital emergency department, *Ann Emerg Med* 13:900-904, 1984.
56. Lowery RB, Calhoun JH: Fractures of the calcaneus. Part II: treatment, *Foot Ankle Int* 17:360-366, 1996.
57. Quill GE: Fractures of the proximal fifth metatarsal, *Orthop Clin North Am* 26:353-361, 1995.
58. Myerson M, Manoli A: Compartment syndromes of the foot after calcaneal fractures, *Clin Orthop* 290:142-150, 1993.
59. Rockwood CA Jr., Green DP, Bucholz RW: *Fractures in adults,* ed 4, Philadelphia, 1996, Lippincott-Raven.
60. Kumagai S, et al: Chopart's fracture dislocation: a case report and review of the literature, *Nebr Med J* 81:116-119, 1996.
61. Koch J, Rahimi F: Nutcracker fractures of the cuboid, *J Foot Surg* 30:336-339, 1991.
62. Nyska M, et al: Fractures of the body of the tarsal navicular bone: case reports and literature review, *J Trauma* 29:1448-1451, 1989.
63. Sangeorzan BJ, Mayo KA, Hansen ST: Intraarticular fractures of the foot: talus and lesser tarsals, *Clin Orthop* 292:135-141, 1993.
64. Sangeorzan BJ, Swiontkowski MF: Displaced fractures of the cuboid, *J Bone Joint Surg* 72B:376-378, 1990.
65. Myerson M: The diagnosis and treatment of injuries to the Lisfranc joint complex, *Orthop Clin North Am* 20:655-664, 1989.
66. Vuori JP, Aro HT: Lisfranc joint injuries: trauma mechanisms and associated injuries, *J Trauma* 35:40-45, 1993.
67. Ross G, et al: Plantar ecchymosis sign: a clinical aid to diagnosis of occult Lisfranc tarsometatarsal injuries, *J Orthop Trauma* 10: 119-122, 1996.
68. Englanoff G, Anglin D, Hutson HR: Lisfranc fracture-dislocation: a frequently missed diagnosis in the emergency department, *Ann Emerg Med* 26:229-33, 1995.
69. Graeme KA, Jackimczyk KC: The extremities and spine, *Emerg Med Clin North Am* 15:365-379, 1997.
70. Kaplan JD, et al: Lisfranc's fracture-dislocation: a review of the literature and case reports, *J Am Podiatr Med Assoc* 81:531-539, 1991.
71. Vogler HW, et al: Fifth metatarsal fractures: biomechanics, classification and treatment, *Clin Podiatr Med Surg* 12:725-747, 1995.
72. Jones R: Fracture of the base of the fifth metatarsal by indirect violence, *Ann Surg* 35:697-700, 1902.
73. Rettig AC, Shelbourne D, Wilckens J: The surgical treatment of symptomatic nonunions of the proximal (metaphyseal) fifth metatarsal in athletes, *Am J Sports Med* 20:50-54, 1992.
74. O'Malley MJ, Hamilton WG, Munyak J: Fractures of the distal shaft of the fifth metatarsal. "Dancer's fracture", *Am J Sports Med* 24:240-243, 1996.

Penetrating Extremity Trauma and Peripheral Vascular Injury

30

MICHAEL A. GIBBS, WILLIAM S. MILES, AND JOSEPH MESSICK

With the striking increase in civilian violence, there has been a parallel rise in the incidence of penetrating cardiovascular trauma. Mattox et al[1] reviewed the Houston experience between 1958 and 1988. More than half of the 5760 reported cases occurred in the last decade of the study, representing a 400% increase in incidence over this 30-year period. In most series 40% to 75% of these injuries involve the extremities.[1-3]

Most vascular injuries of the extremity result from penetrating trauma. In a recent review of 220 operatively-explored patients, the mechanism of injury was gunshot wounds in 54%, stab wounds in 15%, shotgun wounds in 12%, blunt trauma in 15%, and iatrogenic in 3%.[2]

ANATOMY

Upper Extremity

Major vessels include the axillary, brachial, radial, and ulnar arteries. The lateral border of the first rib defines the beginning of the axillary artery. The axillary artery courses distally and becomes the brachial artery at the inferior border of the teres major muscle. The brachial artery continues to just below the antecubital fossa, where it divides into the radial and ulnar arteries. In the palm the ulnar and radial arteries supply the superficial and deep palmar arches, respectively. There are numerous important collateral arteries arising along the course of these vessels, including the thyrocervical trunk, thoracoacromial artery, subscapular artery, posterior circumflex humeral artery, profunda brachii, and superior and inferior ulnar collateral arteries (Fig. 30-1).

Lower Extremity

The lower extremity begins at the inguinal ligament anteriorly and the inferior gluteal fold posteriorly. Major vessels include the femoral artery, popliteal artery, anterior and posterior tibial artery, and peroneal artery. As the external iliac artery courses under the inguinal ligament, between the pubic symphysis and the anterior superior iliac spine, it becomes the common femoral artery. The common femoral artery then bifurcates into the superficial femoral artery (SFA) and the profunda femoral, also known as the deep femoral artery (DFA). The DFA serves as the major source of blood to the muscular thigh. *Injuries to the DFA are associated with significant blood loss, and will not result in a pulse deficit or abnormal arterial pressure index (API).* The SFA, which serves as a conduit to the lower leg, passes through the adductor canal near the junction of the middle and distal thirds of the thigh, and emerges as the popliteal artery. The popliteal artery traverses the popliteal fossa and forms the trifurcation, which gives rise to the anterior and posterior tibial arteries and the peroneal artery. These three vessels converge in the foot to form the plantar arch. Important collateral branches include the profunda femoris artery, the medial and lateral circumflex femoral arteries, the genicular anastomosis, and communicating branches distal to the trifurcation (Fig. 30-2).

PATHOPHYSIOLOGY

There are several types of arterial injury that manifest in different ways. A vessel that is completely transected may bleed less than a vessel that is torn.

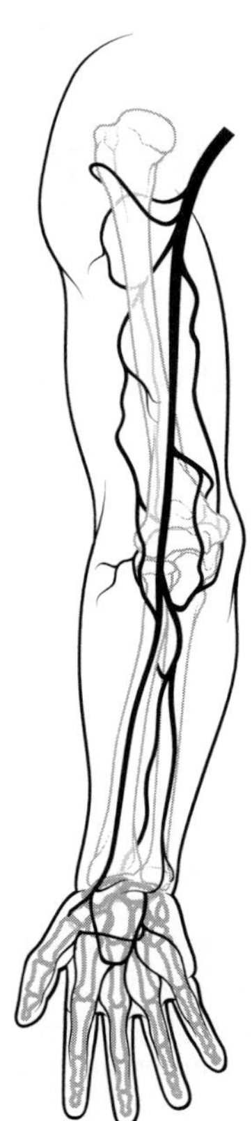

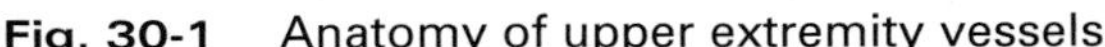

Fig. 30-1 Anatomy of upper extremity vessels.

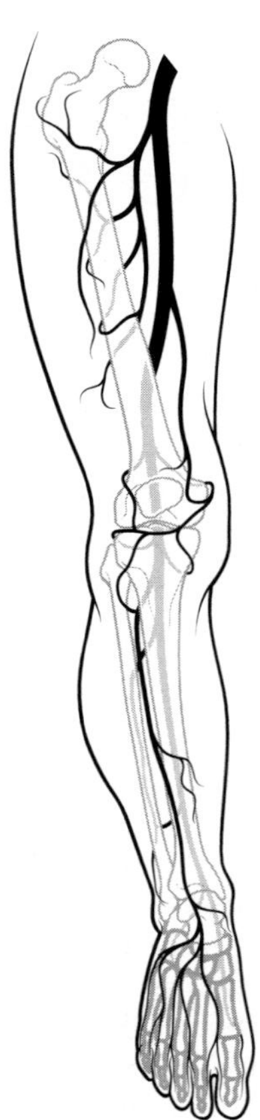

Fig. 30-2 Anatomy of lower extremity vessels.

This outcome is because a transected vessel is more likely to contract, which results in greater hemostasis.

Pulses may remain normal distal to the site of significant arterial injuries in 25% to 49% of cases.[4] Even vessels that are completely severed may generate a distal pulse. This phenomenon may occur through a number of mechanisms. Collateral flow from arteries proximal to the wound may divert blood around the disruption and back into the distal vessel. Alternatively, the proximal and distal stumps of transected vessels may still abut each other after the artery is divided. The proximal stump will beat with the arterial pressure wave and pound the distal stump, yielding a distal pulse despite lack of blood flow. However, a Doppler signal will be abnormal (see the following discussion).

Partial disruption of a vessel can lead to pseudoaneurysm formation, a disruption of all three layers of the artery contained by clot or surrounding tissue. Although a pseudoaneurysm produces few acute complications, it can have long-term consequences. Most importantly, clot can form in the sac months to years after injury and result in distal embolization. Partial disruption can produce an intimal flap. In this injury, an injuring agent produces a small fissure or flap in the intima. This flap may become a nidus for future emboli, or may grow larger over time and occlude the vessel in a delayed fashion. The intimal flap may even cause an arterial dissection.

If penetrating trauma lacerates both the artery and accompanying vein, an arteriovenous (AV) fistula may result. In this case, blood flows from the high-pressure arterial system directly into the low-pressure venous system. Acutely, this shunt may produce a thrill or bruit. Over time, the patient may develop significant limb swelling secondary to an overload of the venous system, and if the shunt is large, persistent tachycardia and high-output congestive heart failure. Compression of the fistula with finger pressure temporarily eliminates the shunt and slows the heart rate (Branham's sign).

Minor trauma to a vessel may result in vascular spasm. These patients demonstrate a pulse deficit that ultimately resolves. Because the diagnosis is based on characteristic findings on duplex sonography or angiography, this diagnosis should be made only *after* an objective test.

PHYSICAL EXAMINATION

Once the ABCs are addressed, the clinician can then turn to a detailed examination of the involved extremity. Examination of the extremity begins at the torso and progresses distally. The axilla, back, and chest should be examined carefully when wounds involve the upper extremity, as should the perineum and buttocks when the lower extremity is involved. Groin injuries, often considered extremity injuries, are especially lethal. Vascular trauma at the inguinal ligament can bleed into the retroperitoneum with little external evidence of hemorrhage. Palpate and stress the extremity to detect associated fractures. Because of the forces involved, a fracture should always raise suspicion for an associated neurovascular injury. Document the location and trajectory of bullets, the presence of foreign bodies or debris, and the degree of tissue devitalization. Drawings and photographs provide useful documentation and a reference for other clinicians involved in the patient's care. Although the location and morphology of the wound may help predict the likelihood of damage to underlying structures, this assumption does not always hold true. It is best to assume that all patients with penetrating extremity trauma have a neurovascular injury until proven otherwise. A diligent search for arterial injury is mandatory. Capillary refill, skin color, temperature, and the strength of distal pulses should be noted and compared with the contralateral extremity. Placing an examination glove over the diaphragm of the stethoscope allows the physician to listen for a bruit over the wound without bloodying his or her equipment.

A careful neurologic examination is also essential. Because of the close association between major arteries and neural structures, the presence of a neurologic deficit in the absence of hard signs for arterial injury increases the likelihood of occult arterial injury. Neurologic and vascular lesions coexist in as many as 50% of cases.[5] In addition, the absence of neurologic function or a deterioration in neurologic function may be an important sign of an evolving compartment syndrome.

The detection of vascular injury in patients with penetrating extremity trauma requires recognition of several important signs. However, the accuracy of the vascular examination is compromised by shock. Clinical signs of vascular injury remain absent or equivocal until the intravascular volume has been normalized and tissue perfusion restored. Most clinically significant extremity vascular lesions manifest unequivocal physical findings, or "hard signs" (Box 30-1). These signs include pulse deficit, distal ischemia, active hemorrhage, an expanding or pulsatile hematoma, or the presence of a bruit or thrill. One or more hard signs reliably predict the presence of arterial injury requiring repair.

"Soft signs" represent more equivocal physical findings, which should alert the physician to potential vascular injury (Box 30-2). These signs include small but stable hematomas, injury to an anatomically related nerve, unexplained hypotension, and a history of hemorrhage in the field. "Proximity" defines a penetrating wound in which the path of the penetrating agent potentially crosses the normal position of a major artery.

An important test in penetrating forearm injuries is the Allen test. This maneuver evaluates the arterial flow in the radial and ulnar arteries. To perform the test, the patient should elevate his or her arm and repeatedly clench his or her fist while the physician occludes both the radial and ulnar arteries at the wrist. Once the hand is blanched, release of the radial artery should result in rapid return of normal color.

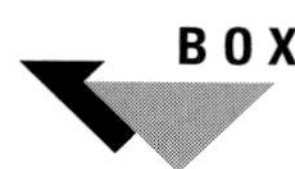

BOX 30-1
Hard Signs of Vascular Injury

- Absent or diminished distal pulses
- Active hemorrhage
- Large, expanding, or pulsatile hematoma
- Bruit or thrill
- Signs of distal ischemia
  - –Pain
  - –Pallor
  - –Paresthesia
  - –Paralysis
  - –Poikilothermy

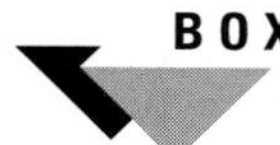

BOX 30-2
Soft Signs of Vascular Injury

- Small, stable hematomas
- Injury to an anatomically related nerve
- Unexplained hypotension
- History of hemorrhage no longer present
- Proximity of injury to a major vessel

The test is then repeated, this time releasing the ulnar artery. An abnormal Allen test (delayed return of blood to the hand compared with the opposite limb) is evidence of arterial injury.

CONTROVERSIES IN DIAGNOSTIC EVALUATION

The management of patients sustaining penetrating extremity trauma has evolved considerably during the past three decades. The pendulum has swung towards expectant management for the majority of these injuries, with far less reliance on surgical exploration and diagnostic testing. This change is well supported by the medical literature, and it provides advantages for both physician and patient. However, the bulk of research in this arena has been conducted at large trauma centers possessing special personnel, technology, experience, and resources. The management strategies suggested in the following discussion may not be immediately applicable to all clinical practice settings. Patient-specific factors that influence diagnostic strategies include the presence and severity of other injuries, location of the penetrating extremity wound, allergies to contrast, and co-morbid disease. Other considerations are local resources, including adequate number of expert personnel and the availability of diagnostic tools.

The presence of hard signs of vascular injury is diagnostic of arterial trauma requiring surgical repair. In the vast majority of cases, the presence of hard signs mandates immediate surgery without time-consuming (and therefore limb-threatening) evaluation. The risk of prolonged ischemia and ongoing hemorrhage, or both, outweighs the benefit of arteriography. In rare circumstances, arteriography in the patient with hard signs of vascular injury is useful. These circumstances include the following:

1. Injuries with multiple possible sites of vascular disruption (e.g., shotgun wounds)
2. Injuries associated with extensive bony or soft tissue destruction
3. Injuries in patients with preexisting vascular disease

In these situations, a limited intraoperative arteriogram may serve as a reasonable and timely alternative to formal multiplanar studies in the angiography suite. Traditionally, soft signs of vascular injury were considered an appropriate trigger for screening arteriography. However, recent studies suggest that they do not accurately predict the presence or absence of vascular injury.[6,7] Although soft signs are certainly not diagnostic of clinically significant vascular trauma, the authors believe that their presence merits further evaluation with noninvasive testing (e.g., API and/or duplex Doppler ultrasonography).

The assessment of penetrating extremity trauma with "proximity" to major vessels, but without clinical signs of vascular injury, remains an area of controversy. During the Korean conflict and Vietnam War, mandatory surgical exploration for all penetrating proximity wounds was recommended.[8-10] This approach was reasonable given the severity of soft tissue destruction associated with high-velocity military wounds. However, this practice was applied to the civilian population with little regard for the clinical distinction between civilian and military ballistics.[11-13] Although this practice decreased the incidence of missed arterial injuries, it came at the expense of a large number of negative explorations (up to 84% in one series), with attendant cost and significant morbidity.[14]

As arteriography became increasingly available, this technique was widely used to identify occult vascular trauma in patients with proximity injury, avoiding the consequences of negative exploration. Arteriography rapidly became the diagnostic gold standard.[14-16] Using arteriography to exclude vascular injury in patients with proximity wounds also has several important shortcomings, which include the following:

1. Low yield. Predictably, arteriography in patients without other signs of vascular injury is associated with a high percentage of negative studies. When proximity is the only indication for arteriography, roughly 1 in 10 to 1 in 20 studies are abnormal.[17,18]
2. Clinically insignificant findings. The majority of angiographic abnormalities identified in this patient population do not require surgical intervention (e.g., focal narrowing, small intimal defects, small pseudoaneurysms, and AV fistulas). The self-limited natural history of these clinically occult nonocclusive arterial injuries has been documented both retrospectively and prospectively.[7,18-20]
3. Limited accuracy. Arteriography is not a perfect test. False-negative and false-positive studies occur in between 1.8% and 3% of cases.[21]
4. Complications. Groin hematomas, AV fistulas, contrast dye reactions, and renal damage occur in up to 5% of patients.[14,22]
5. Expense. The cost of arteriography is roughly $1500 to $2000, an expense difficult to justify when the majority of studies are normal, and most abnormal cases are managed nonoperatively.

This reasoning suggests that a policy of routine screening arteriography for proximity alone is expensive, of limited clinical benefit, and associated with nontrivial complications. More recently, several authors have suggested that clinically important arterial injuries can be effectively ruled by other means.

DIAGNOSTIC APPROACH TO PROXIMITY INJURIES

A spectrum of clinical findings should prompt an appropriate graded response, from immediate surgical exploration to expectant management. Patients with hard signs of vascular injury should undergo immediate operative exploration and repair without further testing. Those with soft signs of vascular injury or with wounds in proximity to major vessels require a detailed physical examination and measurement of the arterial pressure index. These tests should direct further evaluation and management. Fig. 30-3 provides an algorithmic approach to the diagnosis of vascular injury.

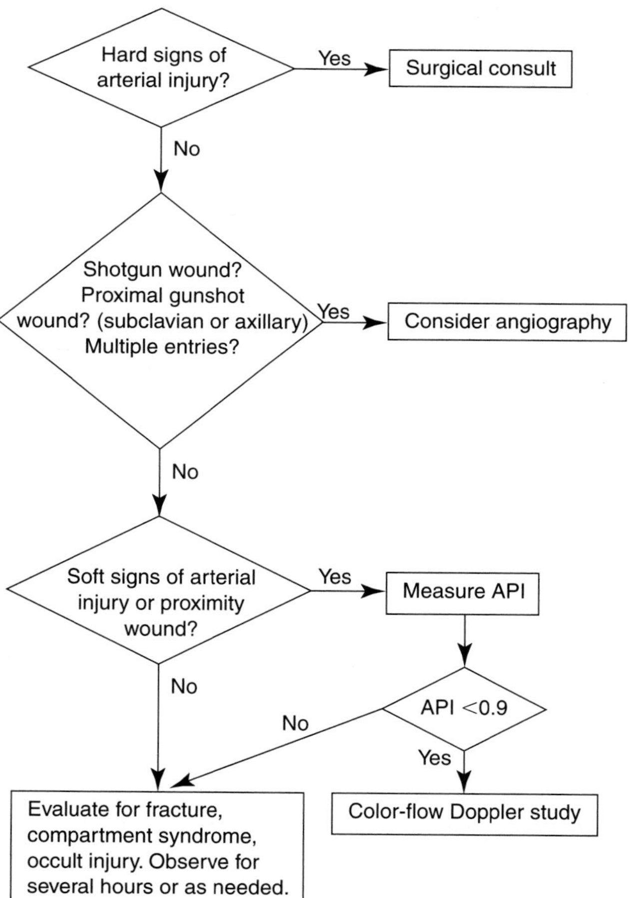

Fig. 30-3 Management of penetrating extremity trauma (after initial stabilization).

Use of Physical Examination Alone

The results of several recent studies suggest that in many cases vascular injury in patients with proximity wounds can be excluded using the physical examination alone. Frykberg et al[23] have demonstrated that a careful physical examination can identify or rule out vascular trauma in patients with proximity injury. In a large cohort of patients with proximity injury, they performed serial examinations during a 24-hour period of observation. Patients with shotgun wounds, thoracic outlet injuries, and a history of chronic vascular disease were excluded. The positive and negative predictive values of a normal physical examination were 100% and 99.3%, respectively. A recent long-term follow-up study has validated the safety of this approach.[24]

The arterial pressure index (API) is an integral part of the physical examination. It should be routine for patients with proximity injury who lack absolute indications for immediate surgery. A standard manual blood pressure cuff and a vascular (or fetal) Doppler are all the tools necessary to perform an API. The API is determined by obtaining Doppler pressures in the distal vessels of the injured extremity (posterior tibial/dorsalis pedis or radial/ulnar) and dividing this number by the Doppler pressure in an uninjured limb. A value of <0.90 is considered abnormal.

Several studies have assessed the accuracy of the API in patients with penetrating extremity trauma. Lynch et al[25] calculated the API in 93 consecutive patients with 100 limb injuries. There were 21 arterial injuries, and an API <0.90 had a sensitivity of 95% and a specificity of 97%. Johansen et al[26] evaluated 100 traumatized limbs in 96 consecutive patients, and found the negative predictive value of an API >0.90 to be 99%. Others have reported similar findings.[27-29] The API does has several important limitations (Box 30-3). Occasionally, severe extremity injuries will not permit API determination because of an inability to apply a blood pressure cuff. Hypovolemia may cause

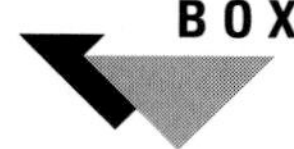

BOX 30-3
Conditions That Render Arterial Pressure Index or Duplex Sonography Less Accurate

- Proximal injuries (axillary and groin)
- Subclavicular injuries
- Popliteal injuries
- Shotgun wounds
- Multiple wounds in the same extremity
- Shock

an initially low API value that normalizes following resuscitation.[30] Rarely, arterial spasm may result in a transiently abnormal API in the absence of vascular injury.[25,26] In addition, nonocclusive lesions that do not reduce flow (small intimal flaps, pseudoaneurysms, or arteriovenous fistulas) may not alter the API. Finally, the dynamics of lower extremity blood flow ensure that injury to the deep femoral artery yields a normal API. For these reasons, it is still advisable to follow patients with proximity wounds and a normal API with either observation and serial measurements or duplex Doppler ultrasonography.

Duplex Doppler Ultrasonography

Unless they have hard signs of arterial injury and require angiography or surgery, duplex scanning is indicated in all patients with proximity injury and an API of less than 0.9.[31] It is accurate, noninvasive, and allows for serial evaluations. Duplex imaging gives real-time assessments of flow velocities and waveform characteristics that identify specific injuries. Intimal flaps, thrombosis, complete arterial disruption, and AV fistula produce unique flow signatures that are well described.[32,33]

Several studies have addressed the use of duplex scanning in proximity injury. Bynoe et al[34] applied this technology to 198 consecutive patients with penetrating extremity trauma. The results of ultrasonography were compared with arteriography, surgical exploration, or clinical follow-up. Duplex scanning had a sensitivity and specificity of 95% and 99%, respectively. Of note, there were three situations where duplex imaging had higher false-negative or equivocal results (Box 30-3): shotgun wounds, and popliteal and subclavicular injuries. In a study of 175 patients with 20 documented injuries, Fry et al[35] found duplex scanning to have a sensitivity of 100%, specificity of 97%, and accuracy of 97%. Knudson et al[36] prospectively studied 77 patients with 86 extremity injuries using color-flow Doppler and then angiography. Four patients had positive study results, and all were confirmed with angiography. There were no false-negative studies. Bergstein et al[37] compared duplex scanning with arteriography in 67 patients with 75 penetrating injuries. There were four angiographically demonstrated injuries, two of which were detected by ultrasonography (sensitivity 50%). Two missed injuries were small pseudoaneurysms of an axillary artery and an aberrant radial artery. The authors recommended cautious interpretation of negative studies with wounds of the axilla or in proximity to bifurcating arteries. Because the number of true-positives in this series was small, the sensitivity of the test is not accurately represented.

Duplex Doppler has limitations. State-of-the-art equipment is expensive and not widely available. The technology is sophisticated and requires skill in operation and interpretation. A learning curve is required for clinicians to become proficient with its use.

EVALUATION OF SHOTGUN WOUNDS

Shotgun injuries are ballistically and clinically very different from gunshot wounds. Extremity wounds caused by shotgun blasts typically have a much higher degree of tissue destruction.[13,38] Deitch et al[39] reviewed 85 patients with 112 extremity shotgun wounds and found major soft-tissue injuries in 59%, bone and joint injuries in 44%, nerve injuries in 21%, and vascular injuries in 26%. The presence or absence of neurologic injury was the major predictor of long-term function. Because of the extensive wounding capacity of these weapons and the potential for vascular injury at multiple levels, screening arteriography is recommended for significant injuries, even when soft signs of vascular injury are absent.

MANAGEMENT PRIORITIES

The first priority in the management of the patient with penetrating extremity trauma is to control ongoing hemorrhage and restore intravascular volume. Control external hemorrhage by direct manual pressure. The use of a blood pressure cuff as a proximal tourniquet is ill-advised, since it may worsen venous bleeding and leads to compartment hypertension. Blind clamping of actively bleeding vessels in the wound is strongly discouraged, since this maneuver invariably causes further injury to neurovascular structures. Gunshot wounds to the extremities can penetrate into the chest or abdomen. An apparently simple shoulder wound may hide a tension pneumothorax. The greatest potential for death in this setting is from unrecognized and under-appreciated shock (see Chapter 8).

The next priority in the patient with known or suspected vascular injuries is to identify significant injury and expedite definitive repair. Early surgical consultation is essential, and steps should be taken to avoid inertia. There is no need to complete an extensive diagnostic work-up before consultation, since unnecessary delays pose an immediate threat to limb viability and function. All patients with hard signs of vascular injury require *immediate* consultation. The often-quoted window of "6 hours to revascularize an extremity" may be excessively liberal. Some patients suffer significant functional loss despite revascularization before 6 hours.

Because of collateral flow, certain distal vascular injuries do not require repair. Consequently, penetrating trauma to these areas does not need an extensive evaluation. Injuries to the arteries of the leg distal to the midcalf do not generally require surgery or vascular studies. Patients with a possible radial or ulnar artery injury distal to the midforearm should be first evaluated with the Allen test. If either the radial or ulnar artery is injured, adequate collateral flow through the remaining intact artery yields a normal Allen test. Patients with good collateral flow may not require vascular repair of an injured radial or ulnar artery. However, because local practices vary, consult a vascular surgeon in such cases.

Patients with penetrating extremity trauma may sustain a compartment syndrome. This complication is more likely in patients who suffer a high-velocity gunshot wound, a shotgun wound, or an associated fracture. Pain on passive range of motion of a distal joint is an important early finding; absent pulses are a late and ominous sign.

Once vascular injury has been ruled out, the treating physician should adhere to the sound principles of wound care. Patients with low-velocity wounds and isolated soft-tissue injuries can usually be treated as outpatients.[40] Débride obviously devitalized tissue. The value of wound irrigation in small penetrating wounds is unclear.

Most wounds caused by a knife or gun require little intervention. The development of infection in minor gunshot wounds is rare. In a study of over 3000 such patients treated and released from the ED *without* antibiotic therapy, the infection rate was 1.8%.[41] Infection was most likely in patients with multiple injuries, gross wound contamination, significant tissue devitalization, large wounds, or delays in treatment.

No randomized controlled trial has demonstrated which penetrating extremity wounds (if any) benefit from antibiotic therapy. Suggested indications for antibiotics include the following:

1. Wounds more than 12 hours old, especially of the hands and the lower extremities
2. Devitalized tissue
3. Significantly contaminated wounds
4. Wounds involving joint spaces, tendons, or bones*

Although antibiotic therapy is not routinely recommended, a single dose of a parenteral agent (e.g., first-generation cephalosporin), followed by 5 to 7 days of outpatient oral therapy appears reasonable.[41,42]

*American College of Emergency Physicians: Clinical policy for the initial approach to patients presenting with penetrating extremity trauma, *Ann Emerg Med* 23(5):1147-1156, 1994.

Orthopedic consultation is appropriate in patients with fractures associated with gunshot wounds. Subsequent management depends on the site and nature of injury. Although some patients require hospitalization for surgical debridement and intravenous antibiotics, there is growing evidence that many patients with extraarticular long-bone fractures not requiring surgical fixation can be treated with immobilization and outpatient antibiotic therapy.[43-45] Patients discharged from the ED should have timely follow-up with the consulting orthopedic surgeon. All wounds with suspected or obvious joint penetration should be admitted for wound irrigation and intravenous antibiotic therapy.[46,47] Gunshot wounds to the foot are also considered high-risk, and some authors suggest admission for this injury,[48] despite the lack of definitive evidence for this recommendation.

Disposition

Patients with evidence of vascular injury on physical examination or diagnostic studies require admission to a surgeon. Patients with a negative evaluation may be discharged if no significant injury is found. Others benefit from a period of observation. Patients with swelling, persistent bleeding, and those with significant pain can be followed clinically in the ED for a period of several hours. Patients who are discharged following penetrating extremity trauma should be instructed to return immediately for increased pain, swelling, numbness, or weakness. A wound check in several days may detect complications.

CONCLUSION

Patients with penetrating extremity trauma may sustain limb-threatening vascular injury. Certain physical findings such as an absent pulse or signs of distal ischemia are sufficient grounds for surgical intervention. Other patients have "soft signs" that require further evaluation. The API is an important maneuver, and a ratio of less than 0.90 should prompt duplex sonography. Angiography is best reserved for a select few with positive duplex sonography or patients with proximal wounds.

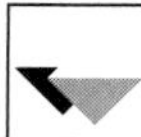

PEARLS & PITFALLS

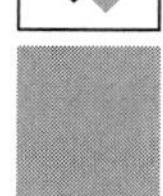

- ◆ Pulses may remain normal distal to the site of significant arterial injuries in 25% to 49% of cases.

- Placing an examination glove over the diaphragm of the stethoscope allows the physician to listen for a bruit over the wound without bloodying his or her equipment.
- The diagnosis of vascular spasm should be made only *after* duplex sonography or arteriography demonstrates an intact vessel.
- Hard signs of vascular injury are diagnostic of arterial trauma requiring surgical repair.
- Routine screening arteriography for proximity alone is expensive, of limited clinical benefit, and associated with complications.
- Injuries to the DFA are associated with significant blood loss and will not result in a pulse deficit or abnormal arterial pressure index (API).
- Duplex scanning is indicated in all patients with proximity injury and an API of less than 0.9—unless patients have hard signs of arterial injury and require angiography or surgery.
- Screening arteriography is recommended for significant injuries resulting from shotgun wounds.
- There is no evidence to suggest antibiotics are necessary in penetrating extremity wounds.

REFERENCES

1. Mattox KL, et al: Five thousand seven hundred sixty cardiovascular injuries in 4459 patients: epidemiologic evolution 1958 to 1987, *Ann Surg* 209:698-705, 1989.
2. Feliciano DV, et al: Management of vascular injuries to the lower extremities, *J Trauma* 28:319-328, 1988.
3. Menzoian JO, et al: Management of vascular injuries to the leg, *Am J Surg* 144:231-234, 1982.
4. Stein JS, Strauss E: Gunshot wounds to the upper extremity: evaluation and management of vascular injuries, *Orthop Clin North Am* 26:29-35, 1995.
5. Sitzmann JV, Ernst CB: Management of arm arterial injuries, *Surgery* 96:895-901, 1984.
6. Frykberg ER, et al: A reassessment of the role of arteriography in penetrating proximity extremity trauma: a prospective study, *J Trauma* 29:1041-1050, 1989.
7. Frykberg ER, et al: Nonoperative observation of clinically occult arterial injuries: a prospective evaluation, *Surgery* 109:85-96, 1991.
8. Hughes CW: Arterial repair during the Korean War, *Ann Surg* 147:555-561, 1958.
9. Rich NM, Baugh JH, Hughes CW: Acute arterial injuries in Vietnam: 1,000 cases, *J Trauma* 10:359-369, 1970.
10. Inui FK, Shannon J, Howard JM: Arterial injuries in the Korean conflict (experience with 111 consecutive injuries), *Surgery* 37: 850-857, 1955.
11. Sinkler WH, Specer AD: The value of peripheral arteriography in assessing acute vascular injuries, *Arch Surg* 80:300-304, 1960.
12. Kelly GL, Eiseman B: Civilian vascular injuries, *J Trauma* 15:507-514, 1975.
13. Perry MO, Thal ER, Shires GT: Management of arterial injuries, *Ann Surg* 173:403-408, 1971.
14. Geuder JW, et al: The role of contrast arteriography in suspected arterial injuries of the extremities, *Am Surg* 51:89-93, 1985.
15. Snyder WH 3d, et al: The validity of normal arteriography in penetrating trauma, *Arch Surg* 113:424-426, 1978.
16. Sirinek KR, et al. Reassessment of the role of the routine operative exploration in vascular trauma, *J Trauma* 21:339-344, 1981.
17. Reid JD, et al: Assessment of proximity of a wound to major vascular structures as an indication for arteriography, *Arch Surg* 123:942-946, 1988.
18. Stain SC, et al: Selective management of nonocclusive arterial injuries, *Arch Surg* 124:1136-1141, 1989.
19. Panetta TF, et al: The natural history of nonoperative vascular injuries, *Am J Surg* 25(abstract):708, 1985.
20. Frykberg ER, Vines FS, Alexander RH: The natural history of clinically occult arterial injuries: a prospective evaluation, *J Trauma* 29:577-583, 1989.
21. Richardson JD, Vitale GC, Flint LM Jr: Penetrating arterial trauma: analysis of missed vascular injuries, *Arch Surg* 122:678-683, 1987.
22. Earnest F 4th, et al: Complications of cerebral angiography: prospective assessment of risk, *AJR* 142:247-253, 1984.
23. Frykberg ER, et al: The reliability of physical examination in the evaluation of penetrating extremity trauma for vascular injury: results at one year, *J Trauma* 31:502-511, 1991.
24. Dennis JW, et al: Validation of nonoperative management of occult vascular injuries and accuracy of physical examination alone in penetrating extremity trauma: 5- to 10-year follow-up, *J Trauma* 44:243-252, 1998.
25. Lynch K, Johansen K: Can Doppler pressure measurement replace "exclusion" arteriography in the diagnosis of occult extremity arterial trauma? *Ann Surg* 214:737-741, 1991.
26. Johansen K, et al: Non-invasive vascular tests reliably exclude occult arterial trauma in injured extremities, *J Trauma* 31:515-519, 1991.
27. Nassoura ZE, et al: A reassessment of Doppler pressure indices in the detection of arterial lesions in proximity penetrating injuries of the extremities: a prospective study, *Am J Emerg Med* 14:151-156, 1996.
28. Weaver FA, et al: Is arterial proximity a valid indication for arteriography in penetrating extremity trauma? A prospective analysis, *Arch Surg* 125:1256-1260, 1990.
29. Schwartz MR, et al: Refining the indications for arteriography in penetrating extremity trauma: a prospective analysis, *J Vasc Surg* 17:116-122, 1993.
30. Belcaro G, Nicolaides AN: Pressure index in hypotensive or hypertensive patients, *J Cardiovasc Surg* 30:614-617, 1989.
31. Meissner M, Paun M, Johansen K: Duplex scanning for arterial trauma, *Am J Surg* 161:552-555, 1991.
32. Mitchell DG, et al: Femoral artery pseudoaneurysm: diagnosis with conventional duplex and color Doppler, *Radiology* 165:687-690, 1987.
33. Helvie MA, et al: The distinction between femoral artery pseudoaneurysms and other causes of groin masses: value of duplex Doppler sonography, *AJR* 150:1177-1180, 1988.
34. Bynoe RP, Miles WAS, Bell RM, et al: Noninvasive diagnosis of vascular trauma by duplex ultrasonography, *J Vasc Surg* 14:346-352, 1991.
35. Fry WR, et al: The success of duplex ultrasonographic scanning in diagnosis of extremity vascular proximity trauma, *Arch Surg* 128:1368-1372, 1993.
36. Knudson MM, et al: The role of duplex ultrasound arterial imaging in patients with penetrating extremity trauma, *Arch Surg* 128:1033-1038, 1993.

37. Bergstein JM, et al: Pitfalls in the use of color-flow duplex ultrasound for screening of suspected arterial injuries in penetrated extremities, *J Trauma* 33:395-402, 1992.
38. Meyer JP, et al: Peripheral vascular trauma from close-range shotgun injuries, *Arch Surg* 120:1126-1131, 1985.
39. Deitch EA, Grimes WR: Experience with 112 shotgun wounds of the extremities, *J Trauma* 24:600-603, 1984.
40. Brouker ME: Outpatient antibiotic treatment of uncomplicated gunshot wounds: ramifications for military use, *Mil Med* 162: 266-267, 1997.
41. Ordog G J, et al: Infection in minor gunshot wounds, *J Trauma* 34:358-365, 1993.
42. Ordog G J, et al: Civilian gunshot wounds—outpatient management, *J Trauma* 36:106-111, 1994.
43. Knapp TP, et al: Comparison of intravenous and oral antibiotic therapy in the treatment of fractures caused by low-velocity gunshots. A prospective, randomized study of infection rates, *J Bone Joint Surg* 78-A:1167-1171, 1996.
44. Hansraj KK, et al: Efficacy of ceftriaxone versus cefazolin in the prophylactic management of extra-articular cortical violation of bone due to low-velocity gunshot wounds, *Orthop Clin North Am* 26:9-17, 1995.
45. Joshi A, Labbe M, Lindsey RW: Humeral fracture secondary to civilian gunshot injury, *Injury* 29(suppl 1):13-17, 1998.
46. Brannon JK, et al: Gunshot wounds to the elbow, *Orthop Clin North Am* 26:75-84, 1995.
47. Perry DJ, et al: Gunshot wounds to the knee, *Orthop Clin North Am* 26:155-163, 1995.
48. Boucree JB Jr, Gabriel RA, Lezine-Hanna JT: Gunshot wounds to the foot, *Orthop Clin North Am* 26:191-197, 1995.

31 Soft-Tissue Injuries

JOEL M. BARTFIELD AND RONALD L. STRAM

Teaching Case

A 30-year-old man had a beer bottle smashed against his right lower thoracic back. He presented with a 5-cm jagged laceration in this region. His wound was anesthetized with lidocaine, irrigated with normal saline, and sutured after debriding the wound edges. He returned to the emergency department (ED) 5 days later with increasing pain at the suture site, and purulent drainage was evident. A radiograph revealed a 3-cm-long piece of glass imbedded deep within the wound. His wound was reopened and irrigated, and the glass foreign body (FB) was removed. His wound was then packed open. ■

Emergency physicians (EPs) frequently manage patients with a variety of wounds ranging from simple lacerations to complex bite wounds. This chapter discusses many aspects of wound management, including initial inspection and examination, methods of closure, and anesthetic administration. It also offers suggested guidelines for antibiotic treatment and admission criteria.

WOUND PHYSIOLOGY

Wounds that violate the epithelium heal through a process of scar formation followed by maturation. The immediate response to a break in the skin is reflex vasoconstriction, platelet aggregation, and subsequent clot formation. Clots further contract, dehydrate, and form an eschar that affords protection from external contamination.[1]

Within the actual wound, the following processes occur: inflammation, epithelialization, fibroplasia, and contraction. Inflammation is initially beneficial in that it removes contamination from bacteria, foreign debris, and devitalized tissue. Granulocytes peak within 12 hours to control bacteria and suppress infection. Macrophages appear within 24 to 48 hours and control debris, recycle reusable substrates, and play critical roles in fibroblast replication and angiogenesis. As white blood cells within the wound die, their contents are released and an exudate is formed. A surplus of exudate interferes with epithelialization and fibroplasia and is the characteristic of early wound infection.[2,3]

Within 24 to 48 hours, epithelial cells rise to the surface to begin to cover the surface defect. This process makes the wound impermeable to water. Although there is initially some adhesiveness between the wound edges in the first 3 days, by the fourth day collagen synthesis begins and scar formation is initiated through fibroplasia. This process of collagen formation through fibroplasia begins to provide tensile strength to wounds by the fifth day following injury and is almost completed by the twenty-eighth day.[4]

The process of contraction is the movement of skin edges towards the center of the defect. Contraction occurs primarily in the direction of underlying muscle fibers and is the most important process in wound healing by secondary intention.[5]

INITIAL TEN-MINUTE EVALUATION

The patient should be placed in a supine position before examining any wound. Even the most stoic-appearing individuals may have a vasovagal reaction to this initial evaluation, and the physician must therefore ensure that the patient sustains no further injury.

Before considering alternatives to closure or further wound care, bleeding must be controlled. Direct pressure usually suffices. If a large arterial bleed is suspected, decide whether the vessel can be ligated or if repair is mandated. Careful exposure and knowledge of anatomy answers this question. Control bleeding by either direct pressure or proximal pressure of the arterial source if repair is deemed necessary. Tourniquets are rarely required to control bleeding. However, a blood pressure cuff applied above the wound may be useful to visualize FBs or damage to deep structures. It is crucial to continue to limit ongoing blood loss while arrangements are being made for definitive repair.

Nonvital small peripheral vessels that are actively bleeding can often be managed by simple ligature or cauterization. It is mandatory to obtain direct visualization of underlying structures to achieve this goal. Blind application of hemostats should never be done, since this action may damage underlying nerves, tendons, and other structures.

Simple lacerations should be covered with saline-soaked dressings if there is an expected delay of greater than 2 to 3 hours until wound closure. However, wounds that are at high risk for subsequent infection, such as crush injuries or contaminated wounds, should be copiously irrigated without delay.

History should include the following: past medical history with attention to significant co-morbidities, medications (especially corticosteroids, warfarin, aspirin), allergies, tetanus status, and circumstances surrounding the injury. Co-morbidities that may decrease wound healing include diabetes mellitus, advanced age, peripheral vascular disease, alcoholism, uremia, collagen vascular disease, chronic corticosteroid use, and end-stage chronic obstructive pulmonary disease.[6] Special attention should be paid to the age of the wound and mechanisms of injury that may warrant further evaluation (e.g., syncope, motor vehicle crash).

Physical examination should focus on the potential for injury deep to the skin. Perform a thorough functional examination to rule out tendon injury. Patients with a tendon injury may have distal range of motion but reduced strength. Careful wound exploration rules out the presence of FBs with special attention to reactive substances such as organic material. Potential joint violation should be excluded in all wounds that are in proximity to joints. Obtain radiographs for any suspected bony injury or radiopaque FBs. Ultrasound, computed tomography (Fig. 31-1), or magnetic resonance imaging may identify other FBs if there is a high clinical suspicion.[7]

TYPES OF CLOSURE

Primary Closure

Before considering techniques for wound closure, the care provider must determine whether or not primary closure is indicated. This decision involves two issues: condition of the wound and age of the wound.

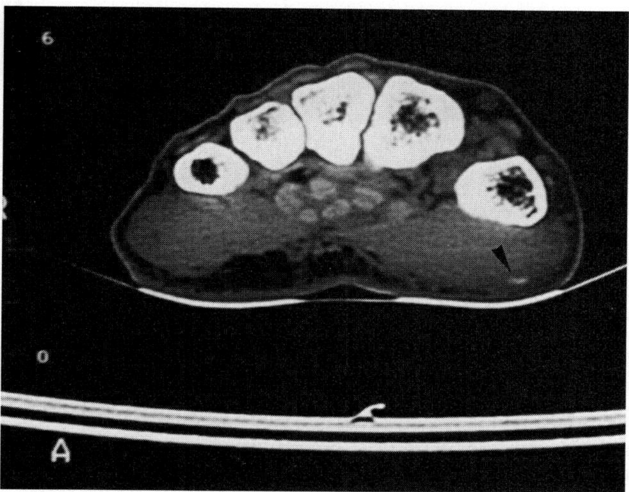

Fig. 31-1 Computed tomography of right hand with wood foreign body not seen by plain-film radiographs *(arrowhead)*.

Wounds that appear vital after cleaning, irrigation, and debridement can be considered for primary closure. Most wounds can be closed without significantly increased risk of infection or poor healing within 6 to 8 hours, except for those wounds involving the distal extremities. The chance for bad outcomes increases after as little as 3 hours for foot lacerations and 4 to 5 hours for hand lacerations.[8] Face and scalp lacerations, however, can safely be closed despite a 24-hour delay.[9]

Healing by Secondary Intention

Wounds that are at high risk for infection, such as grossly contaminated wounds or puncture wounds, should not be repaired primarily. However, initial wound management remains the same; instead of performing primary closure, these high-risk wounds are simply dressed. Dressings must be kept clean and dry and changed at least once a day. Wounds subsequently heal by granulation and reepithelialization.[5,6]

Delayed Primary Closure (Tertiary Closure)

Delayed primary closure is a good option for those wounds that would have an unacceptable cosmetic outcome or delay in healing by secondary closure. This technique is also useful for grossly contaminated wounds and high-velocity missile wounds.[2,10,11]

Initial wound management consists of copious irrigation and debridement followed by gauze packing and subsequent dressing with petrolatum (Xeroform) or saline-soaked micropore gauze. Dressings are changed at least once daily with special attention to maintaining moisture. The patient may return to the ED for wound closure in 4 to 5 days if there is no evidence of infection.[11,12] Because the process of epithelialization will have already begun and could impair wound healing, the EP should "freshen" the wound edges by gently shaving them with a scissors or scalpel.

ANATOMY OF WOUND CLOSURE

Wounds that are under high tension or contain devitalized tissue are at higher risk for poor healing. Undermining, multiple-layer closure, vertical mattress sutures, or some combination minimizes tension on the wound (Fig. 31-2). Undermining is performed by gently separating the dermal-fascial plane of the wound edge by blunt dissection with a straight or curved hemostat. "Sharp" undermining may be accomplished using a scalpel. Multiple-layer closure should involve minimal use of absorbable suture to approximate the deep fascial plane.

Typical wounds that contain devitalized tissue include crush injuries and stellate lacerations. Damaged tissue should be removed by careful debridement, accomplished by simple or wide excision, depending on the amount of damaged tissue. Fig. 31-3 emphasizes the need for making beveled edges during debridement to allow eversion of the epidermal margins. If a wide excision is necessary to ensure proper approximation, an elliptic excision is performed parallel to natural skin tension lines where the length-to-width ratio is approximately 3:1.[13,14]

Once tension is minimized and devitalized tissue removed, wounds can be closed utilizing basic wound closure techniques. These techniques include layer matching, wound-edge eversion, and minimizing dead space.

PROPHYLACTIC ANTIBIOTIC USE

Although prophylactic antibiotics are commonly used in a large variety of settings, justification for this practice is difficult to reference. The numerous trials on prophylactic antibiotics frequently yield conflicting results. Antibiotics are not generally indicated for a wound that presents late to the ED (more than 12 hours) unless the wound appears infected.

Certain high-risk wounds (Box 31-1) *might* benefit from prophylactic treatment with antibiotics. Treatment should be directed towards skin flora or towards any species that are suspected contaminants; generally, a first-generation cephalosporin (such as cephalexin 500 mg q 6h) is chosen. Parenteral antibiotics are rarely indicated for prophylaxis. If they are given for a clenched fist injury or open fracture, they should be administered less than 3 hours after injury; otherwise, effectiveness is diminished.[14-16] Again, a first-generation cephalosporin such as cefazolin 1 to 2 gm may be appropriate. A more broad-spectrum agent such as ampicillin/sulbactam provides greater activity against oral pathogens that may be present in a bite wound. It is unclear how long a subsequent course of oral prophylactic antibiotics should be continued; however, a 3- to 5-day course is probably adequate.[17]

TETANUS PROPHYLAXIS

Tetanus status should be assessed in all patients who have sustained wounds that violate the epithelial barrier. Patients who have had tetanus immuniza-

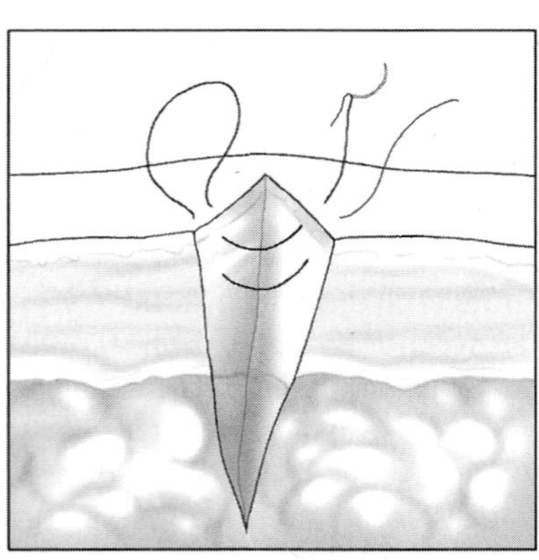

Fig. 31-2 Vertical mattress suture.

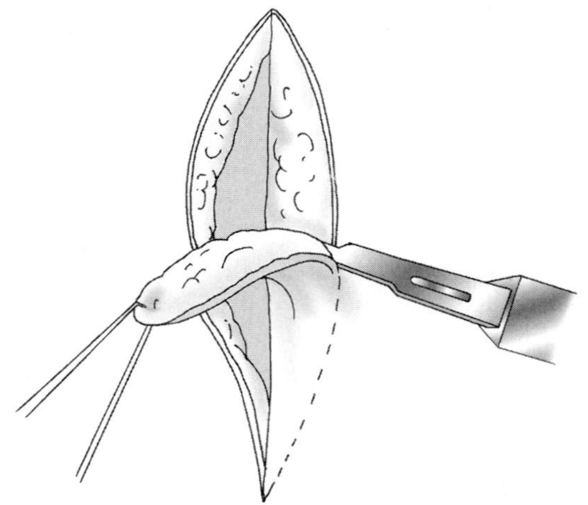

Fig. 31-3 Debridement and excision of damaged tissue.

tion in the past consisting of at least three properly timed immunizations should receive a tetanus toxoid booster if they have not done so within 10 years for uncontaminated or minor wounds and within 5 years for all other wounds. Those patients who have not been properly immunized before their injury should receive their first tetanus toxoid at the time of their injury for minor uncontaminated wounds, and tetanus toxoid plus tetanus immune globulin (250 to 500 units intramuscularly) for all other wounds. Patients who have not been properly immunized before their injury should also be referred for completion of their immunization series. The second immunization should be given at least 4 weeks after the first and the final immunization given 6 months later.[18,19]

GUNSHOT AND STAB WOUNDS

The most important aspect in the management of gunshot wounds (GSWs) and stab wounds is management of underlying injury. The surface wound is usually best managed conservatively. Debride any obviously devitalized tissue and determine if a bullet entrained any pieces of wadding or clothing in the wound. All such foreign objects should be removed. Bullets themselves may safely remain in the soft tissues, but can be removed if they are very superficial and especially if they are tenting the skin. Unless a knife wound has slashed the patient and left a large defect, most stab wounds and wounds caused by bullets can be covered with a sterile dressing without need for repair. (This approach does not apply, of course, to sucking chest wounds.)

The development of infection after minor GSWs is rare. In a study of over 3000 such patients treated and released from the ED *without* antibiotic therapy, the infection rate was 1.8%. Infection was most likely in patients with multiple injuries, gross wound contamination, significant tissue devitalization, large wounds, or delays in treatment.[20]

BOX 31-1
Situation in Which Prophylactic Antibiotics May Be Considered

WEAK EVIDENCE IN FAVOR OF ANTIBIOTICS

- Puncture wounds to the foot
- Mutilating injuries that require extensive revision
- Lacerations in areas of lymphatic obstruction
- Amputation injuries, especially if reimplantation is being considered
- Extensive ear lacerations involving cartilage
- Wounds older than 10 to 12 hours, especially wounds involving the hands and the lower extremities
- Patients with co-morbid disorders (diabetes mellitus, immunosuppression, peripheral vascular disease)

MODERATE EVIDENCE IN FAVOR OF ANTIBIOTICS

- Grossly contaminated wounds
- Open fractures and joint involvement
- Extensive and/or distal extremity bite wounds (moderate *and* conflicting evidence)

BITES

Epidemiology

Between 500,000 and 2 million animal bites occur in the United States per year.[8,21-23] Dogs account for approximately 80%, with 10% occurring from cats, 5% from humans, with the remainder being accounted for by various mammals, including rodents and monkeys.[23,24] The peak incidence is in children between 5 and 14 years of age.[23,24] Most animal bites are traceable to the owners; however, many bites go unreported. Approximately 5% to 15% occur from wild or untraceable animals, which often necessitates the need for rabies prophylaxis.[23]

Approximately 75% of animal bite wounds occur on the upper extremity; the hand being the most commonly involved. However, in children under the age of 9 the predominant location is the face and head.[25,26] In one study,[26] 30% of all dog bite wounds to the hand became infected. In contrast, 65% to 70% of human bite wounds to the hand became infected. Wounds to the face are least likely to become infected, with an incidence of less than 5%.

Microbiology of Bite Wounds

Although multiple organisms can be cultured from the mouths of animals, only a few of these organisms are implicated as pathogens in bite wounds. The most frequent aerobic pathogens found in dog bite infections are *Staphylococcus aureus, Staphylococcus epidermidis, Enterobacter,* and other various unidentifiable gram-negative rods. Occasionally, anaerobic species are identified, but no one species predominates.[21,23,27] Another pathogen commonly identified is *Pasteurella multocida,* found in approximately 50% of all dog bites and 70% of all cat bites.[28,29] *P. multocida* must be suspected if signs of infection develop in less than 24 hours following the bite, whereas infections caused by staphylococcal and streptococcal species tend to manifest in 48 to 96 hours following the bite.[29]

In contrast to animal bites, infections caused by human bites more often contain multiple pathogens.

Three patterns of pathogens related to human bites occur: mixed pathogens, gram-negative and gram-positive aerobes with a predominance of *S. aureus*, or pure cultures of *S. aureus*.[30] Infections related to mixed pathogens that include *Enterobacter spp., Klebsiella spp., Streptococcus spp., Proteus spp., Escherichia coli*, and *Pseudomonas spp.* are the most common.[22,30,31] Over 70% of the *S. aureus* found in this setting are resistant to penicillin.[22,30,31] Another common organism found in human bites *is Eikenella corrodens*, a facultative gram-negative anaerobe. *E. corrodens* is isolated in approximately 30% of all human bite hand wounds.[32] *E. corrodens* is resistant to cephalosporins.

Risk Factors for Infection

Wounds involving the hand, wrist, and foot or any joint are at high risk for developing infection. Additionally, puncture wounds and crush injuries, especially those that contain damaged tissue that cannot be easily debrided, are likely to suppurate. Cat bites have a higher incidence of infection as compared with dog and human bites. This risk is related both to the high incidence of *P. multocida* and the characteristic puncture-type wounds, which deeply inoculate bacteria. Human bites have a higher incidence of infection as compared with dog bites.

There are several predisposing factors that place patients at higher risk for the development of wound infections from animal bites. Patients greater than 50 years of age are at increased risk. Additionally, those patients with premorbid conditions that alter immune response, such as diabetes mellitus, alcoholism, and asplenism, are at increased risk.[6,25]

Management of Bite Wounds

GENERAL CONSIDERATIONS

For large wounds that violate epidermis and dermis, standard wound care techniques should be carried out. Careful attention should be made to adequately debride and copiously irrigate the wound. Cultures should be obtained from wounds that present late and appear infected. Radiographs should be obtained on any wound that has suspected underlying bony injury, joint space involvement, or retained FB. Assess the need for passive tetanus immunization and rabies prophylaxis. Wounds at high risk for rabies inoculation include those incurred from skunks, bats, foxes, and raccoons. Consult the local health department for local recommendations regarding rabies prophylaxis, since these recommendations vary with regional incidence of infected animals.

Wounds involving the face that are not grossly contaminated and less than 12 hours old can be repaired primarily after adequate wound management. This concept is particularly true of dog bites because of their lower incidence of infection as compared with human and cat bites. It may not be appropriate to primarily close bites on the extremities, particularly the hand, because of the high incidence of subsequent infection.[24,30,33] Puncture wounds do not require closure and, in addition, wound closure may increase the incidence of infection.

PROPHYLACTIC ANTIBIOTICS

Prophylactic antibiotics are given before any signs of wound infection. Although data are conflicting, it has been suggested that prophylaxis for animal bites that are at high risk for developing infection is a prudent practice. These high-risk situations include cat and human bites and those wounds involving the hand, wrist, foot, or any suspected joint. Additionally, a lower threshold for prescribing antibiotics is needed for patients prone to infection because of immunosuppression or for those patients who have prosthetic heart valves or joints.[31-33]

Human bite wounds in proximity to the metacarpophalangeal joints deserve special attention. This "clenched-fist injury" often causes serious joint infection and unless specifically questioned patients may not reveal the true mechanism of injury. ("I just cut it Doc.") The management of clenched-fist injuries differs between locales. Some physicians place the patient on antibiotics and schedule a mandatory recheck the following day. Other practitioners admit such patients to the hospital for subspecialty consultation and intravenous (IV) antibiotics.[30,31] All agree that these wounds should not be closed primarily because of the high risk for subsequent infection.

INFECTED WOUNDS

Wounds that already show signs of infection on presentation to the ED should be treated with antibiotics directed at the most likely pathogens. Those patients with established infections involving the hand or foot often require admission to the hospital and treatment with IV antibiotics. Although some infected wounds on other locations may be managed with antibiotics on an outpatient basis, adequate follow-up is essential. Patients with significant co-morbidities are best managed as inpatients.

MINIMIZING PAIN OF WOUND ANESTHESIA

Physicians should maintain a calm demeanor and minimize pain associated with anesthesia administration as outlined in the following discussion. One study reports the calming influence of music during suture repair.[34] Although it may not be possible to provide music in many emergency settings, physicians should minimize patient anxiety. For example, anesthesia preparation and the attendant large needles are best performed out of the eyesight of patients.

Several factors affect the degree of patient discomfort including the type of anesthetic,[34,36] needle size,[37,38] pH,[36,39-41] temperature of the solution,[42-44] and speed and depth of injection.[37,38,45,46] Local anesthetics are weak bases that are slightly acidified to increase their shelf-life. Adding small amounts of sodium bicarbonate (9:1 dilution, that is, 9 cc of anesthetic to 1 cc sodium bicarbonate) to anesthetics decreases pain of infiltration.[36,37,39-43] The buffered agent can be used for up to 1 week after preparation with no loss in efficacy.[47] Although some studies have suggested that warming solutions decrease pain of infiltration, data are conflicting.[42-44] Additionally, two clinical trials have demonstrated that pain of infiltration is lessened by inserting the needle within the wound rather than through intact skin.[48,49] Finally, one recent study has suggested that pretreatment of wounds with topical tetracaine reduces pain of infiltration.[50]

ALTERNATIVES TO NEEDLE INFILTRATION

Topical Agents

Several different agents and combination of agents have been studied as topical anesthetics. The agent that has been studied and used most extensively is TAC, a combination of tetracaine (0.5 %), adrenaline (1:2000), and cocaine (11.8%).[51] However, TAC has been found to be inferior to lidocaine infiltration on wounds other than those involving the face and scalp.[51] In the largest published series comparing TAC with lidocaine infiltration, TAC was inferior to lidocaine even for facial lacerations.[52] TAC is less effective for large lacerations, and in adults as compared to children.[51] Additionally, like other topical anesthetics, the agent needs to be left in place for at least 10 to 15 minutes (or until the wound edges blanch) to achieve anesthesia. The agent is contraindicated on areas supplied by end arterioles as a result of its vasoconstrictive properties.[51,52] Importantly, TAC cannot be used on mucous membranes or burns because of enhanced cocaine absorption.[51] Inappropriate use of TAC on or adjacent to mucous membranes has been associated with seizures and death.[53-57]

Other topical anesthetic combinations are as effective and safer than TAC. Topical 5% lidocaine with epinephrine[58] and lidocaine, epinephrine, and tetracaine (LET)[59] compare favorably to TAC. LET has replaced TAC in many EDs for reasons of safety, cost, and storage. (LET is not a controlled substance like TAC.)

EMLA cream is a eutectic mixture of lidocaine and prilocaine and has been used successfully as an anesthetic on intact skin before invasive procedures such as phlebotomy, intravenous insertion, and lumbar puncture.[60-66] The agent is currently FDA approved for use with intact skin only. Additionally, it can require up to 1 hour for anesthesia to be achieved.

SELECTION OF ANESTHETICS

Local and regional anesthetics are generally either amide or esters of the "caine" family. Esters were the first to be developed, of which procaine (Novocain) is the prototype. Unlike amide anesthetics that are metabolized by the liver, ester anesthetics are metabolized in plasma by pseudocholinesterases. Additionally, esters have a relatively high incidence of allergic reactions compared with amides. Generally, amides such as lidocaine are used.

Maximum Safe Dosages of Local Anesthetics

Like all medications, local anesthetics have dosage-related toxicities. Although mg/kg dosing is useful in pediatric patients, the maximum safe dosages for adults are generally expressed in absolute terms, since weight does not correlate well with peak anesthetic drug levels.[67] The maximum safe amount of plain lidocaine in an adult patient is 4 mg/kg (300 mg in an average-sized adult). Since a 1% solution contains 1000 mg per 100 ml or 10 mg/ml, this dose would represent 30 cc of 1% lidocaine. Table 31-1 provides generally accepted maximum dosages for commonly used local anesthetics. It is important to emphasize that these dosages refer to subcutaneous or intradermal injections only. Systemic toxicity may occur at much lower doses if anesthetics are injected intravascularly.

Several options can be considered if volumes that approach toxicity are required, including selection of a less toxic agent, dilution of the agent, provision of anesthesia as a nerve or field block that often requires less volume that simple local anesthesia, and the addition of epinephrine. Epinephrine at a concentration of approximately 1:100,000 can be added to anesthetics or is commercially available for some anesthetics. In addition to increasing the maximum volume that can be administered safely, the vasoconstrictive properties of epinephrine help provide a more bloodless field and thus assist in wound closure. However, the EP should wait 8 to 10 minutes after injection before closing the wound to achieve the full vasoconstrictive

TABLE 31-1
Maximum Safe Dosages for Selected Anesthetics

GENERIC NAME	TRADE NAME	CLASSIFICATION	ADULT DOSAGE	PEDIATRIC DOSAGE
Lidocaine	Xylocaine	Amide	300 mg	4 mg/kg
Lidocaine w/epi*	Xylocaine w/epi*	Amide	500 mg	7 mg/kg
Bupivacaine	Marcaine	Amide	175 mg	1.5 mg/kg
Bupivacaine w/epi*	Marcaine w/epi*	Amide	225 mg	3 mg/kg
Procaine	Novocain	Ester	500 mg	7 mg/kg
Procaine w/epi*	Novocain w/epi*	Ester	600 mg	9 mg/kg

**epi*, Epinephrine.

effect. Although there is a theoretic risk of increase in incidence of infection because of vasoconstriction, this risk does not appear clinically significant. In some studies, anesthetics containing epinephrine have been shown to cause more pain with infiltration than anesthetics without epinephrine.[35,36] The advantages and disadvantages of epinephrine-containing anesthetics should be considered before using an anesthetic containing epinephrine. Anesthetics containing epinephrine should be avoided in regions of the body with end-arteriolar supply, such as digits, penis, ear lobes, and nose.

Alternative Agents for Patients Who Report Allergy to Local Anesthetics

True anaphylaxis to local anesthetics, particularly amides, is extremely rare.[68-70] Skin testing among patients with a reported lidocaine allergy has shown that very few reactions represent true allergies.[69,70] Nonetheless, anaphylaxis is a potentially lethal complication that is obviously best avoided.

Unfortunately, patients are often unable to distinguish a history of a true allergic reaction from a vasovagal reaction. Furthermore, even if there is a history of a true allergic reaction, patients may be unable to report as to which class of anesthetics they are allergic. Anesthetics from an alternate class could be used if the specific allergy was known. The situation is further complicated by the fact that patients who report a true allergy to "lidocaine" are most often allergic to methylparaben, the preservative used in multidose vials, rather than to lidocaine itself. The traditional alternatives to the amide anesthetics (e.g., lidocaine, bupivicaine, mepivacaine) are the ester anesthetics (e.g., procaine, tetracaine). Their degradation product is para-amino benzoic acid (PABA), a chemical that is closely related to methylparaben, which could possibly induce the same allergic reaction. If the caregiver knew with certainty that a given patient was allergic to methylparaben rather than to lidocaine itself, a reasonable alternative would be to use single-dose lidocaine that contains no preservatives. However, it is difficult for physicians and patients alike to make this distinction. Therefore alternatives to traditional anesthetics have been sought.

Diphenhydramine (Benadryl) is an antihistamine with local anesthetic properties.[71-74] The chemical structure of antihistamines is closely related to that of local anesthetics, but dissimilar enough to avoid cross-reactivity.[71] This agent has been studied by a number of different researchers over the last decade, using volunteers and patients.[69-73] One percent diphenhydramine (prepared by making a 4:1 dilution of 4 cc of normal saline with 1 cc of 5% diphenhydramine) provides anesthesia comparable to 1% lidocaine, but the solution is considerably more painful to administer than lidocaine.[71-73] In an effort to reduce pain of infiltration, Ernst et al[73] compared 0.5% diphenhydramine with 1% lidocaine, but found the former less effective. Furthermore, sedation, local irritation, erythema, vesicle formation, tissue necrosis, and prolonged anesthesia have all been reported by patients or study participants.[71,72,74,75] Adding buffer to diphenhydramine does not ameliorate these effects.[75] Given the relative discomfort of diphenhydramine infiltration and potential side effects, an alternative noncaine anesthetic would be desirable for patients who are allergic to lidocaine.

Benzyl alcohol has such potential.[35,76,77] Anecdotal reports and research protocols show that 0.9% benzyl alcohol (as found as a preservative in multidose normal saline) yields minimal pain of infiltration, provides good anesthesia,[35,76-78] and has low toxicity [79,80] Wightman and Vaughan[35] compared benzyl alcohol and five other anesthetics and found that benzyl alcohol was the least painful. Unfortunately, the duration of anesthesia for benzyl alcohol was only a few minutes.[34] By adding epinephrine to the solution, benzyl alcohol can provide long-term anesthesia, though less adequately than lidocaine with epinephrine.[76] A comparison of benzyl alcohol with epinephrine, lidocaine with epinephrine, and placebo found that benzyl alcohol with epinephrine was the least painful on administration. Its anesthetic potential was greater than placebo but not as great as lidocaine with epinephrine.[76] Bartfield et al[81] compared 0.9% benzyl alcohol with epinephrine 1:100,000, 1% diphenhydramine, and 0.9% buffered lidocaine and reported that benzyl alcohol with epinephrine was the least painful of the three anesthetics. Although benzyl alcohol with epinephrine was somewhat less effective than buffered lidocaine, it provided adequate anesthesia for the majority of subjects tested in this volunteer study.

LOCAL VERSUS REGIONAL ANESTHESIA

Local Anesthesia

Anesthesia for most wounds is accomplished through local infiltration of anesthetics directly into the wound. This technique has several advantages. It is easy to accomplish, reliable and, as long as proper amounts and technique are utilized, quite safe. Additionally, local infiltration, particularly with anesthetics containing epinephrine, provides local hemostasis.

Local anesthesia has several noteworthy disadvantages. Infiltration of anesthetics in and around wounds distorts anatomy and can make subsequent repair of lacerations more difficult. As compared with nerve blocks, local anesthesia often requires larger volumes of anesthetic. Additionally, local infiltration requires multiple injections.

Field Blocks

Some areas of the body lend themselves to anesthesia via field blocks. This technique involves infiltration of anesthetic in an area that either surrounds the area that has been injured or interrupts the nerve supply to the area. Advantages of this technique include providing reliable anesthesia without disrupting anatomy. One disadvantage is that relatively large volumes of anesthetic are required. Common areas that can be anesthetized by field blocks include the forehead, ear, and nose.

Nerve Blocks

Nerve blocks offer several advantages over local anesthesia including the fact that they often require smaller volumes of anesthetic, can often be given as a single injection, and do not distort anatomy. A good working knowledge of anatomy is critical for successful performance, and proper antiseptic technique is essential. Care should be taken to identify landmarks. Patients should be told that they might feel paresthesias during the technique (in fact, paresthesias indicate that the anesthetic is being delivered in an area very close to the nerve). If paresthesias are elicited, the needle should be withdrawn slightly before injecting the anesthetic. Since vascular structures tend to be located near many nerves, it is important to aspirate and make sure that the tip of the needle is not in an artery or vein before injecting. Deliver an adequate amount of anesthetic in the area of the nerve and following infiltration, gently massage the area to diffuse the anesthetic. Nerve blocks may take 10 to 15 minutes to take effect. Bupivacaine provides a longer duration of activity than lidocaine. If a block has been unsuccessful, the practitioner has the option of attempting the block again or resorting to local anesthesia, remembering not to exceed the maximum allowable amount of local anesthetic.

SPECIFIC NERVE BLOCKS

An exhaustive review of all nerve blocks is beyond the context of this text. This discussion therefore is limited to the most commonly used and helpful including digital nerve blocks and blocks involving nerves supplying sensation to the hand, foot, and face.

Digital Nerve Blocks

Digital nerve blocks are the most commonly performed nerve block. Hand and finger injuries are relatively common and the technique is easily learned. There are two sets (palmar and dorsal) of digital nerves and each runs along the lateral aspect of the digit. The palmar nerves supply most of the sensation to the fingertip and block at this location is generally all that is required. The dorsal set must also be infiltrated for the thumb and fifth finger. Since digital arteries provide end arterial circulation to the finger and toe tips, anesthetics with epinephrine should never be used for digital nerve blocks.

There are several techniques for performing digital nerve blocks. The nerve can be blocked anywhere along its course proximal to the injury or at the metacarpophalangeal (MCP) joint. MCP blocks are performed by inserting a needle into the web space between the digits on either side of the digit and depositing the anesthetic opposite the joint. Although the technique is relatively easy to learn, in one study involving 30 volunteers, it was found to be less reliable (23% failure rate versus 3% failure rate) and to have a slower onset (6.35 minutes versus 2.82 minutes) compared with digital blocks performed at the proximal phalanx.[82] Conventional digital blocks can be performed by introducing the needle through the dorsal or ventral surface of the digit (blocks performed through the ventral surface tend to be more painful).

Nerve Blocks of the Hand

An appreciation for the sensory innervation of the hand is essential when choosing appropriate nerve blocks for hand injuries (Fig. 31-4). The innervation of the hand is somewhat variable. Depending on the location of the injury, more than one block may be required. However, local anesthesia in the hand, especially the thick skin of the palm, can be particularly painful and difficult to administer. The ability to perform these nerve blocks is therefore useful.

ULNAR NERVE

The ulnar nerve is best blocked at the wrist. At the wrist, the ulnar nerve lies between the flexor carpi ulnaris tendon and the ulnar artery. Access to the nerve can be achieved by either introducing the needle between these two structures or by introducing the needle underneath the flexor carpi ulnaris tendon at the ulnar aspect of the wrist. With either technique take care to avoid injecting the block into the ulnar artery by aspirating before injection. A total of 5 to 7 cc of agent is injected to achieve anesthesia.[83]

MEDIAN NERVE

The median nerve travels between the palmaris longus and the flexor carpi radialis tendons. The palmaris longus can be located by having the patient oppose the thumb and fifth finger and flex the wrist against resistance. If the tendon is congenitally absent (approximately 20% the time), the location of the nerve is approximately 1 cm ulnar to the flexor carpi radialis. The nerve is blocked by puncturing the flexor retinaculum between the two wrist creases at the location of the nerve and injecting 5 to 8 cc of agent at this site.[83]

RADIAL NERVE

The radial nerve follows the radial artery and then fans out dorsally distal to the wrist. Inject into the anatomic snuffbox and lay a 6- to 8-cm wheel of anesthetic across the dorsal portion of the radial aspect of the wrist.

Ankle Blocks

There are five different nerves that can be blocked at the level of the ankle to provide foot anesthesia. Since the anatomy is variable, the nerves are often blocked in groups. The sole of the foot is supplied by the tibial nerve (which branches into the medial and lateral plantar nerve) and the sural nerve (Fig. 31-5). The most lateral aspect of the dorsum of the foot is supplied by the sural nerve with the remainder supplied by the superficial and deep peroneal nerves and the saphenous nerve (Fig. 31-6). These blocks are somewhat more difficult to perform than blocks at the wrist or face.

TIBIAL NERVE (MEDIAL AND LATERAL PLANTAR NERVES)

The tibial nerve runs between the medial malleolus and the Achilles tendon in close proximity to the tibia. The block is accomplished by injecting 5 cc of

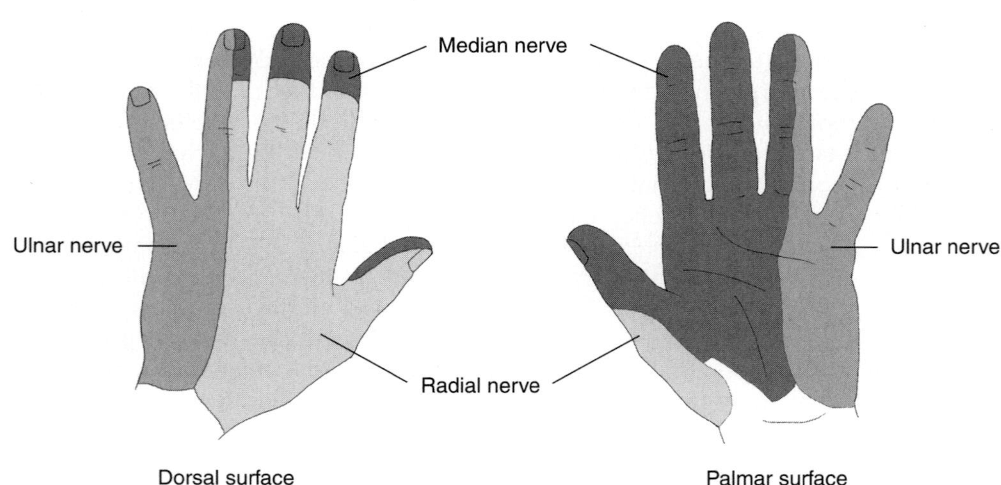

Fig. 31-4 Sensory innervation of the hand.

anesthetic agent between the posterior tibial artery and the Achilles tendon just posterior to the medial malleolus.[83] This block is best achieved with the patient in the prone position with the foot in slight dorsiflexion.

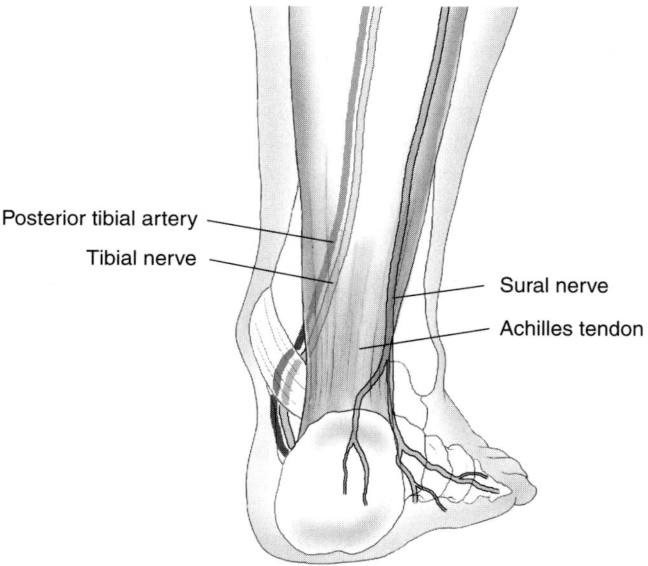

Fig. 31-5 Sensory innervation of the plantar aspect of the foot.

SURAL NERVE

The sural nerve is located between the lateral malleolus and the Achilles tendon. As compared with the tibial nerve, it is relatively superficial. The nerve is blocked just lateral to the Achilles tendon at the top of the lateral malleolus by injecting 5 cc of agent superficially in a fanlike distribution.[83]

SUPERFICIAL PERONEAL, DEEP PERONEAL, AND SAPHENOUS NERVES

To achieve an anterior ankle block, all three nerves must be anesthetized. With the patient in a supine position, the skin is entered between the extensor hallucis longus and anterior tibial tendons at a point parallel to the superior aspect of the medial malleolus. The deep peroneal nerve is blocked by a deep injection between the two tendons, whereas the other two nerves are blocked by superficial injections. The needle is then withdrawn and redirected subcutaneously toward the lateral malleolus to block the superficial peroneal nerve and then medially to block the saphenous nerve.[83] A total of 15 cc of agent is usually required to block all three nerves.

Blocks Involving Facial Nerves

Since they do not distort anatomy, nerve blocks in this location are often preferable to local anesthesia. The

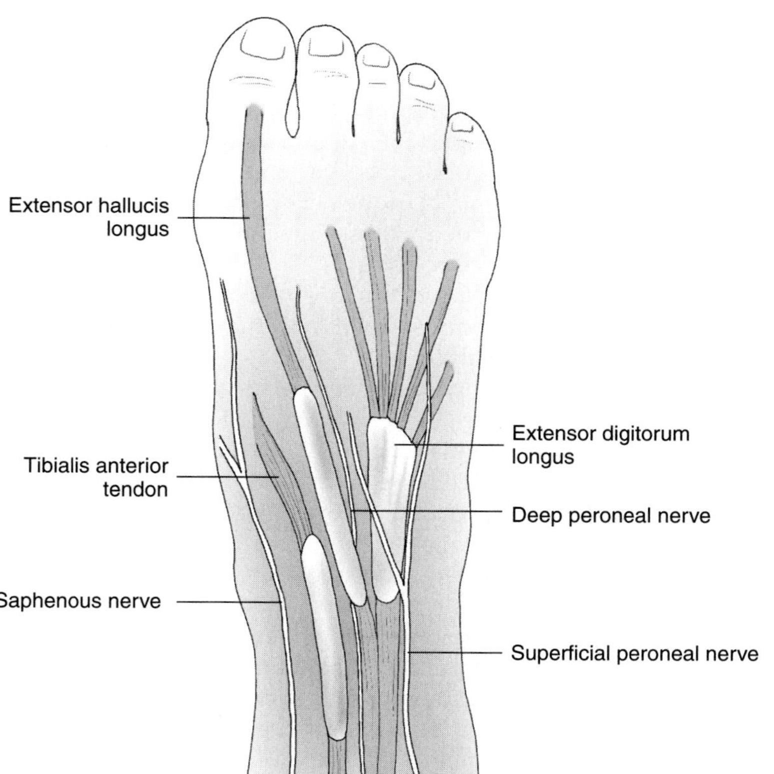

Fig. 31-6 Sensory innervation of the dorsum of the foot.

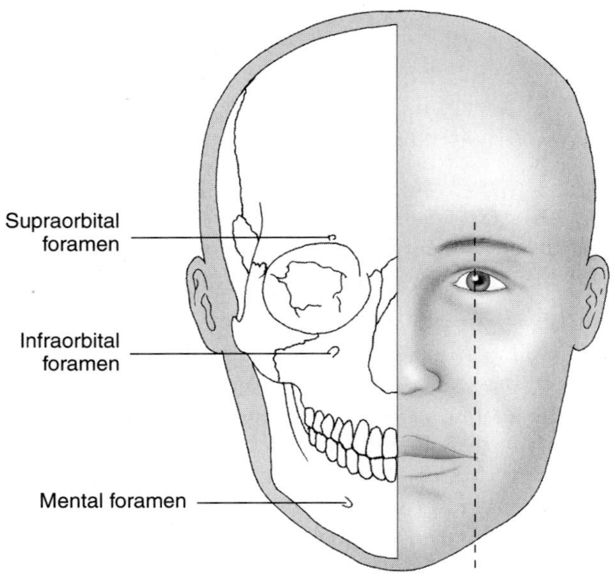

Fig. 31-7 Landmarks for facial nerve blocks.

trigeminal nerve supplies sensation to the face. The three branches of this nerve that are most commonly blocked are the supraorbital, infraorbital, and mental nerves. These nerves have very reliable anatomic locations, making nerve blocks easy and reliable. The foramina that these three nerves exit from all fall along a line that connects the medial aspect of the pupil with the corner of the mouth (Fig. 31-7).

SUPRAORBITAL AND SUPRATROCHLEAR NERVES

The supraorbital nerve supplies sensation to most of the forehead with the area near the bridge of the nose supplied by the supratrochlear nerve. Since these nerves supply the scalp as far back as the lambdoidal suture, these blocks are useful for cleansing road-rash injuries to the forehead.[84] The supraorbital nerve exits at the supraorbital foramen, and the supratrochlear nerve exits 5 to 10 mm medial to it. Both nerves can be blocked with a wheal of anesthetic across the brow. These techniques should be avoided in patients with open skull fractures to prevent cranial and bulbar palsies.[84]

INFRAORBITAL NERVE

The infraorbital nerve exits through the infraorbital foramen that is easily palpated along the line previously described, just below the inferior border of the orbit. The nerve supplies sensation to the medial aspect of the midface, including the upper lip. The infraorbital nerve can be blocked by injection either through intact skin or through the intraoral route. The latter method involves inserting a ¾-inch needle to the hub into the buccal-mucosal sulcus opposite the upper canine and palpating the foramen as the anesthetic is introduced. Care must be taken to introduce the needle along the surface of the maxilla and a ¾-inch long needle should be used to avoid penetrating the globe. This latter technique was shown to be more reliable and less painful in volunteers.[85]

MENTAL NERVE

The mental nerve supplies sensation to the superior chin and lower lip. The nerve exits through the mental foramen, which can be palpated along the previously described line in the midchin. The nerve can be blocked by either transcutaneous or intraoral injection. The latter is performed by inserting a ¾-inch needle to the hub into the buccal-mucosal fold opposite the lower canine and palpating the foramen as the anesthetic is introduced. The intraoral technique was shown to be more reliable and less painful in volunteers.[86]

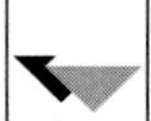

PEARLS & PITFALLS

- Use delayed primary closure for contaminated wounds or crush wounds with devitalized tissue.
- When exploring wounds of the hand, visualization of deep structures is key. Use a blood pressure cuff to obtain a bloodless field.
- Test tendon strength against resistance.
- Prophylactic antibiotics are rarely indicated in uninfected wounds.
- Suspect *P. Multocida* infection in animal wounds that become infected within the first 24 hours. This organism should be treated with penicillin and is resistant to erythromycin.
- Suspect human bite wounds for those wounds involving the metacarpophalangeal joints.
- Do not use anesthetics containing epinephrine in areas supplied by end-arteriolar circulation.
- LET has replaced TAC in many emergency departments for reasons of safety, cost, and storage.
- Buffered anesthetics reduce pain of infiltration.
- Obtain radiologic studies in wounds with suspected FB contamination.
- Document well. Record the search for foreign bodies and the status of underlying structures.

REFERENCES

1. Trott A: Mechanisms of surface soft tissue trauma, *Ann Emerg Med* 17:1279-1283, 1988.
2. Hunt JK, Van Winkle W: *Wound healing: normal repair: fundamentals of wound management in surgery,* South Plainfield, NJ, 1976, Chirurgecom.
3. Ordman LJ, Gillman T: Studies in the healing of cutaneous wounds I. The healing of incisions through the skin of pigs, *Arch Surg* 93:857-882, 1966.
4. Timberlake GA: Wound healing: the physiology of scar formation, *Curr Concepts Wound Care* 9:4, 1986.
5. Zitelli JA: Secondary intention healing: an alternative to surgical repair, *Clin Dermatol* 2:92-106, 1984.
6. Hunt TK: Disorders of wound healing, *World J Surg* 4:271-277, 1980.
7. Flom LL, Ellis GL: Radiologic evaluation of foreign bodies, *Emerg Med Clin North Am* 10:163-177, 1992.
8. Edlich RF, et al: Principles of emergency wound management, *Ann Emerg Med* 17:1284-1302, 1988.
9. Hotter AN: Physiologic aspects and clinical implications of wound healing, *Heart Lung* 11:522-531, 1982.
10. Bryant WM: Wound healing, *Clin Symp* 29:1-36, 1977.
11. Edlich RF, et al: Studies in the management of the contaminated wound. I. Optimal time for closure of contaminated open wounds. II. Comparison of resistance to infection of open and closed wounds during healing, *Am J Surg* 117:323-329, 1969.
12. Dimick AR: Delayed wound closure: indications and techniques, *Ann Emerg Med* 17:1303-1304, 1988.
13. Kirk RM: *Basic surgical techniques,* Edinburgh, 1978, Churchill Livingston.
14. Haley RW, et al: Identifying patients at high risk of surgical wound infection: a simple multivariate index of patient susceptibility and wound contamination, *Am J Epidemiol* 121:206-215, 1985.
15. Burke JF: The effective period of preventive antibiotic action in experimental incisions and dermal lesions, *Surgery* 50:161-168, 1961.
16. Rutherford WH, Spence RA: Infection in wounds sutured in the accident and emergency department, *Ann Emerg Med* 9:350-352, 1980.
17. Haughey RE, Lammers RL, Wagner DK: Use of antibiotics in the initial management of soft tissue hand wounds, *Ann Emerg Med* 10:187-192, 1981.
18. Diphtheria, tetanus, and pertussis: guidelines for vaccine prophylaxis and other preventive measures, *MMWR* 34:405-414, 419-426, 1985.
19. Centers for Disease Control: Recommendations of the Immunization Practices Advisory Committee (ACIP): rabies prevention, *MMWR* 29:265-280, 1980.
20. Ordog GJ, et al: Infection in minor gunshot wounds, *J Trauma* 34:358-365,1993.
21. Goldstein EJ: Bite wounds and infection, *Clin Infect Dis* 14:633-638, 1992.
22. Goldstein EJ, et al: Bacteriology of human and animal bite wounds, *J Clin Microbiol* 8:667-672, 1978.
23. Kizer KW: Epidemiologic and clinical aspects of animal bite injuries, *J Am Coll Emerg Phys* 8:134-141, 1979.
24. Dire DJ: Emergency management of dog and cat bite wounds, *Emerg Med Clin North Am* 10:719-736, 1992.
25. Goldstein EJ, Richwald GA: Human and animal bite wounds, *Am Fam Phys* 36:101-109, 1987.
26. Lindsey D, et al: Natural course of the human bite wound: incidence of infection and complications in 434 bites and 803 lacerations in the same group of patients, *J Trauma* 27:45-48, 1987.
27. Ordog GJ: The bacteriology of dog bite wounds on initial presentation, *Ann Emerg Med* 15:1324-1329, 1986.
28. Goldstein EJ, Citron DM, Finegold SM: Dog bite wounds and infection: a prospective clinical study, *Ann Emerg Med* 9:508-512, 1980.
29. Arons MS, Fernando L, Polayes IM: Pasteurella multocida: the major cause of hand infections following domestic animal bites, *J Hand Surg Am* 7:47-52, 1982.
30. Malinowski RW, et al: The management of human bite injuries of the hand, *J Trauma* 19:655-659, 1979.
31. Farmer CB, Mann RJ: Human bite infections of the hand, *South Med J* 59:515-518, 1966.
32. Goldstein EJ, Barones MF, Miller TA: Eikenella corrodens in hand infections, *J Hand Surg Am* 8:563-567, 1983.
33. Callaham ML: Treatment of common dog bites: infection risk factors, *J Am Coll Emerg Phys* 7:83-87, 1978.
34. Menegazzi JJ, et al: A randomized, controlled trial of the use of music during laceration repair, *Ann Emerg Med* 20:348-350, 1991.
35. Wightman MA, Vaughan RW: Comparison of compounds used for intradermal anesthesia, *Anesthesiology* 45:687-689, 1976.
36. Christoph RA, et al: Pain reduction in local anesthetic administration through pH buffering, *Ann Emerg Med* 17:117-120, 1988.
37. Arndt KA, Burton C, Noe JM: Minimizing the pain of local anesthesia, *Plast Recon Surg* 72:676-679, 1983.
38. Berk WA, Welch RD, Bock BF: Controversial issues in clinical management of the simple wound, *Ann Emerg Med* 21:72-80, 1992.
39. Bartfield JM, et al: Buffered versus plain lidocaine as a local anesthetic for simple laceration repair, *Ann Emerg Med* 19:1387-1389, 1990.
40. Bartfield JM, Ford DT, Homer PJ: Buffered versus plain lidocaine for digital nerve blocks, *Ann Emerg Med* 22:216-219, 1993.
41. Orlinsky M, et al: Pain comparison of unbuffered versus buffered lidocaine in local wound infiltration, *J Emerg Med* 10:411-415, 1992.
42. Brogan GX Jr, et al: Comparison of plain, warmed, and buffered lidocaine for anesthesia of traumatic wounds, *Ann Emerg Med* 26:121-125, 1995.
43. Mader TJ, Playe SJ, Garb JL: Reducing the pain of local anesthetic infiltration: warming and buffering have a synergistic effect, *Ann Emerg Med* 23:550-554, 1994.
44. Bartfield JM, et al: The effects of warming and buffering on pain of infiltration of lidocaine, *Acad Emerg Med* 2:254-258, 1995.
45. Krause RS, et al: The effect of injection speed on the pain of lidocaine infiltration, *Acad Emerg Med* 4:1032-1035, 1997.
46. Scarfone RJ, Jasani M, Gracely EJ: Pain of local anesthetics: rate of administration and buffering, *Ann Emerg Med* 31:36-40, 1998.
47. Bartfield JM, et al: Buffered lidocaine as a local anesthetic: an investigation of shelf life, *Ann Emerg Med* 21:16-19, 1992.
48. Kelly AM, Cohen M, Richards D: Minimizing the pain of local infiltration anesthesia for wounds by injection into the wound edges, *J Emerg Med* 12:593-595, 1994.
49. Bartfield JM, Sokaris SJ, Raccio-Roback N: Local anesthesia for lacerations: pain of infiltration inside versus outside the wound, *Acad Emerg Med* 5:100-104, 1998.
50. Bartfield JM, et al: Topical tetracaine attenuates the pain of infiltration of buffered lidocaine, *Acad Emerg Med* 3:1001-1005, 1996.
51. Grant SA, Hoffman RS: Use of tetracaine, epinephrine, and cocaine as a topical anesthetic in the emergency department, *Ann Emerg Med* 21:987-997, 1992.
52. Hegenbarth MA, et al: Comparison of topical tetracaine, adrenaline, and cocaine anesthesia with lidocaine infiltration for repair of lacerations in children, *Ann Emerg Med* 19:63-67, 1990.
53. Dailey RH: Fatality secondary to misuse of TAC solution, *Ann Emerg Med* 17:159-160, 1988.
54. Jacobson S: Errors in emergency practice, *Emerg Med* 19(20):106-109, 1987.
55. Daya MR, et al: Recurrent seizures following mucosal application of TAC, *Ann Emerg Med* 17:646-648, 1988.

56. Wehner D, Hamilton GC: Seizures following topical application of local anesthetics to burn patients, *Ann Emerg Med* 13:456-458, 1984.
57. Dronen SC: Complications of TAC (letter), *Ann Emerg Med* 12: 333, 1983.
58. Blackburn PA, et al: Comparison of tetracaine-adrenaline-cocaine (TAC) with topical lidocaine-epinephrine (TLE): efficacy and cost, *Am J Emerg Med* 13:315-317, 1995.
59. Ernst AA, et al: LAT (lidocaine-adrenaline-tetracaine) versus TAC (tetracaine-adrenaline-cocaine) for topical anesthesia in face and scalp lacerations, *Am J Emerg Med* 13:151-154, 1995.
60. Buckley MM, Benfield P: Eutectic lidocaine/prilocaine cream: a review of the topical anesthetic/analgesic efficacy of a eutectic mixture of local anesthetics (EMLA), *Drugs* 46:126-151, 1993.
61. Michael A, Andrew M: The application of EMLA and glyceryl trinitrate ointment prior to venipuncture, *Anaesth Intens Care* 24:360-364, 1996.
62. Young SS, Schwartz R, Sheridan MJ: EMLA cream as a topical anesthetic before office phlebotomy in children, *South Med J* 89: 1184-1187, 1996.
63. Vaghadia H, al-Ahdal OA, Nevin K: EMLA patch for intravenous cannulation in adult surgical outpatients, *Can J Anaesth* 44:798-802, 1997.
64. Sharma SK, et al: EMLA cream effectively reduces the pain of spinal needle insertion, *Reg Anesth* 21:561-564, 1996.
65. Juarez Gimenez JC, et al: Anesthetic efficacy of eutectic prilocaine-lidocaine cream in pediatric oncology patients undergoing lumbar puncture, *Ann Pharmacother* 30:1235-1237, 1996.
66. Lee JJ, Rubin AP: EMLA cream and its current uses, *Br J Hosp Med* 50:463-466, 1993.
67. Scott DB, et al: Factors affecting plasma levels of lignocaine and prilocaine, *Br J Anaesth* 44:1040-1049, 1972.
68. Chandler MJ, Grammer LC, Patterson R: Provocative challenge with local anesthetics in patients with a prior history of reaction, *J All Clin Immunol* 79:883-886, 1987.
69. Incaudo G, et al: Administration of local anesthetics to patients with a history of prior adverse reaction, *J All Clin Immunol* 61: 339-345, 1978.
70. Adriani J, Zepernick R: Allergic reactions to local anesthetics, *South Med J* 74:694-699, 703, 1981.
71. Green SM, Rothrock SG, Gorchynski J: Validation of diphenhydramine as a dermal local anesthetic, *Ann Emerg Med* 23:1284-1289, 1994.
72. Ernst AA, et al: Lidocaine versus diphenhydramine for anesthesia in the repair of minor lacerations, *J Trauma* 34:354-357, 1993.
73. Ernst AA, et al: 1% lidocaine versus 0.5% diphenhydramine for local anesthesia in minor laceration repair, *Ann Emerg Med* 23: 1328-1332, 1994.
74. Dire DJ, Hogan DE: Double-blinded comparison of diphenhydramine versus lidocaine as a local anesthetic, *Ann Emerg Med* 22:1419-1422, 1993.
75. Singer AJ, Hollander JE: Infiltration pain and local anesthetic effects of buffered vs plain 1% diphenhydramine, *Acad Emerg Med* 2:884-888, 1995.
76. Martin S, Wilson L: Benzyl alcohol with epinephrine as an alternative local anesthetic, *Acad Emerg Med* 3(abstract):493-494, 1996.
77. Thomas DV: Saline with benzyl alcohol prevents pain of needle insertion (letter), *Anesth Analg* 63:882-883, 1984.
78. Nuttall GA, Barnett MR, Smith RL, et al: Establishing intravenous access: a study of local anesthetic efficacy, *Anesth Analg* 77:950-953, 1993.
79. Novak E, et al: The tolerance and safety of intravenously administered benzyl alcohol methylprednisolone sodium succinate formulations in normal human subjects, *Toxicol Appl Pharmacol* 23:54-61, 1972.
80. Kimura ET, et al: Parenteral toxicity studies with benzyl alcohol, *Toxicol Appl Pharmacol* 18:54-61, 1971.
81. Bartfield JM, Weeks Jandreau S, Raccio-Robak N: A randomized trial of diphenhydramine vs benzyl alcohol with epinephrine as an alternative to lidocaine local anesthesia, *Acad Emerg Med* 5(abstract):466, 1998
82. Knoop K, Trott A, Syverud S: Comparison of digital versus metacarpal blocks for repair of finger injuries, *Ann Emerg Med* 23:1296-1300, 1994.
83. Ferrera PC, Chandler R: Anesthesia in the emergency setting. Part I. Hand and foot injuries, *Am Fam Physician* 50:569-573, 1994.
84. Ferrera PC, Chandler R: Anesthesia in the emergency setting. Part II. Head and neck, eye and rib injuries, *Am Fam Physician* 50:797-800, 1994
85. Lynch MT, et al: Comparison of intraoral and percutaneous approaches for infraorbital nerve block, *Acad Emerg Med* 1:514-19, 1994.
86. Syverud SA, et al: A comparative study of the percutaneous versus intraoral technique for mental nerve block, *Acad Emerg Med* 1:509-13, 1994.

Trauma in Pregnancy

32

LAWRENCE E. KASS AND JEAN T. ABBOTT

Emergency care of the injured pregnant female involves two organisms. Fortunately, the conundrum is simplified when one realizes that survival of the fetus depends on the care given to the mother. If the mother is unstable, the fetus is always in jeopardy. Changes in maternal physiology affect both evaluation and resuscitation, and obscure the presence of shock. Other gravid phenomena, such as the supine vena caval syndrome, also influence prehospital and emergency department (ED) care.

After 24 weeks gestation, the emergency physician (EP) must consider fetal welfare somewhat separately from that of the mother. At this age, the fetus can live apart from the mother if an emergency cesarean section (C-section) is indicated. An assessment of the fetus's well-being is an integral part of the secondary survey. Fetal monitoring is the best means of detecting fetal distress, and is mandatory in the injured pregnant patient with a viable fetus. Before 24 weeks gestation, the fetus has almost no chance of a life outside the womb, and maternal resuscitation is all that matters to its survival. Therefore, before 24 weeks, fetal monitoring serves no useful purpose.

EPIDEMIOLOGY OF TRAUMA IN PREGNANCY

Trauma is the leading cause of death in reproductive-age women, and it is the most common "nonmaternal" cause of death during pregnancy.[1] In two recent series, trauma surpasses even direct and indirect maternal causes as the most important cause of maternal mortality.[2,3] Pregnancy itself does not affect the risk of traumatic death from a particular injury. The major causes of *maternal* death are the same as those in nonpregnancy: head injuries and hypovolemia.[4]

Injury in the pregnant patient may be intentional or unintentional. Although motor vehicle crashes (MVCs) and falls are the most common causes of injury overall, homicide and suicide deaths account for one third to one half of fatalities.[1,2] In MVCs, direct blows to the steering wheel or dashboard are associated with abruptio placenta that may well be prevented by proper use of restraints.[5,6] Airbags have only been studied anecdotally in pregnancy, but have not been reported to cause problems when used in conjunction with properly applied three-point restraint systems.[7]

Intentional injury is common in pregnancy, and up to one third of all trauma seen during pregnancy may be a result of such.[8] Homicides account for fully one third of maternal trauma deaths, and the rate is particularly high in urban centers.[1] Suicide accounted for 9% of maternal deaths in the series by Fildes et al[2] and 14.4% in the CDC series.[1] Domestic violence occurs in at least 8% to 17% of women during pregnancy.[9] Pregnant teens are especially likely to be abused. Single blows or kicks to the abdomen in late pregnancy are associated with abruptio placenta and fetal loss.[10,11]

FETAL INJURY AND DEATH

Maternal death and severe maternal hypovolemia are the leading causes of fetal demise (Box 32-1). The central principle in obstetric trauma is that aggressive resuscitation of the mother is likely to save the baby. In general, fetal death correlates with severe maternal injuries. However, fetal death in severe maternal trauma is not certain, and a few authors dispute the association between maternal injury and fetal mortality.[5,12,13,15] In both blunt and penetrating trauma, fetal mortality generally exceeds maternal death rates.[16] Although most fetal deaths occur at the time of injury, late and potentially preventable deaths have been reported.[10,17]

On occasion, the fetus may die after minimal maternal trauma. Most of these reports involve isolated blows to the abdomen, or relatively trivial maternal injuries such as a fall or minor MVC. Premature uterine contraction is the most common nonlethal complication of maternal trauma. Abruptio placenta, uterine rupture, direct fetal injury, and maternal-fetal hemorrhage with sensitization are also potential morbidities.[16,18,19]

PHYSIOLOGY OF PREGNANCY

Pregnancy is a hyperdynamic, hypermetabolic state. An outline of the normal laboratory values and physiologic changes in pregnancy are included in Tables 32-1 and 32-2.

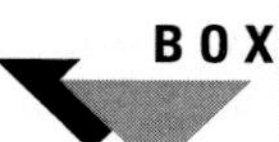

BOX 32-1
Major Causes of Fetal Death After Maternal Trauma[13,14]

Maternal death
Maternal hypotension/major injuries
Placental abruption
Placental laceration
Uterine rupture
Direct fetal trauma (head, trunk, extremities)
Maternal-fetal hemorrhage
Fetal anemia

Cardiovascular

Cardiovascular changes during pregnancy conceal the presence of shock. Cardiac output (CO) increases by 20% to 30%. Most of this increase occurs in the first trimester, resulting in a CO of 6 to 7 liters/minute by week 12.[20] Plasma volume increases disproportionately, resulting in a "physiologic anemia." Because of this increase in blood volume, signs of shock may not be manifest despite significant maternal hemorrhage. A pregnant woman may lose 35% of her blood volume before the vital signs change. Hypotension and tachycardia are late and ominous findings.

Although baseline pulse rate is 80 to 95 beats/minute in late pregnancy, rates over 100 should be considered abnormal. Patients usually experience a 5 to 15 mmHg drop in systolic pressure during the second trimester, secondary to decreased vascular tone and impaired venous constriction during the first two trimesters.[23] Nonetheless, hypotension in the pregnant trauma patient should be considered abnormal until proven otherwise. Because the diaphragm rises during late pregnancy, the electrocardiogram shows a leftward shift of the heart and T wave inversion (most commonly V2). Premature atrial contractions are common.

When a woman in the second half of pregnancy lies supine, the uterus compresses her inferior vena cava and impairs blood return to the heart. This situation can lead to a 20% decrease in CO and is responsible for the **supine hypotensive syndrome,** seen in 20% of

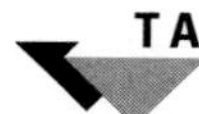

TABLE 32-1
Physiologic "Normals" in Pregnancy[20-22]

Most changes occur by tenth or twelfth week of pregnancy

TEST	COMMENTS
Hematocrit	32%-34% (with iron supplementation)
White blood count	Gradual increase: 18,000/(mm^3)[26] third trimester 25,000/(mm^3)[26] at delivery
Fibrinogen	300 to 600 mg/dl (versus 200-400 in nonpregnancy)
Prothrombin time	No change
Partial thromboplastin time	No change
Arterial pCO_2	30-32 mmHg
A-a gradient	Up to 24
Systolic blood pressure	Slightly lower first and second trimesters; position dependent
Diastolic blood pressure	Low with possibly widened pulse pressure
Heart rate	Gradual increase to 80-95 bpm
Central venous pressure	Normal to low

women after 20 weeks gestation.[24] Susceptibility varies widely, but is more likely to occur with hypovolemia.[25] The increase in venous pressures below the level of the uterus may also cause major blood loss from leg and pelvic wounds. Late in pregnancy, pelvic fractures are likely to produce dangerous hemorrhage because of the increase in venous pressures.

During hemorrhage, blood is shunted away from the "nonessential" uterus to support the maternal circulation. Profound fetal hypoperfusion may coexist with an apparently innocuous clinical presentation in the mother. The astute clinician can exploit this phenomenon by detecting fetal distress as a subtle sign of compensated shock in the mother.

Respiratory

Respiratory changes also impact trauma management. Since the diaphragm is pushed upwards by the growing uterus, lung volumes decrease. During the second half of pregnancy, the diaphragms rise about 4 cm cephalad. As a result, respiratory reserve is severely limited, and the pregnant mother becomes especially vulnerable to the effect of acute lung injury. Seemingly trivial rib fractures, pneumothoraces, or small pulmonary contusions may cause significant respiratory distress, and these injuries must be treated aggressively. Intubation of the pregnant patient poses a unique challenge, and rapid desaturation following paralysis is the norm. The EP should also keep these anatomic changes in mind when tube thoracostomy is required. The tube should be inserted above the standard position, high in the axilla, to avoid an inadvertent biopsy of the liver or spleen.

In the pregnant patient the respiratory center is more sensitive to changes in pCO_2 than in the nonpregnant state.[21] Respiratory rate and minute ventilation typically increase, and the pCO_2 drops to 30 to 32 mmHg even at sea level. This decreased pCO_2 results in a compensatory renal excretion of sodium bicarbonate. For this reason, maternal buffering capacity is impaired, and patients are more likely to develop lactic acidosis following hemorrhage.

Abdominal and Genitourinary

Pregnant women with gross hemoperitoneum may have a relatively benign abdominal examination. Since the mass

TABLE 32-2
Physiologic Changes That Affect Resuscitation in Pregnancy

CHANGES	CONSEQUENCES
CARDIOVASCULAR	
Increase in cardiac output	
Increase in heart rate	
Decrease in systemic vascular resistance	Failure to recognize shock (30%-35% blood loss before changes in vital signs)
Venous hypertension in the retroperitoneum and lower extremities	Life-threatening retroperitoneal hemorrhage with pelvic fractures
Paradoxic response to shock in first and second trimester	
Compression of vena cava by the gravid uterus	Supine hypotension syndrome
PULMONARY	
Elevated diaphragms	Misplaced chest tube in liver or spleen
Decreased functional reserve	Predisposition to fetal hypoxia
Chronic respiratory alkalosis	Rapid desaturation during intubation
	Decreased buffering capacity
GASTROINTESTINAL	
Concentration of intestines in upper abdomen during third trimester	Increased risk of bowel injury with penetrating upper abdominal wounds
Decreased gastrointestinal motility	Increased risk of aspiration
Decreased peritoneal irritation	Decreased reliability of abdominal examination

Adapted from Colucciello SA: *Emerg Med Rep* 16(18):171-182, 1995.

of the uterus fills the abdomen, viscera are rearranged and pain patterns become less predictable. Peritoneal irritation from blood in the peritoneal cavity is less likely because the parietal peritoneum is lifted off the visceral organs and the chronically stretched membrane is less sensitive. Attenuation of the rectus muscles prevents guarding. Decreased muscle tone causes prolonged gastric emptying and slowing of peristalsis, making emesis during rapid sequence intubation more likely.

The glomerular filtration rate is increased, and smooth muscle tone of the ureter is decreased. In the third trimester of pregnancy the dome of the bladder is pushed out of the pelvic cavity by the enlarging uterus, making it more vulnerable to injury following abdominal injury.

Hematologic

Because the plasma volume increases disproportionately, a physiologic anemia occurs during pregnancy. Hematocrits run from 32% to 34%, even with iron supplementation. The white count progressively rises in normal pregnancy, reaching as high as 18,000 cells/mm^3 in the third trimester, and 25,000 cells/mm^3 during delivery.[26] Because of the increased plasma proteins, the sedimentation rate increases to 70 to 80 mm/hr. Fibrinogen levels increase to 400 to 600 mg/dl.[27] Although the prothrombin time (PT) and partial thromboplastin time (PTT) do not change, levels of multiple other proteins involved in the coagulation cascade increase, resulting in hypercoagulability of late pregnancy and the peripartum period.

Physiologic Response to Hypovolemia In Pregnancy

The maternal circulation is protected at the expense of the fetal circulation during hypovolemia; however, shunting within the fetus itself can compensate for hypoxia, protecting vital fetal organs[28] (Table 32-2). Because of the mother's expanded intravascular volume, maternal tachycardia and hypotension occur late in shock, often only after a 30% to 35% blood volume loss. At low volumes, blood pressure is also extremely position dependent, and the supine hypotension syndrome is important and aggravated by hypovolemia.

The uterus is extremely sensitive to vasopressors, hypercarbia, and hypoxia, all of which impair placental circulation. In addition, the placental vascular bed does not autoregulate, and blood flow to the fetus varies with mean arterial blood pressure.

INJURIES UNIQUE TO PREGNANCY

Premature Contractions

Frequent uterine contractions are the most common finding after nonfatal maternal trauma. These contractions may indicate contusion to the uterus or blood irritating the uterine musculature, as in abruption. Although these contractions rarely progress to preterm delivery, obstetricians recommend that the mother should be monitored until contractions cease.[18,29-31] The utility of tocolysis in the trauma situation is unproven and such decisions are best left to the obstetrician.

Fetal Distress

Fetal distress may be signaled by several means, the most reliable being fetal monitoring (cardiotocographic monitoring). The normal fetal heart rate is 120 to 160 beats/minute, and slower or faster rates are worrisome. In addition, decelerations occurring after uterine contractions (late decelerations), variable decelerations, and loss of beat-to-beat variability of the fetal heart tracing indicate fetal distress.

Nonspecific fetal distress manifested by abnormal cardiotocographic monitoring is probably the most common fetal morbidity seen after maternal trauma. Although these abnormalities, along with premature labor, may be a sign of abruptio placentae, they may spontaneously resolve.[29] Fetal distress may arise from a variety of insults, from direct fetal injury, transient fetal hypoxia, maternal hypovolemia, or placental abruption.

Late in pregnancy, direct uterine forces can injure the fetus, producing skull fractures and intracranial hemorrhage. This situation is especially likely in the last weeks of gestation when the fetal head has "engaged" the pelvis. Fetal long-bone fractures are rare. Penetrating trauma to the gravid uterus may rarely be associated with fetal injuries to the chest, abdomen, or extremities.

Abruptio Placentae

Abruptio placentae occurs when there is separation of the placenta from the underlying uterine wall. In the trauma patient abruption is thought to be the result of the different elastic properties of the uterus and placenta—resulting in a "shearing" effect when the elastic uterus is deformed by external forces, causing separation from the relatively inelastic placenta. Abruptio placentae is common following blunt abdominal trauma, being reported in 1% to 3% of minor or non–life-threatening maternal injuries, and up to 50% of life-threatening maternal injuries.[32,33]

Vaginal bleeding is common. Although abdominal pain is also frequent, abruption may be clinically occult. Cardiotocographic detection of fetal distress is the most *sensitive* means of detecting abruption, although it is nonspecific. Ultrasound (US) detection of placental abruption is *specific,* but lacks sensitivity, detecting only 50% of cases. Therefore it is recommended that the patient be continuously monitored to detects signs of fetal distress, and that the injury then be defined using US.[28]

Uterine Rupture

During the first trimester, the gravid uterus is protected by the bony pelvis and is rarely subject to direct injury. However, after this period it becomes an intraabdominal organ and is at risk. Direct trauma resulting in uterine rupture is a rare event, reported in only about 0.6% of cases of severe direct abdominal trauma.[18] Physical manifestations vary from minimal abdominal tenderness to obvious peritonitis and shock. While prior uterine surgery (e.g., cesarean section or myomectomy) increases the risk of uterine rupture, rupture can occur in the normal uterus as well.

Diagnosis may be suggested by a difficult to palpate uterine fundus or, more specifically, by palpation of fetal parts outside the uterus. Ultrasound may demonstrate extended fetal extremities, an oblique fetal lie, or evidence of extrauterine fetal parts. If US is unavailable and suspicion for uterine rupture is high, an abdominal radiograph may show an "uncoiled" fetus.

Maternal-Fetal Hemorrhage

Mixing of maternal and fetal blood (**maternal-fetal hemorrhage** or **MFH**) is associated with maternal trauma. MFH occurs 4 to 5 times more commonly in injured pregnant women than in noninjured controls and can result in fetal anemia, fetal death, or isoimmunization of the mother.[18] The **Kleihauer-Betke** (**K-B**) test can estimate the volume of fetal blood in the maternal circulation, but cannot predict other complications such as uterine irritability or abruptio placenta. It should not replace fetal monitoring and US.[19]

The K-B test should not be used to determine *the need* for Rh immune globulin (RhoGAM), but may be of some value in determining *the amount* of immune globulin needed. The test is insensitive to maternal-fetal hemorrhage. As little as 0.01 to 0.03 cc of fetal blood will sensitize 70% of Rh-negative women, whereas 5 cc of fetal blood is required to produce a positive K-B test. The physician can limit K-B testing to patients who sustain severe blunt abdominal trauma in the second half of pregnancy. This approach will detect the rare patient who requires additional RhoGAM because of massive (i.e., greater than 30 cc) transfusion of fetal blood into the maternal circulation.[30]

PREHOSPITAL CONSIDERATIONS

Because of the changes described earlier, prehospital providers must always consider occult hemorrhage and shock in the pregnant patient suffering significant trauma. Women with all but the most minor of injuries should have supplemental oxygen and an intravenous (IV) line started en route. If a women who is more than 24 weeks gestation has a critical injury, medics should notify the ED early during transport. Advanced notice allows the EP to prepare for a possible emergency C-section and neonatal resuscitation.

Prehospital providers should transport women greater than 20 weeks estimated gestational age (EGA) in a left lateral decubitus position to displace the gravid uterus off the inferior vena cava and prevent supine hypotension. Women who do not require spinal immobilization can simply rest on their left side or have a pillow placed under their right buttock. If the patient requires spinal immobilization, a wedge or rolled blanket under the backboard should elevate the right side 15 degrees.[16] It is also possible to manually displace the uterus towards the left.[24]

The use of pneumatic anti-shock garments (PASG) during pregnancy is controversial. A position paper published in 1997 by the National Association of EMS Physicians lists pneumatic antishock garments as a class III intervention (inappropriate, possibly harmful) in pregnancy.[34] Others advocate PASG use for stabilizing pelvic fractures in the first trimester, for tamponade of bleeding from leg injuries (inflating leg compartments only), or, possibly, treatment of shock unresponsive to intravenous fluids.[26,35-37] Although there are no clear data in the literature to support either position, the authors recommend that PASG be *avoided* in situations where inflation of the abdominal compartment may cause compression of the uterus and vena cava, and increase the risk of supine hypotension.

EVALUATION AND DIAGNOSTIC STUDIES

History

The first priority during the history, as in all other trauma patients, is to rapidly collect information about mechanism of injury, known or suspected injuries, and the prehospital clinical status. Questions should be asked about direct blows to the abdomen that may injure the fetus. Also of importance in the pregnant female is to ask gestational age and any pregnancy-related complications such as hypertension or diabetes.

In patients suffering assaults, stab wounds, or gunshot wounds, domestic violence must always be considered. The EP must recognize the clues of domestic violence and explore the patient's safety and risk of repeated injury. The patient should be directly asked, "Did someone hurt you?" Although only very few women report abuse on standard medical history forms, many more of these same women admit to abuse when directly questioned by a healthcare provider. In addition, pregnancy can be a time of significant stress and it is important to ask questions about depression and suicide risk when appropriate.

Physical Examination

The "ABCs" of the primary survey are virtually unchanged during pregnancy and are directed at the mother. Remember that maternal pulse and blood pressure can be misleading. Since pregnancy is a low-resistance, hyperdynamic state, mild tachycardia may be normal; the blood pressure is normal to low for a healthy young woman, with a somewhat widened pulse pressure (see Table 32-2). The physiologic hypervolemia of pregnancy and the ability to shunt blood flow away from the gravid uterus may result in a normal heart rate and blood pressure despite life-threatening hemorrhage. *Normal vital signs do not rule out occult blood loss or injury.*

Once the mother's airway, breathing, and circulatory status are assessed and primary management is started in the critical patient, immediate recognition of pregnancy must occur. Evaluation of the fetus occurs during the secondary survey. The gestational age is pivotal to determine the further course of fetal resuscitation. After 24 weeks of gestation, the fetus is potentially viable and emergent delivery may be the next step in resuscitation of both the mother and fetus. Measurement of fundal height is essential to fetal resuscitation and obstetric consultation (Fig. 32-1). Between 24 and 36 weeks, the fundal height in centimeters approximates the gestational age in weeks. A fundus that rises above the umbilicus may contain a fetus that might be viable outside the uterus. If fetal parts can be palpated outside the uterus, suspect uterine rupture. Fundal height should be measured repeatedly during the ED stay; a fundus that is large-for-dates or increasing may represent bleeding within the uterus, usually as a result of placental abruption.

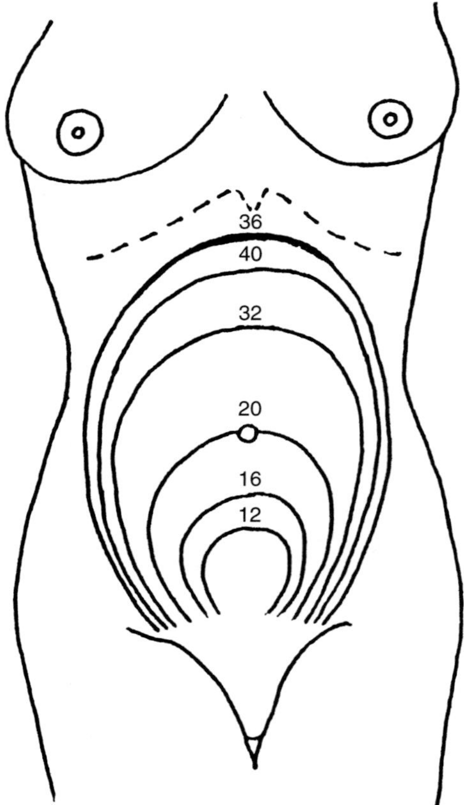

Fig. 32-1 Approximate fundal height for various gestational ages.

Thus there is an added "D" for consideration of delivery in the primary assessment of the pregnant trauma victim.

The secondary evaluation of the pregnant patient differs from the nongravid patient in the following ways:

1. The physical examination of the abdomen is less reliable for detecting signs of peritoneal irritation
2. Vital signs and laboratory values must be interpreted with knowledge of the different "normal ranges" during pregnancy
3. The diagnosis of a pelvic fracture takes on added significance because the hypertrophic vasculature increases the risk of significant retroperitoneal hemorrhage

The emergency physician should both visually and manually inspect the vulva and outer vaginal vault for bleeding, mucosal tears, bony fragments, or secretions. The need for further gynecologic examination should be driven by the physician's clinical suspicion of injury. If there is no bleeding, or if there is bleeding in a woman less than 20 weeks gestation, the EP may safely perform a speculum examination as indicated. However, after 20 weeks of gestation, examination and palpation of the cervix may precipitate uncontrollable bleeding in the presence of placenta previa. Therefore, if blood is present on the perineum and the uterus is at or above the umbilicus, consult an obstetrician. The EP may perform a partial speculum examination (placing the speculum tip partially in the vagina) to differentiate rectal, vulvar, vaginal, or cervical bleeding. Do not evaluate the cervix either digitally or with ring forceps in the vaginally bleeding patient who is greater than 20 weeks. In general, pelvic examinations after 20 weeks should only be done for specific indications (e.g., pelvic fracture). Vaginal bleeding is a poor predictor of abruptio placenta and other pregnancy complications. Cardiotocographic (C-T) monitoring is the mainstay of pregnancy assessment.[29]

Laboratory Studies

Serum laboratory studies should be performed as in a nonpregnant individual. As noted in Box 32-1, many of the "normal" values for laboratory tests may differ slightly from those of the nonpregnant individual. The EP should test for pregnancy in all significantly traumatized women of childbearing potential. A bedside urine pregnancy screen in the trauma room can significantly affect clinical decision-making. The last menstrual period, use of birth control or history, and reports of sexual activity are inadequate to eliminate the diagnosis of pregnancy. On the other hand, while a woman may think she is pregnant, only a definitive test such as fetal heart tones, US, or beta-hCG can determine the gravid state.

Acidosis is an important clue to occult shock. Lactate rises as tissue perfusion falls, long before a change in the vital signs is clinically evident. Lactate levels or a base deficit from an arterial blood gas are among the most valuable blood tests in obstetrical trauma.

The physician should test all pregnant women who present with blunt trauma (or penetrating uterine trauma) for Rh type. Rh typing is more important than the K-B test, which can be left to the obstetric consultant.

Fluid in the vaginal vault may reflect ruptured membranes and should be tested by either Nitrazine paper (which turns purple on contact with the alkaline amniotic fluid) or by the appearance of "ferning" as it dries on a microscope slide. Note that the Nitrazine test may be falsely positive for amniotic fluid in the presence of blood or urine.[35,38]

Because of the high concentration of thromboplastin in the placenta and plasminogen activator in the uterus, injury to the gravid uterus or abruptio placenta can trigger a consumptive coagulopathy. In patients with significant trauma, particularly to the abdomen, baseline coagulation studies are helpful: platelet count, fibrinogen degradation products, PT and PTT. However, such tests are unnecessary in patients with minor injuries. Serial levels of hemoglobin or hematocrit are more valuable than an isolated value.

Radiologic Studies

PLAIN FILMS

Any radiograph that is indicated should be performed and not withheld out of concern for fetal radiation exposure. The concerns about fetal irradiation are threefold: organ malformation, childhood malignancies, and small head size.[39]

The fetus is most vulnerable to radiation-induced malformation from the tenth day through the tenth week after conception. Exposure to less than 5000 to 10,000 mrd (millirads) during this time is not associated with a significant increase in the 4% to 6% background incidence of congenital defects. Exposures to greater than 15,000 mrd are clearly associated with an increased incidence of developmental abnormalities. After the twentieth week of gestation, radiation is unlikely to cause fetal malformation.[39]

Exposure to radiation is associated with an increased risk of cancer fatality before 14 years of age. For exposures of up to 100 mrd during the second or third trimester, the risk may be approximately 1 in 15,000 children. For an exposure of 5000 mrd, the risk may be about 1 in 300. For exposures during the first trimester, the risk may be higher, but the data are inadequate for accurate risk assessment.[39]

Based on animal studies and evaluation of the survivors of the atomic bomb explosions at Hiroshima and Nagasaki, there appears to be an increased risk of small head size from fetal irradiation, without a necessarily associated intellectual deficit. This complication can occur with exposure during the second through fifteenth week of gestation, if the dose is between 5000 and 10,000 mrad.[39]

For standard trauma radiographs, the exposure to the unshielded ovary ranges from less than 1 mrd for a cervical spine or extremity film to up to approximately 200 to 1300 mrd for a lumbosacral series (Table 32-3).

When possible, the EP should limit the scope of the examination, shield the abdomen, and collimate the x-ray beam. The use of clinical decision rules such as the Ottawa ankle and knee rules may result in fewer unnecessary films.

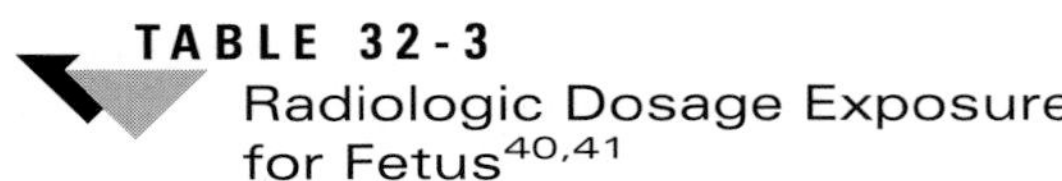

TABLE 32-3 Radiologic Dosage Exposure for Fetus[40,41]

EXAMINATION	ESTIMATED DOSE TO UTERUS/FETUS (MRDS)
Cervical spine (series)	0.0-1.0
Extremity (per view)	0.0-1.0
Chest (PA portable)	0.0-5.0
Head/chest CT scan	<50
Pelvis	200-300
Lumbar spine (AP and lateral)	200-1300
Abdominal CT scan	3000-10,300

CT, Computed tomography; *AP,* anteroposterior.

COMPUTED TOMOGRAPHY

Wagner et al[42] found that fetal exposure to computed tomography (CT) radiation ranged from 3000 to 10,300 mrd and varied with patient size, the number of cuts obtained, and whether the fetus was in, or adjacent to, the field. CT scanning of the maternal head or chest exposes the unshielded gravid uterus to minimal radiation (<50 mrd).[20,43] If abdominal CT scanning is performed before 20 weeks gestation, the EP should shield the uterus with a lead apron and scan the upper abdomen to look for liver or spleen injury. After 20 weeks, a standard scan may be safe. Intravenous contrast has little or no deleterious effect on the fetus.

Ultrasound

In the pregnant patient, US can identify hemoperitoneum without the risks of needle/catheter injury associated with diagnostic peritoneal lavage (DPL) or fetal radiation from CT. In the critical patient who is also pregnant, it provides timely and important information about fetal age and viability. Timely US can assist in determining whether emergent C-section is indicated.

Ultrasound is used routinely in obstetric practice to estimate gestational age, fetal activity (general and cardiac), fetal tone, fetal breathing movements, amniotic fluid volume, position and integrity of the placenta, and the presence of intrauterine blood.[12,44] However, sonography should not be used to exclude abruptio placenta. Although some subplacental hematomas can be visualized, a significant number cannot.[18,32] In the nonemergent trauma victim, sonographic fetal assessment should be performed after maternal assessment and stabilization.

Diagnostic Peritoneal Lavage

Diagnostic peritoneal lavage has often been cited as being relatively contraindicated in advanced pregnancy.[45] A review of the literature reveals mostly case series, but suggests that DPL remains a useful tool in the evaluation of blunt abdominal trauma.

Rothenberger et al[46] reported a case series of 12 patients evaluated by DPL (8 infraumbilical, 4 supraumbilical, all by open technique) and found 100% sensitivity for the 8 who had internal bleeding confirmed by laparotomy and 100% specificity for the 4 without injury. There were no significant complications from the procedure.

Esposito et al[47] studied 40 pregnant patients who were victims of blunt abdominal trauma. Thirteen underwent DPL, and they found DPL had a 100% positive predictive value (PPV) and a 92% overall accuracy in this small series.

Despite the accuracy of DPL, CT and US are better choices to evaluate pregnant patients who are hemodynamically stable. However, in hypotensive patients, immediate laparotomy is essential for patients with hemoperitoneum. In such cases, a bedside test such as DPL or US is essential. If DPL is chosen, it should be performed using an open supraumbilical approach to minimize the risk of uterine injury.

EMERGENCY DEPARTMENT MANAGEMENT

General Principles

1. Take care of the mother. Resuscitation of the mother maximizes fetal survival. In general, what is good for the mother is good for the fetus.
2. Think shock. Signs and symptoms of shock are late and ominous in the pregnant trauma victim. Therefore pay close attention to optimizing oxygen delivery and intravascular volume. Consider early blood administration to patients who remain unstable despite fluids. Rapidly assess for hemoperitoneum (using DPL or US) and determine their need for immediate laparotomy.
3. Prevent or treat the supine hypotensive syndrome. Women greater than 20 weeks EGA should be managed in a left lateral decubitus position or on a backboard tilted 15 degrees with a wedge or pillow. Manually deflecting the uterus to the left has also been described.
4. Do not hesitate to obtain indicated radiographs. Never withhold indicated radiographs because of concerns for fetal irradiation. Accurate determination of maternal injury is essential. If uterine shielding is feasible, it will decrease fetal radiation exposure significantly.
5. Objectively evaluate the abdomen with US in pa-

Airway
Assess and control
Preoxygenation and Sellick's maneuver especially important before intubation

↓

Breathing
Assess and manage
Place chest tubes in fourth intercostal space

↓

Circulation
Assess maternal circulation
Intravenous access
Tilt to left if thought to be greater than 20 weeks estimated gestational age
Consider measurement of lactate
Liberal abdominal ultrasound

Fig. 32-2 Algorithm for resuscitation of the pregnant patient.

tients with serious mechanisms or subtle abdominal findings. Consider the use of lactate levels or base deficit (from an ABG) in patients at risk for occult bleeding.

6. Determine gestational age and fetal well-being after the primary survey.
7. Cardiotocographic monitoring should be initiated as early as feasible and continued for at least 4 hours in fetuses greater than 20 to 24 weeks gestational age. Monitoring is indicated even in cases of minor mechanisms of injury and no abdominal pain.
8. Administer RhoGAM to any Rh-negative woman presenting with trauma. For pregnancies of 13 weeks EGA or greater, give 300 μg intramuscularly (IM). For earlier pregnancies, 50 μg IM is sufficient. Even minor abdominal injury appears to increase the incidence of MFH, and isoimmunization should be prevented by treatment with RhoGAM.[48] The K-B test may be useful in detecting and quantifying MFH in the very small percentage with large-volume transfusion who require additional doses of RhoGAM.[30] RhoGAM is effective when administered up to 72 hours after antigenic exposure.[30]

Initial Maternal Resuscitation (Fig. 32-2)

AIRWAY AND BREATHING

Respiratory reserve is compromised in late pregnancy, because the uterus is enlarged and the diaphragm is elevated to the level of the nipple line. Early intubation may be required to maintain a patent airway and adequate ventilation. Because of delayed gastric emptying and an increased risk of aspiration, it is important to maintain cricoid pressure during intubation and to place a nasogastric tube in the seriously ill patient. If a chest tube is indicated in the third trimester, use the open technique to place it higher in the chest (fourth intercostal space).[38] An exploratory finger placed in the incision prevents intubating the liver or spleen.

CIRCULATION AND SHOCK

The initial treatment of shock mandates decompressing the inferior vena cava by turning the patient on her left side or deflecting the uterus to the side. If the patient remains hypotensive, resuscitate with volume, first with isotonic crystalloid then with blood as needed. The EP must rapidly search for causes of shock, usually hemothorax, hemoperitoneum, and pelvic or long-bone fracture. They must also consider impairment of cardiac contraction as a result of cardiac tamponade or tension pneumothorax. Avoid vasopressors in pregnancy (and in nonpregnancy as well) since they severely compromise uterine blood flow.[35,49] Persistently hypotensive patients are best served by blood administration and surgery, not by vasoactive drugs.

Hemodynamically significant cardiac dysrhythmias can be treated electrically. Cardioversion and defibrillation are safe in all stages of pregnancy and do not harm the fetus or induce premature labor.[50,51]

MEDICATIONS

Give tetanus immunizations to the pregnant female in the same dose and for the same indications as in the nonpregnant adult. Both tetanus toxoid and tetanus immune globulin are safe in pregnancy. As tetanus antibodies can cross the placenta, proper immunization of the mother decreases the risk of neonatal tetanus.[52,53] Consult appropriate drug references as needed before giving medications to pregnant women.

The EP or obstetrician should give a routine dose (300 μg) of RhoGAM to any injured Rh-negative expectant mother.[29,30] RhoGAM is effective if given within 72 hours of MFH.

The Hemodynamically Unstable Mother (Fig. 32-3)

The pregnant female who remains hemodynamically unstable despite resuscitation should have an emergent bedside abdominal US to assess fetal gestational age and viability. If US is unavailable, a fundal height above the umbilicus combined with a fetal Doppler will suffice.

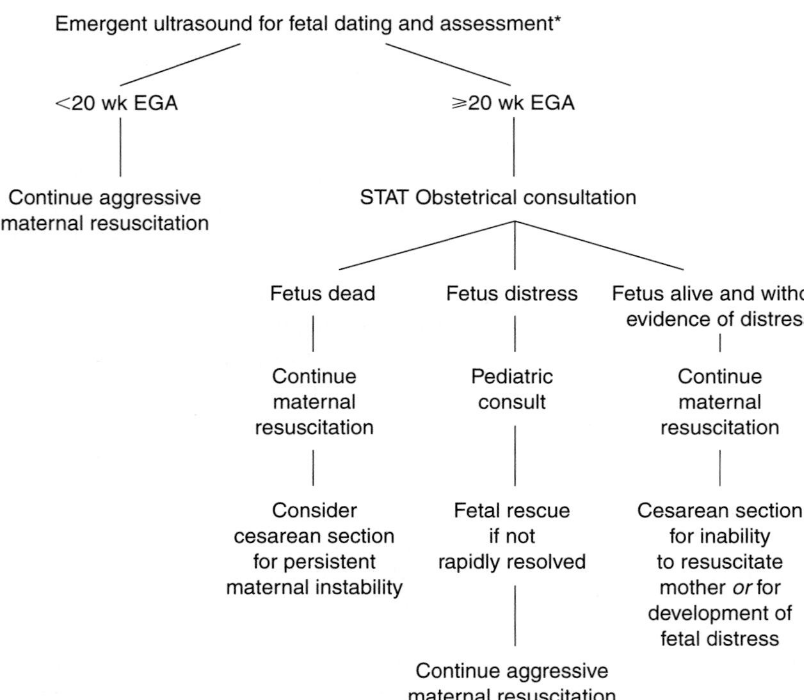

Fig. 32-3 Algorithm for the management of the unstable pregnant patient.

If the fetus is judged to be less than 20 weeks EGA, devote attention exclusively to the mother. Delivery of such a previable fetus is not an option, and the small uterus has little hemodynamic significance in regards to cardiac filling.

If the fetus is determined to be of 20 weeks EGA or greater, assess fetal well-being and obtain emergent obstetric consultation. When fetal death occurs after trauma, it is frequently immediate and before evaluation in the ED. If the fetus is dead, again focus on the mother. Fetal demise is not an indication for emergent cesarean delivery, since the mother will usually deliver spontaneously within 1 week. The only indications for emergent cesarean delivery of a dead fetus are persistent maternal instability (in which case delivery may improve maternal venous return and CO), uterine rupture, and situations in which the gravid uterus physically impairs the ability to evaluate or repair internal maternal injury.

If the older fetus is able to survive outside the mother, ascertain the degree of distress. Ominous findings include a heart rate of less than 120 or greater than 160, or cardiotocography demonstrating abnormalities such as late decelerations or decreased beat-to-beat variability. In such cases, the obstetrician will consider emergent cesarean delivery. The EP should perform an emergency C-section only in the moribund patient and not for fetal distress. Continued maternal resuscitation must persist during fetal assessment.

If the greater than 24-week fetus is alive and without signs of distress, continue fetal monitoring during further maternal resuscitation. Call the labor and delivery nurse to bring a cardiotocographic monitor to the resuscitation room. This nurse can be invaluable in interpreting the strips before the obstetrician's arrival.

The Hemodynamically Stable Mother

The hemodynamically stable pregnant female (Fig. 32-4) should undergo fetal evaluation by determining fundal height and using a Doppler device to measure fetal heart rate. In more seriously injured women, the EP should consider US for a more complete assess-

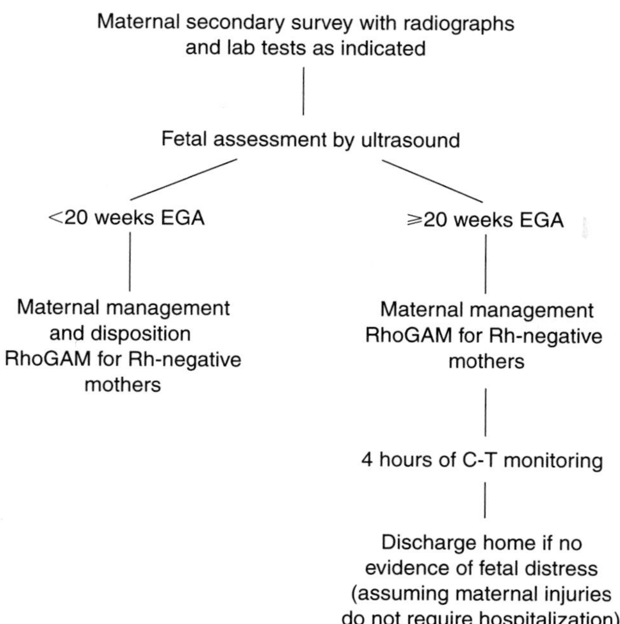
Maternal secondary survey with radiographs and lab tests as indicated
Fetal assessment by ultrasound
<20 weeks EGA
≥20 weeks EGA
Maternal management and disposition RhoGAM for Rh-negative mothers
Maternal management RhoGAM for Rh-negative mothers
4 hours of C-T monitoring
Discharge home if no evidence of fetal distress (assuming maternal injuries do not require hospitalization)

Fig. 32-4 Algorithm for the management of the stable pregnant patient.

ment, including EGA, fetal activity (general and cardiac), fetal tone, fetal breathing movements, amniotic fluid volume, position and integrity of the placenta, and the presence of intrauterine blood.

The central concern regarding fetal monitoring relates to EGA. If the fetus could survive outside the uterus (generally 24 weeks EGA or more), fetal distress may prompt an emergency C-section. For this reason, pregnant females who are over 24 weeks EGA with relatively minor injuries require at least 4 hours of fetal monitoring to detect distress or fetal demise.[10,17,54-56] Some authorities advocate initiating C-T monitoring as early as 20 weeks EGA, noting that if premature contractions are noted in this previable period, the pregnancy can sometimes be supported and delivery delayed for several weeks.[33,57] Monitoring simultaneously records continuous fetal heart rate (FHR), as well as uterine contractions. Detection of contractions, or signs of fetal distress such as an abnormal baseline heart rate, decreased heart rate variability (beat-to-beat or long term), or late decelerations require emergent consultation with an obstetrician.[36] As in the case of the unstable mother, the discovery of fetal demise is not an indication for a C-section.

If the fetus is found to be less than 20 weeks EGA, the secondary survey and subsequent management are essentially unchanged from the nongravid patient. Radiographic and laboratory studies should be ordered as needed to evaluate the mother.

SPECIAL TRAUMA CONSIDERATIONS

Penetrating Abdominal Trauma

Pregnancy may be an exception to the general rule that gunshot wounds to the abdomen require exploratory laparotomy. In mid to lower abdominal wounds during late pregnancy, the gravid uterus protects the other viscera. As a result, associated visceral injuries occur in only 19% of women with gunshots to the gravid uterus and maternal morbidity is rare.[58] Exploratory laparotomy is required for maternal indications, and for a distressed but alive fetus. Surgery is also necessary for abdominal wounds above or lateral to the gravid uterus.

Franger et al[58] reported on 3 cases and developed guidelines for the management of abdominal gunshot wounds during pregnancy. They propose observation without surgical exploration if (1) the mother is stable, the fetus is either alive and healthy, or dead; (2) the entrance wound is below the fundus; (3) the bullet is within the uterus on radiograph; (4) the abdominal examination is unremarkable; and (5) there is no blood in the urinary or gastrointestinal tract. Since these recommendations are based on case reports only, some authorities still advocate laparotomy for all gunshot wounds. They argue that without exploration it is impossible to determine the extent of uterine injury, and that the late risks of either infection or uterine rupture remain unknown.[37] During exploration, conservative management of the uterus without evacuation or cesarean delivery is possible if there is no fetal distress or injury. In cases of fetal demise, vaginal delivery can be accomplished at a later time.[16,58,59]

Stab wounds to the gravid uterus are rare, with only 19 reported in the literature.[43,60] Though successful observation of the stable patient with uterine penetration has been reported,[34] some authorities recommend exploratory laparotomy for all cases of stab wounds to the abdomen with known peritoneal penetration.[37,43] Other approaches may combine DPL with fetal ultrasound to determine need for laparotomy. Upper abdominal wounds are more likely to injure the bowel, which is crowded between the fundus and diaphragm.

Electrical and Thermal Injuries

ELECTRICAL INJURY

Accidental electrical injury can cause fetal death or later complications (oligohydramnios or growth retardation), even when the mother appears well. The case reports of fetal demise occur mainly in women in whom the current passes through the uterus or who suffer major electrical insults, such as lightning strikes. Fetal injury is attributed to the good conductive properties of both amniotic fluid and the highly vascular uterine bed.[61,62] Using prospective data, Einarson et al[63] criticize former reports of high risk of fetal demise because of reporting bias towards adverse outcomes. These authors found no difference in pregnancy outcomes between exposed women and pregnant controls. They noted that electrical exposures are usually to 110V household current and that current crossed the uterus in only a minority of cases. Because a small risk to the fetus does exist and reassurance is important, it is still recommended that all women who have experienced electrical shocks be examined and that fetal well-being be assured. Patients with normal fetal heart rates may be discharged without a period of monitoring since fetal death appears to occur at the time of injury only.[16,63]

THERMAL INJURY

Risk of maternal death after major burns is not altered by pregnancy. However, fetal mortality exceeds maternal death, and rises with increasing burn size. Fetal survival is uncommon when maternal burns exceed 50% total body surface area (TBSA).[64] Fetal demise often occurs in the early post-burn period because of maternal hypovolemia resulting from a capillary leak syndrome.

Pregnant victims of burn injuries should be managed in a similar fashion as their nonpregnant counterparts. However, there is no evidence to suggest the adequacy of "burn formulas," such as the Parkland equation, during pregnancy. Because "third spacing" results in decreased uterine blood flow, the physician should closely observe urine output, vital signs and, possibly, central venous pressure, to ensure adequate resuscitation. Burn victims, especially those injured in enclosed space fires, should be evaluated for carbon monoxide (CO) poisoning. The physician should order a CO level in patients at risk, and not rely on pulse oximetry, which is falsely normal in CO poisoning. Because of the increased fetal binding of CO, most authorities recommend immediate hyperbaric oxygen therapy for all symptomatic patients and any asymptomatic patients with CO levels greater than 15 to 20 mmHg.[65]

Perimortem Cesarean Section

Though successful perimortem cesarean sections have been reported as far back as 237 BC, less than 190 cases have been reported in the modern literature. The reports are case series, and mainly involve women with nontrauma arrests in the operating suite with anesthetic complications at the time of induction for cesarean section—a very different patient population than that seen in the ED. Many EPs will go their entire career without ever being involved in one. However, in the presence of a traumatic cardiac arrest, early perimortem section may save both the fetus and the mother.

Successful outcome is a function of two factors: an EGA of greater than 24 to 25 weeks[66] and a prepared staff capable of performing a ***prompt*** delivery. Speed means everything in a perimortem C-section. An expedient US or Doppler heart rate to confirm fetal life is useful, but *should not delay intervention* for lack of this equipment. Of note, determining EGA by US is particularly difficult in fetuses less than 29 weeks EGA[67] and often subject to 1 to 2 weeks of uncertainty.

Katz et al[68] reviewed 61 perimortem sections and demonstrated the strong correlation between time after maternal arrest and fetal outcome. Seventy percent of all survivors were delivered within 5 minutes of maternal arrest, and all of them were neurologically intact. After 15 minutes, only six (5%) survived, usually with severe neurologic sequelae. In the only case series of pregnant trauma patients, four of five fetuses requiring immediate cesarean section on arrival survived.[4]

Preparation for a perimortem cesarean section begins with advance warning by the paramedics, who should estimate the EGA. A fundal height below the umbilicus obviates perimortem section, since such a small fetus cannot survive. In the ED, the EP should continue maternal CPR, ventilation, and fluid resuscitation. They should anticipate and prepare for an immediate resuscitation of the neonate. **Call for help**. Pediatric/neonatal consultation should be requested as soon as possible, optimally before patient arrival. Three teams are useful if resources allow. One team can resuscitate the mother, another can perform the cesarean section, while the third will resuscitate the baby.

Thoracotomy with open cardiac massage has been suggested by some, but the aorta should not be cross-clamped before fetal rescue. Thoracotomy should not delay fetal rescue unless the mother has suffered a penetrating wound to the heart. In such a case, release of a pericardial tamponade and internal cardiac massage may be lifesaving to mother and child.

The cesarean section should be performed by the most experienced physician present—preferably an obstetrician. However, time constraints may require the EP or trauma surgeon to act.

The approach is a classic, midline vertical incision, using a large (e.g., #10) scalpel, extending from the epigastrium to the symphysis pubis, and carried through all layers to the peritoneal cavity. The uterus is identified and incised vertically from the fundus to the reflection of the bladder. Retraction may be helpful, but is not crucial. If an anterior placenta is encountered, it should be incised to reach the fetus. Promptly clamp and cut the cord following the delivery of the child. Delivery will suddenly increase venous return to the heart and possibly promote maternal survival.

CONTROVERSIES/CUTTING EDGE

Who Gets Monitored, and for How Long?

Cardiotocographic monitoring for 4 hours detects almost all fetal-maternal complications.[18] If signs of uterine irritability or fetal distress are noted during this period, obstetric consultation and admission for a 24-hour monitoring is indicated.

What Is the Risk of Maternal-Fetal Hemorrhage and How Should It Be Managed?

Infusion of Rh-positive fetal red blood cells may sensitize the mother and complicate future pregnancies. Because the K-B test is insensitive to MFH, all Rh-negative women sustaining blunt trauma, or penetrating uterine trauma should receive RhoGAM within 72 hours. The K-B test is indicated only for later management of women with significant abdominal trauma or obstetric complications who may have sustained massive MFH (i.e., >30 cc fetal blood). Neither the K-B test nor RhoGAM is required in the first few hours of maternal resuscitation. In addition, the K-B test cannot predict fetal complications.[29,30]

When Should You Suspect Domestic Violence?

Domestic violence is a common cause of trauma in pregnant, as well as in nonpregnant, women. There are no subgroups without risk. Therefore all women with non–motor vehicle–related trauma should be asked questions to determine the exact mechanism of their injuries.[9] The EP should directly ask, "Did someone hurt you?"

What Are the Indications for Perimortem Cesarean Section?

Perimortem cesarean section is a heroic and infrequent procedure for fetal and maternal rescue. It is indicated when the mother is either dead or moribund and there is a viable fetus (>24 weeks gestation) with signs of life. A skill that cannot be taught with models, it is unlike any other emergent procedure we perform. It requires cooperation with trauma surgery and obstetrics for ongoing management.

At What Gestational Age Should the Asymptomatic Patient Be Admitted to the Hospital for Fetal Monitoring?

Some authors note that fetal survival is unlikely before 24 weeks and therefore do not recommend monitoring before this point.[26] Others argue for monitoring after 20 weeks, noting that tocolysis and fetal transfusions can increase the likelihood of a near-viable fetus reaching maturity.[33,57] However, tocolysis is of uncertain benefit in traumatic premature labor and fetal transfusions unlikely in the vast majority of U.S. hospitals.

DISPOSITION

Admission criteria are no different between pregnant and nonpregnant patients. Disposition to an operating suite, intensive care unit, or ward bed is also unchanged. All admitted patients over 20-weeks EGA should have obstetric consultation and continuous C-T monitoring during their hospital stay. Local practice may determine whether the obstetrician or trauma surgeon admits the mother, but both should be active with in-house care.

Patients over 20 weeks gestation who do not have other indications for admission, but who have sustained injury from a fall, assault, or MVC are at risk for premature labor or abruption. They should have at least 4 hours of C-T monitoring on the labor floor. If premature contractions, vaginal bleeding, or fetal distress occurs during this time, monitoring is usually continued for at least 24 hours.[18,29,30]

Patients less than 20 weeks EGA who do not require admission for maternal trauma can be safely discharged. Documentation of normal fetal heart tones is reassuring. Fetal loss is rare with minor trauma in this population.[69] Under 12-weeks EGA, spontaneous miscarriage is a common event, and there is no evidence that the miscarriage rate is increased in the first trimester with less than severe maternal trauma.[16]

Prevention and patient education are also important during discharge of the pregnant trauma victim. Mothers should return to the ED for abdominal cramping, decreased fetal movement, or if they pass blood or fluid from their vagina. The EP should inform mothers that three-point seat belts should be worn in pregnancy. Although insufficient data exist to demonstrate confidently that seat belts save lives in the pregnant patient, there is no evidence that they are detrimental.[6,70] In one recent survey,[71] only 66% of pregnant patients use their seatbelts; patients frequently do not know that the correct usage is with a lap belt low across the pelvis and the shoulder strap across the chest above the uterine fundus.

It is believed that they protect by preventing ejection from the motor vehicle, just as in the general population.

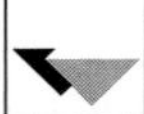

PEARLS & PITFALLS

- Failure to recognize maternal shock resulting from normal vital signs and a benign abdomen.
- Failure to recognize and treat the supine hypotensive syndrome.
- Failure to objectively evaluate the abdomen with ultrasound or DPL in patients with a history suggestive of significant abdominal trauma.
- Failure to order needed tests such as indicated radiographs, serial hemoglobins, or lactates.
- Failure to ask about intentional trauma in pregnant patients.
- Missing the opportunity to teach the pregnant patient how and why to wear seat belts.
- Discharge of a patient because of minor maternal injuries with a potentially viable fetus without a period of cardiotocographic monitoring.

REFERENCES

1. Koonin LM, et al: Maternal mortality surveillance, United States, 1980-1985, *MMWR* 37(SS-5):19-29, 1988.
2. Fildes J, et al: Trauma: the leading cause of maternal death, *J Trauma* 32:643-645, 1992.
3. Sachs BP, et al: Maternal mortality in Massachusetts: trends and prevention, *N Engl J Med* 316: 667-672, 1987.
4. Esposito TJ, et al. Trauma during pregnancy: a review of 79 cases, *Arch Surg* 126:1073-1078, 1991.
5. Biester EM, et al. Trauma in pregnancy: normal revised trauma score in relation to other markers of maternofetal status: a preliminary study, *Am J Obstet Gynecol* 176:1206-1212, 1997.
6. Hendey GW, Votey SR: Injuries in restrained motor vehicle accident victims, *Ann Emerg Med* 24:77-84, 1994.
7. Sims CJ, Boardman CH, Fuller SJ: Airbag deployment following a motor vehicle accident in pregnancy, *Obstet Gynecol* 88:726, 1996.
8. Poole GV, et al: Trauma in pregnancy: the role of interpersonal violence, *Am J Obstet Gynecol* 174:1873-1878, 1996.
9. Helton AS, McFarlane J, Anderson ET: Battered and pregnant: a prevalence study, *Am J Public Health* 77:1337-1339, 1987.
10. Farmer DL, et al: Fetal trauma: relation to maternal injury, *J Pediatr Surg* 25:711-714, 1990.
11. Ribe JK, Teggatz JR, Harvey CM: Blows to the maternal abdomen causing fetal demise: report of three cases and a review of the literature, *J Forensic Sci* 38:1092-1096, 1993.
12. Drost TF, et al. Major trauma in pregnant women: maternal/fetal outcome, *J Trauma* 30:574-578, 1990.
13. Kissinger DP, et al: Trauma in pregnancy: predicting pregnancy outcome, *Arch Surg* 126:1079-1086, 1991.
14. Lane PL: Traumatic fetal deaths, *J Emerg Med* 7: 433-435, 1989.
15. Scorpio RJ, et al: Blunt trauma during pregnancy: factors affecting fetal outcome, *J Trauma* 32:213-216, 1992.
16. Lavery JP, Staten-McCormick M: Management of moderate to severe trauma in pregnancy, *Obstet Gynecol Clin North Am* 22:69-90, 1995.
17. Stafford PA, Biddinger PW, Zumwalt RE: Lethal intrauterine fetal trauma, *Am J Obstet Gynecol* 159:485-489, 1988.
18. Pearlman MD, Tintinalli JE, Lorenz RP: A prospective controlled study of outcome after trauma during pregnancy, *Am J Obstet Gynecol* 162:1502-1510, 1990.
19. Towery R, English TP, Wisner D: Evaluation of pregnant women after blunt injury, *J Trauma* 35: 731-736, 1993.
20. van Oppen AC, et al: A longitudinal study of maternal hemodynamics during normal pregnancy, *Obstet Gynecol* 88: 40-46, 1996.
21. Weinberger SE, et al: Pregnancy and the lung, *Am Rev Resp Dis* 121:559-581, 1980.
22. Abbott J. Emergency management of the obstetric patient. In Burrows GN, Duffy TP (editors): *Medical complications during pregnancy,* ed 5, Philadelphia, 1998, Saunders.
23. Duvekot JJ, et al. Early pregnancy changes in hemodynamics and volume homeostasis are consecutive adjustments triggered by a primary fall in systemic vascular tone, *Am J Obstet Gynecol* 169:1382-1392, 1993.
24. Milsom I, Forssman L: Factors influencing aortocaval compression in late pregnancy, *Am J Obstet Gynecol* 148:764-771, 1984.
25. Kinsella SM, Lohmann G: Supine hypotensive syndrome, *Obstet Gynecol* 83:774-88, 1994.
26. Agnoli FL, Deutchman ME: Trauma in pregnancy, *J Fam Prac* 37:588-592, 1993.
27. Barclay ML. Critical physiologic alterations in pregnancy. In Pearlman MD, Tintinalli JE (editors): *Emergency care of the woman,* New York, 1998, McGraw-Hill.
28. Parer JT, Livingston EG: What is fetal distress? *Am J Obstet Gynecol* 162:1421-1427, 1990.
29. Dahmus MA, Sibai BM. Blunt abdominal trauma: are there any predictive factors for abruptio placentae or maternal-fetal distress? *Am J Obstet Gynecol* 169:1054-1059, 1993.
30. Goodwin TM, Breen MT: Pregnancy outcome and fetomaternal hemorrhage after noncatastrophic trauma, *Am J Obstet Gynecol* 162:665-671, 1990.
31. Williams JK, et al: Evaluation of blunt abdominal trauma in the third trimester of pregnancy: maternal and fetal considerations, *Obstet Gynecol* 75:33-37, 1990.
32. Fleming AD: Abruptio placentae, *Crit Care Clin* 7:865-875, 1991.
33. Lee RB, Wudel JH, Morris JA Jr: Trauma in pregnancy, *J Tenn Med Assoc* 83:74-76, 1990.
34. Domeier RM, et al: Position paper: National Association of EMS Physicians: use of pneumatic antishock garment (PASG), *Prehosp Emerg Care* 1:32-35, 1997.
35. Esposito TJ: Trauma during pregnancy, *Emerg Med Clin North Am* 12:167-199, 1994.
36. Henderson SO, Mallon WK: Trauma in pregnancy, *Emerg Med Clin North Am* 16:209-228, 1998.
37. Neufeld JD: Trauma in Pregnancy. In Rosen P, ed: *Emergency medicine: concepts and clinical practice,* ed 4, St Louis, 1998, Mosby.
38. Colucciello SA. The challenge of trauma in pregnancy: guidelines for targeted assessment, fetal monitoring, and definitive management, *Emerg Med Reports* 16:171-181, 1995.
39. Goldman SM, Wagner LK: Radiologic management of abdominal trauma in pregnancy, *AJR* 166:763-767, 1996.

40. Eliot G: Pregnancy and radiographic examination. In Haycock CE (editor): *Trauma and pregnancy,* Littleton, MA, 1985, PSG Publishing.
41. Rosenstein M: Handbook of selected organ doses for projections common in diagnostic radiology. HEW publication (FDA) 89-8031. Rockville, MD. US Dept. of Health and Human Services, Center for Devices and Radiologic Health, 1988.
42. Wagner LK, Archer BR, Zeck OF: Conceptus dose from two state-of-the-art CT scanners, *Radiology* 159:787-792, 1986.
43. Sakala EP, Kort DD: Management of stab wounds to the pregnant uterus: a case report and a review of the literature, *Obstet Gynecol Surv* 43:319-324, 1988.
44. Ma OJ, Mateer JR, DeBehnke DJ: Use of ultrasonography for the evaluation of pregnant trauma patients, *J Trauma* 40:665-668, 1996.
45. ACS: *Advanced trauma life support student manual,* Chicago, 1993, American College of Surgeons.
46. Rothenberger DA, et al: Diagnostic peritoneal lavage for blunt trauma in pregnant women, *Am J Obstet Gynecol* 129:479-481, 1977.
47. Esposito TJ, et al: Evaluation of blunt abdominal trauma occurring during pregnancy, *J Trauma* 29:1628-1632, 1989.
48. Bowman JM: Controversies in Rh prophylaxis: who needs Rh immune globulin and when should it be given? *Am J Obstet Gynecol* 151:289-294, 1985.
49. Lee RV, et al: Cardiopulmonary resuscitation of pregnant women, *Am J Med* 81:311-318, 1986.
50. Cullhed I: Cardioversion during pregnancy: a case report, *Acta Med Scand* 214:169-172, 1983.
51. DeSilva RA, et al: Cardioversion and defibrillation, *Am Heart J* 100:881-895, 1980.
52. Briggs GG, Freeman RK, Yaffe SJ: *Drugs in pregnancy and lactation: a reference guide to fetal and neonatal risk,* ed 5, Baltimore, 1998, Williams & Wilkins.
53. Holmdahl MH, Thoren L: Tetanus in pregnancy, *Am J Obstet Gynecol* 84:339,1962.
54. Agran PF, et al: Fetal death in motor vehicle accidents, *Ann Emerg Med* 16:1355-1358, 1987.
55. Fries MH, Hankins GD: Motor vehicle accident associated with minimal maternal trauma but subsequent fetal demise, *Ann Emerg Med* 18:301-304, 1989.
56. Kettel LM, Branch DW, Scott JR: Occult placental abruption after maternal trauma, *Obstet Gynecol* 71:449-453, 1988.
57. Pimentel L: Mother and child: trauma in pregnancy, *Emerg Med Clin North Am* 9:549-563, 1991.
58. Franger AL, Buchsbaum HJ, Peaceman AM: Abdominal gunshot wounds in pregnancy, *Am J Obstet Gynecol* 160:1124-1128, 1989.
59. Kirshon B, Young R, Gordon AN: Conservative management of abdominal gunshot wound in a pregnant woman, *Am J Perinatol* 5:232-233, 1988.
60. Grubb DK: Nonsurgical management of penetrating uterine trauma in pregnancy: a case report, *Am J Obstet Gynecol* 166:583-584, 1992.
61. Fatovich DM: Electric shock in pregnancy, *J Emerg Med* 11:175-177, 1993.
62. Leiberman JR, et al: Electrical accidents during pregnancy, *Obstet Gynecol* 67:861-863, 1986.
63. Einarson A, et al. Accidental electric shock in pregnancy: a prospective cohort study, *Am J Obstet Gynecol* 176:678-681, 1997.
64. Rayburn W, et al: Major burns during pregnancy: effects on fetal well-being, *Obstet Gynecol* 63: 392-395, 1984.
65. Seger D, Welch L: Carbon monoxide controversies: neuropsychologic testing, mechanism of toxicity, and hyperbaric oxygen, *Ann Emerg Med* 24:242-248, 1994.
66. Allen MC, Donohue PK, Dusman AE: The limit of viability—neonatal outcome of infants born at 22 to 25 weeks' gestation, *N Engl J Med* 329:1597-1601, 1993.
67. Hadlock FP, Harrist RB, Martinez-Poyer J: How accurate is second trimester fetal dating? *J Ultrasound Med* 10:557-561, 1991.
68. Katz VL, Dotters DJ, Droegemueller W: Perimortem cesarean delivery, *Obstet Gynecol* 68:571-576, 1986.
69. Rothenberger, D, et al: Blunt maternal trauma: a review of 103 cases, *J Trauma* 18:173-179, 1978.
70. Wolf ME, et al: A retrospective cohort study of seatbelt use and pregnancy outcome after a motor vehicle crash, *J Trauma* 34:116-119, 1993.
71. Pearlman MD, Phillips ME: Safety belt use during pregnancy, *Obstet Gynecol* 88:1026-1029, 1996.

Pediatric Trauma

33

ALFRED D. SACCHETTI, ROBERT BELFER, AND EDWARD DOOLIN

Teaching Case

A 4-year-old male was ejected from the front seat of a fast-moving truck that struck a tree. On arrival to the emergency department (ED), he is being bag-valve-mask ventilated. Pulse and blood pressure are within normal limits for his age. His Glasgow Coma Scale (GCS) is 6. Examination reveals scalp and facial injuries with displaced midface and mandibular fractures and no gross response to pain below C6. Because of his severe facial injuries a surgical airway is required and a needle cricothyrotomy is performed successfully. Chest, pelvis, and cervical radiographs reveal no abnormalities. Abdominal ultrasound (US) shows no free fluid. A computed tomography (CT) scan of his brain shows cerebral hyperemia and subarachnoid hemorrhage (SAH), but no mass lesions. Cervical CT scanning from the skull base to T1 is normal. He is taken to the operating suite for formation of a tracheostomy. A cervical magnetic resonance imaging (MRI) study performed postoperatively shows a cord contusion at C6. The methylprednisolone protocol is initiated.

This case illustrates some of the differences encountered with the management of a pediatric trauma victim when compared with an adult. Surgical cricothyrotomy should not be attempted in children younger than 8 years of age to avoid the complication of subglottic stenosis. However, needle cricothyrotomy provides effective ventilation until a definitive airway can be established. Cerebral hyperemia and SAH are more common on the CT scans of young brain-injured trauma patients, with fewer patients showing mass lesions. In addition, spinal cord injuries may be encountered without plain-film or CT evidence of vertebral injury (spinal cord injury without radiologic abnormality, or SCIWORA).

Trauma is a young person's disease and the number one killer of children under 18 years of age. The statistics for pediatric trauma are sobering. Annually, 20,000 children are killed as a result of trauma, whereas another 30,000 suffer some form of permanent disability. Most pediatric injuries occur between the ages of 5 and 9 years (29%), followed by 1 to 4 years of age (25%), 10 to 14 (25%), 15 to 19 (17%), and finally infants (5%).[1] These statistics from the National Pediatric Trauma Registry may underestimate the true extent of the problem since many patients are seen and treated without entry into any trauma registry. The most dangerous location for a child is on the road, the site of 43% of injuries. The second most dangerous location is the home, the site of another 34% of injuries. Falling is the leading cause of injuries, accounting for 26% of all trauma to children and is the predominate mechanism in infants and toddlers. Motor vehicle crashes (MVCs) with children as occupants represent 19% of injuries, while auto-pedestrian impacts account for another 16%. Alarmingly, violence is a rapidly growing source of injury in urban children, with 68% of gunshots to children being intentional.[1-14] This chapter reviews the unique characteristics of pediatric trauma and emphasizes the important differences in the management of injured children.

PATHOPHYSIOLOGY

Anatomic and physiologic differences lead to corresponding variations in the types of injuries suffered and the child's response to the injury. The most obvious difference between children and adults is size and body proportion. It is these anatomic differences that produce the specific injuries unique to children. For instance, young children's higher center of gravity places them at increased risk for head injuries from falls and MVCs, whereas their relative short stature places them at the right height to suffer chest and abdominal injuries when struck by an automobile. Children also incur a higher incidence of multiple-organ injury from trauma than adults because the kinetic injury generated by any impact is dissipated into a smaller body mass.

Body Temperature

Maintenance of core body temperature is more difficult in a child than in adults as a result of a child's larger relative body surface area and smaller muscle mass. This mass difference results in increased loss of heat through radiation, convection, and conduction. This heat loss is poorly tolerated in critically traumatized pediatric patients and the resultant hypothermia can contribute to hypoxia, dysrhythmias, metabolic acidosis, and increased oxygen consumption.

Airway

There are multiple anatomic differences unique to the pediatric airway that may make it difficult to evaluate and manage an injured child. In the supine child, the relatively large size of the occiput tends to flex the neck, leading to potential airway obstruction. The position of the larynx in the child is more cephalad and anterior than in the adult airway, which complicates alignment of the visual axis from the mouth to the vocal cords. Other sources obstructing a clear view of the larynx include the infant's large tongue, the preschooler's hypertrophied tonsillar tissue, and the relatively compliant tissue of the child's oral cavity. In children the epiglottis is longer, narrower, and protrudes farther into the pharynx than in adults, making it more difficult to manipulate with a laryngoscope blade. Finally, the trachea in a child is short, approximately one half the length of the adult trachea, leading to inadvertent mainstem bronchus intubation in the pediatric trauma patient. In a child <8 years old, the subglottic area below the vocal cords is the narrowest part of the airway. Surgical access to the cricothyroid space is relatively contraindicated in children <8 years because of the propensity to subglottic stenosis. In older children, similar to adults, the vocal cords represent the narrowest area.

Gastric

Aerophagia is a much greater problem in pediatric trauma victims than in adults. This gastric distention leads to decreased lung volume and an added potential for emesis and aspiration. Stomach distention may mimic a surgical abdomen in the pediatric trauma victim.

Cardiovascular

Differences exist in the pediatric cardiovascular system compared with adults. The most obvious variation between these populations is in vessel size and blood volume. A child's blood volume is related directly to body weight and is approximately 80 cc/kg body weight. Because of the resilient cardiovascular system in children, acute blood loss of 10% to 15% of circulating blood volume is generally well-tolerated. Dynamic changes in the child's vascular tone allow rapid compensation via peripheral vasoconstriction and increased heart rate. Systolic blood pressure is maintained at the expense of increased cardiac output and preferential internal perfusion. Compensatory abilities are so efficient in children that up to 30% of circulating blood volume can be lost before a decrease in blood pressure is noted. Hypotension is a late and ominous clinical sign of hemorrhage. Hypotension occurs after all a child's compensatory mechanisms are exhausted and often heralds irreversible shock. One of the more frightening observations in injured children is that they appear stable up to the moment they die.

APPROACH TO THE INJURED CHILD

Assignment of prehospital trauma scores should not dictate ED care of an injured child.[15] The specific injuries present determine the treatment a child requires. Trauma scores have been used in prehospital determinations of transport destinations, need for interhospital transfer, and in determining expected outcomes. Trauma scores designed to reflect the physiologic and anatomic difference between children and adults have been developed and are listed in Table 33-1.[15,16]

The overall ED approach to an injured patient does not change with the patient's age. The physician should still obtain as detailed a history of the event as possible while assessing the ABCs and performing a primary survey. Cervical spine precautions are maintained as permitted by the behavior of the child until the neck can be cleared either clinically or radiographically. Direct particular attention to the child's airway in patients with altered mental status or respiratory distress. Because of the relatively larger tongue in children, there is an increased risk of passive airway occlusion if the face and neck musculature becomes too lax. The smaller diameter of the oropharynx and trachea makes obstruction secondary to blood, hematoma, or anatomic disruption a greater risk.[2,3]

Airway and Breathing

Small children are more dependent on their diaphragms for respirations, so any intraabdominal in-

TABLE 33-1
Pediatric Trauma Score

VARIABLE	+2	+1	−1
Airway	Normal	Maintainable	Unmaintainable
Central nervous system	Awake	Obtunded/LOC	Coma
Body weight	>20kg	10-20 kg	<10 kg
Systolic blood pressure	>90 mmHg	90-50 mmHg	<50 mmHg
Open wound	None	Minor	Open/multiple
Skeletal injury	None	Closed fracture	Open/multiple fractures

Glasgow Coma Scale score less than 8 is indicative of significant trauma.

Revised Trauma Score

CATEGORY	4	3	2	1	0
Glasgow Coma Score	13-15	9-12	6-8	4-5	3
Systolic blood pressure (mmHg)	>89	76-89	50-75	1-49	0
Respiratory rate (bpm)	10-20	>29	6-9	1-5	0

Glasgow Coma Scale score less than 11 is indicative of significant trauma.

jury that limits diaphragmatic excursion can severely compromise breathing. Even gastric distention from excessive air swallowing can compromise a small child's ventilatory capacity. If there is compromise of the patency of the airway or a child's ability to breathe adequately, that child may require endotracheal intubation if clearing the airway fails to improve the respiratory status. Endotracheal intubation should be performed with a Rapid Sequence Intubation (RSI) technique to assure the greatest chance of successful intubation while preserving oxygenation and addressing potentially elevated intracranial pressures. The selection of which paralytics and sedatives to use in any given child depends on physician preference and the individual patient's clinical scenario.[15] The different options for use in RSI are contained in Table 33-2.

Because of the narrowed subglottic trachea, cuffed endotracheal (ET) tubes have not generally been used in children <8 years old. However, some centers have safely used cuffed tubes in the very young patients.[17]

A rapid method of estimating the size of the pediatric ET tube is:

ETT size (in mm) = [16 + age (years)]/4

Alternatively, the size of the endotracheal tube can be estimated by approximating the size of the child's external nares or fifth finger. Optimally some form of chart- or length-based reference should be available in the resuscitation room for rapid selection of equipment before intubation.

If orotracheal intubation cannot be successfully achieved, ventilation may be provided with a laryngeal mask airway (LMA).[15] Children <8 years of age in whom a surgical airway is required should be managed with a needle cricothyrotomy with transtracheal jet ventilation (see Chapter 51). This procedure allows for adequate oxygenation until a definitive surgical airway is obtained.

Circulation

Because children have different cardiovascular responses to hypovolemia, careful monitoring is required. Normal blood pressure must be considered as only one (sometimes unreliable) factor in the entire clinical picture. Capillary refill is another indicator of a child's cardiovascular status, and in a normal state should be <2 seconds. Environmental conditions such as cold temperatures can produce peripheral vasoconstriction and lead to falsely elevated refill times.

The best indications of an adequate circulation are normal mentation, well-perfused and warm extremities, a capillary refill of <2 seconds, and a urine output of 1 to 2 cc/kg/hr. Persistent tachycardia and tachypnea may indicate intravascular depletion, shock, acidosis, or a severe painful condition and should never be attributed solely to anxiety or fear.

TABLE 33-2
Sedation and Analgesia Options

ACUTE ANALGESIA	FENTANYL (0.001-0.002 MG/KG)	MORPHINE (0.05-0.1 MG/KG)	DEMEROL (1-2 MG/KG)
Painful procedure*	Ketamine (0.5-1.5 mg/kg)	Fentanyl (0.001-0.002 mg/kg) and Midazolam (0.01-0.05 mg/kg)	Morphine (0.1 mg/kg) and Midazolam (0.01-0.05 mg/kg)
Painless diagnostic study	Pentobarbital (2.5-5 mg/kg)	Propofol infusion (0.3-3.0 mg/kg/hr) titrated as needed	Midazolam (0.01-0.1 mg/kg)
Fracture care	Peripheral nerve block	Bier block	Ketamine* (0.5-1.5 mg/kg)

Rapid Sequence Intubation Options

CLINICAL SCENARIO	OPTIONS		
Normal blood pressure/no head injury	Etomidate (0.3 mg/kg)	Ketamine (1 mg/kg)	Propofol (0.5-1 mg/kg)
Low blood pressure/no head injury	Etomidate (0.3 mg/kg)	Ketamine (1 mg/kg)	Fentanyl (0.002 mg/kg)
Head injury/normal blood pressure	Propofol (0.5-1 mg/kg)	Thiopental (3-5 mg/kg)	Etomidate (0.3 mg/kg)
Head injury/low blood pressure	Etomidate (0.3 mg/kg)	Thiopental (1-2 mg/kg)	Fentanyl (0.2 mg/kg)

*Avoid ketamine with head injury.
All medications listed include an average dosage for a child's weight. However, each dose must be individualized for any given child's response. Doses should be titrated to the child's reaction to the medication and not simply by the recommended milligrams per kilogram. Hypotensive children and neonates should receive decreased doses of medication.

Even though vital signs may be misleading, all significantly injured children should be followed with continuous pulse oximetry, cardiac monitoring and blood pressure measurements. Blood pressure recordings in infants can be difficult and are most accurately obtained through use of an automated blood pressure device. If proper-sized automated equipment is unavailable, an estimate of a child's systolic blood pressure can be gauged by inflating a blood pressure cuff on an extremity containing a pulse oximetry probe until the pulse oximetry wave or readings disappear. The cuff is then slowly deflated and the pressure at which the probe again begins to monitor capillary blood flow is noted as the child's systolic blood pressure.

In a child with a compromised circulation, initial fluid management should begin with a 20 cc/kg bolus of crystalloid solution. If shock persists, a second bolus may be administered. Hypovolemia refractory to a total of 40 cc/kg indicates either a large acute blood loss or ongoing hemorrhage. Subsequent fluid challenges should consist of 10 cc/kg boluses of type-specific or crossmatched packed red blood cells if time warrants; otherwise uncrossmatched blood may be used.[3] Avoid iatrogenic hypothermia by infusing fluids through a fluid warmer. Devices such as the military anti-shock trousers (MAST) may be used in children to temporarily stabilize pelvic fractures, but should never be used to treat hypovolemia or shock.

General Principles

Weight estimates are essential for appropriate pediatric drug and fluid therapy. Because it is difficult to weigh a traumatized child, length-based weight conversions are generally substituted. Commercial devices such as the Broselow tape system provide not only a quick estimate of a child's weight, but also list appropriate equipment sizes and drug dosages. Children are categorized into various colors painted on the tape that correspond to their size. Color-coded bags containing size-appropriate equipment such as nasogastric and endotracheal tubes may be stored in the trauma room as an adjunct to the tape system.

As noted, children are more prone to heat loss if left exposed in a 72° room. Warming lights, warm blankets, or other measures of heat preservation must be used.[2,3]

Intravenous (IV) access can generally be accomplished in infants and small children within two attempts 90% of the time.[18] If vascular access cannot be secured quickly in a severely injured child, then an intraosseous (IO) needle should be placed in children up to age 6 years. IO needles are most frequently inserted into the anterior tibia, but may also be placed in the femur and humerus. IO lines should never be placed in a bone with a known fracture because infused fluids will leak through the ruptured cortex into the surrounding soft tissue, leading to potential compartment syndrome.

Consider alternative sites for venous access in cases of failed peripheral vein cannulation. The umbilical vein may remain viable in infants, but is unreliable for rapid fluid infusion. Other sites used in pediatric patients include a percutaneous approach to the external jugular veins, subclavian veins, or femoral veins. Saphenous vein cut-downs at the ankle may be required if other efforts fail.

Unless contraindicated because of suspected urethral disruption, a Foley catheter should be placed to monitor urine output in any severely injured child. In infants a 5 to 8 French feeding tube can monitor urine flow instead of a Foley catheter. Because of increased aerophagia with crying, place a nasogastric tube in any child with a significant truncal injury. Aerophagia leading to gastric distention may mimic an acute abdomen.

Children's pain is underestimated and appropriate use of analgesics is encouraged. Morphine and fentanyl provide excellent analgesia, although benzodiazepines may be the best drugs for simple sedation for diagnostic studies and for anxiolysis.[19] One protocol for sedation for CT scanning and MRI uses a titrated dose of pentobarbital.[20] This drug is used in children with isolated head trauma and should not be given to those who may have compensated shock. An initial dose of 2.5 mg/kg IV is given; if the child is not sleeping in 5 minutes, two additional doses of 1.25 mg/kg may be administered 5 minutes apart. Table 33-2 summarizes the different analgesic and sedative options in children. As much as possible, family members should be permitted to remain with their child, even during treatment in the resuscitation room. There is ample evidence that such a presence is beneficial to both the child and the parents and is most valuable in cases where the child dies.[21]

HEAD INJURIES

Epidemiology

Head injuries are a major source of traumatic morbidity in children and the leading cause of death, accounting for up to 70% of the mortality in this population. The heads of children are proportionately larger than those of adults and are more susceptible to injury. MVCs are the most common cause of head injuries in children >2 years of age, accounting for up to 90% of injuries, whereas falls are the most common cause of injuries in younger children. **Nonaccidental trauma (NAT)** is a major cause of head injuries in infants and small children, accounting for up to 95% of severe neurologic injuries in this group.[22,23]

Pathophysiology

A child's head responds differently to blunt injuries than does an adult's. The brain of an infant or child has a higher water content, less myelin and more ligamentous attachments, and as a result is more susceptible to shear forces and diffuse axonal injuries. In children the brain also fills a larger portion of the calvarium with less potential spaces for surrounding CSF buffer.[23] Mass lesions such as epidural hemorrhages (EDHs) and subdural hemorrhages (SDHs) are relatively rare.

Subarachnoid hemorrhage occurs in up to 79% of children with severe head trauma and is the most common intracranial abnormality found on CT scans. Diffuse cerebral swelling is the next most common injury. Severe head injury in adults is generally associated with a mass lesion in 46% of cases, whereas SDHs and EDHs appear in only 25% of children with severe head injury. SDHs shows a bimodal distribution with a small peak in the 0- to 4-year-old group (6% to 20%), followed by a decline in the ages 5 to 15 (3% to 7%) and a steady rise as children become adults (25% to 30%). In contrast, EDHs have a constant rate of about 6% to 7% across all age groups. Cerebral contusions are more common in children, but hemorrhagic contusions are more frequently visualized in adults (33% versus 16%).[23-26]

An intracranial injury unique to children is the parafalcine SDH seen in severely shaken infants. These injuries result from the tearing of the bridging veins seen in abuse. Such children with the "**shaken baby syndrome**" also demonstrate occipital cerebral contusions and intracerebral hemorrhages. Retinal hemorrhages are considered nearly pathognomonic. Shaken babies are also at risk for direct impact type injuries if the skull hits an object while being shaken. Box 33-1 summarizes some commonly encountered signs of child abuse.

Skull fractures occur in 29% to 46% of severely head-injured children. Linear skull fractures involving the parietal bone are the most common fractures. Skull fractures in infants whose skull growth is not complete can present a unique problem. Because of the continued expansion of the calvarium, a fracture that extends through to the subdural space has the potential to develop into a "**growing fracture**," the so-called "**leptomeningeal cyst**." These "growing fractures" arise as an underlying dural tear enlarges,

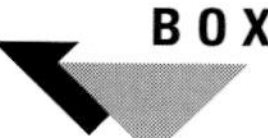

BOX 33-1
Signs of Nonaccidental Trauma

- Presence of immersion burns of buttocks and genitals
- Burns with pattern of object causing burn (e.g., cigarettes, curling iron)
- Presence of strap marks
- Multiple bruises in various stages of healing
- Metaphyseal fractures
- Spiral long bone fractures, especially in non-ambulatory children
- Multiple rib fractures
- Duodenal hematomas and pancreatic pseudocysts
- Retinal hemorrhages

forming a cranial defect (Fig. 33-1). The overall incidence of these fractures is <1% and presents as a pulsatile mass, months to years after the initial trauma.[27]

The "**ping-pong ball**" fracture is a depressed skull fracture unique to very young children (Fig. 33-2). Blunt trauma to the head of a child can result in a depression of the skull with the formation of a pucker similar to a dented ping-pong ball. These fractures are rarely associated with underlying brain or dural injury and these patients have excellent outcomes.[28]

Unlike adults, children may develop hemorrhagic shock from head trauma. Because of the relatively larger head size, it is possible for a child to become acutely hypovolemic from an isolated skull fracture. With the exception of newborns, most intracranial bleeding will not produce acute hypovolemia or shock. However, if the massive bleeding from a fracture extends into the subgaleal space it may impact the child's circulation.[22,29,30]

Infant brains have a higher concentration of excitatory neurotransmitter receptors than adults, which diffuse more easily through the infant brain. It is the activation of these receptors that permits the sodium and calcium ion influxes, which lead to neuronal damage and death following an injury. The increased diffusion may explain why infants suffering severe neurologic insults have a worse outcome than older children.[22,23,26]

Blood flow and intracranial pressure (ICP) control also differs between children and adults. Adults tend to develop transient vasoconstriction following a head injury, whereas children dilate their cerebral vessels leading to hyperemic cerebral blood flow (CBF). This increase in CBF increases the intracranial blood volume and elevates the ICP. Unlike cerebral edema in adults, in which it is the brain tissue itself that swells,

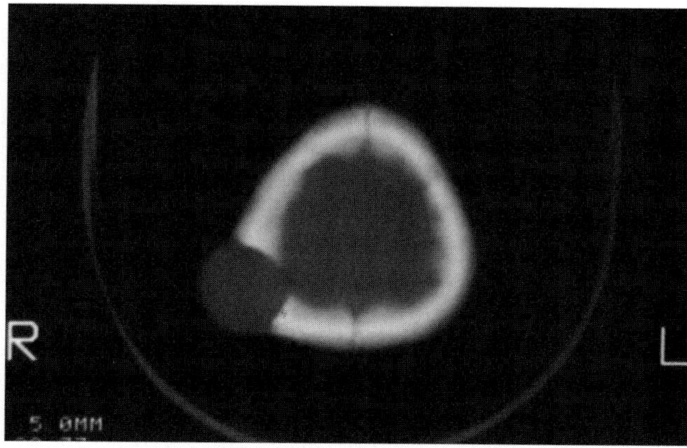

Fig. 33-1 Right parietal growing skull fracture in a 4 year old.

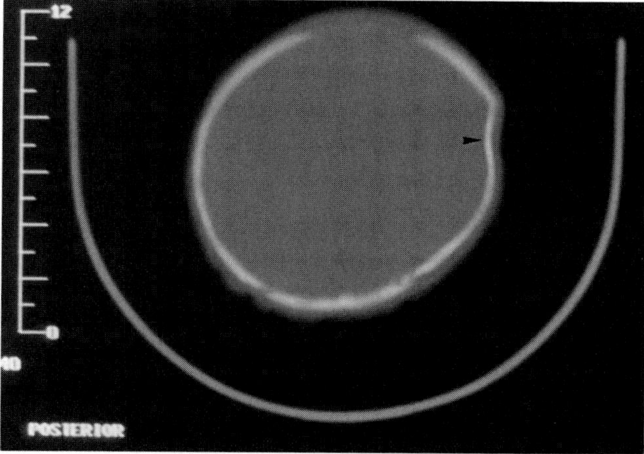

Fig. 33-2 Left parietal ping-pong ball fracture *(arrowhead).*

this process in children is more accurately described as brain swelling or "**malignant hyperemia**."[31,32] Brain swelling can be found in up to 70% of head-related pediatric deaths as opposed to 15% of head-related deaths in adults. Cerebral hyperemia can occur rapidly following minor head injury and, if allowed to proceed unchecked, can produce profound neurologic deficits and death. This model of cerebral hyperemia and its effects on neuronal metabolism is now being reexamined.[31,33,34] After 1 day increased CBF does not contribute significantly to elevated ICP in injured children, and CBF appears to change to match neuronal oxygen demands. The role of increased CBF in the immediate posttraumatic period has not been clearly delineated.

Other causes of increased ICP in children include true cerebral edema, space-occupying lesions, and anatomic obstruction of cerebrospinal fluid egress. As ICP increases, not only can cerebral perfusion pressure drop, but herniation of the brain may occur.

Children with penetrating head trauma generally suffer the same type of injuries as adults. Infants and young children have thinner skulls that can more easily be penetrated. Weapons such as knives, BB pellets, dog teeth, and even pointed sticks can traverse the calvarium of a child. Emergency personnel caring for such children should have a much higher suspicion of intracranial injury in these settings.

Trauma-related seizures occur in 9% to 15% of all head-injured children and up to 39% of those severely injured.[23,35] Seizures occurring immediately after an injury (impact seizures) are generally brief with little or no long-term effects. Early posttraumatic seizures appear in the first week following the injury and are secondary to focal injuries to the brain. Finally, late seizures occur >1 week after a head injury and are the result of scarring in the brain after an injury heals.[22,23]

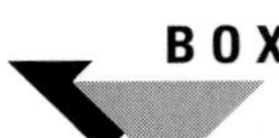

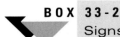

BOX 33-2
Signs of Elevated Intracranial Pressure

Headache
Lethargy
Irritability
Vomiting
Seizures
Bulging fontanelle (if under 1 year of age)
Pupillary dilation
Cushing triad (premorbid finding)
Head tilt
Ataxia
Visual disturbances (post-traumatic blindness)

Emergency Department Evaluation

HISTORICAL CLUES

Injuries that affect the level of consciousness are termed **concussions**. A child need not suffer a complete loss of consciousness (LOC), but may have only been confused for a brief period of time and still have a concussion. The duration of the altered consciousness is indicative of the degree of central nervous system (CNS) trauma. Brief LOCs of a few seconds to <1 minute generally indicate a mild concussion with a good prognosis. Any alteration >1 minute is significant and warrants a careful ED evaluation.[22,26]

Vomiting is a common finding after pediatric head injury in children. The significance of post–head injury vomiting remains controversial. Vomiting has been reported in up to 25% of infants with linear skull fractures.[23,24] Many children cry, swallow air, and distend their stomachs after trivial head injuries. Such scenarios are extremely typical of many childhood injuries, prompting some to regard post-traumatic emesis as a nonspecific finding at best.[36,37] However, children with persistent vomiting beyond the immediate period of injury should be suspected of having a possible intracranial problem. Although not all children who vomit after head injury have increased ICPs, many children with elevated ICPs vomit.[23,24] No individual number has ever been assigned to the number of emesis episodes that effectively identify a CNS problem, but one report has established 3 as the number for which a CT scan should be obtained.[24] Vomiting that persists even after the stomach is empty is also a marker for an intracranial cause of emesis.[22]

PHYSICAL EXAMINATION

Early elevations in ICP can be extremely subtle in presentation. A child's behavior and quality of interaction with the physician or parents is the best clue to intracranial injury. Focal or hard neurologic signs and symptoms may not appear until cerebral herniation occurs, making a high degree of suspicion important in the care of these children.[38] Box 33-2 contains some of the signs and symptoms seen with traumatic elevation of ICP in children. One differentiating characteristic of aware children is that they will exhibit some directed activity, even through their crying. These children may continue to explore their environment, bury their face in a parent's shoulder, or display other actions that require an intact and functional CNS. A child with a constant cry that is unvarying, even in the face of noxious stimuli, has a higher risk of CNS injury. Of course, even more worrisome is the child who does not cry or respond to noxious stimuli.

Children with intracranial injury are more likely to have alterations in level of consciousness or behavior than focal deficits. However, anatomic lesions can also produce focal neurologic findings such as cranial nerve palsies, extremity weakness, or seizures. A decrease in spontaneous activity on one side or failure in one of the extraocular movements may be the only detectable signs of a hemiparesis in a child too frightened to follow commands. Pupillary and deep tendon reflexes are present even in terrified children. Asymmetry of any type should be considered a red flag and aggressively pursued.

The signs of increased ICP can be subtle as noted in Box 33-2. In the infant, the fontanelles will be tense to palpation. Once the increase in ICP reaches the point where herniation occurs, a definitive constellation appears. The most common type of cerebral herniation involves the supratentorial herniation of the uncus of the temporal lobe. Uncal herniation involves compression of the third cranial nerve and upper brainstem, leading to coma, dilation of the ipsilateral pupil, loss

TABLE 33-3
Pediatric Glasgow Coma Scale

Eye opening	
Spontaneous	4
Response to speech	3
Response to pain	2
No response	1
Best motor response	
Normal spontaneous movement	6
Withdraws to touch	5
Withdraws to pain	4
Flexion to pain (decorticate)	3
Extension to pain (decerebrate)	2
No response	1
Best verbal response	
"Coos, babbles, smiles, follows objects"	5
"Irritable and cries, but consolable"	4
Cries/screams no reason	3
Moans/grunts	2
No response	1

of medial eye movement, ptosis, decerebrate posturing, and contralateral hemiparesis.[22,23,38,39] It is important to recognize increased ICP before this stage is reached, since children with overt signs of herniation have a generally poor prognosis.

Clinical findings of skull fractures in infants are quite reliable. Soft tissue swelling over the fracture site can be seen in up to 96% of skull fractures in this age group.[40] As with adults, periorbital and mastoid ecchymoses (raccoon eyes and Battle's sign, respectively), as well as the presence of hemotympanum, imply a basilar skull fracture.

Most trauma evaluations involving the head employ the GCS as a universal CNS assessment tool. The standard GCS can generally be applied to children >3 years old with good validity. Occasionally, it may be necessary to have a parent make the requests of a frightened child to completely evaluate the motor or verbal functions. For younger children, a pediatric GCS has been developed.[22,41,42] Table 33-3 contains a pediatric GCS.

DIAGNOSTIC STUDIES

Radiographic studies in the management of pediatric head trauma must rapidly identify treatable causes of CNS pathology. The optimal study in any child with a significant head injury is a CT scan. This study not only identifies acute intracranial masses, but can also provide evidence of increased ICP. Elevated ICP appears as small compressed ventricles referred to as "slit-like" ventricles; effacement of the basilar cisterns may also be present. CT scans of children with cerebral hyperemia demonstrate a "ground glass" appearance to the brain tissue in association with other signs of elevated ICP. Mass lesions appear the same as in adult patients.[33,38]

Indications for posttraumatic head CT in children remain controversial.[23,36,38,43] Liberal protocols have a very high sensitivity, but will result in performance of a large number of normal studies. More restrictive criteria limit the number of negative studies, but at the expense of missing a percentage of children with significant abnormalities. At a minimum, any child with a LOC >5 minutes, abnormal mental status, seizures, or focal neurologic findings should undergo prompt CT evaluation.[36] CT studies of ambulatory patients with mild-to-moderate complaints are less well-defined. A completely normal neurologic examination, including a GCS score of 15, in an isolated head trauma patient has been demonstrated to be 100% sensitive in eliminating the possibility of intracranial bleeding in some studies.[37,44] Other studies have documented intracranial injuries in up to 5% of patients with GCS scores of 15, 1% of which required neurosurgical intervention.[39,42,43] The decision to obtain CT imaging on these patients must be individualized and should include not only the physician's clinical impressions, but also historical events. Clinical predictors of positive CT scans are contained in Box 33-3.

Plain skull radiographs are rarely indicated in the evaluation of head injuries in children less than age 2 years. In children whose fontanelles are open, skull radiographs may document a fracture in those with a suggestive physical examination. Plain skull films are the most accurate study to define fractures in these children. CT scans miss up to 15% of infants with nondepressed skull fractures, compared with only a 4% miss rate for plain films.[40] Plain films may play a role in determination of child abuse when a minor fall results in a skull fracture. *Do not use skull films in an attempt to predict the presence of underlying intracranial hemorrhages. Order skull films only if the diagnosis of skull fracture needs to be excluded.*

MANAGEMENT

The management of patients with head injuries has been extensively covered in great detail in Chapter 11 and the reader is referred to this section. The ED management of the head-injured child is determined by

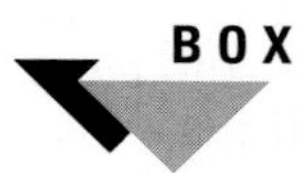

BOX 33-3

Indications for Head Computed Tomography Scan

- Abnormal mental status
- LOC >5 minutes
- High-speed motor vehicle accident
- Fall from a height
- Unwitnessed injury
- Child abuse
- Multiple cranial injuries
- Vomiting three or more times
- Persistent H/A greater than 24 hours after injury
- Clinical skull fracture
- Multiple trauma with head injury
- Neurologic deficit
- Penetrating injury
- Change in mental status or behavior
- Coagulopathy
- PGCS <15

the child's mental status. Children with depressed mental functions are assumed to have an acute intracranial process and treated as such. Even without radiographic confirmation, either cerebral hyperemia or some other cause of elevated ICP should be presumed and aggressively treated. Immediate controlled endotracheal intubation followed by eucapnia is indicated in the presence of a GCS ≤8 or if the patient's airway is in peril. Children experiencing herniation syndromes may be hyperventilated to a pCO_2 of 30 to 35 mmHG to decrease CBF and acutely lower ICP.

Generalized seizures in head-injured children should be treated promptly and aggressively since any seizure activity will increase ICP and exacerbate cellular cytotoxic cascades. Benzodiazepines (diazepam, lorazepam) are generally the drugs of choice for immediate seizure control in children.[22,23] Phenytoin (or fos-phenytoin) is the drug of choice for maintenance control or as a second line drug for failed treatment with benzodiazepines. Evidence for prophylactic use of phenytoin is nonconclusive. Some studies suggest that in children with a GCS ≤8, prophylactic phenytoin may prevent early posttraumatic seizures.[35] Phenobarbital may be used in children refractory to the first line agents.[2,3] Most recently, the use of propofol appears to be a viable alternative in children with status epilepticus unresponsive to benzodiazepines or barbiturates. Propofol is administered as a continuous infusion following an initial bolus. The short half-life of this drug, 8 to 10 minutes, allows the physician to stop the infusion, examine the patient and then restart the infusion if additional sedation or seizure control is needed.[45,46]

DISPOSITION

Disposition of the head-injured child is a function of the nature and severity of the injury, the child's parents or caretakers, the local hospital practices, and the treating physician. Certainly, any child suspected of being a victim of nonaccidental trauma should not be sent home until his or her safety is assured. Infants with isolated skull fractures may be discharged home if they have normal head CT scans and normal neurologic examinations, since they are at low risk for progressive neurologic deterioration.[39,40]

Adolescents and adults with the same presentations also have been shown to have a low risk of delayed deterioration, although no universal discharge criteria have ever been developed.[47,48] At the very least, a GCS of 15, no vomiting, a normal neurologic examination and a reliable home environment are essential before discharging any head-injured child. Those children with more significant injuries but with normal neurologic examinations and negative CT scans have also been safely discharged home.[48]

SPINAL INJURIES

Epidemiology

Spinal trauma is less common in pediatric patients compared with adults, with <10% of spinal cord injuries (SCI) occurring in children under 16 years of age. Trauma-related paralysis in children is rarely associated with spinal column fractures and vertebral fractures generally account for <0.2% of all pediatric fractures and approximately 3% of spinal injuries. Most cervical spine injuries (60% to 70%) occur in children over 12 years of age with <10% to 15% appearing before the age of 8.[2,3,49,50] If the mechanism of injury is consistent with a possible SCI, a full investigation is warranted.[51-53]

Pathophysiology

The spine of the infant and young child demonstrates some anatomic differences from an adult. In addition to the presence of growth plates, the ligamentous attachments of the pediatric spine are more lax than in an adult. The resulting hypermobility permits greater extension and flexion of the spinal column at the extremes. The area of greatest mobility centers around the C1-C2-C3 vertebrae. More horizontally oriented wedge-shaped vertebral bodies and underdeveloped occipital condyles also permit subluxation following anterior-posterior trauma.[49]

Spinal injuries in children result from the hypermobility of the cervical spine and, as a result, are most common at the anatomic fulcrum around the upper cervical vertebrae. The C1-C2 interface is the primary location of cervical spine injuries in children and includes rotatory subluxations, odontoid fractures, fractures of the neural arch of C2 and dislocations without fractures. The younger the child the more likely a C1-C2 dislocation without a fracture is to occur. Surprisingly, because of the space within the neural arches of C1 and C2, many of these dislocations do not present with immediate spinal cord symptoms.[50,51] In contrast, most patients with odontoid fractures have neurologic findings on admission. Other bony spinal injuries seen include anterior compression injuries of the thoracic and lumbar spines in children with lap belt injuries.[50,54-56]

SCIWORA

Children are much more likely to develop the phenomenon termed "**S**pinal **C**ord **I**njury **W**ithout **R**adiologic **A**bnormality" (**SCIWORA**).[50,51,57] This phenomenon has ranged from 4% to 67% in various studies of pediatric SCI patients. The exact cause of SCIWORA has not been defined and may represent a combination of a number of injuries. The most widely held explanation holds that the increased laxity of the spinal ligaments permits the bony components of the vertebral column to distract beyond the capacity of the spinal cord. In cases of SCIWORA, extreme subluxations and distractions stretch the spinal ligaments without creating any permanent deformity. During this event the spinal cord is compromised, either by direct injury to the spinal tracts themselves or injury to the feeding blood vessels. The net result of these events is the presentation of a child with a spinal neurologic deficit and no plain film or CT scan abnormality.

Children who develop SCIWORA may be neurologically normal at the time of the ED presentation and only develop paralysis hours to days later. In these instances an initial injury results in a myelopathy, which evolves after a delay of hours to days. An alternate explanation holds that an unstable condition occurs following the initial injury and remains undetected. With the weakened support, a later minor movement of the spinal column results in direct cord damage.[49,51] Box 33-4 lists reasons why children are at increased risk for SCIWORA.

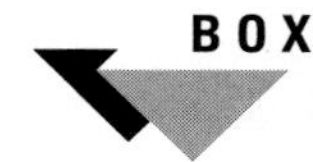

BOX 33-4

Anatomic Reasons for Increased Susceptibility to SCIWORA in Children

- Increased elasticity and hypermobility of pediatric spinal cord
- Relatively larger head size in children places center of gravity higher than in adults
- Horizontal orientation of facet joints
- Poor development of neck musculature

Presentation

Children with spinal injuries present the same as adults. Children with adequate speech skills may complain of neck pain unless an altered mental status or other distraction is present. The history is extremely important in those children with neck pain, and those with normal radiographic studies who are at risk for delayed SCIWORA. Most verbal patients describe transient paresthesias in their extremities if carefully questioned.[51] If a detectable SCI is present, focal weakness or paralysis will be noted, as well as a discrete sensory level. Partial cord syndromes such as central cord, anterior, or Brown-Sequard syndromes also occur.[51]

Neurologically intact children should have their neck palpated to search for any tenderness. If no tenderness is present, the child may be asked to move his or her head through a range of motion. If pain is encountered, the examination is stopped, and the child is immobilized and studied radiographically. Avoid passive range of motion by the physician.

Management

Initially immobilize any child with a potential neck injury to limit any exacerbation of a cervical spine injury. Because of the larger relative head size in a child, supine placement on a backboard does not result in neutral positioning of the child's neck. Both kyphotic and lordotic variations in the angle between C2 and C6 (Cobb angle) of up to 27 degrees occur in children on a flat spine board. Sixty percent of patients in one series had >5 degrees of flexion or extension when held in the standard position.[58] Elevation of the shoulders and trunk with blankets can be used to align the neck in a neutral position. Use of padding to raise the torso 27 mm aligned the spine in children <4 years of age, whereas 22 mm produced the same effect in older children. Rigid collars applied to children also result in nonneutral positioning.

Immobilization in children must also account for the combative behavior that may occur with restraints and separation from parents. An alert quiet child who becomes combative when placed on a backboard should not be forced to use this restraint. Even though

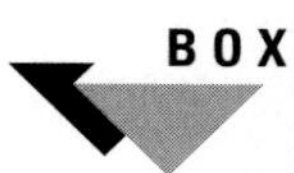

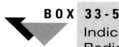

BOX 33-5

Indications for Cervical Spine Radiograph

- Mechanism of injury consistent with potential cervical spine injury
- "Unable to verbalize"
  (Head injury, too frightened, inconsolable, preverbal, substance abuse)
- Neck pain or tenderness
- Motor deficit
- Sensory deficit

the backboard may represent ideal positioning, the fighting and erratic movements of such a child are a much greater risk to an unstable cervical spine than the lack of immobilization. Log-roll the child off the board using cervical spine stabilization and have the parents at the bedside to help ease the child's fears, as well as to avoid the discomfort of the rigid backboard.

Diagnostic Studies

High-risk criteria for cervical radiographs have been developed for children. A summary of these criteria is contained in Box 33-5.[59] It is interesting that the presence of a head injury does not increase the incidence of a cervical spine injury over that found in a multiply traumatized child without a head injury.[59]

Accurate interpretation of pediatric spine films requires experience. The films differ from adult studies in a number of ways. Children may have increased prevertebral tissue that varies with respiration. This prevertebral thickness that occurs during expiration may be misinterpreted as soft-tissue swelling secondary to a fracture. If a film can be timed to inspiration, soft tissue anterior to the vertebral body should be no more than two thirds the width of the C2 vertebral body (approximately 7 mm) for those vertebrae above the glottis and equal to the width of the C3 body (approximately 14 mm) for those below the glottis.[49,60] Children <12 also often present with "**pseudosubluxation**," a normal variant where the upper cervical vertebrae (usually C2 on C3 or C3 on C4) are subluxed anteriorly (Fig. 33-3). Subluxations of up to 3 mm can be considered normal in a child's cervical spine radiograph. In pseudosubluxation, a smooth line should connect the spinolaminar junctions of the upper three vertebrae (**Swischuck's line**). The same difference, 3 mm, can be seen between the anterior and posterior heights of the vertebral bodies.

Radiographic views are similar to those in adults. A screening cross-table lateral (CTL) view with the child

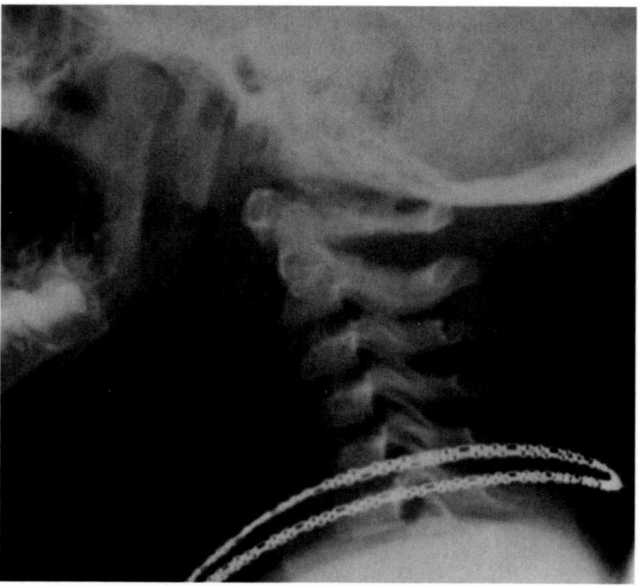

Fig. 33-3 Pseudosubluxation of C2 on C3.

immobilized is the initial film obtained. Most spinal injuries are seen on this view, but 5% to 10% of unstable fractures are missed if anteroposterior (AP) and odontoid views are not obtained.[50] Although the AP and CTL views are easy to obtain, a good odontoid view may be problematic. Considering that most pediatric fractures occur in the first three cervical vertebrae, some clinicians now feel that CT scanning of the upper cervical spine in conjunction with a head CT is actually more efficient in the seriously injured child.[50,54,61]

MRI may detect injuries not obvious on plain films or by CT scanning. Certainly any child with clinical evidence of SCIWORA should undergo urgent MRI studies to identify correctable lesions.[51,62]

Children with clinical or radiographic evidence of SCI should have continued immobilization and emergent consultation with a spine specialist. Although the clinical effects of steroid treatment have been criticized, any child with suspected or proven SCI should receive the methylprednisolone protocol outlined in Chapter 12.[3,63] Ideally, the drug should be administered in the first 8 hours after injury for maximal benefit, along with a gastric acid blocker.

FACIAL TRAUMA

Pediatric facial lacerations are amongst the top five pediatric ED diagnoses, yet significant pediatric facial trauma is relatively rare. Pediatric maxillofacial injuries account for between 1.5% to 15% of all facial fractures, with an incidence of between 1% to 1.5% in children <5 years of age.[64] The most common facial fractures overall involve the nasal bones, whereas the most common fractures requiring hospitalization involve the mandible. Compared with adults, children are more likely to sustain fractures of the forehead and less likely to have maxillary injuries. In children the condyle is the most frequently injured portion of the jaw and is fractured in 40% to 70% of cases. Midface trauma is unusual, with orbital fractures appearing in 20% to 25%, zygomatic fractures in 10% to 15%, and Le Fort fractures in 1% to 3% of children; in some series, Le Fort fractures never occur in children <5 years old. The child's unique anatomy may account for the low incidence of serious midface injuries. In a child the bones are relatively pliable and elastic, making them less susceptible to fracture following blunt injuries. In addition, the lack of air-filled paranasal sinuses and the presence of unerupted teeth strengthen the midface.[64,65]

Axial and coronal CT scanning for orbital and midface fractures is the most useful diagnostic study, since plain films are often difficult to interpret.[64] Mandible fractures can also be detected by CT scanning, but panoramic (Panorex) views are the most helpful imaging technique for mandible injuries.[64]

The ED management of midface trauma focuses on preservation of a patent airway, cervical spine precautions and a careful search for associated neurologic and orthopedic injuries which may be present in up to 30% of these patients.[64] Dental trauma in a child is managed differently than in an adult in that avulsed deciduous ("baby") teeth are not replaced.[66] Laryngeal and anterior neck trauma in children has an increased potential to produce airway obstruction. Children with facial fractures need early follow-up, since facial bones knit more quickly than in adults. Younger children with mandibular fractures have the potential for significant cosmetic deformities resulting from growth arrest and subsequent asymmetric development of the face.

THORACIC TRAUMA

Epidemiology

Thoracic injuries are the second most deadly injuries suffered by children and often appear in conjunction with closed head trauma. Blunt chest trauma (BCT) occurs in 4% to 23% of pediatric trauma cases, with mortality rates between 7% and 26%. Deaths in patients with BCT are dramatically affected by associated extrathoracic injuries. Fatality rates in children with isolated BCT are as low as 4% compared with 29% in children with associated extrathoracic injuries. In those children with multisystem injuries, the death is attributed to the thoracic injury in only 14% of cases. Most BCT in children results from MVCs. Depending on the series, either vehicle-pedestrian (33% to 54%) or vehicle occupant (41%) crashes are the most common mechanisms of injury.

By contrast, penetrating thoracic injuries are much less common, accounting for between 20% and 35% of chest injury cases, with a mortality rate of 14%. Unlike BCT, 97% of deaths in penetrating cases are related directly to the chest injury. Gunshot wounds are the most common cause of penetrating chest injuries, occurring in 60% of cases.[3,4,67-71] Penetrating chest trauma results in similar injuries compared with adults. Pneumohemothoraces tend to predominate, occurring in 64% of patients. Cardiac and great vessel injuries are more common in penetrating injuries, appearing in up to 23% of cases and accounting for most of the mortality in this group.[69]

Pathophysiology

The injuries caused by BCT in children differ significantly from those seen in adults. Thinner ribs, less calcification, and a greater cartilage composition lead to a more pliable chest wall in children. As a result, applied traumatic forces may deform the chest wall and be transmitted directly through to the underlying organs. Damage to the lungs, respiratory tree, heart, and great vessels can occur easily in children with no external evidence of a chest wall injury. **Pulmonary contusions** are the most common injuries in children, occurring in 49% to 68% of BCT victims. Most contusions are posteromedial in location, reflecting compression of the lung by the relatively free anterior chest wall against the fixed posterior thoracic ribs. The crescent shape of most of the contusions conforms to the overall shape of the posterior thorax.[67-69,72]

Pulmonary contusions located in the lower segments are associated with a high incidence of intra-abdominal injuries. Up to 68% of children with right lower or right middle lobe contusions have associated liver or kidney injuries, whereas 36% of children with left lower lobe contusions have splenic or kidney injuries. Conversely, children with splenic or hepatic injuries have a high incidence of pulmonary contusions.[72,73]

Rib fractures are relatively uncommon and the vast majority are found in adolescents. Rib fractures in small children are in fact a significant marker of serious injury, with mortality rates of 20% to 56%. In some series, isolated rib fractures had a fatality rate of 0%, two fractures a rate of 60%, and four or more fractures a rate of 71%.[73-75] Posterior rib fractures in young children may be secondary to nonaccidental trauma and occur when a child is slammed against a wall or thrown on to the floor.

Pneumothoraces (24%), **hemothoraces** (5%), and

lung lacerations (1%) do occur in children, although not with the same frequency as in adults. The flexible chest wall also allows compression of the cartilaginous respiratory tree. The sudden rise in intraluminal pressure that occurs with such compression can result in rupture of the posterior tracheal wall or bronchi. The relatively mobile mediastinum in children makes them much more susceptible to tension pneumothoraces.[4,73]

Injuries to the heart and great vessels are rare occurrences in children. Blunt cardiac injuries in children surviving to reach the ED are frequently nonfatal in nature, with **myocardial contusions** accounting for 95% of such cases. As with adults, pediatric patients with cardiac contusions who are in normal sinus rhythm, with normotension and no dysrhythmias have excellent outcomes.[76] **Traumatic aortic injury** is uncommon in children and presents in a fashion very similar to that seen in adults. Mediastinal widening and abnormalities of the aortic contour are sensitive (100%) but not specific (50%) findings.[77-79]

A particularly lethal pediatric cardiac injury is **commotio cordis**, which is a cause of organized sports-related deaths in children and results when a small object such as a baseball strikes the anterior chest. The belief is that the impact occurs at a vulnerable time in the child's cardiac cycle and produces a nonperfusing dysrhythmia.[76,80]

Traumatic asphyxia resulting from a dramatic pressure wave in the upper body's venous system can also occur in pediatric blunt trauma. Generally considered rare, this condition has been reported to occur in as many as 20% of pediatric blunt trauma patients. Children present with petechiae on the neck and face, often associated with subconjunctival hemorrhage. **Diaphragmatic injuries** also follow the same pattern as in adults, with the majority involving the left hemidiaphragm.[73]

Presentation

Patients with adequate verbal skills and isolated thoracic injuries will generally complain of chest pain. Intrathoracic injuries may produce dyspnea, which may manifest as inability to speak in full sentences. Preverbal children may exhibit the classic symptoms of dyspnea including nasal flaring, retractions, seesaw respirations, grunting, and gasping. A frightened and crying child will swallow air, inflating the stomach and elevating the diaphragm, exacerbating any existing dyspnea.[3,4]

Children with significant parenchymal lung injuries may present with no external signs of trauma. It is important to carefully palpate the chest wall in injured children to identify a thoracic lesion that may not be visible. Absent or decreased breath sounds imply a pneumohemothorax or hemothorax. However, because of the excellent transmission in an infant's or child's chest, the presence of normal breath sounds does not eliminate such an injury. Multiple rib fractures are unusual in infants and small children and a true flail chest is rarely observed in this age group. Hard physical findings such as hypoxia, hemoptysis, or subcutaneous emphysema are highly predictive of significant injuries and must be quickly investigated.[73]

Diagnosis

Radiographic evaluation is the cornerstone of diagnostic studies in chest-injured children. Plain-chest radiographs (CXR) generally reveal significant parenchymal injury, but lack sensitivity early in the course of some patients. Pulmonary contusions may not appear on initial CXR. On average, it takes several hours before a pulmonary contusion becomes radiographically apparent. Chest CT scanning is more sensitive for pulmonary injuries, detecting most immediately after trauma.[81] Pneumohemothoraces are also seen more clearly with CT scanning. In one series the CT identified 62% of pneumothoraces not seen on the plain CXR.[72] CT evaluation also has the advantage of delineating the cause of a widened mediastinum, but only high-resolution helical CT can exclude aortic injury.

Diagnostic adjuncts in the evaluation of chest trauma include continuous pulse oximetry and arterial blood gas (ABG) analysis. Pulse oximetry may alert the physician to unrecognized hypoxia and help monitor the progress of resuscitation, while ABGs provide direct measurements of the patient's acid-base status. The pH identifies those patients with perfusion deficits producing lactic acidosis.[82] Measurement of the arterial pCO_2 helps the physician recognize children who are tiring and in need of endotracheal intubation.

Management

Treatment of pediatric chest injuries is the same as adult injuries. Significant pneumohemothoraces, or pneumothoraces in the setting of positive pressure ventilation, should be quickly drained through tube thoracostomies to prevent development of tension and displacement of the mediastinum. Autotransfusion is valuable in cases of large hemothoraces. Use of positive airway pressure (PAP) systems to limit development of pulmonary contusions has been described in young adults, but not children. PAP may be valuable in children who remain persistently hypoxic despite high-flow O_2 or intubation.[83] ED thoracotomy has the same indication (i.e., penetrating chest trauma with signs of life in the field) and outcomes as in adults with thoracic injuries.

ABDOMINAL TRAUMA

Epidemiology

Abdominal injuries in children are 30% more common than thoracic injuries, but account for 20% less pediatric deaths. The overall mortality rate for pediatric abdominal trauma is 9% to 14%, but most of these patients have associated injuries. Blunt trauma is the most common cause of pediatric abdominal injuries, accounting for 86% of cases, compared with 14% for penetrating injuries. Motor vehicle-related trauma is the leading mechanism of blunt injuries (57%), followed by falls (13%) and bicycle-related trauma (12%). Of MVCs, slightly more than half of the children injured are occupants, whereas the others are pedestrians. The height of the typical car bumper coincides almost perfectly with the height of a small child's abdomen, explaining the high incidence of abdominal injuries in these patients. The protuberant stomach, lack of abdominal musculature, and relatively larger abdominal organs combine to make intraabdominal injuries such a large source of morbidity in children.[4,84,85]

Handlebar injuries and lap-belt restraints are major sources of morbidity in pediatric abdominal injury patients. Both these mechanisms are the leading causes of pancreatic and gastrointestinal (GI) injuries, accounting for anywhere from 27% to 75% of such injuries.

Solid organ injuries predominate, accounting for 68% to 90% of intraabdominal pathology. The liver and spleen are involved about equally, occurring in between 27% and 30% of children. The kidney is the next most commonly injured solid organ, with injuries noted in 17% to 27% of children. The vast majority of kidney injuries are simple contusions or hematomas (50% to 62%) and rarely require operative or angiographic intervention. Pancreatic injuries are relatively rare, appearing in only 2% to 3% of cases, but representing a major source of morbidity. Laceration of the gland can occur in up to 70% of cases, with transection of the duct occurring in another 12% to 14%.[2-4,84-87]

Gastrointestinal injuries are found in up to 14% of intraabdominal injuries in children. Lap belt and handlebar injuries are the most common causes of GI injury, with abuse being the third major cause. The jejunum is the most common site of injury. Unlike the jejunum in which perforation is the most common complication, approximately 50% of duodenal injuries are simply hematomas or contusions.[4,86-93]

Penetrating abdominal trauma produces a completely different pattern of injuries from blunt trauma. Although liver injuries still account for approximately 30% of injuries, splenic and renal injuries decrease to 10%, whereas GI injuries increase to 70%.[3,4]

Presentation

Serial clinical examination is the most important component in the evaluation of a child with an abdominal injury. On presentation, pancreatic injuries and hollow viscus ruptures are difficult to diagnose. Careful serial examinations and radiographic studies are essential to prevent morbidity. Abdominal wall evidence of an intraabdominal injury is extremely variable.[94] Abused children may have absolutely no external evidence of trauma, although many children with lap-belt injuries have abdominal wall ecchymosis.[4,87,95,96] Auscultation of the abdomen generally reveals decreased bowel sounds, even in the absence of an intraabdominal injury, and is not generally helpful. Palpation of the traumatized abdomen remains the most important diagnostic tool in these patients. Children with solid organ injuries leading to intraperitoneal bleeding frequently have tenderness, guarding, and peritoneal signs. The polytraumatized child may have an unremarkable abdominal examination despite a hemoperitoneum, particularly in the presence of extraabdominal injuries or altered mental status.

A gentle touch must be used in the evaluation of infants and small children to detect the relatively subtle signs of guarding presented by their thin abdominal musculature. Children with occult injuries such as jejunal or duodenal injuries may have benign examinations on presentation to the ED. Duodenal hematomas usually manifest as persistent vomiting that begins 12 hours or more after trauma. Diagnoses of GI injuries are often overlooked early on even by experienced pediatric surgeons.[96] *The importance of repeated examinations of the abdomen in children sustaining blunt abdominal trauma (BAT) cannot be overstated.* There is no increase in morbidity or mortality in children with bowel injuries undergoing delayed diagnosis when followed carefully.[93,96-98]

Diagnosis

Baseline hemoglobin and hematocrits are useful in the conservative management of solid organ injuries, whereas serial white blood cell count levels may help follow children with occult bowel injuries, although these tests are very nonspecific and insensitive. Serum amylase levels do not correlate well with pancreatic injury and are generally not necessary.[85,87] Unlike in adults, hepatic enzymes will elevate in response to liver injuries. Elevations in aspartate aminotransferase (AST) and alanine aminotransferase (ALT) have been shown to have sensitivities up to 100% with 92% specificities in patients with liver trauma. In some instances of child abuse, elevated liver function tests were the only indicators of occult abdominal injuries.[99,100] Again, the presence of elevated enzymes only indicate potential hepatic injury but does not predict patient management.

The presence of microscopic hematuria is an important marker for intraabdominal injury in children. Injuries to the kidneys (26%), liver (33%) and spleen (37%) have all been associated with microscopic hematuria. Microscopic hematuria should trigger consideration of an abdominal CT scan in children, not just to examine the kidneys but the other solid organs as well. The exact cut-off for performance of further diagnostic studies in the presence of microscopic hematuria varies between 20 and 50 red blood cells (rbc) per high-powered field (hpf). Most studies demonstrate that in the face of normal hemodynamic parameters a finding of <50 rbc/hpf has a 2% incidence of a significant renal injury. Other studies have shown that even <20 rbc/hpf can have up to a 28% incidence of renal findings, although most of these injuries represented conservatively managed renal contusions or congenital abnormalities.[101-110]

Diagnostic laboratory studies cannot substitute for a good physical assessment. The routine use of admission trauma panels does not appear to identify any more injuries than a careful physical examination and an urinalysis.[111]

Radiographic studies in evaluation of BAT in children are more important than in adults. Unlike adults, in whom the presence of intraperitoneal blood is likely to prompt performance of a laparotomy, hemoperitoneum in children is frequently managed conservatively. In children, it is not the presence of blood in the abdominal cavity, but the cause and extent of the bleeding that helps determine the clinical management. As a result, diagnostic peritoneal lavage (DPL) has little role in the evaluation of abdominal trauma in children.[112,113] However, DPL may be indicated in a child with refractory hypotension who has several possible sources of blood loss. A positive lavage (or abdominal ultrasound) in such a child indicates the need for laparotomy.

The indications for abdominal diagnostic imaging include significant findings on physical examination or a suspicious mechanism of injury. Abdominal tenderness, guarding, peritoneal signs, lap-belt ecchymosis, abdominal wall contusions, and gross hematuria are all findings suggestive of an intraabdominal problem.

Abdominal CT scanning is generally regarded as the diagnostic procedure of choice for evaluation of BAT. This test is capable of identifying the underlying injury causing intraabdominal bleeding and can help determine a management plan for the injured child. Abdominal CT scans are best performed with both oral and IV contrast. Diagnostic accuracy for abdominal CT scans is excellent for detection of renal, splenic, and liver injuries, but limited for pancreatic and bowel injuries. Abdominal CT scans have false-negative rates as high as 26% for GI injuries and 15% for pancreatic trauma.[85,95]

A nonspecific but ominous finding on CT examination is termed "**shock bowel syndrome**" (Fig. 33-4). Generally associated with low perfusion states, the CT findings include diffuse dilation of the intestines, abnormally increased enhancement of the abdominal structures with contrast, greater and lesser peritoneal sac collections, and a diminished caliber of the aorta and vena cava. Findings of hypoperfused bowel generally indicate a poor prognosis, with mortality rates as high as 85%.[95]

In the United States, ultrasound is an evolving diagnostic tool in pediatric trauma patients. In Europe, it is a primary diagnostic tool.[114] Like DPL, it is very sensitive in detecting abdominal fluid or blood, but its ability to explain the exact organ injured is limited. In addition, US is very user dependent, with the success rates from different series being a reflection of not only the technology but also the capabilities of the ultrasonographers. In some series, US was as accurate as CT, with 90% to 100% sensitivity, whereas in other series the sensitivity was as low as 62%. The true utility of US clearly depends on the skills of the examiners using the test. It is an excellent screen for intraperitoneal fluid, but its ability to delineate solid organ injuries is less precise.[95,115-118]

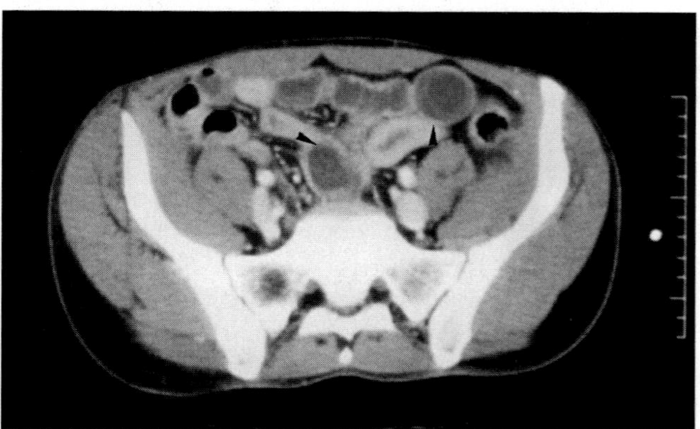

Fig. 33-4 Fluid-filled loops of bowel with thickened walls, indicative of shock bowel *(arrowheads)*.

GENITOURINARY TRAUMA

Epidemiology

Despite the fact that the bladder is an intraabdominal organ in infants, it is rarely injured in BAT. Bladder and proximal urethral injuries occur in <4% of all blunt trauma patients, and external urethral injuries occur in <1% of cases. Most urethral injuries in children occur in males and involve the prostatic and membranous urethra as in adults. The relatively flexible pelvic wall and low incidence of pelvic fractures (<1%) account for the low incidence of this injury. Testicular trauma is also relatively rare in children and is most commonly related to sports trauma, including straddle injuries from bicycles and impact injuries from high-velocity balls.[4,115,117]

Presentation

Clinical evaluation of the child with genitourinary (GU) trauma generally occurs in the later portion of the secondary survey. *Always suspect lower tract GU trauma in the presence of pelvic fractures.* Careful palpation of the suprapubic abdomen may reveal tenderness, and a rectal examination in a male may demonstrate a high-riding prostate. A retrograde urethrogram, followed by a cystogram, are the studies needed to evaluate these injuries.

Scrotal and testicular injuries frequently present with ecchymoses, hematomas, and swelling, making careful palpation difficult. If a discrete nontender testicle can be palpated and delineated, then testicular rupture is less likely, but not completely eliminated. Testicular US with Doppler blood flow is the diagnostic study in evaluation of these patients. Once a testicular injury has been ruled out, the patient may be discharged with instructions for ice, rest, and analgesics. One cautionary note in the management of young males with testicular injuries is the possibility of testicular torsion. Although trauma is a very infrequent cause of torsion, a child with this problem may erroneously attribute it to a temporally related event such as a fall or sports activity.

ORTHOPEDIC TRAUMA

Epidemiology

Skeletal injury occurs in approximately 20% of all trauma sustained by children. In children 2 years old through adolescence, fractures of the upper extremities outnumber fractures of the lower extremities 7:1, with fractures of the radius being the most common. The primary mechanism of skeletal injury to children in the United States is blunt trauma secondary to MVCs and pedestrian-automobile accidents.[119-122]

Pathophysiology

Anatomic, physiologic, and biochemical differences exist between fractures in adults and those in growing children. The child's bone is made up of the diaphysis, metaphysis, physis, and epiphysis. The physis, or growth plate, is the weakest site in a child's bone. Many pediatric fractures occur through the physis, creating the potential for either partial or total growth arrest. The biochemical properties of the immature skeleton also make a child's bone more porous, allowing for incomplete fractures such as **torus**, **bowing**, or **greenstick** fractures (Figs. 33-5 and 33-6). A torus (buckle) fracture results from failure of the bone in compression at the metaphyseal region of long bones. Bowing results from a plastic deformation in a bone bent beyond its elastic limits and is most commonly seen in the radius, ulna, and fibula. A greenstick fracture represents bending of immature bone, resulting in a fracture of half of the cortex of the bowed bone, resembling a broken young tree branch.[120]

Classification

The **Salter-Harris (SH) classification** is used to describe fractures involving the epiphyseal portion of the bone and is useful in determining mechanism of

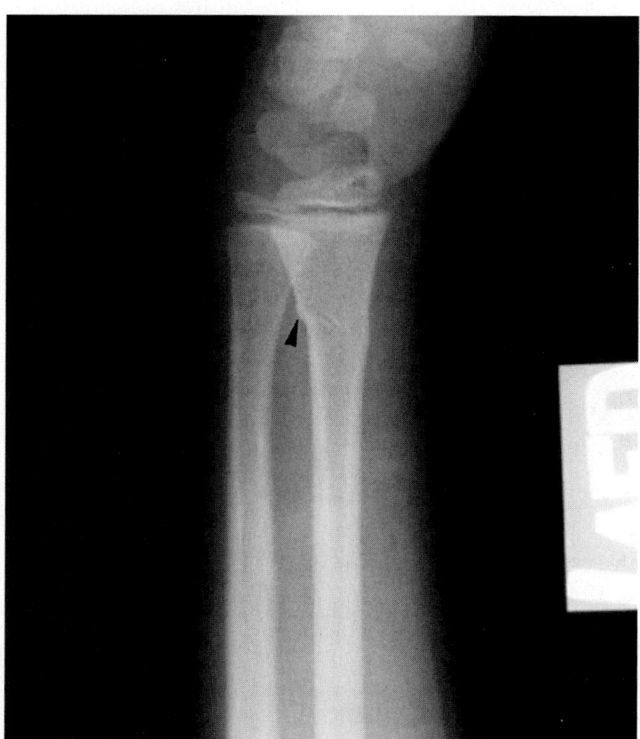

Fig. 33-5 Left radial torus (buckle) fracture *(arrowhead).*

injury, appropriate treatment, and prognosis. There are five major SH fractures, with the higher numbers representing more severe injuries (Fig. 33-7). **Type I fractures** (Fig. 33-8) are secondary to a shearing force, with separation of the metaphysis from the epiphysis through the zone of cartilage transformation. Radiographs may or may not show displacement. If undisplaced, radiographs may appear normal and the only clinical indication of injury is point tenderness over the growth plate. Treatment usually consists of closed reduction by gentle manipulation, with open reduction reserved for unstable fractures. The prognosis for future growth is excellent. If a type I SH fracture is suspected but not confirmed radiographically, the patient should be splinted and referred for repeat radiographs within 1 to 2 weeks.

Type II injuries (Fig. 33-9) result in a fracture fragment consisting of the physis and a triangular piece of the metaphysis, referred to as the **Thurston-Holland sign** on radiographs. Displacement is variable, and the risk of growth disturbance is low, since the germinal layer of the growth plate is usually spared. Treatment is usually by closed reduction.

A **type III fracture** line (Fig. 33-10) passes though a portion of the open growth plate, then through the epiphysis. If the fracture line extends to the end of the

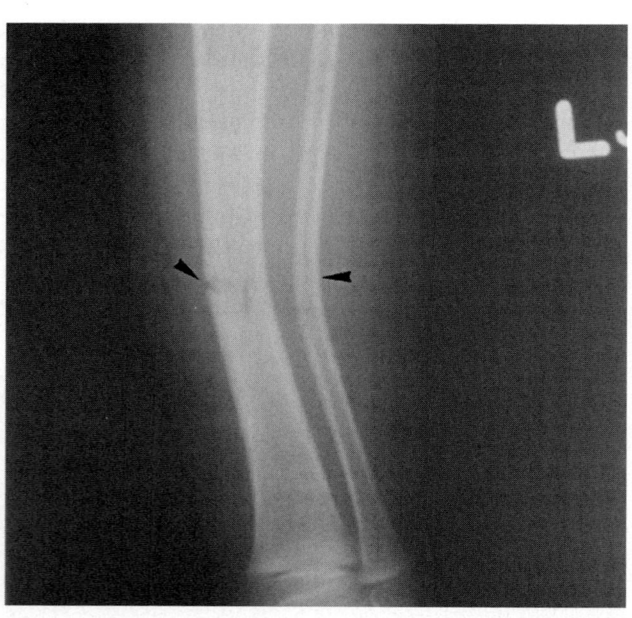

Fig. 33-6 Greenstick fracture of left tibia and bowing fracture of left fibula *(arrowheads).*

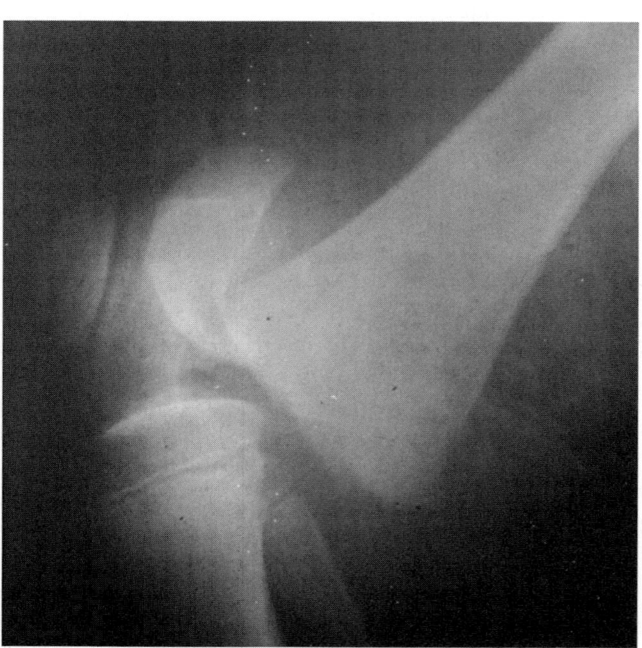

Fig. 33-8 Salter-Harris type I fracture of distal femur.

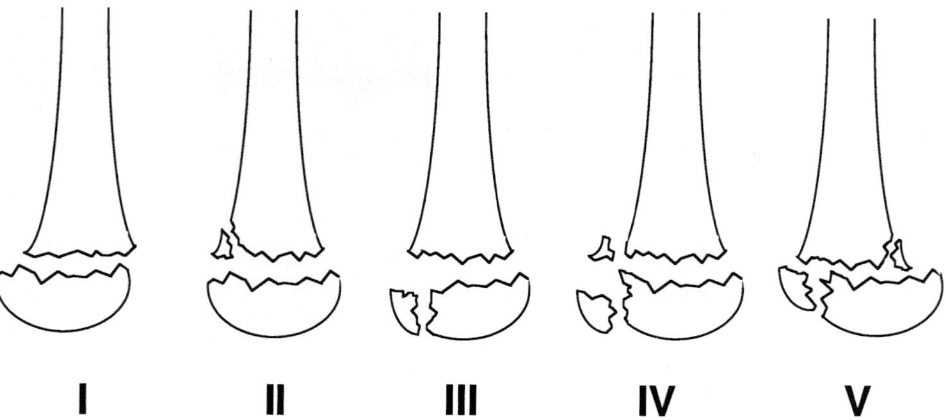

Fig. 33-7 Salter-Harris classification of growth plate fractures.

bone it becomes an intraarticular fracture. The most common site for a type III injury is the distal tibia. Open reduction and internal fixation to restore joint congruity and minimize the risk of growth disturbance may be required for displaced fractures. Nondisplaced fractures are treated with closed reduction. The prognosis for future growth is good.

Type IV fractures (Fig. 33-11) involve portions of the epiphysis, metaphysis, and physis. Open reduction and internal fixation is usually required to obtain accurate reduction. Long-term morbidity approaches 10%.

A **type V fracture** represents a crush injury of the growth plate. This injury is rare and the diagnosis is commonly made in retrospect. Morbidity approaches 100% and treatment is aimed at reversal of growth arrest.[121-123]

In general, the younger the child the greater the amount of remodeling that can be expected in fractures that involve the growth plate. Remodeling, though, does not occur in displaced intraarticular fractures (SH types III and IV), hence the need for aggressive orthopedic reduction. About 85% of epiphyseal fractures are associated with normal long-term growth; in the remaining 15%, partial or complete premature growth cessation may occur, most commonly in the distal humerus and femur.

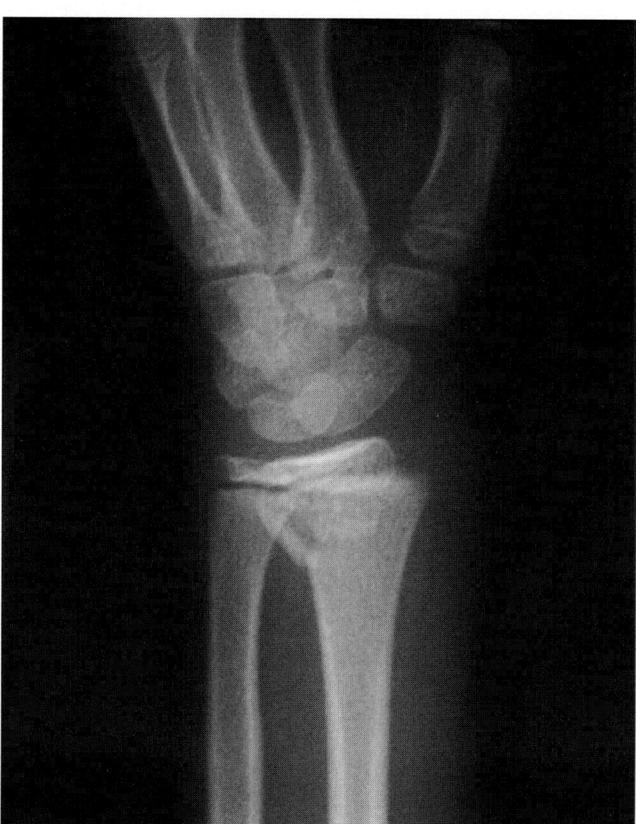

Fig. 33-9 Salter-Harris type II fracture of left distal radius.

Specific Injuries

Specific injuries tend to produce characteristic fractures in children. The presentation and initial therapies for traumatic skeletal injuries are determined by the bone involved and the type of trauma.

CLAVICLE

The clavicle is the most commonly fractured bone in children, with midshaft fractures accounting for 85% of all these fractures. The typical mechanism to produce this injury is a fall onto the shoulder. The clavicle is also the most commonly fractured bone in newborns. These children may present to the ED with pseudoparalysis or lack of spontaneous movement of the affected limb. Examination of the child with a clavicle fracture generally reveals crepitus, swelling, and tenderness, with variable deformity of the clavicle. Management with either a figure-of-eight apparatus or a sling both produce excellent results. Slings are generally preferred since they do not require periodic adjustment, are more easily removed for bathing and dressing and are better tolerated. Clavicle fractures may occur at the medial border and are usually of the SH type I or II. These fractures have an excellent ability to remodel and surgical treatment is rarely re-

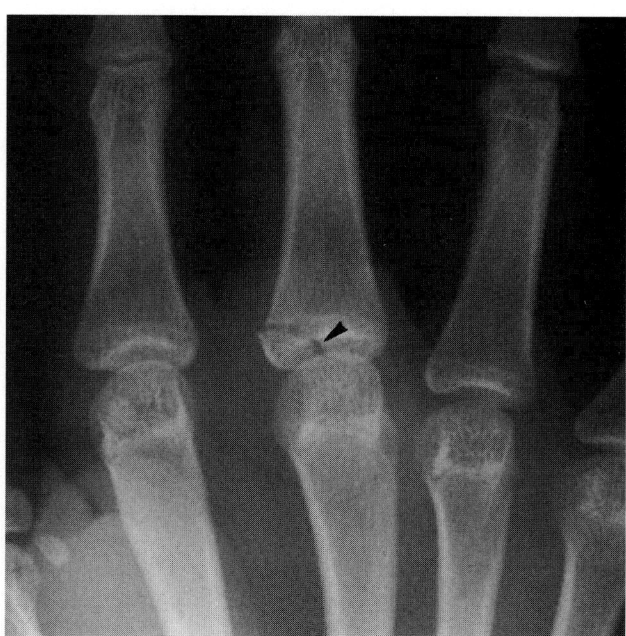

Fig. 33-10 Salter-Harris type III fracture of right third finger *(arrowhead).*

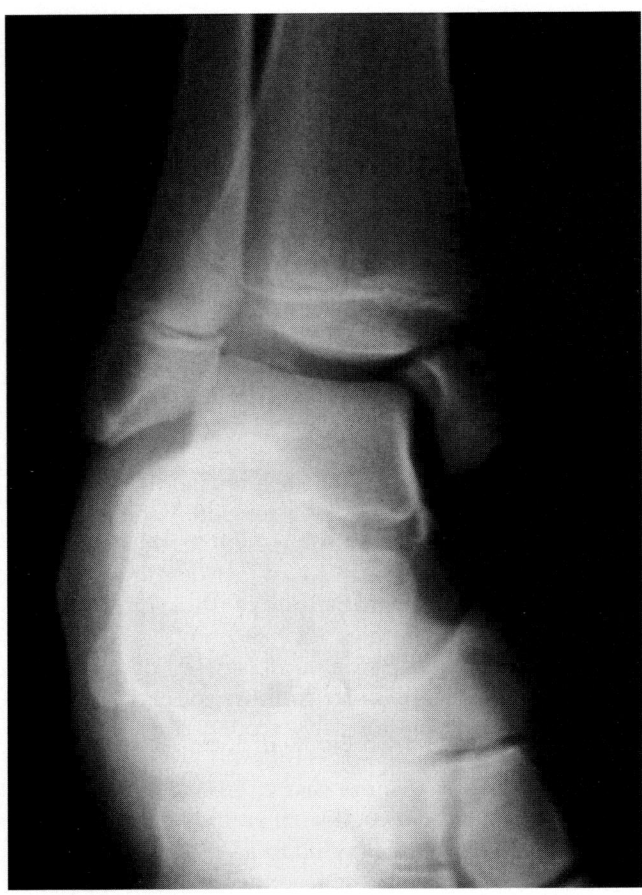

Fig. 33-11 Salter-Harris type IV fracture of distal tibia.

quired. Complications of any type of pediatric clavicle fracture are rare despite the close proximity of the subclavian neurovascular structures, although a careful examination of the chest and neck is indicated in any child with this fracture to rule out associated pneumothorax or vascular injury.

HUMERUS

Fractures of the proximal humerus usually occur after a backward fall onto the outstretched hand or secondary to direct trauma to the shoulder. In children <6 years old, SH type I fractures predominate, whereas in children older than 6 years of age, SH type II fractures are the most common. Radiographs may be difficult to interpret as a result of lucency of the physis; comparison views of the uninjured shoulder or oblique views are helpful. These fractures are generally managed with immobilization with a sling and swathe type device. Humeral shaft fractures are quite rare in children and are often the result of child abuse or direct trauma from a MVC. The risk of radial nerve injury is less common in children than in adults. A sling or swathe incorporating a plaster splint or long-arm cast is useful for fracture immobilization in these injuries.[122]

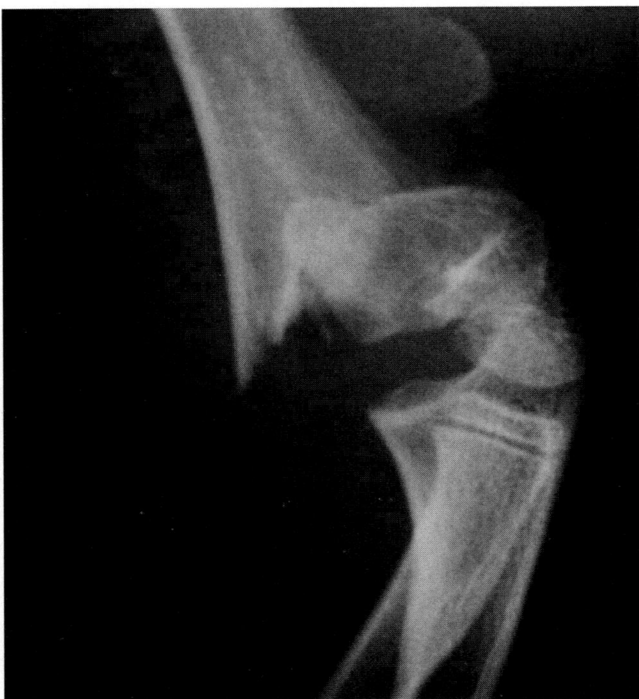

Fig. 33-12 Supracondylar humerus fracture.

ELBOW

Supracondylar fractures (Fig. 33-12) are the most common fractures involving the elbow in children. No pediatric fracture poses more difficulties in management or holds a greater threat of complication than a displaced fracture of the distal humerus. Supracondylar fractures are common in the first decade of life, with the usual mechanism of injury being a fall onto an outstretched hand or extended elbow. The minimal radiologic examination includes an AP view of the elbow in as much extension as possible, and an anatomic lateral view with the elbow flexed. Comparison views of the opposite elbow are useful if a subtle fracture is suspected. The presence of a **fat-pad sign** secondary to joint effusion increases the suspicion of an occult fracture (Fig. 33-13).

Supracondylar fractures are classified into three groups: Type I fractures are nondisplaced with intact anterior periosteum and are treated with simple immobilization. Type II fractures show posterior displacement of condyles with a disrupted anterior periosteum and intact posterior periosteum. Management usually requires manipulation or reduction by percutaneous pinning. Type III fractures are completely displaced without continuity of the periosteum. Treat-

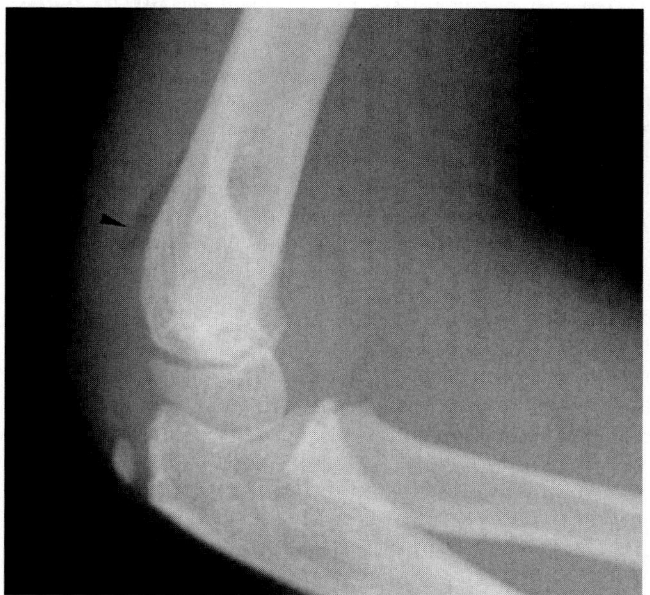

Fig. 33-13 Posterior fat pad sign *(arrowhead).*

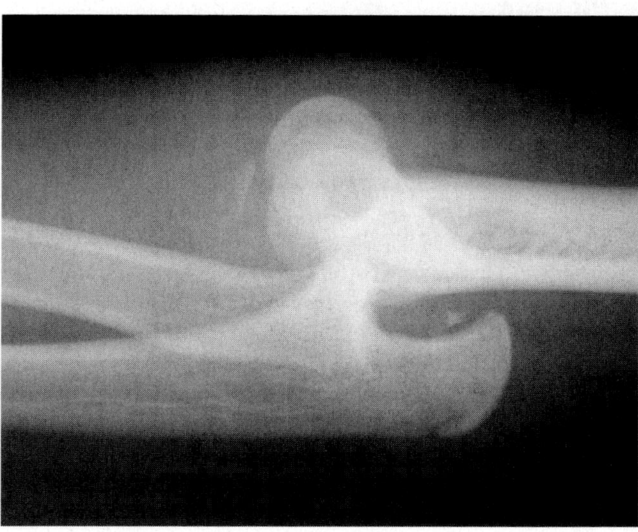

Fig. 33-14 Elbow dislocation.

ment for type III fractures is performed in the operating suite with closed reduction and percutaneous pinning. Displaced fractures (types II and III) are associated with neurovascular injuries to the median or radial nerves or to the brachial artery. **Cubitus varus** (i.e., varus deformity of the elbow) is the most frequent complication, occurring in up to 57% of cases.[124] **Volkmann's ischemic contracture** is a dangerous complication that occurs in 0.5% of cases as a result of increased compartment pressures.[124] All types of supracondylar fractures require urgent orthopedic consultation.

Lateral condyle fractures of the humerus are frequently SH type II, and although stable, these injuries are at risk for fibrous nonunion. If the fracture is displaced, pinning and possibly open reduction and internal fixation may be needed to prevent long-term diminished range of motion in the elbow.

The elbow is a difficult area to assess radiographically in skeletally immature children. Normal growth plates are frequently misinterpreted as fractures, whereas mildly displaced fractures may not be readily apparent. The appearance of six secondary ossification centers about the elbow, each with variable times to their appearance and closure, contribute to this confusion. In general, the secondary ossification centers of the elbow appear in this order: capitulum (lateral condyle), radial head, medial epicondyle, trochlea (medial condyle), olecranon, and lateral epicondyle, starting from about age 1.5 years for the capitulum to 10 years for the lateral epicondyle.

Dislocation of the elbow (Fig. 33-14) tends to occur in the older pediatric age group with a peak incidence of approximately 13 years of age. The majority of elbow dislocations are of the posterior type. Diagnosis is confirmed by radiographs, and treatment is with prompt reduction.

Radial head subluxation (**nursemaid's elbow**) is a very common orthopedic injury in children that is generally diagnosed clinically and readily corrected with closed reduction in the ED. The child presents with a history of being lifted by one arm and subsequently refuses to use the extremity. If the clinical picture is clear, radiographs are unnecessary and the arm is reduced through extension of the elbow and supination of the forearm, followed by elbow flexion; reduction is usually palpable.

FOREARM

Forearm fractures are also common in children secondary to falls onto outstretched arms. Seventy-five percent of these fractures involve the distal one third. All forearm radiographs should contain the entire radius and ulna, the elbow, and the wrist. Isolated fracture of the ulna may be accompanied by dislocation of the radial head (**Monteggia fracture**), while isolated radial fractures may be accompanied by disruption of the distal radio-ulnar joint (**Galeazzi fracture**). Shaft fractures of the pediatric radius and ulna are quite frequent and include torus, greenstick, and complete fractures. Fractures of the distal radius and ulna are most common in childhood because of the relative weakness of metaphyseal bone in this area. In addition, many are physeal fractures, usually of the SH I and II types. Treatment is generally accomplished through closed reduction and casting for even significantly displaced fractures. Operative intervention may be needed for unstable fractures.

HIP

The mechanism of injury of hip fractures in children is usually secondary to severe trauma from high-impact MVCs or falls. Pediatric complications of hip fractures include avascular necrosis (AVN), coxa vara, nonunion or malunion, and premature epiphyseal growth arrest. The presence of the physis and vascularity of the upper femur plate in growing children places them at greater risk of AVN (Fig. 33-15) and growth arrest than in skeletally mature adults. Overall prognosis is determined by both fracture level and the degree of displacement. The more proximal the fracture, the higher the risk of AVN and greater the likelihood of growth disturbance. Treatment includes prompt identification and immobilization, usually with internal fixation. In the ED, immobilization is best accomplished with bed rest and buttressing of the leg with pillows to prevent lateral motion until traction can be established. Traction splints should not be used in hip fractures because the proximal bar frequently sits just under the fracture site. Hip dislocations are most commonly posterior and require emergency reduction.

Slipped capital femoral epiphysis (SCFE) (Fig. 33-16) can occur following minimal trauma in overweight children early in adolescence. These injuries may be very subtle and should be carefully investigated in any child at risk for this injury.

PELVIS

Pelvic fractures are uncommon in injured children. Genitourinary (GU) injuries occur in 5% to 10% of children with pelvic fractures, and abdominal injuries are noted in 10% to 20%. The likelihood of GU/abdominal injuries increases when there are multiple fracture sites in the pelvis. Unlike adults, children are not prone to life-threatening hemorrhage and death in association with multiple fracture sites in the pelvis because their thicker periosteum frequently contains any fracture bleeding. The primary mechanism of pelvic fractures is related to motor vehicles (90%). Pelvic fractures can be classified as fractures involving the pelvic ring, avulsion fractures of the apophyses, and fractures involving the acetabulum. Management of pelvic fractures and accompanying GU/abdominal injuries requires coordination between the trauma, urologic, and orthopedic surgeons and needs to be individualized based on the severity of the injuries.

FEMUR

Femoral shaft fractures frequently result from trauma caused by motor vehicles. Concomitant injury to the head and chest are common. Hemorrhage owing to femoral shaft fractures in children is usually less se-

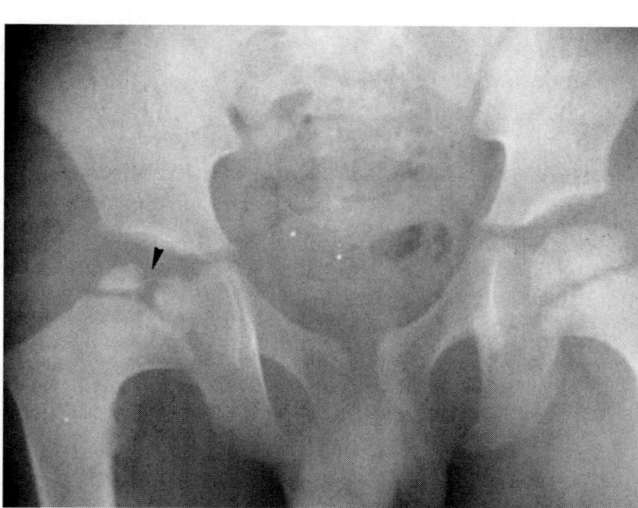

Fig. 33-15 Avascular necrosis of the right hip *(arrowhead).*

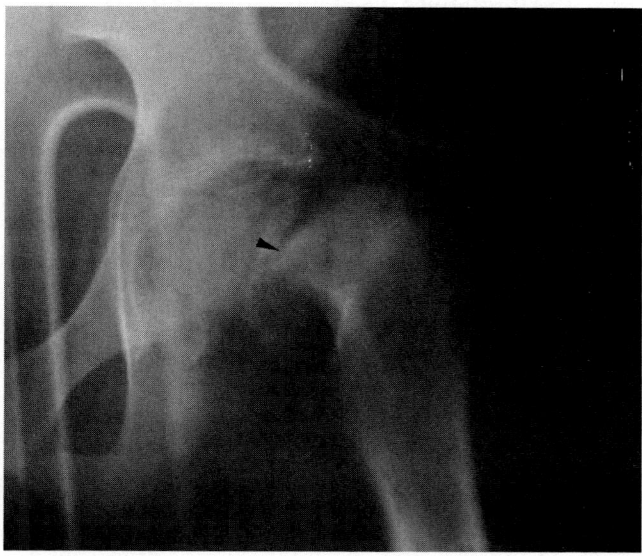

Fig. 33-16 Left slipped capital femoral epiphysis *(arrowhead).*

vere than in adults and may contribute to, but not cause, shock. Immobilization of the femur with a Hare traction splint or Buck's traction provides comfort and may decrease bleeding into the thigh. Femur fractures are very easily anesthetized with femoral nerve blocks and children should have such a block placed before placement of the traction splint whenever possible. Definitive treatment depends on the age, severity of injury, and the child's general condition and includes spica cast application or traction with delayed casting. Open reduction and internal fixation is rarely indicated. Overriding of midshaft fracture fragment ends is desirable due to the phenomenon of overgrowth, whereby the fracture end sites stimulate growth of the bone. Children between the ages of 2 and 12 years are most likely to experience overgrowth.[125]

KNEE

Fracture sites for knees include SH epiphyseal fractures of the distal femur, fractures of the proximal tibia, and avulsion fractures of the tibial spine and anterior tibial tubercle. The distal femoral physis is the most active in longitudinal growth, contributing 70% of the femoral length and 40% of the overall leg length. Fractures in this area may cause major growth abnormalities, making anatomic reduction imperative. Avulsion fractures of the knee involve ligamentous injury in the child. If undisplaced, closed treatment is indicated; separation or delayed union of undisplaced fractures requires open reduction. Children with SCFE often present with complaints of knee pain only. Therefore any child with pain in the knee should undergo a thorough hip evaluation as well.[122]

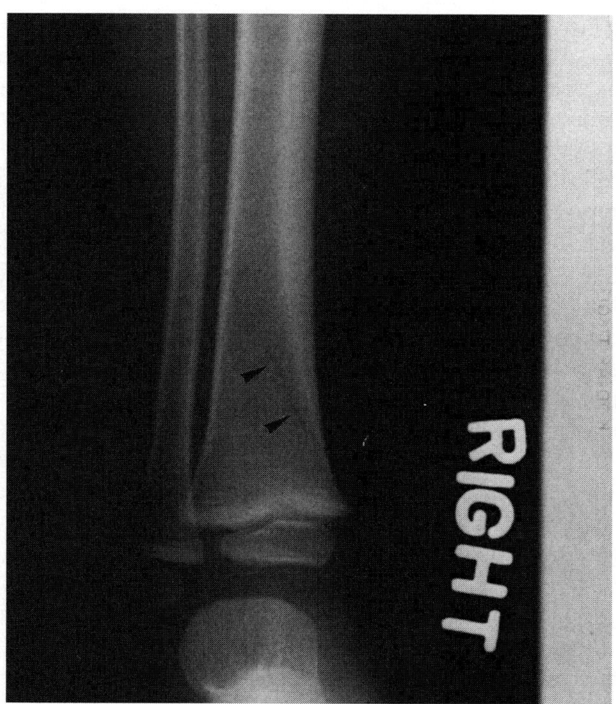

Fig. 33-17 Toddler's fracture *(arrowheads).*

TIBIA/FIBULA

Tibial fractures are the most common injuries of the lower extremities in children. Nondisplaced fractures require short- or long-leg casting. Displaced tibial fractures require immobilization of the knee and ankle in long leg casts. Neurovascular injuries with associated compartment syndrome are seen more commonly with displaced tibial fractures. The distal tibial physis contributes approximately 20% of the overall leg length. Most fractures are SH type II. Less frequently, SH type III or IV fractures are present.

Toddler's fractures (Fig. 33-17) are spiral fractures of the distal tibia produced by torsion of the foot. Children will present with refusal to bear weight. The initial injury may not be seen on early radiographs, but films taken several days to 2 weeks later may show the fracture line. Long-leg casting for 3 to 4 weeks is the treatment.

THORACIC AND LUMBAR VERTEBRAE

Thoracic and lumbar spine fractures are relatively uncommon injuries in children. However, lap-belt injuries increase the risk of posterior element fractures of the lower thoracic and upper lumbar vertebrae (**Chance fractures**).[88] The presence of a Chance fracture from a seatbelt injury is closely associated with hollow viscus injuries (see Chapter 19).

NONACCIDENTAL INJURIES IN CHILDREN

Epidemiology

Physical abuse accounts for 70% of all forms of child abuse. Over 4000 children die annually as a result of physical abuse, the majority younger than 3 years of age. Fatalities and serious injuries appear more common in younger children and their injuries are more likely to lead to a worse prognosis. Physical abuse may be the greatest killer of children between 6 and 12 months of age when compared with any specific cancer, malformation, or infectious disease. Boys are twice as likely as girls to be victims of physical abuse. It is estimated that 1% to 2% of U.S. children are victims of **nonaccidental trauma (NAT)** and that 10% of all ED visits of injured children <5 years old are the result of abuse. Consider the possibility of abuse in every child who presents with a serious injury. Many of the physical findings described in the following section are pathognomonic for NAT.

Burns

Burns are the second leading cause of accidental death among children in the United States, accounting for approximately 10% of all cases of physical abuse. Up to 15% of all children presenting to the ED with burn injuries received them deliberately. The scald burn is the most common type of burn injury resulting in hospitalization. Scald burns can be the result of immersion or splashing with hot liquid, most commonly water. Many cases of immersion burns involve a history in which the child allegedly fell into the bathtub. The mechanism for these burns generally involves a child who was dipped or dunked into hot water while being held in the caretaker's arms. Immersion burns occur when the child's knees are forcibly flexed and the buttocks and genitals are submerged. Physical examination reveals characteristics indicative of intentional injury, including well-demarcated burns with a circumferential configuration, absence of splash marks, and deep second- and third-degree burns. These sites are almost always chosen as punishment for enuresis or toilet training resistance, most commonly occurring in 2 to 3 year olds. If an extremity is immersed into scalding water, the area of the burned skin may resemble a stocking or a glove and splash marks or satellite burns are conspicuously absent. Conversely, spill burns or inadvertent immersions characteristically have splash marks.[126]

Dry contact burns, the second most frequent cause of abusive burns, occur with many different objects. These burns have a particular pattern resembling the hot surface of the object involved, such as a curling iron or radiator. These burns result from forcibly holding a heat source in contact with a child. Such objects cause second-degree burns without any blister formation and usually involve only one surface of the body. The shapes of the burns are pathognomonic for the object used to inflict the injury. Intentional cigarette burns are usually multiple and located on the palms, soles, back, buttocks, abdomen, or forearms. The imprints are 7 to 8 mm in diameter and sharply circumscribed.

Fractures

Fractures account for 10% to 15% of childhood injuries and are a frequent component of child abuse. Fractures are present in 10% to 36% of physically abused patients. Greater than half of the fractures in infants <1 year of age are the result of abuse. Injury characteristics suggestive of child abuse include fractures that occur in the metaphyses of the long bones, rib fractures, multiplicity of lesions, and multiple fractures in different stages of healing. Metaphyseal/epiphyseal fractures are virtually diagnostic of physical abuse since forces needed to produce these injuries are rarely generated by accidental trauma. Sudden traction of the extremity, such as shaking, stretching, or shearing of a limb, pulls away a portion of the metaphysis, leading to an avulsion, corner or bucket-handle fracture visible on radiographs of the involved extremity. Nonaccidental diaphyseal fractures are more common than metaphyseal fractures, although the latter are more specific to child abuse. Transverse diaphyseal fractures may be produced by a bending type of force or result from a direct blow. Spiral diaphyseal fractures result from torsional forces in which the limb is twisted (Fig. 33-18). This type of injury may be seen after an incident in which a caretaker has diapered an infant; the thigh is grasped vigorously and then twisted, causing the femur to sustain a spiral fracture. Both spiral and transverse fractures are common in accidental injuries; however, spiral fractures should be regarded as inflicted in infants and children <2 years old because of the extreme degree of force required to produce such injuries.[127,128] Toddler's fractures of the distal tibia must also be kept in the differential in ambulatory children.

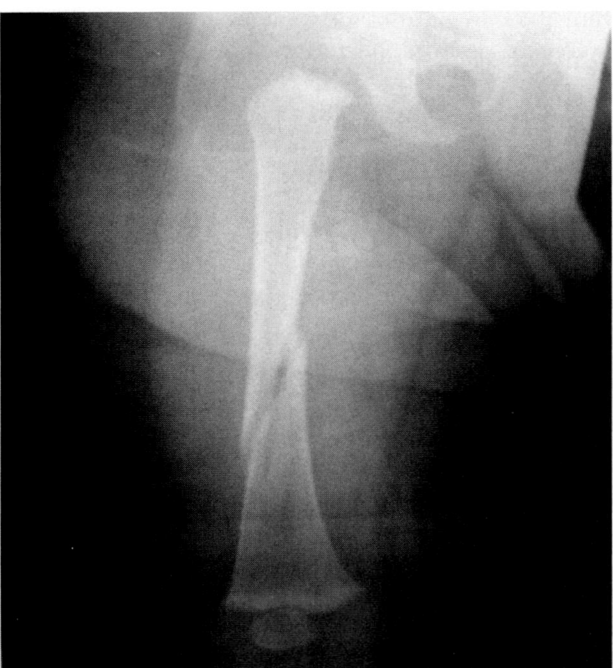

Fig. 33-18 Spiral fracture of right femur.

Rib fractures are frequently present in the abused child (Fig. 33-19). They are often bilateral or multiple, and may be noted when skeletal surveys are performed. All rib fractures in children <5 years old should be viewed with a suspicion of child abuse. In

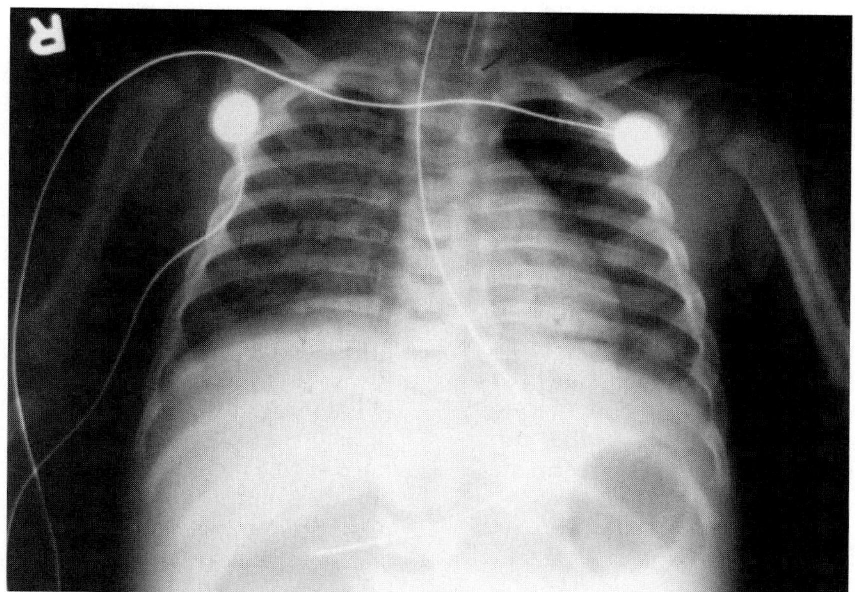

Fig. 33-19 Multiple old bilateral rib fractures.

infants and toddlers, rib fractures are usually posterior or lateral, and occur from violent compression of the chest as the child is shaken or thrown against the floor or wall. Vigorous CPR has not been found to fracture ribs in infants and children.[126]

Abdominal Trauma

Abdominal trauma is a serious form of child abuse, having significant morbidity and mortality (up to 50%). Intraabdominal injuries are the second most common cause of death in battered children, although they are not frequent injuries. These injuries are the result of being punched or kicked forcefully. Because of developmental differences, weak abdominal musculature, and less dense mesenteric attachments, children are more susceptible than adults to serious injuries from abdominal trauma. The increased mortality rate appears to be related both to the severity of initial injury and to delay in seeking treatment. Intraabdominal visceral injuries are more commonly found in children 2 years of age or older. Despite major abdominal injuries, external bruises are manifested infrequently, and may be present in only 10% to 50% of cases, leading to delayed presentation and delayed diagnosis. Specific abdominal injuries include ruptured liver or spleen, intestinal perforations, duodenal hematoma, pancreatic injury, and kidney laceration. Trauma to the abdomen is routinely denied in these cases. If there is no explanation for the injury, the physician must consider abuse in any abdominal crisis of undetermined etiology.[126]

Skin and Soft-Tissue Injury

The skin and soft tissues are the most common sites of manifestations of intentional injuries. Bruises account for >80% of injuries seen in the abused child. Inflicted bruises are so common at certain sites that finding them there is virtually pathognomonic for abuse. Bruises that predominate on the buttock and lower back almost always relate to punishment. Mongolian spots in African-American or Asian children can be confused with intentional injury at these sites. Genital area or inner thigh bruises are usually inflicted for toilet mishaps. Strap marks, loop marks, or other bizarre-shaped bruises are almost never accidental. Bruises found at multiple stages of healing are diagnostic and imply repeated beatings. The differential diagnosis of skin markings is broad. All bruises should be recorded as to size, shape, position, and color. Normally active children are likely to have bruises over bony prominences such as knees, elbows, and shins; bruises over soft tissues are more likely to be intentionally inflicted.

Bruises will go through various stages after they are inflicted. They will appear reddish-blue for the first 1 to 2 days after injury due to local hemorrhage.

A blue-purplish hue then develops at 3 to 5 days after injury. A greenish discoloration then develops secondary to release of biliverdin following lysis of red blood cells at 6 to 8 days post-injury. A yellowish-brown pigmentation then occurs at 8 to 10 days after injury. Bruising resolves within 21 days.

Shaken Baby Syndrome

Shaken baby syndrome is composed of the classic triad of intracranial injury, retinal hemorrhage, and long-bone fractures in young infants (frequently without external signs of abuse). More recent studies demonstrate that a direct blow or impact to the head probably contributes to the severity of the injury in this syndrome. The high mortality (50%) and morbidity (15%) seen in this syndrome emphasize the importance of early identification and prompt treatment.[129]

Emergency Department Management

In all 50 states in the United States, the physician must report suspected child abuse to the local **Child Protective Service (CPS)** agency. However, unless the physician considers the diagnosis, such a report can never occur. Physicians are protected from civil liability when they report a suspected case of child abuse in good faith. Reluctance to report can lead to recurrence of injuries or even death. More than 2.5 million children in the United States are reported to state CPS agencies as possible victims of abuse annually. The highest priority of treatment is to protect the child. If abused children are returned to the parents without intervention, 35% are seriously injured and 5% are killed. In about 20% of cases, the child must be temporarily placed in a foster home while the natural home is made safe.

A **skeletal survey** is indicated in young children when NAT is suspected. Fractures involving the posterior ribs (old or new) or metaphyses should raise serious consideration for NAT. Every bone in the body is imaged on a skeletal survey.

TRAUMA SYSTEMS FOR PEDIATRICS

In addition to the medical science involved in treating children, trauma management must also address access to care, injury sequelae, patient demographics, and programs for education, research, and prevention. When an injury occurs, the victim must be entered into the system. Because of the variability in training and abilities of first responders to a scene, any pediatric trauma system must be able to accommodate multiple access parameters. Police, fire department personnel, paid and volunteer rescue, BLS, or ALS providers all compose first responders in some portion of any geographic area involved in a pediatric trauma system. Regardless of background, these first responders must be able to assess the injured and decide if the patient is a candidate for trauma system management. Decisions to triage the patient into the program must be safe, accurate, efficient, consistent, and applicable by many different care providers. As with adult triage criteria, too liberal a set of standards results in over-triage to the trauma center, whereas restrictive triage criteria lead to inappropriate transport to an under-prepared facility. Any triage criteria must allow for some degree of judgment on the part of the personnel tending to an injured child. Gray-area decisions are best resolved with on-line communications with a command physician. As always, if there is any question it is probably best to over-triage to the pediatric trauma center.

No consensus pediatric triage criteria have been developed. Box 33-6 contains the initial New Jersey State Pediatric Trauma Triage criteria. Like any medical document, these criteria are continually reexamined in the light of changing technology and hospital capabilities in an effort to develop the most sensitive and specific pediatric trauma triage criteria.

Transportation of the injured child within a pediatric trauma system depends on the condition and location of the child, the surrounding facilities, and the transport equipment available. Small children do not require a stretcher or multiple attendants to move them from an injury scene to a hospital facility. It is not unusual for these children to be carried into an ED after transport by a private vehicle or police. However, the prehospital care providers must pay proper attention to spinal immobilization when indicated. In some medical models, this approach has been shown to be a more rapid means of establishing endotracheal intubation in a critically ill child.[130] Regardless of the scenario, any pediatric trauma system should be designed to maximize the speed with which a child receives definitive care.

In the adult system the term the "Golden Hour" refers to the consequences of untreated injuries following some form of trauma. In the pediatric population the term the "**Platinum 20 Minutes**" has been coined to recognize the increased metabolic rate and the potential for rapid unexpected deterioration in children. The exact mode of transportation selected for a given child depends on the accident scene, its location with respect to the trauma center, the nature of the injuries, and the availability of resources. The key function in any pediatric trauma triage scenario is to provide the child with the most immediate access

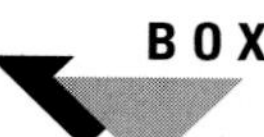

BOX 33-6

New Jersey Pediatric Trauma Triage Guidelines Indications for Transport to Trauma Center

- Altered mental status
- Poor perfusion
  - Pallor
  - Weak pulses
  - Mottling
  - Cyanosis
- Heart rate
  - ≤5 years old: <80 or >180
  - >5 years old: <60 or >160
- Respirations
  - >60
  - Labored
  - Apnea
- Cap refill >2 second
- Penetrating injuries
  - Head/torso
  - Proximal extremities
- Flail chest
- Airway difficulty
- Multiple long-bone fractures
- Pelvic fracture
- Paralysis
- Amputation
- Burns with trauma
- Seat belt marks on torso
- Ejection from motor vehicle
- Fall >3 times patient's height
- Extrication >20 minutes
- High-voltage injury
- Unrestrained in rollover
- Auto versus pedestrian/bicycle
- Front seat passenger with air bag

to airway stabilization, vascular support, and CNS treatment without delaying arrival at a definitive care center.

Within the trauma center model there exists the concept of a pediatric trauma center. The American College of Surgeons suggests that specific centers that treat children should have capabilities above those of a general trauma center. Such centers are recognized by the ACS as trauma centers with a commitment to children or level I pediatric centers. Whether triage systems direct all children to a pediatric trauma center remains unclear. There are little comparative outcome data on each component of trauma systems, although criteria have been created to try to measure the effectiveness of various facilities. The variability of the patient population, the overall good outcomes, and the measurement of crude variables (e.g., death) make these data difficult to interpret.

PREVENTION

Trauma is unique in the setting of the twentieth century in that it is a disease that is largely man-made and to a great degree preventable. Prevention may occur in the form of passive restraints in automobiles or fences around swimming pools, or it may be active as with bike helmets or life vests. Prevention can also take the form of education and behavior modification to teach children and their caretakers how to avoid situations that place a child at risk for a serious injury.[131]

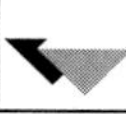

PEARLS & PITFALLS

- ◆ Vital signs are late predictors of shock in children.
- ◆ Persistent tachycardia and tachypnea may indicate intravascular depletion, shock, acidosis, or a severe painful condition and should never be solely attributed to anxiety or fear.
- ◆ Hypothermia is a common problem in pediatric resuscitations.
- ◆ Gastric distention may mimic an acute abdomen–consider early nasogastric decompression.
- ◆ Avoid cricothyroidotomy in children under 8 years of age to avoid subglottic stenosis.
- ◆ Consider SCIWORA in children with motor or sensory deficits in the face of normal plain or CT radiographs.
- ◆ Rib fractures are markers for serious intrathoracic injury in children.
- ◆ Seat belt abrasions should prompt investigation for hollow viscus injuries and Chance fractures.
- ◆ Microscopic hematuria in children is common but also may indicate intraabdominal solid organ injury.
- ◆ Consider the potential for growth plate injuries–splint and refer for orthopedic consultation if child is tender along the site of a growth plate, even if radiographs are normal.
- ◆ Consider the possibility of child abuse if the history given by the caretakers is not consistent with the injuries sustained by the child.

REFERENCES

1. National Pediatric Trauma Registry Home Page: http://www.nemc.org/rehab/factshee.htm.
2. Moront ML, Eichelberger MR: Advances in the treatment of pediatric trauma, *Curr Opin Gen Surg* 41-49, 1994.
3. Jaffe D, Wesson D: Emergency management of blunt trauma in children, *N Engl J Med* 324:1477-1482, 1991.
4. Harris BH, et al: American Pediatric Surgical Association principles of pediatric trauma care, *J Pediatr Surg* 27:423-426, 1992.
5. Lescohier I, DiScala C: Blunt trauma in children: causes and outcomes of head versus extracranial injury, *Pediatrics* 91:721-725, 1993.
6. Cooper A, et al: Epidemiology of pediatric trauma: importance of population-based statistics, *J Pediatr Surg* 27:149-153, 1992.
7. Durkin MS, et al: Epidemiology and prevention of severe assault and gun injuries to children in an urban community, *J Trauma* 41:667-673, 1996.
8. Mazurek AJ: Epidemiology of paediatric injury, *J Accid Emerg Med* 11:9-16, 1994.
9. Mosenthal AC, et al: Falls: Epidemiology and strategies for prevention, *J Trauma* 38: 753-756, 1995.
10. Wright MS: Update on pediatric trauma care, *Curr Opin Pediatr* 7:292-296, 1995.
11. Teanby DN, et al: Regional review of blunt trauma in children, *Br J Surg* 81:53-55, 1994.
12. Zavoski RW, et al: A population-based study of severe firearm injury among children and youth, *Pediatrics* 96:278-282, 1995.
13. Choi E, Donoghue ER, Lifschultz BD: Deaths due to firearms injuries in children, *J Forensic Sci* 39:685-692, 1994.
14. Vane DW, Shackford SR: Epidemiology of rural traumatic death in children: a population-based study, *J Trauma* 38:867-870, 1995.
15. Gerardi MJ, et al: Rapid-sequence intubation of the pediatric patient, *Ann Emerg Med* 28:55-74, 1996.
16. Eichelberger MR, et al: A comparison of the trauma score, the revised trauma score, and the pediatric trauma score, *Ann Emerg Med* 18:1053-1058, 1989.
17. Deakers TW, et al: Cuffed endotracheal tubes in pediatric intensive care, *J Pediatr* 125:57-62, 1994.
18. Sacchetti AD, Carraccio CA: Subcutaneous lidocaine does not affect the success rate of intravenous access in children less than 24 months of age, *Acad Emerg Med* 3:1016-1019, 1996.
19. Sacchetti A, et al: Pediatric analgesia and sedation, *Ann Emerg Med* 23:237-250, 1994.
20. Strain JD, et al: IV Nembutal: safe sedation for children undergoing CT, *AJR* 151:975-979, 1988.
21. Sacchetti A, et al: Family member presence during pediatric emergency department procedures, *Pediatr Emerg Care* 12:268-271, 1996.
22. Goldstein B, Powers KS: Head trauma in children, *Pediatr Rev* 15:213-219, 1994.
23. Mansfield RT: Head injuries in children and adults, *Crit Care Clin* 13:611-628, 1997.
24. Dietrich AM, et al: Head trauma in children with congenital coagulation disorders, *J Pediatr Surg* 29:28-32, 1994.
25. Masson F, et al: Characteristics of head trauma in children: epidemiology and a 5-year follow-up, *Arch Pediatr* 3:651-660, 1996.
26. Stein SC, Spettell CM: Delayed and progressive brain injury in children and adolescents with head trauma, *Pediatr Neurosurg* 23:299-304, 1995.
27. Muhonen MG, Piper JG, Menezes AH: Pathogenesis and treatment of growing skull fractures, *Surg Neurol* 43:367-373, 1995
28. Ersahin Y, et al: Pediatric depressed skull fractures: analysis of 530 cases, *Child's Nerv Syst* 12:323-331, 1996.
29. Kleinman PK, Spevak MR: Soft tissue swelling and acute skull fractures, *J Pediatr* 121:737-739, 1992.
30. Ros SP, Cetta F: Are skull radiographs useful in the evaluation of asymptomatic infants following minor head injury? *Pediatr Emerg Care* 8:323-330, 1992.
31. Skippen P, et al: Effect of hyperventilation on regional cerebral blood flow in head-injured children, *Crit Care Med* 25:1402-1409, 1997.
32. Bruce DA, et al: Diffuse cerebral swelling following head injuries in children: the syndrome of "malignant brain edema", *J Neurosurg* 54:170-178, 1981.
33. Muizelaar J, et al: Cerebral blood flow and metabolism in severely head-injured children. Part 1: Relationship with GCS score, outcome, ICP, and PVI, *J Neurosurg* 71:63-71, 1989.
34. Sharples PM, et al: Cerebral blood flow and metabolism in children with head injury. Part 1: Relation to age, Glasgow coma score, outcome, intracranial pressure and time after injury, *J Neurol Neurosurg Psychiatry* 58:145-152, 1995.
35. Lewis RJ, et al: Clinical predictors of post-traumatic seizures in children with head trauma, *Ann Emerg Med* 22:1114-1118, 1993.
36. Vera M, et al: Computed tomography imaging in children with head trauma: utilization and appropriateness from a quality improvement perspective, *Infect Control Hosp Epidemiol* 14:491-499, 1993.
37. Davis RL, et al: Cranial computed tomography scans in children after minimal head injury with loss of consciousness, *Ann Emerg Med* 24:640-645, 1994.
38. Jamjoon A, Cummins B, Jamjoon ZA: Clinical characteristics or traumatic extradural hematoma: a comparison between children and adults, *Neurosurg Rev* 17:277-281, 1994.
39. Stein SC, Doolin EJ: Management of minor closed head injury in children and adolescents, *Pediatr Surg Int* 10:465-471, 1995.
40. Greenes DS, Schutzman SA: Infants with isolated skull fractures: What are their clinical characteristics, and do they require hospitalization? *Ann Emerg Med* 30:253-259, 1997.
41. Reilly PL, et al: Assessing the conscious level in infants and young children: a paediatric version of the Glasgow coma scale, *Child's Nerv Syst* 4:30-33, 1988.
42. Pietrzak M, Jagoda A, Brown L: Evaluation of minor head trauma in children younger than two years, *Am J Emerg Med* 9:153-156, 1991.
43. Moreea S, Jones S, Zoltie N: Radiography for head trauma in children: What guidelines should we use? *J Accid Emerg Med* 14:13-15, 1997.
44. Atabaki SM, et al: A prospective study of pediatric closed head injury: Can clinical signs predict CT findings? *Pediatr Emerg Care* 14(abstract):83-84, 1998.
45. Mitchell WG: Status epilepticus and acute repetitive seizures in children, adolescents, and young adults: etiology, outcome, and treatment, *Epilepsia* 37(suppl 1):S74-S80, 1996.
46. Kuisma M, Roine RO: Propofol in prehospital treatment of convulsive status epilepticus, *Epilepsia* 36:1241-1243, 1995.
47. Kadish HA, Schunk JE: Pediatric basilar skull fracture: Do children with normal neurologic findings and no intracranial injury require hospitalization? *Ann Emerg Med* 26:37-41, 1995.
48. Davis RL, et al: The use of cranial CT scans in the triage of pediatric patients with mild head injury, *Pediatrics* 95:345-349, 1995.
49. Bonadio WA: Cervical spine trauma in children: Part I. General concepts, normal anatomy, radiographic evaluation, *Am J Emerg Med* 11:158-165, 1993.
50. Givens TG, et al: Pediatric cervical spine injury: a three-year experience, *J Trauma* 41:310-314, 1996
51. Kriss VM, Kriss TC: SCIWORA (spinal cord injury without radiographic abnormality) in infants and children, *Clin Pediatr* 35:119-124, 1996.

52. Manary MJ, Jaffe DM: Cervical spine injuries in children, *Pediatr Ann* 25:423-428, 1996.
53. Orenstein JB, Klein BL, Ochsenschlager DW: Delayed diagnosis of pediatric cervical spine injury, *Pediatrics* 89:1185-1188, 1992.
54. Lui TN, et al: C1-C2 fracture-dislocations in children and adolescents, *J Trauma* 40:408-411, 1996.
55. Dietrich AM, et al: Pediatric cervical spine fractures: predominately subtle presentation, *J Pediatr Surg* 26:995-999, 1991.
56. Bonadio WA: Cervical spine trauma in children: Part II. Mechanisms and manifestations of injury, therapeutic considerations, *Am J Emerg Med* 11:256-278, 1993.
57. Pang D, Wilberger JE Jr.: Spinal cord injury without radiographic abnormalities in children, *J Neurosurg* 57:114-129, 1982.
58. Curran C, et al: Pediatric cervical-spine immobilization: achieving neutral position? *J Trauma* 39:729-732, 1995.
59. Laham JL, et al: Isolated head injuries versus multiple trauma in pediatric patients: Do the same indications for cervical spine evaluation apply? *Pediatr Neurosurg* 21:221-226, 1994.
60. Schwartz GR, et al: Pediatric cervical spine injury sustained in falls from low heights, *Ann Emerg Med* 30:249-252, 1997.
61. Etzwiler LS, Smith ER, Lelyveld S: Cervical spine injuries, *Pediatr Emerg Care* 12:233-235, 1996.
62. Grabb PA, Pang D: Magnetic resonance imaging in the evaluation of spinal cord injury without radiographic abnormality in children, *Neurosurgery* 35:406-414, 1994.
63. Bracken MB, et al: A randomized, controlled trial of methylprednisolone or naloxone in the treatment of acute spinal-cord injury. Results of the Second National Acute Spinal Cord Injury Study, *N Engl J Med* 322:1405-1411, 1990.
64. Koltai PJ, Rabkin D: Management of facial trauma in children, *Pediatr Clin North Am* 43:1253-1275, 1996.
65. Division of Injury Control, Center for Environmental Health and Injury, Centers for Disease Control: Childhood injuries in the United States, *Am J Dis Child* 144:627-646, 1990.
66. Nelson LP, Shusterman S: Emergency management of oral trauma in children, *Curr Opin Pediatr* 9:242-245, 1997.
67. Rielly JP, et al: Thoracic trauma in children, *J Trauma* 34:329-331, 1993.
68. Black TL, et al: Significance of chest trauma in children, *South Med J* 89:494-496, 1996.
69. Reinhorn M, et al: Penetrating thoracic trauma in a pediatric population, *Ann Thorac Surg* 61:1501-1505, 1996.
70. Peclet MH, et al: Thoracic trauma in children: an indicator of increased mortality, *J Pediatr Surg* 25:961-965, 1990.
71. Stafford PW, Harmon CM: Thoracic trauma in children, *Curr Opin Pediatr* 5:325-332, 1993.
72. Manson D, et al: CT of blunt chest trauma in children, *Pediatr Radiol* 23:1-5, 1993.
73. Sarihan H, et al: Blunt thoracic trauma in children, *J Cardiovasc Surg* 37:525-528, 1996.
74. Garcia VF, et al: Rib fractures in children: a marker of severe trauma, *J Trauma* 30:695-700, 1990.
75. Lee RB, et al: Three or more rib fractures as an indicator for transfer to a level I trauma center: a population-based study, *J Trauma* 30:689-694, 1990.
76. Abrunzo TJ: Commotio cordis: the single, most common cause of traumatic death in youth baseball, *Am J Dis Child* 145:1279-1282, 1991.
77. Eddy AC, et al: The epidemiology of traumatic rupture of the thoracic aorta in children: a 13-year review, *J Trauma* 30:989-991, 1990.
78. Ali IS, et al: Blunt traumatic disruption of the thoracic aorta: a rare injury in children, *J Pediatr Surg* 27:1281-1284, 1992.
79. Spouge AR, et al: Traumatic aortic rupture in the pediatric population: role of plain film, CT and angiography in the diagnosis, *Pediatr Radiol* 21:324-328, 1991.
80. Bromberg BI, et al: Recognition and management of nonpenetrating cardiac trauma in children, *J Pediatr* 128:536-541, 1996.
81. Schild HH, et al: Pulmonary contusion: CT vs plain radiograms, *J Comput Assist Tomogr* 13:417-420, 1989.
82. Kharasch SJ, et al: The routine use of radiography and arterial blood gases in the evaluation of blunt trauma in children, *Ann Emerg Med* 23:212-215, 1994.
83. Hurst JM, DeHaven CB, Branson RD: Use of CPAP mask as the sole mode of ventilatory support in trauma patients with mild to moderate respiratory insufficiency, *J Trauma* 25:1065-1068, 1985.
84. Shilyansky J, et al: Diagnosis and management of duodenal injuries in children, *J Pediatr Surg* 32:880-886, 1997.
85. Arkovitz MS, Johnson N, Garcia VF: Pancreatic trauma in children: mechanisms of injury, *J Trauma* 42:49-53, 1997.
86. Graham JS, Wong AL: A review of computed tomography in the diagnosis of intestinal and mesenteric injury in pediatric blunt abdominal trauma, *J Pediatr Surg* 31:754-756, 1996.
87. Takishima T, et al: Characteristics of pancreatic injury in children: a comparison with such injury in adults, *J Pediatr Surg* 31:896-900, 1996.
88. Anderson PA, et al: The epidemiology of seatbelt-associated injuries, *J Trauma* 31:60-67, 1991.
89. Sivit CJ, et al: Safety-belt injuries in children with lap-belt ecchymosis: CT findings in 61 patients, *AJR* 157:111-114, 1991.
90. Powell EC, Tanz RR, DiScala C: Bicycle-related injuries among preschool children, *Ann Emerg Med* 30:260-265, 1997.
91. Smith MD II, et al: Pediatric seat belt injuries, *Am Surg* 63:294-298, 1997.
92. Voss M, Bass DH: Traumatic duodenal hematoma in children, *Injury* 25:227-230, 1994.
93. Bensard DD, et al: Small bowel injury in children after blunt abdominal trauma: Is diagnostic delay important? *J Trauma* 41:476-483, 1996.
94. Saladino R, Lund D, Fleisher G: The spectrum of liver and spleen injuries in children: failure of the pediatric trauma score and clinical signs to predict isolated injuries, *Ann Emerg Med* 20:636-640, 1991.
95. Taylor GA: Imaging of pediatric blunt abdominal trauma: What have we learned in the past decade? *Radiology* 195:600-601, 1995.
96. Moss RL, Musemeche CA: Clinical judgment is superior to diagnostic tests in the management of pediatric small bowel injury, *J Pediatr Surg* 31:1178-1181, 1996.
97. Newman KD, et al: The lap belt complex: intestinal and lumbar spine injury in children, *J Trauma* 30:1133-1138, 1990.
98. Albanese CT, et al: Is computed tomography a useful adjunct to the clinical examination for the diagnosis of pediatric gastrointestinal perforation from blunt abdominal trauma in children? *J Trauma* 40:417-421, 1996.
99. Hennes HM, et al: Elevated liver transaminase levels in children with blunt abdominal trauma: a predictor of liver injury, *Pediatrics* 86:87-90, 1990.
100. Coant PN, et al: Markers for occult liver injury in cases of physical abuse in children, *Pediatrics* 89:274-278, 1992.
101. Abou-Jaoude WA, et al: Indicators of genitourinary tract injury or anomaly in cases of pediatric blunt trauma, *J Pediatr Surg* 31:86-89, 1996.
102. Stalker HP, Kaufman RA, Stedje K: The significance of hematuria in children after blunt abdominal trauma, *AJR* 154:569-571, 1990.

103. Sweeney RL, Doolin EJ, Ross SE: Hematuria in injured children: Is emergency radiographic evaluation mandatory? *Ann Emerg Med* 20(abstract):473, 1991.
104. Swischuk LE: Abdominal trauma and hematuria, *Pediatr Emerg Care* 10:181-182, 1994.
105. Stein JP, et al: Blunt renal trauma in the pediatric population: Indications for radiographic evaluation, *Urology* 44:406-410, 1994.
106. Middlebrook PF, Schillinger JF: Hematuria and intravenous pyelography in pediatric blunt renal trauma, *Can J Surg* 36:59-62, 1993.
107. Knudson MM, et al: Hematuria as a predictor of abdominal injury after blunt trauma, *Am J Surg* 164:482-485, 1992.
108. Hashmi A, Klassen T: Correlation between urinalysis and intravenous pyelography in pediatric abdominal trauma, *J Emerg Med* 13:255-258, 1995.
109. Miller KS, McAninch JW: Radiographic assessment of renal trauma: our 15-year experience, *J Urol* 154:352-355, 1995.
110. Morey AF, Bruce JE, McAninch JW: Efficacy of radiographic imaging in pediatric blunt renal trauma, *J Urol* 156:2014-2018, 1996.
111. Isaacman DJ, et al: Utility of routine laboratory testing for detecting intraabdominal injury in the pediatric trauma patient, *Pediatrics* 92:691-694, 1993.
112. Sivit CJ, et al: Blunt trauma in children: significance of peritoneal fluid, *Radiology* 178:185-188, 1991.
113. Hermier M, et al: role of imaging in the management of abdominal trauma in children, *Arch Pediatr* 2:273-285, 1995.
114. Akgur FM, et al: Initial evaluation of children sustaining blunt abdominal trauma: ultrasonography vs. diagnostic peritoneal lavage, *Eur J Pediatr Surg* 3:278-280, 1993.
115. Krupnick AS, et al: Use of abdominal ultrasonography to assess pediatric splenic trauma. Potential pitfalls in the diagnosis, *Ann Surg* 225:408-414, 1997.
116. Akgur FM, et al: Prospective study investigating routine usage of ultrasonography as the initial diagnostic modality for the evaluation of children sustaining blunt abdominal trauma, *J Trauma* 42:626-628, 1997.
117. Katz S, et al: Can ultrasonography replace computed tomography in the initial assessment of children with blunt abdominal trauma?, *J Pediatr Surg* 31:649-651, 1996.
118. Akgur FM, et al: The place of ultrasonographic examination in the initial evaluation of children sustaining blunt abdominal trauma, *J Pediatr Surg* 28:78-81, 1993.
119. Ogden JA: Skeletal growth mechanism injury patterns, *J Pediatr Orthop* 2:371-377, 1982.
120. Kao SC, Smith WL: Skeletal injuries in the pediatric patient, *Radiol Clin North Am* 35:727-746, 1997.
121. Landin LA: Epidemiology of children's fractures, *J Pediatr Orthop–B* 6:79-83, 1997.
122. Blasier RD, Aronson J: Fractures in children, *Curr Opin Pediatr* 6:85-89, 1994.
123. Brown JH, DeLuca SA: Growth plate injuries: Salter-Harris classification, *Am Fam Physician* 46:1180-1184, 1992.
124. Smith JT, Morrissy RT: Preventing complications of supracondylar fractures in children, *Complic Orthop* Sept/Oct:135-145, 1989.
125. Scoles PV: *Pediatric orthopedics in clinical practice,* ed 2, St Louis, 1988, Mosby.
126. Gothard TW, Runyan DK, Hadler JL: The diagnosis and evaluation of child maltreatment, *J Emerg Med* 3:181-194, 1985.
127. Sills RM, Pena ME: Bones, breaks, and the battered child: Is it unintentional or is it abuse? *Pediatr EM Rep* 3:1-10, 1998.
128. Merten DF, Carpenter BL: Radiologic imaging of inflicted injury in the child abuse syndrome, *Pediatr Clin North Am* 37:815-837, 1990.
129. American Academy of Pediatrics Committee on Child Abuse and Neglect: shaken baby syndrome: Inflicted cerebral trauma, *Pediatrics* 92:872-875, 1993.
130. Sacchetti A, Carraccio C, Feder M: Pediatric EMS Transport: Are we treating children in a system designed for adults only? *Pediatr Emerg Care* 8:4-8, 1992.
131. Stylianos S, Eichelberger MR: Pediatric trauma: prevention strategies, *Pediatr Clin North Am* 40:1359-1368, 1993.

34 Geriatric Trauma

CARL C. D'ANDREA

Teaching Case

An 85-year-old woman was the belted front seat passenger in a high-speed, head-on motor vehicle crash (MVC). The passenger windshield was starred. She had a 5-minute loss of consciousness and is complaining of mild right chest and upper abdominal pain. Her systolic blood pressure is 120 mmHg and her pulse is 60 bpm. Her medical history includes hypertension and atrial fibrillation and her medicines are warfarin, digoxin, and metoprolol. She has a normal chest film and normal hemoglobin, and is considered stable enough to undergo serial examinations. She is found moribund an hour later, with a blown pupil and a blood pressure of 60.

The elderly trauma victim may appear stable on arrival, only to decompensate with little warning. A blood pressure of <140 mmHg in any elderly person, let alone one with a history of hypertension, should be considered relative hypotension. Lack of tachycardia is not reassuring, since patients on β-blockers cannot mount a tachycardic response to blood loss. Warfarin allows for continued bleeding and should prompt a careful search for intracranial or intraabdominal bleeding.

Geriatric trauma is a growing national concern. As the population ages, the percentage of injuries incurred by the elderly increases, and the need for proper triage, resuscitation, and disposition is imperative. The elderly, defined as people 65 years of age or older, currently comprise 12% of the U.S. population, but account for a disproportionately high 28% of injury fatalities. They use over 30% of all healthcare cost expended on injury.[1,2] With these current statistics, and the estimation that the elderly population will grow to over 68 million by the year 2040,[2] the significance of geriatric trauma is profound. Although multiple research projects and multicenter studies concentrate on trauma, very few focus on the elderly.

An early study by Oreskovich et al[3] cast a dim light on the benefits of aggressive management of geriatric trauma. This widely quoted article examined the outcome of 100 consecutive geriatric trauma victims. Before injury, 96% were independent, but at discharge 88% did not return to their previous level of independence; 72% required full nursing home care. Although the mortality rate was only 15%, the authors concluded that there is little hope of returning to an independent existence for the majority of geriatric trauma victims. Opposing this assumption were studies by both van Aalst et al[4] and DeMaria et al,[5] which showed that aggressive management can restore the majority of elderly patients to their preinjury status.

Certain principles recur in geriatric traumatology. Although advancing years reduce physiologic reserve, the premorbid status is more important than chronologic age. Pitfalls abound in emergency resuscitation. Initial assessment frequently overlooks significant injury for many reasons, one of the most important of which is the fact *that vital signs are insensitive in shock.*

EPIDEMIOLOGY

Trauma is the most common cause of death in people under 45 years of age and is currently the seventh leading cause of death in the geriatric population.[6] The incidence of trauma mortality among the elderly, however, might be underestimated.[7] Data from the Major Trauma Outcome Study[8] (MTOS) revealed that motor vehicle crashes (MVCs) were the most common cause of death for people under the age of 65, but falls predominated for those 65 years of age and older. Following falls were MVCs, pedestrian-MVCs, stab wounds, gunshot wounds, and others. The elderly have a mortality rate and hospital length of stay nearly double that of younger patients, and a significantly higher complication rate.[9] The Diagnosis-Related Group (DRG) payment system grossly underestimates the cost for elderly patient care.[9-11] The financial cost of geriatric trauma in the United States exceeds 20 billion dollars a year.[12]

MECHANISM OF INJURY

The mechanism of injury has profound implications for all trauma patients, but in the elderly it has special significance. The emergency physician (EP) must determine why the injury occurred—"what were the precipitating events?" The initial precipitant such as syncope, hypoglycemia, or cardiac dysrhythmia may be more significant to the patient's course than the actual injury.

Falls

Falls are the most common cause of injury in the United States[13] and the most common cause of injury-related deaths in the elderly.[14] About one in three elderly people fall each year,[15-17] and of those who fall, 20% to 30% suffer moderate to severe injuries.[16-18] Sattin et al[19] showed that for elderly patients who fell and required medical attention, 42% required hospital admission and 50% of those admitted were ultimately discharged to a nursing home. Falls are usually from a flat surface or relatively low heights (e.g., stepladder, stairs) and occur most commonly at home.[20] Fractures and soft-tissue injuries occur 5% to 20% of the time, but more serious injuries (e.g., cervical fractures, subdural hematomas) are also caused by this apparently benign mechanism.[17,21,22]

The cost for treatment and rehabilitation of fall-related injuries in the elderly is extreme. In a study based on all admitted elderly patients in Washington state in 1989, 5.3% were admitted due to injuries from falls, and the cost for treatment was over 53 million dollars.[18] This study did not include the long-term costs for recurrent falls, rehabilitation, and nursing home care.

Why elderly people fall has been the subject of much research.[16,23,24] Hazards, such as stairs or loose floor rugs, are not a major etiology; instead, co-morbid conditions, medications, and the deterioration of vision, strength, and coordination that come naturally with aging were more highly predictive for falls (Box 34-1).[16,17,24,25]

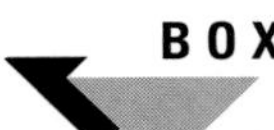

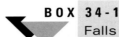

BOX 34-1
Falls in the Elderly: Medical Reasons

1. **Cardiac**
   a. Dysrhythmia
   b. Valvular disease (e.g., aortic stenosis)
   c. Myocardial ischemia, infarction
2. **Neurologic**
   a. Transient ischemic attack
   b. Cerebrovascular accident
   c. Dementia
   d. Parkinson's disease
   e. Seizure
   f. Intracranial hemorrhage
3. **Toxic/Metabolic**
   a. Hypokalemia
   b. Hypernatremia/hyponatremia
   c. Hyperglycemia/hypoglycemia
   d. Ethanol
   e. Iatrogenic (medication-induced)
      i) Anticholinergic
      ii) Antipsychotic
      iii) Diuretics
      iv) Antihypertensives
4. **Miscellaneous**
   a. Degenerative joint disease
   b. Gastrointestinal hemorrhage
   c. Infection, sepsis

Adapted from Baraff LJ, et al: *Ann Emerg Med* 30:480-492, 1997.

A study by Riggs[26] examined the mortality rate for accidental falls between 1962 and 1988 and showed a significant decrease in the elderly. The sharp decline was attributed to improved evaluation, resuscitation, and trauma management.

EMERGENCY DEPARTMENT MANAGEMENT

Because prior falls are the most important risk factor for further falling, the EP should discuss possible instigating factors with the patient, family, or caregiver. Problems with vision, gait, and proprioception are common, and are often easily remedied. Simple things such as a new eyeglass prescription, hearing aid, proper footwear and adequate lighting can all decrease the chances for further falling and the morbidity and mortality that accompanies it. Polypharmacy, especially with sedatives such as benzodiazepines or barbiturates, is a widespread and preventable cause.

Motor Vehicle Crashes

While falls are the overall leading cause of injury-related deaths in persons over the age of 65, motor vehicle crashes (MVCs) are the number one cause of trauma-related deaths in those aged 65-74.[6] There are over 22 million licensed drivers over the age of 65 in the United States, comprising about 13% of all licensed drivers.[27] Although older drivers drive less miles than younger drivers, their risk of crash involvement is higher per mile driven and they are responsible for the majority of the crashes in which they are involved.[6,28] Older drivers are more likely to crash in seemingly favorable conditions (e.g., close to home, during daylight, and in good weather). Alcohol also plays a much less important role in geriatric MVCs compared with the younger age groups, the latter having alcohol use implicated up to 52% of the time.[29]

As with elderly fallers, elderly drivers have impaired vision, hearing, and coordination. Situational confusion and frank syncope have also been implicated in elderly victims of MVCs.[28,30,31] A comparison of young and old victims of MVCs showed that 74% of elderly drivers found to be at fault in a MVC had significant underlying medical conditions, compared with 15% of the younger drivers at fault. Using victim accounts, witness accounts, and police records, investigators determined that the elderly driver was at fault in 80% of the crashes. Importantly, syncope was deemed responsible in 18% of the cases. In 30% of the elderly MVCs, no cause for the crashes was found, but in those cases, 75% of the drivers had significant underlying medical conditions.[28]

Not only are the elderly more likely to cause MVCs, they are also more likely to be severely injured as a result. Although the distribution of injuries is similar for both the elderly and young victim of a MVC, the elderly have a higher severity for any given injury. One exception is sternal fracture from the use of seat belts, where the elderly are more likely to sustain these injuries, perhaps related to decreased bone density from osteoporosis.[32] However, major cardiopulmonary complications are less likely.

Pedestrian-Motor Vehicle Crashes

Pedestrian-Motor Vehicle Crashes (PMVCs) are the most devastating mechanism of injury in the elderly population.[27,33] PMVCs involve the elderly more than any other age group, including children.[34] Over 20% of PMVCs involve elderly people, causing the highest case fatality rate in any age group.[34] Most of the accidents occur at crosswalks, where vision, hearing, coordination, and gait all play important roles.[27,33] The aged person may suffer from kyphosis, making it difficult to see traffic lights, street signals, and oncoming vehicles.[33] In addition, the time allotted for crossing a street during a red light is insufficient for a significant portion of the elderly.[27]

McCoy et al[32] also showed that the elderly were more likely to be involved in a PMVC as a result of walking directly into the path of an oncoming car. Confusion, combined with vision and hearing difficulties, was found to be the primary cause for these occurrences.

Penetrating Trauma

In 1990, there were approximately 5000 deaths resulting from penetrating trauma in people over the age of 65.[6] There are few studies, however, dealing specifically with penetrating trauma in the elderly. Many studies deal with different forms of geriatric trauma, but limit the descriptions to "assault" or "other" when discussing injury other than falls, MVCs, or burns. The incidence and mortality for gunshot wounds in the elderly is 5.5% and 52%, respectively, whereas in the younger group the incidence and mortality is 13% and 19.5%.[8,9] Likewise, stab wounds had a much lower incidence but a much higher mortality rate for the elderly.

Elder Abuse

Always consider the possibility of intentional injury in the elderly trauma victim.[35,36] Elder abuse is less recognized than child or spousal abuse.[37,38] In 1980 the U.S. Senate Special Committee on Elder Abuse estimated that there are between 500,000 and 2,500,000 cases each year in the United States.[35,39] In the most widely cited study on the topic, the occurrence rate was 32 per 1000 adults over the age of 65.[36]

A recent survey looking at emergency evaluation and reporting of suspected geriatric abuse showed only a 50% report rate.[38] Only 31% of the EPs responding knew of a protocol at their hospital dealing with elder abuse.

A comprehensive review identified several risk factors for both the victim and abuser.[40] In families a "generation inversion" occurs in which the elder becomes increasingly dependent, occasionally leading to stress in the caregiver. When the stress becomes unbearable, the caregiver may strike out at the victim or refuse to help with the victim's activities of daily living (ADL). Risk factors associated with abusers include a history of anxiety or depression, alcohol abuse, or social dysfunction.[36,39,40] Abusers are most commonly the spouse or children of the victim, and there is no definite sex predominance.[39,40] For the victims of elder abuse, risk factors include dementia, physical disability, and female sex (although this last factor has been disputed).[36,40]

The EP confronted by a suspected case of elder

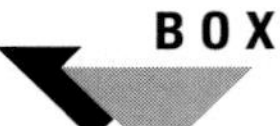

BOX 34-2
Indicators of Potential Elder Abuse

PHYSICAL
Occult fractures
Bruises of varying ages
Immersion pattern of injury
Genital/anal trauma

PSYCHOSOCIAL
Inconsistent histories
Overly/Underly concerned caregiver
Poor hygiene, bedsores
Clothing inappropriate for season/situation
Dehydration, malnutrition

abuse (Box 34-2) should contact social services and report the abuse to the appropriate state agency. As of 1990, 43 states have mandated the reporting of elder abuse.[40] If the physician believes that the victim is at significant risk for further abuse, and social services cannot provide emergency shelter, admission is justified.

Burns

The elderly suffer disproportionate mortality from burns. Approximately 2.5 million people are burned each year in the United States and 12,000 of those burned die.[22] Victims 65 years of age or older account for 10% of these deaths and 13% of all admissions to burn centers.[41-43] Most elderly patients are burned at home.[41-43]

As early as 1902, mortality from burns was considered dependent on burn size and the patient's age.[44] A widely used formula suggests that mortality can be estimated by the addition of those two figures.[44] The Baux Index calculates mortality as:

mortality = age + Total Body Surface Area (TBSA) burned

The TBSA is based only on second- and third-degree burns and does not take into account first-degree injury. In the elderly there is 100% mortality when the patient has greater than 70% TBSA burns.

Regionalization of burn care, improvements in fluid resuscitation and nutrition, and aggressive treatment of burn wounds have decreased mortality for burn victims over the last few decades. In the 1940s, burns greater than 10% TBSA were usually fatal, but today survival is likely even with burns approaching 50% TBSA.[45] Unfortunately, the elderly do not fare as well. Current statistics estimate a 50% mortality for a victim over the age of 60 with full-thickness burns of 10% to 14% TBSA.[46] The TBSA is the single highest predictor of mortality, but age and the presence of an inhalation injury also predict a poor outcome.[22] The older the patient, the greater the likelihood of inhalation injury. Lower extremity burns, excessive fluid requirements over the first 24 hours, and the development of pneumonia are also associated with higher mortality in the elderly burn victim.[44]

The geriatric risk for burns and burn complications involve the same factors that place them at risk for other injuries. The elderly are more likely to have co-morbid conditions and to take medications that predispose to transient confusion, dizziness, and syncope. Dementia and coordination difficulties can be especially dangerous to the geriatric smoker. The older person has diminished senses and slower reaction times, putting them at risk for deeper burns.[41,44,45] In addition, elderly people have skin atrophy and a thinner dermis, leading to more severe, full thickness injury.[41,44-46] Since elderly people are more likely to delay seeking medical care for a burn[41] and have a decreased immune response,[47] they are at risk for secondary infection and sepsis.

EMERGENCY DEPARTMENT MANAGEMENT

The initial treatment of the elderly burn victim differs little from that of their younger counterparts. Fluid resuscitation using standard calculation formulas, analgesia, tetanus prophylaxis, and monitoring of urine output are the same. Consider cervical spine injury and carbon monoxide poisoning. Determine the need for endotracheal intubation early in the evaluation. Reserve antibiotics for documented infection.[48] The American Burn Association suggests that patients older than 50 years of age with burns greater that 20% TBSA be considered for burn center transfer. Before transfer, always evaluate the need for definitive airway management.

The treatment of burns in the elderly has undergone changes over the last several years. Initially it was thought that as a result of poor or delayed healing, conservative management was advocated, including frequent dressing changes, topical antibiotics, hydrotherapy, blunt debridement, and delayed skin grafting.[41,46] This approach was challenged because of the high rates of burn wound sepsis and multisystem organ failure seen with delayed excision and grafting.[45] More recent investigations have shown an increased survival and decreased complication rate and hospital stay with early excision and skin grafting of burns less than 20% TBSA.[45]

Although the elderly have a higher mortality rate for burn injury than their younger counterparts, 50% of those who survive can return to a partially independent existence.[42] Survivors have a life expectancy equal to that a person of similar age and health status.[42]

Finally in the case where the burn is severe and death is certain (>70% TBSA in one study[44]), involve the family early-on in a decision to withhold futile resuscitative efforts. In such cases, consider a morphine drip to control pain and avoid heroic interventions that only prolong suffering.

PHYSIOLOGY OF AGING

Normal aging affects all physiologic processes. Subtle irreversible changes that begin in the thirties leads to progressive deterioration with increasing age.[49] Although the rate of change may differ among organ systems, for a given system the rate of deterioration is fairly constant.[49]

Cardiovascular

As a result of cardiovascular changes, an elderly patient in shock can exhibit normal vital signs. During a geriatric trauma resuscitation, a normal pulse and blood pressure may lull the EP into dangerous complacency.

The cardiac output (CO) declines about 1% a year starting after the third decade, so that the CO of an 80-year-old person is roughly half that of a 20 year old.[49] The reason for this decline is unknown, but several factors may be involved including coronary artery disease and left ventricular hypertrophy.[9,50] Over a quarter of MVCs in the elderly may be associated with acute changes in cardiac status, and in the majority of these crashes the change in cardiac status was the precipitating cause.[51]

A number of changes impair the tachycardic response and blunt increases in CO in the elderly trauma patient. These changes include a diminished response to both endogenous and exogenous catecholamines,[52] myocardial fibrosis, decreased compliance, and decreased cardiac filling.[49] With age, stiffening of the arteries leads to an increased cardiac workload.[53] Finally, amyloidosis has been found in as many as 78% of subjects over the age of 70.[44,49] Amyloid deposits stiffen the heart, cause conduction defects and lead to congestive heart failure.

In addition to these age-related cardiovascular changes, medications such as β-blockers, calcium channel blockers, and digoxin can diminish the cardiac response to stress.

MANAGEMENT CONCERNS

In the case of suspected hemorrhage, consider early transfusion to maximize oxygen delivery. A hematocrit of 30% in a patient with suspected ongoing blood loss should prompt blood replacement. Early involvement with a trauma or general surgeon is essential.

Pulmonary

Aging also exerts important changes in the structure and function of the respiratory system. Adult respiratory distress syndrome and alveolar collapse are common final pathways in geriatric chest trauma.

Loss of chest wall compliance occurs as a result of calcification of the costal cartilage and kyphosis. Rib fractures are frequent and lead to splinting and alveolar collapse. A decrease in the alveolar elastic recoil leads to airway collapse and hypoxemia.[54] This hypoxemia reduces pulmonary surfactant, causing further alveolar collapse.[54] Loss of pulmonary surfactant may contribute to the adult respiratory distress syndrome (ARDS), a common cause of death in the elderly trauma victim.[54] Elderly patients have diminished pulmonary reserve, which causes further airway collapse.[49] Air trapping, seen most notably in chronic obstructive pulmonary disease (COPD), dilutes inspired air, decreases the PaO_2, and compresses the diaphragm, limiting tidal volume.[55]

MANAGEMENT CONCERNS

COPD can also complicate resuscitation of the elderly patient. Although oxygen is universally accepted as being beneficial in trauma, high-flow oxygen may suppress the hypoxic ventilatory drive in a patient with COPD. A Venturi mask can control the FiO_2,while frequent arterial blood gases (ABGs) help assess oxygenation and ventilation. A persistent SaO_2 below 90% or evidence of increasing CO_2 (e.g., somnolence, lethargy, stupor) mandate endotracheal intubation and mechanical ventilation.

Renal

With aging, there is a decrease in both the renal mass and number of functional glomeruli, which results in declining creatinine clearance and overall renal function.[46,56] This deterioration in function has significant implications for the elderly trauma patient. Many drugs (e.g., aminoglycosides, penicillins, and digoxin) that are renally cleared have a prolonged half-life. The decline in renal blood flow and glomerular filtration rate increases the risk of renal failure from hypotension and contrast agents.[56]

Finally, one of the classic assessments used in the trauma victim is the adequacy of urine output. Standard trauma guidelines often use 50 cc/hr in an adult as the minimal urine output to ensure adequate fluid replacement. In the elderly, however, adequate urine output does not necessarily mean adequate resuscitation. The geriatric patient not only has a decreased ability to concentrate urine, but also frequently uses diuretics. These factors make urine output a less sensitive indicator of proper resuscitation and perfusion.[56]

MANAGEMENT CONCERNS

When a good alternative exists, avoid the use of nephrotoxic drugs in the elderly. Parenteral hydration before contrast studies may reduce contrast-induced acute renal failure.

Immune System

A significant portion of elderly trauma patients die as a result of infectious complications.[3,57] The elderly have both a diminished cough reflex and decreased clearance of secretions by the mucociliary apparatus.[49] These mechanical difficulties, combined with a higher colonization of the oropharynx with gram-negative bacilli, make aspiration, pneumonia, and sepsis particularly common in the elderly.[49] Unfortunately, with the increased risk of infectious complications comes a decline in immune function. Aging produces a decrease in cell-mediated and humoral response to foreign antigens, and an increase in the immune response to autoantigens. These phenomena have been linked to the involution of the thymus gland and the altered balance between T-lymphocytes.[47] For these reasons, the elderly are unable to mount an effective response to an infectious agent, and generate immune complexes that deposit in various tissues and organs, leading to decreased function. This failure to recognize self has been theorized as a possible cause for the aging process itself.[47] In regards to surgical stress, the immune response of the elderly lags behind that of younger patients.[58]

Endocrine/Metabolic

OSTEOPOROSIS

Orthopedic injuries are common in the elderly, whether from a fall or from major trauma, primarily resulting from the changes associated with osteoporosis.[59,60] Osteoporosis, a decrease in bone density, is a multifactorial problem related to age, hormonal status, ancestry, and body habitus.[49,61] As many as 15% of Caucasian women over the age of 65 have significant osteoporosis, and 30% of these women will suffer a fracture as a result of osteoporosis by the age of 75.[61] Falls may result in a fracture approximately 5% to 20% of the time and typically occur in the wrist, humerus, hip, and pelvis.[17] Compression fractures of the lumbar spine are particularly common, often without a history of trauma.[61]

METABOLIC RESPONSE TO STRESS

Elderly patients may develop an oxygen debt early during trauma, from which they never recover. This debt is reflected in rising levels of lactate and increasing acidosis secondary to anaerobic metabolism in shock.

Elderly patients are also susceptible to the problems associated with the hypermetabolic, hypercatabolic state associated with severe injury.[62,63] Investigations of the metabolic response to stress began with the classic description by Cuthbertson[64] regarding the "ebb" and "flow" phases of metabolism following injury. The initial, or "ebb," phase is marked by a decrease in cardiac output, temperature, and oxygen consumption. When homeostasis is regained and tissue perfusion has been restored, the body undergoes the "flow" phase of hypermetabolism. During this phase the energy needs of the cardiac and pulmonary system increase, as does the need for substrate to provide this energy. Additional energy is needed for cell proliferation and immune defense.[63,65] Initially, the body responds by breaking down protein and releasing amino acids to serve as precursors for gluconeogenesis and cellular proliferation. Fat stores are mobilized for energy expenditure, and serum levels of catecholamines and cortisol are increased.[12]

When comparing the catabolic response to injury between young and old patients, several differences are apparent. First, the elderly have less lean muscle mass and more adipose tissue. During muscle breakdown for gluconeogenesis, critically ill patients can lose a great deal of their muscle mass, and in the elderly this loss results in a higher percentage lost of their total body mass.[63] This loss of muscle mass results in a severe depletion of strength, and the inability to move or effectively deep breathe and cough. These changes place the elderly at high risk for pneumonia, deep venous thrombosis, and possible pulmonary embolus. Second, metabolic stress leads to hyperglycemia and insulin resistance in the elderly.[49,62,63,65] Hyperglycemia combined with an age-related inability to maximally resorb glucose in the kidney leads to an osmotic diuresis, dehydration, and further muscle breakdown.[49] The treatment of the endocrine and metabolic changes associated with stress and the nutritional needs of the elderly trauma patient are the subject of much research. Early parenteral and enteral nutrition, optimizing glucose calories, and infusion of insulin to facilitate uptake of glucose are all under investigation.[63,65] The use of human growth hormone, shown to be particularly diminished in the geriatric population, might have a role in meeting the catabolic needs of the elderly trauma patient in the future.[63]

APPROACH TO THE GERIATRIC TRAUMA PATIENT

Prehospital

In regards to the prehospital management of geriatric trauma patients, there is little difference compared with a younger adult. Given the higher likelihood of preexisting medical conditions in the elderly population and their possible contribution to the cause of the accident, it is critical for the prehospital personnel to explore the events leading up to the injury, if time allows.

The elderly are the most commonly under-triaged group and suffer increased morbidity and mortality as a result of under-resuscitation.[66] Traditional trauma triage using trauma scores is insufficient in the elderly. Pellicane et al[67] found that in an elderly trauma population, 52% of the deaths occurred in patients with a prehospital trauma score of 15 and 16. Medics should consider trauma center transport for adults older than 55 years of age, especially if they have co-morbid disease.

Emergency Department Evaluation

As with prehospital care, the initial resuscitation of the elderly trauma victim differs little from that of other adults. During the initial evaluation, someone associated with the case should be gathering information on the patient's medical history, current medications, and primary doctor. The medical history can often alter management and has been shown to predict morbidity, mortality, and length of hospital stay (Fig. 34-1).[68]

Although measurement of pulse rate, respirations, and blood pressure are routine, temperature monitor-

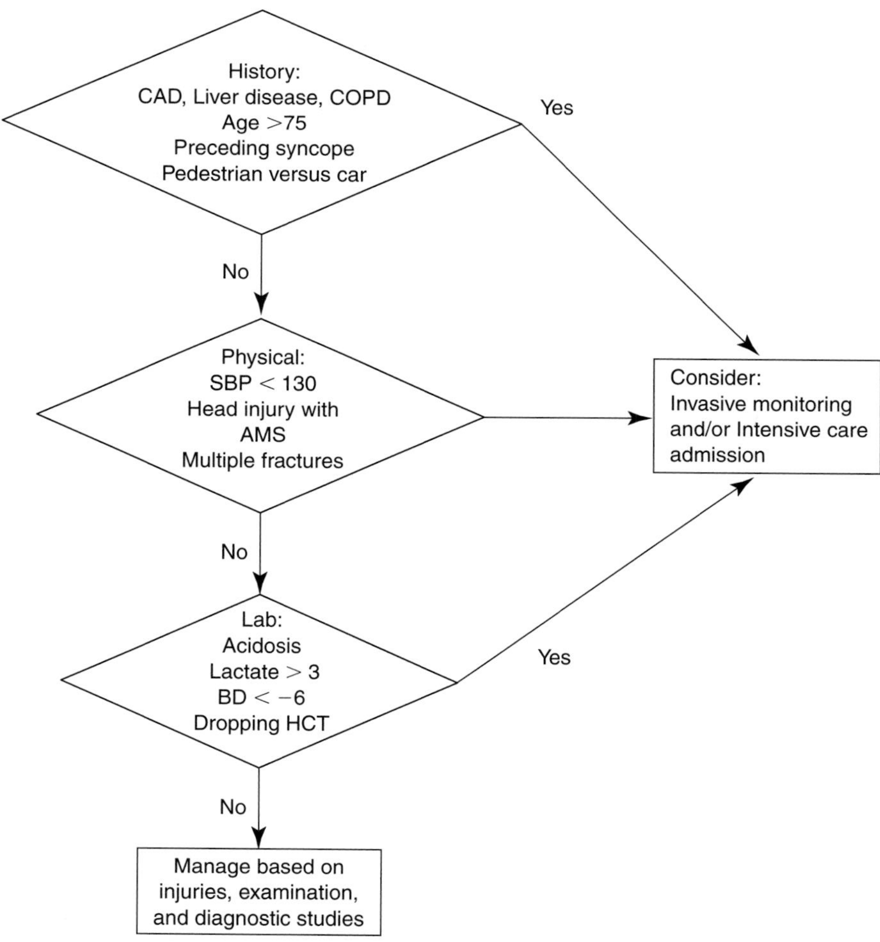

Fig. 34-1 Criteria for intensive care in geriatric trauma.

ing is a critical but often overlooked aspect of trauma care. It is particularly important in the elderly, because of slowed metabolism and difficulty in maintaining core temperature.[59]

Management of the airway poses several unique concerns. The most vital concept in this regard is that elderly patients have limited cardiopulmonary reserve. Early intubation is essential to decrease the work of breathing and avoid progressive respiratory failure and cardiovascular collapse. There should be a much lower threshold for early endotracheal intubation in the elderly patient with traumatic brain injury, blunt chest injury, or hemodynamic instability, compared with the younger patient. During the assessment be sure to examine and clear the airway of dentures and recognize their potential for airway compromise.[60] Remember that elderly patients with limited cardiovascular reserve or acute volume loss are particularly vulnerable to the hypotension that may be caused by induction agents (e.g., benzodiazepines, barbiturates). Reduced doses should be used in this setting. Also recognize that elderly patients with limited pulmonary reserve and/or blunt chest trauma may be difficult to preoxygenate, and desaturate rapidly during intubation. In summary, be aggressive, but be gentle!

The EP should send blood for hemoglobin and hematocrit, type and crossmatch, electrolytes, blood urea nitrogen (BUN), and creatinine. ABGs are helpful in the seriously injured to determine respiratory compromise and adequacy of resuscitation. The pH and base deficit may be the most illuminating numbers on the ABG profile. Acidosis is a sensitive indicator of occult shock. It is more sensitive than a patient's vital signs, or urine output. A base deficit of less than (more negative than) or equal to -6 predicts severe injury and mortality in the elderly.[69] Recent evidence has shown that both the initial serum lactate level and the time to normalization can accurately predict survival in multisystem trauma.[70,71]

Vital signs are insensitive to physiologic stress and invasive monitoring may improve outcome of elderly trauma victims. Invasive monitoring shows that 43% of hemodynamically stable geriatric trauma victims may have inadequate cardiac output.[72] In a landmark study, Scalea et al[72] used invasive monitoring in 60 multisystem trauma patients over the age of 65. They enrolled all elderly trauma patients who presented with risk factors predictive of mortality (i.e., SBP under 130, acidosis, multiple fractures, or head injury). Arterial lines, pulmonary artery catheterization, and rapid transport to the intensive care unit (ICU) were performed on all patients, regardless of injury severity. Scalea's group achieved a significant increase in survival by using these data to optimize oxygen delivery. They employed volume infusion, inotropes, and afterload reduction to maximize oxygen delivery.

Further evidence supporting poor clinical correlation with actual physiologic reserve came from Del Gurcio and Cohn.[73] In a study of elderly patients "cleared" for surgery by physical examination, chest radiographs, electrocardiogram, and basic laboratory studies, a full 64% of them showed abnormalities increasing risk of surgery, and 23% were deemed inoperable after invasive monitoring (i.e., arterial lines and pulmonary artery catheterization). All patients who were deemed inoperable but underwent surgery died.

The elderly trauma patient, in general, requires a higher level of vigilance to maximize good outcome. Initial hypotension, a Glasgow Coma Scale of less than 7, or evidence of head injury all predict a poor outcome and require emergent evaluation and treatment.[4] Normalization of vital signs and an apparently benign physical examination can grossly underestimate the severity of injury, physiologic reserve, and the need for further resuscitation.

Another area of concern is oligoanalgesia in the elderly. For a variety of reasons, physicians either neglect pain control in elderly trauma victims, or give inadequate medication.[74,75] Titration of intravenous narcotics is both safe and humane (see Chapter 10).

INJURY EVALUATION

Head and Cervical Spine. The striking difference in the elderly are the types of head injury that occur and the amount of force needed to produce injury.[76] As the brain ages, the dura mater becomes firmly adherent to the skull, making epidural hematomas unlikely.[60,77,78] Brain atrophy in a fixed cranium puts strain on the emissary (bridging) veins that travel from the brain surface to the various dural sinuses.[76] Head trauma in this setting often leads to a subdural hematoma (SDH), which is three times more likely in the elderly population.[59] Significant head injury in the elderly can be caused by minimal or no apparent trauma and can present with little or no neurologic deficit. With brain atrophy, intracranial hemorrhages can also grow to large sizes before causing compressive effects.

Liberal use of cranial computed tomography (CT) is essential in the elderly victim of head trauma. Indications may include the following:

1. Multisystem injuries
2. A history of loss of consciousness
3. Abnormal neurologic examination
4. Dementia or intoxication
5. Focal neurologic findings
6. Any head trauma in the setting of oral anticoagulant use

Early neurosurgical involvement is the rule, and transfer necessary if either a neurosurgeon is not available or a CT scan cannot be done on an emergent basis. Craniotomy with decompression is the treatment of choice for a SDH, although individual differences may alter management.[78-80] Although the patient is in the ED, careful neurologic checks should be frequent and repeat CT scans performed for deterioration.

Just as CT scanning in head injury should be used liberally, so too should plain radiographs of the cervical spine. The elderly spine is more susceptible to fracture resulting from degenerative change and osteoporosis. In the setting of a fracture with minimal or no trauma, consider a pathologic process (e.g., neoplasm or rheumatoid arthritis).[81] As with the younger population, neck pain, tenderness to palpation, altered mentation, distracting injuries, or neurologic deficit should prompt complete radiologic examination. Cervical spine films are not indicated in the alert, unintoxicated patient who has no spinal tenderness, neurologic deficit, and no painful distracting injuries.[82]

Much has been reported about the "occult" cervical spine injury, although close scrutiny of these cases reveals that most do not meet the above criteria and that cervical films were warranted.[83-88] Further evaluation of a suspected cervical spine injury might include CT, magnetic resonance imaging (MRI), or bone scans.

The treatment of cervical spine injury in the elderly is similar to that in the young and includes rigid collar, halo vest, or surgical stabilization, depending on the type and severity of injury. The need for early mobilization is unique to the elderly to promote respiratory function and maintain mental health.[85]

Because of age-related narrowing of the cervical canal and vascular disease of spinal arteries, the elderly are more susceptible to the central cord syndrome. In this syndrome, injury or ischemia to the central portion of the cervical cord produces a deficit of upper extremity motor strength and sensation. Tingling or burning sensation in the arms and particularly the hands is typical. Motor weakness is variable. Central cord syndrome typically occurs in the absence of a demonstrable vertebral fracture, making the diagnosis clinical. The EP should specifically question the older patient regarding such arm symptoms and examine the upper extremities for subtle weakness or sensory deficit. MRI is the imaging modality of choice to demonstrate a central cord injury, since it provides the best anatomic definition of the spinal cord and will delineate edema or hematoma. In patients with suspected or proven central cord syndrome neurosurgical consultation is mandatory. Those with demonstrable weakness should receive high-dose corticosteroids (see Chapter 12).

Chest. The elderly have a higher mortality and complication rate from chest trauma as a result of both the injury itself and secondary pulmonary insults.[89-91] Rib fractures are the most common injury, with hemothorax, pneumothorax, flail chest, and pulmonary contusions occurring with lesser frequency.[91,92] Of interest to note is that the use of 3-point restraint belts, although improving overall mortality rates in all age groups, increases the risk for chest injury in the elderly, including aortic lacerations and myocardial contusions.[93] Although the authors certainly do not recommend that elderly patients avoid restraint use, the EP should recognize that these devices may not provide the protection given to a younger patient.

An elderly patient with chest trauma or injuries possibly requiring mechanical ventilation presents a dilemma to an EP. Endotracheal intubation and mechanical ventilation, although immediately life saving, can increase the risk of death resulting from aspiration, pneumonia, or ARDS.[3,94] Pulmonary complications are a major factor in the mortality of the elderly trauma victim and intubation should not be routine.[3,5,89,94,95]

Intubation is indicated in the treatment and stabilization of hypoxemia associated with pulmonary contusion and flail chest. However, in the patient with normal mental status, and adequate oxygenation and ventilation, begin management with supplemental oxygen and aggressive pulmonary toilet. Analgesia in the form of parenteral narcotics, or intercostal or epidural nerve blocks allow adequate chest wall movement.[92,96] One recent study showed a significant decrease in the mortality and infection rate with internal fixation of flail segments compared with prolonged mechanical ventilation.[97]

Associated with the possibility of pulmonary injury is the potential for both aortic and cardiac injury. The "broken halo" sign is a disruption in a calcified aortic knob, and is associated with aortic rupture.[98] A recent study comparing operative repair in the young and old showed a 163-fold increased likelihood of mortality in the elderly.[99] The authors suggested that perhaps nonsurgical or delayed surgical management should be considered in the elderly because of comorbidities or coexisting injuries.

The diagnosis of cardiac contusion continues to be difficult and at best, inexact. The elderly patient, given a decreased cardiac output, poor myocardial compliance, and atherosclerosis, is more sensitive to the effects of a myocardial contusion. Despite its limitations, the ECG is the most sensitive screening tool to predict short-term cardiac complications. An abnormal ECG (whose changes are not known to be old) should prompt admission and cardiac monitoring. A

2-D echocardiogram may be helpful in such patients. If the echocardiogram shows evidence of contusion, admit the patient to the ICU.[100] Further studies, including possible radioisotope scanning,[100] can be chosen in conjunction with the admitting service.

Abdomen and Pelvis. Significant abdominal injury occurs in approximately one third of elderly patients with multisystem trauma.[60] The abdominal examination is often unreliable,[27,57,60] and serious injury can occur with seemingly minor trauma.[101] Therefore, the ED evaluation should include liberal use of diagnostic studies. The elderly do not tolerate laparotomy as well as the young, but hypotension is the greater stressor, and is highly predictive of mortality.[3,94,102] The choices of diagnostic peritoneal lavage (DPL), ultrasound (US), and abdominal CT scanning are the same as with younger patients, but with some caveats. DPL should be used with caution in those with a history of previous abdominal surgeries. CT scans are contraindicated in the hypotensive patient. Such patients must be first stabilized or undergo DPL or US in the resuscitation suite if they do not meet criteria for immediate laparotomy. Ensure adequate intravenous hydration if contrast agents are used to lessen the risk of renal failure.

Pelvic fractures are common in the elderly and cause significant mortality.[103,104] Several classification systems exist, and the risk of mortality is increased for certain fracture types.[25,103,105] In the setting of a pelvic fracture and hypoperfusion, mortality rate can approach 50%, and may reach 90% if the fracture is open.[103] Massive transfusion of blood and blood products are also often required, and complications such as ARDS and coagulopathies are frequent.

A recent study showed a positive yield of 64% in unstable trauma patients who underwent pelvic angiography and a 100% success rate of embolization.[106] However, 50% of patients died of multisystem organ failure (MSOF) or coexisting head injury despite successful embolization. The average age of nonsurvivors was 63 compared with 38 for survivors.

Extremity Trauma. Common fractures include hip, Colles' and Smith's fractures in the wrist, and proximal humeral fractures. The cumulative lifetime incidence of hip fracture in the United States in people reaching the age of 90 is approximately 32% for females and 17% for males.[19] Fractures of the wrist usually occur in the setting of a fall on the outstretched hands.

Although physical examination may often be adequate to rule out a fracture in the younger adult population, it will often underestimate significant injury in the elderly.[59] Although patients with hip fractures usually present with pain over the hip or inability to walk, some elderly patients are able to bear weight on a fractured hip. Liberal use of radiographs is necessary to assess for bony injury and immobilization should be considered for all but the mildest of injuries. On occasion, CT scans or MRI may be necessary, particularly in the elderly trauma patient with significant hip pain with ambulation but normal plain films.

In the case of serious isolated extremity injury or extremity injury in the setting of multisystem trauma, immediate reduction and splinting is essential with frequent evaluation of neurovascular status to check for either direct injury or ischemia secondary to increased compartmental pressures.

In general, the elderly do well after isolated extremity injury.[107] Depending on the injury, treatments include immobilization, closed reduction and casting, or open reduction and internal fixation. Co-morbid conditions have been shown to increase complication rates as does prolonged bed rest.[107,108] Early ambulation, if possible, is critical in the postoperative period to prevent early complications associated with immobilization (e.g., atelectasis, pneumonia, DVT).

DISPOSITION

There is very little research on geriatric patients with seemingly mild trauma regarding potential complications and morbidity.[109] Any injury to an elderly patient that was caused by a syncopal event requires admission for cardiac monitoring. An injury either proven to be or suspected of being caused by abuse justifies admission, if the safety of the patient cannot be ensured. Admission would also be required in an elderly patient without a support system at home. In some systems with excellent home health care, a visiting nurse or aide could substitute for hospitalization. Many authors advocate admission for elderly patients with chest wall injury (e.g., isolated 1 to 2 rib fractures) to ensure adequate pulmonary toilet and lessen the risk of atelectasis and pneumonia immediately following injury.[67,76]

With intensive care and invasive monitoring, elderly trauma patients who survive fare comparably well to their younger counterparts.[110-112] But when does an elderly patient require intensive care? It has been theorized that elderly trauma patients who die suddenly in the hospital often might have been developing subclinical MSOF before cardiovascular collapse and that intensive care with invasive monitoring would allow earlier detection and intervention.[72] However, in the age of cost containment it would be prohibitive to admit all elderly trauma patients to the ICU. In Scalea et al's study,[72] 29% of the population was found to have "no significant injury." Further research regarding specific types of trauma, pretrauma health, in-hospital care[113] and complications may further define those elderly who would benefit from intensive care for seemingly non–life-threatening injuries.

The decision to transfer an elderly trauma patient to a level I trauma center can be difficult. Scoring systems, although predictive of outcome, help little in the initial resuscitation phase.[114-117] The American College of Surgeons has suggested that elderly patients, in general, be considered for transfer to a trauma center.[118] This recommendation has been supported in the literature in studies that have shown that the elderly population are frequently under-triaged, resulting in preventable complications and delays in definitive care.[66,115,119] Certain triage guidelines based on the trauma score and type and severity of injury are well known but fail to take age into account.[114] The Geriatric Trauma Score (GTS) was developed to adjust outcome based on age and cardiac health, but requires infectious complications as the third variable.[95] Obviously, this score can only be calculated on a retrospective basis. Other scoring systems using age as a factor have failed to gain wide acceptance.[120] Elderly patients can have high mortality despite favorable triage scoring and can have severe injury with minimal mechanism or physical findings. For these reasons prudence dictates early involvement with both the hospital surgeon and level I referral center as needed.

CONCLUSION

The elderly have higher mortality rates, incidence of complications, and length of hospital stay for any given injury compared with the younger trauma population. Geriatric trauma is a growing national concern and will become more common as the U.S. population ages. Using current trends, it has been estimated that the elderly will comprise 40% of all trauma victims by the year 2050.[121] Detailed knowledge of the differences between the young and old will only become more important with the passage of time. With the high likelihood of coexisting disease conditions and decreased physiologic reserve, geriatric trauma victims require liberal use of diagnostic studies, possible invasive monitoring, and frequent admission.

Vigilance is required for all healthcare professionals involved in the geriatric trauma victim's care. Triage scoring systems are often inadequate and can grossly underestimate severity of injury. With proper management and careful attention to the pathophysiology of aging, a high percentage of surviving geriatric trauma victims can lead productive and fulfilling lives.

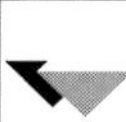

PEARLS & PITFALLS

- Premorbid status is more important than chronologic age.
- Consider early transfer to trauma center.
- Consider why the accident occurred. Syncope may be responsible for almost 20% of MVCs in the elderly. Vital signs and urine output are often unreliable to detect shock.
- Physical examination may underestimate injury. Hemoperitoneum and chest pathology are often overlooked.
- Use lactate to aid decision-making.
- Use invasive monitoring for high-risk patients.
- Be liberal in admission criteria.
- Admit to adequate level of care—trauma center referral, admission to ICU.

REFERENCES

1. Covington DL, Maxwell JG, Clancy TV: Hospital resources used to treat the injured elderly at North Carolina trauma centers, *J Am Geriatr Soc* 41:847-852, 1993.
2. DeMaria EJ: Evaluation and treatment of the elderly trauma victim, *Clin Geriatric Med* 9:461-471, 1993.
3. Oreskovich MR, et al: Geriatric trauma: injury patterns and outcome, *J Trauma* 24:565-572, 1984.
4. van Aalst JA, et al: Severely injured geriatric patients return to independent living: a study of factors influencing function and independence, *J Trauma* 31:1096-1102, 1991.
5. DeMaria EJ, et al: Aggressive trauma care benefits the elderly, *J Trauma* 27:1200-1205, 1987.
6. Accident Facts. National Safety Council. Chicago, 1993.
7. Fife D: Injuries and deaths among elderly persons, *Am J Epidemiol* 126:936-941, 1987.
8. Champion HR, et al: Major trauma in geriatric patients, *Am J Public Health* 79:1278-1282, 1989.
9. Finelli FC, et al: A case control study for major trauma in geriatric patients, *J Trauma* 29:541-548, 1989.
10. DeMaria EJ, et al: Do DRG payments adequately reimburse the costs of trauma care in geriatric patients? *J Trauma* 28:1244-1249.
11. MacKenzie EJ, Morris JA Jr, Edelstein SL: Effect of pre-existing disease on length of hospital stay in trauma patients, *J Trauma* 29:757-765, 1989.
12. Johnson CL, et al: Trauma in the elderly: an analysis of outcomes based on age, *Am Surg* 60:899-902, 1994.
13. Lambert DA, Sattin RW: Deaths from falls, 1978-1984, *MMWR* 37:SS-1, 21-26, 1988.
14. Hogue CC: Injury late in life: Part I. Epidemiology, *J Am Geriatr Soc* 30:183-190, 1982.
15. Baraff LJ, et al: Practice guideline for the ED management of falls in community-dwelling elderly persons, *Ann Emerg Med* 30:480-492, 1997.
16. Tinetti ME: Factors associated with serious injury during falls by ambulatory nursing home residents, *J Am Geriatr Soc* 35:644-648, 1987.

17. Tinetti ME, Williams TF, Mayewski R: Fall risk index for elderly patients based upon number of chronic disabilities, *Am J Med* 80:429-434, 1986.
18. Alexander BH, Rivara FP, Wolf ME: The cost and frequency of hospitalization for fall related injuries in older adults, *Am J Public Health* 82:1020-1023, 1992.
19. Sattin RW, et al: The incidence of fall injury events among the elderly in a defined population, *Am J Epidemiol* 131:1028-1037, 1990.
20. Mosenthal AC, et al: Falls: epidemiology and strategies for prevention, *J Trauma* 38:753-756, 1995.
21. Goldschmidt MJ, et al: Craniomaxillofacial trauma in the elderly, *J Oral Maxillofac Surg* 53:1145-1149, 1995.
22. Smith DL, et al: Effect of inhalation injury, burn size, and age on mortality: a study of 1447 consecutive burn patients, *J Trauma* 37:655-659, 1994.
23. Nickens H: Intrinsic factors in falling among the elderly, *Arch Intern Med* 145:1089-1093, 1985.
24. Tinetti ME, Speechley M, Ginter SF: Risk factors for falls among elderly persons living in the community, *N Engl J Med* 319:1701-1707, 1988.
25. Tinetti ME, Speechley M: Prevention of falls among the elderly, *N Engl J Med* 320:1055-1059, 1989.
26. Riggs JE: Mortality from accidental falls among the elderly in the United States, 1962-1988: demonstrating the impact of improved trauma management, *J Trauma* 35:212-219, 1993.
27. Schwab CW, Kauder DR: Trauma in the geriatric patient, *Arch Surg* 127:701-706, 1992.
28. Rehm CG, Ross SE: Elderly drivers involved in road crashes: a profile, *Am Surg* 61:435-437, 1995.
29. Santora TA, Schinco MA, Trooskin SZ: Management of trauma in the elderly patient, *Surg Clin North Am* 74:163-186, 1994.
30. Carr DB: Assessing older drivers for physical and cognitive impairment, *Geriatrics* 48:46-51, 1993.
31. Martin RE, Teberian G: Multiple trauma and the elderly patient, *Emerg Med Clin North Am* 8:411-420, 1990.
32. McCoy GF, Johnstone RA, Duthie RB: Injury to the elderly in road traffic accidents, *J Trauma* 29:494-497, 1989.
33. Kong LB, et al: Pedestrian-motor vehicle trauma: an analysis of injury profiles based by age, *J Am Coll Surg* 182:17-23, 1996.
34. Sklar DP, Demarest GB, McFeeley P: Increased pedestrian mortality among the elderly, *Am J Emerg Med* 7:387-390, 1989.
35. Lachs MS, et al: ED use by older victims of family violence, *Ann Emerg Med* 30:448-454, 1997.
36. Pillemer K, Finkelhor D: The prevalence of elder abuse: a random sample survey, *Gerontologist* 28:51-57, 1988.
37. Bradley M: Elder abuse, *BMJ* 313:548-550, 1996.
38. Jones JS, et al: Elder mistreatment: national survey of emergency physicians, *Ann Emerg Med* 30:473-479, 1997.
39. Jones J, et al: Emergency department protocol for the diagnosis and evaluation of geriatric abuse, *Ann Emerg Med* 17:1006-1015, 1988.
40. Kleinschmidt KC: Elder abuse: a review, *Ann Emerg Med* 30:463-472, 1997.
41. Desai MH: Care of geriatric patients. In Herndon DN (editor): *Total burn care,* Philadelphia, 1996, Saunders.
42. Manktelow A, et al: Analysis of life expectancy and living status of elderly patients surviving a burn injury, *J Trauma* 29:203-207, 1989.
43. Ostrow LB, et al: Burns in the elderly, *Am Fam Phys* 35:149-154, 1987.
44. Anous MM, Heimbach DM: Causes of death and predictors in burned patients more than 60 years of age, *J Trauma* 26:135-139, 1986.
45. Burdge JJ, et al: Surgical treatment of burns in elderly patients, *J Trauma* 28:214-217, 1988.
46. Kara M, et al: An early surgical approach to burns in the elderly, *J Trauma* 30:430-432, 1990.
47. Weksler ME: Senescence of the immune system, *Med Clin North Am* 67:263-272, 1983.
48. Schwartz LR: Thermal burns. In Tintinalli JE, Ruiz E, Krome RL (editors): *Emergency medicine: a comprehensive review,* ed 4, New York, 1996, McGraw-Hill.
49. Boss GR, Seegmiller JE: Age-related physiological changes and their clinical significance, *West J Med* 135:434-440, 1981.
50. White NK, Edwards JE, Dry TJ: The relationship of the degree of coronary atherosclerosis with age, in men, *Circulation* 1:645-654, 1950.
51. Rodstein M, Camus AS: Interrelation of heart disease and accidents, *Geriatrics* 28:87-96, 1973.
52. Lakatta EG: Age-related alterations in the cardiovascular response to adrenergic mediated stress, *Fed Proc* 39:3173-3177, 1980.
53. MacSweeney ST, Powell JT, Greenhalgh RM: Pathogenesis of abdominal aortic aneurysm, *Br J Surg* 81:935-941, 1994.
54. Levitzky MG: Alveolar ventilation. In *Pulmonary physiology,* ed 2, New York, 1986, McGraw-Hill.
55. Braun SR: Chronic obstructive pulmonary disease. In Braun SR (editor): *Concise textbook of pulmonary medicine,* New York, 1989, Elsevier Science Publishing.
56. Papper S: The effects of age in reducing renal function, *Geriatrics* 28:83-87, 1973.
57. Lonner JH, Koval KJ: Polytrauma in the elderly, *Clin Orthop Rel Res* 318:136-143, 1995.
58. Linn BS, Jensen J: Age and immune response to a surgical stress, *Arch Surg* 118:405-409, 1983.
59. Demarest GB, Osler TM, Clevenger FW: Injuries in the elderly: evaluation and initial response, *Geriatrics* 45:36-42, 1990.
60. Levy DB, Hanlon DP, Townsend RN: Geriatric trauma, *Clin Geriatr Med* 9:601-620, 1993.
61. Miller MD: Orthopedic trauma in the elderly, *Emerg Med Clin North Am* 8:325-339, 1990.
62. Desai D, March R, Watters JM: Hyperglycemia after trauma increases with age, *J Trauma* 29:719-723, 1989.
63. Robinson A: Age, physical trauma and care, *Canad Med Assoc* J 152:1453-1455, 1995.
64. Cuthbertson DP: Post-shock metabolic response, *Lancet* 1:433-437, 1942.
65. Jeevanandam M, Petersen SR, Shamos RF: Protein and glucose fuel kinetics and hormonal changes in elderly trauma patients, *Metab Clin Exper* 42:1255-1262, 1993.
66. Zimmer-Gembeck MJ, et al: Triage in an established trauma system, *J Trauma* 39:922-928, 1995.
67. Pellicane JV, Byrne K, DeMaria EJ: Preventable complications and death from multiple organ failure among geriatric trauma victims, *J Trauma* 33:440-444, 1992.
68. Zietlow SP, et al: Multisystem geriatric trauma, *J Trauma* 37:985-988, 1994.
69. Davis JW, Kaups KL: Base deficit in the elderly: a marker of severe injury and death, *J Trauma* 45:873-877, 1998.
70. Abramson D, et al: Lactate clearance and survival following injury, *J Trauma* 35:584-588, 1993.
71. Milzman DP, Rothenhaus TC: Resuscitation of the geriatric patient, *Emerg Med Clin North Am* 14:233-244, 1996.
72. Scalea TM, et al: Geriatric blunt multiple trauma: improved survival with early invasive monitoring, *J Trauma* 30:129-136, 1990.
73. Del Guercio LR, Cohn JD: Monitoring operative risk in the elderly, *JAMA* 243:1350-1355, 1980.
74. McNinch M. Age as a risk factor for inadequate emergency department analgesia, *Am J Emerg Med* 14(2):157-160, 1996.

75. Wilson JE, Pendleton JM: Oligoanalgesia in the emergency department, *Am J Emerg Med* 7(6):620-23, 1989.
76. Gennarelli TA, Thibault LE: Biomechanics of acute subdural hematoma, *J Trauma* 22:680-686, 1982.
77. Amacher AL, Bybee DE: Toleration of head injury in the elderly, *Neurosurgery* 20:954-958, 1987.
78. Ellis GL: Subdural hematoma in the elderly, *Emerg Med Clin North Am* 8:281-294, 1990.
79. Seelig JM, et al: Traumatic acute subdural hematoma: major mortality reduction in comatose patients treated within four hours, *N Engl J Med* 304:1511-1518, 1981.
80. Wilberger JE Jr, Harris M, Diamond DL: Acute subdural hematoma: morbidity and mortality related to timing of operative intervention, *J Trauma* 30:733-736, 1990.
81. Chan L, Snyder HS, Verdile VP: Cervical fracture as the initial presentation of multiple myeloma, *Ann Emerg Med* 24:1192-1194, 1994.
82. Mower WR, et al: Selective cervical spine radiography of blunt trauma victims: Results of the National Emergency X-radiography Utilization Study (NEXUS), *Academ Emerg Med* 6:451, 1999.
83. Bresler MJ, Rich GH: Occult cervical spine fracture in an ambulatory patient, *Ann Emerg Med* 11:440-442, 1982.
84. Haines JD Jr: Occult cervical spine fractures: illustrative cases and x-ray guidelines, *Postgrad Med* 80:73-77, 1986.
85. Lieberman IH, Webb JK: Cervical spine injuries in the elderly, *J Bone Joint Surg* Br 76:877-881, 1994.
86. Mace SE: Unstable occult cervical-spine fracture, *Ann Emerg Med* 20:1373-1375, 1991.
87. McKee TR, Tinkoff G, Rhodes M: Asymptomatic occult cervical spine fracture: case report and review of the literature, *J Trauma* 30:623-626, 1990.
88. Ogden W, Dunn JD: Cervical radiographic evaluation following blunt trauma, *Ann Emerg Med* 15:604-605, 1986.
89. Horst HM, et al: Factors influencing survival of elderly trauma patients, *Crit Care Med* 14:681-684, 1986.
90. Peterson RJ, et al: Pediatric and adult thoracic trauma: age-related impact on presentation and outcome, *Ann Thorac Surg* 58:14-18, 1994.
91. Shorr RM, et al: Blunt chest trauma in the elderly, *J Trauma* 29:234-237, 1989.
92. Allen JE, Schwab CW: Blunt chest trauma in the elderly, *Am Surg* 51:697-700, 1985.
93. Martinez R, Sharieff G, Hooper J: Three-point restraints as a risk factor for chest injury in the elderly, *J Trauma* 37:980-984, 1994.
94. Osler T, et al: Trauma in the elderly, *Am J Surg* 156:537-543, 1988.
95. DeMaria EJ, et al: Survival after trauma in geriatric patients, *Ann Surg* 206:738-743, 1987.
96. van der Sluis CK, et al: Major trauma in young and old: what is the difference? *J Trauma* 40:78-82, 1996.
97. Ahmed Z, Mohyuddin Z: Management of flail chest injury: internal fixation versus endotracheal intubation and ventilation, *J Thorac Cardiovasc Surg* 110:1676-1680, 1995.
98. Perchinsky MJ, et al: 'The broken halo sign': a fractured calcified ring as an unusual sign of traumatic rupture of the thoracic aorta, *Injury* 25:649-652, 1994.
99. Camp PC Jr, et al: Blunt traumatic thoracic aortic lacerations in the elderly: an analysis of outcome, *J Trauma* 37:418-423, 1994.
100. Rosenthal MA, Ellis JI: Cardiac and mediastinal trauma, *Emerg Clin North Am* 13:887-902, 1995.
101. Cross JJ, et al: Ureteric rupture in an elderly patient following minor trauma: case report, *J Trauma* 36:594-596, 1994.
102. Knudson MM, et al: Mortality factors in geriatric blunt trauma patients, *Arch Surg* 129:448-453, 1994.
103. Naam NH, et al: Major pelvic fractures, *Arch Surg* 118:610-616, 1983.
104. Trunkey DD, et al: Management of pelvic fractures in blunt trauma injury, *J Trauma* 14:912-923, 1974.
105. Eastridge BJ, Burgess AR: Pedestrian pelvic fractures: 5-year experience of a major urban trauma center, *J Trauma* 42:695-700, 1997.
106. Agolini SF, et al: Arterial embolization is a rapid and effective technique for controlling pelvic fracture hemorrhage, *J Trauma* 43:395-399, 1997.
107. Pereles TR, et al: Open reduction and internal fixation of the distal humerus: functional outcome in the elderly, *J Trauma* 43:578-584, 1997.
108. Sartoretti C, et al: Comorbid conditions in old patients with femur fractures, *J Trauma* 43:570-577, 1997.
109. Ferrera PC, Bartfield JM, D'Andrea CC: Geriatric trauma: outcomes of elderly patients discharged from the ED, *Am J Emerg Med* 17:629-632,1999.
110. Carrillo EH, et al: Long term outcome of blunt trauma care in the elderly, *Surg Gynecol Obstet* 176:559-564, 1993.
111. Day RJ, Vinen J, Hewitt-Falls E: Major trauma outcomes in the elderly, *Med J Aust* 160:675-678, 1994.
112. Shabot MM, Johnson CL: Outcome from critical care in the "oldest old" trauma patients, *J Trauma* 39:254-260, 1995.
113. Taheri PA, et al: Physician resource utilization after geriatric trauma, *J Trauma* 43:565-569, 1997.
114. Baker SP, et al: The injury severity score: a method for describing patients with multiple injuries and evaluating emergency care, *J Trauma* 14:187-196, 1974.
115. Cottington EM, et al: The utility of physiological status, injury site, and injury mechanism in identifying patients with major trauma, *J Trauma* 28:305-311, 1988.
116. Knaus WA, et al: APACHE II: a severity of disease classification system, *Crit Care Med* 13:818-829, 1985.
117. Le Gall JR, et al: A simplified acute physiology score for ICU patients, *Crit Care Med* 12:975-977, 1984.
118. American College of Surgeons Committee on Trauma: *Advanced trauma life support,* ed 5, Chicago, 1993, Academic Press.
119. Hedges JR, Osterud HR, Mullins RJ: Adult minor trauma patients: good outcome in small hospitals, *Ann Emerg Med* 21: 402-406, 1992.
120. Boyd CR, Tolson MA, Copes WS: Evaluating trauma care: the TRISS method, *J Trauma* 27:370-378, 1987.
121. MacKenzie EJ, et al: Acute hospital costs of trauma in the United States: implications for regionalized systems of care, *J Trauma* 30:1096-1103, 1990.

PART FOUR

MECHANISMS OF INJURIES

35 The Management of Burns

THOMAS J. RUSSELL

Teaching Case

A 35-year-old electrician presents to the emergency department (ED) with severe burns to the arm, chest, neck, back, and feet. He touched a high-voltage wire, which then set the room on fire. He is awake but confused with second-degree burns to his entire chest, partial back, and partial neck. He had a combination of second- and third-degree burns encircling the right arm. He also has third-degree burns to the right palm and both feet.

He was intubated after discovery of singed nasal hairs, carbonaceous sputum, and a carboxyhemoglobin level of 30%. The emergency physician (EP) began fluid resuscitation for the 30% second and third degree burns, and administered opiate analgesics. The patient's urine appeared dark and oily, and he was alkalinized for treatment of myoglobinuria and for rhabdomyolysis. Before transport to the regional burn center, he lost Doppler signals in his right wrist, and an EP performed an escharotomy, which restored vascular flow. ■

Despite being mostly preventable, burns cause significant injury, disability, and mortality. Nearly 500,000 Americans visited EDs in 1991 for burns.[1] However, the vast majority of burn patients sustain minor injuries and can be treated in the ED and discharged home.[2,3]

Burns frequently affect children and young adults, and the personal toll is often devastating. Even minor burns can cause significant long-term disability if they affect crucial areas of the body such as the hands, face, or feet. The financial cost of burn care is also significant. It includes both direct treatment costs, as well as loss of productivity.

As with most types of traumatic injury, recovery in burn patients is dependent on many factors. The type of burn, initial care, host factors, patient motivation, and eventual rehabilitation all contribute to outcome.

EPIDEMIOLOGY

There are between 1.25 and 2 million burns per year in the United States.[1] Improved prevention (especially smoke detectors) and medical progress have decreased burn deaths and hospitalization by 50% over the twenty-year period of 1971-1991.[1] Still, approximately 6000 people die from burns each year.[1,4]

The elderly are particularly likely to die of burns. Geriatric burn mortality may be calculated by the Baux formula—age plus percent body surface area (BSA) burned equals mortality.[5] This formula is less accurate at extremes of age and a significant number of patients survive despite Baux scores greater than 100.[6,7,8] However, when more than 70% of the body surface area is burned, or if the Baux score is greater than 130, nearly all elderly patients die.

Burns are also a common cause of death in childhood, and younger children (under age 4) are affected disproportionately.[9] Scald burns are particularly common. Children are burned by accident and as the result of abuse.[10]

Although drug and alcohol intoxication is rarely reported with minor burn wounds,[11] it occurs in 6.9% to 50% of burns that require hospitalization.[12,13] Nearly one half of major burns occur at home, whereas almost two thirds of minor burns occur outside of the home.[11,14] Non-Caucasian ethnic groups have a 76% higher incidence of major burns.[14]

PATHOPHYSIOLOGY

The skin is the largest organ in the human body and accounts for 15% of its weight.[15] The skin protects from infection, regulates heat, and acts as a vapor barrier. The skin contains three layers: epidermis, dermis, and subcutaneous tissue. The epidermis is the outermost layer and is made of stratified epithelial cells that protect against infection and toxins while conserving moisture. It has the regenerative capability to cover wounds. The dermis is the middle layer made up of an outer papillary dermis and an inner reticular dermis. The thickness of the dermal layer is 1 to 4 mm depending on body location, with the thickest areas being the back and thigh and the thinnest being on the genitals and eyelids. The dermal layer is thinner in the very old and the very young. This layer connects the three layers of the skin, and provides stability and nutrients to the epidermis. Skin appendages (i.e., nerves, sweat glands, hair follicles, sebaceous glands, and blood vessels) are contained within the dermis. Because skin appendages are lined with epithelium, burns that extend to the dermis may still regenerate. The final subcutaneous layer is composed of adipose and connective tissue. This layer does not possess any regenerative capability if the above layers are destroyed.

Burn wounds are classified into three zones.[16] Each zone is three-dimensional and may extend deep into the tissues.

1. *Zone of Coagulation:* irreversible cell death; blood flow is absent.
2. *Zone of Stasis:* surrounds the zone of coagulation; blood flow is impaired. This ischemia can easily progress to cell death if the wound sustains additional insults such as crush, infection, or desiccation.
3. *Zone of Hyperemia:* surrounds the zone of stasis and is a minimally injured; this area is characterized by an inflammatory response.

Thermodynamics of Burn Injury

There are many types of burns, including scald, thermal, chemical, and electrical. Burn severity depends on energy transfer to the skin. Heat transfer is a function of multiple factors including the temperature of the substance, its heat capacity, the duration of contact with the skin, and efficiency in transferring heat.

Scald burns account for up to 30% of burn injuries, and this proportion is larger in the pediatric population.[15] Scald burns can result from immersion into or splashes from water, grease, or oil. Water at temperatures of 44° C (110° F) will not injure the skin until hours of contact. However, water at 51° C (123° F) can cause burns in seconds. Water ≥70° C (160° F) can cause instantaneous full thickness burns.[17] Immersion burns typically produce deeper injury, since the contact time is greater than with splash exposures.

Superheated steam may result in injury similar to that of a scald burn. These injuries are likely to cause airway problems if the head and neck are involved.

Thermal burns include flame, flash, and contact burns. Flames account for up to 50% of burn injuries[15] and frequently involve structure fires or some type of combustible material, such as gasoline. Although flames are high temperature and transfer significant heat, the duration of contact varies widely. Flash burns are the third most common type of burn and result from proximity to an explosion. These burns are of high temperature but brief duration. Because air conducts heat so poorly, patients exposed to flash burns usually injure unprotected skin only. However, if the flash ignites clothing, more serious burns may occur. On occasion, flash burns may compromise the airway.

Contact burns result when the skin touches hot objects such as metals, plastic, or glass and account for less than 5% of burns.[15] Often these wounds are deep although small in overall size. The duration of the contact, heat capacity of the substance, and the heat transfer capability determine severity of injury.

Chemical burns account for 3% of burn injuries.[15] They occur when a strong acid or alkali contacts the skin. In contrast to other contact burns, chemicals progressively damage the skin until inactivated or removed. High chemical viscosities may result in prolonged duration of contact. The chemical agent causes an exothermic reaction. Although the temperature of this reaction is low, there is significant heat transfer to the skin.

Acid burns are relatively self-limited. They cause a coagulation necrosis, which generally limits deep-tissue injury. Alkaline burns cause a liquefaction necrosis, which results in deep-tissue damage. Hydrofluoric acid violates the rule of superficial acid burns and can cause significant deep-tissue damage. Therapeutic interventions attempt to mitigate the depth of injury by neutralizing the acid with magnesium or calcium compounds.

Electrical burns account for 10% of burn injuries.[15] The resistance of body tissues to the flow of electrical current generates heat. Temperature is directly related to amperage and duration of contact, and the tissue susceptibility to electrical current is an important aspect of electrical injury.

The extent of damage caused by electrical injury is often under-appreciated. Although the patient may only have a tiny entry or exit wound, internal damage may be profound.

EMERGENCY DEPARTMENT EVALUATION

History

An accurate history improves care of the burn victim. Determine if the fire was in enclosed space and ascertain the nature of burning substances. Smoke inhalation is a major cause of mortality. Industrial fires may expose the patient to particularly toxic fumes. Ask about pulmonary symptoms, cough, and shortness of breath.

Interview medics and available witnesses. Determine loss of consciousness, prehospital vital signs, and the patient's response to prehospital interventions. In the case of burned children, determine if the caretaker's story is plausible.

The type of burn (thermal/scald/chemical/electricity) predicts injury patterns and complications. For example, electrical burns are associated with myoglobinuria, whereas immersion burns are generally deep-tissue injuries. The history may suggest further injuries besides the obvious burns, especially when a fall, explosion, or vehicular crash is involved.

Past medical history also influences prognosis. Renal, cardiac, and immunosuppressive diseases complicate healing. Determine the patient's tetanus status and identify any allergies. A sulfa allergy precludes the use of Silvadene in burn treatment. The patient's current medications may play a significant role in the physiologic response to burns, especially beta-blockers and antihypertensives. Patients who either use illicit opiates or are on methadone maintenance therapy may require titanic doses of narcotics to control pain.

Physical Examination

Unlike many forms of trauma, burns are truly quantifiable and are best described in terms of depth and in extent of body surface area (BSA) involved. A burn is a dynamic process. A wound that initially appears to be only moderately severe may evolve into a serious injury over the next 24 to 48 hours.

DEPTH OF BURNS

Burn severity increases with burn depth. Progressively deeper burns are classified as first, second, third, and fourth degree (see Tables 35-1 and 35-2).

First-degree burns are superficial and involve the epidermis. Local pain and erythema *without blister formation* characterize this type of burn. Sunburn represents a prototypical first-degree burn. Systemic response is mild or absent in most cases. These wounds heal spontaneously without complication, although the injured epithelium may desquamate several days later.

Second-degree burns are divided into superficial partial thickness, and deep partial thickness. **Superficial partial thickness** burns involve the entire epidermis and the superficial dermis. The wounds are warm and moist, and blisters may be present on arrival to the ED or may develop hours later. Because patients retain sensation, the burn is quite painful. Flash burns, brief contact burns, and scalds are typical causes.

TABLE 35-1
Depth of Burns Classification

BURN SEVERITY	DEFINITION
First degree	Superficial; involves epidermis; without blister
Second degree	Superficial partial thickness and deep partial thickness Epidermis and superficial dermis; blisters, systemic response
Third degree	Entire epidermis and dermis Waxy, blisters, lesions; hypertrophic scarring; wound contracture; white, cherry, red, black thrombosed capillaries; leathery
Fourth degree	All epidermis, dermis, subcutaneous tissue, underlying muscle, fascia, bone Myoglobinuria/renal failure Reconstructive surgery

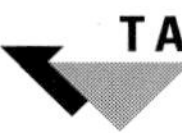

TABLE 35-2
Depth of Burn and Examination Findings

First degree	Local pain and erythema without blister formation
Second degree	*Superficial partial thickness:* painful, warm, moist with blister formation *Deep partial thickness:* molted, waxy-white, with ruptured blisters; pain sensation absent but pressure sensation intact
Third degree	Insensate white, black, or cherry red; pressure sensation and two-point discrimination are lost
Fourth degree	Charred wounds involving muscle, bone, or fascia

Moderate or large second-degree burns may produce a systemic response. Most second-degree burns heal in 14 to 21 days with little or no scarring, although some degree of hypopigmentation is common in darker-skinned individuals. New epidermis forms from the surrounding edges and the intact skin appendages.

Deep partial thickness burns involve the entire epidermis and the dermis, leaving intact deep skin appendages. The wounds appear waxy, and blisters may be flaccid or ruptured. These wounds are occasionally less painful than superficial burns because of damage to nerve endings; however, patients usually

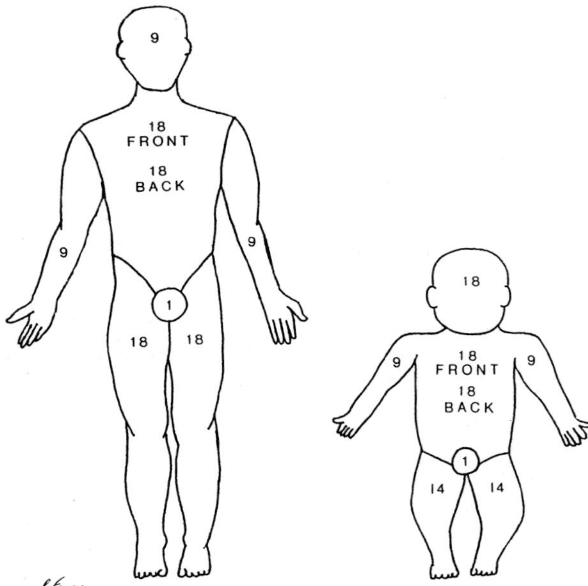

Fig. 35-1 Rule of Nines.

retain pressure sensation. These burns become more painful as the wound heals. Initially, these lesions may be difficult to distinguish from third-degree burns. Intact sensation, to any degree distinguishes these burns from third-degree injuries. However, further trauma or infection can cause these burns to progress in severity. Scalds, brief flame contact, or longer direct contacts are frequent etiologies. Deep partial thickness burns heal in 4 to 6 weeks, as new epidermis develops from intact skin appendages. Hypertrophic scarring and wound contracture may complicate healing and may require skin grafting.

Third-degree burns destroy the epidermis and dermis, as well as injure the subcutaneous tissue. The wounds are insensate; however, surrounding tissues may be extremely painful. These burns appear white, cherry, red, or black. Thrombosed capillaries are frequently seen histologically and deep blisters may be present. Patients lose sensation to pressure and pin prick, and the skin feels leathery secondary to destruction of tissue elasticity in the dermis and subcutaneous layers. Third-degree burns are often caused by high-intensity flash exposure, flames, chemicals, electrical injury, or prolonged contact with hot surfaces. Healing is slow and new epidermis grows only from peripheral epithelial migration. Wound contracture and scarring are common, and skin grafting is often necessary.

Fourth-degree burns not only destroy the epidermis, dermis, and subcutaneous tissue, but underlying muscle, fascia, or bone as well. The skin is charred and the wound depth is difficult to assess in the ED. Molten metal, electrical injury, or prolonged contact with flames often results in fourth-degree burns. Because of the damage to the muscle, there is great potential for myoglobinuria and subsequent renal failure. Extensive reconstructive surgery is generally required.

EXTENT OF BURNS

Estimation of burn size is crucial to management. Burn size is usually measured in terms of percent of total body surface area (BSA) burned. *Only second-degree, third-degree, and fourth-degree burns are counted.* First-degree burns are not considered when estimating burn size.

The "**rule of nines**" is a valuable technique to estimate burn size (Fig. 35-1). Although it often leads to overestimation of burn size, it remains an effective tool. The rule of nines must be adapted to the pediatric patient to account for the proportionately larger head and smaller lower extremities of children. When evaluating smaller burns, the area of an individual's palm (not counting the fingers) approximates 1% of his or her body surface area. The Lund and Browder chart allows for a more accurate estimation of total BSA for both children and adults.[18] These charts divide the body into smaller zones to facilitate calculation of burn size.

BURN SEVERITY CLASSIFICATION

Burns may be classified into minor, moderate, or severe based on the total BSA affected and the depth of the burns (Table 35-3 and Box 35-1). First-degree burns are not included in determination of burn severity.

Minor burns include second-degree burns of less than 15% BSA in adults or 10% BSA in children or the elderly, and less than 2% full-thickness burns. Addi-

TABLE 35-3
Burn Severity Classification

Minor	Second-degree burns of less than 15% body surface area (BSA) in adults or 10% BSA in children or the elderly; less than 2% full-thickness burns
Moderate	Second-degree burns of 15%-25% BSA in adults or 10%-20% BSA in children or the elderly; less than 10% BSA full-thickness burns
Major severe	Second-degree burns of greater than 25% BSA in adults or greater than 20% BSA in children or the elderly; full-thickness burns greater than 10% BSA

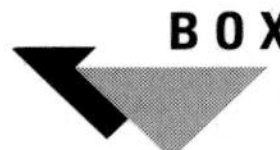

BOX 35-1
Classification of Burn Severity[3]

MAJOR BURNS

1. Partial-thickness burns >25% BSA in adults or >20% BSA in children or the elderly.
2. Full-thickness burns >10% BSA.
3. All burns involving the face, eyes, ears, hands, feet, or perineum that may result in functional or cosmetic impairment.
4. Burns caused by caustic chemical agents.
5. High-voltage electrical injury.
6. Burns complicated by inhalation injury, major trauma, or poor-risk patients.

MODERATE BURNS

1. Partial-thickness burns 15% to 25% BSA in adults and 10% to 20% BSA in children or the elderly.
2. Less than 10% BSA full-thickness burns.
3. Not involving risk to areas of specialized function such as the face, eyes, ears, hands, feet, or perineum.

MINOR BURNS

1. Burns <15% BSA in adults or 10% BSA in children or the elderly.
2. Less than 2% full-thickness burns.
3. No functional or cosmetic risk to areas of specialized function.

Adapted from the American Burn Association Injury Severity Grading System.

tionally, there can be no significant burns to functional or cosmetically at-risk areas involved such as the face, genitals, or hands.

Moderate burns are second-degree burns of 15% to 25% BSA in adults or 10% to 20% BSA in children or the elderly, and less than 10% BSA full-thickness burns. Moderate burns may include minor but not major injury to cosmetically at-risk areas or specialized function areas such as the hands, feet, eyes, head, neck, or perineum.

Major burns are second-degree burns of greater than 25% BSA in adults or greater than 20% BSA in children or the elderly and any full-thickness burns greater than 10% BSA. Severe chemical burns, high-voltage burns, as well as burns complicated by inhalation injury are considered major burns. Patients with concomitant major trauma or those with significant underlying disease are also at risk for significant morbidity and mortality. Any burns of the face, eyes, ears, hands, feet, or perineum that are likely to result in functional or cosmetic impairment are included in this category.

EMERGENCY MANAGEMENT

Prehospital Treatment

Prehospital personnel must rapidly remove the patient from the burn environment. They should look for signs of inhalation injury such as dyspnea, singed nasal or facial hair, periorbital burns, black sputum, or brassy cough. All patients with possible inhalation injury require high-flow oxygen. Those who are in respiratory distress may require intubation in the field.

Medics should remove clothing and jewelry, brush off gross debris, and cover the patient with a sterile or clean sheet. In the case of chemical injury, medics must brush off the dry powder and, assuming the chemical is identified and there is no contraindication, copiously irrigate the patient during transport. Although hot tar burns should be cooled with water, medics should not attempt to remove the tar. Instruct prehospital care providers to apply moist dressings to cool burn surfaces. However, they should use caution and closely monitor the patient if the total BSA of the burn is more than 15%, since cooling of large burns may produce hypothermia.

In patients with significant burns, medics should begin an intravenous (IV) line in an upper extremity. If possible, they should avoid putting the needle through burned skin. Lactated Ringer's and normal saline are the best resuscitative fluids, and hypotensive patients should receive a fluid challenge. Early hypotension may be from the intravascular fluid loss from the burn itself or the result of an injury and bleeding sustained at the time of the burn. Medics may administer opiate analgesia in the prehospital setting if the patient is hemodynamically stable.

Treatment of Minor and Moderate Burns

Emergency physicians are the first and sometimes only physicians to treat many burn injuries. Early wound care has great impact on outcome. Undertreatment of burns may result in a partial thickness burn progressing into a full thickness burn.

COOLING

Since the second century, physicians have used wound cooling to treat burns.[19,20] Prompt wound cooling, usually by moist dressing or immersion in room temperature water, has multiple salutatory effects. It decreases tissue temperature, pain, histamine release, prostaglandins, thromboxane, wound edema, and overall severity of the burn.[20-22] Burns that are not cooled may suffer continued cell death and release of oxygen free radicals. These radicals promote injury to cell membranes, accelerate arachidonic acid release, and increase local ischemia.[23] Although rapid cooling of the burn gives the best response,[21] even a 60-minute delay will inhibit prostaglandins and thromboxane and provide pain relief.[22] The majority of the benefit from cooling is usually accomplished in the prehospital phase of care.

Burn wounds are considered tetanus prone, and EPs should follow standard prophylaxis guidelines (see Chapter 31).

Clean wounds with normal saline or tap water, and some authorities recommend a mild antiseptic soap or detergent. If soaps are used, rinse the wound with sterile saline before applying a dressing. Although some authors have suggested shaving the hair around the burn before cleaning,[2,24] this recommendation is not universally accepted. Unless the burn surgeons ultimately caring for the patient request shaving off hair, this practice should be avoided. Patients often require additional analgesia during wound cleansing.

MANAGEMENT OF BLISTERS

Physicians have debated management of burn blisters for years; "to pop or not to pop, that is the question." It is likely that when a medical debate continues for so long and is so polarized, neither camp is correct.

The proponents of leaving blisters intact argue that these provide comfort and act as a natural biologic dressing, which promotes wound healing. Acutely débriding blisters is painful, and opens the wound to bacterial colonization.

Others argue that burn blister fluid suppresses the body's bactericidal activity,[25-28] since some research suggests that blister fluid impairs leukocyte activity. Those who take the "middle of the road" approach agree that if there are no signs of infection, small blisters with thick epithelial coverings should be left intact.[2,3,24,29] Aspirators recommend removal of the blister fluid to prevent infection,[30] while leaving the epithelial covering intact.[23,31] Epithelial blisters that are loose or over joints may be debrided. Barring no signs of infection, small blisters with thick epithelial coverings may initially be left intact.[2,3,24,25]

An aggressive camp argues for removing all blister fluid and their epithelial covering.[30,33] They believe that burn blister fluid may inhibit wound healing and result in burn progression.[25,30] The ultimate approach to blister management must be done in concert with the expectations of the burn surgeons who will ultimately care for the patient over the course of the wound healing. Intuitively, *primum non nocera* should apply, with minimal initial debridement in the ED, restricted to those blisters that are already ruptured.

Regardless of initial management, whether leaving blisters intact, aspirating them, or removing blisters, there is consensus on follow-up care. The patient should be instructed to return to the ED or see the burn surgeon within 24 to 48 hours for additional evaluation and debridement. The epithelium covering of ruptured or aspirated blisters may need to be removed on follow-up visits. To remove sloughed skin or blisters, the EP may use scissors, forceps, or gentle traction with a gauze pad.

BURN DRESSINGS

The goal of burn dressing is to promote healing by controlling the fluid balance and keeping the surface moist.[34] The dressing should avoid pooling of liquid. Burn dressing may be open or closed, depending on burn extent, location, and the patient's activity level and preference.

Open wound care involves a topical agent but no overlying dressing. Once the burn has been cleaned and débrided, the wound should be covered with a topical agent. The wound is washed with soap and water two to three times a day and the topical agent reapplied. The continuous inspection of the wound and frequent range of motion exercise makes this dressing desirable for head, neck, and hand burns. Because this type of wound care permits environmental contamination, a child or an individual returning to a work environment would benefit from a closed dressing.

A closed dressing may also employ a topical burn agent. Once the burn has been cleaned and débrided, fine mesh gauze is placed over the wound. This gauze may be soaked with saline before application for patient comfort.[24] Over this layer a large layer of absorbent gauze is placed (at least one-half inch thick) to absorb fluids from the wound surface. This dressing can be used without topical therapy for most minor burns (i.e., second degree burns of less than 15%

BSA in adults). If the dressing involves the digits of the hands or feet, then each individual digit must be wrapped, and padding placed between the digits prevents further injury. The entire dressing should be wrapped snugly with gauze wrap. The EP must take care to avoid excess pressure when wrapping the wound, and if possible, avoid placing tape on the skin.

TOPICAL ANTIMICROBIAL THERAPY

Nearly all physicians involved in burn care use topical antimicrobial therapy. Although most minor burns are not at risk for infection,[2] requiring the patient to apply a topical antimicrobial agent daily forces the patient to look at the wound at least once a day. Because topical agents are less effective in the presence of proteinaceous exudate, burn wounds should be washed between applications.

Normal skin harbors few pathogenic bacteria.[3] Although most burns are initially sterile, they become easily soiled. A multitude of pathogens infect burns including normal skin flora. *Pseudomonas* infections may be devastating.

Topical therapy is no substitute for wound cleansing, and initial therapy is prophylactic.[19] Because third-degree burns are prone to infection, topical antimicrobial therapy is nearly always indicated. Deep partial thickness second degree burns also benefit from topical antimicrobial agents. Because epithelial growth arises from deep skin appendages, infection can convert a partial thickness wound to a full-thickness wound. If a wound becomes infected while using a topical agent, the wound must be cultured, and the agent changed.

Several factors affect the choice of a topical agent. Patient compliance, clinical efficacy, ease of use, cost, availability, toxicity, and side effects all play important roles. Certain agents may have a particular advantage in select circumstances.

Silver Sulfadiazine. *Silver sulfadiazine (Silvadene)* is the most commonly used topical antimicrobial. It is a compound of silver nitrate with sodium sulfadiazine commercially available in a "micronized" 1% water-soluble cream. It is painless and well tolerated as a once- or twice-a-day application.

The in vitro antimicrobial spectrum of silver sulfadiazine is appropriately wide and includes *S. aureus*, Enterobacteriaceae spp., *E. coli*, and *Candida albicans*. A comparison of eight topical agents found it to be the most effective.[35] Silver sulfadiazine delays gram-negative colonization of burn wounds by 10 to 14 days.[36]

Systemic absorption is minimal and slow,[37] and toxicity is rare. For this reason, it is used for burns covering large BSAs. Although some organisms may be resistant, resistance is not a significant issue in minor burns. There has been some concern that silver sulfadiazine may retard burn wound healing by a mechanism other than inhibiting epithelial growth.[38] It can combine with the wound exudate to form a pseudomembrane, which can be painful to remove in the first day. However, the membrane can be easily stripped after 72 hours. Because silver sulfadiazine contains a sulfur moiety, it should be avoided in patients with a sulfur allergy. Some believe that silver sulfadiazine should not be applied to sun-exposed skin, since the silver may precipitate and stain the epithelium.

Mafenide Acetate. *Mafenide acetate (Sulfamylon)* is commercially available in a water-miscible cream. A carbonic anhydrase inhibitor, it penetrates even the most deeply burned skin, and has a broad spectrum of antimicrobial activity. It inhibits common gram-negative burn pathogens, including *Pseudomonas aeruginosa,* and gram-positive organisms, including *Clostridia spp,* but has little antifungal activity.[36] Because mafenide is readily absorbable, it can produce metabolic acidosis when applied to burns covering large BSAs (15%). It is rapidly absorbed, and must be applied at least every 12 hours, often causing significant pain on application. Because of these limitations, it is rarely used in the outpatient setting.

Chlorhexidine. *Chlorhexidine* is commercially available as Hibiclens solution. This effective skin antiseptic has a broad coverage of wound pathogens,[35] but little is known about its toxicity and absorption characteristics.[39] It is not recommended for use as a topical antimicrobial agent.

Aloe Vera. *Aloe vera* is commercially available in a >50% concentration combined with a preservative. It is readily available, inexpensive, easy to use, and painless. Aloe inactivates bradykinin and decreases thromboxane.[40] Its antimicrobial activity includes *Pseudomonas aeruginosa, Enterobacter aerogenes, S. aureus,* and *Klebsiella pneumoniae.*[41] Many patients find this "natural" agent appealing. Because of its limited antimicrobial activity, EPs should continue to recommend topical agents with broader antimicrobial coverage and those topical agents that are consistent with the recommendations of the burn specialists in the medical community.

Other Agents. Topical nonprescription antimicrobial creams or ointments may also be employed for burn wound treatment. Bacitracin zinc ointment, polymyxin B-bacitracin (Polysporin), and polymyxin B-neomycin-bacitracin (Neosporin) are examples of soothing antiseptics. They also are cosmetically acceptable when used as open dressings on the hands or face. Neomycin-containing compounds may lead to skin sensitization.

There are numerous "home remedies" for burn care. Surprisingly, agents such as honey and potato peels are used to good effect in third world countries. The high osmolarity of honey inhibits bacterial growth and keeps the burn moist. Unfortunately, the lack of clinical research with these home remedies makes any recommendation for their use suspect.

The standard approach to the outpatient management of minor burns is to apply an antimicrobial topical therapy and follow the patient closely with a 24-hour return visit. In the absence of evidence-based medicine data the choice of topical antimicrobial agent should be based on the consensus of the burn specialist in the medical community and in consideration of the patient's allergies.

SYNTHETIC BURN DRESSINGS

Synthetic burn dressings are most appropriate for second-degree burns, but can also be applied to third-degree burns before surgical repair. These dressings are cut to fit the burn and must be carefully applied to avoid collecting air or fluid under the dressing. Do not use these dressings if the burn wound is contaminated. Synthetic dressings are left in place for 10 to 14 days and are allowed to separate spontaneously. At this point, most burn healing should be complete. If fluid collects under the dressing it must be aspirated or the dressing removed to prevent infection. Synthetic dressings prevent further mechanical wound trauma that results from daily cleaning and dressing changes. At the same time, they provide a protective barrier. Synthetic dressings are not suitable for wounds that occur over joints or areas that require frequent range of motion such as fingers.

Many types of synthetic dressings are available and many more are under development. Most are somewhat costly and clinical trials are limited. Once again it is essential for the EP to work in concert with the burn surgeons in the medical community to arrive at a comprehensive care plan for these patients.

A list of some of the more common types of burn dressings includes the following:

1. *Biobrane* (Winthrop Pharmaceuticals, New York) is a biosynthetic bilaminar membrane dressing that consists of a knitted nylon fabric mechanically bonded to an ultrathin silicone membrane. It provides a vapor barrier and prevents wound desiccation. Biobrane limits bacterial penetration but allows topical antimicrobial agents to penetrate to the wound. In comparison to 1% silver sulfadiazine, it significantly reduced both healing time and pain and was associated with decreased wound care.[42] Biobrane is difficult to use and may prematurely separate from the wound.
2. *DuoDerm* (Convatec, Inc., Arlington Heights, IL) is an occlusive dressing impermeable to moisture and gases. It is composed of outer polyurethane foam and an inner hydrocolloid layer that adheres to the skin. The dressing interacts with the wound bed and exudate collects beneath the foam, forming a barrier between the wound and the dressing. Burn wounds heal faster using DuoDerm when compared with 1% silver sulfadiazine.[43,44] It is opaque, has no inherent antimicrobial properties, and can be left in place for 5 days. Because of its opaque nature, physicians are unable to directly visualize the burn.
3. *Op-Site* (Smith and Nephew Medical, Massillon, OH) is a polyurethane film permeable to gases, and permits the passage of both carbon dioxide and oxygen. A clear, impermeable dressing, fluid frequently collects beneath it.[43]
4. *Sildimac* (Marion Laboratories, Kansas City, KN) is an elastic, flexible, and conformable synthetic sheet that contains a sustained-release delivery system for silver sulfadiazine. It is opaque and adheres to dry surfaces while conforming to body contours. Sildimac requires dressing changes only every 4 to 7 days.

Allografts, xenografts, and amniotic membranes[45] are effective biologic dressings but are beyond the scope of ED treatment. Decisions about what patients are candidates for these types of dressings can only be made after consultation with the burn specialists.

Treatment of Major Burns

Initial resuscitation must emphasize airway management, maintenance of circulation, and prevention of hypothermia (Box 35-2). In a patient with multiple injuries, the burn wound may take lower priority. Early recognition of criteria for burn center transport expedites care (see Box 35-5).

AIRWAY AND RESPIRATORY

The EP must aggressively manage any patient with signs of airway injury. Patients who inhale superheated steam, while rare, develop rapid airway swelling. If intubation is not accomplished early in the clinical course, it may soon become impossible. Some chemical burns and severe thermal injury may also preclude oral intubation, and cricothyroidotomy may be necessary.

Inhalational injury to the lungs is much more common than upper airway problems. Such patients may cough up black (carbonaceous) sputum or may have singed nasal hairs. Massively burned lips are an ominous sign. A history of being trapped in an en-

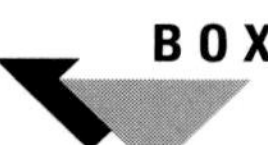

BOX 35-2

Interventions for Major Burns

INTERVENTIONS
Airway management
Fluid resuscitation
Determine burn size
Prevent hypothermia
Pain management
Tetanus as indicated
Determine need for burn center transfer

TUBES
100% oxygen
Nasogastric tube
Foley catheter with urinometer
2 Large-bore IVs with Ringer's lactate

MONITORS
Pulse oximetry
Cardiac monitor
Noninvasive BP

LABORATORY STUDIES
CBC
Electrolytes and renal studies (basic metabolic panel)
CO level if closed-space fire or patient symptomatic
CPK if third- or fourth-degree burns or electrical injury with entry or exit wounds
Urinalysis and urine myoglobin
Coagulation studies if massive burns
Pregnancy test if female of childbearing age

OTHER DIAGNOSTIC STUDIES
CXR
ECG

closed space also suggests inhalation injury. Fiberoptic scopes can visualize the airway and determine the extent of the injury.[46] This procedure should be done liberally on burn patients where there is any suspicion of inhalation injury. Patients with visible signs of airway injury (i.e., erythematous and edematous vocal cords) should undergo early oral intubation. A conscious patient with no respiratory distress, normal oxygenation, and no injury noted with a fiberoptic scope, is unlikely to require urgent intubation.

A victim of a fire in an enclosed space may inhale various toxins. Many products of combustion produce bronchospasm, pulmonary edema, and ventilation-perfusion mismatch.[3,47,48] Pulmonary complications cause or directly contribute to death in 77% of burns

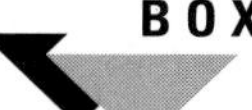

BOX 35-3

Indications for Hyperbaric Oxygen (HBO) for Carbon Monoxide (CO) Exposure

NOTE: There are little empiric data to base firm recommendations on regarding the use of HBO for CO poisoning. The following represents some commonly found suggestions regarding indications.

CO level of >15% in pregnant women
Ischemic chest pain
Syncope or seizures
Neurologic abnormalities
Initial COHb levels ≥25% to 30%
Failure to improve with high-flow oxygen

accompanied by inhalation injury.[49] All patients at risk require 100% oxygen until a carboxyhemoglobin (COHb) level is known to be less than 10%. Consider hyperbaric oxygen therapy for pregnant women, very young and very old patients, and patients with cardiovascular or neurologic signs or symptoms (Box 35-3). Empiric hyperbaric oxygen therapy is recommended for COHb levels ≥25% if a hyperbaric chamber is at the treating facility; transfer these patients to a hyperbaric facility if the COHb levels >40%. Cyanide is also present in smoke and can lead to death if not recognized and treated. Patients with marked metabolic acidosis, normal arterial oxygen content, and high-venous oxygen content may have cyanide toxicity. Some poison centers recommend routine treatment of cyanide poisoning for patients who have altered mental status, coma, or acidosis after a structural fire, *using only the sodium thiosulfate portion* of the cyanide antidote kit. Contact your local poison center for more information regarding this approach.

All patients with major burns require an initial chest radiograph even if inhalation injury is not clinically suspected. The film establishes an important baseline for comparison with future studies.

FLUID MANAGEMENT

Patients with significant burns require immediate IV access. If possible, place large-bore peripheral catheters through intact (nonburned) tissue. However, if no other sites are available, catheters can be placed through a burn. Elderly patients with large burns, those with significant co-morbid disease (renal failure, cardiac disease, liver disease), or patients requiring high ventilator pressures may require invasive cardiac monitoring to gauge adequate volume resuscitation.

Central venous catheters pose a significant infection risk in burn patients and should not be routine. If used, place central catheters early in the burn treatment since landmarks are soon lost secondary to tissue edema.

Major burns lead to intravascular fluid depletion. Burns of this size cause direct vascular injury and release vasoactive mediators, which increase vascular permeability. Generalized edema develops with maximal plasma loss in the first 8 to 12 hours. After 24 hours, fluid shifts begin to stabilize and plasma levels start to normalize.[3,48,50]

Numerous clinical trials have tried to define the best fluid choice for initial burn therapy. A dizzying array of different formulas, crystalloids, colloids, and isotonic and hypertonic fluids confront the EP. Regardless of the formula chosen, clinical parameters and not calculated numbers should guide initial treatment. A normal blood pressure and heart rate less than 120 beats per minute may indicate adequate fluid levels in a young and otherwise healthy adult. Patients at the extremes of age and those on cardiac medications may suffer intravascular depletion despite a near-normal blood pressure and heart rate. *A urine output of 0.5 ml/kg/hour for adults and 1.0 ml/kg/hour for children is the best clinical indicator of adequate fluid resuscitation in burn victims.* Increased fluid requirements occur with electrical injuries, escharotomies, chronic diuretic therapy, alcohol/drug use, inhalation injury, delayed fluid resuscitation, or mannitol use for myoglobinuria.[48] Although excessive fluids may promote body edema and, on occasion, pulmonary edema, most errors lie in under-resuscitation.

The most popular burn fluid formulas, Parkland and Modified Brooke, call for lactated Ringer's solution (LR) given at 2 to 4 ml/kg/% BSA burn over 24 hours. The Parkland formula uses for 4 ml/kg/% BSA burn, whereas the Modified Brooke employs 2 ml/kg/% BSA burn (Box 35-4). The percent burned area is calculated by adding the total of second-degree, third-degree, and fourth-degree burns sustained. In both formulas, one half of the fluid is given over the first 8 hours *from the burn—not from time of arrival in the ED.* The remaining one-half volume is given over the next 16 hours. This unequal administration compensates for the fact that most of the vascular fluid leaks occur in the first 8 to 12 hours.[51]

Pediatric patients may require fluids in addition to those provided by the Parkland formula. Begin resuscitation with both normal maintenance fluids *plus* the Parkland formula fluids. Children may become hypoglycemic with the large fluid loads. If blood glucose falls, give 5% dextrose LR in place of LR.

Some centers use hypertonic saline (HS) in an effort to decrease the edema associated with burns and to increase organ perfusion. Further experience is needed with this approach, since HS can markedly increase body sodium while minimally increasing cardiac output.[51] Although some studies showed that HS improved outcome, other research demonstrated no improvement over resuscitation using LR.[52-54] In most EDs, LR remains the resuscitation fluid of choice.

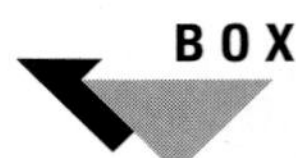

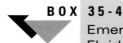

BOX 35-4
Emergency Department Burn Fluid Resuscitation

FIRST 24 HOURS
Fluid of choice: lactated Ringer's

Adults
2 to 4 ml/kg/% BSA burned (excluding first-degree burns)
One half of fluid to be infused in the first 8 hours after the injury
One half of fluid to be infused over the next 16 hours

Pediatrics
4 ml/kg/% BSA burned (excluding first-degree burns)
One half of fluid to be infused in the first 8 hours after the injury
One-half of fluid to be infused over the next 16 hours
Add normal maintenance fluids to burn resuscitation fluid

The above calculations are only a guide. Adjust fluids to maintain urine output of 0.5 ml/kg/hour in adults and 1 ml/kg/hour in children.

CARDIOVASCULAR

Major burns affect most organ systems in the body. Vascular fluid shifts decrease preload, whereas sympathetic drive increases afterload, thus compromising cardiac output. Major electrical burns may affect the cardiac conduction system causing rhythm disturbances. Most patients admitted to the hospital with electrical burns receive at least 24 hours of cardiac monitoring. Electrocardiograms (ECGs) should be obtained on all admitted burn patients as a baseline study.

RENAL

In victims of major burns, the kidneys suffer from decreased perfusion, whereas muscle breakdown can deposit myoglobin in the renal tubules. Both of these insults may lead to renal insufficiency or even renal failure. Although a standard urine dipstick often turns positive for blood in the presence of myoglobin, this test is insensitive for muscle breakdown. Measure the total CPK to determine the risk of this complication; serial levels of CPK in conjunction with successive determinations of BUN and creatinine will herald pigment-induced renal injury.

Although fluid therapy corrects the decreased perfusion, management of myoglobinuria is more complex. Whereby alkalinization of the urine and administration of mannitol may decrease pigment deposition in the tubules, each therapy has its own risks. Burn center consultation may be helpful in this regard. Maintaining a brisk urine output also treats myoglobinuria.

Obtain a urinalysis and renal function studies in patients with major burns. A Foley catheter attached to a urinometer accurately monitors urine output and prevents outflow obstruction.

GASTROINTESTINAL

Vasoconstriction in the gastrointestinal tract often leads to ileus and increased mucosal permeability. Stress ulcers frequently arise in the stomach (Curling ulcers). Place a nasogastric tube and consider administering an H_2-receptor antagonist such as cimetidine.[55]

IMMUNE SYSTEM

Major burns depress the immune response by impairing immunoglobulin production, neutrophil chemotaxis, phagocytic activity, and cell-mediated response.[48,56,57] Despite the suppressed immune system, *systemic antibiotics are not recommended unless the patient has an established infection.*[15,58] Topical antimicrobial therapy is recommended for major burns since they are otherwise likely to become infected.[3] However, many burn centers prefer that acute burn patients transferred to their facility not be covered with topical antimicrobials. Thick lotions and cream impair the initial evaluation and the topicals are usually removed on the patient's arrival. Consult with the accepting burn center to determine their preference before applying topical antimicrobial therapy.

ANALGESIA

Burn pain is inversely proportional to the depth of burn, and analgesia and patient comfort are critical in initial treatment of serious burns. In conscious patients, have them rate their pain on a scale of 1 to 10. Changes in the pain score over time determines efficacy of pain management.

Intravenous opioids also facilitate the examination and evaluation of burn wounds. Avoid intramuscular and oral analgesics, since absorption is erratic in those with significant burns. Intravenous morphine at 0.1 to 0.2 mg/kg is a reasonable initial dose in both children and adults. Opioids often require frequent titration depending on the clinical circumstances. Physicians must remember to use analgesics before wound cleaning, debridement, or dressing changes.

ESCHAROTOMY

Full-thickness or third-degree burns produce an eschar that will not stretch or expand. During fluid resuscitation, tissues swell secondary to capillary leak and the resultant edema increases pressure beneath the skin. As edema progresses, the eschar acts like a tourniquet and constricts distal blood flow. In such cases, the EP must be prepared to perform emergency escharotomy.

Circumferential third-degree burns to extremities are most likely to cause ischemia, but occasionally even partial-circumferential burns require emergent release. Elevation of the affected extremity and frequent active range of motion may be helpful in these instances. Burns that encompass the entire chest cavity adversely affect ventilation before causing tissue damage. Circumferential full-thickness neck burns and resultant progressive tissue swelling may even obstruct the airway.

Indications for escharotomy are clinical. A patient with vascular embarrassment may complain of pain, paresthesias, or progressive loss of sensation. However, these findings are variable and sometimes difficult to elicit in the burned patient. Motor function and pulses persist despite significant vascular impairment on the capillary level. Measuring arterial flow by ultrasound Doppler reliably detects decreased flow, and compartment pressure monitoring also indicates the need for escharotomy. A local reduction in arterial oxygen saturation measured with a pulse oximeter also points to vascular embarrassment. In general, the EP must consider escharotomy early on for patients with circumferential full-thickness burns that begin to manifest neurovascular compromise.

Escharotomy requires no anesthesia and should be relatively bloodless, since the incision is performed through insensate skin with coagulated blood vessels. Each cut should penetrate to the level of subcutaneous fat. The incisions may be made with electrocautery if immediately available, or with a simple scalpel. Although life- or limb-saving, escharotomy incisions are potential sources of infection. After the procedure, dress the wounds in a sterile fashion with antimicrobial agents.

Limb Escharotomy. Incise the lateral and medial aspects of the affected limb to the level of the subcutaneous fat. With a proper, deep incision, the skin should spring open; a small amount of blood may issue from the wound base when living tissue is

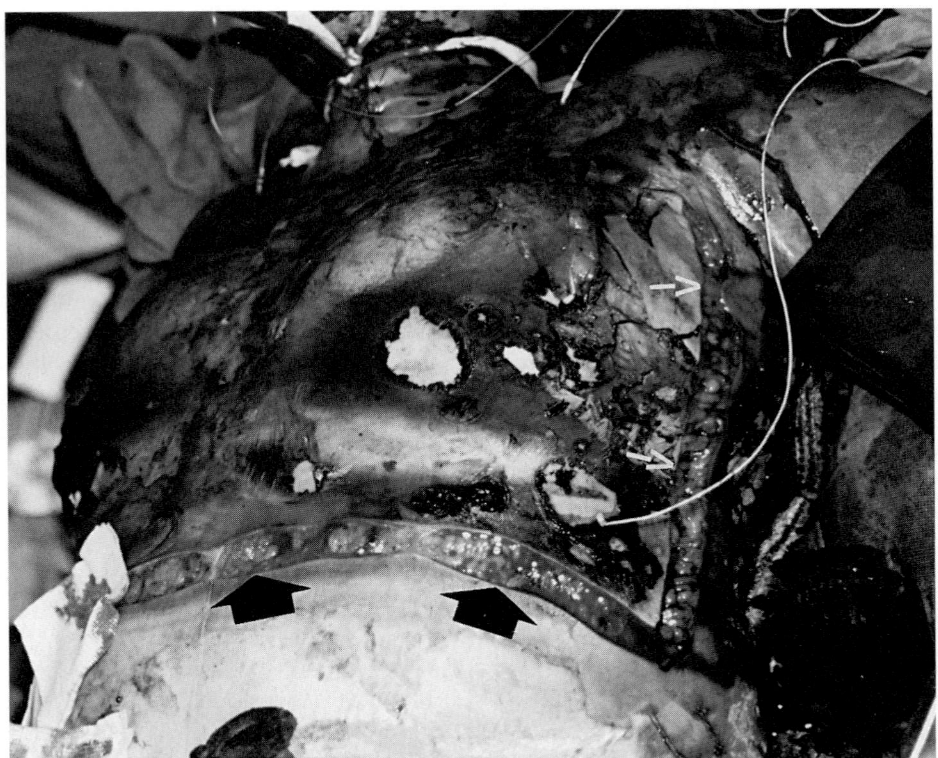

Fig. 35-2 Chest escharotomy.

reached. Incisions should be carried out over affected joints as well. Every effort should be made to avoid injuring superficial nerves during the process.

Chest Escharotomy. Burns that impair respiration by constricting the chest wall require immediate escharotomy. The incision should extend from the clavicle to the costal margin in the anterior axillary line bilaterally and be joined by transverse incisions (Fig. 35-2).

Neck Escharotomy. Burns that compromise the airway must be released. Make the incision posterolaterally to avoid the great vessels of the neck.

Genital Escharotomy. Perform a *penile escharotomy* midlaterally to avoid the dorsal vein.

Special Circumstances

HOT TAR BURNS

Tar used in roofing and road paving comes in two forms: coal-pitched tar and petroleum-derived asphalt. Tar is heated to 120° to 135° C (275° to 300° F) for paving roads and 218° to 245° C (450° to 500° F) for roofing. When tar splashes onto the skin it becomes enmeshed in the hair on the skin and causes burns. The longer the time hot tar is in contact with the skin, the deeper the burn.

Tar must be rapidly cooled to stop the heat transfer. Cooling is usually accomplished at the scene by using copious amounts of cold water. To prevent further damage, *tar should not be removed at the scene.*

Ultimately, tar must be removed to gain access to the burned tissue. Tar forms an occlusive barrier and may lead to bacterial overgrowth. However, pulling tar off without softening may denude skin appendages and worsen the injury. If underlying burns are not significant, tar removal may be delayed for 24 to 36 hours. Apply an emulsifying agent such as a petroleum-based antibiotic ointment under a bulky dressing. Common antibiotic ointments such as bacitracin zinc ointment, polymyxin B-bacitracin (Polysporin), and polymyxin B-neomycin-bacitracin (Neosporin) can soften tar for safe removal. Petroleum jelly is an inexpensive alternative, and mayonnaise or butter are effective, although pungent home remedies. Other surface-acting agents including polyoxyethylene sorbitan (Tween 80), polysorbate (De-Solu-it), and Shur-Clens also soften tar for removal. The patient may return the next day for tar removal. Although gasoline is readily available, it should not be used, since it can further damage skin and increase burn depth.

ELECTRICAL BURNS

Electrical burns result from high-intensity heat generated when a current passes through body tissues. The heat produced is directly proportional to amperage and the resistance of the tissue through which it passes. Electrical injury is described as low voltage if the current source is less than 1000 volts, and high voltage if greater than 1000 volts. (Although some authorities consider 500 volts as the limit for low-voltage injuries.) Electricity may be direct current (DC) or alternating current (AC).

Electrical burns are deceiving and exhibit the "tip of the iceberg" phenomenon. Patients may have only small cutaneous lesions but massive deep tissue injury. Electrical injuries have several components: source (entry), ground (exit) burns, and underlying tissue injury. Current typically enters the body through the hands or head and exits through the soles of the feet or opposite arm.

The entry and exit wounds are small areas of full-thickness burns. They may appear as a small white area, only millimeters across, often with a charred central punctum. There may be more than one source site, as well as multiple ground sites, on a victim. Because current takes the shortest path, electricity may arc across a flexed joint, such as the anterior elbow, leaving "kissing burns." These burns are the result of temperatures up to 2500° C (4500° F).

The tissues with the greatest resistance, such as skin and bone, generate the most heat. Wet skin has one tenth the resistance of dry skin. As bones heat, deep tissues surrounding the bones become damaged. Nerves, blood vessels, and muscle have the lowest resistance.[59,60]

Electrical injuries are often associated with blunt trauma and other cutaneous burns. The discharge of electricity can fling the victim or cause muscle contraction and subsequent bone fractures or joint dislocations. Household current at 60 cycles causes tetanic contractions of muscles. If a person grabs a live wire, these contractions prevent him or her from releasing his or her grip. Electrical burns may also ignite clothing, causing further injury.

The heat generated as current passes through high-resistance tissues causes burns on the skin and accompanying damage to fingers and limbs. Smaller volume tissues (e.g., fingers, arms) are unable to dissipate the heat and sustain greater damage than the chest or abdomen, which disperse heat over a greater area. In major electrical injuries, fingers and arms frequently require full or partial amputation.[61]

Current passing through the chest can affect the heart, particularly the conduction system. The electrical shock may cause the heart to go into asystole (seen more often with DC) or ventricular fibrillation (seen more often with AC). The heart muscle may suffer burns or infarction from electrical injury.

Electricity can damage the nervous system in several ways. Current that passes directly through the head may cause brain damage or death. Spinal cord injuries may occur with electrical current that passes from one side of the body to the other.[62] Peripheral nerves can also be damaged and some injuries are delayed.

Muscles are frequently injured by electrical injuries. As the muscle cells are damaged, they release myoglobin (see the previous discussion). High-voltage electrical injuries are especially prone to rhabdomyolysis. Muscle swelling can lead to compartment syndrome, and the EP must determine if fasciotomy is required before the patient is transported to a burn center.

Current that passes through the eyes may cause cataracts, and this complication is particularly likely with lightning injuries. Cataract formation may be delayed. High-voltage injury is associated with a 6% incidence of cataract formation.[63]

The most common type of electrical burn in toddlers is a mouth burn from chewing on electrical cords.[64] This injury can cause life-threatening and delayed hemorrhage from the labial artery when the eschar separates from the burn wound. This complication is likely 3 to 5 days after injury.

The initial management of electrical burns is familiar, and the standard priorities apply. A good neurologic examination is essential to ascertain peripheral nerve injury. Laboratory studies should include cardiac markers and liver function tests. An ECG and cardiac monitoring are essential. Myoglobinuria should be ruled out because of the high likelihood of massive muscle damage in electrical burns.

Patients with high-voltage injuries should be monitored for at least 24 hours to detect and treat any cardiac dysrhythmias. Those with entry or exit wounds may benefit from a burn center. Admit patients with otherwise nonsignificant electrical burns if the patient is at high risk for complications. Risk factors include a history of loss of consciousness or prior cardiac disease, an abnormal cardiac rhythm or ECG, hypoxia, or chest pain.

Patients with minor electrical injuries may be safely discharged from the ED if they have no entry or exit wounds. Some authors suggest obtaining an ECG and to test the urine for hemoglobin, a surrogate marker for myoglobin. Discharged patients should return for cardiac symptoms. All patients should be warned about possible late neurologic and eye symptoms.

CHEMICAL BURNS

Chemicals progressively damage the skin until inactivated or removed from the skin. With few exceptions, the mainstay of treatment for chemical burns is water irrigation. Immediate irrigation can decrease burn depth and pain.[65] Water not only cleanses the wound and removes particulate matter in the wound but also dilutes the chemical remaining on the skin. However, chemical powders should be brushed off before wash-

TABLE 35-4
Chemical Burn Treatment

Water lavage	Chromic acid Potassium permanganate Cantharides Lyes (hydroxide salts) Chlorox Dichromate salts Pieric acid	Tannic acid Tungstic acid Sulfosalicylic acid Trichloracetic acid Cresylic acid Acetic acid Formic acid
Calcium salt injection	Oxalic acid Hydrofluoric acid	
Oil immersion	Sodium metal White phosphorus Mustard gas	
Avoid water lavage	Sodium metal Potassium metal Lithium metal	
Specific approaches	Sodium metal Lyes (hydroxide salts) Hydrofluoric acid White phosphorus	Excision Weak acid lavage (vinegar) Calcium gluconate injection Copper sulfate solution

ing. Clothing can be removed while water is applied to the wound. Lavage should continue until the effluent has a neutral pH; this procedure may take more than 1 hour with certain alkalis.

The issue of neutralizing agents is complex. Neutralizing agents create heat on inactivation of the chemical and may accelerate injury. It is best to consult a toxicology text or a poison center regarding the use of such agents. In any event, do not use a neutralizing agent before copious water irrigation. If neutralization is used, water will carry away the excess heat.

Water lavage should not be used in treating alkali metals such as sodium, potassium, and lithium. These metals burn and even explode on contact with water. Cover these metals with oil and then carefully remove the particles. Table 35-4 lists which chemicals should be treated with water lavage, oil immersion, or have other specific approaches.

HYDROFLUORIC ACID

Hydrofluoric acid (HF) is used for glass etching, semiconductor manufacture, and production of plastics. It is often used in the home as a rust remover. A potent inorganic acid, it causes significant burns in small amounts and relatively low concentrations.

Hydrofluoric acid contact gives the skin a tough coagulated appearance, and causes progressive tissue destruction and severe pain. Initial injury derives from liberated hydrogen ions, but the subsequent harm results from the fluoride ions. Stopping fluoride ion destruction requires binding to either calcium or magnesium. HF can penetrate fingernails with little destruction to the nail but significant ruin to the nail bed.

Treatment for HF burns consists of immediate water irrigation. If pain persists, then the fluoride ion can be inactivated with calcium salt. Apply topical calcium gluconate to stop any surface fluoride activity. The hospital pharmacy can prepare a gel by combining 3.5 grams of calcium gluconate with 150 ml of water-soluble lubricant. This mixture is then applied with an occlusive cover. If the burns are on the hand, fill a latex glove with the calcium gluconate gel and place the glove on the hand. Continuing pain after topical application requires either direct calcium injection or an intraarterial infusion.

For minor burns resistant to topical therapy, inject 10% calcium gluconate subcutaneously with a small-bore needle into the affected area; the maximum dose is 0.5 ml/cm^2. Calcium chloride is caustic and should not be used in this situation. It is helpful to have the patient outline the painful area before injection. When injecting into digits, the maximum volume may be reached before all of the fluoride ions are bound.

Intraarterial infusion of calcium gluconate can also counteract the fluoride ion and is useful in patients with extensive hand burns.[66,67] To employ this therapy, place a catheter in the radial artery and infuse a solution of 10 ml of calcium gluconate diluted into 50 ml of dextrose and water over 4 hours. If the pain persists, repeat this infusion. Complications such as arterial spasm or thrombosis can arise from the arterial cannulation and infusion.

Large surface exposures may cause death by hypocalcemia, and IV calcium is indicated in this circumstance.

PHOSPHORUS BURNS

White phosphorus is commonly found in fireworks, insecticides, and military weapons. It spontaneously ignites when it comes into contact with air. White phosphorus is lipid soluble and easily penetrates the dermis. This yellowish burn is extremely painful and emits a garlic odor.[68]

Treatment involves removing any nonburning phosphorus, followed by water irrigation or immersion. Water will stop the burning of phosphorus, allowing debridement. A 1% copper sulfate solution applied to the wound turns the phosphorus black, making it easier to see and remove. After the phosphate is removed, irrigate the wound to wash away the copper sulfate solution.

DISPOSITION

Most minor burns and some moderate burns can be treated in the outpatient setting with close follow-up. Moderate burns may often require short-term hospitalization, with the bulk of the wound treatment and healing done at home. Major burns usually require transport to a regional burn center for proper care.

Some patients require admission to the hospital even if the affected BSA is small. The elderly, children, and patients with underlying medical or psychiatric problems are more likely to suffer complications. Some patients may require admission for pain control, monitoring of co-morbid diseases, frequent dressing changes, and patient education. If the physician doubts the patient has the resources to care for his or her burn as an outpatient, a short admission is preferable to treatment failure.

The American Burn Association has developed guidelines for transfer to a regional burn center (Box 35-5). Under these guidelines, patients with major burns and some with moderate burns should be transferred to a burn center. The guidelines suggest that burns >10% BSA in the elderly or young, as well as any burn >20% BSA at any age, should be treated in a burn center. They believe that full-thickness burns >5% BSA also require a burn center. Any significant electrical, chemical, or inhalation injury or significant burns to the hands, feet, or perineum are high risk and benefit from specialty care.

To ensure proper ongoing care of burn wounds, the EP should provide explicit discharge instructions and follow-up. Initial follow-up should be in 1 to 2 days depending on the severity of the burn. Subsequent visits can range from 1 to 7 days as circumstances warrant.

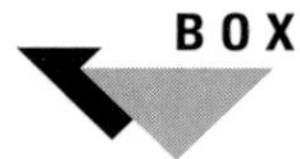

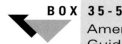

BOX 35-5

American Burn Association Guidelines for Transfer to a Burn Center

Any burn >10% of total BSA in patients <10 and >50 years old
Burns involving >20% of total BSA at any age
Full-thickness burns involving >5% of total BSA
Significant burns of hands, face, feet, genitalia, perineum, or major joints
Significant electric injury
Significant chemical injury
Significant inhalation injury, concomitant mechanical trauma, co-morbidities
Patients with special psychosocial or rehabilitative care needs

Dressing inspection and changes must be done once or twice daily, and patients should take analgesics 30 minutes before dressing change. Whoever changes the dressing should take it down to the fine mesh gauze or to the topical antibiotic level. Fine mesh gauze may remain in place if the gauze is dry and adherent on the wound and no topical antibiotic therapy is being used.[3,24] When using topical agents, the wound must be cleaned once or twice daily with tap water (the shower or bathtub is convenient). A new layer of topical agent and a bulky gauze dressing can then be applied.

Although dressing supplies must be available to facilitate proper wound care, some patients cannot afford or obtain supplies. In these cases, the ED may assist in supplies. The patient often requires medical or lay help for dressing changes.

Patients must elevate burned extremities above heart level to reduce swelling. Range of motion exercises are mandatory to keep skin from stiffening and are best done at dressing change times.

Moisturizing lotion is recommended for wounds after they begin to dry.[2,24] Emollient lotions containing lanolin or aloe vera will keep the wound soft, moist, and pliable for good healing. These lotions should only be applied after the wound has stopped secreting fluids.

Systemic antibiotics have no role in the initial outpatient treatment of burn victims. Overuse of systemic antibiotics in the absence of infection may engender resistant organisms.

Outpatient analgesia is important in all burn types. Pain from burns decreases with burn depth. Some second degree burns have increased pain 24 to 48 hours after injury. Oral opiates should be prescribed for pain control unless contraindicated. Nonsteroidal antiinflammatory medications decrease pain and aid in burn healing. They should be used in conjunction with opiates.

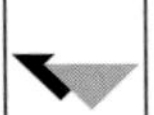

PEARLS & PITFALLS

- Pulmonary complications cause or directly contribute to death in 77% of burns accompanied by inhalation injury.
- Patients with airway injury need emergent management, *before* swelling progresses.
- Measure COHb in symptomatic patients (altered mental status, headache, chest pain, etc.)
- Burn formulas: Adjust fluids according to clinical parameters and not calculated numbers.
  - Parkland Formula: 4 cc/kg/BSA per day. One half of the fluid is given over the first 8 hours *from the trauma* (not from time of arrival in the ED).
  - A urine output of 0.5 ml/kg/hour for adults and 1.0 ml/kg/hour for children is the best clinical indicator of adequate fluid resuscitation in burn victims.
- Systemic antibiotics are not recommended without a source of infection.
- Use NSAID liberally in patients with burns.
- Aggressively manage pain—intravenous opioids are drugs of choice.
- Determine need for burn center transport soon after performing the primary and secondary surveys.

REFERENCES

1. Brigham PA, McLoughlin E: Burn incidence and medical care use in the United States: estimates, trends, and data sources, *J Burn Care Rehabil* 17:95-107, 1996.
2. Warden GD: Outpatient care of thermal injuries, *Surg Clin North Am* 67:147-157, 1987.
3. Griglak MJ: Thermal injury, *Emerg Med Clin North Am* 10:369-383, 1992.
4. Munster AM: Burns of the world, *J Burn Care Rehabil* 17:477-484, 1996.
5. Baux S: Contribution a l'etude du traitement local des brulures thermiques etendues, These, Paris 1961.
6. Wassermann D, Schlotterer M: Survival rates of patients hospitalized in French burns units during 1985, *Burns* 15:261-264, 1989.
7. Bang RL, Ghoneim IE: Epidemiology and mortality of 162 major burns in Kuwait, *Burns* 22:433-438, 1996.
8. Cadier MA, Shakespeare PG: Burns in octogenarians, *Burns* 21: 200-204, 1995.
9. Stuart JD, Kenney JG, Morgan RF: Pediatric burns, *Am Fam Physician* 36:139-146, 1987.
10. Bennett B, Gamelli R: Profile of an abused burned child, *J Burn Care Rehabil* 19:88-94, 1998.
11. Glasheen WP, et al: Epidemiology of minor burn injuries, *Burns* 8:423-432, 1982.
12. Grobmyer SR, et al: Alcohol, drug intoxication, or both at the time of burn injury as a predictor of complications and mortality in hospitalized patients with burns, *J Burn Care Rehabil* 17: 532-539, 1996.
13. Howland J, Hingson R: Alcohol as a risk factor for injuries or death due to fire and burns: review of the literature, *Public Health Rep* 102:475-483, 1987.
14. Glasheen WP, et al: Identification of the high-risk population for serious burn injuries, *Burns* 9:193-200, 1983.
15. Drueck C III: Emergency department treatment of hand burns, *Emerg Med Clin North Am* 11:797-809, 1993.
16. Jackson DM: The diagnosis and the depth of burning, *Br J Surg* 40:588-596, 1953.
17. Moritz AR, Henriques FC Jr: Studies of thermal injury. Part II. The relative importance of time and surface temperature in the causation of cutaneous burns, *Amer J Pathol* 23:695-720, 1948.
18. Lund CC, Browder NC: The estimate of areas of burns, *Surg Gynecol Obstet* 79:352-358, 1944.
19. Alexander JW: Burn care: a specialty in evolution-1985 presidential address, American Burn Association, *J Trauma* 26:1-6, 1986.
20. Davies JW: Prompt cooling of burned areas: a review of benefits and the effector mechanisms, *Burns* 9:1-6, 1982.
21. Demling RH, Mazess RB, Wolberg W: The effect of immediate and delayed cold immersion on burn edema formation and resorption, *J Trauma* 19:56-60, 1979.
22. Heggers JP, et al: Cooling and the prostaglandin effect in the thermal injury, *J Burn Care Rehabil* 3:350-354, 1982.
23. Phillips LG, Robson MC, Heggers JP: Treating minor burns: ice, grease, or what? *Postgraduate Med* 85:219-231, 1989.
24. Shuck JM: Outpatient management of the burned patient, *Surg Clin North Am* 58:1107-1117, 1978.
25. Rockwell WB, Ehrlich HP: Should burn blister fluid be evacuated? *J Burn Care Rehabil* 11:93-94, 1990.
26. Deitch EA, Smith BJ: The effect of blister fluid from thermally injured patients on normal lymphocyte transformation, *J Trauma* 23:106-110, 1983.
27. Deitch EA: Opsonic activity of blister fluid from burn patients, *Infect Immunol* 41:1184-1189, 1983.
28. Deitch EA, Bubke M, Baxter CR: Failure of local immunity: a potential cause of burn wound sepsis, *Arch Surg* 120:78-84, 1985.
29. Deitch EA, et al: Burn wound sepsis may be promoted by a failure of local antibacterial host defenses, *Ann Surg* 206:340-348, 1987.
30. Garner WL, et al: The effects of burn blister fluid on keratinocyte replication and differentiation, *J Burn Care Rehabil* 14:127-31, 1993.
31. Gowar JP, Lawrence JC: The incidence, causes and treatment of minor burns, *J Wound Care* 4:71-74, 1995.
32. Zhang YB, et al: Burns during pregnancy: an analysis of 24 cases, *Chin Med J* 94:123-126, 1981.
33. Kagan RJ, Warden GD: Management of the burn wound, *Clin Dermatol* 12:47-56, 1994.

34. Quinn KJ: Design of a burn dressing, *Burns* 13:377-381, 1987.
35. Herruzo-Cabrera R, et al: Evaluation of the penetration strength, bactericidal efficacy and spectrum of action of several antimicrobial creams against isolated microorganisms in a burn centre, *Burns* 18:39-44, 1992.
36. Monafo WW, Ayvazian VH: Topical therapy, *Surg Clin North Am* 58:1157-1171, 1978.
37. Aoyama H, Yokoo K, Fujii K: Systemic absorption of sulphadiazine, silver sulphadiazine and sodium sulphadiazine through human burn wounds, *Burns* 16:163-165, 1990.
38. Stern HS: Silver sulphadiazine and the healing of partial thickness burns: a prospective clinical trial, *Br J Plast Surg* 42:581-585, 1989.
39. Krisanda TJ, Bethel CA: Burn care procedures. In Roberts JR, Hedges JR (editors): *Clinical procedures in emergency medicine,* ed 3, Philadelphia, 1998, Saunders.
40. Klein AD, Penneys NS: Aloe vera, *J Am Acad Dermatol* 18:714-720, 1988.
41. Heck E, et al: Aloe vera (gel) cream as a topical treatment for outpatient burns, *Burns* 7:291-294, 1980.
42. Gerding RL, Imbembo AL, Fratianne RB: Biosynthetic skin substitute vs. 1% silver sulfadiazine for treatment of inpatient partial-thickness thermal burns, *J Trauma* 28:1265-1269, 1988.
43. Madden MR, et al: Comparison of an occlusive and a semiocclusive dressing and the effect of the wound exudate upon keratinocyte proliferation, *J Trauma* 29:924-931, 1989.
44. Hermans MH, Hermans RP: Duoderm, an alternative dressing for smaller burns, *Burns* 12:214-219, 1986.
45. Ramakrishnan KM, Jayaraman V: Management of partial-thickness burn wounds by amniotic membranes: a cost-effective treatment in developing countries, *Burns* 23(suppl):S33-S36, 1997.
46. Becker DG, et al: Salvage of a patient with burn inhalation injury and pancreatitis, *Burns* 19:444-446, 1993.
47. Harms BA, et al: Microvascular fluid and protein flux in pulmonary and systemic circulations after thermal injury, *Microvasc Res* 23:77-86, 1982.
48. Morehouse JD, et al: Resuscitation of the thermally injured patient, *Crit Care Clin* 8:355-365, 1992.
49. Darling GE, et al: Pulmonary complications in inhalation injuries with associated cutaneous burn, *J Trauma* 40:83-89, 1996.
50. Ward PA, Till GO: Pathophysiologic events related to thermal injury of skin, *J Trauma* 30(suppl):S75-S79, 1990.
51. Demling RH: Fluid replacement in burned patients, *Surg Clin North Am* 67:15-30, 1987.
52. Gunn ML, et al: Prospective, randomized trial of hypertonic sodium lactate versus lactated ringer's solution for burn shock resuscitation, *J Trauma* 29:1261-1267, 1989.
53. Horton JW, White DJ: Hypertonic saline dextran resuscitation fails to improve cardiac function in neonatal and senescent burned guinea pigs, *J Trauma* 31:1459-1466, 1991.
54. Griswald JA, et al: Hypertonic saline resuscitation: efficacy in a community-based burn unit, *South Med J* 84:692-696, 1991.
55. Wong L, Munster AM: New techniques in burn wound management, *Surg Clin North Am* 73:363-371, 1993.
56. Moran K, Munster AM: Alterations of the host defense mechanism in burned patients, *Surg Clin Nor Am* 67:47-56, 1987.
57. Hansbrough JF, Zapata-Sirvent RL, Peterson VM: Immunomodulation following burn injuries, *Surg Clin Nor Am* 67:69-92, 1987.
58. Boss WK, et al: Effectiveness of prophylactic antibiotics in the outpatient treatment of burns, *J Trauma* 25:224-227, 1985.
59. Jaffe RH: Electropathology: a review of the pathologic changes produced by electric currents, *Arch Pathol* 5:837-870, 1928.
60. Hammond JS, Ward CG: High-voltage electrical injuries: management and outcome of 60 cases, *South Med* J 81:1351-1352, 1988.
61. Hanumadass ML, et al: Acute electrical burns: a 10-year clinical experience, *Burns* 12:427-431, 1986.
62. Koller J, Orsagh J: Delayed neurological sequelae of high-tension electrical burns, *Burns* 15:175-178, 1989.
63. Saffle JR, Crandall A, Warden GD: Cataracts: a long-term complication of electrical injury, *J Trauma* 25:17-21, 1985.
64. Baker MD, Chiaviello C: Household electrical injuries in children: epidemiology and identification of avoidable hazards, *Am J Dis Child* 143:59-62, 1989.
65. Leonard LG, Scheulen JJ, Munster AM: Chemical burns: effect of prompt first aid, *J Trauma* 22:420-423, 1982.
66. Vance MV, et al: Digital hydrofluoric acid burns: treatment with intraarterial calcium infusion, *Ann Emerg Med* 15:890-896, 1986.
67. Pegg SP, Siu S, Gillett G: Intra-arterial infusions in the treatment of hydrofluoric acid burns, *Burns* 11:440-443, 1985.
68. Konjoyan TR: White phosphorus burns: case report and literature review, *Mil Med* 148:881-884, 1983.

36 Domestic Violence

MARIA PELUCIO

Teaching Case

A 25-year-old woman, 18 weeks pregnant, visits the emergency department (ED) for the fourth week in a row for various complaints. Today she complains of mild epigastric pain and appears anxious. Her male partner is in the room and seems overly protective and at times angry. The examiner notices bruises in various stages of healing. She has several facial wounds that are partially concealed by make-up.

How would you proceed with your evaluation? ■

Domestic violence (DV) takes place in the context of an increasingly violent world. Historically, infectious diseases and injury are the two leading causes of premature death in the United States.[1] But although we have made significant strides in reducing mortality from infectious diseases and unintentional injury, casualties from interpersonal violence have escalated. Domestic violence is the leading cause of injury to women aged 15 to 44 years. In the United States, approximately 6 million women per year are assaulted by their partners, and more than twice that number are abused during their lifetime.

Domestic abuse is woven into the tapestry of family violence. More violence occurs inside the home than outside its walls.[2] Seventeen percent of the nation's homicides occur within the family, and 30% to 50% of all female murder victims are killed by a current or former partner.[3-5]

Violence is rarely random and inexplicable; patterns are emerging. Once considered distinct, child abuse, youth violence, DV, and elder abuse prove interrelated and rooted in similar familial struggles.[1] These struggles include fragmented families, alcohol and drug abuse, and limited social and economic resources. It is more important to consider an episode of DV in terms of the context in which a person lives and not merely a specific injury.[2]

HISTORICAL PERSPECTIVE

Domestic violence has become a national epidemic.[2] In the United States, it is nearly as common as childbirth, about 4 million instances per year.[6] Abuse may be the most common cause of injury in women, responsible for more injury than motor vehicle crashes, muggings, and rape combined.[7]

Violence between intimate partners is not new, and transcends eras and cultures.[8] It is difficult to compare the current prevalence with the past, because of recent changes in awareness and willingness to report abuse. Throughout history, men have had dominion over the women and children in their lives. According to English common law, a man was permitted to beat his wife as long as the stick was no greater than the diameter of his thumb.[9] This law was known as the "rule of thumb."[10] Historically, both the legal and the medical professions viewed violence in the home as a private matter.

The first modern reports of wife abuse occurred in the 1960s, and in 1971, the first shelter for battered women appeared in London.[11] One landmark paper that identified the syndrome of battered women came from the emergency medicine literature in 1980.[12] Domestic violence is now recognized as an important consideration in women's and family health issues.

EPIDEMIOLOGY

Domestic violence is a constellation of behaviors that may include repeated battering, psychologic abuse, sexual assault, progressive social isolation, economic control, deprivation, and intimidation (Box 36-1). A current or former intimate partner perpetrates the

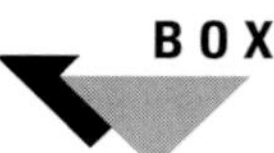

BOX 36-1
Domestic Violence: Its Many Forms

Domestic Violence is an established form of exhibiting control and eliciting fear
- Physical abuse
- Emotional abuse
- Intimidation, coercion, and threats
- Economic manipulation
- Isolation
- Sexual abuse

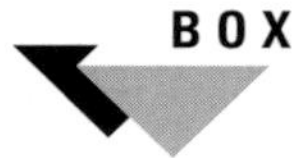

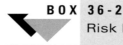

BOX 36-2
Risk Factors for Abuse*

Note: ***Any*** woman may be at risk for abuse
- Age: 17 to 28 years
- History of childhood abuse
- Marital status: single, separated, or divorced
- Homeless
- Pregnant
- Alcohol or drug abuse
- Jealous or possessive partner

*References 3, 13, 41.

abuse. Domestic violence occurs in same-sex relationships as well. Although men can be victims, the vast majority of cases involve women. In addition, women are at much greater risk for sustaining physical injury in abusive situations.[13] Even the process of leaving the abuser carries great risk. Women who leave abusive relationships are at a 75% greater risk of being murdered than those who stay.

Domestic violence occurs in women of all racial backgrounds and socioeconomic classes (Box 36-2).[14] There is no conclusive evidence that poor women are at greater risk than middle- and upper-class women, but middle- and upper-class women have the economic resources to escape.[15]

It is estimated that intimate partner violence results in 5 to 10 billion dollars a year in health care, lost productivity, and criminal justice intervention.[16] Population-based studies suggest that 8% to 12% of women experience some form of partner violence in any given year.[17] Abuse may drive women into the streets, and half of all homeless women and children are refugees of DV.

Patients are more at risk when there is alcohol or drugs involved during the altercation. Alcohol abuse by the male partner is the strongest predictor of injury to the woman (odds ratio, 12:9).[18] Victims and families at a DV scene reported that 92% of the DV assailants had used alcohol the day of the assault, and 67% had used cocaine.[19]

The number of males who are victims of DV is less well known. Although the existence of male victims of DV is acknowledged, most studies indicate that males are more likely perpetrators.[20] In a study of 695 ED patients,[21] 22% identified themselves as victims of DV; 62% of these were female and 38% were male. In another ED study,[20] 14% of men and 22% of women had experienced nonphysical violence, whereas 28% of men and 33% of women had experienced past physical violence.

For the practicing emergency physician (EP), it is also important to consider the children in a DV situation. Child abuse occurs in 50% of homes where the women are beaten. The EP should voice questions concerning the welfare of the children, specifically regarding their immediate safety and the presence of a weapon in the home. Although there is conflicting law concerning the reporting of adult DV nationwide, child abuse laws are liberal and allow the clinician to involve child protective services in any suspicious and concerning situation.

DOMESTIC VIOLENCE AND THE EMERGENCY DEPARTMENT

The EP has a unique role in the recognition and prevention of DV (Fig. 36-1). Statistically, the EP is the most likely professional to interact with DV victims.[22] Interactions with healthcare workers may be the only opportunity for DV victims to obtain professional help, since at least 40% never contact the police.[23] Box 36-3 lists statistics concerning DV.

Victims seek medical care for both assault and nonassault concerns. Abuse is the single most powerful predictor of both total yearly visits to the physician and outpatient healthcare costs. Abuse is more predictive of medical contact than age, ethnicity, self-reported symptoms, and injurious health behaviors.[24] Following the year in which violence occurs, female victims use healthcare services twice as often as nonvictims, and their healthcare costs are 2.5 times as high.

CLINICAL CLUES TO IDENTIFYING VICTIMS OF DOMESTIC VIOLENCE

Many victims of DV present to the ED with a "cover story." They will not admit to abuse, but instead complain of "running into a door" or "falling down the

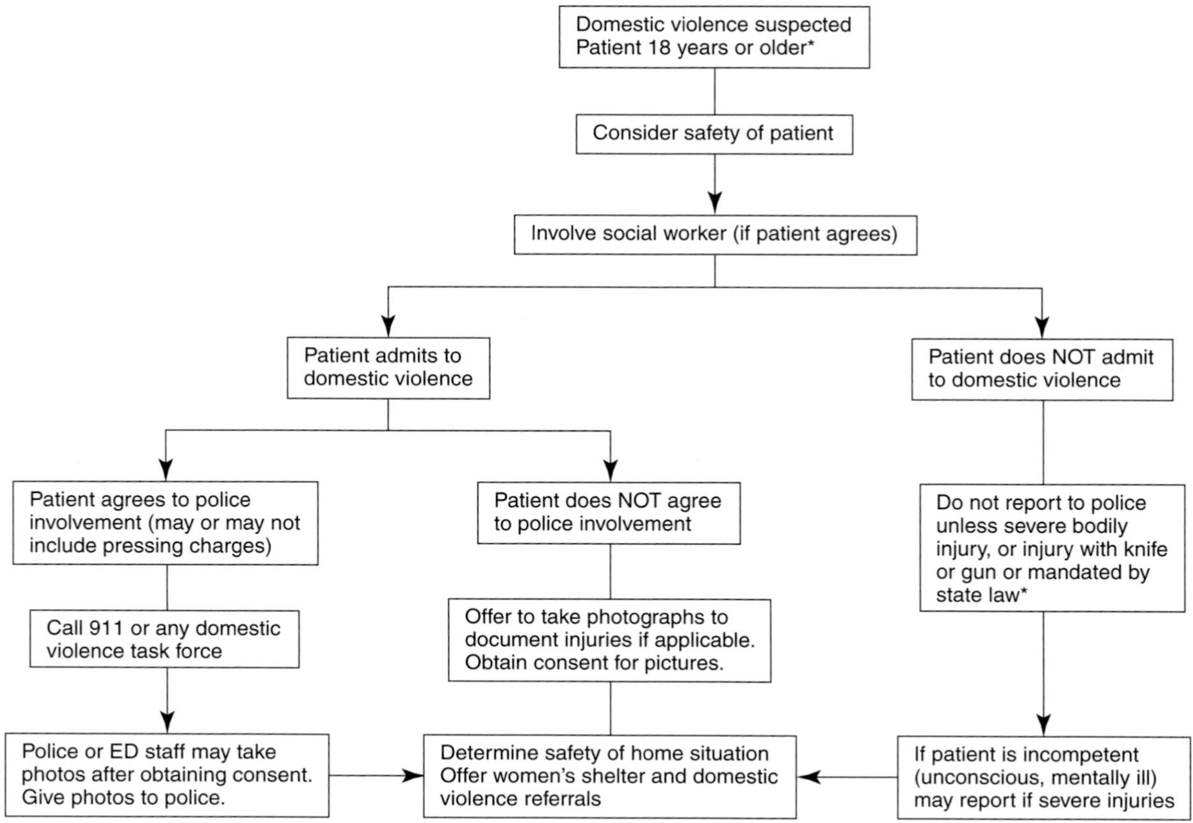

Fig. 36-1 Algorithm for management of domestic violence in the emergency department.

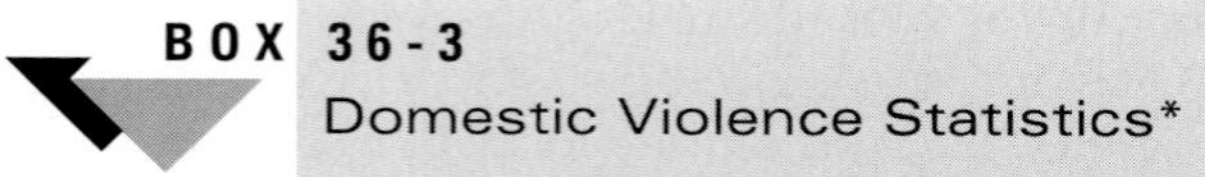

BOX 36-3
Domestic Violence Statistics*

- One million emergency department visits per year for domestic violence (DV)
- 19% to 42% of injured women seen in the emergency department are victims of DV
- One in six women have been victims of DV
- 2000 deaths per year from domestic violence
- 150,000 American men are victims of partner violence
- 15% to 25% of pregnant women are battered and have increased miscarriage rates
- 25% of women who attempt suicide are battered

*References 3, 42, 43.

stairs." It is a natural, but an incorrect impulse to accept the patient's history at face value. Patients must be asked directly, in a safe milieu, "Did someone hurt you?" Clues to DV arise from the history, patient's demeanor, and patterns of medical visits. When interviewing a patient, pay attention to inconsistencies in the history. An ever-present, over-concerned, or domineering partner may also be a clue. Alternatively, the patient may appear isolated, or there may be an unusual delay in seeking treatment. Box 36-4 lists clinical findings suggestive of DV.

Certain injury patterns tend to occur with abuse (Box 36-5). These patterns include injuries in various stages of healing and attempts to disguise bruises with clothing, make-up, or jewelry. Injuries to the ulnar aspect of the forearm (defense wounds), bottom of the feet, and back of the legs are common.[25] In a series of 546 women with maxillofacial trauma, 51 (9%) the injuries were caused by violence from an intimate

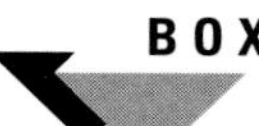

BOX 36-4

Clinical Clues to Identifying Victims of Domestic Violence

PHYSICAL
- Injuries at multiple sites and in multiple stages of healing
- Head and abdomen injuries
- Bruises, lacerations, abrasions, welts on head, face, torso, buttocks, upper thighs, and genitalia
- Injuries to the ulnar/ventral side hands and forearms as if in defense
- Any evidence of choking or strangulation
- Bruises of fingertip imprints or fists
- Marks that have resulted from a belt buckle or household objects
- Human bites
- Fractures of nose and jaw
- Bilateral injuries of legs or arms
- Patches of missing hair
- Burns that have a distinctive pattern such as cigarette, iron, radiator
- Injuries that do not fit the explanation
- Bruised, bleeding, or inflamed external genitalia; injuries from forced sexual intercourse
- Injuries during pregnancy
- History of miscarriages
- Suicide attempt
- Pelvic inflammatory symptoms

EMOTIONAL
- Nervousness
- Passivity
- Repeated requests for tranquilizers
- Insomnia or nightmares
- Hesitance and embarrassment about "accident"
- Depressive or suicidal

OTHER INDICATORS
- Partner accompanies patient and dominates her
- Delay in seeking treatment
- Multiple prior visits (trauma or nontrauma)
- History incompatible with the injuries
- Drug/alcohol dependence
- Isolation from family and friends
- Eating disorder
- Repetitive somatoform symptoms
- Medical records reveals repeated use of emergency department
- Chronic pelvic pain
- Irritable bowel syndrome
- Unintended pregnancy
- Fear of returning home and/or fear for safety of children

male, making it the third most important cause of women's facial trauma in the study.[26]

The pattern of abuse may change in pregnancy, when assaults are directed to the abdomen and genitalia.[25] In some situations, battering may actually begin or increase during pregnancy.[14] Domestic violence may be more common for pregnant women than preeclampsia, gestational diabetes, and placenta previa.[27] Pregnant teenagers are at greatest risk for abuse.[14,28] Both delay in seeking prenatal care, as well as physical mistreatment, may explain the increased rates of miscarriage, stillbirth, and low birth weight infants to these mothers.[14,29]

Depression, anxiety, and substance abuse are common as victims become demoralized by chronic abuse. Abuse can also precipitate drug overdoses and suicide attempts.[11] Patients complain of chronic conditions, such as insomnia, headaches, chronic pelvic pain, gastrointestinal complaints, and vague musculoskeletal complaints rather than admitting to abuse.[3,25,29,30] Eating disorders are common, and

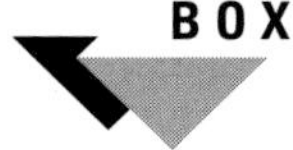

BOX 36-5

Injuries Frequently Associated with Abuse

MOST SENSITIVE
- Tympanic membrane rupture
- Rectal or perineal injury
- Facial contusions
- Neck contusions (finger marks from choking)
- Abdominal lacerations/penetrations

LESS SENSITIVE
- Orbit/zygoma/nasal fracture
- Abdominal contusion
- Dental trauma
- Head/ facial abrasions or lacerations
- Chest abrasion
- Upper extremity abrasion/contusion (look for finger marks)

patients may eventually become labeled as hypochondriacs or neurotics.[14]

Because EPs may not make a clinical association with these complaints and DV, the fundamental problem is often overlooked. Only direct questioning reveals the true source of the problem. Domestic violence is particularly overlooked when a patient uses the ED as her source of primary care. These patients are sometimes difficult and noncompliant, missing appointments and displaying hostile or defensive behavior.[25,29]

Ideally, to optimize the interview, examination, and disposition of women suspected of being victims of DV, the EP should attempt to have some one-on-one time with the patient, which may require the patient to submit to clinically unnecessary radiographs, to separate the patient from the potential abuser. A brief interview in the radiology department allows the EP to ascertain the patient's risk of further harm, offer interventions for rescue, and provide educational material such as palm cards. Each encounter with a victim of DV is an opportunity to provide education and expose the victim to alternatives for rescue.

BARRIERS TO IDENTIFICATION OF DOMESTIC VIOLENCE

Patient Barriers (Box 36-6)

The most difficult and frustrating question concerning DV is why the victims stay in the abusive relationship. The reasons are often complex and variable, and difficult for an outsider to understand. Childhood experiences of physical or sexual abuse, or witnessing DV makes it hard for a battered woman to recognize a relationship as abusive.[31-33] Many are reluctant or unable to seek help, whereas others are held captive in their homes. Others lack the money or means to escape. Cultural, ethnic, or religious background influence a woman's response to abuse and her awareness of options.

Physician Barriers (Box 36-7)

One of the biggest barriers to treatment of DV is lack of recognition. Physicians often accept the cover story without question, and do not probe for abuse. The ironic "Catch 22" is that the very presence of a "cover story" is part of the syndrome of DV.

Traditionally, physicians are not well-trained to identify adult patients who have been victimized.[34,35] In 1989 only 47% of medical schools offered programs of instruction in this area.[36] Overall, physicians may detect only 5% of DV victims.[2,7,21] Several studies in the ED document that EPs and nurses detect spousal abuse in only 10% to 20% of instances.[37]

Until recently, healthcare professionals rarely addressed issues of abuse and violence, even when the signs or symptoms were present. Many physicians are blinded by their misconceptions.[38] Some physicians have trouble recognizing their "peers," that is people of similar race, education, and economic backgrounds, as possible victims of DV. Others are reluctant to approach issues of DV because of the misplaced concerns regarding time constraints and confidentiality. In one study, 71% of physicians considered lack of time the key deterrent to pursuing questions of DV in their practice.[38] Some professionals may "blame the

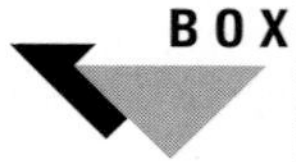

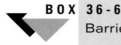

BOX 36-6
Barriers to Seeking Help

- Fear that revelation will jeopardize her safety or the safety of her children
- Hope that things will get better
- Lack of funds, housing, job, child care, emotional support
- Shame and humiliation
- Thinking she deserved the abuse
- Fear that she would not be believed
- Feeling protective of her partner
- Lack of awareness that her physical symptoms are caused by the stress of living in an abusive relationship
- Belief that her injuries are not severe enough to mention

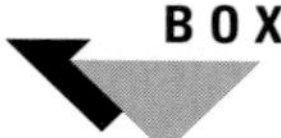

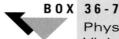

BOX 36-7
Physician Barriers to Domestic Violence Recognition and Management

- Lack of knowledge of domestic violence (DV)
- Thinking it is not the professional's place to intervene
- Believing that the woman must have provoked the abuse
- Not knowing how to intervene
- "Blaming the patient" for not leaving the relationship
- Disbelief because the alleged assailant is present and seems concerned and pleasant
- Concern that identifying and managing DV will take an overwhelming amount of time
- Difficulties dealing with the feelings evoked by listening to stories of abuse

victim," concluding the patient perhaps instigated the abuse. They blame the patient for being "too weak" to leave the relationship and thus undeserving of sympathy. It is sometimes difficult for EPs, who tend to be action-oriented, to understand how a person can stay in an abusive situation. Physicians must realize it requires time for the abused woman to reestablish self-esteem and emotional and financial stability.[29]

Some authors believe that female physicians are more likely than men to be empathetic toward victims of domestic violence. They argue that patients are more likely to disclose information to female physicians.[37] Indeed some male physicians may be less interested in the issue of DV than their female counterparts.[34] However, male physicians can have a great impact by validating a woman's experience and speaking out against abuse.[37]

INTERVENTION

Education and Universal Screening (Box 36-8)

Education is essential to improve physicians' awareness and responsiveness to DV. Yet a recent study of 1521 practicing clinicians from various disciplines documented that more than one third had received no education about child, elder, or spouse abuse.[39] Instruction should begin early in a physician's training. Medical students develop significant awareness of DV after only 3 hours of instruction during the first year of school.[20]

Some researchers suggest screening *all* patients for DV. Proponents of universal screening note that EPs routinely use standard questions to screen for common diseases such as diabetes and high blood pressure. They argue that DV is more common than many other medical problems that affect women aged 15 to 45 years.

The value of universal screening has not been proven in the ED. Currently, we suggest questioning any patient who has sustained non–motor vehicle trauma about the possibility of injury from an intimate partner (Fig. 36-2). In particular, be alert to high-risk patients or those with suspicious injuries (see Boxes 36-2 and 36-4).

Because of time constraints, other hospital personnel can also address these issues with the patient. Protocols are helpful, and may involve social service personnel, police, or victim's assistance representatives. These options vary within specific communities.

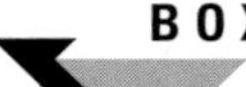

BOX 36-8

Suggestions to Screen Patients for Domestic Violence

1) Realize that women are reluctant to bring up the subject out of fear and denial.
2) Interview the patient alone. Privacy is crucial. Avoid confronting a potential abuser unless a safe strategy is in place for the woman.
3) Ask directly about abuse; however, be sensitive and sympathetic. In the beginning, avoid questions like "Does your boyfriend beat you" or "Are you being abused?" since the patient may not yet see herself as being beaten or abused.
4) Include questions about emotional and sexual abuse.
5) Remember that chronic medical and gynecologic problems, psychiatric illness, and substance abuse may have their roots in abuse.
6) Determine if there is a weapon at home, since this places the woman at greater risk of harm.
7) Assess the current safety of the home situation including whether there are children at risk.
8) Be nonjudgmental and supportive.
9) Encourage her to have the police involved but respect her wishes if she refuses.

(NOTE: Some states have mandatory reporting laws, and all states require reporting of firearm injuries.)

EXAMPLES OF QUESTIONS INCLUDE THE FOLLOWING:

- "Because domestic violence is so common, I ask all my patients about it"
- "I noticed you have a number of bruises. Did someone hurt you?"
- "You seem frightened of you partner. Has he ever hurt you?"
- "Many patients tell me someone close has hurt them. Could this be happening to you?"
- "You mention your spouse loses his temper with the children. Does he lose his temper with you?"
- "You mentioned your partner uses drugs and/or alcohol. How does he act when drinking or using drugs?"
- "Sometimes when someone is over-protective or jealous, he or she hurt the one he or she love. Is this happening to you?"
- "Your partner seems very concerned and anxious. Was he responsible for your injuries?"

Interviewing Process

During the interview, avoid being judgmental. The physician should not compound the abuse and scorn inflicted by the patient's partner. The very fact that the patient has come for help is an important first step. Because few DV victims follow-up with mental health referrals, counseling in the ED becomes especially important.[21] Be direct and clear in question-

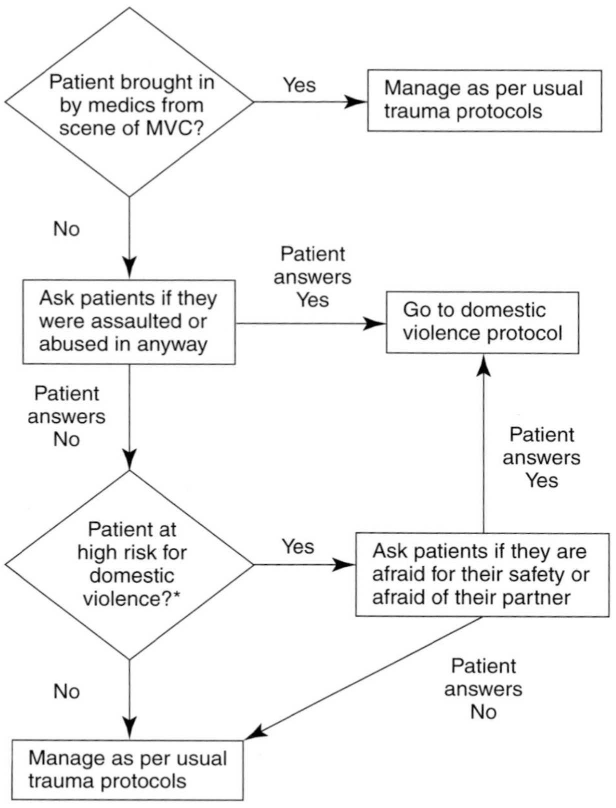

*High risk includes
- Females 17 to 28 years of age
- Homeless
- Pregnant
- Alcohol or drug abuse
- Multiple bruises of various ages
- Geographic bruises like strap marks
- History of multiple ED visits for trauma
- Suspicious cover story (woman with black eye walked into door—bruised lip and fell down stairs)
- Bruises to the neck (fingermarks)
- Dominating partner in room

Fig. 36-2 Algorithm for screening for domestic violence in patients with trauma.

ing. Ask, "Did someone hit you or push you?" or "Are you afraid of your partner?" This directness is not "meddling," but may be life saving.

Studies indicate that although a patient may be reluctant to initiate the discussion of abuse, they are very willing to report it when asked. Patients feel a sense of relief, and less feelings of betrayal, when a healthcare worker brings up the subject. The vast majority of patients favor physicians routinely asking about physical and sexual abuse.[35] However, in practice, only 30% of physicians ask about physical or sexual abuse, and none on a routine basis.[35]

DOCUMENTATION

1. Detail the complete history as described by patient. Using the patient's own words is helpful. "My husband hit me with a bat" is preferable to "Patient has been abused."
2. Determine pregnancy status.
3. Describe the injuries in terms of the following:
   - Location
   - Length, width, depth, shape, and color
   - Age
   - Use body chart or drawing if possible
4. Photograph. Although written documentation can be challenged in court, photographic evidence is difficult to dismiss. Police photography is best if the patient agrees.
   - Obtain consent
   - Take photographs before medical treatment is given if patient is clinically stable
   - Photograph at various angles and distances
   - Take at least two photos of each injury
   - Include the patient's face in at least one photograph
   - Include a ruler or small object next to wounds if possible for scale. Mark photograph on the back with names of women and examiner, medical record number, and date taken. Attach photograph to medical record or turn over to police if present
   - DO NOT give photographs to patient since this breaks the "chain of evidence" and places the patient at risk if the abuser finds them
5. Torn or bloody clothing can be used as evidence (involve police in the chain of evidence).
6. Complete the sexual assault kit if indicated.

THE LEGAL SYSTEM

Laws concerning DV vary between states. EPs should have a basic knowledge of the local statutes and how patients can access legal help. Often times a social worker or patient representative can provide this information. In particular, it is helpful to know or have access to the following:

1. The state statutes concerning mandatory reporting, including various types of assault that require police reporting, such as use of a gun, knife, or other deadly weapon
2. How, when, and for what reasons a patient can obtain a restraining order
3. Local advocacy groups and victim assistance organizations
4. Legal services for low-income or minority victims
5. What constitutes misdemeanor versus felony charges regarding DV cases

6. How to properly file photographs with the police or within the hospital record-keeping system
7. Safe places for victims to relocate, such as women's shelters or churches

MANDATORY REPORTING

Recent efforts among research groups have focused on the impact of various state laws, social programs, and hospital-based advocacy programs. Victims of DV tend to suffer recurrent abuse, and often return to a cycle of violence. Current efforts try to break this cycle. Although the community has embraced the social and medical forces that prompted child abuse reporting standards, similar standards are not easily applied to women involved in intimate partner violence.

One of the most controversial debates among DV activists surrounds mandatory reporting. Almost all states mandate reporting when the patient is injured by a gun, knife, or other deadly weapon.[40] California passed a mandatory reporting law requiring all physicians to report domestic violence cases to the police. Four other states currently have similar statutes. Some believe this mandatory reporting will break the cycle of violence. Others worry that mandatory reporting will be ineffective and prompt reprisals, placing the woman at even greater risks.

Several recent studies demonstrate the lack of effectiveness in these laws. Sachs et al[8] found that the mandatory reporting law in California did not increase medical reports of DV during the 2 years after its implementation. Reasons cited included physician ignorance of the law, noncompliance with the law, reluctance of victims to report, or possibly increased direct police reporting by the victims themselves. The AMA has recently opposed mandatory reporting of DV, instead endorsing state efforts to implement anonymous reporting systems. ED advocacy programs are not always the solution and do not always increase the rate of women willing to seek protective orders. In addition, the programs did not decrease recidivism, although there was a higher rate of shelter use.

PEARLS & PITFALLS

- Although controversy surrounds routine *reporting*, routine *screening* is the best way to identify the victims of DV.
- Do not accept the cover story at face value. Probe for the *real* mechanism of injury, especially in high-risk victims or in the setting of high-risk wounds.
- Physicians should familiarize themselves with the local and state statutes that apply to domestic violence. They or their patient representatives should know what community resources are available, including legal services, restraining order policies, counseling agencies, and shelters.
- Physicians are the best patient advocates, encouraging the victim to seek further help.
- Abuse is recurrent—it occurred before this ED visit—it will most likely occur again.
- Intervention may prevent future and even fatal injury.
- In general, question any patient who has sustained non–motor vehicle trauma about the possibility of injury from an intimate partner.
- Involve police whenever a patient agrees (or automatically in the case of mandatory reporting states).

REFERENCES

1. Muelleman RL, Lenaghan PA, Pakieser RA: Battered women: injury locations and types, *Ann Emerg Med* 28:486-492, 1996.
2. Abbott J: Injuries and illnesses of domestic violence, *Ann Emerg Med* 29:781-785,1997.
3. Flitcraft AH, et al: *Diagnostic and treatment guidelines on domestic violence,* Chicago, 1992, American Medical Association.
4. Arbuckle J, et al: Safe at home? Domestic violence and other homicides among women in New Mexico, *Ann Emerg Med* 27: 210-215,1996.
5. Crime in the US 1983. Washington DC: US Department of Justice, 1984.
6. Shalala D: American Medical Association conference on family violence: health and justice. Conference proceedings. Washington, DC, 9-12,1994.
7. Stark E and Flitcraft A: Spouse abuse. In Surgeon General's Workshop on Violence and Public Health: Source Book. Leesburg, Virginia: October 27-29, 198. Atlanta, GA: Centers for Disease Control, US Public Health Service, SA1-SA43, 1985.
8. Sachs CJ, et al: Failure of the mandatory domestic violence reporting law to increase medical facility referral to police, *Ann Emerg Med* 31:488-494,1998.
9. 1 W Blackstone, 1 *Commentaries on the Law of England** (445-446),1765.
10. *State v Rhodes*, 61 NC (Phil Law) 445, 1868.
11. Ross DS: Adult abuse. In Rosen P, et al (editors): *Emergency medicine concepts and clinical practice,* ed 3, St Louis, 1992, Mosby.
12. Appleton W: The battered woman syndrome, *Ann Emerg Med* 9:84-91,1980.
13. Stets JE, Straus MA: Gender differences in reporting marital violence and its medical and psychological consequences. In: Strauss MA, Gelles RJ (editors): *Physical violence in American families: risk factors and adaptations to violence in 8,145 families,* New Brunswick, NJ, 1990, Transaction Publishers.
14. el-Bayoumi G, Borum ML, Haywood Y: Domestic violence in women, *Med Clin North Am* 82:391-401,1998.

15. Goodman PE: Not in my practice: a look at the pervasive consequences of domestic violence, *N C Med J* 58:310-314,1997.
16. AMA: 4 million American women abused annually, *Hosp Health Net* 20:15, 1994.
17. Witt S, Olsen S: Prevalence of domestic violence in the United States, *J Am Med Womens Assoc* 51:71-82, 1996.
18. Kyriacou DN, et al: Emergency department-based study of risk factors for acute injury from domestic violence against women, *Ann Emerg Med* 31:502-506,1998.
19. Brookoff D, et al: Characteristics of participants in domestic violence: assessment at the scene of domestic assault, *JAMA* 277:1369-1373,1997.
20. Ernst AA, et al: Domestic violence in an inner city ED, *Ann Emerg Med* 30:190-197,1997.
21. Goldberg WG, Tomlanovich MC: Domestic violence victims in the emergency department: new findings, *JAMA* 251:3259-3264,1984.
22. Rounsaville B, Weissman MM: Battered women: a medical problem requiring detection, *Int J Psychiatry Med* 8:191-202,1977-1978.
23. Bachman R, Coker AL: Police involvement in domestic violence: the interactive effects of victim injury, offender's history of violence, and race, *Violence Vict* 10:91-106,1995.
24. Koss MP, Koss PG, Woodruff WJ: Deleterious effects of criminal victimization on women's health and medical utilization, *Arch Intern Med* 151:342-347,1991.
25. McCoy M: Domestic violence: clues to victimization, *Ann Emerg Med* 27:764-765,1996.
26. Zachariades N, Koumoura F, Konsolaki-Agouridaki E: Facial trauma in women resulting from violence by men, *J Oral Maxillofac Surg* 48:1250-1253,1990.
27. Gazmararian JA, et al: Prevalence of violence against pregnant women, *JAMA* 275:1915-1920,1996.
28. McFarlane J, et al: Assessing for abuse during pregnancy. Severity and frequency of injuries and associated entry into prenatal care, *JAMA* 267:3176-3178,1992.
29. Bash KL, Jones F: Domestic violence in America, *N C Med J* 55: 400-403,1994.
30. Shadigian EM: Violence against women, *Female Patient* 19:73-80,1994.
31. Wolfe DA, Korsch B: Witnessing domestic violence during childhood and adolescence: implications for pediatric practice, *Pediatrics* 94:594-599,1994.
32. Groves BA, et al: Silent victims: children who witness domestic violence, *JAMA* 269:262-264,1993.
33. Carlson BE: Children's observations of interparental violence. In Roberts AR (editor): *Battered women and their families*, New York, 1984, Springer.
34. Kellermann AL: Domestic violence and the internist's response: advocacy or apathy? *J Gen Intern Med* 5:89-90, 1990.
35. Friedman LS, et al: Inquiry about victimization experiences: a survey of patient preferences and physician practices, *Arch Intern Med* 152:1186-1190,1992
36. Education about adult domestic violence in US and Canadian medical schools, 1987-1988, *MMWR* 38:17-19,1989.
37. Gremillion DH: Should physicians be required to report domestic violence? *N C Med J* 58:320-322,1997.
38. Sugg NK, Inui T: Primary care physician's response to domestic violence: opening Pandora's box, *JAMA* 267:3157-3160,1992.
39. Tilden VP, et al: Factors that influence clinicians' assessment and management of family violence, *Am J Public Health* 84:628-633,1994.
40. Hyman A, Schillinger D, Lo B: Laws mandating reporting of domestic violence: do they promote patient well-being? *JAMA* 273:1781-1787,1995.
41. McCauley J, et al: Clinical characteristics of women with a history of childhood abuse: unhealed wounds, *JAMA* 277:1362-1368,1997.
42. Campbell JC, et al: Battered women's experiences in the emergency department, *J Emerg Nurs* 20:280-288,1994.
43. McLeer SV, Anwar R: A study of battered women presenting in an emergency department, *Am J Public Health* 79:65-66, 1989.

Motor Vehicle Crashes

37

B. TILMAN JOLLY

The traumatic intersection of human and vehicle is the byproduct of society's growing dependence on ever-faster transportation. Although the automobile has revolutionized American life, it is responsible for the majority of traumatic injuries. A typical emergency department (ED) may see dozens of crash victims daily whose injuries range from minimal to life threatening. A physician who understands the mechanisms of injury can provide better care to the wounded. The savvy emergency physician (EP) anticipates certain injuries based on a description of the crash. This knowledge is also vital to improve vehicle and roadway design and modify other aspects of injury prevention.

In 400 BC, Hippocrates described head injury associated with hitting a hard object after a fall (Fig. 37-1). Centuries later, Hugh de Haven suggested advances in crash protection during World War I. He promoted a crash-protective design and championed the benefits of safety equipment to reduce casualties in plane crashes.[1] In the ensuing years, innovations such as seat belts, laminated glass, crumple zones, and air bags have prevented thousands of injuries. These and other changes in vehicle design have markedly changed the patterns of injuries presenting to EDs.

Of the 150,000 persons who die of injuries each year, over 40,000 die in motor vehicle crashes (MVCs). Approximately 32,000 of these victims are vehicle occupants, with the rest divided among pedestrians, bicyclists, and motorcyclists. In addition to automotive mortality, hundreds of thousands more are injured each year.[2] The sheer volume of cases, coupled with the fact that this disease disproportionately affects the young, demands an understanding of injury mechanisms.

PHYSICS

Transfer of kinetic energy from inanimate to animate objects causes injury in MVCs. Because physical laws govern this transfer of energy, several concepts are essential to understand crash dynamics:

- Kinetic Energy: The amount of energy represented by a moving mass. Kinetic Energy = $\frac{1}{2}mv^2$, where m = mass and v = velocity. This relationship explains why increased velocity is more critical to injury than an increase in mass.
- Newton's First Law: A body continues in a state of rest or uniform motion unless an external force causes a change.
- Newton's Second Law: The rate of change of momentum is proportional to the force producing the change. The change takes place in the direction of the applied force.
- Newton's Third Law: To every active force there is always an equal and opposite reactive force.
- Speed: the change in position with respect to time, independent of direction.
- Velocity: The change in position with respect to time in a specified direction (thus a vector quantity).
- Change in Velocity (ΔV): The ΔV can describe the severity of the crash and may be applied to the vehicle or any other object (such as parts of a human body). The change in velocity is measured from the instant of contact with another object to stopping. Multiple impacts can produce multiple different ΔV's. Importantly, the original speed before braking may be well above the ΔV, since the vehicle may slow significantly before impact. Unfortunately, the unbelted occupant continues to travel at the original velocity and experiences a higher ΔV than the car.
- Angular Velocity: Change of rotation with respect to time.
- Acceleration: Change in velocity with respect to time. Measured in feet per second, or more commonly in g's. The acceleration caused by gravity is one g. Negative acceleration in a crash is calculated by the formula: $g = mph^2/(30 \text{ times } s)$ where s = stopping distance in feet. A 30-mile per hour (mph)

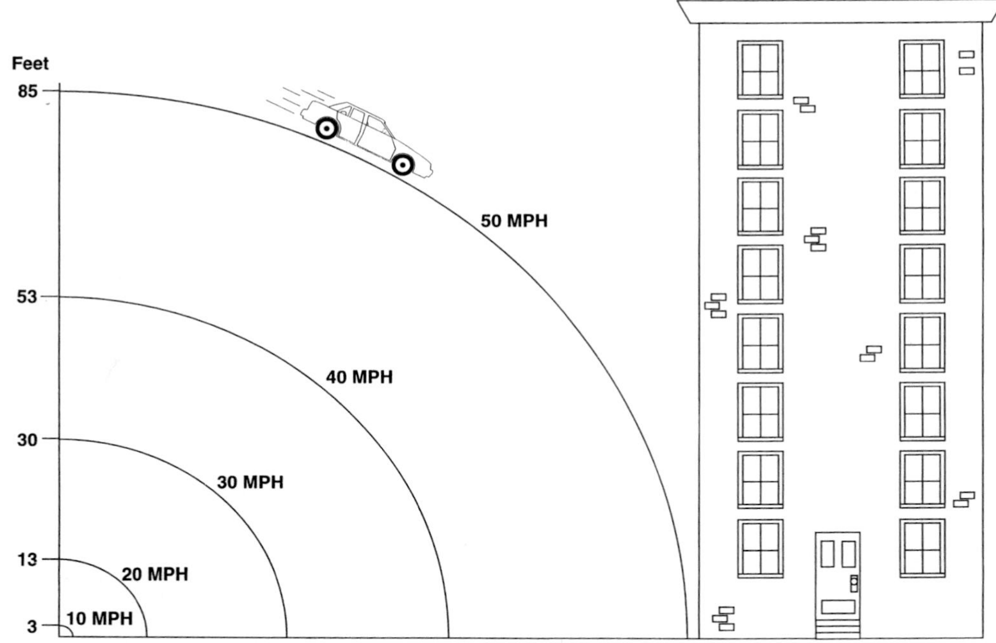

Fig. 37-1 Drop-height equivalents with vehicle miles per hour.

crash into a rigid barrier with a stopping distance (crush) of 2 feet results in a negative acceleration of 15 g.

- Crush: The amount of exterior deformation of the car in a crash. More crush with the same velocity reduces the g forces, and thus reduces the severity of injury.
- Intrusion: The amount of interior deformation in a crash.
- Principal Direction of Force (PDOF): The angle from which one object strikes another. PDOF in a crash is calculated using the vectors traveled by the vehicles along with the point of contact. A vehicle occupant tends to move toward the PDOF.

All of the above concepts are important to understanding crash dynamics and are vital to the science of crash reconstruction. The following sections address specific crash types and typical associated injuries.

CRASH INVESTIGATION

Emergency physicians can use information about the crash to estimate severity of injury and anticipate specific injuries. Knowledge of proper restraint of adults and children allows the EP to recognize errors in restraint use that cause specific injuries.

Professional crash investigators painstakingly examine every detail of a crash scene and the vehicles involved, determining mechanisms of specific injuries and the possibility of defects in materials or systems. This information, when correlated with very specific injury details, provides a better understanding of injury mechanisms. Emergency physicians can use this type of information for clinical decision-making in the ED and in the field.

Scene photography is becoming commonplace in EMS systems. These photographs are now arriving with the patient in the trauma bay. Hunt et al[3] demonstrated that field providers can reliably photograph the scene and depict the area and severity of the crash, even in adverse circumstances. However, these investigators did not use these pictures for clinical decision-making. Unfortunately, physicians not trained in crash investigation may not be able to accurately interpret these pieces of evidence. Ros et al[4] asked EPs to estimate ΔV from standardized photographs. Fewer than 50% were within 10 mph, and 70% overestimated the velocity.

One important area of current investigation involves trauma triage. Standard criteria for trauma center transport include physiologic factors and mechanism of injury. Misuse of these criteria, particularly the mechanism criteria, can result in over-triage and under-triage. Over-triage may occur when the mechanism appears severe, but the patient's injuries are not serious enough to warrant a trauma center. Under-triage may result from personnel on the scene missing clues to severe injury and taking the patient to a hospital that lacks appropriate resources. Better correlation of crash damage and likelihood of injury could reduce both problems.

Jones and Champion[5] used three data sets to attempt to correlate ΔV and vehicle crush with severity of injury. Although recognizing that these data sets are very complex, they recommended that patients be transported to trauma centers from frontal crashes with 20 or more inches of crush, from offset frontal crashes with 28 or more inches of crush, and from side impacts with intrusion of greater than 15 inches. These types of calculations will likely affect future triage criteria in emergency medical services (EMS) systems.

Future technologies may significantly influence triage and care of victims of MVCs. Car sensors combined with computerized wireless communications may permit instant transmission of specific crash location and other information to EMS systems and hospitals. In theory, application of this technology allows earlier localization of events, and transmission of crash-specific information allows dispatch of appropriate EMS response. This information may also affect triage within the trauma system. Video transmission to a medical control officer could assist with triage and on-scene medical care. Some of these technologies are already in place, whereas others are being quickly developed. Two domestic automakers already have cellular crash notification and localization technology available as an option. Proper integration of these advances into EMS systems will be vital in the next decade.

EMERGENCY DEPARTMENT INTERVIEW

The EP should obtain as much information as is clinically appropriate regarding victims of vehicular crashes. In the unstable patient, resuscitation takes precedence over history. The physician should interview medics regarding the condition of the vehicle, amount of vehicular intrusion, seat-belt use, and airbag deployment. Patient ejection is an important historical feature. The ejected occupant is at high risk and should always be considered to have major injuries until proven otherwise. The old saw that it is safer to be thrown clear of the car is simply not true. Ejected trauma victims are among the most horrifically injured.

Instant photographs are perhaps worth a thousand words when describing the incident severity. If the patient is conscious, determine the speed of the crash, point of impact, and other force vectors. Obviously, the medics and patient will provide other valuable information in regards to events preceding the crash, prehospital vital signs, Glasgow Coma Scale, and prehospital interventions.

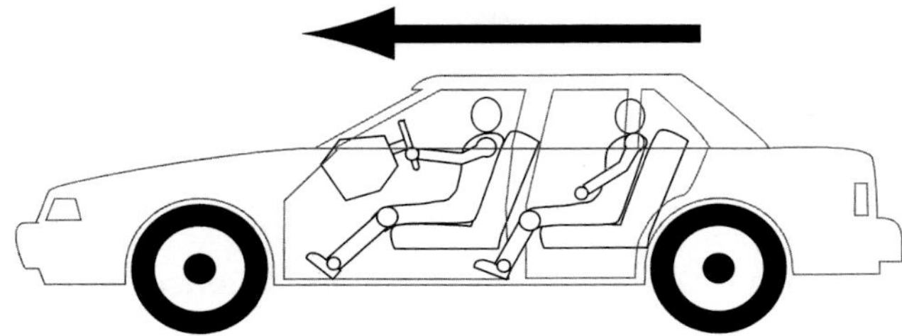

Fig. 37-2 Vehicle in motion.

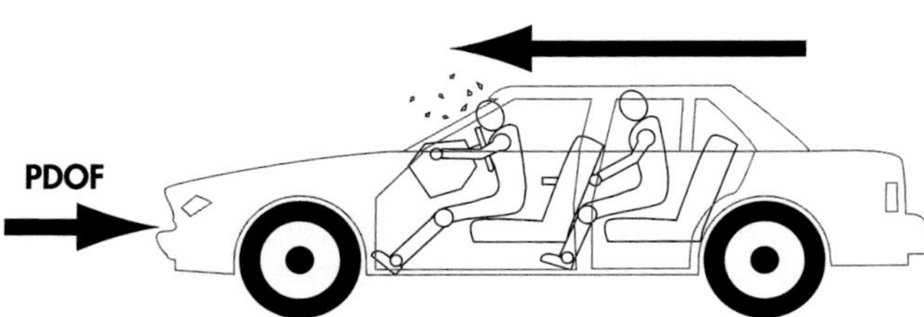

Fig. 37-3 Occupant contact with vehicle.

FRONTAL CRASHES

The frontal crash is the most common type of MVC, and also the type for which the greatest number of safety systems are designed.[1] Air bags, laminated windshields, crush zones, collapsible steering columns, and knee bolsters are designed to protect the vehicle occupant in a frontal crash. Although seat belts provide protection in all types of crashes, their major benefit is to keep occupants from flying forward during a frontal crash.

A MVC consists of three collisions, some of which are not easily apparent. This concept is most easily illustrated during a frontal crash. First, the vehicle strikes an object (Fig. 37-2). The velocity (including directional factors), mass, and rigidity of the objects involved govern the dynamics of this collision. A second collision occurs when the occupant strikes the interior of the vehicle (Fig. 37-3). The timing and severity of this contact relate to the velocity of the vehicle and the occupant and the PDOF of the crash. An occupant tends to move toward the PDOF (Fig. 37-4). Seat belts are a vital factor in the dynamics of the second collision. These restraints allow the occupant to "ride down" the impact, thus lessening the sudden deceleration forces exerted on the body.

The third collision in a crash is internal, and directly causes injuries to the organs involved. The

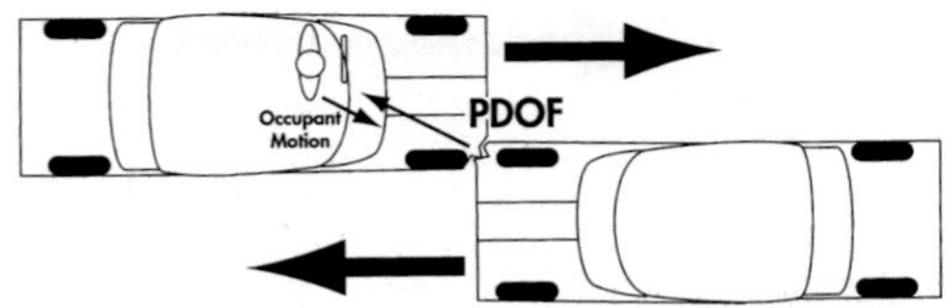

Fig. 37-4 Occupant motion in a frontal offset crash.

brain, intrathoracic organs, and intraabdominal organs decelerate against more rigid structures. Severity of injury depends on forces involved and the tissue characteristics of the individual organs. Brain trauma represents perhaps the most serious injury in frontal crashes. The relationship of focal and diffuse injuries to linear and angular accelerations is complex. Experimentally, crash injury risk to the brain is measured by assessing linear acceleration at the center of gravity of the head. From that number is derived the Head Injury Criterion (HIC). An HIC of 1000 is considered the limit of tolerance and is used for regulatory purposes. Thus all of the features that allow increased stopping distance for the brain, including seat belts, air bags, and vehicle padding, attempt to reduce the HIC, and decrease brain injuries.[1]

Forces on the chest during a crash are also complex. Some investigators have noted a relationship between number of rib fractures and risk of intrathoracic injury. However, rapid loading of the chest may not break ribs but still causes significant pulmonary, cardiac, and vascular injury. Fracture of the ribs dissipates energy, protecting the lungs to some extent. This phenomenon is why children, who have very elastic ribs that easily transmit applied force, are prone to pulmonary contusions. Regulations allow loads as high as 2500 lb during the interaction between chest and steering wheel in a 15-mph test. Crash dummies, which account for the injury tolerance of specific organs, can improve design of vehicle restraint systems and interior structures.[1]

Emergency physicians can anticipate certain injuries based on specific elements of the history obtained from the medics or patient. Certain injuries are characteristic of frontal impacts; others are unique to specific crash conditions. The head and face often strike the roof header or A-pillar (the metal structure between the windshield and the side window). The driver's head hits the A-pillar when the PDOF is near the 11 o'clock position.

Cervical spine injuries are serious sequelae of frontal crashes. Unrestrained occupants move forward and extend the neck after striking the windshield. This extension can be quite dramatic and can produce a "hangman's fracture" of the posterior elements of C2. In contrast, a belted occupant will not typically contact the windshield. Although the head will forcefully flex, the restrained occupant is less likely to sustain serious cervical spine injury.[6]

In the absence of an air bag, a belted driver can still suffer significant head and facial injuries from contact with the steering wheel. Sudden deceleration of the chest into the steering wheel can cause significant chest injuries, most seriously myocardial rupture, aortic disruption, and pulmonary contusion. The seat belt can fracture the sternum in the restrained victim while the steering wheel or dashboard is likely to cause sternal fractures in the unrestrained patient. A number of studies have examined whether sternal fractures signal critical injury. These authors agree that most sternal fractures without clear evidence of other injury do not require extensive workup or monitoring.[7-10]

Posterior hip dislocation is frequent in front seat occupants during frontal crashes. Rosenthal and Coker[11] reviewed 46 patients with this injury. Forty-three were in MVCs, and few, if any, were belted. The mechanism of this injury is direct force on a flexed knee with the hip in flexion. Energy is transmitted down the shaft of the femur as the occupant hits the dashboard. The femoral head is driven down and out of the acetabulum, frequently fracturing the posterior acetabulum. Because of the dramatic forces involved, associated injuries are common. The authors note that 70% of their patients had craniofacial injuries, the average hospital stay was 7 weeks, and no patient with a job that involved standing returned to that position.

Fractures of the lower extremity, particularly below the knee, have come under increasing scrutiny (Fig. 37-5). While representing a low threat to life, ankle and foot injuries can impair standing and walking and thus affect long-term outcome. Mackenzie et al[12] followed a large group of patients with severe isolated lower extremity fractures and found that only 48% returned to work in 6 months. The mechanism of these injuries is still under investigation, but footwell intrusion and brake pedal dynamics play important roles. Although air bags and seat belts reduce head and upper torso trauma, the devices do not reduce lower extremity injury. Interestingly, early investigators noted that women might be at increased risk of lower extremity injury. Dischinger et al[13] examined this question taking into consideration occupant height. These investigators found that shorter occupants, not just females, were at greater risk of lower extremity injury, especially to the foot and ankle. Seat position, leg length, and foot size are all possible factors. Forceful braking may evert the ankle, placing the joint in a vulnerable position for fracture-dislocation. Eversion may also predispose to fracture dislocation of the midfoot, the so-called Lisfranc injury. Future

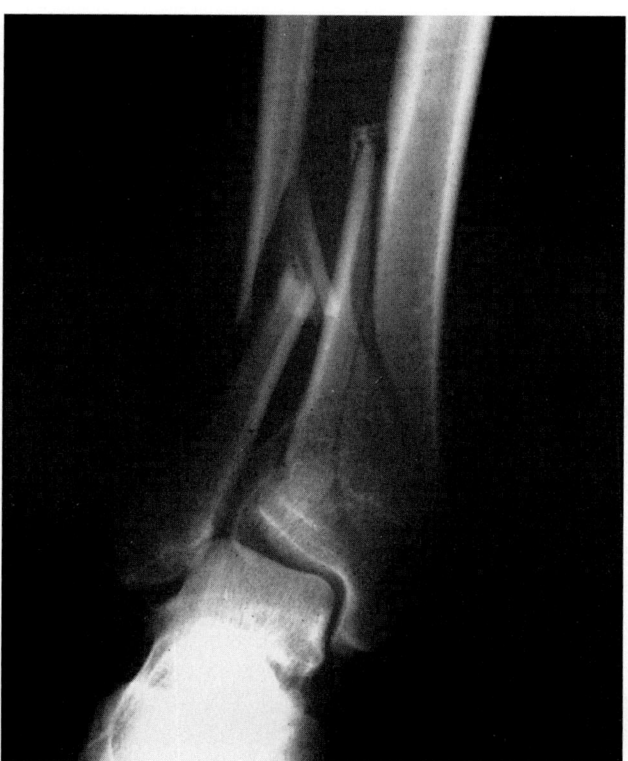

Fig. 37-5 Pilon fracture sustained during forceful braking in frontal crash.

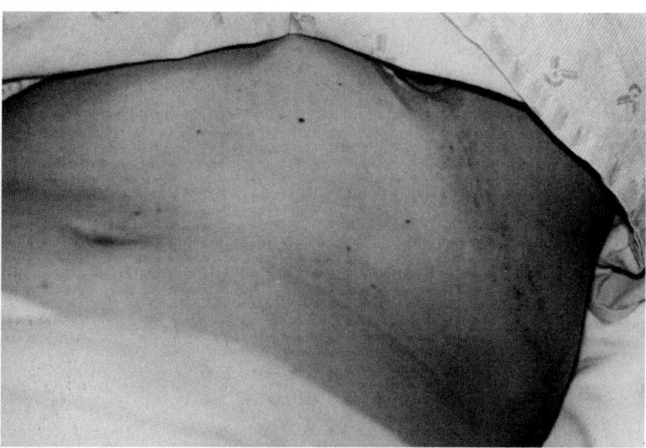

Fig. 37-6 Left upper quadrant seat-belt mark. Patient was a front-seat passenger restrained by only the shoulder belt. She suffered a splenic laceration requiring splenectomy.

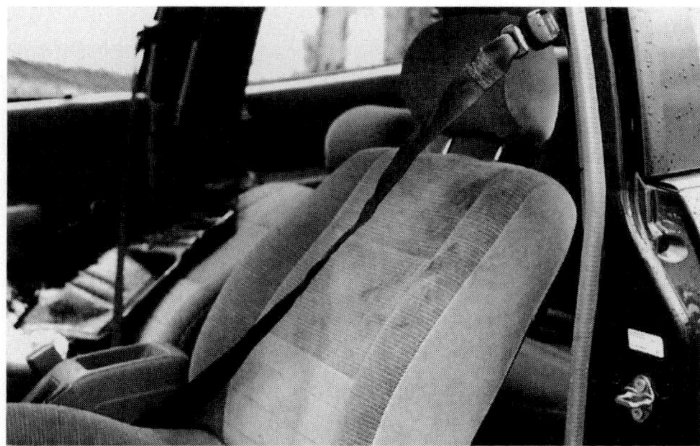

Fig. 37-7 Position of shoulder belt on driver's side of vehicle.

vehicle designs may account for these and other injuries.

SEAT BELTS

Intraabdominal injuries are common in multiple types of impact. Unbelted occupants can sustain almost any injury, frequently catastrophic. Specific types of belts are associated with particular injuries. Some vehicles have automatic shoulder restraints with manual lap belts in the front seat. Approximately 70% of occupants with this type of belt wear only the shoulder restraint.[14] This half-belted practice can result in liver injuries for drivers. In these cases, the liver receives a greater proportion of the energy than it would with three-point restraints. This phenomenon is associated with a PDOF near the 1 o'clock position, which forces the shoulder harness into the right upper quadrant.[15] A front seat passenger wearing only a shoulder restraint may suffer an analogous injury to the spleen. Suspect a liver or spleen injury if there is significant frontal crush and the occupant wore only a shoulder belt and no lap belt (Figs. 37-6 to 37-8).

The original belts in motor vehicles consisted of lap belts. Until recently, lap belts were the only restraints available in the rear seat. Lap belts worn in isolation are associated with lumbar spine fractures and injuries to the small intestine. This pattern of injury relates to the rapid and forceful flexion over the belt, particularly in children. In these cases, the lap belt rides high on the abdomen above the pelvis, creating an axis of flexion on the abdominal wall. One study of 10 children with the lap belt complex of lumbar spine and/or intestinal injuries found that all 10 had seatbelt marks above the pelvis. Lap-belt marks in this position should trigger a search for lumbar spine fractures and occult intestinal injury.[16] These types of injuries are often called "seat-belt syndrome." It is preferable not to use this term, since there are multiple different patterns of injury associated with specific types of seat-belt use and misuse (Figs. 37-9 and 37-10). A "lap-belt syndrome" better describes the constellation of abdominal ecchymosis and intestinal injury with or without a lumbar spine fracture.

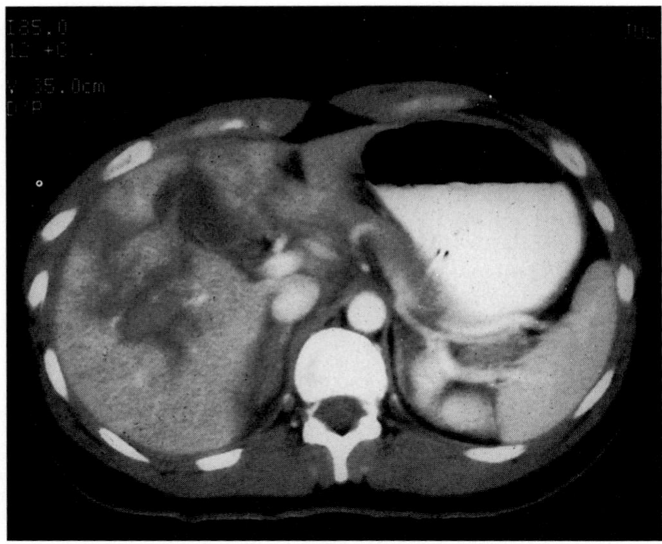

Fig. 37-8 Complex liver laceration in the driver of the car in Fig. 37-7 restrained only by the shoulder belt.

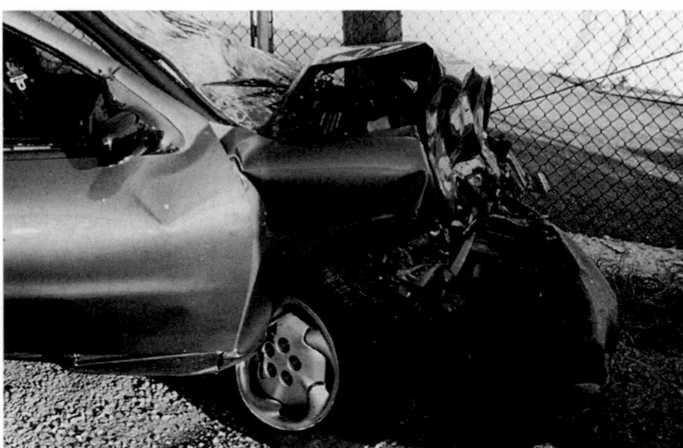

Fig. 37-10 Patient in Fig. 37-9 was in the back seat of this vehicle. Note significant frontal damage.

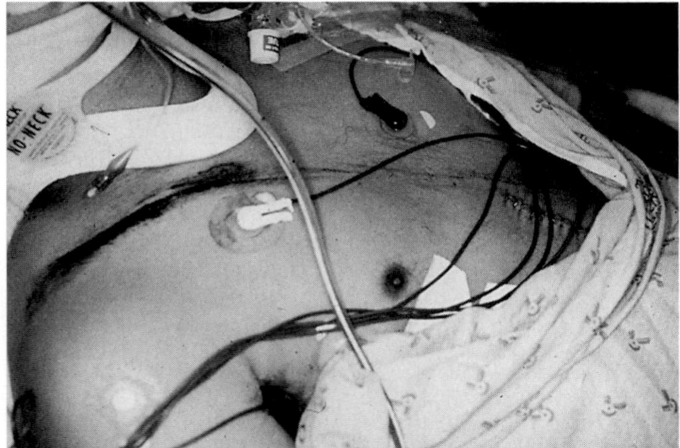

Fig. 37-9 Shoulder-belt mark on patient wearing 3-point restraint. Lap-belt mark not shown. Patient sustained a ruptured left hemidiaphragm in a frontal impact.

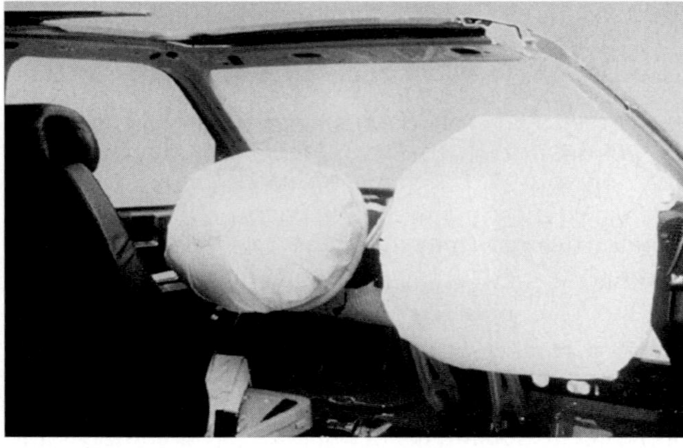

Fig. 37-11 Fully-deployed driver and passenger-side air bags. (Courtesy of the Insurance Institute for Highway Safety.)

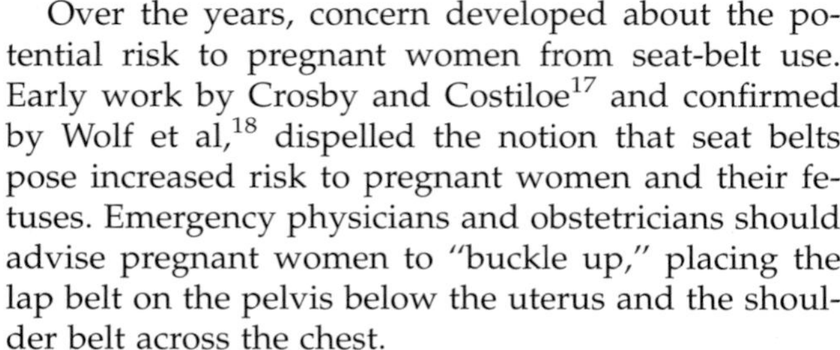

Over the years, concern developed about the potential risk to pregnant women from seat-belt use. Early work by Crosby and Costiloe[17] and confirmed by Wolf et al,[18] dispelled the notion that seat belts pose increased risk to pregnant women and their fetuses. Emergency physicians and obstetricians should advise pregnant women to "buckle up," placing the lap belt on the pelvis below the uterus and the shoulder belt across the chest.

AIR BAGS

Air bags have become an important means of protection for front seat occupants in anterior crashes. The air bag is designed to work as supplemental restraint in frontal crashes (Fig. 37-11). Lack of seat-belt use increases the potential for air bag–related injuries. Air bag deployment is now a common element to consider when caring for patients injured in MVCs. As of model year 1998, driver- and passenger-side air bags are required in every new car sold in the United States. An air bag activates above a preset crash deployment threshold (ΔV). The air bag deploys within milliseconds after a crash, allowing the front seat occupant to decelerate into the device. Optimal protection occurs when the occupant is fully belted (Fig. 37-12).

Injuries and deaths directly related to air bag con-

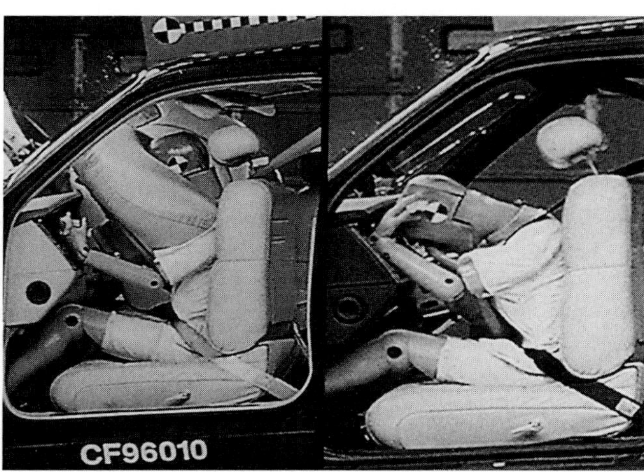

Fig. 37-12 Identical 35 mile per hour crashes. On left, air bag and seat belts. On the right, seat belts alone. (Courtesy of the Insurance Institute for Highway Safety.)

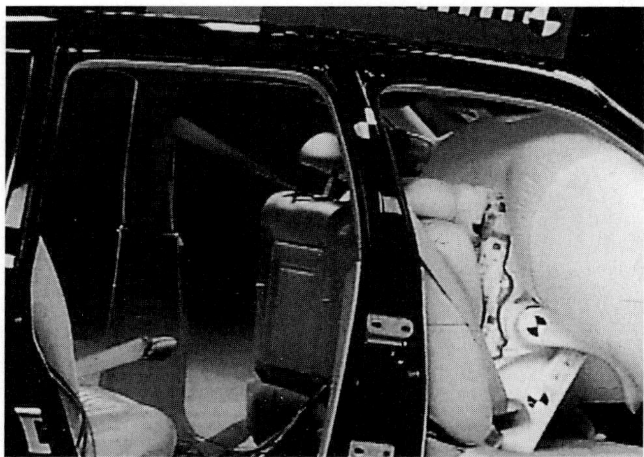

Fig. 37-13 Position of infant and infant seat after impact by air bag in front passenger seat. (Courtesy of the Insurance Institute for Highway Safety.)

tact have occurred. The deaths occur in three general categories. The adult casualties are often unbelted drivers or those slumped over the steering wheel. A second category includes children in the passenger seat, or short adult females in the driver compartment, also mostly unbelted or improperly belted. Both of these types of occupants are subject to preimpact braking. Before impact, braking slows the vehicle, but not the unbelted occupants. The unbelted occupants slide forward on their seats, coming into close proximity to the air bag module. As the air bag deploys at speed approaching 200 mph, it causes lethal head, neck, and chest injuries. The third category of fatal injuries has occurred in infants in rear-facing infant carriers placed in the front seat. In these cases, the infant's head is in such close proximity to the air bag module that death is almost inevitable (Fig. 37-13).

Nonlethal air bag injuries are also common in the ED. Patients may describe "smoke" filling the car after deployment, raising concern about burns. This "smoke" is most commonly powder that is used to coat the surface of the bag to reduce sticking. Some complain of abrasions from contact with the nylon surface of the bag. Burns to the hands occur if the hot chemicals in the bag vent directly onto the hands. Eye injuries include corneal abrasions and burns, as well as retinal detachments and globe ruptures.[19-24] When the driver's arm is held across the steering wheel during deployment, upper extremity fractures can ensue.[25-27] The air bags can also rupture the tympanic membrane.

ANTI-LOCK BRAKES

One recent advance in engineering includes anti-lock brakes. These brakes were designed to reduce skidding and allow drivers to maintain control of vehicles during braking. Theoretically, anti-lock brakes would reduce injury by avoiding crashes. However, studies have not demonstrated an appreciable reduction in injuries. Part of this problem may be as a result of drivers who do not understand how to apply these brakes, which should not be pumped. During surveys, as many as 50% percent of drivers describe incorrect use of these brakes.[28]

SIDE IMPACTS

The second-most common type of crash is side impact ("T-bone"). Approximately 32% to 34% of police-reported crashes are initially side impact, and in 30% of vehicle occupant deaths the primary impact is on the side.[29] Dischinger et al[30] compared injuries among drivers who were victims of frontal and lateral crashes. Drivers over 55 years of age experienced a greater risk of side impact crashes. Investigators also found that injuries to the face and lower extremities were more common in frontal impacts, whereas injuries to the chest, abdomen, and pelvis were more common in left lateral impacts. The mortality rate was higher in the lateral impacts despite the fact that there was no difference in the Injury Severity Score (ISS). This disparity might be explained by the underweighing of severity of injury by ISS that occurs when there are multiple injuries to one body region.

Side impacts make injuries to the torso more likely. As the point of impact is typically directed toward the pelvis or abdomen, anticipate injuries in those regions, particularly to the spleen in a driver or the liver in a front-seat passenger. The head or neck may be injured because of lateral bending of the neck and secondary contact of the head on the striking car (Fig. 37-14). Unbelted occupants may directly injure other occupants as they are thrown across the car.

Farmer et al[29] used a national database to analyze risk of injury in side impacts. Near-side occupants (on the side of the crash) of cars are more likely to be injured than near-side occupants of trucks. However, the far-side occupant in a truck is at greater risk than the far-side occupant of a car. Intrusion plays a great role in injury, particularly to near-side occupants. When there was at least 6 inches of intrusion, occupants seated adjacent to the impact had a 16% risk of significant injury.

The occupant being struck from the side receives less protection from the vehicle than in any other type of collision. Depending on the rigidity of the side of the car, the near-side occupant is subject to a ΔV that approaches the impact speed of the striking vehicle. The best solution for protection in side crashes lies in improving rigidity and padding to doors and frames. This solution increases the effective ride-down distance for the occupant. Although a seat belt has a very small benefit for near-side occupants, seat belts reduce the impact with other occupants or structures in the car, and decrease the risk of ejection.[31]

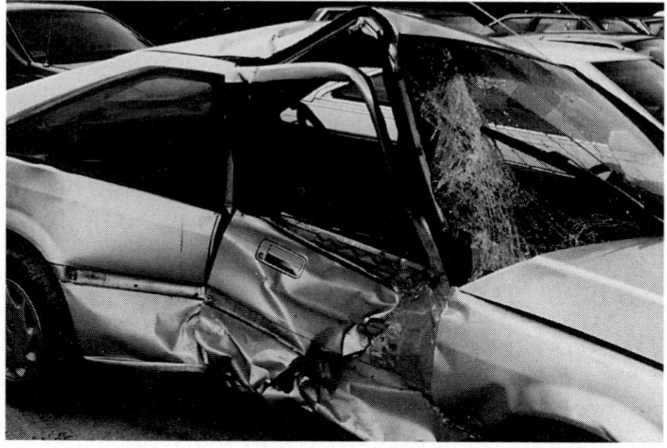

Fig. 37-14 The unbelted driver of this vehicle crossed to the passenger side and sustained a cervical spine fracture.

Side-impact air bags are now becoming part of the auto fleet. Some models deploy from the door or the seat to protect the principal points of impact, the torso and pelvis. Others deploy from the B-pillar (between the two windows), and one model deploys from the roof header (above the window) and remains inflated for a prolonged period. These devices protect the head from the common secondary impact. The overall effect of these devices remains unknown.

REAR-END CRASHES

The rear-end crash is a common mechanism of injury, particularly in heavily congested urban areas. Often one vehicle is stopped at a traffic light and is struck at low-to-moderate speed by another vehicle. Severe rear-end collisions can have devastating effects. Severity of injury is related to restraint use and influenced by design issues such as headrest placement and seat stiffness.

A high-speed rear-end crash will often occur to a parked car, often in poor visibility on a roadside. The unrestrained occupant will "ramp up" the seat and be projected back toward the PDOF (Fig. 37-15).[32] The head and neck can be injured by contact with the roof and objects in the rear of the car. The seat may initially extend backwards, and then spring forwards, slamming the victim against the dash. If the impact is severe enough, the seat back may fail, putting the occupant in a vulnerable position.

In a rear-end collision, the victim's neck will first extend, then flex.[33] A secondary frontal crash may also occur as the car is thrown forward. In this case the occupant may be in a far forward position at impact, and thus exposed to increased risk of injury.

The term *whiplash* is commonly used to describe the cervical strain associated with mild-to-moderate severity rear-end crashes. This term is nonspecific. Extension-flexion injury more appropriately describes

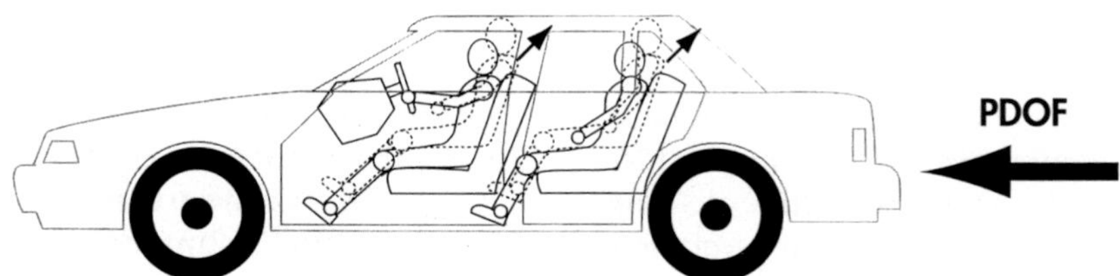

Fig. 37-15 Unbelted occupant motion up and out of seats during rear impact.

the mechanism leading to cervical pain. At impact, the neck extends over the seat back. An appropriately placed headrest may arrest this extension. However, 90% of the time the headrest is in an unfavorable position.[34] The head rebounds and the neck flexes, suddenly stretching the cervical soft tissues. Patients may complain of neck pain, headache, dizziness, and nausea, and cervical films may be negative, or demonstrate only loss of lordosis. The mechanism of this injury and its relationship to diagnosis and outcome are perplexing questions that affect a large proportion of patients injured in MVCs. There is little agreement regarding diagnosis, treatment, outcomes, or the contribution of psychologic and litigation factors for this condition.[35,36]

ROLLOVER CRASHES

Rollovers are the most random and unpredictable of crashes. Ninety percent of rollovers occur off the roadway. Unless there is a single defining impact, such as with a wall, the energy of the crash is dissipated over many minor impacts. This gradual energy dissipation reduces the injury risk of a rollover, assuming that the occupant is not ejected from the vehicle.[1] However, higher speed increases the number of rolls and the number of peak decelerations of the vehicle and increases the chances for occupant injury.[37]

Most rollovers begin when a wheel goes off road, and the driver tries to quickly maneuver back. The car begins to slide and trips over its tires and rolls to the side. The aspect of the rollover most closely related to injury risk is the severity of car-to-ground impacts, not necessarily the quantity of those impacts.[38]

Crash investigators or field providers may report that during a rollover, the roof "came down," hitting the occupant and, causing injury. They may also report that the occupant was trapped between the roof and the seat during the roll. These common theories imply that increasing roof strength of cars will decrease the risk of occupant injury. These misconceptions were tested by Orlowski et al[38] by testing standard roofs against roll cage–reinforced roofs in rollover tests. While the vehicle roll dynamics differed between roof types, there was no correlation with damage to the crash-test dummies. During the roll, the dummies moved out from the center of gravity of the vehicle and hit the roof and upper door. They lost contact with the seat and remained in this position throughout the roll. Orientation of the dummy and the ΔV of the vehicle influenced neck injury. Roll-caged roofs offered no increased protection and there was no correlation between roof deformity and injury.

In a rollover, centrifugal force may drive the patient headfirst into the roof. Thus anticipate head and neck injuries from axial loading. These injuries may include burst fractures of the spine, such as the Jefferson fracture of C1. Extremities suffer significant injuries if they protrude through windows or the windshield.

PEDIATRIC CONSIDERATIONS

Although acute care of injured children is discussed elsewhere in this text, the EP should understand child occupant restraints to appreciate injury risk. A 15-pound child held in a passenger's arms in a 30-mph crash effectively becomes a 300-pound projectile. All children traveling in motor vehicles must be appropriately restrained.

The basic principle of child restraint is the same as for adults: link the occupant to the vehicle. Restraints allow the occupant to "ride down" the crash forces and avoid ejection. Infants, toddlers, and children all require different types of restraints based on height, weight, and age. Children under 12 years of age should always ride in the back seat—back seat occupants are 30% less likely to suffer injury. This rule becomes especially important as passenger air bags enter the vehicle fleet.

Infants less than 1 year old and less than 20 pounds should ride in rear-facing infant seats buckled into a back seat. The rear-facing seat is designed to protect the neck from severe flexion forces normally experienced in a frontal crash. Between 20 and 40 pounds, children should be placed in forward-facing child seats. From 40 pounds to about 60 pounds (until the seat belts fit), children should ride in booster seats.

All states have laws mandating child restraint. Unfortunately, 12% of infants and 30% of toddlers are unrestrained.[39] Roadside checks also typically show that 80% to 90% of the restrained children are improperly restrained. Graham et al[40] documented pediatric injuries related to safety seat misuse. Errors included: harness not strapped around child; improper restraint device; child seat not attached to the automobile; and restraint misuse without a collision. Newer attachment mechanisms may correct some of the problems associated with loosely tethered seats. Emergency physicians should inquire about restraint and anticipate more severe injuries in unrestrained and poorly restrained children.

AUTO-PEDESTRIAN CRASHES

In the United States, pedestrians are second to vehicle occupants in numbers of annual motor vehicle deaths; 6000 to 7000 pedestrians die each year after being struck by cars.[41] However, in other parts of the world, of the 500,000 annual traffic deaths, at least half are pedestrians.[1] Several groups are at high risk. Pedes-

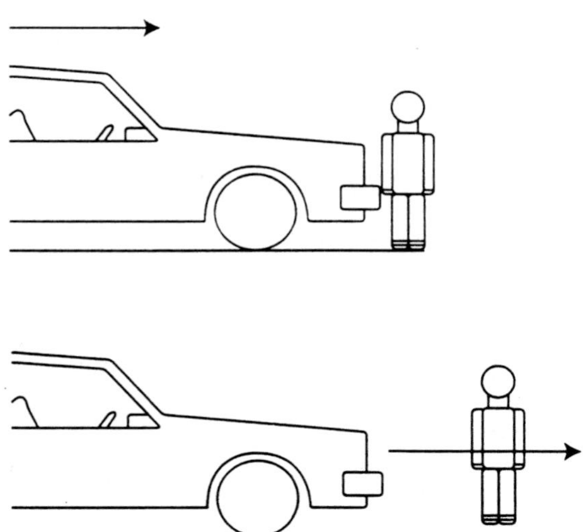

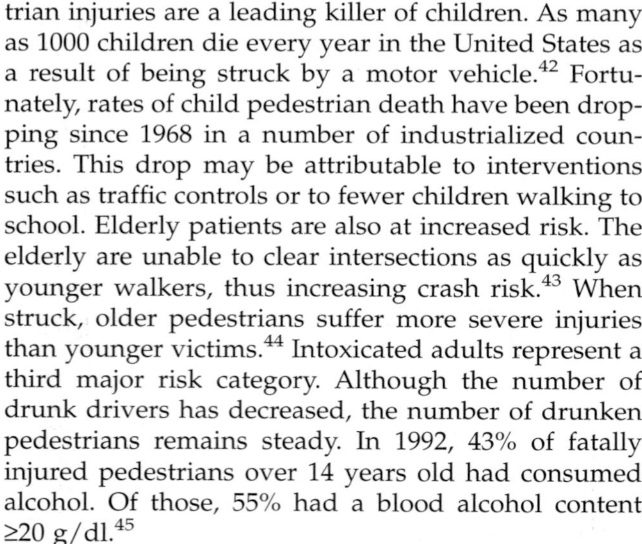

Fig. 37-16 Primary impact with small pedestrian with neutral center of gravity. Initial impact at pelvis and patient pushed forward. (Used with permission of the American College of Emergency Physicians.)

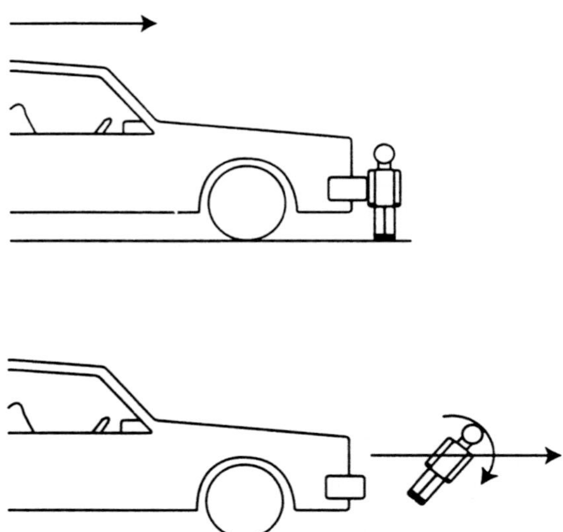

Fig. 37-17 Primary impact with toddler, above the center of gravity. Initial impact on chest with potential for being "run over." (Used with permission of the American College of Emergency Physicians.)

trian injuries are a leading killer of children. As many as 1000 children die every year in the United States as a result of being struck by a motor vehicle.[42] Fortunately, rates of child pedestrian death have been dropping since 1968 in a number of industrialized countries. This drop may be attributable to interventions such as traffic controls or to fewer children walking to school. Elderly patients are also at increased risk. The elderly are unable to clear intersections as quickly as younger walkers, thus increasing crash risk.[43] When struck, older pedestrians suffer more severe injuries than younger victims.[44] Intoxicated adults represent a third major risk category. Although the number of drunk drivers has decreased, the number of drunken pedestrians remains steady. In 1992, 43% of fatally injured pedestrians over 14 years old had consumed alcohol. Of those, 55% had a blood alcohol content ≥20 g/dl.[45]

The mechanism of injury of pedestrians depends on the relationship between the body characteristics of the pedestrian and the geometry of the vehicle. The bumper of a typical passenger vehicle will strike the adult pedestrian in the upper tibia. The victim will rotate onto the front of the vehicle, hitting his or her pelvis on the hood. Depending on the speed of the vehicle and the height of the pedestrian, the patient's head will subsequently strike the hood or windshield. The victim is then thrown to the ground in an unpredictable fashion. Thus most pedestrians are "run under," not "run over" (Figs. 37-16 to 37-18).[30]

This mechanism mostly injures the lower extremities. Lane et al[46] analyzed 65 passenger car (PCS) collisions with pedestrians and 133 light truck and van (LTV) collisions with pedestrians—all of which led to injury. The initial contact with the vehicle was frontal in 90% of the fatal cases and 75% of the nonfatal cases. The PCS cases had a significantly higher number of lower extremity injuries, resulting from contact with the bumper. The LTV cases had a higher incidence of chest and abdominal injuries, resulting from initial contact with the higher front ends of these vehicles. Among the fatalities, serious head injuries were present over 80% of the time. In the PCS cases, the head most frequently contacted the windshield and frame or hood after the pedestrian's body wrapped over the front of the car. In the LTV cases, the pedestrian was most commonly projected forward, causing the head to strike the ground.

Brainard et al[47] reviewed 185 consecutive cases of pedestrians struck, of whom 25 died. The most common fracture site was the tibia-fibula, and 62% of these were open. Forty-nine percent of patients with a femur fracture had an accompanying pelvis fracture, and 44% of those died. Twenty-three of the patients sustained ipsilateral upper and lower extremity fractures, which the authors termed the *ipsilateral dyad*.

Knowledge of these mechanisms can aid the EP in caring for the pedestrian struck. Ask the field providers about the circumstances of the crash, the type of vehicle involved, the impact speed, and the distance the victim was thrown. Remember that the severity of injury is strongly related to the impact speed, but less directly for ground contacts.[1] Patients will frequently arrive with dramatic lower extremity injuries. Al-

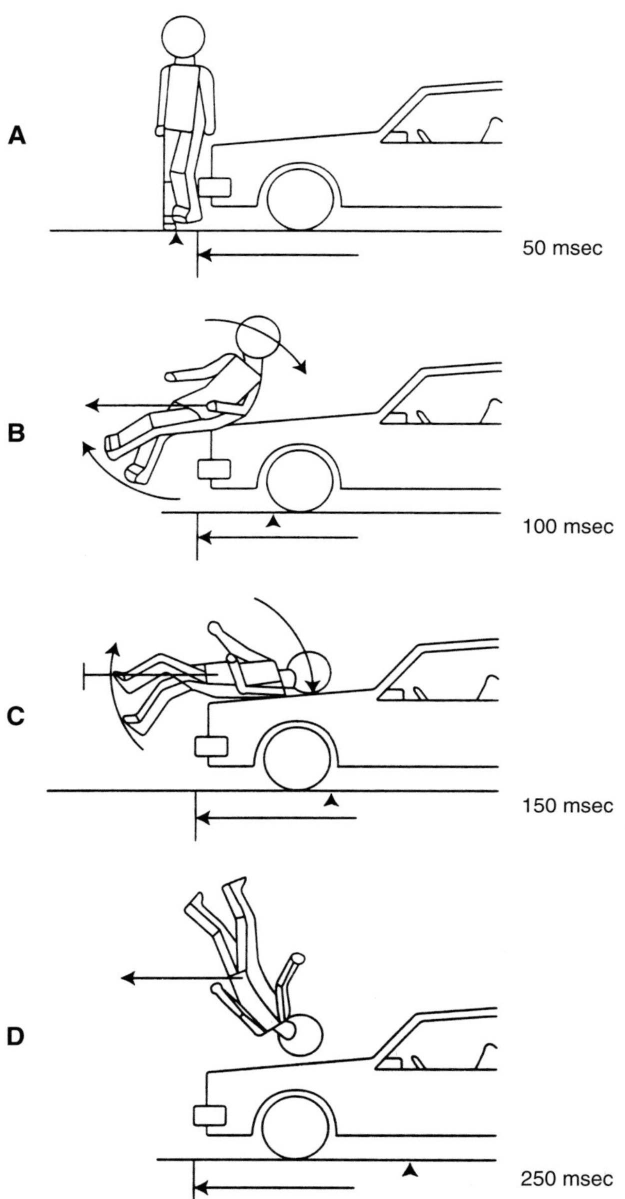

Fig. 37-18 Multiple impacts involving adult struck below the center of gravity. **A,** Primary impact: bumper-lower leg. **B,** Secondary impact: grill edge–pelvis. **C,** Tertiary impact: hood-craniocervical area. **D,** Quaternary impact. (With permission of the American College of Emergency Physicians.)

though these injuries can be debilitating, they are rarely life threatening. Look for the more serious head, chest, and abdominal injuries, using information about the speed of impact and geometry of the vehicle to guide diagnostic decisions. Anticipate upper extremity injuries on the same side as lower extremity injuries.

MOTORCYCLES

Motorcyclists share the highway speed of vehicle occupants without the safety afforded by a protective metal cage. Add to this risk the inherent instability of a two-wheeled vehicle, and it is not difficult to understand why motorcycles have a death rate per 100 million miles of personal travel 35 times that of cars.[48] The frequency of brain death among injured drivers has won this vehicle the morbid appellation of "donor-cycle." The injury patterns of motorcyclists depend on the forces of impact and are heavily influenced by protective gear, particularly helmets.

Motorcyclists who sustain frontal impacts into vehicles are usually thrown forward into those vehicles. Their leading surface is typically the head. After the rider leaves the cycle, the rider's trajectory and subsequent injuries are often unpredictable. What is known, however, is the clear protective effect of motorcycle helmets. Studies of helmet use[49] and helmet use laws[50,51] demonstrate a major decrease in injuries and improved outcomes associated with helmets. For some years, there was concern about potential increases in spinal cord injury because of helmets. This myth has been dispelled. Orsay et al[52] demonstrated no significant change in spinal cord injury with helmet use, and he confirmed that helmets significantly decreased head injury.

Passenger vehicles can also strike riders from the side. The initial impact will crush the lower extremity between the vehicle bumper and the motorcycle. Riders may also "lay down" their bikes to avoid contact with objects or simply after losing control. Without protective clothing, the abrasions resulting from contact between skin and roadway is extensive and severe.

OTHER MOTORIZED VEHICLES

Other motorized vehicles carry specific risks. Motorbikes are popular in certain areas, particularly in tourist resorts and in Europe. One study from Bermuda[53] examined injuries and found frequent abrasions and fractures. Head injuries were much less common, probably as a result of a strict helmet law on the island. The most common mechanism of injury was simply losing control of the bike; striking a fixed object or another vehicle was less common.

Medical research may occasionally lead to a change in federal law. One regulatory success in injury prevention regards all-terrain vehicles (ATVs). Krane et al[54] examined the circumstances of 23 patients admitted after ATV crashes; 10 of the patients were under 16 years old, and only 2 of the 23 patients had helmets. Three-wheel ATVs were most commonly involved, and rollovers and collisions were the most frequent mechanisms of injuries. Three-wheeled ATVs with balloon tires had a particular tendency to overturn. By 1987 ATVs had caused 900 deaths. In 1988, medical reports of this carnage prompted a ban on the sale of new three-wheel ATVs in the United States. However, four-wheel ATVs are still on the market and remain dangerous, particularly when operated by inexperienced drivers.[55]

BICYCLES

Bicycling is not only a popular recreational activity but is used for commuting and primary employment. Each year in the United States there are 800 deaths and 500,000 ED visits for bicycling-related injuries.[41] Although bicyclists do not typically develop the speed of motorcyclists, they are exposed to similar injuries as motorcyclists and benefit from similar safety equipment, especially helmets.

Bicyclists can be injured after contact with a moving object (motor vehicle), a stationary object (tree or parked car), or after a fall. The most common injuries, other than contusions and abrasions, are those to the shoulder joint. These injuries include acromioclavicular separations and glenohumeral dislocations.[56] Although the most common mechanism of injury for cyclists is a fall from loss of balance, clearly the most severe is impact with a moving vehicle.[57]

As with motorcyclists, the most severe trauma in a collision with a motor vehicle occurs with the initial impact. Depending on the geometry and speed of the vehicle, the second major impact may occur with the car or with the ground. Cyclists can become airborne and can travel great distances before hitting the ground.

As is the case with motorcycles, helmets reduce the severity of brain injury, which is the most potentially severe sequelae.[58,59] Rivara et al[60] studied off-road cyclists, who have a higher injury rate than other cyclists. However, because of 80% helmet use, these cyclists have a much lower rate of serious brain injury.

INJURY PREVENTION

Emergency physicians are in a unique position to educate the individuals regarding injury prevention. After suffering the physical and emotional trauma of a crash, victims may be at their most susceptible to advice. The cyclist is apt to agree to future helmet use after receiving a laceration to the forehead. Likewise, a broken jaw is likely to inspire future seat-belt use in a motorist, especially if reinforced by the physician. Written discharge instructions for particular injuries may include counseling on injury prevention.

CONCLUSION

Information about mechanism of injury can assist the EP to care for victims of vehicular crashes. Paramedics use this information to determine the most appropriate destination hospital. Physicians must understand both Newtonian principles and common injury patterns to anticipate occult trauma in an individual patient. In the future, this union of medicine and physics will guide injury control strategies, EMS system design, and ED care.

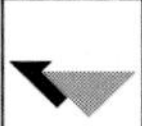

PEARLS & PITFALLS

- Emergency physicians can anticipate certain injuries based on specific elements of the history obtained from the medics or patient.
- Have the patient or medics describe the point of impact, seat belt use, air bag deployment, vehicular intrusion, and other aspects of the crash.
- Even a small amount of intrusion in a direct lateral impact carries significant injury risk.
- Ejection marks a significant mechanism of injury, often associated with multiple trauma.
- Suspect a liver or spleen injury if there is significant frontal crush and the occupant wore only a shoulder belt and no lap belt.
- Injuries to the face and lower extremities are more common in frontal impacts, whereas injuries to the chest, abdomen, and pelvis are more common in lateral impacts.
- A "lap-belt syndrome" describes the constellation of abdominal ecchymosis and intestinal injury, with or without a lumbar spine fracture. The intestinal injury is often occult.
- In bicyclists, the most common injuries, other than contusions and abrasions, are those to the shoulder joint.
- Use discharge instructions to educate all victims of vehicular crashes regarding seat belts, helmets, and child restraints.

REFERENCES

1. Mackay M: Engineering in accidents: vehicle design and injuries, *Injury* 25:615-621, 1994.
2. National Center for Health Statistics: *Health, United States 1996-97 and injury,* Hyattsville, MD, 1997, Chartbook.

3. Hunt RC, et al: Photographic documentation of motor vehicle damage by EMTs at the scene: a prospective multicenter study in the United States, *Am J Emerg Med* 15:233-239, 1997.
4. Ros SP, et al: Can emergency physicians correlate between vehicle damage and velocity change? *Ped Emerg Care* 11:277-279, 1995.
5. Jones IS, Champion HR: Trauma triage: vehicle damage as an estimate of injury severity, *J Trauma* 29:646-653, 1989.
6. Viano DC: Causes and control of spinal cord injury in automobile crashes, *World J Surg* 16:410-419, 1992.
7. Hills MW, Delprado AM, Deane SA: Sternal fractures: associated injuries and management, *J Trauma* 35:55-60, 1993.
8. Roy-Shipara A, Levi I, Khoda J: Sternal fractures: a red flag or a red herring? *J Trauma* 37:59-61, 1994.
9. Wojcik JB, Morgan AS: Sternal fractures: the natural history, *Ann Emerg Med* 17:912-914, 1988.
10. Wright SW: Myth of the dangerous sternal fracture, *Ann Emerg Med* 22:1589-1592, 1993.
11. Rosenthal RE, Coker WL: Posterior fracture-dislocation of the hip: an epidemiologic review, *J Trauma* 19:572-581, 1979.
12. MacKenzie EJ, et al: Physical impairment and functional outcomes six months after severe lower extremity fractures, *J Trauma* 34:528-539, 1993.
13. Dischinger PC, Kerns TJ, Kufera JA: Lower extremity fractures in motor vehicle collisions: the role of driver gender and height, *Accid Anal Prev* 27:601-606, 1995.
14. Reinfurt DW, St.Cyr CL, Hunter WW: Usage patterns and misuse rates of automatic seat belts by system type, *Accid Anal Prev* 23:521-530, 1991.
15. 39th Annual Proceedings of the Association for the Advancement of Automotive Medicine 39:193-212, 1995.
16. Newman KD, et al: The lap-belt complex: intestinal and lumbar spine injury in children, *J Trauma* 30:1133-1140, 1990.
17. Crosby WM, Costiloe JP: Safety of lap-belt restraint for pregnant victims of automobile collisions, *N Engl J Med* 284:632-636, 1971.
18. Wolf ME, et al A retrospective cohort study of seatbelt use and pregnancy outcome after a motor vehicle crash, *J Trauma* 34:116-119, 1993.
19. Campbell JK: Automobile air bag eye injuries, *Nebr Med J* 78: 306-307, 1993.
20. Duma SM, et al: Airbag-induced eye injuries: a report of 25 cases, *J Trauma* 41:114-119, 1996.
21. Gault JA, et al: Ocular injuries associated with eyeglass wear and airbag inflation, *J Trauma* 38:494-497, 1995.
22. Larkin GL: Airbag-mediated corneal injury, *Am J Emerg Med* 9:444-446, 1991.
23. Onwuzuruigbo CJ, et al: Traumatic blindness after airbag deployment: bilateral lenticular dislocation, *J Trauma* 40:314-316, 1996.
24. Sastry SM, et al: Retinal hemorrhage secondary to airbag-related ocular trauma, *J Trauma* 38:582, 1995.
25. Freedman EL, Safran MR, Meals RA: Automotive airbag-related upper extremity injuries: a report of three cases, *J Trauma* 38:577-581, 1995.
26. Huelke DF, et al: Upper extremity injuries related to airbag deployment, *J Trauma* 38:482-488, 1995.
27. Marco F, et al: Bilateral Smith fracture of the radius caused by airbag deployment, *J Trauma* 40:663-664, 1996.
28. Insurance Institute for Highway Safety: Antilocks may not make the difference that many expected, *Status Report* 29(2):1-5, 1994.
29. Farmer CM, Braver ER, Mitter EL: Two-vehicle side impact crashes: the relationship of vehicle and crash characteristics to injury severity, *Accid Anal Prev* 29:399-406, 1997.
30. Dischinger PC, Cushing BM, Kerns TJ: Injury patterns associated with direction of impact: drivers admitted to trauma centers, *J Trauma* 35:454-458, 1993.
31. Mackay M: Mechanisms of injury and biomechanics: vehicle design and crash performance, World *J Surg* 16:420-427, 1992.
32. Viano DC: Restraint of a belted or unbelted occupant by the seat in rear-end impacts. 36th Stapp Car Crash Conference, SAE 922522, Seattle WA, 1992.
33. Mackay M: A review of the biomechanics of impacts in road accidents. In Ambrosio JAC, et al (editors): *Crashworthiness of transportation systems: structural impact and occupant protection*, Netherlands, 1997, Kluwer Academic Publishers.
34. Viano DC, Gargan MF: Headrest position during normal driving: implications to neck injury risks in rear crashes, *39th Annual Proceedings of the Association for the Advancement of Automotive Medicine* 39:215-229, 1995.
35. Hammacher ER, van der Werken C: Acute neck sprain: "whiplash" reappraised, *Injury* 27:463-466, 1996.
36. Mayou R, Bryant B: Outcome of "whiplash" neck injury, *Injury* 27:617-623, 1996.
37. Moffatt EA: Occupant motion in rollover collisions, Proceedings of the 19th Conference of the Association for the Advancement of Automotive Medicine 19:49-58, 1975.
38. Orlowski KF, Bundorf RT, Moffatt EA: *Rollover crash tests: the influence of roof strength on injury mechanics*, Washington, DC, 1985, Society of Automotive Engineers 851734.
39. National Center for Statistics and Analysis: *Traffic safety facts 1995: children*, Washington, DC, 1995, National Highway Traffic Safety Administration.
40. Graham CJ, Kittredge D, Stuemky JH: Injuries associated with child safety seat misuse, *Ped Emerg Care* 8:351-353, 1992.
41. Rivara FP, Grossman DC, Cummings P: Injury prevention: first of two parts, *N Engl J Med* 337:543-548, 1997.
42. Agran PF, et al: The role of the physical and traffic environment in child pedestrian injuries, *Pediatrics* 98:1096-1103, 1996.
43. Hoxie RE, Rubenstein LZ: Are older pedestrians allowed enough time to cross intersections safely? *J Am Geriatr Soc* 42: 241-244, 1994.
44. Kong LB, et al: Pedestrian-motor vehicle trauma: an analysis of injury profiles by age, *J Am Coll Surg* 182:17-23, 1996.
45. CDC: Alcohol involvement in pedestrian fatalities-United States 1982-1992, *MMWR* 42:716-719, 1993.
46. Lane PL, McClafferty KJ, Nowak ES: Pedestrians in real world collisions, *J Trauma* 36:231-236, 1994.
47. Brainard BJ, Slauterbeck J, Benjamin JB: Fracture patterns and mechanisms in pedestrian motor-vehicle trauma: the ipsilateral dyad, *J Orthop Trauma* 6:279-282, 1992.
48. Baker SP, et al: *The injury fact book*, ed 2, New York, 1992, Oxford University Press.
49. Offner PJ, Rivara FP, Maier RV: The impact of motorcycle helmet use, *J Trauma* 32:636-642, 1992.
50. Muelleman RL, Mlinek EJ, Collicott PE: Motorcycle crash injuries and costs: effect of a reenacted comprehensive helmet use law, *Ann Emerg Med* 21:266-272, 1992.
51. Sosin DM, Sacks JJ, Holmgreen P: Head injury-associated deaths from motorcycle crashes: relationship to helmet-use laws, *JAMA* 264:2395-2399, 1990.
52. Orsay EM, et al: Motorcycle helmets and spinal injuries: dispelling the myth, *Ann Emerg Med* 23:802-806, 1994.
53. Carey MJ, Aitken ME: Motorbike injuries in Bermuda: a risk for tourists, *Ann Emerg Med* 28:424-429, 1996.
54. Krane BD, et al: All-terrain vehicle injuries: a review at a rural level II trauma center, *Am Surg* 54:471-474, 1988.

55. Dolan MA, Knapp JF, Andres J: Three-wheel and four-wheel all-terrain vehicle injuries in children, *Pediatrics* 84:694-698, 1989.
56. Nekomoto JS, et al: Bicycle couriers: a unique injury risk group, 41st Annual Proceedings of the Association for the Advancement of Automotive Medicine 41:157-168, 1997.
57. Weiss BD: Bicycle-related head injuries, *Clin Sports Med* 13:99-112, 1994.
58. Spaite DW, et al: A prospective analysis of injury severity among helmeted and nonhelmeted bicyclists involved in collisions with motor vehicles, *J Trauma* 31:1510-1516, 1991.
59. Thompson DC, Rivara FP, Thompson RS: Effectiveness of bicycle safety helmets in preventing head injuries: a case-control study, *JAMA* 276;1968-1973, 1996.
60. Rivara FP, et al: Injuries involving off-road cycling, *J Fam Pract* 44:481-485, 1997.

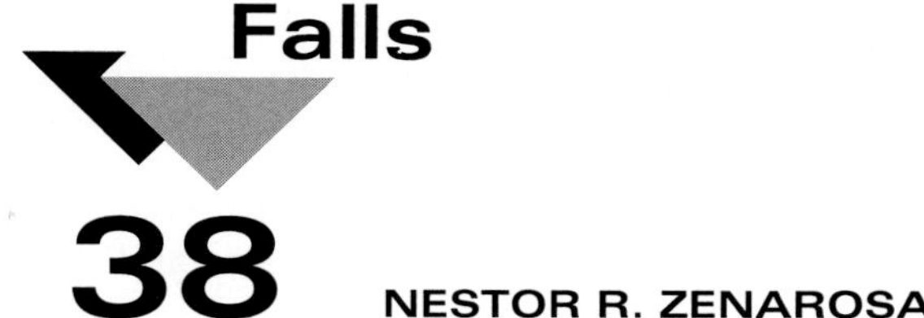

38 Falls

NESTOR R. ZENAROSA

Teaching Cases

Case 1: A 13-year-old girl was walking her dog. As the dog ran, the leash wrapped around the girl's waist and she was thrown to the ground. On arrival to the emergency department (ED), she complained of abdominal pain and nausea. Her abdomen was tender in her right upper quadrant. An abdominal CT scan showed a large liver laceration with free intraperitoneal fluid. She did not require surgery and was discharged home after 5 days.

Case 2: A 21-year-old man was parachuting when his parachute tangled, and only partially opened. On arrival of the medics, he was pulseless and unresponsive. After prehospital resuscitation, he arrived to the ED with weak pulses. His injuries included cerebral edema, interventricular hemorrhage, pubic symphysis diastasis, acetabular fracture, sacroiliac joint diastasis, renal artery intimal tear, and hemorrhage from both internal iliac arteries. Despite intensive resuscitation and angiographic embolization of his pelvic vessels, the patient died. ■

Falls produce a wide spectrum of injuries. Falls from ground level can be deceptively severe. Falls from great heights result in extensive multi-system trauma. An understanding of common injury patterns will allow the emergency physician (EP) to anticipate fall-related trauma. Falls are the most common cause of injury in the United States and lead to 13,000 deaths per year.[1-3]

Falls are a major cause of death in the pediatric trauma population, and are the second leading cause of fatality in the adult trauma population behind motor vehicle crashes.[4-6] The Surgeon General has focused a national prevention and educational campaign on falls. Despite the recent attention, falls still represent a major cause of mortality and morbidity in the United States.[1,3,4] Most falls are preventable.

The old saw, "it wasn't the fall that killed him, it was the sudden stop," represents an important physical law–a body in motion tends to stay in motion. Internal organs, which accelerate with the body, continue to move forward on impact with the ground. Solid organs and bones deform or fracture. Structures that are tethered may tear at the site of fixation, such as the aorta at the ligamentum arteriosum, the jejunum at the ligament of Treitz, and the kidney at the renal pedicle.

EPIDEMIOLOGY

Unlike other forms of trauma, falls affect all patient populations. However, some segments are at increased risk for falling or suffering falls with special characteristics.[4]

The geriatric population is at particular risk. Although the elderly represent a small proportion of patients who fall, they comprise over 50% of fall-related deaths.[4] Fortunately, fall-related mortality has been steadily declining among the elderly.[7] Mosenthal et al[4] found that more than half of all patients over the age of 64 who fall suffer coexisting neuropsychiatric or cardiovascular problems. Factors such as medications, gait and balance disturbances, acute illnesses, prolonged bedrest, and history of falls increase the risk of falling.[4,8,9] Simple environmental issues such as better lighting or securing the flooring may alleviate some peril.[8-10] Physicians can prevent falls by avoiding polypharmacy in the elderly, especially combinations of sedating drugs.

Children also suffer disproportionately from falls. Over half of pediatric falls occur between birth and the age of 4 years. Children are more likely to have a lower injury severity score when compared with adults, and can tolerate greater drops.[4] A fall from 5 to

6 stories (60 to 72 feet) marks the 50% mortality threshold for children, whereas the 50% mortality for adults is 4 stories (48 feet).[11-13]

Some environmental issues play a special role in childhood falls, such as child abuse and unrecognized hazards in the home. African-American males under 5 years of age are in particular danger. Many serious falls occur on stairs or from a window. Child walkers (devices on wheels that train children to walk) should never be located above the first floor—if used at all. The vast majority of defenestrations (i.e., falls out of windows) are from 3 stories or less, and occur between May and September. In New York, legislature that required window guards in all multifamily dwellings reduced the number of falls by 96%.[4]

Men between 25 and 40 years of age comprise many falls.[4] A significant number of these patients are intoxicated with alcohol and/or illicit drugs.[14] Mosenthal et al[4] demonstrated that nearly 20% of patients evaluated for illicit drugs after occupational falls tested positive; 7% tested positive for alcohol. There was a significant incidence of unemployment (52%), associated criminal and violent behavior at the time of the fall (19%), alcohol use (52%), and illicit drug use (59%) in nonoccupational falls.[4]

PATHOPHYSIOLOGY

The extent of injury depends on the height of the fall, the type of surface on which the victim lands, the position of impact, and patient factors.[1] The amount of kinetic energy (KE) transferred to the body also determines the severity of injury. When a person collides with a surface, most KE is converted to mechanical energy that is absorbed by the body.[1] On a soft surface, more energy is transmitted to the surface, which deforms and produces less injury. On a hard surface like concrete, nearly all of the KE is transmitted to the body. Other factors that play a significant role in injury severity include the duration of impact (shorter is worse) and the body surface area of contact at impact. The greater the surface area, the greater the dispersion of the impact force.[1,13,14]

CLINICAL PRESENTATIONS

The position of impact correlates with injury patterns. Other factors include the weight and age of the patient. The heavier and older patients do worse than their younger and slimmer counterparts.

Feet-First

Feet-first landings transmit the force over a fairly small area. The body can absorb some of the force with its joints, tendons, and musculature. A parachutist tries to land on his or her toes, then bend at the ankle, knee, and hips, while simultaneously tumbling toward the side. Patients who land in the feet-first position have a high incidence of lower extremity fractures and intracerebral injuries (60%).[1] Force is transmitted upwards, and patients may present with a constellation of calcaneal, tibial plateau, and hip trauma. There is a lower but significant risk of vertebral fractures, particularly in the lower thoracic and upper lumbar regions. Look for vertebral fractures whenever a patient has a lower extremity fracture. In one series, two thirds of the patients with fractures of the feet had simultaneous fractures of the L1-L3 region.[2,3,14]

Torso injuries are also common. Hepatic lacerations are seen in 20% of feet-first falls,[1] whereas mediastinal injuries occur in 25%.[15] Although aortic rupture certainly occurs in feet-first falls, in one series only 2 of 187 patients had significant vascular injury.[14] This discrepancy may be caused by selecting out patients who died at the scene.

Headfirst

It is not surprising that headfirst landings have a very high incidence of intracerebral injuries (almost all patients in some series), as well as skull fractures (60%). One quarter sustain upper extremity and vertebral fractures. The most common spinal fractures involve the cervical and thoracic spine. Forty percent of those who land headfirst will also have rib fractures, often in association with pulmonary injury. There is a small incidence of aortic or intraabdominal injury with this type of landing (10%).[1-3,14]

Buttock-First

Buttock-first landings offer the least amount of flexion at impact to absorb energy. As a result, 80% incur pelvic fractures.[11] Chest injuries are common, and 66% of the patients in one series had significant pulmonary trauma. In one series, 2 out of 11 patients landing in this position had a cardiac tear and 3 had an aortic disruption.[1,11] Sternal injuries can also occur with this type of landing.[3]

Half of all patients who land on their buttocks after a significant fall from a height suffer vertebral fractures, liver injury, kidney injury, or cerebral hemorrhage (usually as a result of secondary bounces).

Side Impacts

The least common position of impact is on the side. One half of the persons landing in this position have fractures of the upper extremities and ribs. Many of those with rib fractures have underlying pulmonary injury. This type of landing also has the highest incidence of renal injury compared with that of other landing positions (20%).[1] Vertebral fractures are most common in the thoracic area. Fifty percent of deaths in side-impact falls are due to an intracerebral injury.[1]

Children

Children experience different injury patterns than adults. The younger child has a more cephalad center of gravity; nearly 90% of childhood falls from a height result in head injuries. A thorough neurologic examination is particularly important in this age group. Optic nerve injuries occur in association with skull fractures involving the orbits.[16] Children almost always fracture an extremity in these falls, although they have a lower incidence of spine and pelvic fractures. Renal, chest, and lung injuries are present in one third of pediatric falls. Pediatric patients frequently suffer intraabdominal injuries, usually involving the liver or spleen.[1,5,13,16-19]

As a result of radiographic differences between adults and children, assessing the pediatric cervical spine after a fall may be difficult. However, in one series, pediatric patients who fell from a low height (i.e., less than 5 feet) and who had cervical spine injuries had clinical evidence either historically or on physical examination of a cervical spine injury.[18] These injuries usually involve the upper cervical spine.

Children will have lower mortality when compared with adults for similar heights.[1] The lower mortality incurred by children may be explained by (1) their smaller mass and reduced-impact energy, (2) increased cartilaginous structure, (3) increased subcutaneous fat, and (4) better cardiopulmonary reserve.

EMERGENCY DEPARTMENT MANAGEMENT

Primary Survey

The primary survey and resuscitation of an unstable fall victim is similar to that of other multiinjured patient. As with any trauma patient, the first priority is the airway. The emergency physician (EP) will be unable to clinically clear the cervical spine of an obtunded fall patient. For this reason, protect the spine during airway maneuvers.

The fall victim who presents in shock on arrival to the ED is unlikely to survive.[3] Although there is a significant incidence of spinal cord injury in fall patients, do not assume shock is neurogenic until hemorrhage, tension pneumothorax, and cardiac tamponade are excluded. Common causes of hemorrhagic shock in the fall victim include hemoperitoneum or hemothorax, multiple long-bone fractures, an unstable pelvic fracture causing a retroperitoneal bleed, and significant scalp lacerations.

Resuscitation occurs in conjunction with the primary survey. If the patient shows lateralizing neurologic signs, perform an urgent brain computed tomographic scan while maintaining spinal immobilization. Only the ongoing management of shock should take priority over evaluation of the brain.[3]

History

Once immediate life threats are ruled out or managed, the EP should take a detailed history from the patient and witnesses. Determine the height of the fall, the position of impact, the type of surface hit, and events leading up until the fall. Do not just treat the fall. Consider the following scenarios:

A young male is brought from the scene with agonal respirations. You note that there are track marks on his arm and he has pinpoint pupils.

An elderly patient is brought to the ED after falling from a tall ladder while painting his house. You note that he is pale and diaphoretic. In addition to the usual trauma evaluation you get an electrocardiogram and note elevated ST segments in anterior leads.

A worker is found down next to a tall building. He was installing an antenna then fell. On his trauma survey you note burn marks on his hands and on his toes.

A young woman is brought from a high-rise fire after she jumped from the third floor. You note that she has a measured oxygen saturation of 86% on her ABG, but the calculated oximetry reading is 96%.

"Falls" may be intentional (jumps) and are a common method of suicide. Institute suicide precautions for patients at risk.

Falls in children occur with nonaccidental trauma (NAT), either from direct assault or criminal neglect. Significant injury from reportedly low heights is common in NAT. Ask about the landing surface, consider the weight of the child, and who was with the child when they fell. Nonaccidental trauma can produce minor, as well as major, injuries.[5,13,16,18,19]

Secondary Survey

The secondary survey involves a head to toe evaluation. However, if the EP knows the position of landing, they can anticipate certain injuries. In the case of a foot-first landing, look for spinal and extremity fractures, and injuries to the liver, spleen, heart, and lung. In headfirst landings expect skull, upper extremity, cervical and thoracic spinal fractures, as well as pulmonary injuries. Side impacts have a high incidence of rib and upper extremity fractures, thoracic spine, pulmonary, and renal injuries. Buttock landings are likely to produce pelvic fractures (80%) and transverse sacral fractures. These sacral injuries appear as subtle lucencies on plain radiographs. There are a large number of patients who suffer renal injuries with this type of fall (50%).[1] This pattern of landing also has one of the highest incidences of cardiac and aortic injury.

SPECIFIC INJURIES

Spinal injuries are a major concern in the fall patient. A low fall does not exclude a spinal injury. Suspect spinal injury if the patient is impaired, has pain or tenderness to palpation, or has suggestive neurologic findings. In one series, 20% percent of the patients had a spinal fracture. Twenty percent of those with a fracture had either a spinal cord or a cauda equina syndrome. The most common site of fracture was the thoracolumbar region (70% of spinal fractures).[14,17] "Cone-downed" radiographs targeting the thoracolumbar junction may be helpful.

Vascular injuries are surprisingly infrequent in fall victims seen in emergency practice. This apparent discrepancy is probably due to the fact that most with significant vascular injuries die at the scene. However, prompt recognition is imperative to treat aortic disruption or retroperitoneal bleed. Severe extremity injuries may result in peripheral vascular trauma, including intimal tears and pseudoaneurysms. Renal artery avulsions are associated with the buttock landing. These pedicle injuries may demonstrate little or no hematuria, but the patient is likely to demonstrate shock from multiple sources of blood loss. Pelvic fractures, particularly vertical shear injury, may result in massive retroperitoneal hemorrhage. These injuries may require external fixation or angiographic embolization. Spinal artery tears may occur with spinous fractures.[3]

Intraabdominal injury, particularly spleen and liver injuries, are major sites of hemorrhage in falls. A fall victim may be hemodynamically unstable and have a pelvic fracture. Such patients require rapid assessment for hemoperitoneum. Diagnostic peritoneal lavage or emergent beside trauma ultrasonography may be useful in this instance.[1-3,14]

Extremity injuries are especially common in feet-first impacts, and often occur in people who jump from heights. Calcaneal fractures are ubiquitous in "jumpers," and may be difficult to visualize on plain films of the foot. A special calcaneal view will better define the injury. Calcaneal fractures are often associated with knee or hip injuries, as well as thoracolumbar compression fractures.

CONCLUSION

A person who suffers a fall is at risk for multisystem trauma. Even minor falls can produce serious sequelae. Factors that determine the clinical presentation include: (1) height of fall, (2) landing surface, (3) position of body upon impact, and (4) age.[1]

The EP must quickly identify and treat life threats, as well as recognize other, less critical injuries. These tasks are simplified by understanding the biophysics of free falls. Historical factors, as well as specific injuries, allow the EP to anticipate occult trauma.

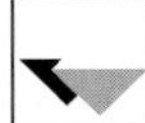

PEARLS & PITFALLS

- Position of impact may predict injury patterns.
  - Feet-first: lower extremity, thoracolumbar spine, torso
  - Headfirst: Head, cervical-spine burst fractures, upper extremity fractures
  - Buttocks-first: chest, pelvic, and abdominal injuries; renal injuries also common
  - Side-first: Chest, head, thoracic spine, upper extremities
- Children are likely to suffer head, chest, and abdominal injuries in falls.
- Consider the cause of a fall, such as suicidal ideation, electrocution, cardiac ischemia, nonaccidental trauma, and drug or alcohol abuse.
- Do not rule out serious injury based on a short fall.
- Anticipate associated injuries: spinal fractures with calcaneal fractures, cervical fractures with head injury.

REFERENCES

1. Warner KG, Demling RH: The pathophysiology of free-fall injury, *Ann Emerg Med* 15:1088-1093, 1986.
2. Richter D, et al: Vertical deceleration injuries: a comparative study of the injury patterns of 101 patients after accidental and intentional high falls, *Injury* 27:655-659, 1996.
3. Buckman RF Jr, Buckman PD: Vertical deceleration trauma. Principles of management, *Surg Clin North Am* 71:331-344, 1991.
4. Mosenthal AC, et al: Falls: epidemiology and strategies for prevention, *J Trauma* 38:753-756, 1995.
5. Roshkow JE, et al: Imaging evaluation of children after falls from a height: review of 45 cases, *Radiology* 175:359-363, 1990.
6. Lambert DA, Sattin RW: Deaths from falls, 1978-1984, *MMWR* 37(SS-1):21-26, 1988.

7. Riggs JE: Mortality from accidental falls among the elderly in the United States, 1962-1988: demonstrating the impact of improved trauma management, *J Trauma* 35:212-219, 1993.
8. Davies AJ, Kenny RA: Falls presenting to the accident and emergency department: types of presentation and risk factor profile, *Age Ageing* 25:362-366, 1996.
9. Dresner-Pollak R, et al: Characteristics of falls in 70 year olds in Jerusalem, *Isr J Med* Sci 32:625-628, 1996.
10. O'Neill TW, et al: Age and sex influences on fall characteristics, *Ann Rheum Dis* 53:773-775, 1994.
11. Steedman DJ: Severity of free-fall injury, *Injury* 20:259-261, 1989.
12. Risser D, et al: Risk of dying after a free fall from height, *Forensic Sci Int* 78:187-191, 1996.
13. Hajivassiliou CA, Azmy A: Physical parameters of free fall in a child, *Injury* 27:739-741, 1996.
14. Velmahos GC, et al: Patterns of injury in victims of urban free-falls, *World J Surg* 21:816-821, 1997.
15. Lopez-Viego MA: *The Parkland trauma handbook,* ed 1, St Louis, 1994, Mosby.
16. Mahapatra AK: Optic nerve injury in children, *J Neurosurg Sci* 36:79-84, 1992.
17. Cooper C, Dunham CM, Rodriguez A: Falls and major injuries are risk factors for thoracolumbar fractures: cognitive impairment and multiple injuries impede the detection of back pain and tenderness, *J Trauma* 38:692-696, 1995.
18. Schwartz GR, et al: Pediatric cervical spine injury sustained in falls from low heights, *Ann Emerg Med* 30:249-252, 1997.
19. Root I: Head Injuries from short distance falls, *Am J Forensic Med Pathol* 13:85-87, 1992.

39 Drowning

JAYNE J. BATTS

Teaching Case

A 4-year-old boy falls through a crack in the ice of a fishing pond in mid-January. He is pulled from the water within 5 minutes, but is apneic and pulseless. He is intubated en route to the emergency department (ED) with cardiopulmonary resuscitation (CPR) in progress. On arrival he has a bradycardia of 40 beats per minute (bpm), with a systolic blood pressure of 70 mmHg. His core temperature is 70° F, and an electrocardiogram (ECG) shows a prominent Osborne wave. Warm, humidified oxygen is placed through the endotracheal tube, warm intravenous (IV) fluids are run through an in-line warmer and a bear-hugger is applied. The cardiopulmonary bypass team is activated and the patient undergoes core rewarming. His blood pressure starts to increase without inotropic agents. After 3 days in the intensive care unit (ICU), the patient appears to be neurologically intact and is discharged home.

More than 100 million Americans participate in water-related activities each year. Submersion injuries constitute a major public health concern with significant morbidity and mortality. Healthcare costs for submersion victims are high, ranging from $2000 for victims who fully recover to over $100,000 per year for those with severe brain damage requiring long-term care.[1]

Drowning is defined as death by suffocation after submersion in water. Over 140,000 drowning deaths occur worldwide each year,[2] and more than 4000 are reported in the United States.[3] ***Near drowning*** is survival, at least temporarily, from submersion.[4] The true incidence of near drowning is unknown since many events go unreported. It has been estimated that for every drowning incident, 500 to 600 near-drowning events occur.[5] The majority of these victims are transported to the ED for evaluation. Although prevention is key, effective on-scene resuscitation and expert care by emergency physicians (EPs) are vital for good outcomes.

EPIDEMIOLOGY

Drowning is a preventable tragedy that primarily affects young, healthy patients. Only motor vehicle crashes cause more accidental deaths in children and young adults.[6] In some states such as California, Arizona, and Florida, drowning is the leading cause of injury-related death in children less than five years of age.[7] Over 90% of drownings occur in fresh water even in coastal areas.[5,8] Drownings peak during the summer months and are most common in the southern and western United States and Alaska.[9]

Overall drowning rates vary depending on sex, race, and age. *Males* are four times more likely to drown than females.[9] The rate of drowning in African-Americans is twice that of Caucasians except in children under 3 years of age, where the ratio is reversed due to residential pool drownings.[10] There is a bimodal age distribution associated with submersion injury. The first peak occurs in *children under 5 years of age* who account for up to 40% of drowning deaths.[11] Most cases of infant submersion occur in the bathtub.[12] Unattended toddlers drown primarily in home swimming pools,[7] but fish tanks, toilets, bathtubs, and washing machines pose serious risks.[5] One previously unrecognized hazard is the 5-gallon industrial bucket used as mop buckets or diaper pails.[13] Since 1984, over 200 children in the United States have drowned in these heavy containers. The use of solar pool blankets is another water hazard.[14] The majority of childhood drowning cases occur during lapses in adult supervision caused by chores, socializing, or phone calls.[7]

A second peak in incidence occurs in *15- to 24-year-old males*[10] who drown in lakes, rivers, canals, and the ocean.[7] Although preschool-aged children have the largest incidence of drowning, adolescents have the highest case fatality rate.[15] In this group, risk-taking behavior such as diving in unsafe water, dangerous boating, trauma, drugs, and alcohol play major roles.[16]

ETIOLOGY

Many cases of adult drowning occur when a swimmer overestimates his or her ability and becomes panicked or fatigued. As many as 90% of drownings occur within 10 yards of safety.[17-19] Drowning may also be a secondary event. Box 39-1 lists some of the factors that are associated with near-drowning episodes.

Trauma

Trauma sustained during water-related activities may cause injuries that prevent victims from resurfacing. Diving into swimming pools or natural bodies of water results in over 1000 spinal cord injuries each year.[20,21] Boating accidents account for approximately 1200 drownings per year.[22] The use of personal watercraft devices, such as jet skies, has resulted in a fourfold rise in associated injuries from an estimated 2860 in 1990 to more than 12,000 in 1995.[23] Sixty percent of the deaths associated with scuba (self-contained underwater breathing apparatus) diving are the result of drowning.[22] Although inexperience and carelessness play major roles in underwater diving accidents, cerebral air embolism and decompression sickness can be contributing factors.

Hyperventilating

Hyperventilating before swimming to increase underwater endurance results in lowering of the $PaCO_2$, without a significant change in the PaO_2. During underwater swimming, the PaO_2 can decrease to 30 to 40 mmHg, while the $PaCO_2$ rises to a level insufficient to stimulate breathing.[24] This phenomenon, known as *shallow-water blackout,* results in a loss of consciousness from hypoxia, which may lead to drowning.[25]

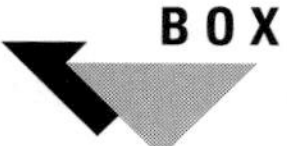

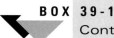

BOX 39-1
Contributing Factors in Near Drowning Events

Inability to swim	Hot tubs/spas
Seizures	Hypothermia
Trauma	Cardiovascular disease
Ethanol	Child abuse/neglect
Hyperventilation	Diabetes
Illicit drugs	Suicide

Hot Tubs and Spas

Hot tubs and spas are also associated with injuries and drowning. Entrapment of hair or body parts in the suction device of the drains is a major cause of accidents.[26] In addition, spas are a drowning hazard when they remain filled with water when not in use. Prolonged use of a hot tub, especially in combination with alcohol or drugs, can lead to a hyperthermia-induced stupor or syncope and subsequent drowning.[27]

Underlying Medical Conditions

Co-morbid conditions such as cardiac disease may result in dysrhythmias, syncope, or myocardial infarction, which can incapacitate a swimmer. Diabetics may become hypoglycemic and disoriented while in the water. Hypothermia and ethanol ingestion may also contribute to hypoglycemia. Epilepsy is associated with a four- to five-fold increased risk of drowning, especially in patients with poorly controlled seizures and in those with a recent change in their drug regimen.[5,28]

Alcohol and Drug Ingestion

Intoxicant ingestion can diminish a swimmer's ability and judgment. Intoxication plays a significant role in adult submersion injuries and is a major contributing factor in 40% to 50% of drownings among adolescent boys.[29] Alcohol-related hypothermia may play a role in some deaths.

Hypothermia

Hypothermia from immersion in cold water can acutely lead to death in three ways. First, a decrease in core temperature leads to confusion and incoordination, which may impair the victim's ability to keep the head above water. Second, cardiac arrest from ventricular fibrillation is seen at core temperatures below 25° C (77° F).[30] Third, the *immersion syndrome* is sudden death following submersion in very cold water (18° C/64° F), felt to be caused by a vagally-mediated asystolic cardiac arrest.[31]

Abuse or Neglect

These factors should be considered in cases of near drowning involving young children. Finally, near drowning may be the result of an unrecognized suicide attempt.

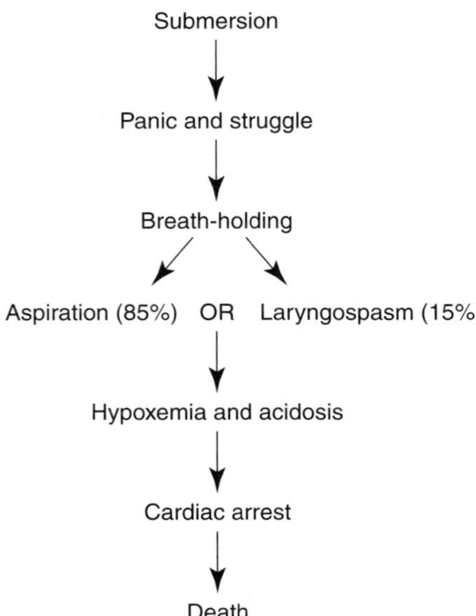

Fig. 39-1 Sequence of events in drowning. (Adapted from Weinstein MD, Krieger BP: *J Emerg Med* 14:462, 1996.)

PATHOPHYSIOLOGY

The classic sequence of drowning is illustrated in Fig. 39-1. After an initial period of panic, there is violent struggling and breath-holding while the victim attempts to reach the surface. Eventually breath-holding is no longer possible and the victim then either inhales water directly or swallows large amounts of water, which is later aspirated when he or she vomits.[32]

Approximately 10% to 20% of victims experience *dry drowning* in which prolonged laryngospasm prevents aspiration but results in death secondary to obstructive apnea.[11] Although only a small percentage of near-drowning victims experience this phenomenon, it is from this subset that 80% to 90% of successful resuscitations occur.[33]

The lethal common denominator in submersion events is hypoxia caused by either laryngospasm or aspiration of water. Struggling accelerates hypoxemia and lactic acidosis and leads to a combined respiratory and metabolic acidosis, ultimately resulting in death.

The organ systems most commonly affected by submersion events are listed in Table 39-1.

TABLE 39-1
Pathophysiology of Near Drowning

ORGAN SYSTEM	FINDINGS
Pulmonary	Noncardiogenic edema, hypoxemia
Cardiac	Myocardial depression, dysrhythmias
Neurologic	Hypoxic encephalopathy, cord injury from trauma
Renal	Acute tubular necrosis, hemoglobinuria
Metabolic	Rare electrolyte changes
Hematologic	Rarely affected

Pulmonary

Pulmonary injury is common in submersion accidents with complications resulting from the aspiration of fluid. Hypotonic fresh water is quickly absorbed through the pulmonary capillary membrane, resulting in a washout of surfactant and the development of atelectasis. Hypertonic saltwater can directly damage the capillary membrane. In addition, the salt will draw capillary fluids into the lungs by osmotic forces, producing noncardiogenic pulmonary edema.[34] The end result of either type of aspiration is decreased lung compliance with intrapulmonary shunting, ventilation-perfusion mismatch, and hypoxemia.

Particulate material such as sand or mud, gastric contents, chemical irritants, or microorganisms may be aspirated along with the water and result in pneumonitis.[35,36]

Secondary drowning is delayed death from the respiratory distress syndrome.[17,37] In up to 5% of victims, secondary drowning may occur hours to days after the initial resuscitation.[38] Unconsciousness at the scene, a history of cyanosis, apnea, or the requirement of CPR are all strong markers for late deterioration.[39] Patients who are intoxicated, have underlying medical conditions, and those at the extremes of age are also at risk.

Cardiac

Primary cardiac problems are unusual in cases of near drowning.[40] Myocardial depression and dysrhythmias including sinus bradycardia or atrial fibrillation may be seen but are usually secondary to hypothermia or acidosis and hypoxemia from pulmonary injury.[41] The "Osborne" or "J" wave is an electrocardiographic manifestation of hypothermia (Fig. 39-2). This hypothermic hump seen at the junction of the QRS and ST segments may appear at temperatures below 32° C (89.6° F), and its size increases with temperature depression.[42-44]

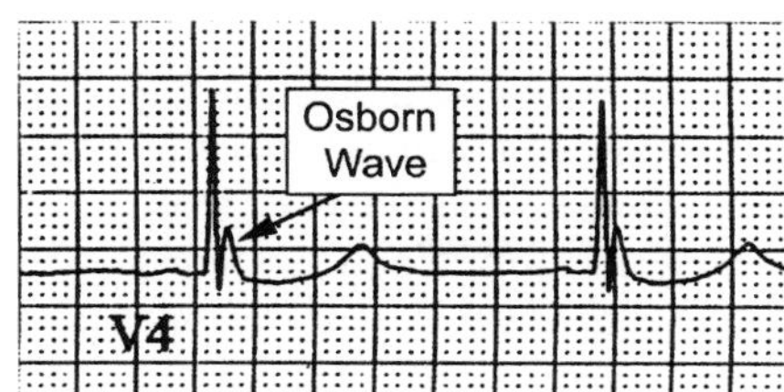

Fig. 39-2 EKG manifestation of hypothermia: "Osborn wave."

Neurologic

Cerebral hypoxia causes the neurologic damage that occurs in near drowning. In the presence of hypoxia, brain tissue becomes acidotic and cerebral edema may develop after circulation is restored.[45-46] Severe anoxic encephalopathy with persistent coma, seizures, delayed language development, spastic quadriplegia, aphasia, and cortical blindness have all been reported as sequelae of submersion events.[47-51] Although hypoxic brain damage is the primary central nervous system (CNS) problem, cervical spine injuries also occur and are frequently associated with diving accidents.[52]

Renal

Renal function is usually normal following a submersion event. Renal failure may occur secondary to acute tubular necrosis from hypoxia or may be precipitated by hemoglobinuria or myoglobinuria.[48,53]

Metabolic

The early literature emphasized major differences between salt-water and fresh-water drownings.[37,54] Authors postulated that hypotonic fresh-water would be drawn out of the alveoli into the circulation, causing vascular overload and diluting serum electrolytes. Conversely, hypertonic salt-water should remain in the lungs, drawing water in by osmotic forces and resulting in pulmonary edema and hypertonic serum. Recent studies have suggested that human near-drowning victims rarely aspirate enough water to cause life-threatening changes in serum electrolytes.[55] Although these changes have occurred in fatal cases, they are rarely seen in victims transported to the ED.[56-59] However, an exception is submersion in extremely concentrated sea water such as the Dead Sea. Significant hypercalcemia and hypermagnesemia contribute to the high fatality rate (40% to 50%) of these near-drowning victims; however, these derangements may be secondary to fluid absorbed from the stomach.[60]

Hematologic

It was previously thought that the aspiration of fresh-water would cause hemolysis and that salt-water aspiration would result in hemodilution.[61,62] However, studies show that following aspiration of either type of water, the hemoglobin and hematocrit remain normal, although a nonspecific leukocytosis may occur.[48,55,63] Disseminated intravascular coagulation (DIC) complicating near drowning is extremely rare.[64]

CLINICAL PRESENTATION

The spectrum of illness after submersion ranges from asymptomatic to full cardiac arrest. Predominant findings relate to hypoxic injury to the lungs and CNS. Specific signs and symptoms vary, depending on such factors as the underlying cause of the accident, length of submersion, temperature of the water, amount of water aspirated, and previous health of the victim.[65]

Respiratory

Complaints of sore throat, hoarseness, coughing, burning in the chest, and dyspnea are common. Tachypnea is the most frequent physical finding.[48,63] Pulmonary examination may also reveal rales, rhonchi, and wheezing. Copious sputum production or cyanosis may precede respiratory failure.

Cardiac

Cardiovascular manifestations include tachycardia, hypotension (from intravascular fluid shifts), and myocardial ischemia.[48,63]

Gastrointestinal

Swallowing large amounts of fluid can distend the abdomen, and vomiting may occur during resuscitation.

Thermoregulatory

Rarely, hypothalamic injury results in fever, but hypothermia is more likely, especially in cold-water submersion events.[48,66]

Neurologic

Cerebral hypoxia manifests as restlessness, lethargy, confusion, seizures, incontinence, hyporeflexia, and coma.

MANAGEMENT

Prehospital Setting

Care of the near-drowning victim starts at the scene of the accident (Box 39-2). Consider the following case scenario: A teenage boy is found by his friends submerged at the bottom of a rock quarry. Apparently, the boys had been diving into the quarry and noticed that their friend did not resurface. When the emergency medical services (EMS) personnel arrive, the teen is unresponsive, cyanotic, and cold. What should be done?

FIRST CONTACT

Treatment of near drowning begins with rapid, cautious removal of the victim from the water. A spinal injury is most likely in those diving from heights, those with physical evidence of trauma, and in victims with an altered level of consciousness. The rescuer should quickly slide the teenager onto a backboard and begin rescue breathing while still in the water.[67] Immediate rescue breathing is the single most important factor influencing survival.[68] In-water chest compressions are difficult to perform, not effective, and may be unsafe for the rescuer.[69]

INITIAL EVALUATION

Once the victim is removed from the water, the medics must rapidly reassess the level of consciousness and check for breathing and a pulse. Peripheral pulses are sometimes difficult to palpate in hypothermic patients. If the victim is pulseless, the medics should begin cardiopulmonary resuscitation (CPR) and then advanced life support (ALS).

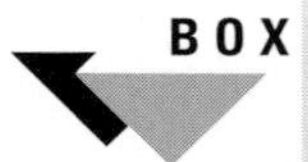

BOX 39-2
Prehospital Management of the Near-Drowning Victim

- Immediate *ventilation and oxygenation*
- Spinal immobilization if indicated
- Intubation if: apneic, altered mental status, or severe respiratory distress
- Intravenous access/fluid resuscitation: if hypotensive
- Treat altered mental status: naloxone, D_{50}, and thiamine
- Cardiac monitoring for dysrhythmias
- Remove wet clothing and wrap in blankets
- Secondary survey
- Obtain history of events from bystanders
- Transfer *all* patients to the emergency department for evaluation

RESPIRATORY

All submersion victims benefit from high-flow oxygen (O_2). If the teenager is apneic, unable to protect his airway, or in severe respiratory distress, intubation and assisted ventilation are indicated. Postural drainage maneuvers to remove water from the lungs are ineffective and not recommended. An appropriate maneuver for airway obstruction should be performed only if healthcare workers suspect a foreign body.[69-71]

CARDIAC

The medics should place the patient on a cardiac monitor. Sinus bradycardia and atrial fibrillation do not require treatment and usually convert spontaneously during rewarming. For hypothermic victims in ventricular fibrillation the recommended approach is one attempt at cardioversion with 2 watt-sec/kg up to 200 watt-sec.[72] Cardioversion is generally unsuccessful if the core temperature is 28° C (82.4° F) or less.

HYPOTHERMIA

Hypothermia can occur even in mildly cool water with prolonged exposure, or in the presence of alcohol, which causes vasodilation.[25] EMS personnel should remove the teen's wet clothing and wrap him in blankets to prevent further heat loss. He should be kept supine and handled as gently as possible by prehospital providers. The onset of ventricular fibrillation has been ascribed to excessive mechanical stimulation, although definitive evidence for this mechanism is lacking.[30,73]

DRUG THERAPY

Indications for pharmacologic intervention in the field are limited. Patients with altered mental status require treatment with 2 mg of naloxone, 50 cc of 50% dextrose (D_{50}) (if a field blood glucose level is unavailable), and 100 mg of thiamine. Medics should initiate a large-bore IV line on all symptomatic patients. Hypotension is treated with a 20 ml/kg fluid challenge of 0.9% normal saline (NS). En route medics should perform a secondary survey to search for other injuries.

HISTORICAL INFORMATION

Bystanders are a rich source of information for prehospital providers. Before leaving the scene, medics should try to determine the time of the incident, period of immersion, type and temperature of the water, circumstances surrounding the submersion, and history of loss of consciousness, apnea, cyanosis, or vomiting.[74] Medics should transport all patients who experience a submersion event, no matter how trivial. The initial appearance of near-drowning victims is deceptive, and they may be at risk for delayed complications.

Emergency Department

When the teenage patient arrives in the ED he is still unresponsive. The medics were unable to intubate him and are assisting his respirations with a bag-valve-mask on 100% O_2. He is fully immobilized and has received naloxone, D_{50}, thiamine, and a 1000 cc bolus of NSS. Vital signs reveal a rectal temperature of 29° C (85.2° F), a pulse of 50 bpm, a shallow respiratory effort with a rate of 12 bpm, and a blood pressure of 80/50 mmHg. His color is gray, his lungs have diffuse rales and expiratory wheezes, his rectal tone is poor, and there is no spontaneous movement of his extremities. The remainder of the examination is unremarkable. A portable chest radiograph (CXR) (Fig. 39-3) shows bilateral perihilar fluffy infiltrates. What is the next step?

Fig. 39-4 outlines the ED management of near-drowning victims. After a trivial episode of submersion in the *asymptomatic* patient, physical examination and pulse oximetry to assess oxygen saturation are

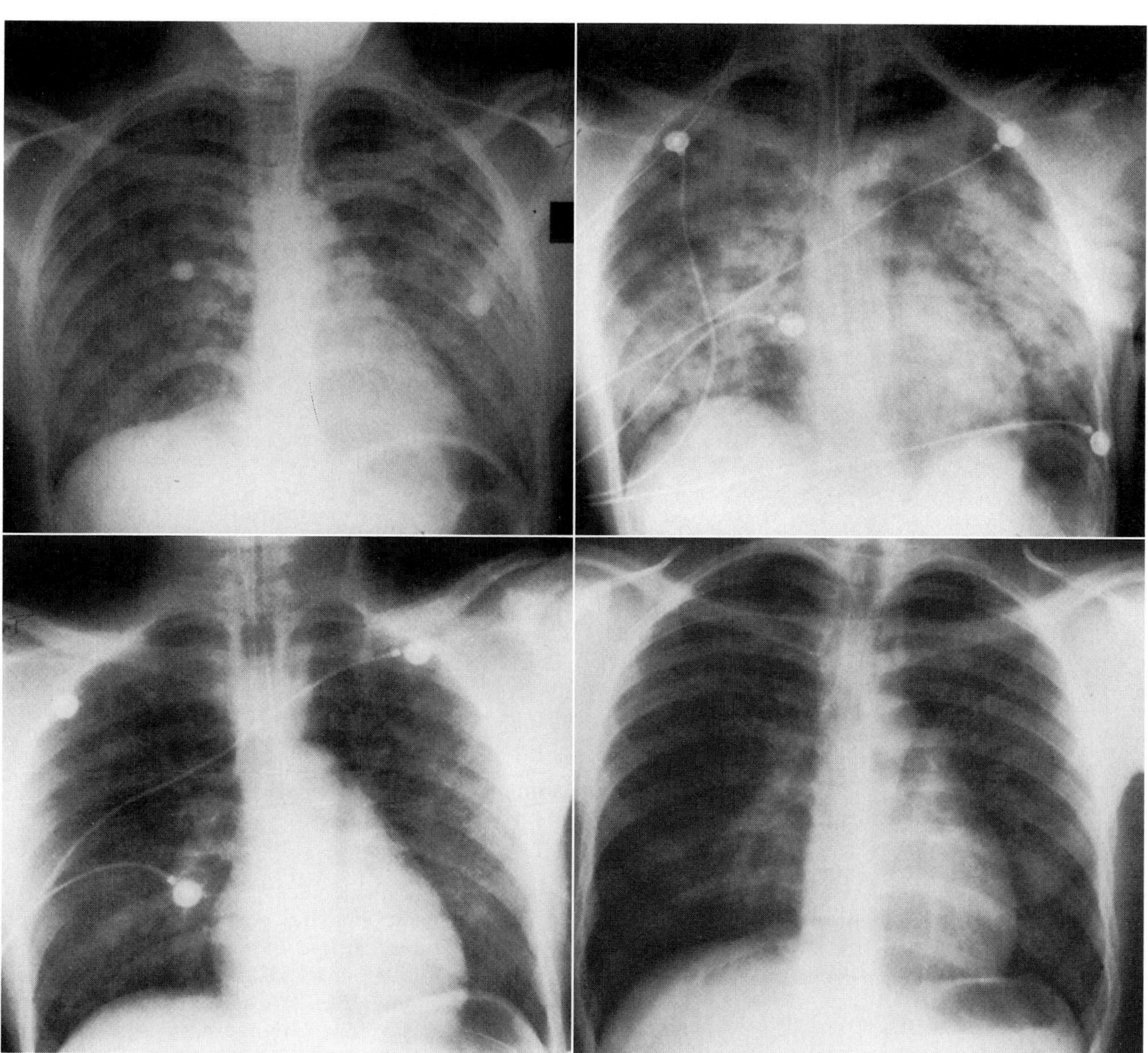

Fig. 39-3 Chest radiograph of near-drowning patient demonstrating diffuse noncardiogenic pulmonary edema. From Holroyd BR, Lesperance RR: Aspiration. In Rosen P, et al: *Diagnostic radiology in emergency medicine,* St Louis, 1992, Mosby.)

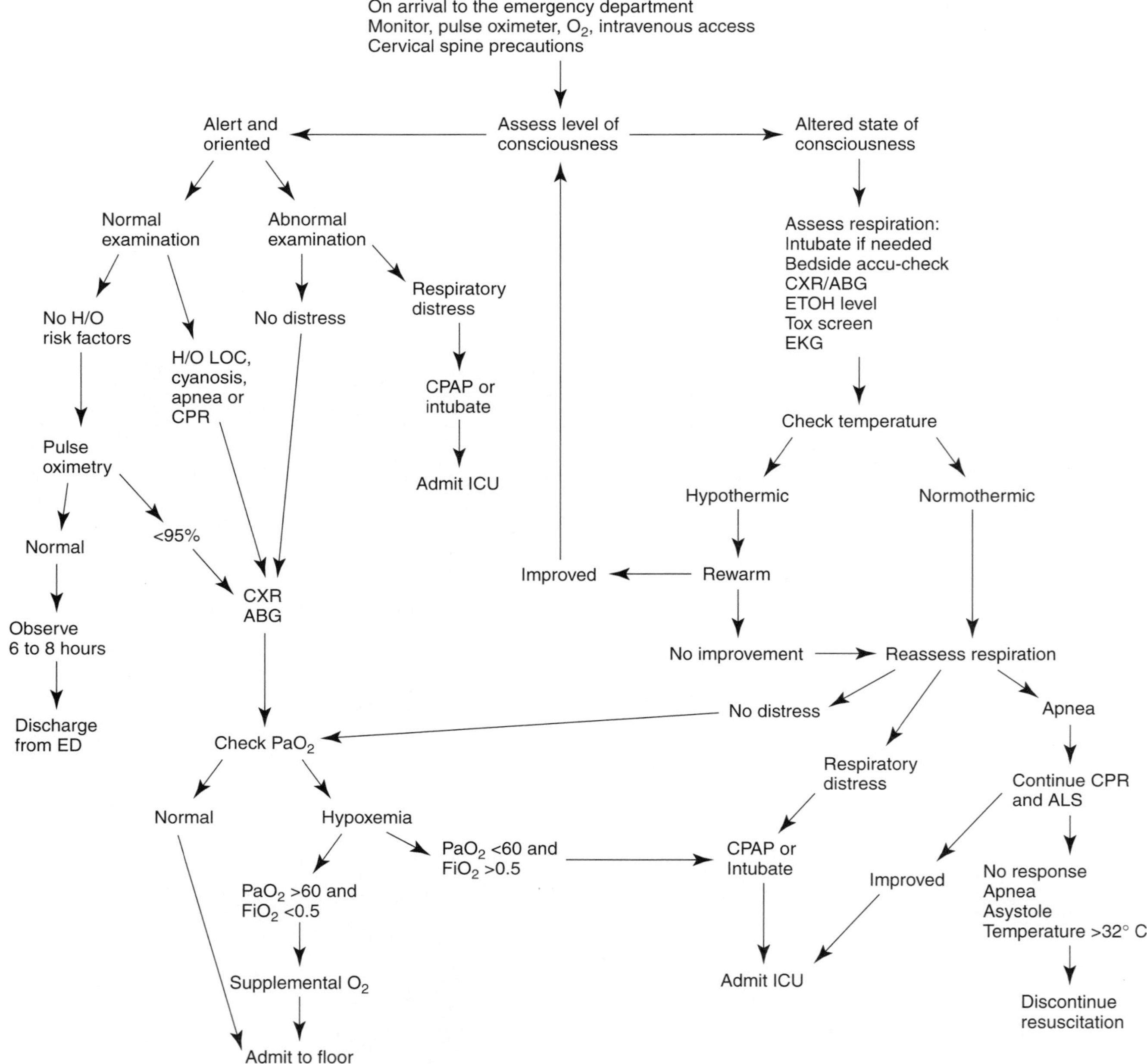

Fig. 39-4 Algorithm for emergency department management of near drowning. (From Shaw KN, Briede CA: *Emerg Med Clin North Am* 7[2]:367, 1989.)

often sufficient for the initial evaluation. Patients who are at risk for late deterioration and those with an abnormal examination or low oxygen saturation should have a more comprehensive evaluation.

GENERAL MEASURES

Management of patients after submersion starts with the ABCs and is then directed at addressing the adverse affects of hypoxia. During the initial primary survey in symptomatic near-drowning victims, the physician should reassess field therapy and ensure a patent airway. Hospital personnel should place the teenager on a cardiac monitor and pulse oximeter, continue supplemental oxygen and establish IV access if not previously done. A stat bedside glucose is required in any victim with altered mental status.

ANCILLARY DATA

Recommended initial studies in symptomatic patients include a CXR and pulse oximetry or arterial blood gas (ABG). An initial normal CXR does not rule out a significant pulmonary injury.[75] A repeat CXR is recommended in any patient with persistent or progressive signs of respiratory distress. The CXR of near-drowning victims may show perihilar infiltrates, varying degrees of pulmonary edema, or may be normal (20%).[75,76] Classic radiographic changes of ARDS may take hours to develop. The typical ABG findings following a significant event reveal hypoxemia with a combined respiratory and metabolic acidosis.

Frequently ordered tests include a complete blood count, electrolytes, blood urea nitrogen, and creatinine.[77,78] Further laboratory testing such as coagulation profile, type and cross, calcium level, magnesium level, serum ethanol, and/or toxicology screens may be indicated depending on the clinical setting.[60,78] An ECG is helpful to evaluate for myocardial ischemia, injury, or conduction defects that may have precipitated the submersion event.

RESPIRATORY

Patients who are spontaneously breathing should remain on humidified oxygen and be monitored closely for signs of respiratory distress, hypoxia, or a decreasing level of consciousness. Persistent hypoxemia on supplemental oxygen is an indication for treatment with continuous positive airway pressure (CPAP).[25,79] Mechanical ventilation is indicated for patients unable to maintain pO_2 >60 mmHg or pCO_2 <50 on 50% oxygen.[79] Intubated patients may require positive end-expiratory pressure (PEEP) starting at 5 mmHg and increasing in 2 to 5 mmHg increments until the patient is adequately oxygenated.[80] Muscle relaxation with paralytics may be useful to prevent muscle straining and improve ventilation and oxygenation.[45,81] A nasogastric tube prevents gastric dilation and decreases the risk of aspiration.

Bronchospasm following submersion usually responds to aerosolized β-agonists such as albuterol.[25] There is no evidence to support the routine use of prophylactic antibiotics in near-drowning victims.[81,82] However, if the aspirated water is known to be grossly contaminated (e.g., sewer water), prophylactic antibiotic therapy has been suggested.[83] In these cases, bronchoscopy may be required to remove particulate matter. Prophylactic steroids are contraindicated, as their use increases mortality.[55,84]

CARDIOVASCULAR

Cardiac dysrhythmias that occur during the course of the resuscitation often resolve with treatment of hypothermia. Persistent hypotension despite crystalloid boluses may require the use of inotropic agents such as dopamine or dobutamine. Critically ill victims will develop a severe lactic acidosis. The primary intervention is to ensure adequate oxygenation, ventilation, and circulation. The use of sodium bicarbonate therapy to correct acidosis is controversial.[16] Place a Foley catheter to monitor urine output in the seriously ill. Arterial lines are helpful to monitor cardiovascular status, especially in those patients who require frequent ABG determinations. More invasive monitoring (central venous pressure and Swan-Ganz catheters) may be indicated in the presence of hemodynamic instability.

CEREBRAL INJURY

The goal in treatment of cerebral injury is to maintain adequate oxygenation and cerebral blood flow and to minimize secondary damage from hypoxia, acidosis, hypotension, fluid overload, and uncontrolled seizure activity.[85] Measures may include elevation of the head of the bed, paralysis (if indicated to treat respiratory failure), and treatment of seizures with standard anticonvulsant therapy. Expectant treatment of cerebral edema with hyperventilation and hyperosmolar agents is unwarranted, since the clinical value of these measures is unproven.[85] Frequent neurologic assessments should be documented in the patient's record.

ASSOCIATED INJURIES

Because trauma is a possibility in all cases of submersion, protect the spine until a spinal injury is ruled out. The teenager was found to have a cervical spine fracture as a result of diving into the rock quarry. Unexplained shock, especially in conjunction with a low hematocrit, suggests the possibility of intraabdominal injury. Hypotension accompanied by bradycardia or priapism provides clues to neurogenic shock. Life-threatening dysbaric injuries may be present in patients involved in scuba diving accidents.

HYPOTHERMIA

Submersion victims often experience some degree of hypothermia, and rewarming is key. Once hypothermia is confirmed with a core temperature, preferably using a low-reading rectal probe thermometer, continuous core temperature monitoring should occur. Methods of rewarming include *passive external rewarming* (PER) achieved by covering the patient with an insulating material and keeping the room temperature >21° C (70° F).[86] This technique is indicated for patients with all levels of hypothermia and is sufficient by itself for mild illness (temperature >34° C/93.2° F).

Moderate hypothermia (temperature 30° to 33° C/86° to 93° F) requires *active rewarming*. External methods (AER) of rewarming include application of radiant light sources, heating blankets, or hot water bottles to the thorax only.[87] Heat application to the extremities may produce thermal injury to vasoconstricted and hypoperfused skin.[88] In addition, leaving the extremities vasoconstricted prevents *core-temperature afterdrop*[89,90] resulting from cold, lactic acid–rich blood being shunted from the periphery to the core.

Profound hypothermia (temperature < 30° C/86° F) requires aggressive treatment with AER in conjunction with *active core rewarming* (ACR) methods. Airway rewarming and heated IV fluids can be administered safely and effectively in all patients. The patient who is clinically stable can receive ACR and vigilant monitoring. If the patient is clinically unstable or in cardiac arrest, cardiopulmonary bypass may be the treatment of choice for core rewarming.[91] Patients who are severely hypothermic may be unresponsive to most drugs and countershock in ventricular fibrillation. Rapid rewarming is the best intervention for those patients resistant to defibrillation. However, the addition of bretylium tosylate may also be useful for ventricular fibrillation in hypothermia.[92] Magnesium sulfate has also been used successfully in the chemical conversion of hypothermic arrest victims.[93] In this setting, lidocaine has little efficacy[94,95] and procainamide has been reported to increase the incidence of ventricular fibrillation[96] and should not be used.

In actual clinical practice, most clinicians use a combination of these rewarming measures. It is not uncommon for a patient with moderate hypothermia to receive airway rewarming, heated IV fluids, radiant light heat, and a warm resuscitation room (>70° F).

It is often difficult to assess hypothermic patients who may appear clinically dead because of marked depression of brain and cardiovascular function. There are documented cases of prolonged submersion under hypothermic conditions with good outcomes, including one case of a child who was successfully resuscitated after a 66-minute submersion in 5° C (42° F) water.[47] Although unusual, full resuscitation with intact neurologic recovery is possible, and rewarming should continue until the patient's core temperature has reached at least 32° C (89.6° F).[97]

CONTROVERSIES

Use of the Heimlich Maneuver

In 1975 Heimlich et al[98] proposed the use of a subdiaphragmatic thrust as the initial treatment in victims of near drowning. Arguments for using the Heimlich maneuver are based on the belief that aspiration of water is the major cause of death because it obstructs the airways and prevents effective ventilation.[99] This belief was primarily based on anecdotal case reports provided to Dr. Heimlich and his colleagues, describing large volumes of fluid being extruded from submersion victims with the use of this maneuver. In some cases, it was reported that ventilation was not successful until the Heimlich maneuver was applied.[99]

Arguments against the use of the Heimlich maneuver are founded in a lack of experimental support. As Modell and Davis[57] have shown, the majority of victims aspirate less than 22 ml/kg. Aspirated fresh water is rapidly absorbed into the circulation and therefore not available for removal.[100] With aspiration of hypertonic sea water, fluid is drawn into the lungs damaging the capillary membrane and resulting in pulmonary edema. There is no evidence that the Heimlich maneuver can remove pulmonary edema fluid or aspirated water from the alveoli.[70,71] Use of this technique may result in vomiting and subsequent aspiration of emesis, compounding the pulmonary injury and interfering with rescue breathing.[101,102] In cases of spinal injury, this technique may be dangerous. Of greatest concern is the fact that it delays the establishment of effective ventilation and oxygenation, which have been shown to be the key to survival.[55,79]

For the above reasons, the American Heart Association has recommended "that the Heimlich maneuver should not be used for victims of near drowning unless obstruction of the airway from foreign body is strongly suspected."[103]

Utility of Cerebral Resuscitation

Because increased intracranial pressure (ICP) and cerebral edema are often seen in comatose patients after near drowning, measures to control ICP have been advocated by some investigators. In 1979 Conn et al[42] proposed a unique therapy to prevent secondary injury to the CNS. The "**HYPER therapy**" consisted of diuresis and fluid restriction (1/3 maintenance), hyperventilation, hypothermia to 30° C, barbiturates, steroids, and muscle paralysis to treat increased ICP guided by invasive monitoring. This recommendation was based on the observation that submersion victims were hyper**H**ydrated, h**Y**perventilating, hyper**P**yretic, hyper**E**xcitable, and hyper**R**igid. In 1980 they reported neurologic survival in a small series of nonflaccid comatose patients who received this therapy.[104]

The argument against aggressive cerebral resuscitation is that multiple studies have shown these interventions have no survival benefit for most patients with increased ICP.[5,105,106] In Bohn et al's[105] series of 40 patients, there was no change in outcome with the use of induced hypothermia or barbiturates. There was also a significantly higher rate of neutropenia and sepsis in those patients treated with induced hypothermia. Additionally, there is no clinical evidence that control of intracranial and cerebral perfusion pressure predicts or improves neurologic outcome. Indeed, there is no consistent relationship between increased ICP and outcome in near drowning.[81,105,107-109] Therefore the use of ICP monitoring, corticosteroids, barbiturates, and controlled hypothermia is no longer recommended.

DISPOSITION

It is tempting to rapidly discharge the *asymptomatic* submersion victim with no evidence of injury. Yet, some authorities have recommended that all patients with a history of submersion be hospitalized.[5,31,110] This recommendation is based on the concern that some victims will develop delayed respiratory complications 12 to 72 hours after the event.[5,38,111]

Although "secondary drowning" has been well documented, it most likely represents evolution of a preexisting lung injury rather than an abrupt phenomenon. In addition, it would be extremely unlikely for a patient sustaining a significant pulmonary insult to present without any signs or symptoms immediately following rescue and initial resuscitation.

More recent literature suggests that most submersion victims can be evaluated and observed for 6 to 8 hours in the ED, then safely discharged if they remain asymptomatic. A 1991 California retrospective review found that 84% of near-drowning victims were discharged home in good condition, most on the same day or after an overnight stay.[112] In a recent review by Noonan et al[113] of 75 hospitalized patients, 98% of patients developed symptoms during the first 4.5 hours after the immersion, with a delay in one victim of 7 hours.

Patients who are discharged from the ED should leave with a responsible adult and a plan for close follow-up. Give strict instructions to return immediately for any respiratory distress including shortness of breath, wheezing, fever, persistent cough, or change in mental status.

Admission is required for victims who have persistent respiratory symptoms (dyspnea, cough, or chest discomfort); physical examination findings such as tachycardia, tachypnea, adventitious lung sounds, respiratory distress, or altered mental status; and for those with an abnormal CXR.[77]

Candidates for ICU admission include those with depressed mental status; hypothermia <32° C (89.6° F); acidosis or persistent hypoxemia; unstable cardiovascular status; those requiring respiratory support including CPAP, PEEP or intubation; or those with rapidly progressing signs or symptoms.[79]

PROGNOSIS

Investigators have studied various prognostic signs and symptoms; however, none is completely reliable. Survival depends on a number of factors, including the age of the victim, water temperature and degree of hypothermia, duration of submersion, and promptness and effectiveness of the initial resuscitation.[68,107,114,115]

Although some studies[48,116] report 12% to 27% of near-drowning victims sustain severe neurologic damage, the prognosis for most *pediatric survivors* is good, with morbidity ranging from 3.5% to 5%.[42,84,117,118] The higher rates of survival in children may be as a result of physiologic differences such as the *diving reflex*.[119,120] This primitive mammalian reflex is triggered by submersion of the face in cold water (<20° C/68° F). The resulting bradycardia and redistribution of blood flow to the heart and brain allow prolonged submersion without CNS damage.[121] Other investigators question the role of the diving reflex. Water temperature and the *degree of hypothermia* also affect survival. The rapid onset of hypothermia decreases the metabolic demands of the body, thus delaying the onset of severe cerebral hypoxia.[122] In Orlowski's review[123] of 17 cases of prolonged submersion followed by good outcomes, water temperature was found to be 10° C (77° F) or colder. Other studies[124-126] have noted a uniformly poor outcome (death or severe neurologic impairment) in all patients who required CPR in the ED after warm water submersion.

The neurologic status of the patient on arrival to the ED has been shown to correlate with outcome. Almost all patients who are alert and fully conscious survive without sequelae, as well as the majority of those who are obtunded but arousable with spontaneous respirations.[84,104] In contrast, patients who present in a coma have mortality rates of 34% to 68%.[81,104,127]

The importance of *rapid rescue and immediate CPR* has been recognized by numerous authorities on the subject of near drowning.[5,70,110,128] A 1990 study by Quan et al[126] demonstrated that prehospital intervention could improve outcome in pediatric submersion victims. Patients receiving advanced cardiac life support (ACLS) for apnea, absent blood pressure and pulse (or severe bradycardia), had a 32% survival rate, and two thirds of these survivors were neurologically intact or only minimally impaired. A bad outcome (death or severe neurologic impairment) was associated with submersion over 9 minutes or CPR longer than 25 minutes (100% risk). This finding correlates with the findings of Orlowski[68] and others[129,130] regarding the importance of *submersion time*.

COMMON PITFALLS

Box 39-3 lists important considerations and potential pitfalls in the management of submersion victims.

Determine the Etiology of the Submersion Event

During the initial evaluation and resuscitation, determine the precipitating cause of submersion. Cerebrovascular accidents, myocardial infarctions, seizures, and substance abuse have all been associated with near drowning. A rapid evaluation of the scene, reports from bystanders, and history from the patient and family may assist in care.

Search for the Underlying Problem in Altered Mental Status

Decreased mental status secondary to hypoxemia is often present in submersion victims. Consider other etiologies, including intracranial injury, hypoglycemia, hypothermia, drug and ethanol intoxication, or a postictal state.

Evaluate for Concomitant Injuries

Diving, boating, surfing, scuba diving, and waterskiing accidents may all cause injuries and place individuals at risk for near drowning. It is imperative to suspect and evaluate patients for occult trauma.

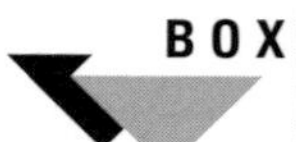

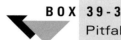

BOX 39-3
Pitfalls in the Management of Submersion Victims Include Failure to:

1. Determine the etiology of the submersion event
2. Search for the underlying problem in altered mental status
3. Consider/evaluate for associated injuries
4. Suspect nonaccidental trauma in cases involving children
5. Promote prevention as the primary health strategy for drowning

Consider Nonaccidental Trauma

In children under 5 years of age, up to 8% of all submersions, and nearly 40% of bathtub submersions may be nonaccidental.[15,131] Any episode involving a bathtub or pool should raise the possibility of child abuse or neglect.

Prevention Is Key to Reducing Morbidity and Mortality

The high case-fatality rate and morbidity associated with near drowning mandate that prevention rather than treatment be the primary health strategy.[48] Multiple approaches to drowning prevention are necessary.

Inadequate fencing is an important factor in swimming pool drownings.[29] The addition of a fence with latched gates may reduce swimming pool drownings by 50% to 90%.[132,133] Because many incidents of young toddler drowning occur during lapses of adult supervision,[15] educating parents about constant vigilance at pools is essential.

Additional factors commonly associated with drowning include alcohol use,[124] poor swimming ability,[134] and absence of persons trained in life-saving techniques, including CPR.[135,136] Encourage parents to install phones near the pool and learn CPR. Advise teenagers and young adults to use personal floatation devices, obtain specific training for personal watercraft devices, and avoid alcohol consumption during water recreation.

Efforts should also be directed to the prevention of drowning in hot tubs, whirlpools, pails, toilets, and other small containers of water.[26,137,138] Advise parents that young children can drown in only 1 to 2 inches of water. Although relatively infrequent, these deaths are easily prevented. Inquiring about a hot tub or whirlpool will alert new parents to this potential hazard. Caution elderly patients of the danger of bathtub falls and encourage patients with medical conditions that may impair consciousness (e.g., seizures) to swim with a partner and shower instead of bathing.

REFERENCES

1. Zamula WW: Social cost of drownings and near-drownings. In: *Submersion accidents occurring to children under five in residential swimming pools,* Washington, DC, 1987, Directorate for economic analysis, US Consumer Product Safety Commission.
2. Plueckhahn VD: Drowning: community aspects, *Med J Aust* 2:226-228, 1979.
3. National Safety Council: *Accident facts, 1993,* Itasca, Il, 1993, National Safety Council.
4. Modell JH: Drown versus near-drown: a discussion of definitions, *Crit Care Med* 9:351-352, 1981.
5. Orlowski JP: Drowning, near-drowning, and ice-water submersions, *Pediatr Clin North Am* 34:75-92, 1987.

6. National Center for Injury Prevention and Control: *Ten leading causes of death tables: 1994,* Atlanta, 1996, Centers for Disease Control and Prevention.
7. Wintemute GJ: Childhood drowning and near-drowning in the United States, *Am J Dis Child* 144:663-669, 1990.
8. Drownings-Georgia, 1981-1983, *MMWR* 34:281-283, 1985.
9. Gulaid JA, Sattin RW: Drownings in the United States, 1978-1984, *MMWR* 37:27-33, 1988.
10. Baker SP, O'Neill B, Karpf RS: *The injury fact book,* Lexington, Ma, 1984, DC Heath & Co.
11. Hazinski MF, et al: Pediatric injury prevention, *Ann Emerg Med* 22:456-467, 1993.
12. Giammona ST: Drowning: Pathophysiology and management, *Curr Probl Pediatr* 1:1-33, 1971.
13. Jumbelic MI, Chambliss M: Accidental toddler drowning in 5-gallon buckets, *JAMA* 263:1952-1953, 1990.
14. Sulkes SB, van der Jagt EW: Solar pool blankets: another water hazard, *Pediatrics* 85:1114-1117, 1990.
15. Quan L, et al: Ten year study of pediatric drownings and near-drownings in King County: lessons in injury prevention, Washington, *Pediatrics* 83:1035-1040, 1989.
16. Knopp R: Near-drowning, *J Am Coll Emerg Phys* 7:249, 1978.
17. Modell JH: *The pathophysiology and treatment of drowning and near-drowning,* Springfield, Il, 1971, Charles C Thomas.
18. Podolsky ML: Action plan for near drownings, *Phys Sportsmed* 9:45, 1981.
19. Press E, Walker J, Crawford I: An interstate drowning study, *Am J Public Health* 58:2275-2289, 1968.
20. Kraus JF. Epidemiological aspects of acute spinal cord injury: a review of incidence, prevalence, causes, and outcome. In Becker DP, Povlishock JT (editors): *Central nervous system trauma status report-1985,* Bethesda, Maryland, 1985, National Institute of Neurological and Communicative Disorders and Stroke, National Institutes of Health.
21. National Coordinating Council on Spinal Cord Injury: Head and spinal cord injury prevention, *NCCSCI Dialogue* (July):3, 1988.
22. Schuman SH, et al: Risk of drowning: an iceberg phenomenon, *JACEP* 6:139, 1977.
23. Branche CM, Conn JM, Annest JL: Personal watercraft-related injuries: a growing public health concern, *JAMA* 278:663-665, 1997.
24. Craig AB Jr: Causes of loss of consciousness during underwater swimming, *J Appl Physiol* 16:583-586, 1961.
25. Olshaker JS: Near drowning, *Emerg Med Clin North Am* 10:339-350, 1992.
26. Monroe B: Immersion accidents in hot tubs and whirlpool spas, *Pediatrics* 69:805-807, 1982.
27. Brown V: Human factor analysis: spa associated hazards-an update and summary, Washington, DC, Division of Human Factors, Directorate for Hazard Identification and Analysis, U.S. Consumer Product Safety Commission, 1981.
28. Orlowski JP, Rothner AD, Leuders H: Submersion accidents in children with epilepsy, *Am J Dis Child* 136:777-780, 1982.
29. Pearn J, Brown J 3rd, Hsia EY: Swimming pool drownings and near-drownings involving children: a total population study from Hawaii, *Milit Med* 145:15-18, 1980.
30. Hegnauer AH, Angelakos ET: Excitable properties of the hypothermic heart, *Ann N Y Acad Sci* 80:336-347, 1959.
31. Martin TG: Near-drowning and cold water immersion, *Ann Emerg Med* 13:263-273, 1984.
32. Ritchie BC: The physiology of drowning, *Med J Aust* 2:1187-1189, 1972
33. Lamphier TA: Current status of treatment of near drowning, *Alaska Med* 21:72-77, 1979.
34. Knopp R: Near drowning. In Rosen P, et al (editors): *Emergency medicine concepts and clinical practice,* St Louis,1983, Mosby.
35. Orlowski JP, Abulleil MM, Phillips JM: Effects of tonicities of saline solutions on pulmonary injury in drowning, *Crit Care Med* 15:126-130, 1987.
36. Sims JK, et al: Marine bacteria complicating near-drowning and marine wounds: a hypothesis, *Ann Emerg Med* 12:212-216, 1983.
37. Levin DL: Near drowning, *Crit Care Med* 8:590-595, 1980.
38. Pearn JH: Secondary drowning in children, *Br Med J* 281:1103-1105, 1980.
39. Bross MH, Clark JL: Near drowning, *Am Fam Phys* 51:1545-1551, 1995.
40. Modell JH: Biology of drowning, *Annu Rev Med* 29:1-8, 1978.
41. Rivers JF, Orr G, Lee HA: Drowning: its clinical sequelae and management, *Br Med J* 2:157-161, 1970.
42. Conn AW, Edmonds JF, Barker GA: Cerebral resuscitation in near-drowning, *Pediatr Clin North Am* 26:691-701, 1979.
43. Martinez-Lopez JI: Induced hypothermia: electrocardiographic abnormalities, *South Med J* 69:1548-1550, 1976.
44. Trevino A, Razi B, Beller BM: The characteristic electrocardiogram of accidental hypothermia, *Arch Intern Med* 127:470-473, 1971.
45. Gonzalez-Rothi RJ: Near-drowning: consensus and controversies in pulmonary and cerebral resuscitation, *Heart Lung* 16: 474-482, 1987.
46. McGillicuddy JE: Cerebral protection: pathophysiology and treatment of increased intracranial pressure, *Chest* 87:85-93, 1985.
47. Bolte RG et al: The use of extracorporeal rewarming in a child submerged for 66 minutes, *JAMA* 260:377-379, 1988.
48. Fandel I, Bancalari E. Near-drowning in children: clinical aspects, *Pediatrics* 58:573-579, 1976.
49. King RB, Webster IW: A case of recovery from drowning and prolonged anoxia, *Med J Aust* 1:919-920, 1964.
50. Reilly K, et al: Linguistic status subsequent to childhood immersion injury, *Med J Aust* 148:225-228, 1988.
51. Sibert JR, Webb E, Cooper S: Drowning and near drowning in children, *Practitioner* 232:439-440, 1988.
52. Kewalramani LS, Orth MS, Taylor RG: Injuries to the cervical spine from diving accidents, *J Trauma* 15:130-142, 1975.
53. Grausz H, Amend WJ Jr., Earley LE: Acute renal failure complicating submersion in sea water, *JAMA* 217:207-209, 1971.
54. Battaglia JD, Lockhart CH: Drowning and near drowning, *Pediatr Ann* 6:270-275, 1977.
55. Modell JH, Graves SA, Ketover A: Clinical course of 91 consecutive near-drowning victims, *Chest* 70:231-238, 1976.
56. Foroughi E: Serum changes in drowning, *J Forensic Sci* 16:269-282, 1971.
57. Modell JH, Davis JH: Electrolyte changes in human drowning victims, *Anesthesiology* 30:414-420, 1969.
58. Modell JH, et al: The effects of fluid volume in seawater drowning, *Ann Intern Med* 67:68-80, 1967.
59. Modell JH, Moya F: Effects of volume of aspirated fluid during chlorinated fresh water drowning, *Anesthesiology* 27:662-672, 1966.
60. Yagil Y, et al: Near drowning in the Dead Sea: electrolyte imbalances and therapeutic implications, *Arch Intern Med* 145:50-53, 1985.
61. Kvittingen TD, Naess A: Recovery from drowning in freshwater, *Br Med J* 1:1315-1317, 1963.
62. Munroe WD: Hemoglobinuria from near-drowning, *J Pediatr* 64:57-62,1964.
63. Hasan S, et al. Near drowning in humans: a report of 36 patients, *Chest* 59:191-197, 1971.

64. Ports TA, Deuel TF: Intravascular coagulation in fresh-water submersion: Report of three cases, *Ann Intern Med* 87:60-61, 1977.
65. Brooks JG. Near drowning, *Pediatr Rev* 10:5-10, 1988.
66. Fuller RH: The clinical pathology of human near-drowning, *Proc R Soc Med* 56:33-38, 1963.
67. Sarnaik AP, Vohra MP: Near-drowning: fresh, salt, and cold water immersion, *Clin Sports Med* 5:33-46, 1986.
68. Orlowski JP: Prognostic factors in pediatric cases of drowning and near-drowning, *JACEP* 8:176-179, 1979.
69. Kizer KW: Resuscitation of submersion casualties, *Emerg Med Clin North Am* 1:643-652, 1983.
70. Ornato JP: The resuscitation of near-drowning victims, *JAMA* 256:75-77, 1986.
71. Ruben A, Ruben H: Artificial respiration-flow of water from the lung and stomach, *Lancet* 1:780-781, 1962.
72. Tacker WA Jr, et al: Transchest defibrillation under conditions of hypothermia, *Crit Care Med* 9:390-391, 1981.
73. Conn AW: Near drowning and hypothermia, *Can Med Assoc J* 120:397-400, 1979.
74. Layon AJ, Modell JH: Drowning and near-drowning. In Tinker J, Zapol W (editors): *Care of the critically ill patient,* ed 2, London, 1991, SpringerVerlag.
75. Hunter TB, Whitehouse WM: Fresh-water near-drowning: radiological aspects, *Radiology* 112:51-56, 1974.
76. Wunderlich P, et al: Chest radiographs of near-drowned children, *Pediatr Radiol* 15:297-299, 1985.
77. Newman AB: Submersion incidents. In Auerbach PS (editor): *Wilderness medicine,* St Louis, 1995, Mosby.
78. Smyrnios NA, Irwin RS: Current concepts in the pathophysiology and management of near-drowning, *J Intens Care Med* 6:26, 1991.
79. Shaw KN, Briede CA: Submersion injuries: drowning and near drowning, *Emerg Med Clin North Am* 7:355-370, 1989.
80. Redding J, Voight GC, Safar P: Drowning treated with intermittent positive pressure breathing, *J Appl Physiol* 15:849-854, 1960.
81. Oakes DD, et al: Prognosis and management of victims of near-drowning, *J Trauma* 22:544-549, 1982.
82. Tabeling BB, Modell JH: Fluid administration increases oxygen delivery during continuous positive ventilation after fresh water near-drowning, *Crit Care Med* 11:693-696, 1983.
83. Modell JH: Drowning, *N Engl J Med* 328:253-256, 1993.
84. Modell JH, Graves SA, Kuck EJ: Near-drowning: correlation of level of consciousness and survival, *Can Anaesth Soc J* 27:211-215, 1980.
85. Modell JH: Treatment of near drowning. Is there a role for H.Y.P.E.R. therapy? *Crit Care Med* 14:593-594, 1986.
86. Ennemoser O, Ambach W, Flora G: Physical assessment of heat insulation rescue foils, *Int J Sports Med* 9:179-182, 1988.
87. Harnett RM, Pruitt JR, Sias FR: A review of the literature concerning resuscitation from hypothermia: Part II. Selected rewarming protocols, *Aviat Space Environ Med* 54:487-495, 1983.
88. Feldman KW, Morray JP, Schaller RT: Thermal injury caused by hot pack application in hypothermic children, *Am J Emerg Med* 3:38-41, 1985.
89. Savard GK, et al: Peripheral blood flow during rewarming from mild hypothermia in humans, *J Appl Physiol* 58:4-13, 1985.
90. Webb P: Afterdrop of body temperature during rewarming: an alternative explanation, *J Appl Physiol* 60:385-390, 1986.
91. Hauty MG, et al: Prognostic factors in severe accidental hypothermia: experience from the Mt. Hood tragedy, *J Trauma* 27: 1107-1112, 1987.
92. Dazyl DF: Bretylium in hypothermia, *Wilderness Med* 4:5, 1987.
93. Buky B: Effect of magnesium on ventricular fibrillation due to hypothermia, *Br J Anaesth* 42:886-888, 1970.
94. Angelakos ET: Influence of pharmacological agents on spontaneous and surgically induced hypothermic ventricular fibrillation, *Ann NY Acad Sci* 80:351-364, 1959.
95. Nielsen KC, Owman C: Control of ventricular fibrillation during induced hypothermia in cats after blocking the adrenergic neurons with bretylium, *Life Sci* 7:159-168, 1968.
96. Dundee JW, Clarke RS: Pharmacology of hypothermia, *Int Anesth Clin* 2:857-872, 1964.
97. Corneli HM: Accidental hypothermia, *J Pediatr* 120:671-679, 1992.
98. Heimlich HJ, Hoffman KA, Canestri FR: Food-choking and drowning deaths prevented by external subdiaphragmatic compression. Physiological basis, *Ann Thorac Surg* 20:188-195, 1975.
99. Heimlich HJ: Subdiaphragmatic pressure to expel water from the lungs of drowning persons, *Ann Emerg Med* 10:476-480, 1981.
100. Moser RH: Drowning: a seasonal disease, *JAMA* 229:563-566, 1974.
101. Modell JH: Is the Heimlich maneuver appropriate as first treatment for drowning? *Emerg Med Serv* 10:63, 1981.
102. Orlowski JP: Vomiting as a complication of the Heimlich maneuver, *JAMA* 258:512-513, 1987.
103. American Heart Association: *Textbook of advanced cardiac life support,* ed 2, Dallas, 1990, American Heart Association.
104. Conn AW et al: Cerebral salvage in near-drowning following neurological classification by triage, *Can Anaesth Soc J* 27:201-210, 1980.
105. Bohn DJ, et al: Influence of hypothermia, barbiturate therapy, and intracranial pressure monitoring on morbidity and mortality after near-drowning, *Crit Care Med* 14:529-534, 1986.
106. Frewen TC, et al: Cerebral resuscitation therapy in pediatric near-drowning, *J Pediatr* 106:615-617, 1985.
107. Allman FD, et al: Outcome following cardiopulmonary resuscitation in severe pediatric near-drowning, *Am J Dis Child* 140: 571-575, 1986.
108. Nussbaum E, Galant SP: Intracranial pressure monitoring as a guide to prognosis in the nearly drowned, severely comatose child, *J Pediatr* 102:215-218, 1983.
109. Sarnaik AP, et al: Intracranial pressure and cerebral perfusion pressure in near-drowning, *Crit Care Med* 13:224-227, 1985.
110. Robinson MD, Seward PN: Submersion injury in children, *Pediatr Emerg Care* 3:44-49, 1987.
111. Dick AE, Potgieter PD: Secondary drowning in the Cape Peninsula, *S Afr Med J* 62:803-806, 1982.
112. Ellis AA, Trent RB: Hospitalizations for near drowning in California: incidence and costs, *Am J Public Health* 85:1115-1118, 1995.
113. Noonan L, Howrey R, Ginsburg CM: Freshwater submersion injuries in children: a retrospective review of seventy-five hospitalized patients, *Pediatrics* 98:368-371, 1996.
114. Jacobsen WK, et al: Correlation of spontaneous respiration and neurologic damage in near-drowning, *Crit Care Med* 11:487-489, 1983.
115. Dean JM, Kaufman ND: Prognostic indicators in pediatric near-drowning, the Glasgow Coma Scale, *Crit Care Med* 9:536-539, 1981.
116. Peterson B: Morbidity of childhood near-drowning, *Pediatrics* 59:364-370, 1977.
117. Pearn JH, Bart RD Jr., Yamaoka R: Neurologic sequelae after childhood near-drowning: a total population study from Hawaii, *Pediatrics* 64:187-191, 1979.
118. Wegener FH, Edwards RM: Cerebral support for near-drowned children in a temperate environment, *Med J Aust* 2:135-137, 1980.

119. Hayward JS, et al: Temperature effect on the human dive response in relation to cold water near-drowning, *J Appl Physiol* 56:202-206, 1984.
120. Ramey CA, Ramey DN, Hayward JS: Dive response of children in relation to cold-water near-drowning, *J Appl Physiol* 63:665-668, 1987.
121. Elsner R, Gooden BA: Reduction of reactive hyperemia in the human forearm by face immersion, *J Appl Physiol* 29:627-630, 1970.
122. Conn AW, Barker GA: Fresh water drowning and near-drowning: an update, *Can Anaesth Soc J* 31:538-544, 1984.
123. Orlowski JP: Drowning, near-drowning, and icewater drowning, *JAMA* 260:390-391, 1988.
124. Biggart MJ, Bohn DJ: Effect of hypothermia and cardiac arrest on outcome of near-drowning accidents in children, *J Pediatr* 117:179-183, 1990.
125. Nichter MA, Everett PB: Childhood near-drowning: is cardiopulmonary resuscitation always indicated? *Crit Care Med* 17: 993-995, 1989.
126. Quan L, et al: Outcome and predictors of outcome in pediatric submersion victims receiving prehospital care in King County, Washington, *Pediatrics* 86:586-593, 1990.
127. Bierens JJ, et al: Submersion in the Netherlands: prognostic indicators and results of resuscitation, *Ann Emerg Med* 19:1390-1395, 1990.
128. Modell JH: Near-drowning. In Callahan ML, editor: *Current therapy in emergency medicine,* St Louis, 1986, Mosby.
129. Pearn J: Survival rates after serious immersion accidents in childhood, *Resuscitation* 6:271-278, 1978.
130. Present P: Child drowning study: a report on the epidemiology of drownings in residential pools of children under age five, Washington, DC, 1987, Division of Hazard Analysis, Directorate for Epidemiology, U.S. Consumer Product Safety Commission.
131. Lavelle JM, et al: Ten-year review of pediatric bathtub near-drownings: evaluation for child abuse and neglect, *Ann Emerg Med* 25:344-348, 1995.
132. Milliner N, Pearn J, Guard R: Will fenced pools save lives? A 10-year study from Mulgrave Shire, Queensland, *Med J Aust* 2:510-511, 1980.
133. Pearn J, Nixon J: Prevention of childhood drowning accidents, *Med J Aust* 1:616-618, 1977.
134. Dietz PE, Baker SP: Drowning: epidemiology and prevention, *Am J Public Health* 64:303-312, 1974.
135. Patetta MJ, Biddinger PW: Characteristics of drowning deaths in North Carolina, *Public Health Rep* 103:406, 1989.
136. Wintemute GJ, et al: Drowning in childhood and adolescence: a population-based study, *Am J Public Health* 77:830-832, 1987.
137. Tron VA, Baldwin VJ, Pirie GE: Hot tub drownings, *Pediatrics* 75:789-790, 1985.
138. Walker S, Middlekamp JN: Pail immersion accidents, *Clin Pediatr* 20:341-343, 1981.

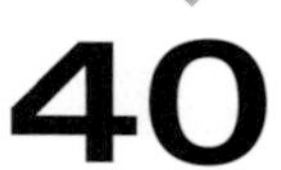

40 Gunshot Wounds

VINCENT N. MOSESSO, Jr. AND PETER C. FERRERA

Firearms pose unique problems in emergency care. Internal injuries range from the inconsequential to disastrous, despite similar entry wounds, and quickly recognizing the difference means life or death for the victim. A basic understanding of ballistics will help the emergency physician (EP) manage patients with gunshot wounds (GSW). Although many of the principles span both military and civilian injuries, this chapter is intended for the civilian practitioner. Treatment of battlefield casualties may differ from the approach to the urban gladiator, mainly because of a disparity in ballistics. The most important aspect in the initial care of patients with bullet wounds is to treat the patient and the wound and not be overly concerned about the weapon that caused the injury.[1]

Diagrammatic representations of standard handgun and rifle cartridges are shown in Fig. 40-1. The metal casing encloses the powder, above which the bullet is seated. The powder is ignited through the flash hole when the primer is struck. A case with a rim is found with revolver and lever action rifle cartridges, and with some bolt action and semiautomatic rifles.

BALLISTICS

Ballistics refers to the movement of a bullet. This movement includes the trajectory down the barrel, through the air, and into a target.[1] Bullets are powered by the expansion of burning gunpowder, which generates pressure (force/area). The "area" in this formula refers to the base of the bullet (equivalent to the diameter of the barrel) and remains a constant for each gun. The energy transmitted to the bullet (with a given mass) depends on mass times force times the time interval over which the force is applied. The last of these factors is a function of barrel length. Bullets accelerate in the gun barrel as the expanding gases push on it. Up to a point, the longer the barrel, the greater the acceleration. For example, rifle bullets have more energy than similar bullets fired from a handgun. Not only is the barrel longer, but more powder is used in rifle cartridges, since the gun chambers withstand greater pressures (70,000 psi versus 40,000 psi for handgun chamber). Although it is difficult to measure the forces in a gun barrel, it is simple to gauge the velocity at which the bullet exits the barrel (**muzzle velocity**).

The movement of a bullet outside the gun barrel is determined by several formulae, the simplest of which is: **Kinetic Energy (KE)** = $1/2\ MV^2$. Velocity (V) is usually measured in feet/second (fps). Mass (M) in pounds is derived from the weight (W) of the bullet in grains divided by 7000 grains per pound times the acceleration of gravity (32 ft/sec). However, with regards to wounds, it is less important to describe KE than how the projectile injures the tissue (i.e., crushing versus tissue tearing by temporary cavitation).

WOUNDING

Cinematic gunfights perpetuate the myth that victims are "knocked down" by the force of a bullet. In reality, real gunshot victims relate that they had no immediate reaction.[2] Incapacitation is primarily a function of where the victim is shot. Gunshot wounds to the brain and upper cervical cord immediately disable the victim, whereas rapid hemodynamic decompensation occurs with massive bleeding from major blood vessels or the heart.[3]

Bullets produce tissue damage in three ways:[4]

1. **Crushing:** Low-velocity bullets (as in handguns) that travel less than 1000 fps damage by crushing.
2. **Cavitation:** Cavitation is significant with projectiles traveling in excess of 1000 fps. The path of the bullet causes a **"permanent" cavity**, whereas a **"temporary" cavity** is formed by acceleration of the medium (air or tissue) in the bullet's wake, causing

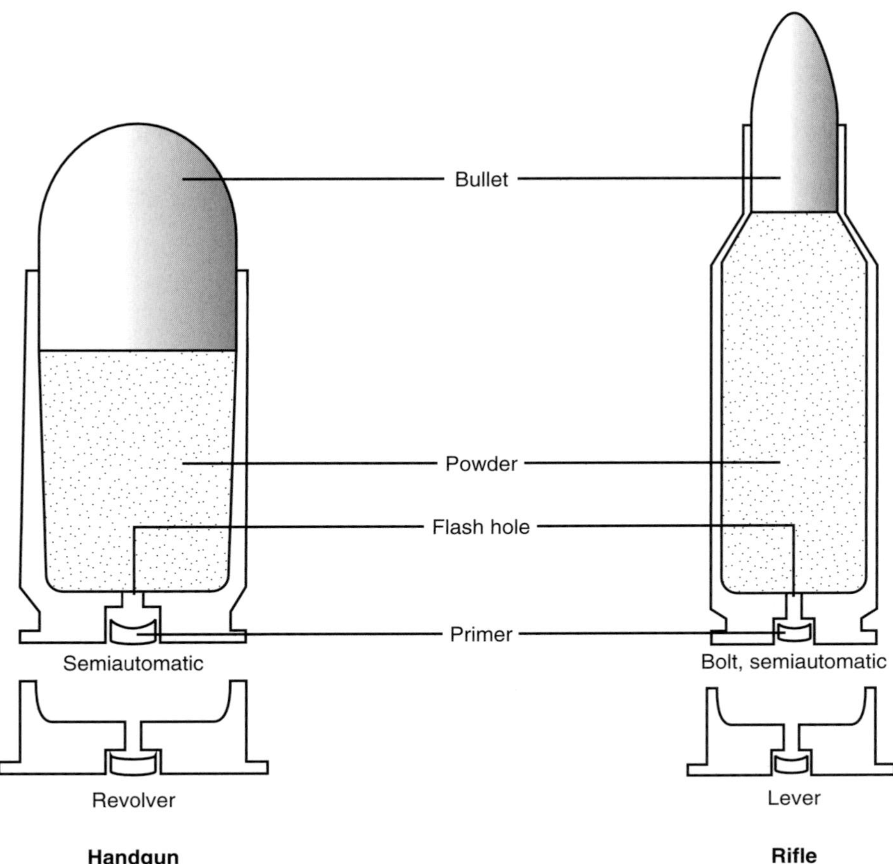

Fig. 40-1 Standard handgun and rifle cartridges. (From the Internet Pathology Laboratory for Medical Education. Copyright 1994-1999, 2000 by Edward C. Klatt, Department of Pathology, University of Utah, Salt Lake City, Utah.)

the wound cavity to be stretched outward. Fractures from cavitation are rare.[1]

3. **Shock waves:** Shock waves (also known as **sonic pressure waves**) represent the projectile's sound striking the surface of an object. These waves compress the tissue and travel ahead of the bullet. The waves last only a few microseconds and at low velocity do not cause profound destruction. At high velocity, generated shock waves can reach up to 200 atmospheres.[5] Still, bone fracture outside the permanent cavity is rare.[1]

Wounding is a complex process dependent on many variables, including bullet size, velocity, shape, spin, distance from muzzle to target, and nature of the injured tissue. These factors interact, and wound severity may be difficult to predict even under controlled testing. A projectile must travel 163 fps to penetrate skin and 213 fps to break bone. Because of these low velocities, other factors are more important in producing damage.[6] Bullet expansion after leaving the muzzle applies to only high-velocity handguns (exceeding 1200 fps).

So-called "**high-velocity**" rounds do not necessarily produce more damage, since they are jacketed and the bullet is smaller. For example, the jacketed bullet of the 6.5 mm high-velocity Mannlicher-Carcano travels for up to 24 inches in soft tissue, leaving small holes that minimally disrupt tissue.[1] Tissue damage is often a function of bullet **yaw**, the tendency of the bullet to turn sideways relative to its path. A fully jacketed 7.62 mm military round creates a much smaller temporary and permanent cavity in tissue than a 7.62 mm civilian "hunting" round (0.308 Winchester) with a soft-point tip, despite the fact that both are high-velocity rounds (Fig. 40-2). The 0.308 Winchester is more destructive because the bullet loses one third of its weight in fragments, which then result in multiple injuries.[1]

Tumbling is important to the injury pattern. The physics of tumble is ironically called **terminal ballistics**. A short, high-velocity bullet tumbles more rapidly in tissue. Tumbling displaces tissue and transfers greater KE to the target. Organ damage is proportionate to the amount of energy a bullet transmits to the

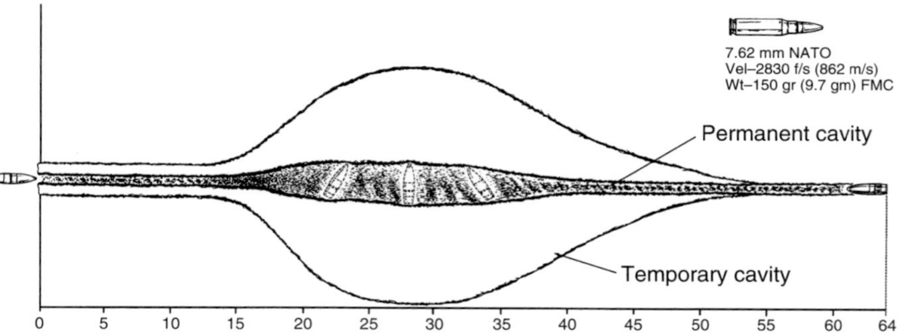

Fig. 40-2 Small temporary and permanent cavity made by military 7.62 NATO bullet. (From Fackler ML: *Ann Emerg Med* 28[2]:194-203, 1996.)

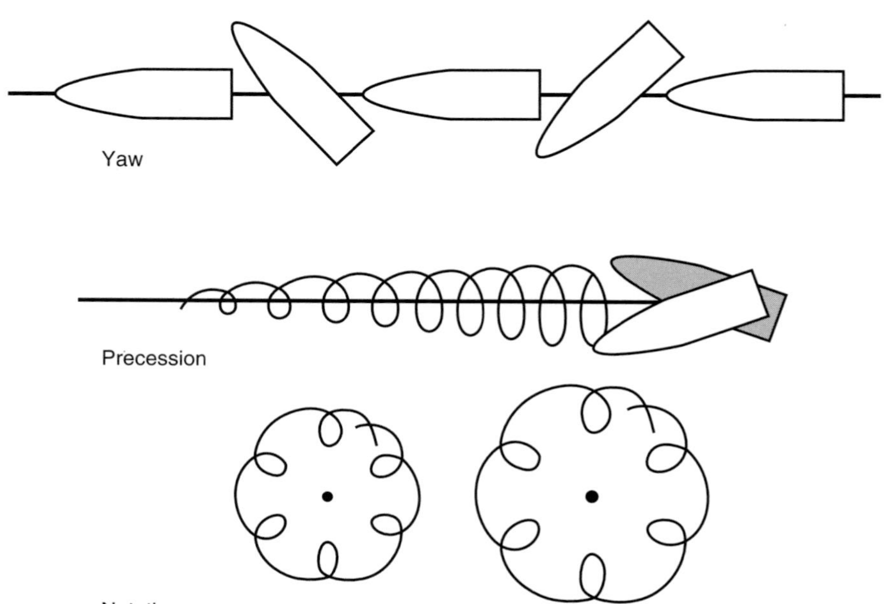

Fig. 40-3 Tumbling may be responsible for significant tissue damage. (From the Internet Pathology Laboratory for Medical Education. Copyright 1994-1999, 2000 by Edward C. Klatt, Department of Pathology, University of Utah, Salt Lake City, Utah.)

tissue. Although a longer, heavier bullet might have more KE, it may pass completely through the target without dissipating its energy. Conversely, a bullet with a low KE will cause significant tissue damage if it transfers all of its force to the target, which is true of handguns at short-range (Fig. 40-3).

Bullet design also determines wounding potential. The Hague Convention of 1899, and subsequently the Geneva Convention, forbade the use of expanding, deformable bullets (**Dum-Dum modification**) during wartime. Therefore military bullets have full metal jackets around the lead core. Modern military assault rifles fire projectiles at such high velocity (>2000 fps) that the bullets need to be jacketed with copper, since lead melts at this speed. Police departments, hunters, and assorted "bad guys" never signed the treaty. They are free to use bullets with a soft lead point or a "hollow-point" designed to deform on impact. These slugs impart their KE to the tissues over a short distance in the body.

The distance from the muzzle to the target also plays a significant role in wounding capacity. Most bullets fired from handguns lose significant KE at 100 yards, whereas high-velocity military 0.308 rounds retain considerable KE at 500 yards. Military and hunting rifles deliver bullets with more KE at a greater distance than handguns and shotguns.

The type of tissue affects both wounding potential and depth of penetration.[4] Tissue density (specific gravity) and elasticity are important factors. The higher the specific gravity, the greater the damage. The greater the elasticity, the less the damage. Thus

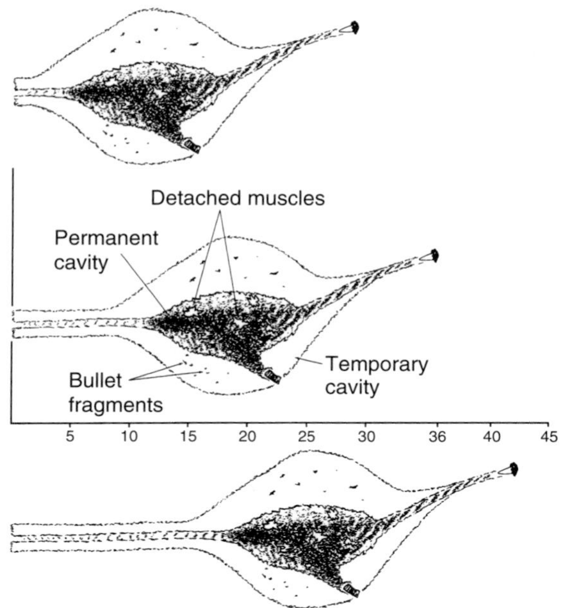

Fig. 40-4 Tissue injury resulting from a M-16 bullet. (From Fackler ML: *Ann Emerg Med* 28[2]:194-203, 1996.)

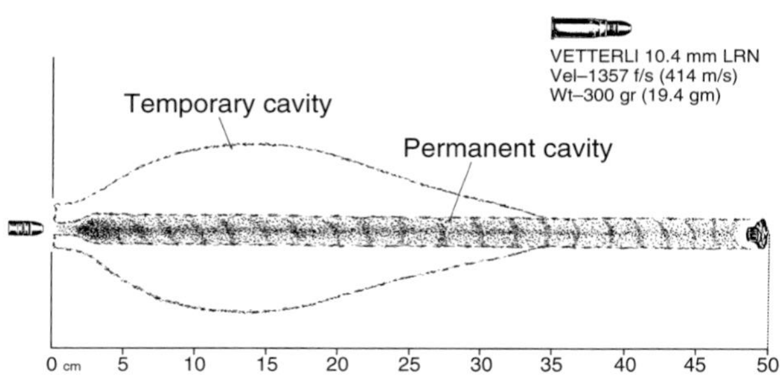

Fig. 40-5 Tissue injury caused by the Vetterli rifle bullet. (From Fackler ML: *Ann Emerg Med* 28[2]:194-203, 1996.)

lung, which is low-density and highly elastic, is damaged less than muscle, which is more dense and less elastic. Liver, spleen, and brain have no elasticity and are easily injured, as is adipose tissue. Fluid-filled organs such as bladder, heart, great vessels, and bowel, can burst when pressure waves are generated. A bullet striking bone shreds the bone and the bullet, generating numerous secondary missiles. Each moving fragment causes additional damage.

An M-16 rifle (0.223 caliber) produces large surface wounds using high-velocity, low-mass bullets that tumble, cause cavitation, and dissipate energy quickly (Fig. 40-4). A hunting rifle (0.308 caliber or greater) has a larger-mass bullet designed to penetrate a large game animal at a distance (Fig. 40-5). Most projectiles above 0.22 caliber can penetrate the relatively thin wallboard of houses and apartments. Bullets fired from a military-style rifle might penetrate several houses.

HANDGUN BALLISTICS

These weapons are easily concealed, but difficult to aim accurately. Most handgun shootings occur at less than 7 yards. Even so, the majority of bullets miss their target. In one study only 11% of assailants' bullets and 25% of bullets fired by police officers hit the intended target.[7] Usually, criminals employ low-caliber weapons because they are cheaper, lighter to carry, and easier to control. Tissue destruction can be increased at any caliber by use of hollow-point expanding bullets. Some law enforcement agencies have adopted such bullets because they are thought to have more "stopping power" at short range. Most handgun bullets, though, deliver less than 1000 ft/lb of KE.[8]

Cartridges

The two major variables in handgun ballistics concern the diameter of the bullet and volume of gunpowder in the cartridge case. In the past, crude design limited the amount of gunpowder, or charge, a cartridge could withstand. Advances in metallurgy have doubled and tripled the maximum pressures to generate more KE. Many different cartridges are available using a variety of loads and bullet designs (Table 40-1).

Comparing the 44 magnum with the 357 magnum demonstrates the impact of bore diameter. The larger area of the 44 magnum creates more force with the same pressure, producing greater energy at the muzzle. Cartridge volume (case capacity) determines the amount of powder and explosive force driving the bullet. Consider the 9-mm parabellum (para) and the 357 magnum. These cartridges have similar diameters and pressures, but the 357 magnum cartridge is much longer. The greater case volume (more powder) delivers more energy. Finally, despite the Colt 45 having the largest bore diameter and one of the longest cases, it does not deliver the maximum energy. The outdated 1873 design of this cartridge case severely handicaps its efficiency.

Bullets

The Glasser "safety slug" consists of a hollow copper jacket filled with #12 birdshot. When the bullet hits the target, the pellets are sprayed over a wide area. However, the pellets quickly decelerate, so they penetrate poorly and are less likely to pass through one person and hit another. They are designed to stop, but not kill, an attacker while avoiding injury to bystand-

TABLE 40-1
Different Types of Cartridges

NAME	COMMENT	CASE LENGTH	CASE DIAMETER	BULLET WEIGHT (GRAINS)	VELOCITY (MUZZLE) IN FPS	ENERGY (MUZZLE) IN FT LBS	ENERGY (AT 100 YD) IN FT LBS
0.22 LR	For inexpensive guns, rimfire (R and A)	0.625	0.222	40	1060	100	75
0.25 auto	Small pocket gun (A only)	0.615	0.251	45	815	66	42
0.380 auto	Popular pocket auto (A only)	0.680	0.355	85	1000	189	140
9 mm para	Popular military handgun (A only)	0.754	0.355	115	1155	391	241
0.38 special	Popular police revolver (R only)	1.155	0.357	110	995	242	185
0.357	Popular police and hunting revolver (R and A)	1.290	0.357	125	1450	583	330
0.44 magnum	Hunting revolver (R only)	1.290	0.430	180	1610	1036	551
0.45 auto	Popular military handgun (R and A)	0.898	0.451	185	1000	411	324
Colt 0.45	Cowboy "sixgun" (R only)	1.285	0.452	225	920	423	352

From Fackler ML: *Ann Emerg Med* 28(2):194-203, 1996.
R, Made for revolver; *A,* made for semiautomatic; velocity in fps.

ers. However, at close range they produce substantial injury. "Shot-shell" cartridges containing pellets are available in a variety of calibers. Speak et al[9] showed that, in handguns, shorter barrel length and larger caliber produced larger pellet patterns.

The Winchester "Black Talon" slug employs a unique notching process that locks the lead core to a copper alloy jacket. This design controls expansion and prevents separation of the core and the jacket on target impact. On impact, six sharp copper points open in a radial fashion, tearing a gaping hole in the target. In one study, Black Talons penetrating plastic sheeting (simulating elasticity of skin) expanded irregularly, whereas those fired into ordinance gelatin (simulating soft tissue) expanded uniformly.[10] The sharp copper points endanger physicians or forensic scientists during bullet removal.

Armor-piercing bullets penetrate soft body armor (such as bulletproof vests worn by law enforcement officers). Though they pierce armor, they wound no more than ordinary bullets of similar size. Some have Teflon coatings to minimize barrel wear with firing. Armor-piercing bullets are illegal to possess and use.

SHOTGUN BALLISTICS

Wounding is a function of the type of shot, or pellets, used in the shotgun shell. Weight, in general, is a constant for a shell: 1 oz of shot would equal either 9 pellets of double O buckshot or 410 pellets of #8 birdshot. A OO or "double ought" pellet is equivalent to a low-velocity 0.38 handgun projectile. The spread of the pellets as they leave the muzzle is determined by both the length of the barrel and the "choke" or constriction of the barrel at the muzzle (from 0.003 to 0.04 inches). More choke means less spread. Full choke gives a 15-inch spread at 20 yards, whereas no choke gives a 30-inch spread at the same distance.[11] A **"sawed-off" shotgun** has a very short barrel and sprays the pellets over a wide area (Fig. 40-6).

At close range (less than 4 feet), the pellets essentially act as one mass and wounds are devastating. A typical shell gives the pellets a muzzle velocity of 1300 fps and KE of 2100 ft/lb. An entrance wound would be about 1-inch diameter, and the wound cavity would contain wadding. At intermediate range (4 to 12 feet) the entrance wound is up to 2 inches diameter, but the borders may show individual pellet markings.

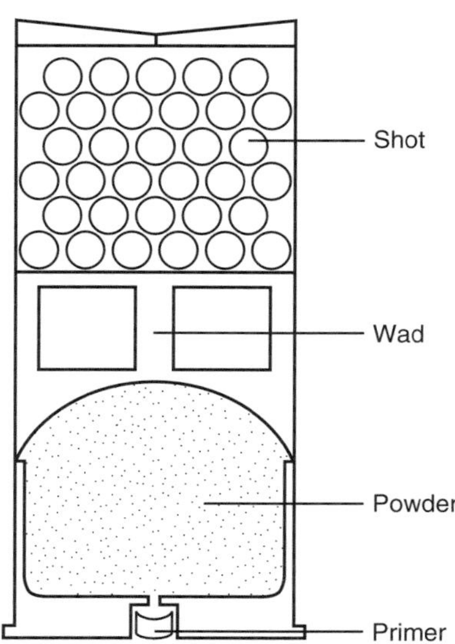

Fig. 40-6 The short barrel of a "sawed-off" shotgun can spray pellets over a wide area. (From the Internet Pathology Laboratory for Medical Education. Copyright 1994-1999, 2000 by Edward C. Klatt, Department of Pathology, University of Utah, Salt Lake City, Utah.)

Wadding may be found near the surface of the wound. Beyond 12 feet, choke, barrel length, and pellet size determine the wounding. If the energy is divided between the pellets, it can be seen that fewer, larger pellets carry more KE, but the spread may disperse them from the target. Pellets, being spherical, are poor projectiles. Most small pellets do not penetrate skin after 80 yards. Although close range wounds are severe, wounding may be minimal at even relatively short distances. Range is the most important factor, and can be estimated in over half of cases, as can the shot size used.[12] A rifled slug fired from a shotgun may have a range of 800 yards.[13]

Shotgun slugs can produce significant injury, because of the slug's size and mass. At close range, survival is rare. In treating shotgun injuries, it is necessary to remember that the plastic shell carrier and the wadding (which may not appear on radiographs) can also cause tissue damage and may need to be found and removed.[14]

Torso Wounds

In patients wounded with multiple superficial pellets, it is easy to overlook the single "deep pellet." Patients with a widely scattered pattern may have most pellets just beneath the skin, but one or more may penetrate vital internal structures. The addition of lateral radiographs and even computed tomographic (CT) scanning in some cases, may identify peritoneal or other deep tissue violation.

Extremity Wounds

As the number of projectiles increase, so does the chance of injury. The ankle-arm index is a valuable means of detecting vascular injury in patients with penetrating extremity trauma (see Chapter 30). However, most studies regarding its utility were limited to patients with a single penetrating wound; individuals with multiple shotgun pellets were generally excluded. Consider the use of color-flow Doppler in such patients.

AIR GUN BALLISTICS

These weapons fire 0.177 or 0.22 round pellets at muzzle velocities of 200 to 900 fps. Though considered of low energy and relatively "safe" for children to use, they can cause severe injury to the eye, soft tissue, superficial blood vessels, and even abdominal organs. The temporal bone is thin and easily pierced. Although air guns are rarely included in gun regulations, homicide and suicide have been reported with their use.[15,16]

MANAGEMENT

Infection

Despite the myth that the bullets are sterilized from high temperatures, all gunshot wounds should be considered heavily contaminated. Bacterial contamination may arise from the bullet, skin organisms, or entrained clothing or wadding. The more devitalized the tissue, the greater the likelihood of contamination and subsequent infection. Abscess may develop, requiring incision and drainage. While β-hemolytic streptococcus remains very sensitive to penicillins,[1] wounds may become infected with β-lactamase–producing organisms. Neovascularization occurs in the region of the wounded tissue within a few days after injury,[1] and the growth of new blood vessels helps to fight bacterial contamination.

Prophylactic Antibiotics

Despite the potential for infection, prophylactic antibiotics do not appear to be valuable in the routine management of extremity gunshot wounds,[17,18] nor do they decrease the rate of infection in low-velocity gunshot wounds that fracture an extremity.[19] If the physician elects to give antibiotics for a low-velocity, extraarticular gunshot wound, the oral route is as effective as intravenous administration.[20] This lack of difference in the two routes may be because antibiotics may not make a difference at all.

Although there are no good placebo-controlled studies examining the issue, most authorities suggest antibiotics for gunshot wounds that penetrate the abdomen. The combination of aztreonam and clindamycin may be useful.[21] Many trauma centers employ a second-generation cephalosporin such as cefotetan, or a combination agent such as ampicillin-sulbactam, usually in association with an aminoglycoside or other agent with gram-negative activity. Lastly, another indication for antibiotics includes GSW that violate the oral cavity.[22]

Wound Care

In military practice, extensive debridement of gunshot wounds is standard. Debridement may be necessary because of the higher velocities and greater tissue destruction seen with martial armament. However, wound debridement and antibiotics are often unnecessary in minor uncomplicated gunshot wounds. It might be useful in those with "multiple injuries, gross wound contamination, significant tissue devitalization, large wounds, or delay in treatment."[23]

Do not suture gunshot wounds.[1] Wounds with small amount of tissue destruction, as is the case with most handgun injuries, usually heal without treatment.[1]

UNUSUAL COMPLICATIONS

Missile Embolization

Missile embolization is an uncommon complication of gunshot wounds. Case reports have described embolization to the pulmonary artery,[24,25] heart,[26] posterior tibial artery,[27] middle cerebral artery,[28,29] and portal vein.[30,31] The initial site of injury may be quite remote from the bullet's ultimate resting place.[26] The bullet may enter through an artery or a vein, and it can take minutes to years to embolize. If no bullet is seen on radiographs of the initial site of injury and there is no exit wound, suspect arterial missile embolization.[30] Of course, a forceful trajectory that carries the bullet to another part of the body is a more common phenomenon.

Missile embolizations are often asymptomatic,[24] and complications depend on its final location. Infarction, thrombosis, and erosion of arterial walls are all potential morbidities.[24,27,31] A chest film that shows a "fuzzy bullet" overlying the heart (a result of motion artifact) suggests missile embolization. Fluoroscopy, computed tomography, and echocardiography are useful in confirming intracardiac location.[26] Missiles that are fixed within the myocardium, intracavitary right-sided missiles, and those missiles within the pericardial space may be managed expectantly.[26] However, some authors feel that all arterial missile emboli should be removed.[27]

Lead Intoxication

The celluloid drama, where the doctors take out a bullet to save a life is a theatrical fantasy. It is standard practice to leave retained bullet fragments within the body. Most often, these fragments do not cause any significant problems as they become encased by fibrinous tissue. Rarely, signs and symptoms of **plumbism** (e.g., anemia, abdominal pain, neuropathies) arise from bullets retained within a synovial cavity.[32,33] Acidic synovial fluid may dissolve lead, promoting absorption into the blood.[34] The onset of symptoms ranges from several days to 40 years after a gunshot wound.[35]

Bullet fragments within joint spaces must be removed to achieve a good outcome and to avoid synovitis.[32,33] Chelation therapy may also be required.[33] In cases of lead polyneuropathy, axonal loss in peripheral nerves is a primary pathologic event.[36]

PEARLS & PITFALLS

- Tissue disruption is determined by the amount of energy the bullet transmits to the tissue.
- The propensity to wound relates to the mass of the projectile, the square of its velocity, and the bullet's ability to deform, fragment, or yaw.
- Treat the wound and not the weapon—a 0.22-caliber weapon can easily kill.
- Antibiotics and extensive debridement are rarely indicated in civilian GSWs.
- Bullet embolization and lead intoxication are rare complications of retained bullets.
- Count the number of bullet holes. An odd number means retained bullets. An even number means either no retained bullets or an even number of retained bullets.
- Always examine the back, axillae, and perineum for unsuspected entry wounds.

REFERENCES

1. Fackler ML: Gunshot wound review, *Ann Emerg Med* 28:194-203, 1996.
2. Fackler ML: Civilian gunshot wounds and ballistics: dispelling the myths, *Emerg Med Clin North Am* 16:17-28, 1998.
3. Karger B: Penetrating gunshots to the head and lack of immediate incapacitation. I. Wound ballistics and mechanisms of incapacitation, *Int J Legal Med* 108:53-61, 1995.
4. Adams DB: Wound ballistics: a review, *Milit Med* 147:831-835, 1982.

5. DiMaio VJ, Zumwalt RE: Rifle wounds from high velocity, center-fire hunting ammunition, *J Forensic Sci* 22:132-140, 1977.
6. Belkin M: Wound ballistics, *Prog Surg* 16:7-24, 1979.
7. Lesce T: Gunfighting tactics, *Survival Guide* 6:28-31, 1984.
8. Ragsdale BD: Gunshot wounds: a historical perspective, *Milit Med* 149:301-315, 1984.
9. Speak RD, Kerr FC, Rowe WF: Effects of range, caliber, barrel length, and rifling on pellet patterns produced by shotshell ammunition, *J Forensic Sci* 30:412-419, 1985.
10. Russell MA, et al: Safety in bullet recovery procedures: a study of the Black Talon bullet, *Am J Forensic Med Pathol* 16:120-123, 1995.
11. DeMuth WE Jr, Nicholas GG, Munger BL: Buckshot wounds, *J Trauma* 18:53-57, 1978.
12. Wilson JM: Shotgun ballistics and shotgun injuries, *West J Med* 129:149-155, 1978.
13. Mattoo BN, Wani AK, Asgekar MD: Casualty criteria for wounds from firearms with special reference to shot penetration–II, *J Forensic Sci* 19:585-589, 1974.
14. Gestring ML, et al: Shotgun slug injuries: case report and literature review, *J Trauma* 40:650-653, 1996.
15. Cohle SD, et al: Suicide by air rifle and shotgun, *J Forensic Sci* 32:1113-1117, 1987.
16. DiMaio VJ: Homicidal death by air rifle, *J Trauma* 15:1034-1037, 1975.
17. Ordog GJ, et al: Infection in minor gunshot wounds, *J Trauma* 34:358-365, 1993.
18. Ordog GJ, et al: Civilian gunshot wounds–outpatient management, *J Trauma* 36:106-111, 1994.
19. Dickey RL, et al: Efficacy of antibiotics in low-velocity gunshot fractures, *J Orthop Trauma* 3:6-10, 1989.
20. Knapp TP, et al: Comparison of intravenous and oral antibiotic therapy in the treatment of fractures caused by low-velocity gunshots: a prospective, randomized study of infection rates, *J Bone Joint Surg* 78-A:1167-1171, 1996.
21. Fabian TC, et al: Superiority of aztreonam/clindamycin compared with gentamicin/clindamycin in patients with penetrating abdominal trauma, *Am J Surg* 167:291-296, 1994.
22. Wallick K IV, Davidson P, Shockley L: Traumatic cavernous sinus fistula following a gunshot wound to the face, *J Emerg Med* 15:23-29, 1998.
23. Ordog GJ, et al: Infection in minor gunshot wounds, *J Trauma* 34:358-365, 1993.
24. Gupta AK, et al: Missile emboli to the pulmonary artery, *Am J Emerg Med* 15:213-214, 1997.
25. Lodder JV: Venous bullet embolism: a case report, *S Afr J Surg* 35:94-97, 1997.
26. Gandhi SK, et al: Selective management of embolized intracardiac missiles, *Ann Thorac Surg* 62:290-292, 1996.
27. Adegboyega PA, Sustento-Reodica N, Adesokan A: Arterial bullet embolism resulting in delayed vascular insufficiency: a rationale for mandatory extraction, *J Trauma* 41:539-541, 1996.
28. Stein M, Mirvis SE, Wiles CE III: Delayed embolization of a shotgun pellet from the chest to the middle cerebral artery, *J Trauma* 39:1006-1009, 1995.
29. Cogbill TH, Sullivan HG: Carotid artery pseudoaneurysm and pellet embolization to the middle cerebral artery following a shotgun wound of the neck, *J Trauma* 39:763-767, 1995.
30. Symbas PN, Symbas PJ: Missiles in the cardiovascular system, *Chest Surg Clin North Am* 7:343-356, 1997.
31. Yates TE, et al: Portal vein embolization following shotgun-pellet injuries to the abdomen, *Am J Forensic Med Pathol* 17:151-154, 1996.
32. Peh WC, Reinus WR: Lead arthropathy: a cause of delayed onset lead poisoning, *Skeletal Radiol* 24:357-360, 1995.
33. Bolanos AA, et al: Lead poisoning from an intra-articular shotgun pellet in the knee treated with arthroscopic extraction and chelation therapy. a case report, *J Bone Joint Surg* 78-A:422-426, 1996.
34. Leonard MH: The solution of lead by synovial fluid, *Clin Orthop Rel Res* 64:255-261, 1969.
35. Linden MA, et al: Lead poisoning from retained bullets: pathogenesis, diagnosis, and management, *Ann Surg* 195:305-313,1982.
36. Wu PB, Kingery WS, Date ES: An EMG case report of lead neuropathy 19 years after a shotgun injury, *Muscle Nerve* 18:326-329, 1995.

41 Stab Wounds

PETER C. FERRERA

Although stab wounds have a lower injury potential than firearm-related injuries, they still are life threatening.[1,2] The external wound can appear trivial, yet the underlying visceral injuries may be grave.[3] This quandary is especially true with narrow knives like stilettos or with ice picks. Both the appearance and direction of the wound may deceive the emergency physician (EP), since the size and direction of the entry wound cannot always predict internal injury.[3] The assailant may twist the knife, or the victim may move his or her body during penetration, resulting in a wound that changes trajectory. Stabbing is the leading cause of penetrating thoracic injuries, with switchblades being the most likely offenders.[3]

GENERAL PRINCIPLES

Antibiotics

There is no convincing data that antibiotics are necessary for patients with simple stab wounds. However, stab wounds to the abdomen that may have inflicted bowel injury warrant preoperative antibiotics. In this case, broad-spectrum coverage against gram-negatives and anaerobes can be accomplished with administration of agents such as cefotetan, or ampicillin/sulbactam. Some centers recommend addition of an agent more active against anaerobes, such as metronidazole or clindamycin.

Suturing

A puncture wound is usually considered deeper than it is wide at the surface. Many stab wounds fall into this category. Unless they are large and gaping, they rarely require closure and may be left to heal by secondary intention. The utility of drains for such wounds remains unproven. Larger wounds are generally closed in the usual manner.

Impalements–Implements In-Situ

Some unfortunates arrive in the emergency department (ED) with a knife sticking out of their body. Although the temptation to tug is great—leave it be! Instruments in the head, neck, and torso may tamponade torn vasculature. Removal in the ED can produce a torrent of internal or external blood.[4] Such items are best left in place for removal in the operating suite *unless* they interfere with resuscitation.[5] Impalement of the extremities can be safely removed in the ED.

In some circumstances, a surgeon may elect to remove an implement in-situ in the ED. They may select this course for patients with severe co-morbid disease in whom general anesthesia may be risky. On other occasions, the surgeon may order a preoperative study to determine the best operative approach, as in the stable patient with possible intraabdominal vascular injury.

CENTRAL CHEST STAB WOUNDS

Patients with stab wounds between the nipples are at great risk for cardiac and mediastinal injury. Patients with penetrating cardiac injuries are much more likely to reach the hospital alive if they are stabbed rather than shot.[6-8] Patients with stab wounds of the heart may be grossly unstable or moribund, whereas in others a lethal injury may be initially occult. Mortality rates vary from 10% to 70% depending on the reporting institution and the geographic locale.[9] Prehospital hypotension does not necessarily portend a bad outcome, and in one series 17% of patients who received field CPR survived.[7] Although pericardial tamponade can kill, it may also delay death by preventing exsanguination from a cardiac wound.[6,9,10,11]

The right ventricle is the chamber most commonly penetrated (>50%), followed by the left ventricle (30%), right atrium (12%), and left atrium (3%).[6,9] The aorta and coronary vessels are rarely injured (1.5%).[9] The majority of cases involve only one chamber.[9] As expected, mortality rises when multiple chambers are involved.[9]

The chest film in patients with cardiac wounds is often normal, and will *not* demonstrate cardiomegaly. Although a few patients with stab wounds to the chest may demonstrate air in the pericardial sac, most patients with acute tamponade from penetrating trauma have a normal cardiac silhouette. A bedside echocardiogram is indicated in patients with stab wounds located between the nipples or those stabbed more peripherally with long objects.[3]

Emergency thoracotomy is more likely to benefit victims of cardiac stab wounds when compared with those who suffer cardiac gunshot wounds.[9,10,12,13] One reason for this difference is the higher rate of multichamber involvement with gunshot wounds.[12]

In cases of combined cardiac and intraabdominal penetrating injuries, the presence of pericardial tamponade, hemothorax, or peritoneal bleeding guides intervention. Obvious cardiac tamponade or massive hemothorax mandates opening the chest first, whereas severe hypovolemic shock with a massive hemoperitoneum justifies a laparotomy before thoracotomy.[14]

PERIPHERAL THORACIC STAB WOUNDS

The chest film remains the single most important test in the patient with penetrating chest trauma. A patient with a hemothorax (HTX) requires a chest tube and admission. Patients with immediate return of more than 1200 cc of blood or those draining more than 200 cc/hour for 4 hours need thoracotomy in the operating suite. Thoracotomy is also indicated for esophageal or tracheobronchial injury.[3]

Management of a pneumothorax (PTX) varies widely. In some centers, observation alone is used for small pneumothoraces, whereas in others, needle aspiration is frequently employed (see Chapter 18). Tube thoracostomy is generally performed for PTX >20% loss of lung volume or for those who fail needle aspiration, for expanding PTX, or for patients with any size PTX who are on positive pressure ventilation.[3]

Disposition of a patient with a thoracic stab wound depends on the location of the wound and clinical presentation. Asymptomatic patients with stab wounds located between the nipples need surgical consultation and, if available, echocardiography. Patients with stab wounds below the nipple line necessitate evaluation for hemoperitoneum (see the following discussion). Patients with hypotension and respiratory distress demand tube thoracostomy if a HTX or PTX is present, and immediate surgical consultation. If a patient has pain on swallowing, consult a surgeon and discuss the need for esophagoscopy or contrast studies of the esophagus.

Some patients with asymptomatic stab wounds to the chest may be safely managed with ED observation. Such patients must have the following:

1. A stab wound that does not endanger the mediastinum (peripheral to the nipples)
2. Be asymptomatic (No shortness of breath, pain with swallowing, abdominal pain, or altered mental status)
3. An initially normal chest radiograph (CXR)

Some authors recommend observation for 6 to 8 hours, at which time a second CXR is obtained. Ordog et al[3] found a 12% incidence of delayed PTX and a 0.6% incidence of delayed HTX in patients with initially negative CXR. Most of these delayed pneumothoraces were managed with simple tube thoracostomy, but those patients with small nonprogressive injuries were observed without intervention. If the follow-up CXR is normal, almost all patients may be discharged to home—as long as the mediastinum or diaphragms are not at risk.[3]

LOWER CHEST STAB WOUNDS

Stab wounds to the lower chest require different management than those of the anterior abdomen or upper chest. Patients with stab wounds below the nipple line (or fourth intercostal space) may have diaphragmatic or intraabdominal injuries.[4] Diaphragmatic injuries occur in as many as 32% of cases of left thoracoabdominal stab wounds.[15] The initial CXR is notoriously inaccurate for these injuries.[15] Obviously, intrathoracic structures are at risk, and HTX, PTX, lung laceration, and cardiac injury must be excluded.

Unlike anterior abdominal stab wounds, formal wound exploration of the chest is dangerous and must be avoided.[4] Local wound exploration in the chest may precipitate uncontrolled intrathoracic bleeding or iatrogenic PTX.[4] However, make sure to carefully inspect the wound. By carefully peeling back the skin edges, the EP may avoid extensive studies in patients with obviously superficial wounds.

Laparoscopy, thoracoscopy, or diagnostic peritoneal lavage (DPL) are reasonable approaches to exclude diaphragmatic penetration and intraabdominal injury. Standard DPL criteria, such as 100,000 rbcs/mm^3 does not detect penetrating diaphragm injuries, since this muscular organ bleeds little when cut. As such, a lower red blood cell count, as low as 5,000/mm^3, will improve sensitivity when evaluating stab wounds to the lower chest.[4]

ABDOMINAL STAB WOUNDS

The management of abdominal stab wounds has been discussed in great detail in Chapter 20. However, some points warrant reinforcement. Unlike firearm-related abdominal injuries, a more selective approach is used with abdominal stabbings.[16,17] Overall survival is 98% for abdominal stab wounds, compared with 88% for abdominal gunshot wounds.[17]

Patients with hypotension or obvious peritonitis following abdominal stab wounds require immediate operation.[18] The only additional investigations might include a stat hemoglobin, a type and crossmatch, and a portable CXR, which is especially important to exclude HTX or PTX. However, the majority of patients with abdominal stab wounds are hemodynamically stable and mandate further evaluation.[18]

Stab wounds of the anterior abdomen violate the peritoneal cavity in only two thirds of cases.[4] Of those with peritoneal violation, only 50% to 75% incur vascular or visceral injury. Since only one third to one half of all patients with abdominal stab wounds need an operation, selective management is warranted.[4,17] Even patients presenting with omental evisceration do not necessarily require laparotomy, since 29% of these patients have no visceral injury.[16,18] Management options include serial physical examinations, local wound exploration, DPL, and laparoscopy.[17,19] All of these methods have their advantages and shortcomings and a combination of procedures may ensure detection of intraabdominal injury.

The liver is the organ most commonly injured (up to 39%), followed by the small bowel (32%).[17,20] Less often, the penetrating object injures the diaphragm (20%), colon (15%), and stomach (13%).[17]

BACK AND FLANK STAB WOUNDS

Most stab wounds to the back and flank do not penetrate the peritoneal cavity or visceral retroperitoneum.[17,21] However, as many as 15% to 40% of stab wounds cause significant injury to these sites.[5] Some patients with serious injuries appear well on ED arrival, since stabbing victims with hollow viscous wounds may lack peritoneal signs on initial evaluation.[21] Diagnostic options include serial examinations, DPL, local wound exploration, and triple contrast-enhanced CT (CE-CT) scans.[17,22] The triple contrast study, which includes PO, IV, and a contrast enema, is useful to identify colorectal injuries and demonstrate both the wound's trajectory and depth.[5] If the CT shows that the wound remains superficial to the deep muscle fascia, the patient may be discharged from the ED.[21] Patients with violation of the deep fascia should be admitted for 24-hour observation.[21] Penetrating ureteral injuries are often missed. The urinalysis is often normal and imaging studies generally unrevealing.

STAB WOUNDS TO THE HEAD

Stab wounds that penetrate the skull carry the risk of immediate vascular laceration and intracranial hemorrhage. These injuries can also lead to pseudoaneurysms and arteriovenous fistulae, which may bleed at a later time.[23,24] Vascular injuries occur in up to 50% of patients sustaining orbital stab wounds.[24] Infections, such as brain abscess and meningitis, are major sequelae. The incidence of infection is highest with stab wounds that pass through a paranasal sinus or the oral cavity.[23]

The EP should determine if the object has penetrated the skull. The patient with a neurologic deficit needs emergent neurosurgical consultation and usually CT evaluation. In the patient with stable vital signs and a normal neurological examination, simple exploration of the wound is usually sufficient to exclude intracranial injury. If the depth of the wound is unclear, or the wound penetrates the skull, a CT scan is usually necessary. Because penetrating head trauma may damage major cranial vessels, angiography may be indicated, especially in patients with zone III neck injuries (above the angle of the mandible). Patients who present with the offending object in place should have it removed in the operating suite.[23]

NECK STAB WOUNDS

Penetration of the platysma mandates surgical consultation. Emergency department exploration of wounds deep to the platysma is a risky endeavor, likely to prompt uncontrolled hemorrhage or worse. The immediate life-threat lies with the airway. An endotracheal tube inadvertently passed into the mediastinum through the wall of a tracheal laceration carries a grave risk of prolonged cerebral anoxia.[25] Hasty thrusting of an endotracheal tube can convert a partial tear of the trachea into a full-thickness injury. Combined esophageal and airway injuries are reported in 20% to 50% of cases of penetrating laryngotracheal injuries.[25,26]

SPINAL STAB WOUNDS

Spinal cord injuries (SCI) secondary to stab wounds are fortunately rare. Neurologic recovery is much higher in patients with SCI due to stab wounds than in those with gunshot wounds.[27] In a series of 18 patients with incomplete injuries due to stab wounds, 70% of patients managed conservatively showed neurologic improvement.[28]

In the ED the physician must perform a detailed neurologic examination and search for additional injuries. Patients with high cervical stab wounds resulting in SCI may have associated vascular, airway, and esophageal injuries.[27] Similarly, those patient with lower thoracic and upper lumbar level SCI may also have concomitant renal and other retroperitoneal lacerations.[27] The methylprednisolone protocol used in patients with blunt cord trauma is not indicated in patients with penetrating spinal cord injuries.[29,30]

Surgery may provide little benefit for both complete and incomplete SCI. In a very large series of spinal stab wounds by Peacock et al,[31] over 50% of the lesions were of the Brown-Sequard type and approximately two thirds of their patients achieved good functional recovery. These authors reserved surgical intervention for retained knife blades, ongoing leakage of cerebrospinal fluid, and abscess drainage.

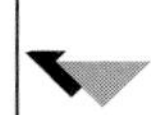

PEARLS & PITFALLS

- Suspect mediastinal injury in patients stabbed between the nipples. Unstable patients require management of HTX and PTX, followed by surgery if they remain unstable.
- Stable patients stabbed between the nipples should undergo echocardiography.
- Initially asymptomatic patients with normal CXR following chest stab wounds occasionally develop a delayed PTX (or rarely, HTX). Obtain a follow-up CXR 6 hours after the initial film.
- Suspect diaphragmatic laceration and intraabdominal injury with stab wounds below the fourth intercostal space (usually at the nipple line).
- The majority of anterior abdominal stab wounds do not cause visceral or vascular injury. Manage such patients selectively.
- Implements-in-situ should usually be removed in the operating suite to avoid uncontrolled hemorrhage.
- Back and flank stab wounds can violate the peritoneum. Triple contrast CT scan demonstrating an intact deep fascia is an auspicious sign.
- Stab wounds to the head may lead to brain injury, pseudoaneurysm, and arteriovenous fistulae formation; obtain consultation early in these cases. Patients may require CT scanning and angiography.

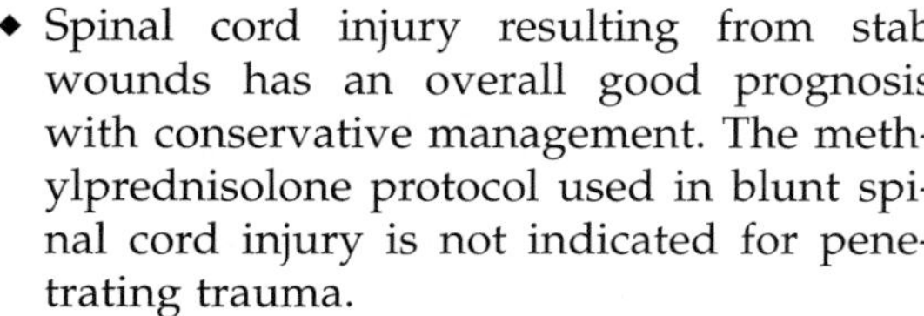

- Spinal cord injury resulting from stab wounds has an overall good prognosis with conservative management. The methylprednisolone protocol used in blunt spinal cord injury is not indicated for penetrating trauma.

REFERENCES

1. Vasquez JC, Castaneda E, Bazan N: Management of 240 cases of penetrating thoracic injuries, *Injury* 28:45-49, 1997.
2. Goins WA, Ford DH: The lethality of penetrating cardiac wounds, *Am Surg* 62:987-993, 1996.
3. Ordog GJ, et al: Asymptomatic stab wounds of the chest, *J Trauma* 36:680-684, 1994.
4. Henneman PL: Penetrating abdominal trauma, *Emerg Med Clin North Am* 7:647-666, 1989.
5. Marx JA: Penetrating abdominal trauma, *Emerg Med Clin North Am* 11:125-135, 1993.
6. Campbell NC, et al: Review of 1198 cases of penetrating cardiac trauma, *Br J Surg* 84:1737-1740, 1997.
7. Rhee PM, et al: Penetrating cardiac injuries: a population-based study, *J Trauma* 45:366-370, 1998.
8. Asensio JA, et al: One hundred five penetrating cardiac injuries: a 2-year prospective evaluation, *J Trauma* 44:1073-1082, 1998.
9. Arreola-Risa C, et al: Factors influencing outcome in stab wounds of the heart, *Am J Surg* 169:553-556, 1995.
10. Branney SW, et al: Critical analysis of two decades of experience with postinjury emergency department thoracotomy in a regional trauma center, *J Trauma* 45:87-94, 1998.
11. Karmy-Jones R, et al: Penetrating cardiac injuries, *Injury* 28:57-61, 1997.
12. Kavolius J, Golocovsky M, Champion HR: Predictors of outcome in patients who have sustained trauma and who undergo emergency thoracotomy, *Arch Surg* 128:1158-1162, 1993.
13. Brown SE, et al: Penetrating chest trauma: should indications for emergency room thoracotomy be limited? *Am Surg* 62:530-533, 1996.
14. Saadia R, Degiannis E, Levy RD: Management of combined penetrating cardiac and abdominal trauma, *Injury* 28:343-347, 1997.
15. Murray JA, et al: Penetrating left thoracoabdominal trauma: the incidence and clinical presentation of diaphragm injuries, *J Trauma* 43:624-626, 1997.
16. Taviloglu K, et al: Abdominal stab wounds: the role of selective management, *Eur J Surg* 164:17-21, 1998.
17. Feliciano DV, Rozycki GS: The management of penetrating abdominal trauma, *Adv Surg* 28:1-39, 1995.
18. Thompson JS, et al: The evolution of abdominal stab wound management, *J Trauma* 20:478-483, 1980.
19. Zantut LF, et al: Diagnostic and therapeutic laparoscopy for penetrating abdominal trauma: a multicenter experience, *J Trauma* 42:825-829, 1997.
20. Lacqua ML, Sahdev P: Effective management of penetrating abdominal trauma, *Hosp Prac* 28:31-38, 1993.
21. Kirton OC, et al: Stab wounds to the back and flank in the hemodynamically stable patient: a decision algorithm based on contrast-enhanced computed tomography with colonic opacification, *Am J Surg* 173:189-193, 1997.
22. Boyle EM Jr., et al: Diagnosis of injuries after stab wounds to the back and flank, *J Trauma* 42:260-265, 1997.
23. Taylor AG, Peter JC: Patients with retained transcranial knife blades: a high-risk group, *J Neurosurg* 87:512-515, 1997.

24. du Trevou MD, van Dellen JR: Penetrating stab wounds to the brain: the timing of angiography in patients presenting with the weapon already removed, *Neurosurgery* 31:905-911, 1992.
25. Grewal H, et al: Management of penetrating laryngotracheal injuries, *Head Neck* 17:494-502, 1995.
26. Minard G, et al: Laryngotracheal trauma, *Am Surg* 58:181-187, 1992.
27. Velmahos GC, et al: Changing profiles in spinal cord injuries and risk factors influencing recovery after penetrating injuries, *J Trauma* 38:334-337, 1995.
28. Simpson RK Jr., Venger BH, Narayan RK: Treatment of acute penetrating injuries of the spine: a retrospective analysis, *J Trauma* 29:42-46, 1989.
29. Prendergast MR, et al: Massive steroids do not reduce the zone of injury after penetrating spinal cord injury, *J Trauma* 37:576-579, 1994.
30. Levy ML, et al: Use of methylprednisolone as an adjunct in the management of patients with penetrating spinal cord injury: outcome analysis, *Neurosurgery* 39:1141-1148, 1996.
31. Peacock WJ, Shrosbree RD, Key AG: A review of 450 stab-wounds of the spinal cord, *S Afr Med J* 51:961-964, 1977.

PART FIVE

ADMINISTRATIVE ISSUES

42 Injury Control

JOHN D. BRODERICK AND DENNIS P. MCKENNA

Every year in the United States, 70,000 people die from unintentional trauma, while millions more are injured. Injuries steal nearly 4 million years of potential life, outstripping the impact of cancer.

Unintentional injury is the epidemic of modern societies and the leading cause of death between 1 and 44 years of age.[1] Motor vehicle crashes (MVCs) are the most frequent cause of unintentional injuries, followed closely by gunshot wounds. Homicide and suicide account for approximately 150,000 deaths in the United States each year.

Injury control endeavors to decrease morbidity and mortality through preventive efforts. Education, legislation, and advances in product safety are essential aspects of injury control. The emergency physician (EP) is in a unique position to recognize the avoidable dangers of modern life. We can intervene on an individual level with each injured patient we see, as well as on a national level through legislative efforts. This chapter reviews injury control issues germane to the practicing EP and highlight opportunities for intervention from the emergency department (ED).

MOTOR VEHICLE CRASHES AND ALCOHOL

Each year in the United States there are 120 million episodes of impaired driving.[2] In 1995 nearly 1 out of 123 drivers were arrested for driving under the influence.[3,4] Driving under the influence is responsible for almost 40% of traffic fatalities,[3] costing our country an estimated 45 billion dollars a year in medical bills and lost productivity.[4] Thirty thousand people will suffer permanent disability from work.[5] In 1997 there were 2 alcohol-related deaths per hour and 315 per week.[6]

Although driving under the influence occurs in all age groups, the younger driver is at special risk. The highest intoxication rates are found in the 21 to 24 year old age group. Twenty six percent within this age group involved in a fatal MVC were intoxicated. The next highest percentage was the 25 to 34 year old group.[5] Although the minimum drinking age is 21 in all 50 states, males age 18 to 20 are as likely to drive while impaired as older males.[2] Fifteen percent of young drivers (16 to 20 years of age) involved in a fatal crash are legally intoxicated.[5] Women are half as likely to be intoxicated when involved in a fatal MVC as men. A 1986 study revealed that 70% of drivers convicted of driving while impaired had a serious drinking problem.[6]

Legislation

Through legislative efforts, there has been a 32% decline in alcohol-related traffic fatalities since 1978. Only part of this reduction can be attributed to restraint devices use. Police agencies have prioritized enforcement of drunk driving laws. In 1995 officers made 1.4 million arrests for drunken driving.[3] If the police pull over someone they suspect may be drinking and driving, there is a 20% chance that they will be correct.[8] A majority (86%) who serve jail time for driving while intoxicated (DWI) have already been through the criminal justice system for a previous DWI or other offense.[9] The median jail term for a DWI conviction is 6 months.[10]

Currently all 50 states and the District of Columbia have a 21-year minimum drinking law. The National Highway Traffic Safety Administration (NHTSA) estimates that since the enforcement of these laws, motor vehicle fatalities have decreased 13% in the 18 to 20 year old age group. This figure correlates to 15,667 lives saved since 1975.[11]

Motor vehicle crashes account for 18% of all deaths and 37% of all injury-related deaths in children between the ages of 0 and 14 years.[12] Several factors contribute to the morbidity and mortality of MVCs, including the speed of the vehicle, the sobriety of the driver, and the use of restraint devices. In 1996 alcohol played a role in almost 25% of fatal MVCs involving children <14 years of age, where either the driver or another car's occupant had a measurable blood alcohol level (BAL) >0.01 g/dl.[13] Injury and death to child passengers and nonintoxicated drivers that were struck by drunk drivers led to a grass roots movement to change public opinion about DWI. Mothers Against Drunk Driving (MADD) and Students Against Drunk Driving (SADD) have educated the public about the dangers of this reckless behavior.

What further interventions can be made to reduce drinking and driving fatalities nationwide? To protect the most vulnerable occupants in MVCs, child advocates want to enact child-endangerment laws, making it a separate violation to drive under the influence of alcohol with a child in the car.

Other measures target high-risk groups. Drivers 21 to 35 years of age who have been arrested for drunk driving are four times as likely to die in an alcohol-related crash compared with their matched cohorts. For those over 35 years of age that risk increases to a factor of 11.[14] For this reason, most states suspend the driving privleges of anyone who drives while intoxicated. This program has been shown to be effective at reducing recidivism.

Another measure adopted in many states is the reduction of the legal BAL to 0.08 g/dl. This limit is recognized by most industrialized nations of the world.[15] One study suggested that lowering the BAL to 0.08 g/dl in all states would decrease alcohol-related deaths by 500 to 600 per year. The direct and indirect healthcare savings could reach 1.5 billion per year.

Because the combination of an inexperienced young driver and alcohol is so deadly, many groups support provisional licenses for drivers under 21 years of age. These drivers would have their licenses upgraded only if they remain free of MVCs or alcohol-related driving offenses. Since a majority of alcohol-related MVCs occurs at night, night curfews for young drivers could also reduce the incidence of crashes.[16]

Unfortunately, 80% of patients who present to the ED with injuries sustained from driving while impaired are not prosecuted for any offense and only a small number are charged with impaired driving. The injury severity is inversely proportional to the chance of being cited, since the severely injured are rarely prosecuted.[17] Although the laws vary by region and state, most EPs are not responsible for reporting impaired drivers to the police.[18]

RESTRAINTS

Seat Belts

Safety restraints are the single most effective means to reduce death and serious injury in MVCs. Proper use of a lap and shoulder harness reduces the chance of death by nearly 50% and prevents moderate to critical injury in a similar percentage. Authorities estimate that safety belts have saved 35,000 lives and prevented 906,000 moderate to critical injuries from 1983 to 1992. Currently, safety belt use is estimated to save 9500 lives annually.[19-22]

Seat belt legislation increases the use of safety restraints. Without restraint laws, seat belt use is traditionally around 15%. However, in states with safety belt laws, their use increased to 68%. In 1984 New York was the first state to pass a safety belt law. Since that time, many states have followed suit. As of the end of 1998, only New Hampshire lacked such a law. [22]

Primary enforcement allows a law officer to issue a citation to drivers not using safety belts. Secondary enforcement requires the police to have a separate reason to stop a driver, who may then be cited for not using a belt.[19] Currently 14 states have primary enforcement laws and 35 have secondary enforcement. Higher compliance is seen in states with primary enforcement laws.

EPs routinely question victims of MVCs regarding seat belt use. Although the primary intent is to judge severity of injury, EPs can use this information to enlighten the patient regarding the value of safety restraints.

Car Seats

In 1996 2172 children were killed as a result of MVCs.[20] Sixty-two percent of these children were passengers in the vehicles, 26% were pedestrians, and 8% were bicyclists. Most child passengers killed were unrestrained (62%).[21] Children who are unrestrained are far more likely to suffer severe injuries and die, especially those under 4 years of age. An important determinant of proper child restraint is the use of a safety belt by the driver. One study found that child passengers of MVCs were restrained 94% of the time when the driver was restrained, but the number of restrained children dropped to 30% when the driver was unrestrained.[23]

A correctly installed and properly used child's seat reduces the risk of death for infants by 71%, whereas for children ages 1 to 4 years mortality is halved. Universal use of child safety seats under the age of 4 years would save 200 lives per year and prevent an additional 20,000 injuries. In addition to the reduction in

TABLE 42-1
Car Seats

INFANTS (BIRTH TO 22 POUNDS)	TODDLERS (20-40 POUNDS)	CHILDREN (CHILDREN OVER 4 YEARS OF AGE OR 40 POUNDS)	CHILDREN OR OLDER CHILD (CHILDREN GREATER THAN 80 POUNDS)
Use rear-facing child seat located in the back seat.	Use forward-facing child seat. Use straps exiting at level of child's shoulder.	Use car booster seat until shoulder and lap belt fit correctly. Shoulder belt should not cross the neck or face.	Use standard seat belt. Children of this age are safest in the back seat.

Caveats:

1. All child seats must be placed in the rear seating compartment.
2. Most automatic seat belts require a safety clip to secure the child seat properly.
3. Convertible seats are designed to accommodate infants and toddlers from birth to 40 pounds. They should face rearward for the infant, forward for the toddler. However, convertible seats may not provide an optimal fitting for infants.

Data from the American Academy of Pediatrics, the American College of Emergency Physicians, and National Highway Traffic Safety Administration.

mortality, child seats would reduce hospitalizations by 69%.[24]

A car seat alone is inadequate. The child must be placed in a correctly fitted seat that is used in the proper manner. As many as 80% of all children who are placed in car seats are improperly restrained.[23] Children under the age of 12 months must have their seats secured in the vehicle's back seat.

The safest place for a child to ride is the back seat, and under ideal circumstances all children under the age of 12 years would always ride in the back seat, using proper car seats or properly fitted seat and lap belts. Children under the age of 12 are 36% less likely to die in a MVC if they are seated in the back seat.[24]

Child restraint seats must be compatible with the age, height, and weight of the child, as well as the vehicle to which it is fitted. These requirements are available at the retail stores, as well as on the Internet (Table 42-1).

The use of child safety seats is lower in rural communities and among the poor, a fact partially attributable to the cost of car seats. However, in that same population, 95% of those who own a car seat are likely to use it.[24] Programs that make car seats available to members of society who cannot afford them provide an enormous service to their communities. EDs should be encouraged to obtain car seats, either through donation or redistribution. If a parent in the ED needs a child seat, it will then be available.

AIR BAGS

Air bags and their safety are currently debated public safety issues, and they have recently received national media exposure. Air bags inflate at a speed approaching 200 mph. They are designed to employ during a collision and serve as a buffer between the person and the windshield and dashboard. Antecedent to their mandated installment, they had been known within the automotive industry to save lives. However, it took federal legislation to force automakers to install them on new vehicles. This legislation allowed the phasing in of the safety device until September 1993, after which compliance had to be 100%. In 1991 Congress passed a law that required passenger cars manufactured after September 1, 1997, to have dual air bags (air bag for driver and right-front passenger) along with manual lap-shoulder belts.

The data on air bags and MVCs on the roadways are compelling. The use of the air bag with a manual lap-shoulder belt has been shown to reduce fatalities by 50%. The reduction in injury risk has been estimated at 60%. The use of air bags alone, without the benefit of lap-shoulder belt, has been shown to reduce the fatality risk by 13%. Air bags have the greatest benefit in head on MVCs. A purely frontal crash with a deployed air bag reduces the risk of fatality by 31%. In frontal impacts, defined as impact from 10 o'clock position to 2 o'clock position (a purely frontal would be 12 o'clock position), the risk of fatal injury is reduced by 19%. Air bags have been estimated to save 1198 lives from 1987 to 1995.[19] Recently, in the popular press there have been reports of children injured by air bags. As of December 1996 there were at least 31 children reportedly killed as a result of injuries sustained from air bags.[13] Accident investigations have revealed that these children were in the front seat and too close to the air bag when it deployed, resulting in fatal head and neck injury injuries. Eleven were infants placed in the front passenger seat in a rear-facing child seat, and 19 out of the remaining 20 were determined to be unrestrained or improperly restrained.

The NHTSA recommends that all children under the age of 12 years sit in the back seat whenever possible. If it is necessary for a child to ride in the front seat he or she should be restrained in a manner that is appropriate for his or her age and size. Such an arrangement would be either a front-facing child safety seat or a properly secured lap and shoulder belt. Rapid deceleration places the child closer to the air bag when it deploys. Therefore the front seat should also be moved as far back from the dashboard, and children should always be prevented from leaning forward against the dashboard. Both of these measures are meant to reduce the likelihood of the air bag injuring or suffocating the child. Under no circumstances should an infant ride in the front seat. They should always be in the back seat in the rear-facing position. The automobile industry is looking into air bags that will not deploy or will deploy with less acceleration when an occupant is nearby. A system currently under production uses a scale on the passenger seat. If there is less than 30 kilograms in the seat, the air bag will not deploy. This type of air bag may, in the future, be legislated into use.[19]

SPEED AND ACCIDENTS

Many fatalities occur in crashes where the vehicle is maintaining a safe and legal speed. However, the risk of serious injury and death is directly related to the speed of the vehicle on impact. Until recently, Congress withheld federal money from states that ignored the national speed limit of 55 mph, a powerful incentive for lower speed limits. When Congress repealed this restriction in 1996, many states increased their maximum speed limits to 70 or 75 mph. From December 1995 to September 1996, 24 states increased their maximum speed limit. During this time, there was reported to be a 15% increase in traffic fatalities.[25] Seven states used as controls that did not change their maximum speed limits during that same time period experienced no change in the mortality rate.

Many public advocates cite these statistics to illustrate the need to reduce speed limits. Others argue that it is not the speed of the vehicle that is responsible for vehicular carnage, but the reckless practices of a small percentage of drivers. Nonetheless, it is clear that many Americans enjoy the increase in speed limits and its impact on travel time.[17] Reducing the speed limit again will potentially be met with resistance from commuters, rural communities, and the trucking industry.

MOTORCYCLES AND HELMETS

Riding a motorcycle is a popular pastime in the United States. In 1996 almost 4 million motorcycles logged nearly 10 billion miles.[26] However, mile for mile a motorcyclist is twenty times more likely to die in a crash than an automobile operator.[27]

Not only does riding a motorcycle have inherent dangers, but many motorcyclists engage in high-risk behavior. In 1997 nearly 29% of fatally injured motorcycle operators had a BAL of 0.10 g/dl or greater. Over 40% of motorcyclists who died after hitting an object other than another vehicle were drinking alcohol.[26] This intoxication rate is higher than in any other type of motor vehicle.

Motorcycle operators involved in a fatal crash are twice as likely to be operating the vehicle with a suspended or revoked license when compared with drivers of fatal automobile crashes. One in five will have an invalid license.[26]

In motorcycle crashes, head injury is the leading cause of death. Wearing a helmet reduces fatalities by 35%.[27] The use of a helmet, although not protecting any other part of the body besides the head, reduces all motorcycle-related injuries by 9%.

Helmets decrease brain injury by two thirds. Because brain injury cases cost more than twice that of non–brain-injured cases,[27] researchers estimate that motorcycle helmets saved 11.3 billion dollars from 1984 to 1997. If all motorcyclists wore helmets this savings would double.[26]

Helmet legislation increases their use. Without helmet laws, usage ranges between 34% and 54%. Helmet laws increase that figure to nearly 100%. In states that have reenacted helmet laws, fatalities are reduced by 30%.[27]

Although seatbelt use is not easily spotted at a distance, a law enforcement officer has no difficulty in detecting a bare head. Twenty-five states, the District of Columbia, and Puerto Rico require all motorcyclists to wear helmets. Forty-seven states require young operators (usually <18) and their passengers to wear helmets.

BICYCLE HELMETS

According to the National Sporting Goods Association, approximately 50 million Americans ride bicycles. Over 150,000 children-cyclists visit the ED each year.[28] In 1975 1003 people died from injuries sustained while riding a bicycle, but by 1997 that number had dropped to 808. Over 95% of all fatalities were not wearing helmets.[29]

The cost to society of all bicycle-related head injuries exceeds 3 billion dollars. The United States would save nearly $140 million per year if just 85% of all children consistently wore a helmet.[30] Unfortunately only 20% of all bicyclists wear their helmets, and increasing their use has become a national goal.[31]

If children aged 4 to 15 always wore their helmets, 150 deaths, 45,000 head injuries, and 50,000 scalp and face injuries would be prevented annually.[30] If everybody who rode a bicycle wore a helmet, one life would be saved every day, and 15 head injuries prevented every hour. A case-control study found that riders who wore helmets reduced their risk of head injury by 85%.[32]

Reducing the number of injuries involves educating the public about the benefits of wearing a bicycle helmet. Children especially are often unable to appreciate these dangers. Some adults will not wear a helmet because they perceive themselves as invulnerable. Other reasons often given for not wearing a helmet include the cost and their perceived unattractive appearance.

Many programs exist on the local, state, or federal level to encourage riders, especially children, to wear their helmets. These measures include education programs for schools and communities, public service announcements, advocacy of helmet use by celebrities and sports figures, vouchers and discount coupons to help with the cost of the helmet, and bicycle rodeos.[29-31]

At least 15 states have enacted bicycle helmet laws that mandate the use of helmets. These laws are often limited to children under the age of 14. There is evidence that the legislative requirement that children must wear a helmet has helped reduce the morbidity and mortality of bicycle-related injuries.[33]

Beyond legislative mandates, there is also a role for the primary care doctor to educate parents and children about the importance of helmet use. Physicians who council parents regarding helmets may double helmet use among those children.[34] The results suggest that physicians still have a very important role in shaping the behavior patterns of their patients.

The EP should recommend a helmet that meets the proper safety standards. A helmet should be certified by an organization such as the American Society for Testing and Materials (ASTM) or the American National Standards Institute (ANSI). Newer helmets have a federal standard sticker inside the helmet and on the box.

The child should try the helmet on in the store to ensure a proper fit. It should fit comfortably when the straps are buckled, sit squarely on the head, and allow little movement forward to back or side to side. A comfortable helmet increases the likelihood of use.

FIREARMS AND INJURIES

EPs and pathologists are keenly aware of the consequences of firearms. The possession of firearms in great numbers is unique to the United States, and the human toll from these weapons is enormous.

In 1994 there were 38,505 deaths from firearms. During the 1980s three times as many people died from firearm-related injuries than from AIDS.[35] Most deaths were from suicides, although homicides were a close second and unintentional deaths a distant third.[36] The U.S. homicide rate is four times that of Scotland, its nearest competitor.[37]

The costs associated with firearm injuries are staggering. In 1990 20.4 billion dollars was spent on direct and indirect medical care related to firearm injuries. The breakdown included 1.4 billion dollars for direct healthcare expenditures, 1.6 billion dollars in lost productivity from injury, and 17.4 billion dollars in lost productivity as a result of death. Since most firearm victims are uninsured, 80% of these costs are borne by the taxpayer.[38]

Although a firearm in the home may provide a sense of security, a gun in the home actually endangers family members; a gun in the home is far more likely to injure or kill a family member than an intruder. Of all firearm fatalities in the home, 2% result from an intruder being shot, 3% are accidental child shootings, 12% are from an altercation resulting in one adult partner shooting another, and 83% are the result of suicide.[39] People who reside in a household that has a gun have a five times greater risk of suicide compared with people who do not have a gun in the home.[40] For every case of self-protection there are 1.3 accidental deaths, 4.6 criminal homicides, and 37 suicides.[41]

Not all firearm injuries are fatal. From June 1992 to May 1993 there were approximately 99,025 nonfatal firearm injuries treated in the United States. Currently firearm injury data is taken from the National Electronic Injury Surveillance System (NEIS), which does not track all hospitals in the United States. Therefore this number probably underestimates total injuries.[42]

The possession of firearms in large numbers disproportionately affects some communities, in particular, inner-city African-American males. Individuals most likely to be victimized by violence are male, young, minority, criminal or delinquent, and have a lower socio-economic status.[43] Homicide is the leading cause of death in African-American men and women aged 15 to 24 years.[44,45] Being shot is predictive of future handgun violence, and one study showed a 44% recurrence rate in a 5-year period following the first shooting.

Unrestricted access to handguns may increase firearm violence. Seattle, Washington, and Vancouver, British Columbia have similar economies and demographics. They also share similar rates of assault and overall criminal activity. Yet, in Seattle there is a 4.8-increased risk of being murdered with a handgun. This difference is thought to be a result of the availability of handguns within each community.[46]

Despite laws that prohibit adolescents from obtaining guns without adult consent, many teens possess and carry firearms. In one study of urban high school students, 34% of those surveyed stated that it was easy to obtain a handgun and 6.4% owned one. One third of the owners had fired the weapon at another person.[47] Data from 1990 indicate that 20% of high school students have carried a weapon at least once during the preceding month, with 5% of those weapons being a firearm, usually a handgun.[48]

The proliferation of firearms continues. However, not all firearms are equal. Sportsmen generally purchase rifles or shotguns for target practice or hunting. These weapons are difficult to conceal and are rarely used in assaults. On the contrary, inexpensive and easy to conceal handguns such as the "Saturday Night Special" are used in 90% of gun-related crimes. Although marketed for self-defense, these weapons are primarily weapons of assault. Current gun laws generally overlook such weapons manufactured in this country.[49] So-called assault weapons, modeled after military hardware, have no conceivable sporting purpose and are used increasingly in violent massacres and drug wars.

The United States has over 20,000 local and state firearm laws, as well as numerous federal ones. The main thrust of these laws is to keep firearms out of the hands of known criminals. However, these laws do nothing to save the lives of most firearm-related deaths, which are suicides and unintentional injury.

In the depressed, suicidal, homicidal, or psychotic patient, the EP must inquire about access to a gun. All patients who present to the ED with suicidal thoughts or a suicidal attempt are at high risk for a self-inflicted gunshot wound. The patient and family must be interviewed as to presence of a gun in the home. If a patient with depression or suicidal thoughts is to be sent home, a responsible adult must remove the gun from the house. A gun in the home is a particularly strong risk factor for successful suicide of an adolescent.

EPs often see children injured by guns in the home. Some states require households with children to have guns stored in a locked cabinet or to be fitted with a trigger lock.

INJURY PREVENTION

To reduce unintentional injuries we must study, educate, and legislate. This broad-based approach involves the government, media, schools, and both the medical and lay community. Professional organizations such as the Society for Academic Emergency Medicine (SAEM) and the American College of Emergency Physicians (ACEP) have dedicated resources to the investigation of injury prevention and control.

Reducing childhood injury rates is an important goal. One of the most successful programs of this kind was undertaken in Sweden. Although the Nordic country's size, demographics and government differ significantly from the United States, Sweden is credited with having the lowest childhood injury death rate in the world.[50] The Swedish death rate for children in MVCs is approximately one half of the United States. Their approach to reducing unintentional injuries is well organized and systematic.[50] The program consists of the following:

1. Injury Surveillance: Comprehensive data collection increases awareness and understanding of unintentional injuries. With this information, epidemiologists and investigators can identify which members of society are at greatest risk. In the United States, the National Center for Injury Prevention and Control (NCIPC) is developing a standardized system of collecting injury-related data from EDs. Information gathered for the Data Elements for Emergency Department System (DEEDS) define patterns of injury in different communities. ACEP, SAEM, American Trauma Society, and National Association of State Emergency Medical Services endorse this effort.[51] Many other organizations track information on injury prevention and control, including the Center for Disease Control and the Injury Control and Emergency Health Service Section of the American Public Health Association. EPs should familiarize themselves with these programs and seek opportunities to support the efforts.
2. Legislation and Regulation: Swedes separate people from "things they would not like to meet." This broad concept keeps bicycle paths away from roads and provides a safer environment inside homes and children's centers.[50] In our own country EPs, who witness first hand the catastrophic consequences of reckless or unsafe behavior, are perfectly suited to lobby lawmak-

ers and help draft laws aimed at reducing unintentional injuries.

3. Safety Education: Information is power. The Swedes demand education on how to avoid injuries and death. Venues include newspapers, radios, televisions, public forums, and communication with physicians and nurses. In the United States pediatric residency programs do not adequately address injury prevention. Of the 17 areas of injury prevention that were surveyed, only 10 (59%) were covered by more than 80% of the programs that responded to the questionnaire. Some topics were broadly and routinely covered, such as the use of car safety seats (99%), seat belts (96%), and bicycle helmets (95%). However, other topics received less attention, such as reducing DWIs (81%), smoke detector use (68%), safety fences around pools (65%), dangers of sports performance–enhancing substances (63%), and safe storage of firearms (56%).[34]

For many patients, the EP acts as a primary care physician and has both a tremendous opportunity and a responsibility to impact behavior. They may be the only healthcare provider to point out areas of risk or negligence. This role will become more important as larger segments of society, including the poor and uninsured, regularly turn to the ED for both their routine and emergent medical care.

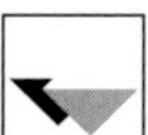

PEARLS & PITFALLS

- Motor vehicle crashes lead to more deaths among children from age 0 to 14 years than any other form of unintentional injury. Emergency physicians should educate patients regarding child restraint devices.
- Safety restraints are the single most effective means to reduce death and serious injury in motor vehicle crashes.
- Everyone in a car should wear seat belts. An air bag is no substitute for a safety harness.
- All motorcyclists and bicyclists should wear helmets. Physicians who council parents regarding helmets may double helmet use among those children.
- A gun in the home is more likely to injure a family member than an intruder. If children are in the home, guns must be kept under lock and key. Storing ammunition separate from guns and the use of locked trigger guards are additional safety measures.
- If a patient is sent home after evaluation for depression, a responsible adult must remove all firearms.
- Homicide is the leading cause of death in African-American men and women aged 15 to 24 years.

REFERENCES

1. National Highway Traffic Safety Administration: *Traffic safety facts, 1997,* Washington, DC, November, 1998, US Department of Transportation.
2. Liu S, et al: Prevalence of alcohol-impaired driving: results from a national self-reported review of health behaviors, *JAMA* 277: 122-125, 1997.
3. Mayhew DR, et al: Youth, alcohol and relative risk of crash involvement, *Accid Anal Prev* 18:273-287, 1986.
4. Crime in the United States: 1009 Uniform Crime Reports, Washington, DC, 1997, Federal Bureau of Investigation.
5. National Highway Traffic Safety Administration: *Traffic safety facts 1997: alcohol,* Washington, DC, 1988, US Department of Transportation.
6. Miller BA, Whitney R, Washousky R: Alcoholism diagnoses for convicted drinking drivers referred for alcoholism evaluation, *Alcohol Clin Exp Res* 10:651-656, 1986.
7. Miller BA, et al: Highway and crash costs in the U.S. by victim age, driver age, restraint use, and blood alcohol level. Association for the Advancement of Automotive Medicine, Fortieth Annual Proceedings, 1996.
8. National Highway Traffic Safety Administration: *Determine reasons for repeat drinking and driving,* Washington, DC, 1996, US Department of Transportation.
9. Bureau of Justice Statistics, Special Report: "Drunk Driving", RL Cohen, U.S. Dept of Justice, September, 1992.
10. SourceBook of Criminal Justice Statistics, 1994, U.S. Dept of Justice, Bureau of Justice Statistics, 1994.
11. National Highway Traffic Safety Administrative Web Site: http: www.nhtsa.dot.gov/
12. National Center for Health Statistics. Health, United States, 1996-97. Hyattsville, MD: CDC, 1997. DHHS publication no. (PHS) 97-1232, 1991.
13. Centers for Disease Control: Alcohol-related traffic fatalities involving children-United States, 1985-1996, *MMWR* 46:1130-1133, 1997.
14. Brewer RD, et al: The risk of dying in alcohol-related automobile crashes among habitual drunk drivers, *N Engl J Med* 331: 513-517, 1994.
15. Hingson R, Heeren T, Winter M: Lowering state legal blood alcohol limits to 0.08%: the effect on motor vehicle crashes, *Am J Public Health* 86:1297-1299, 1996.
16. Insurance Research Council: "Public Attitude Monitor, 1993". Surveys conducted by Roper Starch Worldwide, November, 1993.
17. Cydulka RK, et al: Injured intoxicated drivers: citation, conviction, referral and recidivism rates, *Ann Emerg Med* 32:349-352, 1998.
18. Orsay EM, et al: The impaired driver: hospital and police detection of alcohol and other drugs of abuse in motor vehicle crashes, *Ann Emerg Med* 24:51-55, 1994.
19. National Highway Traffic Safety Administration, Third Report to Congress. "Effectiveness of Occupant Protection Systems and Their Use", Washington, DC, December, 1996, US Department of Transportation.

20. Insurance Institute for Highway Safety: *Facts, 1996 fatalities: children,* Arlington, VA, 1997, IIHS.
21. National Highway Traffic Safety Administration: *Traffic safety facts, 1996-children,* Washington, DC, 1997, US Department of Transportation.
22. National Highway Traffic Safety Administration: *National occupant protection use survey-1996: research note,* Aug 1997. Washington, DC, 1997, US Department of Transportation.
23. National Highway Traffic Safety Administration: *Observed Patterns of misuse of child safety seats, Traffic Tech,* Sept 1996, Washington, DC, 1996, US Department of Transportation.
24. The National SAFEKIDS Campaign: http://www.safekids/org
25. Insurance Institute for Highway Safety: *Motor vehicle deaths on interstates and freeways: 1990-97,* Arlington, VA, 1997, IIHS.
26. National Highway Traffic Safety Administration: *Traffic safety facts 1997,* Washington, DC, 1997, US Department of Transportation.
27. National Highway Traffic Safety Administration: *Motorcycle helmet use laws: state legislative fact sheet,* Washington, DC, Sept 1996, US Department of Transportation.
28. Sosin DM, Sacks JJ, Webb KW: Pediatric head injuries and deaths from bicycling in the United States, *Pediatrics* 98:868-870, 1996.
29. Insurance Institute Highway Safety: *Facts 1996 fatalities: bicycles,* Arlington, VA, 1997,:IIHS.
30. National Safe Kids Campaign. Fact Sheet on Bicycle Injury. Washington, DC: NSKC, 1997.
31. Public Health Service (PHS). Healthy People 2000: Midcourse Review. Washington, DC: PHS, 1996.
32. Thompson RS, Rivara FP, Thompson DC: A case-control study of the effectiveness of bicycle safety helmets, *N Engl J Med* 320: 1361-1367, 1989.
33. Shafi S, et al: Impact of bicycle helmet safety legislation on children admitted to a regional pediatric trauma center, *J Pediatr Surg* 33:317-321, 1998.
34. Zavoski R, et al: Injury prevention in pediatric residency programs, *Arch Pediatr Adol Med* 150:1093-1096, 1996.
35. Mercy JA: The public health impact of firearm injuries, *Am J Prev Med* 9:8-11, 1993.
36. National Summary of Injury Mortality Data, 1987-1994, Atlanta, GA, 1996, Centers for Disease Control and Prevention.
37. Fingerhut LA, Kleinman JC: International and interstate comparisons for homicide among young males, *JAMA* 263:3292-3295, 1990.
38. Max W, Rice DP: Shooting in the dark: Estimating the cost of firearm injuries, *Health Aff* 12:171-185, 1993.
39. Firearms and Suicide, 1998, American Foundation for Suicide Prevention.
40. Kellermann AL, et al: Suicide in the home in relation to gun ownership, *N Engl J Med* 327: 467-472, 1992.
41. Kellermann AL, Reay DT: Protection or peril? An analysis of firearm-related deaths in the home, *N Engl J Med* 314:1557-1560, 1986.
42. Annest JL, et al: National estimates of nonfatal firearm related injuries: Beyond the tip of the iceberg, *JAMA* 273:1749-1754, 1995,
43. Federal Bureau of Investigation. Uniform Crime Reports for the United States, 1992. Washington, DC: Government Printing Office: 31-34, 1993.
44. Kochanek KD, Hudson BL: Advance Report of Final Mortality Statistics, 1992. Onthly Statistics Report; 43 (6). Hyattsville, MD: National Center for Health Statistics, 1995.
45. Cornwell EE III, et al: National Medical Association Surgical Section position paper on violence prevention: a resolution of trauma surgeons caring for victims of violence, *JAMA* 273:1788-1789, 1995.
46. Sloan JH, et al: Handgun regulations, crime, assault and homicide: a tale of two cities, *N Engl J Med* 319:1256-1262, 1988.
47. Callahan CM, Rivara FP: Urban high school youth and handguns: a school-based survey, *JAMA* 267:3038-3042, 1992.
48. Centers for Disease Control: Weapon-carrying among high school students, United States 1990, *MMWR* 40:681-683, 119.
49. Wintemute GJ: *Ring of fire: the handgun makers of Southern Californian,* Sacremento, CA, 1994, Violence Prevention Research Program.
50. Bergman AB, Rivara FP: Sweden's experience in reducing childhood injuries, *Pediatrics* 88:69-74, 1991.
51. Injury Control Update 2:1, A Publication of the National Center for Injury Prevention and Control, 1997.

Total Quality Management for Trauma Care

43

VIVEK TAYAL AND VINCENT P. VERDILE

Long-term commitment to new learning and new philosophy is required of any management that seeks transformation. The timed and the fainthearted, and people that expect quick results are doomed to disappointment.

W. Edward Deming in *Out of the Crisis*

Improving the quality of care to trauma patients is a core objective for any emergency department (ED).[1,2] Currently, certain external forces mandate quality reviews. For instance, the Joint Commission on Accreditation Healthcare Organizations (JCAHO) requires audits of procedural sedation, and many states insist on a variety of reviews to maintain trauma designation. However, the future of trauma quality management programs lies in the continual review and improvement of issues specific to each ED.[3,4] A team effort is the core of Quality Improvement (QI). The multidisciplinary approach allows for a variety of perspectives and will ensure "buy in" from the "stakeholders" (i.e., groups that have input into decisions are more likely to comply with the standards). Emergency physicians (EPs) must work with other medical staff members and the hospital administration to coordinate and standardize the trauma response.[5]

When we think of "trauma" we commonly picture the seriously injured or multiply-injured patient. However, the average EP sees hundreds of injured patients per year outside the trauma resuscitation room. These include, but are not limited to, patients with injuries from minor motor vehicle collisions, assault, falls, domestic violence, sport events, and burns. Although much of the following discussion emphasizes the major trauma patient, the care of less seriously injured patients should also be reviewed and continually improved.

Clinical guidelines, legislative initiatives, and new technologies can improve trauma patient care.[1,2,6,7] Total Quality Management (TQM) programs must analyze the success or failure of these interventions. One important aspect of TQM is the focus on processes rather than the individual. In the past, morbidity and mortality reviews concentrated on individual clinician performance and bad patient outcomes. TQM looks instead at how and why the system promoted or facilitated the care of patients and places the emphasis on meeting or exceeding all of the customers' expectations.[8,9]

QUALITY THEORY AND HISTORY

Quality assurance (QA) began in the early 1900s with the Flexner Report. This document enumerated deficiencies of both medical schools and general medical care. Dr. Ernest Codeman attempted to standardize hospital care in 1912, but few hospitals met basic guidelines. In the 1950s the American Medical Association, American Hospital Association, American College of Physicians (ACP), and the American College of Surgeons (ACS) formed the Joint Commission on Accreditation of Hospitals (JCAH) now known as the JCAHO. Because the mandate was vague, the initial requirements were poorly defined. However, hospitals introduced Morbidity and Mortality (M & M) conferences and began retrospective audits on patient outcome. In 1979 the JCAH moved from audits to QA standards, and in 1985 to the "10-step" process of monitoring and evaluation, which has become the mainstay program of hospital-based QA (Box 43-1). These mandated reviews of certain clinical activities included surgical/trauma cases.[4,10]

By the mid 1980s, the philosophy of TQM was

BOX 43-1
JCAHO 10-Step Process

STEP 1: ASSIGN RESPONSIBILITY
Although the medical director and nurse manager are responsible for ensuring that the 10 steps are successfully accomplished in the emergency department (ED), a team approach is essential.

STEP 2: DETERMINE SCOPE OF CARE AND SERVICE
The ED must identify the scope of care (e.g., will surgeons perform minilaparoscopy in the ED, will emergency physicians use bedside ultrasound).

STEP 3: IDENTIFY GOALS FOR PERFORMANCE IMPROVEMENT
What are the important processes for trauma care in the ED? These processes may include protocols for medical command of paramedics, criteria for trauma team activation, and identifying needed personnel or equipment.

STEP 4: DETERMINE INDICATORS FOR PERFORMANCE MEASUREMENTS
Identify objective measures of performance (e.g., time to consultant arrival for patients in shock and time to completion of CT in cases of severe head trauma).

STEP 5: ESTABLISH NUMERIC THRESHOLDS TO TRIGGER FURTHER INVESTIGATION
These thresholds determine when further evaluation occurs. For instance, one threshold may state that no more than 10% of patients triaged as lowest priority should require chest, abdominal, or cranial surgery in the first 24 hours. More than this number may require revision of triage codes or review of compliance with codes—100% threshold mandates every occurrence be evaluated.

STEP 6: COLLECT AND ORGANIZE DATA
Routine collection and organization of data is a key step for success of the QI program.

STEP 7: INITIATE EVALUATION
An evaluation of the data, processes, thresholds, and outcomes.

STEP 8: TAKE ACTIONS FOR IMPROVEMENT
Analysis should reveal areas for improvement. Recommendations for improvement should involve all members of the team.

STEP 9: REASSESS APPLIED ACTIONS
Retesting and collecting further data after the intervention evaluates success.

STEP 10: COMMUNICATE INFORMATION TO APPROPRIATE PARTIES
Communications with other members of the ED and Trauma team strengthens confidence in the QA/QI process and enhances the process.

spreading throughout industries in the United States. TQM, based on the 1950s work of Deming, Juran, and Donabedian, emphasized analysis of the work process rather than the individual worker. Deming's "Fourteen Points" listed in Box 43-2 serve as a primer in quality and customer service.[11] Although many American businesses quickly adopted the philosophy of TQM, the healthcare industry was slow to respond. Hospitals began applying the principles of TQM in the 1980s.[11-13]

Hospital and physician leadership, which represents the current-day management structure of most hospital organizations, must recognize the need for TQM and implement the philosophy system-wide. The employees, both clinical and nonclinical, must be empowered to utilize TQM to analyze, implement improvements and changes, and reanalyze the systems of care. A top-down micro-management style by the hospital or physician leadership precludes the evolution of TQM within an organization.[8,9]

Although a complete description of the TQM process is beyond the scope of this chapter, suffice it to say that there are key roles for individual members of the TQM team. A leader must be selected from the group, as well as a third-party facilitator who is skilled in the TQM process to educate the team and adhere to the TQM principles. The process, known as "forming, storming, and norming," uses tools to effect change within any system. Samples of these tools are included in Figs. 43-1 to 43-4. Fig. 43-1 is an example of a flowchart used to outline a process of patient care. Fig. 43-2 is a Pareto diagram, which highlights the

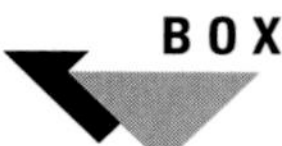

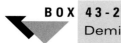

BOX 43-2
Deming Fourteen Points

1. Create constancy of purpose toward improvement of product and service, with the aim to become competitive and to stay in business, and to provide jobs.
2. Adopt the new philosophy. We are in a new economic age. Western management must awaken to the challenge, must learn their responsibilities, and take on leadership for change.
3. Cease dependence on inspection to achieve quality. Eliminate the need for inspection on a mass basis by building quality into the product in the first place.
4. End the practice of awarding business on the basis of price tags; instead, minimize total cost. Move toward a single supplier for any one item, founded on a long-term relationship of loyalty and trust.
5. Improve constantly and forever the system of production and service, to improve quality and productivity, and thus constantly decrease costs.
6. Institute training on the job.
7. Institute leadership. The aim of supervision should be to help people and machines and gadgets to do a better job. Supervision of management needs overhaul, as well as supervision of production workers.
8. Drive out fear, so that everyone may work effectively for the company.
9. Break down barriers between departments. People in research, design, sales, and production must work as a team, to foresee problems of production and in use that may be encountered with the product or service.
10. Eliminate slogans, exhortations, and targets for the workforce, asking for zero defects and new levels of productivity.
11. Eliminate work standards (quotas) on the factory floor. Substitute leadership.
12. Remove barriers that rob the hourly worker of his right to pride of workmanship. The responsibility of supervisors must be changed from sheer numbers to quality.
13. Institute vigorous programs of education and self-improvement.
14. Put everybody in the company to work to accomplish the transformation. The transformation is everybody's job.

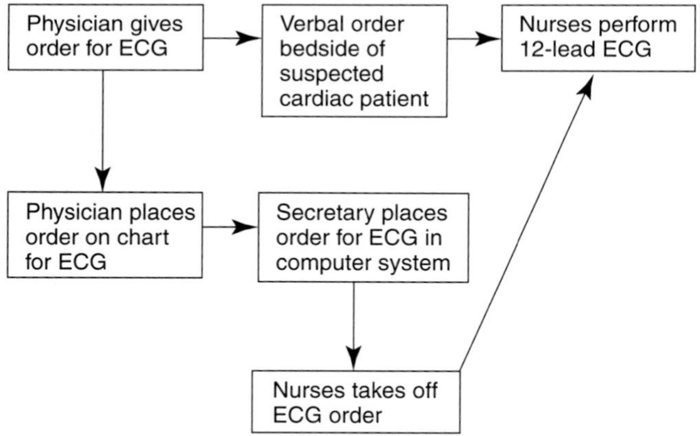

Fig. 43-1 Sample quality improvement tools for Process Improvement Team.

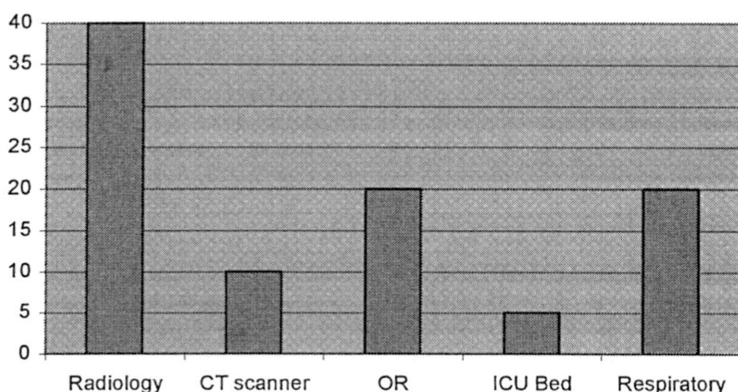

Fig. 43-2 Pareto diagram. Example of delays associated with the movement of the trauma patient through system to emergency department to intensive care unit in minutes.

most frequent issues surrounding the delays in care of a trauma patient in the ED. Fig. 43-3 is a run chart, which displays the average number of patients according to the times of the day. Finally, Fig. 43-4 is a fishbone diagram, which attempts to summarize all of the factors within a process that contributes to the care of the patient. These tools can all be used by the TQM team to analyze a process and seek opportunities for improvement. A sample trauma QI problem, process, and resolution is reviewed in Box 43-3.

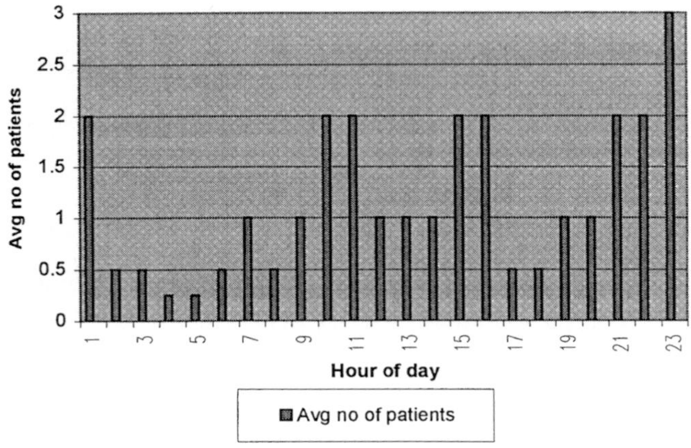

Fig. 43-3 Run chart. Number of trauma-related patients versus time of day.

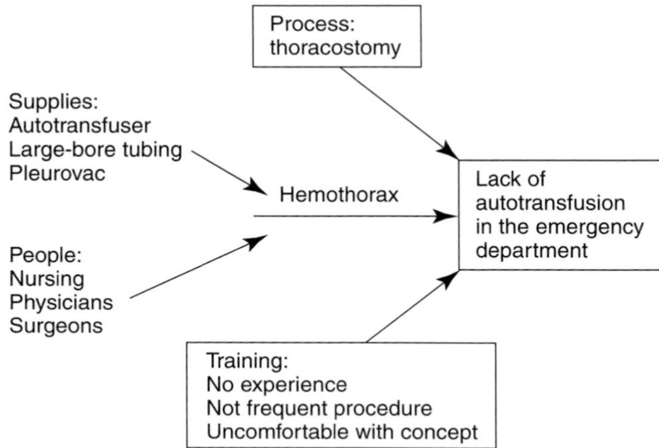

Fig. 43-4 Fishbone diagram. Example of contributing factors to lack of autotransfusion in the emergency department.

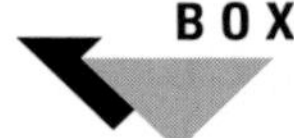

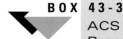

BOX 43-3

ACS Quality Assessment Programs[1,6]

Maintenance of trauma registries
Death audits
Morbidity and mortality reviews
Multidisciplinary trauma conferences
Nursing audits
Prehospital trauma care reviews
Diversion of trauma patients
On-call schedule for trauma-related specialists
Credentialing

EXAMPLE OF QI PROCESS

Rapid Sequence Intubation (RSI) is the preferred method of intubation at County General. However, many other departments, including Anesthesiology and Neurosurgery, are "nervous about the use of these strong drugs in the hands of ED doctors." A QI is set up to monitor intubations for untoward events, missed intubations, deaths, desaturations, and hypotension. However, these reviews do not bring up a significant problem in the trauma room, which is that the drugs and equipment are not readily available. QA may identify problems through a chart review, but QI suggests that a team of emergency physicians, emergency nurses, trauma surgeons, anesthesiologists, and respiratory technicians meet in a focused manner. The team must uncover the problems, determine how often they occur, and how to improve the situation. A box with commonly used intubation drugs is assembled, and an airway cart is placed in the trauma room. An audit to monitor intubations is established. The emergency physician completes an "Airway Sheet" after each intubation documenting drugs used, number of intubation attempts, complications, and outcome. The QI coordinator summarizes the sheets that the team reviews monthly.

ROLE OF TOTAL QUALITY MANAGEMENT IN THE CARE OF THE EMERGENCY DEPARTMENT TRAUMA PATIENT

Regardless of the size of the ED's annual census, TQM must include the care of the trauma patient. Individual EPs are unlikely to see and understand the "whole picture" of ED care without statistical monitoring.[8,14] EDs should evaluate trauma patient care, from both an intradepartmental and an interdepartmental standpoint. A failure to include both the prehospital and post-ED courses in the evaluation of the patient's outcome would be shortsighted. In addition, EDs that are part of a regional or state trauma system must participate in the system-wide evaluation of patient care as well.[15,16]

Fundamental to linking all aspects of the trauma patient's care is the statistical process control (SPC) concept. SPC defines the trauma patient's injury to rehabilitation through numerous measurements including customer satisfaction, cost, outcome, and efficiency.[16-20] SPC is the cornerstone to continuous QI. Therefore TQM through SPC must evaluate emergency medical service (EMS) systems, patient transfers, trauma airway management, the timelines of surgical consultations, and the utilization and effectiveness of diagnostic testing for the trauma patient (Boxes 43-4 to 43-7).[15,16]

Finally, sentinel events (Box 43-8), such as unexpected adverse outcomes and preventable deaths,

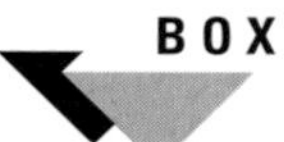

BOX 43-4
ACS 1993 Trauma-Focused Audits

Audit
Ambulance scene >20 minutes
Absence of at least hourly determinations and recording of blood pressure, pulse, respirations, and Glasgow Coma Scale score for any trauma patient beginning with arrival in the emergency department, including time spent in radiology, up to admission to the ward, operating room, or intensive care unit, death, or transfer to another hospital
Patients transferred to another healthcare facility after spending >6 hours in the initial hospital
Any patient requiring reintubation of the airway within 48 hours of extubation
Noncompliance with hospital criteria for trauma center designation

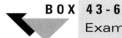

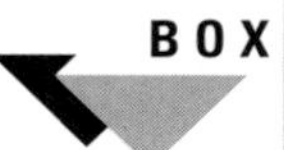

BOX 43-5
Prehospital Audits for the Emergency Department

Equipment audits
Medications audits
Procedures: intubation, intraosseous, deliveries, needle thoracostomies
Response times
Scene times
Transport times
Air vs ground transports

need to be the mainstay of the trauma quality management program. Fundamental to the understanding of the quality review process is familiarization with the definitions commonly used (Box 43-9).

TRAUMA SYSTEM TOTAL QUALITY MANAGEMENT

Regional trauma TQM committees often involve numerous hospitals, EMS agencies, and air medical services and are charged with improving patient care and transfer issues within the transfer system. A fundamentally important role for regional trauma TQM committees is the focus on the transfer process, which involves not only multiple healthcare workers but also multiple healthcare institutions. Important benchmarks include the length of time a patient is held before transfer, an audit of injuries not identified or managed at the referring hospital, and any patients who expire either during transfer or at the receiving facility. Ensuring that the patients arrive at the right resource in a reasonable time frame are all aspects of the process to be evaluated.[21,22]

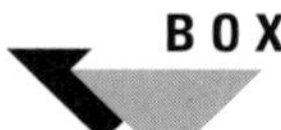

BOX 43-6
Examples of Scheduled Audits

Trauma code designation—monthly
Trauma procedures—monthly or bimonthly
Trauma deaths—monthly
Trauma transfers—quarterly
Trauma imaging: computed tomography, ultrasound, arteriogram ordered from the emergency department—quarterly or biannual
Use of O type blood in trauma room—biannual
Use of MAST trousers in pelvic fractures—whole year
Pediatric fluid, medications, and equipment audit—quarterly or biannual
Pregnancy tests in females of childbearing age—quarterly

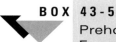

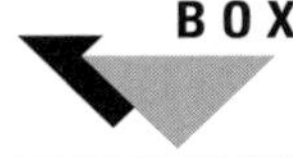

BOX 43-7
Common Emergency Department Procedures for QA in Trauma Patients

RSI
Rescue intubations
Thoracostomies
Thoracotomies
Central lines
Intraosseous lines in children
Blood transfusion
Autotransfusion
External pelvic fixation
Splints

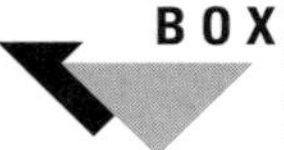

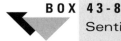

BOX 43-8
Sentinel Events

Missed intubation resulting in anoxic death
Missed abdominal injury resulting in death
Delay of consultant resulting in morbidity
COBRA violation
Iatrogenic injury

EMERGENCY MEDICAL SERVICES

The scope of EMS trauma QI depends on the association of the ED with the EMS agencies. Some EDs sponsor ground or flight programs. These EMS programs should at a minimum evaluate their compliance with national guidelines promulgated by the Department of Transportation (DOT), National Highway Transportation Safety Advisory (NHTSA), American College of Surgeons (ACS), American College of Emergency Physicians (ACEP), and the National Association of EMS Physicians (NAEMSP).[16]

EMS QI programs must evaluate the care, transportation, and triage of trauma patients. Audits may include scene or transport times, appropriate patient destination, and EMS provider's procedural success for intubation, intravenous access, and immobilization. Other topics may include use of blood products, alternative airways, rapid sequence intubation, multicasuality incident and management, and hospital turn-around times.

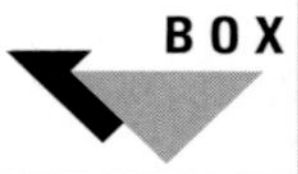

BOX 43-9
Definitions of QA and QI

Quality of Care (adapted from Institute of Medicine's 1990 definition) =
"Quality of care is the degree to which health services for individuals and populations increase the likelihood of desired health outcomes and are consistent with current professional knowledge."[5]
Quality Assurance (QA)—system of standards for patient care using audits or monitors. Those deviations from preset standards usually focus on providers or certain events.[4]
Quality or Process Improvement (QI or PI)—system of improving care through analysis (often statistical) of processes and the system problems, as opposed to the individual provider lapse.[7]

SOCIETY GUIDELINES

The American College of Surgeons (ACS) and the American College of Emergency Physicians (ACEP) have developed position papers on trauma care issues.[1,16] These papers, which may be found both in journals and on web sites, provide important information on quality standards and serve as a starting point for a trauma TQM program.

AMERICAN COLLEGE OF SURGEONS

The Committee on Trauma of the American College of Surgeons (ACS) published the book entitled *Resources for Optimal Care of the Injured Patient*.[16] This publication is an important guide to trauma centers in the United States. It defines resources and responsibilities, and makes recommendations on many aspects of

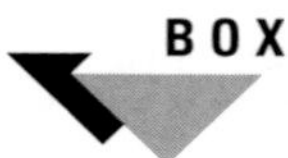

BOX 43-10
ACS 1993 Trauma Audit Filters

Absence of ambulance report on the medical record for a patient transported by prehospital emergency medical service personnel
A patient with a Glasgow Coma Scale (GCS) score of <14 who does not receive a computed tomographic (CT) scan of the head
A comatose trauma patient (GCS <8) leaving the emergency department before a definitive airway is established
Any patient with a gunshot wound to the abdomen managed nonoperatively
Patients with abdominal injuries and hypotension (SBP <90 mmHg) who do not undergo laparotomy within 1 hr of arrival in the emergency department; other patients undergoing laparotomy performed more than 4 hours after arrival in the emergency department
Patients with epidural or subdural brain hematoma receiving craniotomy more than 4 hours after arrival at the emergency department, excluding those performed for intracranial pressure (ICP) monitoring
Interval of >8 hours between arrival and the initiation of debridement of an open tibial fracture excluding a low-velocity gunshot wound
Abdominal, thoracic, vascular, or cranial surgery performed >24 hrs after arrival
A trauma patient admitted to the hospital under the care of an admitting or attending physician who is not a surgeon
Nonfixation of femoral diaphyseal fracture in an adult trauma patient
Selected complications monitored as trends or sentinel events
All trauma deaths

trauma patient care. This book enumerates qualifications of physicians, necessary equipment, scope of EMS care, hospital resources, and expectations for consultants. The ACS strongly promotes QI and the veracity of the QI Program is evaluated during ACS trauma care surveys.[15,23]

The ACS has also suggested audit filters (Box 43-10) and focused audits (see Box 43-5). Emergency physicians should review these audits for appropriate use in their Trauma QI program. Each hospital may tailor these filters for their needs.[8,9]

COMPARISON OF PREDICTED VERSUS ACTUAL MORTALITY

Another useful inquiry is a comparison of actual versus expected trauma mortality based on severity of injury. Injury Severity Scoring (ISS) and Trauma Scoring (TS) provide an estimate of the probability of survival, and permit comparisons between local and national outcomes.[1,24,25]

ISS is an anatomic method of scaling injuries that predicts mortality on an individual case basis. ISS is the sum of the squares of the three most severely injured body regions, each judged by the Abbreviated Injury Scale (AIS). The AIS itself is a numeric scale of injury severity from 1 (minor injury) to 6 (maximal injury–unsurvivable). Although the ISS score attempts to predict mortality, it suffers from several limitations including (1) only the three most severely injured body parts are included; (2) multiple injuries in one body part may not be included, especially bilateral injuries; and (3) the score does not consider age, chronic conditions, and premorbid conditions. Because the ISS is not a physiologic scale and is usually scored after full evaluation of all injuries, it cannot be used in the triage of patients. Scores of greater than 9 to 15 reflect major injury.[10] However, there are several aspects of the ISS system that render it imprecise as a means of analyzing deficiencies in trauma care systems. The utilization of using the ISS tool requires an understanding that observer variation in injury severity scoring and calculations of probability of survival may be substantial.[25,26]

AMERICAN COLLEGE OF EMERGENCY PHYSICIANS CLINICAL POLICIES

ACEP has provided important leadership in trauma QI. Trauma QI begins in the field and extends through the hospital stay and into the rehabilitation phase. ACEP's trauma QI tools for blunt and penetrating trauma are available from the national office.[27]

ACEP has also developed a number of clinical policies pertaining to the care of the trauma patient. The ACEP clinical policy on blunt abdominal trauma includes major trauma patients with multisystem blunt trauma. The committee grades the relevant literature according to an alphabetic score. Grade A includes randomized, controlled, or observational cohort studies or meta-analyses of such studies with appropriate power or confidence limits. Grade B is retrospective cohort studies, whereas grade C is cross-correlational studies, case series, case reports, and consensus statements by expert panels. Recommendations are divided into rules and guidelines. Rules reflect good practice in almost all situations, whereas guidelines are actions that should be considered depending on the circumstance. Any deviations from rules should be explained in writing.[2]

Many ACEP policies also contain QI tools. One such tool documents the presence or absence of particular historical and physical examination findings. Another tool determines the number of rules followed, divided by the number of rules called for according to the policy.

These policies provide a minimal but appropriate standard for trauma patient care in the ED. Emergency physicians should be familiar with these policies.

DATA INFORMATION

TQM is driven by data. Trauma databases may be derived from ED logs, ICD-9 coding (codes for Trauma range from 800 to 959), CPT codes, procedure logs, internal data sheets, EMS logs, transfer sheets, and any other computerized databases. ICD "E" code relates to various injury mechanisms. States or insurance carriers may mandate these codes.

MONITORS

A number of aspects of patient care termed *monitors* provide fertile QI data. These monitors include sentinel events, such as missed intubation or missed injury causing death within 24 hours, and EMS response time. Additional topics involve scheduled focused trauma audits, ED procedures, consultant response times, radiologic procedures and interpretation, nursing documentation, and audits of fluids and blood administration. Targeted ED trauma procedures include high-volume or high-risk intervention such as rapid sequence intubation, thoracostomies, central lines, and trauma ultrasounds. Consultant response times are best measured for surgical emergencies such as abdominal hemorrhage, intracranial hematomas, and unstable pelvic fractures. Prompt radiologic response is also essential for quality of patient care. Audits of

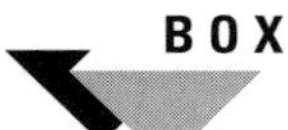

BOX 43-11
Examples of Suggested Trauma Benchmarks

Emergency medical services' time from call notification to arrival (in minutes)
Trauma code designation
Consultant response (in minutes)
Procedural competency (success and complication rates)
Time to computed tomography for traumatic brain injury (in minutes)
Time to operating suite for abdominal injury (in minutes)
Cost of trauma codes (amount per month or year)
Follow-up issues (complication, return visits, missed injuries, deaths)

radiology performance may include the time for radiology technicians to respond to the trauma room, accuracy of computed tomography (CT) reading, and timeliness of special procedures. Nursing benchmarks should also be reviewed.

BENCHMARKING

Outcome indicators and benchmarking are the new quality "buzzwords." Outcome indicators compare similar hospitals with similar case-mixes as measured by mortality and morbidity. These indicators must account for differences in EMS care, percentage of blunt versus penetrating trauma, urban versus rural settings, and the classification of ED. Benchmarking sets standards and goals based on similar settings. Examples of benchmarks include time to CT scan for the comatose patient or the response time of the surgical consultant (Box 43-11).

GETTING STARTED

The first step in developing a trauma QI program requires formation of a Trauma Committee. This committee will include EPs, trauma surgeons, general surgeons, surgical subspecialists, ED nurses, prehospital care providers, floor nurses, and all others involved in the care of the trauma patient.

Identify appropriate guidelines that apply to trauma care. These guidelines may include national standards, state regulations, and hospital policies.

↓

Evaluate existing structure of trauma system and determine how well it meets community needs.

↓

Select monitors to form basis of QA/QI system.

↓

Accumulate data.

↓

Analyze data.

↓

Develop conclusion.

↓

Develop action plan to improve identified problem.

↓

Use process team to change system.

↓

Reaccumulate data and determine degree of success or failure.

CONCLUSION

Trauma TQM must balance local needs and concerns with national and regional standards. Although this process is mandated by a variety of certifying organizations, QI provides an important opportunity to improve patient care. The TQM principle applies science to the management of a trauma system. Data, not personal prejudice or local tradition, must drive decisions. Focus on individual culpability must shift. It is often the system that promotes poor outcomes. Interdepartmental cooperation and communication are essential.

REFERENCES

1. American College of Emergency Physicians: Guidelines for trauma care systems, *Ann Emerg Med* 16:459-463, 1987.
2. American College of Emergency Physicians: Clinical policy for the initial approach to patients presenting with acute blunt trauma, *Ann Emerg Med* 31:422-454, 1998.
3. Eastes L: Toward continuous quality improvement in trauma care. *Crit Care Nurs Clin North Am* 6:451-461, 1994.
4. Weltge AF: Evolution of quality assurance and quality improvement. In Siegel DM, Crocker PJ (editors): *Continuous quality improvement for emergency departments,* Dallas, 1994, American College of Emergency Physicians.
5. Hoelz JJ: Team building: solving problems by multidisciplinary approach. In Salluzzo RF, et al (editors): *Emergency department management: principles and applications,* St Louis, 1997, Mosby.
6. Chassin MR, Galvin RW: National roundtable on health care quality: The urgent need to improve health care quality, *JAMA* 1998; 280:1000-1005.
7. Schwartz CH: Preparation for trauma survey. In Salluzzo RF, et al (editors): *Emergency department management: principles and applications,* St Louis, 1997, Mosby.
8. Mayer TA, Salluzzo RF: Theory of continuous quality improvement. In Salluzzo RF, et al (editors): *Emergency department management: principles and applications,* St Louis, 1997, Mosby.
9. Salluzzo RF, Bartfield JM, Verdile VP: Implementing and evaluating the effectiveness of a quality improvement program. In Salluzzo RF, et al (editors): *Emergency department management: principles and applications,* St Louis, 1997, Mosby.

10. Joint Commission on Accreditation of Health Care Organization: *Accreditation manual for hospitals,* Chicago, 1996, JCAHO.
11. Deming WE: *Out of crisis*, Cambridge, Ma, 1989, Massachusetts Institute of Technology of Press, Center for Advanced Engineering.
12. Juran JM: *Juran on planning for quality,* New York, 1988, The Free Press.
13. Berwick DM: Continuous improvement as an ideal in healthcare, *N Engl J Med* 320:53-56, 1989.
14. Buckley LL, Ellis RS: Interpreting and applying the results of CQI efforts. In Siegel DM, Crocker PJ (editors): *Continuous quality improvement for emergency departments,* Dallas, 1994, ACEP.
15. Nayduch D, et al: American College of Surgeons Trauma Quality Indicators: an analysis of outcome in a statewide trauma registry, *J Trauma* 37:565-575, 1994.
16. American College of Surgeons, Committee on Trauma: *Resources for optimal care of the injured patient: 1993*, Chicago, 1999, ACSC.
17. Davis JW, et al. An analysis of errors causing morbidity and mortality in a trauma system: a guide for quality improvement, *J Trauma* 32:660-666, 1992.
18. Richardson JD, et al: Impact of trauma attendings surgeon case volume on outcome: is more better? *J Trauma* 44:266-272, 1998.
19. Sharp JF, Denholm S: Routine x-rays in nasal trauma: the influence of audit on clinical practice, *J Roy Soc Med* 87:153-154, 1994.
20. Blackstone ME, et al: Lowering hospital charges in the trauma intensive care unit while maintaining quality of care by increasing resident and attending physician awareness, *J Trauma* 39: 1041-1044, 1995.
21. Norwood S, Fernandez L, England J: The early effects of implementing American College of Surgeons level II criteria on transfer and survival rates at a rurally based community hospital, *J Trauma* 39: 240-245, 1995.
22. Sampalis JS, et al: Direct transport to tertiary trauma centers versus transfer from lower level facilities: impact on mortality and morbidity among patients with major trauma, *J Trauma* 43: 288-296, 1997.
23. Mitchell FL, Thal ER, Wolferth CC: American College of Surgeons verification/consultation program: analysis of unsuccessful verification reviews, *J Trauma* 37:557-564, 1994.
24. Cryer HG, et al: Continuous use of standard process audit filters has limited value in a established trauma system, *J Trauma* 41:389-395, 1996.
25. Zoltie N, de Dombal FT: The hit and miss of iss and triss, *Br Med J* 307:906-909, 1993.
26. Yates DW, Woodford M, Hollis S: Trauma audit: clinical judgement or statistical analysis? *Ann Roy Coll Surg* 75:321-324, 1993.
27. American College of Emergency Physicians: Guidelines for trauma care systems: appendix C: quality improvement, *Ann Emerg Med* 22:1096-1100, 1993.

44 Preparing Patient for Transfer

MICHAEL A. GIBBS, MICHAEL H. THOMASON, JOHN A. MARX, AND STEPHEN A. COLUCCIELLO

Although community hospitals provide definitive care for the majority of injured patients, approximately 10% of trauma patients may benefit from the specialized services of regional trauma centers.[1] Both the decision to transfer and the mode of transport should be individualized and based on the patient's injuries, local resources, geography, environmental conditions, and availability of qualified transport personnel. The development of regional trauma systems and well-designed transfer agreements facilitate timely transfer and improve patient outcome.[2-6]

A frequent cause of trauma morbidity arises from delay in transfer. Although a multitude of reasons may account for delay, many delays are a result of over-reliance on diagnostic testing, especially radiographs and computed tomography (CT) scans. Although a trauma patient with a Glasgow Coma Scale (GCS) score of 6 and no lateralizing signs ultimately needs a CT scan, the community hospital is not the optimal place. The reasoning is because all patients with head trauma and a GCS ≤8 require the services of a neurosurgeon *regardless* of CT findings. Unless the community physician intends to drill a burr hole before transfer (a course not indicated in the patient without lateralizing findings) the CT is best deferred to the receiving hospital. Optimal interventions for a comatose (GCS ≤8) trauma patient who arrives at a community hospital include determination of a bedside glucose, intubation using neuroprotective agents for induction, maintaining cerebral perfusion pressure, and calling a trauma center to arrange immediate transfer.

Although a small number of patients require multiple studies to determine the need for transfer, in most cases the need for a trauma center is clinically obvious within minutes of a patient's arrival.

Although scrupulous attention to minor pathology might be acceptable in some aspects of medical practice, it can be a lethal error in trauma. It is not necessary to diagnose all of a patient's injuries before arranging transfer to a trauma center. **As soon as the need for transfer is recognized, the process should be initiated and carried out immediately.** Unnecessary delays in the transfer of severely injured patients remain major causes of preventable mortality. Additional diagnostic studies may be obtained while waiting for the transport team to arrive. Unstable patients should be carefully monitored in a resuscitation area; they do not belong in a CT scanner while awaiting transfer.

Trauma centers and referring hospitals can develop consensus-based guidelines that provide specific recommendations for transfers. These guidelines address the essentials of early management and limit diagnostic and treatment measures to those that affect immediate patient management. Transfer agreements between community hospitals and regional trauma centers developed in advance streamline the transfer of seriously injured patients.

Preparation for transport includes: (1) appropriate clinical stabilization (if possible), (2) communication with the accepting clinical care team, and (3) transfer of appropriate medical documents.

PATIENT STABILIZATION

Begin any appropriate lifesaving measures before interfacility transfer. The essentials of early resuscitation include (1) a secure airway and appropriate intravenous access, (2) volume resuscitation and hemodynamic stabilization, (3) immobilization of the spine and extremities if fracture is suspected, and (4) protection from hypothermia. *This process should not be delayed for laboratory or diagnostic procedures that do not impact the transfer process or the immediate need for resuscitation.*

The Hypotensive Patient

If the patient is hemodynamically unstable, the emergency physician must search for those conditions amenable to emergency department intervention. Patients with external blood loss require direct pressure to bleeding wounds, as well as volume and possibly blood replacement. Other interventions may include placement of a chest tube for tension pneumothorax, and a chest tube and autotransfusion for massive hemothorax. Patients with stigmata of pericardial tamponade on physical examination or on bedside echocardiography will need a needle decompression of the pericardium and perhaps a pericardial window performed by a local surgeon. Patients with unstable pelvic fractures may benefit from application of the pneumatic anti-shock garment (PASG). Traction splints such as the Hare splint may decrease bleeding from femur fractures. Although volume resuscitation for presumed internal bleeding before operation is controversial, it remains standard in most parts of the country.

However, many hypotensive victims of blood trauma will not have tension pneumothorax, massive hemothorax, pericardial tamponade, or unstable pelvic fractures. Other patients remain hemodynamically unstable despite treatment of these conditions. In such cases, intraabdominal injury is likely. If intraabdominal injury is suspected in a hypotensive patient, determine if a local surgeon is *immediately* available to perform a lifesaving laparotomy. If immediate laparotomy is feasible, a bedside diagnostic peritoneal lavage or ultrasound may be appropriate. Transfer may be accomplished after surgery. The decision to perform abdominal surgery at the referring hospital must balance many factors including the timely availability of a willing surgeon, a currently staffed operating suite, the relative stability of the patient, and the time anticipated for the patient to reach the operating suite at the trauma center.

COMMUNICATION

When transfer of a critically ill patient is necessary, nothing replaces direct physician-to-physician communication. A brief dialogue will ensure that the most appropriate mode of transport is used, and that any specialized transport equipment is available. This same physician-to-physician interaction allows the receiving hospital to provide informed medical oversight of the transport team. The referring physician should provide items listed under communication in the following material.

TRANSFER OF INFORMATION

Copies of medical records (notes, orders, medications given, laboratory studies, consent forms, living wills, COBRA forms), radiographs, and any other information important to the delivery of good medical care should always accompany the patient or be transmitted by facsimile to the tertiary care center (Box 44-1).

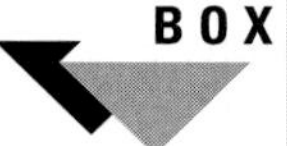

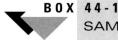

BOX 44-1
SAMPLE TRAUMA TRANSFER GUIDELINES

GENERAL PRINCIPLES

1. Appropriate emergency interventions and expeditious transport to a trauma center may be lifesaving.
2. Perform only those diagnostic studies and therapies that influence immediate patient management before transfer.

RESUSCITATION

1. *Airway:* secure airway (see "Airway Management")
2. *Breathing:* ensure adequate ventilation/oxygenation
3. *Circulation:* maintain adequate organ perfusion

   Adult: Infuse warmed normal saline (NS) or lactated Ringers (LR), up to 2 liters in the hypotensive patient. If patient remains hypotensive, transfuse packed red blood cells (PRBCs). Overaggressive administration of fluids may worsen outcomes in patients with uncontrolled internal hemorrhage. If the patient remains in shock, *and* timely laparotomy is feasible before transfer, perform a DPL or bedside ultrasound.

   Pediatric: Infuse warmed NS or LR (20cc/kg). A second bolus may be given. If patient remains hypotensive, transfuse 10 cc/kg PRBCs and repeat as needed. Intraosseous catheters are indicated if intravenous (IV) access is difficult to obtain. See adult guidelines above if the patient remains in shock.
4. *Disability:* Assess neurologic status (GCS, level of alertness, brief sensory-motor examination, lateralizing focal findings, pupillary reactivity).
5. *Secondary Survey:* Head-to-toe physical examination

Continued

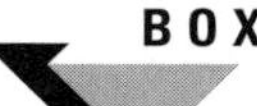

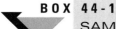

BOX 44-1
SAMPLE TRAUMA TRANSFER GUIDELINES—cont'd

NECESSARY STUDIES

The following recommendations are for patients with multisystem trauma, and may not apply to those with isolated injuries. Although cervical spine radiographs, stat hemoglobin, and pelvic films are listed as optional, they are desirable if time permits. Radiographic evidence of an unstable cervical spine will inspire greater care in immobilization, whereas a hemoglobin of 7 should prompt blood administration. A pelvic fracture seen on radiograph may initiate application of the PASG.

Essential: Anteroposterior (AP)-supine chest radiograph
*Optional:** Cervical spine radiographs
AP pelvis radiograph
STAT hemoglobin
Avoid:† CT scanning
Extremity radiographs

Although it has not been specifically studied as a tool to determine the need for transfer, a serum lactate is a reliable measure of occult shock (see Chapter 9). An immediate bedside base deficit or serum lactate may provide important clues to extent of internal injuries. A lactate greater than 3 or a base deficit more negative than –6 are both associated with increased morbidity. A hypotensive patient does not need a lactate level, since shock is clinically evident.

AIRWAY MANAGEMENT

Indications for Endotracheal Intubation

1. Airway compromise (e.g., facial trauma, inhalation injury)
2. Inadequate ventilation/oxygenation
3. Severe brain injury (GCS ≤8)

Rapid Sequence Induction (RSI)

RSI is a suggested approach to endotracheal intubation in the trauma patient. Variations may be appropriate, depending on the individual patient. In addition, consider the following:

1. Only physicians familiar with the use of neuromuscular-blocking agents should perform RSI.
2. The physician should determine a GCS and perform a brief motor examination before performing RSI.
3. Short-acting sedatives and neuromuscular-blocking agents will facilitate the neurologic examination on arrival to the receiving facility.

PREOXYGENATE
↓
MAINTAIN IN-LINE CERVICAL SPINE STABILIZATION THROUGHOUT PROCEDURE
↓
If concern for increased ICP
ADMINISTER LIDOCAINE (1.5mg/kg IV)
↓
ADMINISTER INDUCTION AGENT‡
(e.g., Etomidate 0.3 mg/kg IV)
↓
APPLY CRICOID PRESSURE
↓
ADMINISTER SUCCINYLCHOLINE (1.5mg/kg IV)§
↓
PERFORM OROTRACHEAL INTUBATION
↓
VERIFY TUBE PLACEMENT
(End-tidal CO_2 detector, Esophageal detector device)
↓
OBTAIN POST-INTUBATION CXR

GENERAL INTERVENTIONS

Procedures

1. Maintain adequate airway and provide supplemental oxygen.
2. Insert a chest tube in patients with a significant pneumothorax or hemothorax, or in patients with a pneumothorax on positive pressure ventilation.
3. Secure two large-bore IV lines. Use warmed IV fluids whenever possible.
4. Apply direct pressure to all sites of external hemorrhage.
5. Immobilize spine (rigid cervical collar, spinal board).
6. Immobilize extremity fractures in anatomic position if possible, and check pulses.
7. Reduce extremity dislocations if neurovascular compromise is present.
8. Apply Pneumatic Anti-Shock Garment (PASG) or similar device in patients with unstable pelvic fractures. A bed sheet tightly wrapped around the pelvis may serve if other options are unavailable.
9. Apply saline-soaked gauze to all open wounds.
10. Insert a Foley catheter and gastric tube in all severely injured patients without contraindications.
11. Rapidly stitch (running O-nylon) bleeding scalp lacerations.

*Patient transport should *not* be delayed to obtain these studies.
†If transfer is already deemed necessary based on clinical findings alone, these studies may cause significant delays and should be avoided. If transfer has already been arranged, the studies may be obtained while waiting for the arrival of transport team.
‡Induction agents should be used with caution in hypotensive patients (BP <90 mmHg).
§Endotracheal intubation itself or succinylcholine may cause bradycardia in children under 8 years old. Administer atropine 0.02 mg/kg IV (minimum of 0.1 mg/dose).

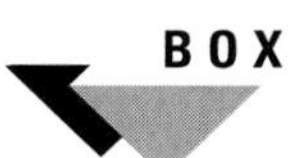

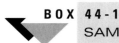

BOX 44-1

SAMPLE TRAUMA TRANSFER GUIDELINES—cont'd

Pharmacology

When paralysis or sedation is required, always use short-acting agents to allow for timely neurosurgical evaluation. All patients who are paralyzed must be sedated. Suggested doses (may repeat as needed):

Sedation: Midazolam (*Versed*): 0.05 mg/kg every 15 to 30 minutes

Paralysis: Vecuronium (*Norcuron*): 0.1 mg/kg every 30 to 45 minutes

HEAD INJURY

1. Secure a stable airway. If endotracheal intubation is required, document a brief neurologic assessment *before* sedative or paralytic agents are given.
2. Use short-acting sedatives and paralytics. **Document time and dosage of all drugs given.**
3. CT scanning of the head is unnecessary in patients with clinical evidence of severe head injury (e.g., coma, focal deficits).
4. When volume resuscitation is required, use only NS, LR, or PRBCs (avoid dextrose-containing solutions).
5. In patients with progressive neurologic deterioration and those with lateralizing findings (e.g., pupillary asymmetry, asymmetric posturing) hyperventilate (16 to 18 breaths per minute) and administer mannitol (1 gram/kg IV over 20 minutes).

COMMUNICATION

1. Once the need for patient transfer is established, the referring physician should call the trauma center as soon as possible.
2. Have the following information available for patient report:
   A. Name and age of patient
   B. Time and mechanism of injury
   C. Most recent vital signs
   D. Lowest recorded blood pressure
   E. Most recent GCS
   F. Status of patient's airway
   G. Medications received
   H. Volume of resuscitation fluids/blood received
   I. List of known and suspected injuries

COMMON PITFALLS

1. Delaying patient transfer to obtain diagnostic studies that will not alter immediate patient management.
2. Failure to perform endotracheal intubation when indicated.
3. Failure to recognize and aggressively treat compensated hemorrhagic shock.
4. Failure to insert a chest tube in a patient with a significant pneumothorax or hemothorax.
5. Failure to recognize, stabilize, and rapidly transport patients with unstable pelvic fractures.
6. Using long-acting paralytic agents and sedatives that delay timely neurosurgical evaluation.
7. Failure to anticipate, recognize, and treat hypothermia in the trauma patient.
8. Failure to sedate patients receiving paralytic agents

THESE GUIDELINES WERE DEVELOPED TO FACILITATE THE RAPID ASSESSMENT, STABILIZATION AND TRANSFER OF THE SEVERELY INJURED PATIENT. THEY ARE ONLY MEANT TO BE GUIDELINES, AND MAY NOT APPLY TO ALL SITUATIONS.

REFERENCES

1. Champion HR, Sacco WJ, Copes WS: Improvement in outcome from trauma center care, *Arch Surg* 127:333-338, 1992.
2. Bazzoli GJ, et al: Progress in the development of trauma systems in the United States. Results of a national survey, *JAMA* 273:395-401, 1995.
3. Cales RH, Trunkey DD: Preventable trauma deaths: a review of trauma care systems development, *JAMA* 254:1059-1063, 1985.
4. Esposito TJ, et al: Analysis of preventable trauma deaths and inappropriate trauma care in a rural state, *J Trauma* 39:955-962, 1995.
5. Maio RF, et al: A study of preventable trauma mortality in rural Michigan, *J Trauma* 41:83-90, 1996.
6. Shackford SR, et al: The effect of regionalization upon the quality of trauma care as assessed by concurrent audit before and after institution of a trauma system: a preliminary report, *J Trauma* 26:812-820, 1986.

Legal Requirements for Transferring Trauma Patients

45

ROBERT A. BITTERMAN

Trauma patients are usually transferred because the transferring facility lacks the capability or the resources necessary to treat the patient's injuries. Examples include head-injured patients in a hospital without a neurosurgeon on staff, patients with an extremity amputation who need the expertise of a hand surgeon, or multiple-trauma patients treated initially in a rural emergency department (ED) who require treatment at a level I trauma center.

Federal law, The Emergency Medical Treatment and Active Labor Act (EMTALA, a.k.a. COBRA) defines such transfers as "medically indicated transfers," because the purpose is to obtain a higher level of medical care necessary to treat the patient's condition.[1] EMTALA governs every aspect of medically indicated transfers, from requiring hospitals to adopt and enforce policies that comply with federal transfer laws,[2] to mandating specific actions by both the transferring hospital and the receiving hospital.[1,2] The "bite of the COBRA" is painful indeed, and failure to comply with these transfer laws carries significant financial penalties for both the physician and hospital alike, penalties not covered by the physician's malpractice insurance.

The Joint Commission on Accreditation of Healthcare Organizations (JCAHO) also requires hospitals to maintain written policies and procedures governing the transfer of patients.[3] Finally, some states have enacted their own transfer laws.[4] Most parallel EMTALA, but some are more burdensome. Physicians responsible for patient transfers should be aware of controlling state laws and regulations, as well as federal law.

DUTIES OF THE TRANSFERRING HOSPITAL

To effect a medically indicated trauma transfer, the physician must first legally 'certify' that the benefits to the patient from the transfer outweigh the risk of the transfer; second, obtain the patient's informed consent; and third, arrange an "appropriate transfer" as defined by law.[5]

Complete a Physician Certification of Transfer

The transferring physician must certify that the hospital's EMTALA obligations and the risks and benefits of the transfer were explained to the patient, and that the transfer is in the patient's best interest. Exceptions are made for the comatose patient (see the following discussion).

The certificate must be in writing and must be signed by the transferring physician. The risks and benefits should be expansively documented; failure to include foreseeable risks could invalidate the patient's consent. Also, the certification must be based on information available *at the time of transfer*, not based on the physician's earlier examination of the patient. Thus the transferring physician needs to reevaluate the patient just before transfer to ensure the transfer is still medically indicated.[6]

Although certification is not legally required for stable patients, a certificate should be completed on *any* trauma transfer regardless of whether the patient is stable or unstable at the time of transfer. This policy ensures uniformity and compels the physician to complete the appropriate documentation, should HCFA or a court later rule that the patient was not stable at the time of transfer.[7]

A physician should certify the transfer as medically indicated only when needed equipment or physician resources are not available at the referring facility. The transfer of an unstable patient to a facility with lesser capabilities, or capabilities equivalent to the transferring facility, violates EMTALA because the transferring hospital should have stabilized the patient with its own staff and available resources.

If the hospital does not have a physician on duty at the time of the transfer, then a "qualified medical person" may sign the certification. However, this person must consult with a physician who accepts responsibility for deciding that the benefits of the transfer outweigh the risks of transfer. The physician must later countersign the certificate.[8]

Obtain the Patient's Informed Consent to the Transfer

The hospital should obtain the patient's informed consent and signature before the transfer. Besides the medical risks and benefits, the consent should also explain the risks associated with helicopter or ambulance transport. If the patient is incapacitated or incompetent to give consent, then the physician should seek consent from the patient's family. If neither the patient nor the family is able to consent to the transfer, then the physician should proceed with the transfer, assuming that a reasonable person in the patient's circumstances would consent to the transfer—what the law refers to as implied consent under the "emergency doctrine."[9]

Arrange an "Appropriate Transfer"

The medically indicated transfer of a trauma patient must follow these four parameters set out in EMTALA's definition of an "appropriate transfer."[10]

STABILIZE THE PATIENT, IF POSSIBLE

The hospital must do everything within its capability to treat and stabilize the patient before transfer. Stabilization may include using a computed tomography (CT) scan to diagnose a subdural hematoma if a neurosurgeon is available at the referring hospital. (However, a CT is *not* necessary if there is no neurosurgeon available to the referring hospital.) Stabilization may also involve requesting the surgeon on-call to perform an emergent laparotomy, if the transferring physician determines this procedure is in the patient's best interest. The transfer may then be completed after the operation if necessary.

The timing of the transfer depends on the condition of the patient and the judgement of the examining physician. *The hospital does not have to stabilize the patient before transfer; it is **not** illegal to transfer an unstable patient under EMTALA.* The law actually requires hospitals to transfer unstable patients if they lack the capacity to stabilize the patient and the patient's best interest is served by moving to a facility that can stabilize the emergency condition.[11]

ARRANGE FOR ANOTHER HOSPITAL TO ACCEPT THE PATIENT IN TRANSFER

Before a hospital can transfer a patient, another hospital must agree to accept the patient in transfer and provide appropriate medical treatment.[10] EMTALA does not require that a physician accept the patient in transfer; the accepting facility may designate nurses, a transfer team, or even the admitting office to accept transfers on its behalf. However, it is prudent to always speak with an accepting physician who can provide advice regarding medical aspects of the transport.

The referring facility must also determine that the receiving hospital has available space and qualified personnel necessary to treat the individual.[10] This information is best obtained during the consultation with the accepting physician. A head-injured patient should not be transferred to a hospital without a neurosurgeon or when the CT scanner is down for repairs.

Ideally, hospitals should prearrange standing transfer agreements with a designated tertiary facility to accept trauma transfers they are unable to manage.

SEND APPROPRIATE DATA TO THE ACCEPTING FACILITY

EMTALA and HCFA's accompanying regulations dictate what data the transferring hospital must send to the receiving facility.[10,12] These data include appropriate medical records related to the emergency condition, recordings of observation of signs or symptoms, preliminary diagnosis, treatment provided, results of any tests that have been performed, the informed written consent, and a copy of the written certification that the transfer is medically indicated.

At times a hospital may transfer a patient because it can't reach its on-call physician or the on-call physician refuses to come in to help care for the patient. In this case the transferring hospital ***must*** send the name and address of the on-call physician who refused or failed to appear within a reasonable time to provide the necessary stabilizing treatment.[10] The definition of a "reasonable time" is often contained in the hospital bylaws. Failure to send this information with the transfer is itself a violation of EMTALA.

A. Examinations and Treatment

__ 1. Medical screening examinations (MSE) performed, to the extent possible considering the emergency department's capabilities and ancillary services and/or on-call physicians available, to determine if the patient is suffering from an emergency medical condition (MSE is only for ED cases), and/or

__ 2. Treatment provided, including any necessary stabilizing treatment, to the extent possible within the resources and physician personnel available to our facility.

B. Interaction with Accepting Facility

__ 1. Transfer accepted by appropriate physician and documented on the Patient Transfer Order form.

__ 2. Transfer accepted by receiving facility.

__ 3. Receiving hospital has adequate space and qualified personnel to appropriately handle the patient's medical condition.

C. Forms To Complete Before Transfer (sample transfer forms are available; see references):

__ 1. If this is a **patient requested transfer:**

__ 1a. Complete the **Transfer Requested By Patient** form

and

__ 1b. Complete the **Patient Transfer Order** form

OR

__ 2. If this is a **medically indicated transfer:**

__ 2a. Complete the **Medically Indicated Transfer** form

and

__2b. Complete the **Patient Transfer Order** form

D. Transfer Procedure:

__ 1. Arrange transfer of the patient through qualified personnel and transfer equipment as appropriate to the patient's condition.

__ 2. Send copies of pertinent patient records with patient to receiving facility.

__ a. Tests: __ Labs __ X-rays __ EKGs

__ Monitor Strips __ ABGs __

Others __________

__ b. Medical records

__ c. Transfer forms

__ 3. Obtain patient's vital signs and reassess patient's medical condition just before the time of transport and document in medical record.

__ 4. Give nursing report to receiving hospital.

__ 5. Send patient's belongings with the patient.

__ 6. Notify patient's family.

Imprint patient's ID here

______________________________ R.N. ______________________________

Signature Name

Date: __________________ Time: __________________

Send completed checklist to Q/A.

Fig. 45-1 Sample patient transfer check list.

State law may require exchange of additional transfer information. For example, Texas and New York require that a memorandum of transfer, which must include the name of the physician authorizing the transfer and must be signed by both the sending and receiving physicians, be sent with the patient.[13]

The American College of Surgeons also expects more detailed information to be contained in the transfer report, such as the patient's Glasgow Coma Scale score and the type and volume of fluids administered before transfer.[14] The use of transfer checklists helps ensure the appropriate data and forms accompany all transfers (Fig. 45-1). Transferring hospitals should also complete appropriate transfer forms that document the presence or absence of an emergency medical condition, whether or not stabilization was achieved, the risks and benefits to the patient regarding transfer, and the patient's informed consent.[1] (Sample forms are also available in reference 7.)

EFFECT THE TRANSFER THROUGH QUALIFIED PERSONNEL AND TRANSPORTATION EQUIPMENT

The transferring hospital is responsible for the patient until the patient arrives at the accepting facility. The hospital should transfer the patient by helicopter, BLS/ALS ambulance, or private car as dictated by the patient's medical condition. It must also choose medical personnel to accompany the patient in transfer who can provide the necessary foreseeable medical measures during transfer.[10] Usually paramedics are adequate, but if airway compromise is likely to occur en route, then the hospital would be obligated to send along a physician or other person capable of surgically securing the airway. In such cases however, the airway is best secured before transfer.

Managed Care Considerations

A hospital should not transfer an *unstable* patient to a hospital mandated by a managed care organization (MCO) unless all of the following conditions are met:

1. The transferring hospital is unable to stabilize the patient's injuries.
2. The MCO facility has the resources necessary to manage the patient's condition and foreseeable complications.

Thus transfers of an unstable patient to a MCO facility are guided by the same principles that determine other transfers. Failure to follow these guidelines makes the transferring hospital liable under EMTALA.

Maintain Records of All Transfers

Hospitals must maintain all records related to transfers both into and out of the hospital for 5 years. These records include patients transferred from the in-patient setting, not just transfers from the ED.[15]

Patient Refusal of a Medically Indicated Transfer

If the trauma patient refuses to consent to a medically needed transfer to a hospital capable of managing the patient's acute injuries, after the hospital informs the patient of the risks and benefits of refusing the offered transfer, then the hospital will not be liable under EMTALA. However, the hospital must ascertain that the patient is competent to refuse medical care and, according to HCFA, the hospital "must take all reasonable steps to secure the individual's written informed consent to refuse such transfer."[16]

DUTIES OF RECEIVING HOSPITAL

EMTALA forces hospitals capable of specialized care to accept patients who require their services. Hospitals that can stabilize the patient's injuries are required to accept the patient in transfer. This nondiscrimination clause states:

> *Hospitals with specialized capabilities or facilities shall not refuse to accept appropriate transfers of individuals who require such specialized capabilities or facilities if the hospital has the capacity to treat the individual.*[17]

"Specialized Capabilities or Facilities"

The law does not define the term *specialized*, but it almost certainly applies to any hospital that has the resources or physician expertise needed to manage the patient's emergency that are not available to the transferring hospital. *The only legal reason for refusing a transfer is the physical inability to properly treat the patient.* Congress expressly forbids hospitals to refuse patients on any other basis, including lack of insurance. When a trauma center is asked to accept a trauma patient from a referring hospital, the best answer is always "Yes." There are few exceptions to this rule.

Capacity

A hospital may, and should, refuse a transfer if it does not have the capacity to treat the patient's condition. However, HCFA defines capacity very generously to include the hospital's past practices of accommodating additional patients in excess of its occupancy limits.[18] In one case an on-call neurosurgeon refused a requested transfer of an emergency neurosurgical case, stating the intensive care unit (ICU) was full. However, the hospital was holding one unit bed open in case of an in-house emergency. HCFA deemed this refusal a violation of EMTALA, stating that if the hospital had an open ICU bed for possible in-house needs, then that bed was available to accept an emergency transfer.[19]

Similarly, if a hospital is not closed to its local EMS system, it may not be at capacity under EMTALA. Trauma centers may be an exception, and may keep beds or operating suites available for acute trauma patients while declining to accept transfers of trauma patients who are in-patients or who could be managed at other area facilities. The goal is to remain available to meet the immediate trauma needs of the community.

Appropriate Transfers

Hospitals only have to accept "appropriate transfers." If it is not clearly in the patient's best medical interest to be transferred at that time, or to that facility, then the hospital is not required to accept the patient. For example, if the transferring hospital clearly has the staff and resources to handle the patient's problem or if it needs to accomplish partial stabilizing treatment before transferring the patient, then the requested hospital may refuse the transfer. It is appropriate to refuse a multiple trauma patient with a tension pneumothorax until the transferring hospital places a chest tube, assuming the transferring hospital is capable of inserting chest tubes. Generally it is safest to recommend how to manage the patient before transfer while simultaneously accepting the patient, thus avoiding unnecessary delay for appropriate transfers.

Inappropriate reasons to refuse trauma patients in transfer include (1) the patient lacks insurance, (2) the hospital does not participate in the patient's managed care plan, (3) the patient's physician is not on staff at that hospital, (4) the patient received services at a different hospital previously, or (5) physician convenience. Hospitals may also not refuse patients because they are out-of-county, out-of-state (including out of state Medicaid patients), or outside the hospital's defined referral service area. The law does not provide such territorial safe harbors. However, hospitals do not have to accept transfers from facilities outside the United States.[20]

Who Accepts Patients on Behalf of the Hospital?

Hospitals should formally designate, in writing, who may accept or refuse transfers on its behalf. If hospitals allow on-call surgeons to decide whether to accept trauma transfers, the surgeons act as agents of the hospital, not their private practice, and must accept appropriate transfers under EMTALA.[21] Illegal refusals are attributed to the hospital also, so both the hospital and the surgeon would be liable for violating federal law.[7]

Hospitals should consider designating the emergency physician (EP) on duty responsible for accepting trauma transfer requests from other EDs. The emergency staff generally knows what resources and personnel are available to the hospital at any given time and have experience arranging such transfers. Also, patients may be advertised to need a certain sub-specialist, when in fact they need a different sub-specialist. The EP can speak to the transferring physician, or evaluate the patient first, then timely assemble the appropriate on-call specialists and other hospital personnel and resources needed to manage the patient's condition.

Managed Care Considerations

Hospitals must accept unstable patients in transfer even if the patient's insurance or managed care plan will not authorize payment for care at that facility.[22] Refusals of unstable transfers on the basis of the patient's insurance status are illegal.[19]

Furthermore, a receiving hospital cannot ask a transferring hospital to delay the transfer until it obtains authorization from the MCO for payment at the receiving hospital. Delaying the transfer of unstable patients to obtain payment authorization is also illegal.[23]

Mandatory Reporting of EMTALA Transfer Violations

A hospital that has reason to believe it received a patient transferred in an unstable condition, in violation of EMTALA, must report the transferring hospital to HCFA.[24] The duty to report rests with the hospital, so EPs or surgeons who receive unstable transfers should inform the hospital's legal counsel, who can then determine the appropriate action.

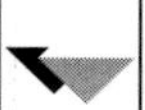

PEARLS & PITFALLS

- Determine the need for transfer *early* after a patient's arrival.
  - Consider the use of a trauma score, clinical presentation, serum markers of shock (lactate or base deficit), Glasgow Coma Scale score, and underlying medical disease in this decision.
- Order only those tests necessary to effect transfer.
- "Package" the patient for transport before arrival of transport services.
  - Secure the airway, treat pneumothorax, establish intravenous access, and immobilize the spine.
- Use a pneumatic anti-shock garment or even a sheet tightly wrapped around the pelvis to treat unstable pelvic fractures.

- Referring Physicians:
  - Contact trauma center.
  - Fill out EMTALA paperwork and send required documents.
  - Use a checklist to avoid mistakes.
- Receiving Physicians:
  - Just say "Yes."

REFERENCES

1. 42 USC 1395dd, The Emergency Medical Treatment and Active Labor Act (EMTALA, a.k.a. COBRA).
2. 42 USC 1395cc(a)(1)(I)(i).
3. Joint Commission on Accreditation of Healthcare Organizations (JCAHO): Emergency Services Standard ER.5.1.2.6, 1998.
4. E.g., California Health & Safety Code Section 1317.5 (West 1990).
5. 5.42 USC 1395dd(c)(1).
6. 42 USC 1395dd(c)(1)(A)(ii).
7. Bitterman, RA: EMTALA. In Henry GL, Sullivan DJ, (editors): *Emergency medicine risk management: a comprehensive review,* ed 2, Chicago, 1997, American College of Emergency Physicians.
8. 42 USC 1395dd(c)(1)(A)(iii).
9. Siegel DM: Consent and refusal of treatment, *Emerg Med Clin North Am,* 11:833-840, 1993.
10. 42 USC 1395dd(c)(2).11.
11. 42 USC 1395dd(b)(1)(B).
12. 42 USC 1395dd(c)(2)(C); 42 CFR 489.24.
13. E.g., Texas Dep't. Health, Hospital Licensing Regulations, Ch. 11, Section 2.10; N.Y. Comp. Codes R. and Regs. Title 4, Section 405.22(j)(2)(i).
14. American College of Surgeons: *Resources for optimal care of the injured patient,* 62, 1990.
15. 42 USC 1395cc(a)(1)(I)(ii); 42 CFR 482.20(r)(1).
16. 1395dd(b)(3); 42 CFR 489.24(c)(2).
17. 42 USC 1395dd(g).
18. 42 CFR 489.24(b).
19. Frew SA, Clarifications, examples of how hospitals can violate COBRA, *Med Malprac Law Strategy* 1:5, 1994.
20. 59 Fed. Reg. 32,105 (1994).
21. 42 USC 1395cc(a)(1)(I)(iii).
22. 59 Fed. Reg. 32,116 (1994).
23. 42 USC 1395dd(h).
24. 42 CFR 489.20(m).

46 Cost-Effective Trauma Care

ANDREW W. ASIMOS

The annual expenditure for acute trauma care in the United States exceeds $16 billion per year.[1] When the indirect costs associated with disability, lost wages, and deaths are added to the direct medical costs, the annual toll escalates to over $150 billion.[2] Although emergency department (ED) diagnostic testing comprises only a fraction of this sum, in aggregate these costs remain staggering, with level I trauma centers spending an estimated $172 million annually for routine laboratory testing alone.[3]

Certain characteristics of trauma patients encourage liberal utilization of both laboratory and radiographic testing. Foremost is alcohol intoxication, which compromises both the history and physical examination. Even in the cooperative patient, a distracting injury or discomfort from a rigid backboard can obscure the clinical picture, making it difficult to identify the need for a radiograph.

Many of the initial tests performed on a trauma patient are routine or "standing orders."[3] Advocates of routine panels believe that they foster consistency in patient care, legitimize verbal orders, and achieve the best outcome.[4] The typical "trauma panel" consists of some constellation of the studies listed in Table 46-1.

Before addressing details of "cost-effective" testing, the term must be defined. Cost effectiveness attempts to minimize costs while at the same time achieving a desired outcome, such as independent living. In the multiply-injured trauma patient, cost effectiveness represents a particular challenge, since undesired outcomes include significant morbidity or mortality. Some medical economics experts advocate formal calculation of cost effectiveness ratios, such as the "cost per year of life gained" or "cost per patient encounter" for given tests. However, in the trauma literature such formal analyses are extremely rare. Even when these more rigorous studies are attempted, the accounting models used are often woefully incomplete, making interpretation treacherous.[5-8] An example of conflicting interpretations is represented by two studies on aortic rupture. One analysis determined that computed tomography (CT) was the most cost-effective strategy for diagnosing aortic rupture in a patient with multisystem injury and a high probability of rupture.[9] Conversely, another study concluded that aortography is the most cost-effective screening tool for patients with blunt chest trauma.[10] Such divergent conclusions dramatize the fact that minor assumptions critically alter cost-effectiveness analysis. Even more difficult to interpret are alleged cost-effective studies that use charges as a proxy for economic costs. The hospital charge for a particular test may bear little relationship to actual cost.

Any rigorous cost study must answer the fundamental question: What test(s) and what results will change a trauma patient's management or outcome? Unfortunately, few well-designed prospective studies have tackled this question. Although most experts consider clinical outcome to be the most powerful demonstration of test utility, this endpoint can be difficult to establish. Because multiple factors influence the outcomes, it is difficult to correlate the impact of a single test or panel obtained early in a patient's course. For example, consider the difficulty in determining the impact of a specific test in the context of dozens of diagnostic studies. The analysis is compounded when decisions based on that test are delayed. Lastly, there is the philosophic question as to the value of a diagnostic test that only increases a physician's certainty but does not change interventions. Such nuances illustrate the challenge of cost-effective analysis.

Despite these concerns, this chapter makes evidence-based recommendations on cost-effective testing, and suggests ways to promote appropriate use of basic laboratory and radiographic diagnostic tests during the ED evaluation of major trauma patients.

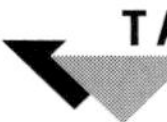

TABLE 46-1
Laboratory Components of Routine Testing Panels for Trauma Patients

DIAGNOSTIC TEST	FREQUENCY IN PANEL
Complete blood count (CBC)	88%
Electrolytes	89%
BUN	89%
Creatinine	89%
Glucose	89%
Amylase	72%
Prothrombin (PT)	81%
Partial thromboplastin time (PTT)	81%
Blood type & screen (T&S) or type & crossmatch (T&C)	90%
Urinalysis (UA)	83%
Ethanol level	80%
Toxicology screen	54%
Arterial blood gas (ABG)	54%
Lactate	Not available

Adapted from Burton JH, Wolfson AB, Rockoff S: *Acad Emerg Med* 2:408, 1995.

LABORATORY EVALUATION

Complete Blood Count

The complete blood count (CBC) is undoubtedly among the most frequently ordered laboratory tests for ED patients. Nonetheless, in the acute management of trauma data suggest that the CBC rarely affects resuscitation or operative management.[11,12] Although the hemoglobin or hematocrit level is of primary interest, its impact on patient management, including emergent blood transfusion, is questionable.[13] A low hemoglobin level observed after injury is usually an indicator of serious ongoing hemorrhage, but it is an insensitive marker for acute blood loss.[14] Beyond the hemoglobin or hematocrit, the only other component of the CBC of demonstrated utility in acute trauma is the platelet count for severely head injured patients.[13] The white blood cell level has no relation to intraabdominal injury in trauma patients[13] and cannot predict the severity or specific nature of injury.[15] Although it is frequently elevated in trauma, it is neither sensitive nor specific for diagnosis or prognosis.

Based on these observations, most experts agree that a baseline hemoglobin or hematocrit is the only component of a CBC that should be routinely obtained in all major trauma patients. However, patients with major head trauma may benefit from a platelet count as well. The baseline hemoglobin or hematocrit can provide a useful starting point for patients thought or known to have ongoing hemorrhage. Additionally, a surprisingly low level will occasionally alert the emergency physician (EP) or surgeon to occult hemorrhage.

Electrolyte Panels

The other ubiquitous ED laboratory test is the electrolyte panel. Several investigators have evaluated the utility of a standard electrolyte panel in the management of trauma victims.[12,13,16-18] The potassium (K^+) level is considered to be among the most clinically important electrolytes; nonetheless, there have been no convincing studies that demonstrate its utility. Although hypokalemia is the most commonly cited potassium abnormality, many referenced studies addressing this topic have been retrospective. Most patients with hypokalemia were not treated, and suffered no significant sequelae. Interestingly, one study found hypokalemia to be more prevalent in hypotensive patients, those with an Injury Severity Score (ISS) ≥9, and those requiring emergent surgery; however, the clinical significance of this finding is unclear.[13]

The glucose value is of frequent interest in trauma patients; however, a bedside glucose-measuring device exists in virtually every ED. The use of such a device, versus a multichannel analyzer, is certainly appropriate to exclude profound hypoglycemia or hyperglycemia in the trauma patient. Because hypoglycemia can masquerade as mental status changes from head trauma, the bedside measurement of glucose is prudent in any victim of multiple trauma with altered consciousness. Although drivers with diabetes suffer accidents during an insulin reaction, the comatose victim is unlikely to give this history. The EP faced with a trauma patient with altered mental status is likely to concentrate on obtaining a CT scan. When hypoglycemia is finally recognized in trauma patients, glucose administration may be too late. Nothing is quite so embarrassing as rushing to the CT scanner to administer an amp of D_{50}.

Two groups conducted regression analyses and identified historical or physical criteria associated with clinically significant abnormal electrolyte values.[17,18] Those criteria are compiled in Box 46-1. Although some of these criteria were derived from and prospectively validated with medical patients, if any of these criteria apply to a major trauma victim, electrolytes seem justified. However, beyond extreme glucose or K^+ abnormalities, it is unlikely that other electrolyte values affect the ED evaluation of the trauma patient.

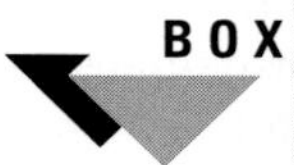

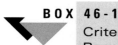

BOX 46-1
Criteria for Ordering Electrolyte Panels in Trauma Patients

- Hypertension
- Age >50
- Glasgow Coma Scale score of ≤10
- Vomiting
- Taking diuretic medication
- Recent seizure
- Muscle weakness
- Alcoholism
- Abnormal mental status
- Recent history of electrolyte abnormality
- History of renal failure (Dialysis patient)

Adapted from Tortella BJ, Lavery RF, Rekant M: *Acad Emerg Med* 2:190-194, 1995.

Indices of Renal Function

One reason patients undergo testing of renal function is because the radiologists want to know. Trauma patients frequently undergo emergent radiographic examinations, including CT scanning and angiography, which require the administration of contrast media. Since chronic renal insufficiency is a major risk factor for acute contrast-mediated kidney disease, measurement of serum creatinine, and to a lesser extent blood urea nitrogen (BUN), is routine. Fortunately, the incidence of clinically overt acute renal failure is rare, with an estimated occurrence in 0.15% of contrast media administrations.[19] Nonetheless, knowledge of a patient's creatinine level before contrast media administration seems ideal in patients at risk for renal insufficiency. These risk factors are listed in Box 46-2.[20] Since factors are cumulative, a creatinine or a BUN measurement may be useful in such patients. Alternatively, modalities such as ultrasound or the use of low osmolar contrast should be considered in the presence of borderline renal function.

Although these recommendations *seem* reasonable, there is little empiric evidence for measurement of renal function in the trauma patient. One study identified 10 trauma patients with elevated BUN or creatinine levels, including 6 patients with prior chronic renal failure, hypertension, or diabetes mellitus.[13] All four patients with elevated BUN or creatinine levels without premorbid renal dysfunction were hypotensive on arrival, but had return to normal renal function, including two who received intravenous (IV) contrast for "one-shot" pyelography. These limited data question the need to test renal function, even if contrast material is needed.

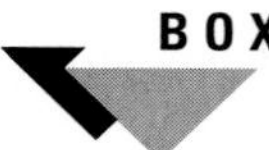

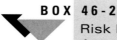

BOX 46-2
Risk Factors for Developing Acute Contrast Media-Induced Renal Insufficiency

MAJOR
- Chronic renal insufficiency (serum creatinine >1.5 mg/dl)
- Diabetes mellitus with renal insufficiency
- Dehydration

MINOR
- Multiple myeloma
- Age >70 years
- Hypertension
- Cardiac disease
- Long-term use of diuretics
- Large contrast media dose
- Repeated contrast media exposure within 72 hours

From Cochran ST: *JAMA* 277:517-518, 1997.

Coagulation Profiles

Coagulation studies are important for patients with severe head trauma, because they are at risk for rapid development of disseminated intravascular coagulation (DIC). One study showed that 67% of patients with a Glasgow Coma Scale (GCS) score of <8 had a low platelet count or prolonged PT/PTT, with abnormalities proportional to the severity of the head injury.[13] Another study found that either one or both of PT and PTT were abnormal in 59% of trauma patients studied, of whom 5% were given fresh frozen plasma.[16] Abnormal PT and PTT were associated with each of a low SBP (<90 mmHg), RR (<10/minute) and GCS (<12). Based on these combined findings, proposed criteria for measuring coagulation indices are listed in Box 46-3. In addition, patients who need intracranial pressure monitors will also need coagulation studies; the monitor should not be placed until a coagulopathy has been corrected.

Amylase

Because there are several sources of amylase in the body, most importantly the pancreas and salivary glands, the presence of an elevated amylase is nonspecific. Several studies have evaluated the value of serum amylase in suspected intraabdominal injury.[13,16,21-24] All studies have found low sensitivity, specificity, and predictive value, regardless of associated craniofacial trauma. Isoenzymes of amylase fare no better. One study concluded that although hyper-

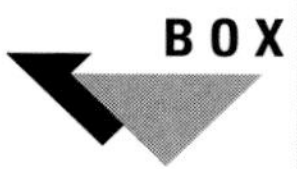

BOX 46-3
Criteria for Performing Coagulation Studies

PLATELET COUNT
- GCS ≤8

PT/PTT
- Systolic blood pressure <90 mmHg
- Respiratory rate <10/minute
- Glasgow Coma Scale score <12
- Suspected liver disease
- Recent or current use of heparin or warfarin
- Patients who will need intracranial pressure monitors

Adapted from Frankel HL, et al: *J Trauma* 37:728-736, 1994, and Namias N, McKenney MG, Martin LC: *J Trauma* 41:21-25, 1996.

amylasemia was found in 7% of trauma patients, it did not correlate with intervention.[16] The overwhelming data indicate that serum amylase should *not* be used as a screening test in the multiple-trauma patient.

Blood Bank Testing

Many consider the most important blood test in a trauma patient to be a type and crossmatch (T&C). However, blood bank testing represents perhaps the least cost-effective area in trauma patients. This lack of cost effectiveness is due to a poor understanding of blood compatibility tests, along with the minimal likelihood of serious transfusion reactions by using abbreviated compatibility testing. Multiple factors have fostered liberal utilization of blood bank testing. Some physicians falsely believe that converting a type and screen (T&S) to a type and crossmatch (T&C) usually takes longer than 10 minutes. In addition, the ATLS manual recommends that blood should be sent for a type and screen in the hemodynamically normal patient.[25] This recommendation is not supported by the medical literature.

A T&S is more likely to conserve a hospital's blood supply than a T&C, which increases the rate of blood wastage.[26] When a crossmatch is performed, the units are reserved for an individual patient for up to 2 days and are taken out of the available blood pool.

Several retrospective studies of ED transfusions in trauma patients have been conducted. One study concluded the best predictor of blood use was the trauma score (TS).[27] Seventy percent of patients with a TS of <14 required a transfusion. This study was performed before the development of the Revised Trauma Score (RTS)[28] and no one has evaluated the association between the RTS and blood usage. Another retrospective review of not only trauma victims, but all types of patients, concluded that any one of four criteria predicted transfusion:[29]

- Shock (defined as SBP <90 mmHg or SBP <100 mmHg and pulse >120 beats per minute ([bpm], unless a tilt test was negative **OR** SBP <110 mmHg with a pulse >140 bpm, unless the tilt test was negative **OR** a positive tilt test)
- Hematocrit <30%
- Observed blood loss of at least 500 cc or grossly visible gastrointestinal bleeding
- Emergency operation with anticipated blood loss

However, there has been no prospective validation of these criteria. Another retrospective study found that significantly more trauma victims with a prehospital SBP <100 mmHg required transfusion.[30] Although this criterion was prospectively evaluated, it failed to identify 7% of patients who received blood. Nonetheless, it concluded that prehospital blood pressure is a useful adjunct to clinical judgment in determining the need for crossmatch. Another study linked base deficit (BD) to blood transfusion and concluded that patients with a BD more negative that –6 should undergo a T&C versus a T&S.[31] In this series, 72% of patients with a BD more negative than –6 versus only 16% of patients with BD more positive than –6 received transfusions within 24 hours of admission. However, this study has several methodological flaws.[32] Finally, another group concluded that only 8.5% of trauma patients required a blood transfusion within 48 hours of admission, 90% of whom received uncrossmatched blood emergently during resuscitation.[13] This group suggested that a T&S should not be routine in trauma patients. It is notable that none of these guidelines have met widespread use.

A main priority in hypotensive trauma patients should be to ensure the availability of type-specific blood as soon as possible.[25,33] Beyond ABO/Rh typing, the likelihood of blood transfusion needs to be considered, along with its urgency and the time required by the blood bank to perform a T&S and convert it to a T&C. Although several criteria for performing a T&C have been suggested, none have been adequately prospectively validated or adopted. Given the remote likelihood of a serious transfusion reaction with blood that is compatible based on the T&S and realizing that a screen can be converted to a crossmatch usually within 10 minutes, a T&S will suffice in most trauma scenarios.

For similar reasons, the EP can usually order only two crossmatched units at a time. That blood can be infusing while the blood bank crosses the next two units. However, patients who have massive hemorrhage may benefit from a cross match of 4 to 6 units at a time.

Urinalysis

BLUNT TRAUMA

Adults. Several prospective and retrospective studies have investigated the utility of urinalysis after blunt trauma.[34-39] *All studies conclude that radiographic evaluation is warranted in adult blunt trauma patients with gross hematuria or in patients with the combination of microscopic hematuria and shock.* Adult blunt trauma victims without shock (<90 mmHg) do not require dipstick or microscopic examination of their urine. A visual examination of the urine for gross blood is adequate to rule out surgical injury in such patients. Although adult patients with microscopic hematuria and no shock may have a renal contusion, they will not require intervention.

Children. In children, however, the threshold to search for a genitourinary injury should be lower. Based on review of the literature, children sustaining blunt trauma with >50 red blood cells per high power field should be evaluated by a renal imaging study.[40,41] Curiously, the finding of hematuria in a child is most closely associated with splenic injury than with demonstrable kidney trauma (see Chapter 33).

PENETRATING TRAUMA

No combination of urinary parameters can predict a severe injury in patients with penetrating renal trauma. All such patients require urinalysis if the bullet or knife wound is in proximity to the urinary tract. Microscopy may be more sensitive to small amounts of blood than dipstick, but the assertion that microscopy is favored over dipstick analysis has not been subject to scientific scrutiny.

Urine Pregnancy Tests

Some centers test for pregnancy in all female trauma victims of childbearing potential. A positive test may influence the choice of further diagnostic studies and medications. It should also prompt shielding of the abdomen where possible when radiographs are ordered.

At least 2% of female trauma victims of childbearing age have unrecognized pregnancy.[42] Furthermore, a woman's history regarding last menstrual period, birth control use, or even sexual activity are unreliable when determining the possibility of pregnancy.[43] In one unusual case a comatose woman with head trauma was found to have an ectopic pregnancy.[44]

Ethanol Level

The link between alcohol (ETOH) use and trauma is well-established, and almost half of all trauma patients admitted to hospitals have detectable ethanol in their blood.[45,46] This finding begs the question "What use are alcohol levels to the EP?" Although "legal" blood draws are important for prosecution of drunk drivers, measurement of ETOH has no clear role in the acute management of trauma.

POSSIBLE ROLES OF ALCOHOL LEVELS IN THE EMERGENCY DEPARTMENT

Evaluation of Head Trauma. Possible benefits include a more aggressive search for brain injury in intoxicated patients with altered mental status if their blood alcohol level is relatively low. A bedside Breathalyzer provides rapid information in such a case; however, the reliability of this device is dependent on the patient's ability to forcefully exhale.

Substance Abuse Intervention. A broader question regarding the routine measurement of blood alcohol content (BAC) in trauma patients entails the use of the ETOH level to identify patients with drinking problems. Such patients could be targeted for rehabilitation programs.[47] A substance abuse consultation team may enroll 60% of hospitalized trauma patients with substance abuse disorders into alcohol treatment programs.[48] Unfortunately, long-term outcome data are lacking. If such interventions decrease recidivism of alcohol abuse, such counseling would likely be cost effective to society. However, one study suggests that BAC testing within 6 hours of injury does not identify patients with current alcohol abuse or dependence.[49] Conversely, another study of motor vehicle collision patients showed that an elevated ETOH level (≥100 mg/dl) was associated with having been stopped for drinking, having a restricted license, having a "driving while intoxicated" arrest, using illegal drugs, and having a previous admission to the hospital.[50]

ALCOHOL TESTING AND TRAUMA CENTERS

Based on the prevalence of ETOH use by trauma victims, the American College of Surgeons' Committee on Trauma recommends routine a BAC in trauma patients.[25] However, a survey indicated that despite available resources, only 64% of level I and 48% of level II trauma centers routinely perform BAC testing on trauma patients.[51] The primary explanation for omitting a BAC was that it was considered "clinically not important." Those who advocate routine testing believe it aids in anesthetic management of pain, predicts withdrawal, and explains altered sensorium. No data, however, have demonstrated benefits of a BAC in the management of these scenarios. In trauma patients with an ISS of 1 to 15, alcohol intoxication has been associated with an increased rate of endotracheal intubation, diagnostic peritoneal lavage, and head CT scanning.[52] One group has suggested a simple demographic model that could be used to decide whether or not to test for ethanol based on a high probability that a given patient would test positive for alcohol.[53] The predictive model uses attributes, such as sex, age, race, injury type (intentional versus unintentional), and time of injury (night versus day and weekend versus weekday), to characterize patients as being at low-, medium-, or high-risk for having a BAC ≥50 mg/dl. Such a model may represent a cost-effective screen for more selective ordering of a BAC if it is ultimately demonstrated that knowledge of the ETOH level contributes to management.

BOTTOM LINE

Based on the prevailing data, it is unclear as to the value of a BAC measurement in both the initial management of trauma patients and in contributing to the rehabilitation. If routine testing is performed, consider using a bedside Breathalyzer. Although formal cost-effectiveness analyses of such devices versus a centralized lab are lacking, the acquisition and reusable costs associated with these devices are minimal.[54]

Toxicology Screen

Many of the issues that apply to BAC testing apply to toxicology screens in the trauma patient. Less than half of all level I and level II trauma centers routinely perform drug screens on trauma patients, despite the ACS Trauma Committee's recommendations.[51] It is of no surprise that the primary reason cited was that they are "clinically not important." Those in support of routine screening argue that, similar to routine ETOH screening, toxicology screens are important for epidemiologic reasons and for substance abuse intervention. However, no data suggests an increased rate of successful substance abuse intervention with routine toxicology screening. From an ED perspective, toxicology screens cannot predict overall ISS or the need for an emergent airway, laparotomy, or a neurosurgical procedure.[55] Nonetheless, some authorities suggest that the directed use of such testing is warranted, because the finding of negative levels in a lethargic or comatose trauma patient prompts the more rapid investigation of neurosurgical etiologies of altered mental status. However, no data demonstrates that routine toxicology testing is cost effective.

Arterial Blood Gas and Lactate

The arterial blood gas (ABG), in particular the pH and base deficit (BD), has been extensively investigated to determine its association with both initial patient management and outcome. Several studies suggest that pH and BD results are important for guiding resuscitation or indicating ongoing blood loss.[56-61] Two base deficit thresholds are markers for significant risk of mortality: (1) >15 mmol/l in a patient <55 years of age without a head injury, (2) >8 mmol/l in elderly patients (>55 years) without a head injury or a young patient with a head injury.[59] Based on such findings, it is recommended that BD be used to guide resuscitation and prompt early invasive monitoring in trauma patients. In addition to aiding in management decisions, BD can also be of diagnostic benefit. A study concluded that a BD more negative than −6 has greater predictive value for indicating intraabdominal injuries requiring surgical repair than the presence of hypotension or chest or pelvis injuries.[62] Another prospective study evaluated the contribution of routine laboratory, radiographic findings and electrocardiographic data to the anesthetic management of trauma patients. The authors concluded that only the ABG gave information additional to that obtained by the clinical examination.[11]

It is ironic that serum lactate, which is not routinely obtained in most trauma panels, is one of the most useful tests in the acute management of trauma patients. The association between serum lactate levels and hypovolemic shock has been well documented for several years,[63-66] and, as with ABG parameters, admission lactate level correlates with outcome in a number of studies.[57,60,67-71] A retrospective study shows that lactate level predicts blood and fluid needs in trauma patients.[72] Finally, admission lactate is a better triage tool than standard triage criteria over a wide range of ISS scores.[73]

Because published data suggests ABG parameters and lactate levels help guide resuscitation and outcome projections, their inclusion in a "standard" major trauma panel may be justified, particularly if results are rapidly available. However, prospective studies are needed to determine whether their routine use is cost effective.

Point-of-Care Testing

Point-of-care testing represents the latest phenomenon of laboratory testing. It refers to any testing performed outside the hospital's main laboratory. Many of the diagnostic tests discussed thus far are available on POCT analyzers, which afford nearly instant results compared with an institution's centralized lab. In general, POCT is more expensive than centralized lab testing.[74-79] Despite this increased cost-per-test, proponents of POCT emphasize having results available sooner ultimately decreases overall patient care costs. They opine that earlier and more accurate diagnoses reduce morbidity, decrease overall testing, and shorten the length of stay.

One study of a POCT panel in trauma patients, which included a hematocrit, electrolyte, and ABG parameters, concluded that the sheer number of abnormal values warranted measurement. However, it is unclear how abnormal values obtained via POCT affected patients' management.[13] Furthermore, in cases where management was changed on the basis of abnormal values (e.g., treating hypokalemia), no comparison was made between the outcomes of patients who were treated versus those who were not. Finally, although it has been argued that the POCT laboratory values measured are of special interest in the most critically injured, their impact on management is debatable.[11]

Because of their ability to rapidly provide results, POCT analyzers have considerable potential in the evaluation of trauma patients. If the POCT analyzer improves outcome or patient management, it may be cost effective, despite increased cost per test compared with traditional centralized testing.

PEDIATRIC DIAGNOSTIC TESTING

Most cost-effective studies regarding diagnostic testing in pediatric trauma mirror results of adult investigations. One exception involves the contribution of the urinalysis (UA).[80-82] Virtually all children sustaining blunt trauma should undergo microscopic urinalysis, since the finding of >50 red blood cells per high power field should prompt an investigation for a clinically significant renal injury.[40,41] Another study advocates adding a hemoglobin or hematocrit and a T&S to a routine testing panel for pediatric trauma patients.[82] However, as in adults, most children who undergo crossmatch are never transfused. One group demonstrated that transfusions are uncommon in children with a Pediatric Trauma Score of >7.[83] In summary, the prevailing data suggest that for pediatric blunt trauma patients, hemoglobin or hematocrit and a urinalysis are the only diagnostic tests that are routinely cost effective.[81,84]

ELECTROCARDIOGRAMS

The electrocardiogram (ECG) in trauma patients is most useful to detect a *clinically significant* myocardial contusion or more rarely a myocardial infarction. Myocardial contusion is complicated by the lack of a consistent "gold standard" for diagnosing this entity. However, the initial ECG is an important predictor for complications of myocardial contusion.[85-91]

Commonly associated ECG findings include premature ventricular contractions, unexplained sinus tachycardia, atrial fibrillation, bundle branch block (usually right), and ST segment changes.[25] Some studies have shown that a normal initial ECG does not preclude significant delayed dysrhythmias,[87,90] whereas others suggest that an abnormal ECG does not guarantee subsequent cardiac complications.[92] Despite these controversies, further diagnostic evaluation for myocardial contusion in blunt trauma patients should be reserved for those patients with demonstrable dysrhythmias and hemodynamic compromise.[93]

The ECG may be valuable when the trauma was preceded by syncope or chest pain; however, the contribution of routine ECGs in trauma patients is unknown. Certainly, a dysrhythmia or a myocardial infarction can precipitate a motor vehicle crash. Suspect cardiac precipitants of trauma in the elderly, particularly if it is a one-vehicle incident. One study found that 86% of ECGs in trauma patients were normal, but the study did not correlate treatment, outcome, injuries, or examination with the ECGs.[12] For medical patients, a retrospective evaluation of predetermined criteria has outlined criteria for obtaining an admission ECG.[94] Those criteria are listed in Box 46-4, but it must be emphasized that they were not developed for, nor prospectively applied to, trauma patients. Nonetheless, these criteria represent reasonable guidelines for determining in which trauma patients to perform an

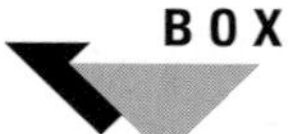

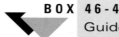

BOX 46-4
Guidelines for Performing an ECG In Trauma Patients

- Suspected myocardial contusion
- History of coronary artery disease, dysrhythmia, congestive heart failure (CHF), conduction disturbance, cor pulmonale, pericarditis, or cardiomyopathy
- Palpitations
- Syncope or coma
- Symptom complex suggestive of angina or CHF
- Suspected cardiotoxic overdose
- Irregular pulse
- Pulse >120 or <60 beats per minute
- Systolic blood pressure >200 or <90 mmHg or diastolic blood pressure >120
- Serum K^+ >5.7 or <3

Adapted from Garland JL, Wolfson AB: *Ann Emerg Med* 23:275-280, 1994.

ECG. In general, many trauma centers obtain an ECG on seriously injured patients over the age of 50, as well as those with chest pain, significant chest trauma, or syncope.

RADIOGRAPHIC EVALUATION

Cervical Spine

Perhaps no area of diagnostic testing for trauma victims has received as much attention as that of cervical spine (C-spine) radiography. To complicate the issue, there is even controversy regarding what constitutes an adequate C-spine radiographic series. Although it is recognized that a majority of patients who even present with the symptoms of C-spine pain or tenderness will not have serious cervicospinal injuries, the sequelae associated with missing a serious injury have fostered a conservative approach.[95] Furthermore, none of the studies conducted thus far suggesting a more liberal policy have had a sufficient number of injuries to achieve an acceptable statistical power. Finally, the use of different "gold standards" among studies, along with interpretation of radiographs by a range of specialists, make the interpretation of the literature challenging.

The first cost-effective hurdle of C-spine radiography concerns who needs radiography. Institutions and individual physicians vary considerably when ordering C-spine radiography, even in alert and stable trauma patients.[96] A Musculoskeletal Task Force convened by the American College of Radiology unanimously agreed that asymptomatic, alert patients with normal physical examinations did not require radiographs.[97] In the recently published National Emergency X-Radiography Utilization Study (NEXUS) the following criteria were prospectively validated in a cohort of 27,389 low-risk patients at 22 academic and nonacademic emergency departments:[98]

- Midline cervical tenderness on palpation
- Altered mental status because of CHI, intoxication, or metabolic derangement
- Neurologic deficits
- Distracting injuries considered severe enough to "distract" patients from cervical spine pain or tenderness.

Using these criteria, only 15 fractures (0.05%) were missed, of which 1 (0.004%) required surgical intervention; none of the injuries were unstable. These criteria have been corroborated in several smaller studies.[99-103] Other data suggests that neck pain or neurologic signs or symptoms also predict C-spine injury.[102,104,105]

The ATLS Manual states that "patients with maxillofacial or head trauma should be presumed to have an unstable cervical spine injury, and such injury should be presumed until a complete cervical spine radiographic series is reviewed."[25] This presumption is unsupported by scientific evidence. Even in the presence of blunt head trauma, the C-spine can be cleared clinically if the patient is alert, sober, and without distracting injuries.[106-108] Many retrospective studies fail to establish a special relationship between facial and C-spine injury.[109-115] However, several pediatric studies have concluded that any neck pain in the setting of trauma warrants radiographs.[116-118]

The second hurdle is to determine what constitutes the "complete" C-spine series. Opinions on the minimal number of plain radiographs necessary to evaluate the C-spine in trauma patients range from two films (anteroposterior [AP] and lateral; lateral and odontoid) to seven (lateral, odontoid, AP, obliques, flexion, and extension views). Although no randomized controlled trial exits, the literature suggests the following points:

1. *It is never appropriate to "clear the C-spine" based on a lateral view alone.* A lateral view, with visualization of C7-T1, cannot detect all significant fractures, dislocations, or subluxations. Since the mid 1980s, it has been recognized that up to 25% of fractures can be missed on the lateral view, particularly those at the upper and lower extremes of the C-spine.[104,119-121] Although most undetected fractures on the lateral will be identified with the addition of an odontoid view,[121,122] most groups advocate adding the AP to comprise a "three-view series," with inclusion of the swimmer's view as needed to visualize the C7-T1 region.[95,123] However, there is data to suggest that the AP view is not routinely necessary for initial C-spine clearance.[124]
2. *The value of CT in visualizing the cervico-thoracic junction.* Regarding adequate visualization of the C7 and T1 region, new methods in digital radiography may improve the ability to clear the lateral view. These methods should ultimately decrease the number of films or views required in some cases and over time may decrease the cost of clearing the CS.[125] Until such technology becomes more readily available, CT may be more cost-effective than repeated and inadequate plain radiographs.[126]
3. *The choice of a three-view versus five-view series appears to be a matter of local preference.* Routine oblique views are advocated by some to identify posterior laminar fractures, pedicle fractures, unilateral facet dislocations, and subluxation.[127-129] However, others conclude that oblique views rarely (1 out of 100), if ever, delineate additional significant abnormalities not seen on the three-view series.[130,131] After a review of the literature, a task force from the American College of Radiology was unable to reach consensus on the appropriateness of routine

oblique views.[97] The C-spine radiographic series controversy expands with the issue of flexion-extension views. These views are endorsed by some to investigate suspected laxity suggested by the standard views or in all patients with considerable neck pain, but an unremarkable initial standard C-spine series.[132] Ultimately, until a large series with sufficient statistical power is completed, the question of what views comprise the most cost-effective C-spine series remains unresolved. A three-view series consisting of lateral, open-mouth, and AP views are an accepted minimum.

Chest Radiograph

The ATLS manual states "a chest x-ray should be obtained on all patients who have sustained torso trauma (blunt or penetrating) and who are unconscious, going to the operating room, and/or are in respiratory distress."[25] Yet there are no evidence-based criteria that direct the cost-effective use of chest radiography. Despite the lack of randomized controlled trials (RCTs) addressing this issue, most authorities consider the chest radiograph (CXR) the single most important film used to evaluate the victim of trauma. It is inarguably the most frequent.

Consider the diagnostic limitations of supine AP CXRs when choosing the chest film technique. Both hemothorax and pneumothorax, undetectable on a supine film, may appear on the upright view.[133] For this reason, consider an erect film as the initial CXR in hemodynamically stable patients who sustain penetrating trauma to the chest. Although supine chest radiography remains the first line radiographic study of choice for almost all multiply-injured blunt trauma patients, this view may falsely suggest aortic injury, caused by physiologic widening of the mediastinum.[9,134] An upright film taken in full inspiration reveals a normal mediastinum in most of these patients.[135]

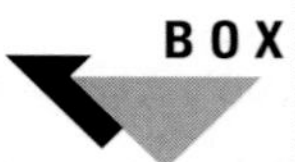

BOX 46-5

Criteria for Obtaining Thoracolumbar Radiographs

- Back pain and tenderness
- Fall of ≥10 feet
- Ejection from a motorcycle
- Motor vehicle crash of >50 miles per hour
- Deformity or neurologic deficits referable to the thoracolumbar spine
- Major distracting injuries (including cervical spine fractures)
- Injury severity score >15

Thoracolumbar Radiographs

Although ATLS guidelines recommend AP and lateral screening views of the thoracic and lumbar spine in patients sustaining significant trauma,[25] the scientific evidence in this area does not support such a liberal policy.[136] Several groups describe criteria for surveillance thoracic and lumbar radiographs (Box 46-5).[137-139] Unfortunately, these criteria remain to be validated.

Pelvis Radiograph

Many studies conclude that routine pelvis radiographs are not indicated in awake patients without pelvic pain or a suspicious physical examination.[140-143] This approach contradicts the unreferenced ATLS manual's recommendation that "a pelvic x-ray should be obtained on all patients who sustain blunt trauma to the torso."[25] Several prospective studies evaluated a total of 1614 awake blunt trauma patients and found 111 pelvic fractures. Only five fractures were missed in the absence of pelvic pain or positive physical examination findings, none of which required intervention. The evidence supports the dictum that pelvis films should be reserved for patients who meet the criteria listed in Box 46-6.

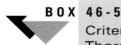

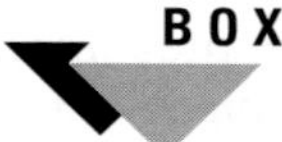

BOX 46-6

Criteria for Performing a Pelvis Radiograph in Blunt Trauma Patients

- Hemodynamically unstable
- Physical examination unreliable based on level of consciousness
- Ecchymosis, swelling, laceration (pelvis, perineum, genitalia, sacrum, lower lumbar, medial thigh), blood at urethral meatus, gross hematuria
- Pain with palpation of pubis and iliac spines
- Pain with palpation of sacrum and lower lumbar spine
- Lower extremity sensory or gross motor abnormalities
- Rectal examination with abnormal tone or prostate, or with blood or bony deformity
- Joint pain with external and internal rotation of hips

SPECIAL CIRCUMSTANCES

Wide Mediastinum

Angiography is among the most expensive and invasive diagnostic tests in trauma patients. Although several studies propose that *helical* CT (not static CT) can limit the necessity for aortic angiography,[9,144-147] this position is not universally accepted.[10] Central to this issue of CT versus angiography is the bias of the operating surgeon. If a surgeon will not operate based on the results of CT, all positive studies must be confirmed with angiography. In general, the best evidence shows that a normal helical CT rules out aortic disruption, and has the advantage of imaging other body parts in the multiply-injured patient.

Penetrating Extremity Trauma

Regarding penetrating extremity trauma, two studies suggest that physical signs and duplex sonography can eliminate the need for angiography in most cases.[148,149] A normal ankle-brachial index may obviate the need for further studies (see Chapter 30).

Abdominal Trauma

Although the merits of ultrasonography in the diagnosis of abdominal trauma are discussed elsewhere in this text, a few general comments are warranted. As EPs and trauma surgeons become proficient in trauma ultrasonography, it may begin to replace diagnostic peritoneal lavage (DPL) and CT. Some analyses suggest that abdominal ultrasonography costs the same as DPL and is less than one fourth the cost per test of CT.[150,151] These comparisons, however, depend on important cost assumptions, including equipment, training, and reimbursement.[152] Nonetheless, prevailing evidence suggests that ultrasound will soon be standard in all ED trauma resuscitation rooms. Many authors already promote algorithms that rely on ultrasound to screen for abdominal injury, replacing CT or DPL in most instances.[153-157]

CONCLUSIONS

Because of the heterogeneity of trauma patients, few diagnostic studies should be routine. Before adopting universal cost-effective measures, our specialty must conduct scientifically valid, prospective studies. However, based on the prevailing evidence, we propose a few recommendations (Box 46-7). Although a normal hematocrit or hemoglobin level does not exclude significant hemorrhage, a low value should alert the EP to potential blood loss. For this reason, some early measurement of hemoglobin or hematocrit is valuable in virtually all victims of major trauma. Secondly, several studies suggest that base deficit and/or a lactate level are reliable and early predictors of injury severity and assist in early management of trauma patients. Bedside tests, although more expensive than traditional central lab analysis, may be cost effective. Factors such as age, acuity level, mechanism of injury, premorbid disease, anatomic injury, and hemodynamic stability must be considered in cost-effective decisions.

With regards to radiography, these studies can usually be obtained selectively based on the physical examination. Patients with midline neck tenderness, altered mentation, neurologic deficit, or a severe distracting injury should have cervical radiography (at least a three-view series). When these findings are absent, radiography can be safely deferred. A similar approach can be applied to the thoracolumbar spine. Pelvic radiography can also be obtained selectively, based on the presence or absence of pelvic compression tenderness and/or instability. Chest radiography should be obtained in all patients suffering significant deceleration, even in the absence of external chest trauma, and an upright radiograph can be very useful to define the mediastinum.

Special mention should be made of the blunt trauma patient presenting in shock. In this situation it imperative for the EP to identify potential sites of life-threatening hemorrhage within minutes. A single AP film of the chest and pelvis should be taken as soon as the secondary survey is completed without wasting time to obtain these films using the clinical criteria described earlier. These films will immediately identify major intrathoracic bleeding, and rule out a pelvic ring injury as a source of retroperitoneal hemorrhage.

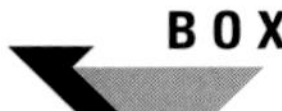

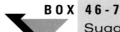

BOX 46-7

Suggested "Standard" Laboratory Studies for Major Trauma Patients

- Hemoglobin or Hematocrit
- Base deficit and/or lactate
- Visual examination of the urine (hemodynamically stable adult patients)
- Dipstick analysis or microscopic examination (children or hemodynamically unstable adults)
- Bedside glucose for altered mental status—even if obvious head trauma
- Pregnancy test for women of childbearing potential

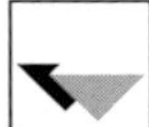

PEARLS & PITFALLS

- Age, acuity level, mechanism of injury, premorbid disease, anatomic injury, and hemodynamic stability must be considered in cost-effective decisions.
- Hemoglobin or hematocrit is valuable in virtually all victims of major trauma.
- Base deficit or lactate levels are reliable and early predictors of injury severity.
- Point-of-care test, although more expensive than traditional central lab analysis, may be cost effective.
- Patients with midline neck tenderness, altered mentation, neurologic deficit, or a severe distracting injury should have cervical radiography. When these findings are absent, radiography can be safely deferred.
- Pelvic radiography can also be obtained selectively based on the presence or absence of pelvic tenderness.
- Chest radiography should be obtained in all patients suffering significant deceleration.

REFERENCES

1. Harlan LC, Harlan WR, Parsons PE: The economic impact of injuries: a major source of medical costs, *Am J Public Health* 80:453-459, 1990.
2. Position Papers for the Third National Injury Control Conference: Setting the national agenda for injury control in the 1990's, *Morb Mortal Wkly Rep* 41(RR-6):1-38, 1992.
3. Burton JH, Wolfson AB, Rockoff S: Routine laboratory testing in emergency department trauma patients at level 1 trauma centers: a national survey, (abstract) *Acad Emerg Med* 2:408, 1995.
4. Myers MB, Norwood SH: Standing orders for trauma care, *J Emerg Nurs* 20:111-117, 1994.
5. Balas EA, et al: Interpreting cost analyses of clinical interventions, *JAMA* 279:54-57, 1998.
6. Keffer JH: Economic considerations of point-of-care testing, *Am J Clin Pathol* 104(suppl 1):S107-S110, 1995.
7. Udvarhelyi IS, et al: Cost-effectiveness and cost-benefit analyses in the medical literature. Are the methods being used correctly? *Ann Intern Med* 116:238-244, 1992.
8. Weinstein MC, Stason WB: Foundations of cost-effectiveness analysis for health and medical practices, *N Engl J Med* 296: 716-721, 1977.
9. Hunink MG, Bos JJ: Triage of patient to angiography for detection of aortic rupture after blunt chest trauma: cost-effectiveness analysis of using CT, *AJR* 165:27-36, 1995.
10. Brasel KJ, Weigelt JA: Blunt thoracic aortic trauma: a cost-utility approach for injury detection, *Arch Surg* 131:619-626, 1996.
11. Roux A, Lourens L, Richards E: Contribution of preoperative investigations to the anaesthetic management of adult trauma patients, *Injury* 24:17-20, 1993.
12. Nelson E, et al: The use of baseline investigations in patients admitted from an accident and emergency department, *Irish Med J* 85:100-102, 1992.
13. Frankel HL, et al: Minimizing admission laboratory testing in trauma patients: use of a microanalyzer, *J Trauma* 37:728-736, 1994.
14. Knottenbelt JD: Low initial hemoglobin levels in trauma patients: an important indicator of ongoing hemorrhage, *J Trauma* 31:1396-1399, 1991.
15. Callaham M: Inaccuracy and expense of the leukocyte count in making urgent clinical decisions, *Ann Emerg Med* 15:774-781, 1986.
16. Namias N, McKenney MG, Martin LC: Utility of admission chemistry and coagulation profiles in trauma patients: a reappraisal of traditional practice, *J Trauma* 41:21-25, 1996.
17. Tortella BJ, Lavery RF, Rekant M: Utility of routine admission serum chemistry panels in adult trauma patients, *Acad Emerg Med* 2:190-194, 1995.
18. Lowe RA, Arst HF, Ellis BK: Rational ordering of electrolytes in the emergency department, *Ann Emerg Med* 20:16-21, 1991.
19. Byrd L, Sherman RL: Radiocontrast-induced acute renal failure: a clinical and pathophysiologic review, *Medicine* 58:270-279, 1979.
20. Cochran ST: Determination of serum creatinine level prior to administration of radiographic contrast media, *JAMA* 277:517-518, 1997.
21. Boulanger BR, et al: The clinical significance of acute hyperamylasemia after blunt trauma, *Can J Surg* 36:63-69, 1993.
22. Mure AJ, et al: Serum amylase determination and blunt abdominal trauma, *Am Surg* 57:210-213, 1991.
23. Takahashi M, et al: Hyperamylasemia in critically injured patients, *J Trauma* 20:951-955, 1980.
24. Olsen WR: The serum amylase in blunt abdominal trauma, *J Trauma* 13:200-204, 1973.
25. Advanced trauma life support program for doctors. In American College of Surgeons: *Advanced trauma life support program for doctors*, Chicago, 1997, American College of Surgeons.
26. Feng CS, Ng AK: An analysis of donor blood wastage due to outdating in a large teaching hospital, *Pathology* 23:195-197, 1991.
27. West HC, et al: Immediate prediction of blood requirements in trauma victims, *South Med J* 82:186-189, 1989.
28. Champion HR, et al: A revision of the Trauma Score, *J Trauma* 29:623-629, 1989.
29. Clarke J, et al: Optimal blood ordering for emergency department patients, *Ann Emerg Med* 9:2-6, 1980.
30. Hooker EA, et al: Do all trauma patients need early cross-matching for blood? *J Emerg Med* 12:447-451, 1994.
31. Davis JW: Admission base deficit predicts transfusion requirements and risk of complications, *J Trauma* 41:769-774, 1996.
32. Asimos AW, Gibbs M: Admission base deficit predicts transfusion requirements and risk of complications, *J Trauma* 42(Letter):571-573, 1997.
33. Gervin AS, Fischer RP: Resuscitation of trauma patients with type-specific uncrossmatched blood, *J Trauma* 24:327-331, 1984.
34. Eastham JA, Wilson TG, Ahlering TE: Radiologic assessment of blunt renal trauma, *J Trauma* 31:1527-1528, 1991.
35. Mee SL, et al: Radiographic assessment of renal trauma: a 10-year prospective study of patient selection, *J Trauma* 141:1095-1098, 1989.
36. Klein S, et al: Hematuria following blunt abdominal trauma. The utility of intravenous pyelography, *Arch Surg* 123:1173-1177, 1988.
37. Hardeman SW, et al: Blunt urinary tract trauma: identifying those patients who require radiological diagnostic studies, *J Urol* 138:99-101, 1987.

38. Nicolaisen GS, et al: Renal trauma: re-evaluation of the indications for radiographic assessment, *J Urol* 133:183-187, 1985
39. Guice K, et al: Hematuria after blunt trauma: when is pyelography useful? *J Trauma* 23:305-311, 1983.
40. Ahn JH, Morey AF, McAninch JW: Workup and management of traumatic hematuria, *Emerg Med Clin North Am* 16:145-164, 1998.
41. Morey AF, Bruce JE, McAninch JW: Efficacy of radiographic imaging in pediatric blunt renal trauma, *J Urol* 156:2014-2018, 1996.
42. Lippmann S, Bordador B, Shaltout T: Detection of unknown early pregnancy: a matter of safety, *Postgrad Med* 83:129-131,135, 1988.
43. Ramoska EA, Sacchetti AD, Nepp M: Reliablity of patient history in determining the possibility of pregnancy, *Ann Emerg Med* 18:48-50, 1989.
44. Lipton JD, Thomason MH: Ectopic pregnancy in a blunt trauma patient, *J Emerg Med* 12:343-346, 1994.
45. Erstad BL, Harlander DK, Daller JA: Hematologic effects of ethanol consumption in trauma patients, *Ann Pharmacother* 27:889-891, 1993.
46. Rice DP, Kelman S, Miller LS: Estimates of the economic costs of alcohol and drug abuse and mental illness, 1985 and 1988, *Public Health Rep* 106:280-292, 1991.
47. Cherpitel CJ: Screening for alcohol problems in the emergency room: a rapid alcohol problems screen, *Drug Alcohol Depend* 40:133-137, 1995.
48. Fuller MG, et al: The role of a substance abuse consultation team in a trauma center, *J Stud Alcohol* 56:267-271, 1995.
49. Maio RF, et al: Alcohol abuse/dependence in motor vehicle crash victims presenting to the emergency department, *Acad Emerg Med* 4:256-262, 1997.
50. Mancino M, et al: Identification of the motor vehicle accident victim who abuses alcohol: an opportunity to reduce trauma, *J Stud Alcohol* 57:652-658, 1996.
51. Soderstrom CA, Dailey JT, Kerns TJ: Alcohol and other drugs: An assessment of testing and clinical practices in U.S. trauma centers, *J Trauma* 36:68-73, 1994.
52. Jurkovich GJ, et al: Effects of alcohol intoxication on the initial assessment of trauma patients, *Ann Emerg Med* 21:704-708, 1992.
53. Soderstrom CA, et al: Predictive model to identify trauma patients with blood alcohol concentrations > or = 50mg/dl,. *J Trauma* 42:67-73, 1997.
54. Gibb K: Serum alcohol levels, toxicology screens, and use of the breath alcohol analyzer, *Ann Emerg Med* 15:349-353, 1986.
55. Sloan EP, et al: Toxicology screening in urban trauma patients: drug prevalence and its relationship to trauma severity and management, *J Trauma* 29:1647-1653, 1989.
56. Davis JW, Kaups KLMD, Parks SN: Base deficit is superior to pH in evaluating clearance of acidosis after traumatic shock,. *J Trauma* 44:114-118, 1998.
57. Sauaia A, et al: Early predictors of postinjury multiple organ failure, *Arch Surg* 129:39-45, 1994.
58. Falcone RE, et al: Correlation of metabolic acidosis with outcome following injury and its value as a scoring tool, *World J Surg* 17:575-579, 1993.
59. Rutherford EJ, et al: Base deficit stratifies mortality and determines therapy, *J Trauma* 33:417-423, 1992.
60. Siegel JH, et al: Early physiologic predictors of injury severity and death in blunt multiple trauma, *Arch Surg* 125:498-508, 1990.
61. Davis JW, et al: Base deficit as a guide to volume resuscitation, *J Trauma* 28:1464-1467, 1988.
62. Davis JW, et al: Base deficit as an indicator of significant abdominal injury, *Ann Emerg Med* 20:842-844, 1991.
63. Mizock BA, Falk JL: Lactic acidosis in critical illness, *Crit Care Med* 20:80-93, 1992.
64. Dunham CM, et al: Oxygen debt and metabolic acidemia as quantitative predictors of mortality and the severity of the ischemic insult in hemorrhagic shock, *Crit Care Med* 19:231-243, 1991.
65. Cady LD, et al: Quantitation of severity of critical illness with special reference to blood lactate, *Crit Care Med* 1:75-80, 1973.
66. Vitek V, Cowley RA: Blood lactate in the prognosis of various forms of shock, *Ann Surg* 173:308-313, 1971.
67. Grzybowski M, et al: Prevalence of lactic acidosis on ED presentation and association with hospitalization rates, *Acad Emerg Med* 3(abstract):479, 1996.
68. Milzman DP, et al: Admission lactate: a rapid predictor of survival following traumatic injury, *Ann Emerg Med* 21(abstract): 596, 1992.
69. Abou-Khalil B, et al: Hemodynamic responses to shock in young trauma patients: need for invasive monitoring, *Crit Care Med* 22:633-639, 1994.
70. Aduen J, et al: The use and clinical importance of a substrate-specific electrode for rapid determination of blood lactate concentrations, *JAMA* 272:1678-1685, 1994.
71. Abramson D, et al: Lactate clearance and survival following injury, *J Trauma* 35:584-589, 1993.
72. Milzman D, et al: Admission lactate predicts fluid requirements for trauma victims during the initial 24 hours, *Crit Care Med* 22(abstract):A73, 1994.
73. Livingston DH, Slomovitzet al: Lactate identifies major trauma better than standard triage criteria, *Acad Emerg Med* 3(abstract): 532, 1996.
74. Lindsley J, Eble JN: Cost analysis of point-of-care laboratory testing in a community hospital, *Am J Clin Pathol* 104(Letter): 107-108, 1995.
75. Maclin PE, Mahoney WC: Point-of-care testing technology, *J Clin Ligand Assay* 18:21-33, 1995.
76. Nosanchuk JS, Keefner R: Cost analysis of point-of-care laboratory testing in a community hospital, *Am J Clin Pathol* 103: 240-243, 1995.
77. Tsai WW, et al: Point-of-care versus central laboratory testing: an economic analysis in an academic medical center, *Clin Ther* 16:898-910, 1994.
78. Kiechle FL, Ingram-Main R: Bedside testing: beyond glucose, *MLO* May;65-68, 1993.
79. Salem M, et al: Bedside diagnostic blood testing: its accuracy, rapidity, and utility in blood conservation, *JAMA* 266:382-389, 1991.
80. Isaacman DJ, et al: Utility of routine laboratory testing for detecting intra-abdominal injury in the pediatric trauma patient, *Pediatrics* 92:691-694, 1993.
81. Ford EG, et al: Emergency center laboratory evaluation of pediatric trauma victims, *Am Surg* 56:752-757, 1990.
82. Bryant MS, et al: Impact of emergency room laboratory studies on the ultimate triage and disposition of the injured child, *Am Surg* 54:209-211, 1988.
83. Grupp-Phelan J, Tanz RR: How rational is the crossmatching of blood in a pediatric emergency department? *Arch Pediatr Adolesc Med* 150:1140-1144, 1996.
84. Kharasch SJ, et al: The routine use of radiography and arterial blood gases in the evaluation of blunt trauma in children, *Ann Emerg Med* 23:212-215, 1994.
85. Maenza RL, Seaberg D, D'Amico F: A meta-analysis of blunt cardiac trauma: ending myocardial confusion, *Am J Emerg Med* 14:237-241, 1996.
86. Cachecho R, Grindlinger GA, Lee VW: The clinical significance of myocardial contusion, *J Trauma* 33:68-73, 1992.

87. Fabian T, et al: A prospective evaluation of myocardial contusion: correlation of significant arrhythmias and cardiac output with CPK-MB measurements, *J Trauma* 31:653-660, 1991.
88. Foil MB, et al: The asymptomatic patient with suspected myocardial contusion, *Am J Surg* 160:638-643, 1990.
89. Norton MJ, Stanford GG, Weigelt JA: Early detection of myocardial contusion and its complications in patients with blunt trauma, *Am J Surg* 160:577-582, 1990.
90. Wisner DH, Reed WH, Riddick RS: Suspected myocardial contusion: triage and indications for monitoring, *Ann Surg* 212(1): 82-86, 1990.
91. Baxter BT, et al: A plea for sensible management of myocardial contusion, *Am J Surg* 158:557-562, 1989.
92. Healey MA, Brown R, Fleiszer D: Blunt cardiac injury: is this diagnosis necessary? *J Trauma* 30:137-146, 1990.
93. Mattox KL, et al: Blunt cardiac injury, *J Trauma* 33:649-650, 1992.
94. Garland JL, Wolfson AB: Routine admission electrocardiography in emergency department patients, *Ann Emerg Med* 23:275-280, 1994.
95. Davis JW, et al: The etiology of missed cervical spine injuries, *J Trauma* 34:342-346, 1993.
96. Stiell IG, et al: Variation in emergency department use of cervical spine radiography for alert, stable trauma patients, *Can Med Assoc J* 156:1537-1544, 1997.
97. Kathol MH: Cervical spine trauma. What is new? *Radiol Clin North Am* 35:507-532, 1997.
98. Hoffman JR, et al: Selective cervical spine radiography in blunt trauma: the National Emergency X-radiographic Utilization Study (NEXUS), *Ann Emerg Med* 32(2)(abstract):S1, 1998.
99. Velmahos GC, et al: Radiographic cervical spine evaluation in the alert asymptomatic blunt trauma victim: much ado about nothing, *J Trauma* 40:768-774, 1996.
100. McNamara RM, Heine E, Esposito B: Cervical spine injury and radiography in alert, high-risk patients, *J Emerg Med* 8:177-182, 1990.
101. Kreipke DL, et al: Reliability of indications for cervical spine films in trauma patients, *J Trauma* 29:1438-1439, 1989.
102. Ringenberg BJ, et al: Rational ordering of cervical spine radiographs following trauma, *Ann Emerg Med* 17:792-796, 1988.
103. Roberge RJ, et al: Selective application of cervical spine radiography in alert victims of blunt trauma: a prospective study, *J Trauma* 28:784-788, 1988.
104. Bachulls BL, et al: Clinical indications for cervical spine radiographs in the traumatized patient, Am *J Surg* 153:473-478, 1987.
105. Roth BJ, et al: Roentgenographic evaluation of the cervical spine: a selective approach, *Arch Surg* 129:643-645, 1994.
106. Bayless P, Ray VG: Incidence of cervical spine injuries in association with blunt head trauma, *Am J Emerg Med* 7:139-141, 1989.
107. Neifeld GL, et al: Cervical injury in head trauma, *J Emerg Med* 6:203-207, 1988.
108. Fischer RP: Cervical radiographic evaluation of alert patients following blunt trauma, *Ann Emerg Med* 13:905-907, 1984.
109. Hills MW, Deane SA: Head injury and facial injury: is there an increased risk of cervical spine injury? *J Trauma* 34:549-554, 1993.
110. Andrew CT, et al: Is routine cervical spine radiographic evaluation indicated in patients with mandibular fractures? *Am Surg* 1992;58:369-372.
111. Oller DW, et al: The relationship between face or skull fractures and cervical spine and spinal cord injuries: a review of 13,834 patients, *Accid Anal Prev* 24:187-192, 1992.
112. Williams J, et al: Head, facial, and clavicular trauma as a predictor of cervical-spine injury, *Ann Emerg Med* 21:719-722, 1992.
113. Davidson JS, Birdsell DC: Cervical spine injury in patients with facial skeletal trauma, *J Trauma* 29:1276-1278, 1989.
114. O'Malley KF, Ross SE: The incidence of injury to the cervical spine in patients with craniocerebral injury, *J Trauma* 28:1476-1478, 1988.
115. Sinclair D, et al: A retrospective review of the relationship between facial fractures, head injuries, and cervical spine injuries, *J Emerg Med* 6:109-112, 1988.
116. Laham JL, et al: Isolated head injuries versus multiple trauma in pediatric patients: do the same indications for cervical spine evaluation apply? *Pediatr Neurosurg* 21:221-226, 1994.
117. Dietrich AM, et al: Pediatric cervical spine fractures: predominately subtle presentation, *J Pediatr Surg* 26:995-1000, 1991.
118. Lally KP, et al: Utility of the cervical spine radiograph in pediatric trauma, *Am J Surg* 158:540-542, 1989.
119. Blahd WH Jr, Iserson KV, Bjelland JC: Efficacy of the posttraumatic cross table lateral view of the cervical spine, *J Emerg Med* 2:243-249, 1985.
120. Streitwieser DR, et al: Accuracy of standard radiographic views in detecting cervical spine fractures, *Ann Emerg Med* 12:538-542, 1983.
121. Shaffer MA, Doris PE: Limitation of the cross table lateral view in detecting cervical spine injuries: a retrospective analysis, *Ann Emerg Med* 10:508-513, 1981.
122. Ehara S, El-Khoury GY, Clark CR: Radiologic evaluation of dens fracture: role of plain radiography and tomography, *Spine* 17:475-479, 1992.
123. Ross SE, et al: Clearing the cervical spine: initial radiologic evaluation, *J Trauma* 27:1055-1060, 1987.
124. Holliman CJ, et al: Is the anteroposterior cervical spine radiograph necessary in initial trauma screening? *Am J Emerg Med* 9:421-425, 1991.
125. Janchar T, et al: New methods in digital radiography improve the ability to clear the cross-table lateral cervical spine in trauma patients, *Acad Emerg Med* 4(abstract):395, 1997.
126. Borock EC, et al: A prospective analysis of a two-year experience using computed tomography as an adjunct for cervical spine clearance, *J Trauma* 31:1001-1006, 1991.
127. Murphey MD: Trauma oblique cervical spine radiographs, *Ann Emerg Med* 22:728-730, 1993.
128. Turetsky DB, et al: Technique and use of supine oblique views in acute cervical spine trauma, *Ann Emerg Med* 22:685-689, 1993.
129. Doris PE, Wilson RA: The next logical step in the emergency radiographic evaluation of cervical spine trauma: the five-view trauma series, *J Emerg Med* 3:371-385, 1985.
130. MacDonald RL, et al: Diagnosis of cervical spine injury in motor vehicle crash victims: how many x-rays are enough? *J Trauma* 30:392-397, 1990.
131. Freemyer B, et al: Comparison of five-view and three-view cervical spine series in the evaluation of patients with cervical trauma, *Ann Emerg Med* 18:818-821, 1989.
132. Lewis LM, et al: Flexion-extension views in the evaluation of cervical-spine injuries, *Ann Emerg Med* 20:117-121, 1991.
133. Chan O, Hiorns M: Chest trauma, *Eur J Rdiol* 23:23-34, 1996.
134. Mirvis SE, et al: Value of chest radiography in excluding traumatic aortic rupture, *Radiology* 163:487-493, 1987.
135. Schwab CW, et al: Aortic injury: comparison of supine and upright portable chest films to evaluate the widened mediastinum, *Ann Emerg Med* 13:896-899, 1984
136. Samuels LE, Kerstein MD: 'Routine' radiologic evaluation of the thoracolumbar spine in blunt trauma patients: a reappraisal, *J Trauma* 34:85-89, 1993.
137. Durham RM, et al: Evaluation of the thoracic and lumbar spine after blunt trauma, *Am J Surg* 170:681-685, 1995.

138. Terregino CA, et al: Selective indications for thoracic and lumbar radiography in blunt trauma, *Ann Emerg Med* 26:126-129, 1995.
139. Frankel HL, et al: Indications for obtaining surveillance thoracic and lumbar spine radiographs, *J Trauma* 27:673-676, 1994.
140. Yugueros P, et al: Unnecessary use of pelvic x-ray in blunt trauma, *J Trauma* 39:722-725, 1995.
141. Koury HI, Peschiera JL, Welling RE: Selective use of pelvic roentgenograms in blunt trauma patients, *J Trauma* 34:236-237, 1993.
142. Salvino CK, et al: Routine pelvic x-ray studies in awake blunt trauma patients: a sensible policy? *J Trauma* 33:413-416, 1992.
143. Civil ID, et al: Routine pelvic radiography in severe blunt trauma: is it necessary? *Ann Emerg Med* 17:488-490, 1988.
144. Morgan PW, et al: Evaluation of traumatic aortic injury: does dynamic contrast-enhanced CT play a role? *Radiology* 182:661-666, 1992.
145. Raptopoulos V, et al: Traumatic aortic tear: screening with chest CT, *Radiology* 182:667-673, 1992.
146. Richardson P, et al: Value of CT in determining the need for angiography when findings of mediastinal hemorrhage on chest radiographs are equivocal, *AJR* 156:273-279, 1991.
147. Fenner MN, et al: Evaluation of possible traumatic thoracic aortic injury using aortography and CT, *Am Surg* 56:497-499, 1990.
148. Ordog GJ, et al: Extremity gunshot wounds: Part 1. Identification and treatment of patients at high risk of vascular injury, *J Trauma* 36:358-368, 1994.
149. Frykberg ER, et al: The reliability of physical examination in the evaluation of penetrating extremity trauma for vascular injury: results at one year, *J Trauma* 31:502-511, 1991.
150. Rozycki GS, et al: Prospective evaluation of surgeons' use of ultrasound in the evaluation of trauma patients, *J Trauma* 34:516-527, 1993.
151. Shackford SR: Focused ultrasound examinations by surgeons: the time is now, *J Trauma* 35:181-182, 1993.
152. Thomas B, et al: Ultrasound evaluation of blunt abdominal trauma: program implementation, initial experience, and learning curve, *J Trauma* 42:384-390, 1997.
153. Branney SW, et al: Ultrasound based key clinical pathway reduces the use of hospital resources for the evaluation of blunt abdominal trauma, *J Trauma* 42:1086-1090, 1997.
154. McElveen TS, Collin GR: The role of ultrasonography in blunt abdominal trauma: a prospective study, *Am Surg* 63:184-188, 1997.
155. Nordenholz KE, et al: Ultrasound in the evaluation and management of blunt abdominal trauma, *Ann Emerg Med* 29:357-366, 1997.
156. Boulanger BR, et al: Emergent abdominal sonography as a screening test in a new diagnostic algorithm for blunt trauma, *J Trauma* 40:867-874, 1996.
157. McKenney MG, et al: 1000 consecutive utltrasounds for blunt abdominal trauma, *J Trauma* 40:607-612 1996.

47 Medicolegal Issues: Brain Death, Organ and Tissue Transplantation, Confidentiality, and Restraints

CHRISTINE MILOSIS AND ROBERT E. O'CONNOR

BRAIN DEATH

For most of recorded history, cessation of breathing meant death. Today, medical advances allow for the prolonged mechanical support of patients by maintaining essential organ functions. In these cases, the absence of brain function determines death. Although an individual without a functioning brain eventually dies regardless of artificial support, there are several ethical and practical reasons to declare death in a timely manner. These reasons include maintaining patient dignity, decreasing the suffering of loved ones, and optimizing resource utilization. Medical personnel must also determine brain death before tissue death to consider organs for transplantation.

The decision to cease acute medical interventions during trauma resuscitation does not depend on brain death criteria. The emergency physician (EP) may stop resuscitation when he or she deems the patient clinically dead, or when he or she believes that further intervention would be futile. In many trauma centers, cardiac arrest from blunt trauma precludes resuscitative interventions, since survival from blunt trauma arrest is so dismal.

The most authoritative document regarding brain death comes from the *President's Commission on the Guidelines for the Determination of Death.*[1] This report, the *Uniform Determination of Death Act,* first outlined the standard of care for determining death in the United States. The Determination of Death Act requires the following criteria: (1) irreversible cessation of circulatory and respiratory functions, or (2) irreversible cessation of all functions of the entire brain, including the brainstem. It specifies that these determinations should be made in accordance with accepted medical standards.

Both the *Harvard Criteria*[2] and the *Special Communication by the President's Commission*[3] represent currently accepted medical standards to determine brain death. The discussion presented in this chapter is based largely on the *Special Communication by the President's Commission,* since it best defines the current standard of care.

The determination of death requires the establishment of the irreversible loss of vital functions. The physician must assess responsiveness, breathing, and circulation. In many cases, clinical examination is sufficient. The trauma victim with no signs of life and no cardiac activity is dead. However, a patient with a heartbeat but no immediately obvious neurologic function may require additional investigations before the determination of brain death.

Similarly, the declaration of brain death in an artificially supported person requires sophisticated clinical testing and, in the minority of cases, sophisticated confirmatory testing unfamiliar to most physicians.[4,5] Consequently, determining brain death is often within the domain of neurologists, intensivists, and neurosurgeons and rarely EPs.

The first step in determining brain death requires a well-defined etiology of coma, such as structural or metabolic causes. The second step requires that no specific interventions can reverse the comatose state. The third step entails excluding reversible conditions that produce deep coma. Some examples of reversible conditions that cause deep coma include hypothermia, intoxication, hypotension, and the Guillain-Barré syndrome. The last step includes serial examinations that allow sufficient time to elapse between examinations. It is suggested to allow 6 hours between examinations for coma resulting from structural causes, and 12 to 24 hours between examinations for patients with toxic or metabolic causes of coma. Ethchlorvynol and meprobamate, for instance, may cause prolonged coma and flat-line electroencephalograms (EEGs). If these agents are suspected, the interval between examinations should be quite lengthy.

Examination of Cerebral Function

The Glasgow Coma Scale (GCS) is the first step in assessing a patient with coma. Brain death is characterized by a GCS score of 3. However, if a response is elicited to voice or pain, some cerebral function is intact. Decerebrate and decorticate movements also indicate some level of brainstem functioning and are thus inconsistent with the diagnosis of brain death. However, it is acceptable to have "lower" functions such as spinal cord reflexes, shivering, and piloerection and make the determination of brain death.

Confirmatory testing for brain death is only necessary in the rare instance where clinical findings are equivocal, or when the cause of coma is unknown despite a thorough search for the etiology. In these cases, the physician may use an EEG or a blood flow study. The most sensitive and specific blood flow study is four-vessel cerebral arteriography. Other tests of cerebral blood flow are available but are either less sensitive (e.g., digital subtraction angiography and transcranial Doppler ultrasound) or less specific (e.g., brainstem acoustic evoked potential). EEG used in this setting determines neuronal activity. Confirmatory testing never substitutes for clinical testing of both cerebral and brainstem functions.[5]

Examination of Brainstem Function

The loss of brainstem functioning requires an absence of each of these six reflexes: corneal, pupillary, gag, cough, oculocephalic, and oculovestibular. It also requires an absence of an integrated response to pain and lack of respiratory efforts on apnea testing.

In brain death, pupils are midposition, unreactive, and between 3 and 7 mm in diameter. Always test pupillary response in a darkened room by shining a very bright light sequentially into both eyes. Some medications, such as atropine and barbiturates, may alter the pupillary response. Any interpretation of the pupillary response must be done in the context of the patient's prescribed medications or potential toxins ingested.

To test corneal reflexes, firmly touch the cornea of both eyes with a cotton-tipped applicator. If testing results in no lid movement, then corneal reflexes are absent. Make certain that contact lenses are removed before testing.

The gag reflex is tested by stimulation of the posterior pharyngeal tissues with a tongue depressor. Rapidly pulling and pushing on the endotracheal tube is a variant of this test. In the brain dead patient, the maneuvers should not result in a gag or cough (ventilator "clutching" response).

Elevating the patient's head to 30 degrees and sequentially instilling ice water into each ear canal with a syringe will assess the oculovestibular reflex. Before testing, check that the tympanic membrane is intact and the external ear canal is patent. The test involves squirting approximately 50 ml of ice water into each ear. Instill the water into one ear and then wait 5 minutes to inject water into the opposite ear. With an intact brainstem, the eyes will deviate towards the ear with water. A negative reflex occurs when there is no eye movement during testing.

The oculocephalic reflex is inappropriate in the trauma patient, since it requires movement of the neck. It is impossible to "clear" the cervical spine in the comatose patient.

Apnea testing determines spontaneous respiratory effort with discontinuation of mechanical ventilation. During apnea testing, the pCO_2 is allowed to climb to approximately 60 mmHg. This action should stimulate the respiratory drive in a patient with a functioning brainstem and no history of chronic obstructive pulmonary disease.[6] Begin testing by adjusting the ventilator settings to achieve a pCO_2 of 40 mmHg and a pO_2 of greater than 300 mmHg as confirmed by arterial blood gas (ABG). Use 100% FiO_2. Once these levels are achieved, ventilate the patient for 30 minutes, then disconnect the ventilator and use 100% oxygen via blow-by. In approximately 7 minutes, the pCO_2 should reach 60 mmHg. Observe the patient for any respiratory effort. If respiratory effort is noted, the test is not consistent with brain death; immediately reattach the ventilator. If no respiratory effort is noted by 7 minutes, draw another ABG and reattach the ventilator. If the ABG reveals that indeed a pCO_2 of at least 60 mmHg is achieved without respiratory effort observed, then the test is positive and consistent with brain death. To document brain death, two such tests have to be done separated by an appropriate period. If there are no respiratory efforts observed during the second apnea test, the patient may be declared dead.

Determining Brain Death in Children and Neonates

Although the definition of brain death is the same for children and neonates as for adults, it is more difficult to determine brain death in this group. According to the *Presidential Commission*, the previously discussed guidelines are appropriate for ages 5 years and older. The *Task Force for the Determination of Brain Death in Children*[7] suggests the following guidelines for younger children:

- Premature infants: brain death criteria do not apply
- Newborns at or near term (>38 weeks gestation): brain death criteria may be used 7 days after the initial insult

- Infants aged 7 days to 2 months: two clinical examinations and two EEGs separated by 48 hours
- Infants aged 2 months to 1 year: two clinical examinations and two EEGs separated by at least 24 hours
- Children aged greater than 1 year: observation period of at least 12 to 24 hours

Brain Death in Pregnant Patients

Whether or not a pregnant, brain dead mother should be sustained to support the fetus to delivery is a vexing ethical dilemma. The literature reports several cases where brain dead mothers were supported for greater than 2 months just for this purpose. The authors suggest that if the gestational age of the fetus is approximately 24 weeks, then treating physicians should consider maternal support.[8] Obviously, the older the gestational age, the greater the likelihood of fetal viability. Clearly, this decision must involve the next of kin, as well as a neonatal intensivist, adult intensivist, obstetrician, and an ethics committee or expert. Sustaining the vital functions of a pregnant mother for the short period of time needed to give steroids to aid in fetal lung maturation is far different from maintaining a pregnant mother for months to reach a near-term fetus. There is no easy answer to this dilemma and each case needs to be addressed on an individual basis within the context of the patient's family and medical community's understanding and expectation.

Perimortem cesarean section is a very clinically challenging situation that is covered in more detail in Chapter 32. The EP, when confronted with a futile resuscitation of a pregnant patient and a fetus beyond 24 weeks gestation, must perform a cesarean section in the emergency department (ED) to offer any chance of survival to the fetus.[8]

ORGAN AND TISSUE TRANSPLANTATION

Whole organs suitable for transplant include kidneys, liver, lungs, heart, and pancreas. Patients, once declared brain dead, become candidates for organ donation. It is essential that the potential organ grafts are adequately perfused until the time of harvesting to have a successful transplantation. Transplant tissues include eyes, bones, skin, ligaments, tendons, cartilage, rotator cuff, fascia lata, thoracic aorta, nerves, pericardium, heart valves, and saphenous veins. Tissue grafts can survive for a finite period of time without perfusion, so even those patients who have died from cardiopulmonary arrest may donate tissue. It is essential that the EP get the local or regional organ and tissue procurement team involved early on after clinical death or brain death is established so that optimal harvesting can occur.

It is the physician's responsibility to determine whether a brain dead or newly dead patient is a potential organ or tissue donor. Certain infectious and neoplastic diseases preclude transplantation. Patients with the human immunodeficiency virus and metastatic neoplastic disease, for example, are not suitable. However, patients with hepatitic viral disease or cytomegalovirus may be suitable donors, and it is important to discuss suitability with the regional organ and/or tissue banks.

The apnea test previously described is performed last in the second battery of brain death testing. If there is no response to apnea testing, the patient may be declared dead and mechanical ventilation is not reapplied. If, however, the patient is to be an organ donor and there is no response to apnea testing, the patient is still declared dead but the mechanical ventilator is reapplied to support organ function until harvesting can occur. Intensive support then becomes crucial to avoid tissue hypoxia and hypotension. Brain dead patients who sustain periods of hypotension may become unsuitable donors.[4,5,9]

Once the determination has been made regarding suitability as a donor, the next of kin may be approached regarding organ donation *before* the second battery of brain death tests. The interval of time between the declaration of death and the retrieval of the organs should be kept to a minimum and not exceed 12 hours.[9] Informing the local procurement office of a possible organ donor before the declaration of death is acceptable to expedite organ harvesting. *It is crucial that the family of the donor understand that death has already occurred when the patient fails the second apnea test, and that organ procurement has no bearing on this fact.* The family is not responsible for the costs incurred after the declaration of death, and the organ bank typically underwrites the transplant-associated costs.[9]

Recent studies show that success in obtaining consent for donation is dramatically increased if the issue of donation is not broached until after the declaration of brain death. Families have difficulty understanding the concept of brain death despite careful explanation. They may erroneously believe that consent for organ donation is a decision regarding life versus death. Many procurement organizations recommend that issues of donation are best understood after death has been declared (i.e., *after* the second negative apnea test). Historically, these issues were discussed before the second apnea test.

Because of the interval of time required to establish brain death, identification and medical support of organ donors are not usually within the domain of the

EP. Ideally, the physician requesting organ donation should not be the same physician declaring death. Usually, the intensivist is the appropriate physician to determine the suitability of an organ donor and to determine or declare brain death. Many trauma centers have organ procurement teams, expert at determination of donor suitability and experienced in interacting with grieving families. When available, the EP should alert the organ procurement team regarding a possible donor. If clear guidelines are provided regarding donor suitability, EPs may request tissue or organ donation from the family of the decedent. In fact, in some states, a discussion with the family about organ donation is required by law.

Ideally, all persons would have advanced directives regarding organ and tissue donation in the form of a donor card or personal will. Unfortunately, most patients do not have advanced directives, and usually the next of kin is asked to consent regarding donation. In many states, the next of kin may authorize an anatomic gift. This responsibility falls with the spouse, adult child, either parent, adult sibling, legal guardian or another authorized person depending on the family's situation and the surviving members.

Ethical Issues

A physician is ethically bound to comply with the reasonable wishes of rational patients. If a person has stated through advanced directive that they wish to be an anatomic donor and they are suitable, then harvesting may legally proceed regardless of the wishes of the next of kin. In reality, however, if the family is opposed to donation, the procurement is less likely for fear of "bad press" or suggestions of "organ stealing." Likewise, if a person through advanced directive has stated that he or she do not wish to be an anatomic donor, then harvesting cannot be undertaken regardless of the suitability of the donor or the wishes of the next of kin to the contrary.

If there are no advanced directives to guide anatomic donation, the physician must decide to request donation of organs or tissues if the patient is suitable. In most cases, the physician should make this request, but certain family dynamics might preclude this discussion. In the case of an extremely hostile family who blames the physician for the death, or a family that will not accept the notion of brain death, the request for donation may be counterproductive. However, some hospitals or local laws may mandate an automatic request for donation (see the following discussion).

When requesting a donation, the physician may state that the gift may be of benefit to others. The physician should not badger or coerce the family to consent by inducing guilt or projecting his or her own beliefs.

Transplant science is technically and physiologically complex. The act of donation itself does not guarantee a successful outcome. Families need to understand that although the donation may save another person, the desired outcome cannot be guaranteed. It is appropriate to inform families of an estimate of success based on previous results.

Legal Issues

All physicians are encouraged to review the laws regarding transplantation in the state in which they practice. Physicians must realize that they are legally bound to request organ donation from the families of suitable donors if they work in a hospital receiving federal funds through Medicare and Medicaid programs. The National Organ Procurement and Transplantation Network (NOPTN) and its regional and local subsidiaries determine and organize the disbursement of anatomic gifts and the individual physician has no role in this process.

CONFIDENTIALITY

Confidentiality is implicit to the physician-patient relationship. Patients understand that physicians will not reveal their personal information to other persons or institutions without patient consent. This definition is explicit in the Hippocratic Oath, the American Medical Association Principles of Medical Ethics, the American College of Physicians Ethics manual, and the American Hospital Association Patient's Bill of Rights.

Why is confidentiality important? The assumption of confidentiality in physician-patient relationships is important because it increases the likelihood that the patient will reveal sensitive information that may relate to his or her health.[10] Transmitting this information to others without the permission of the patient not only jeopardizes this essential trust but may also cause the patient harm. For example, a patient is accompanied to the ED by his or her supervisor because of shortness of breath at work. If the ED physician reveals to the supervisor that this may be the result of heart disease, then this information may affect future employment. Similarly, if the physician relates the same information to a nurse in an indiscreet manner and is overheard by the patient's supervisor, then the physician has also failed in maintaining the patient's confidentiality. Physicians can breach confidentiality both directly and indirectly. Breach of confidentiality can tarnish the medical profession and may cause the patient harm and embarrassment.

There are circumstances that override the requirement of confidentiality. When a patient poses a threat to himself or herself, or to others, then the right to confidentiality is abrogated by a higher moral, and sometimes legal, obligation.[11] For example, a patient presents to the ED after a motor vehicle crash (MVC) and confides to the physician that she drove her car into a tree in a suicide attempt. Regardless of the fact that she has told the physician this information in confidence, the physician must pursue a psychiatric evaluation to protect the patient.

Another common trauma scenario relates to the evaluation of a patient in an MVC who crashed as a result of a seizure disorder. In some states, the physician is legally obligated to report this information to the proper authorities. Other recognized areas in which the physician is legally obligated to breach confidentiality include cases of suspected child abuse and any wound sustained as a result of the use of a gun.[11] In some states, the physician must report cases of suspected domestic violence, regardless of the patient's wishes.

Maintaining patient confidentiality is paramount unless there is an identified and vulnerable party disclosed by the patient to the physician in the course of the clinical encounter. In the suicide example, the patient is the identified and vulnerable party. In the seizure case, any person on the road may be injured as the result of an impaired driver. Contrast these examples with a case in which a physician tells a patient's neighbor that the patient has AIDS. This disclosure is an indefensible breach of confidentiality, since the physician would be unjustified in assuming that AIDS poses a threat to the neighbor.[11]

The special circumstance of treating adolescent minors requires separate consideration. As minors, adolescents are not able to consent for or refuse treatment. This situation changes, of course, once the adolescent seeks medical attention for problems regarding contraception, pregnancy, substance abuse, and sexually transmittable diseases. In most states, these clinical conditions define an emancipated minor and the patient is treated as if he or she were an adult. The EP may treat such conditions without the parent's knowledge unless the patient consents to informing the parents. In these circumstances, the patient is entitled to the tenet of confidentiality for the greater social good. The EP must be familiar with the state statutes governing the care and treatment of minors and especially what circumstances change that legal definition.

With the advent of electronic communication and the storage of sensitive information on computers, the challenge of maintaining patient confidentiality becomes far more difficult. In specific, the environment of the ED poses special challenges concerning confidentiality. Consider the fishbowl environment and the staggering number and variety of people who may populate the ED at any one time. It is not unusual to find paramedics, BLS crews, police officers, detectives, state troopers, chaplains, clerical staff, housekeeping staff, x-ray technicians, volunteers, medical students, consulting physicians and residents, transport staff, security personnel, and, of course, patients and their family members. Also unique to the ED is the transmission of patient information from paramedics to base stations via radio bands.

How can we safeguard the confidentiality of patients in the ED? The layout should encourage patient privacy. Close curtains and doors and discourage family members from using the phones, or speaking with the doctors in the core area where other patients are easily visible. All members of the healthcare team should examine the patient in privacy and use a discreet tone of voice in obtaining a patient's history and speaking among themselves and on the telephone. Patient charts should be in specified locations and no information discernible to a passerby. Manual patient tracking systems, or "greaseboards," should be located out of sight of the general ED population, or at least the ED staff should use abbreviations to limit the amount of information that can be garnered by interlopers or other patients about patients undergoing an evaluation. Finally, paramedics and police officers should complete their reports in an area separate from the treatment area.

When emergency medical services communicate with base stations, paramedics must not reveal the name or location of the patient, since laypersons may monitor these radio bands. There is no circumstance imaginable when the patient's name, malady, or location will benefit the EP before the patient's arrival in the ED.

The trauma patient is at exceedingly greater risk of having his or her basic rights infringed on because of the multidisciplinary effort and high drama surrounding such events. It is important to protect the trauma patient from curious onlookers, who may go unnoticed amidst all the activity in the trauma bay. The EP should ensure that only those individuals directly involved in the patient's care are in the trauma bay.

Many people may attempt to obtain information or access to the patient's medical records. Interested parties include police officers, insurance carriers, media, family members, and friends of the patient. With the exception of parents of unemancipated minors, these parties do not have the right to access the medical record or obtain information regarding the patient's medical condition without a subpoena or the expressed consent of the patient. If asked, it is generally acceptable for the physician to use general terms describing the patient's condition, such as "critical," "guarded," or "stable." It is impossible for a physician to know the wishes of a patient who is unconscious or incapable of decision-making as a result of an altered mental status. In this case, the physician should provide information to the family, especially if it appears that the patient may never regain consciousness. Be careful divulging information over the telephone, particularly regarding a sensational trauma case or one with legal implications. Unscrupulous parties may falsely identify themselves as family members to obtain otherwise confidential information. Encouraging family members to come to the ED whenever possible, asking for a call back number if visitation is not possible, and involving the ED's social service support system are essential steps to maintain confidentiality.

RESTRAINTS

Physical restraint of the trauma patient may be necessary to protect healthcare workers, to facilitate patient evaluation, or to protect the patient from injury. Because of the potential for physical harm and litigation, physical restraint must not be applied solely for staff convenience, and the patient must not be restrained any longer than is required for safety. Frequent reassessment is mandatory, with removal of the restraints being done once the crisis has passed.

Once the decision has been made to restrain the patient, adequate personnel (5 at a minimum) should be assembled with each given an assigned task. A team leader should instruct each member regarding his or her duties, preferably with members restraining a preassigned extremity. The patient should be restrained in a manner intended to reduce the chance of accidental injury to all parties.

The physician should document that the restrained patient posed a risk to self or others, and that less aggressive measures have failed. Ongoing documentation should include a description of behavior every 15 minutes, assessment of circulation and skin integrity every 2 hours, and release of a single extremity periodically if the patient's condition permits. The physician should reevaluate and document the need for restraints every 4 hours. If prolonged physical restraint is anticipated, consider pharmacologic restraint using benzodiazepines, droperidol, haloperidol, or other agents (see Chapter 10). In extreme cases, paralysis by neuromuscular blockade with endotracheal intubation and mechanical ventilation may be required.

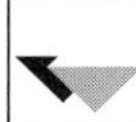

PEARLS & PITFALLS

Brain Death

- Confirmatory testing never substitutes for clinical testing of both cerebral and brainstem functions.[5]
- The loss of brainstem functioning requires an absence of each of these six reflexes: corneal, pupillary, gag, cough, oculocephalic, and oculovestibular. It also requires loss of response to pain and no respiratory efforts on apnea testing.

Organ Donation

- Many procurement organizations recommend that the family be approached regarding donation *after* death has been declared (i.e., after the second negative apnea test).
- Some situations may *demand* that the family be approached for organ donation. Consult the local organ procurement team for details.

Confidentiality

- Confidentiality is difficult to maintain in the trauma situation. Efforts should include clearing the trauma room of unauthorized individuals, speaking discretely, and keeping the charts safe from bystanders.
- Involve the patient if possible before releasing any information beyond his or her status (critical, serious, or stable). In case of the unconscious trauma victim, family members deserve more information.

Restraints

- Physicians may restrain patients to protect the patient and others.
- Always document the need for restraints and failure of less restrictive measures.
- Use a flow sheet to document the condition of the restrained patient at defined intervals.

REFERENCES

1. Report of the Medical Consultants on the Diagnosis of Death to the President's Commission for the Study of Ethical Problems in Medicine and Biomedical and Behavioral Research: Guidelines for the determination of death, *JAMA* 246:2184-2186, 1981.

2. Report of the Ad Hoc Committee of the Harvard Medical School to Examine the Definition of Brain Death: A definition of irreversible coma, *JAMA* 205:337-340, 1968.
3. President's Commission for the Study of Ethical Problems in Medicine and Biomedical and Behavioral Research: Defining Death: A Report on the Medical, Legal and Ethical Issues in the Determination of Death, Washington, DC, 1981, U.S. Government Printing Office.
4. Bernat JL, Taylor RM: *Clinical neurology: ethical issues in neurology,* Philadelphia, 1997, Lippincott-Raven.
5. Bernat JL: Ethical and legal aspects of the emergency management of brain death and organ retrieval, *Emerg Med Clin North Am* 5:661-675, 1987.
6. Report of the Quality Standards Subcommittee of the American Academy of Neurology: Practice parameters for determining brain death in adults, *Neurology* 45:1012-1014, 1995.
7. Task Force for the Determination of Brain Death in Children: Guidelines for the determination of brain death in children, *Arch Neurol* 44:587-588, 1987.
8. Loewy EH: The pregnant brain dead and the fetus: Must we always try to wrest life from death? *Am J Obstet Gynecol* 157: 1097-1101, 1987.
9. Bernat JL: Ethical issues in brain death and multiorgan transplantation, *Ethic Issues Neurol Prac* 7:715-728, 1989.
10. American College of Physicians: American College of Physicians ethics manual: third edition, *Ann Intern Med* 117:947-960, 1992.
11. Iverson KV, et al: *Ethics in emergency medicine,* Baltimore, 1986, Williams & Wilkins.

Legal Issues Concerning Informed Consent in Trauma Care

48

ROBERT A. BITTERMAN

The doctrine of "informed consent" is rooted in the fundamental principle of the American legal system that "every human of adult years and a sound mind has a right to determine what should be done with his own body."[1] Physicians may not examine or treat persons, including trauma victims, without their consent. Furthermore, consent must be informed; the patient must be told certain material information concerning the nature, risk, and alternatives of the treatment before he or she can be deemed to have effectively consented to the medical intervention.

Physicians should always endeavor to obtain informed consent, but must remain cognizant of the significant limitations and number of exceptions to the doctrine, especially in the emergency setting. *Delaying treatment in an emergency to obtain informed consent is a much more serious and a much more common medical-legal problem than failure to obtain proper informed consent.*

The objectives of this chapter are two-fold: first, to teach the general rules of consent regarding common scenarios in the management of the trauma patient; second, and perhaps more importantly, to help the practicing physician know when and how to cast aside the general rules. We must recognize situations that demand an exception, and act in a manner not only legally appropriate but also consistent with sound medical judgment.

"WHEN IN DOUBT" RULE

Like medicine, the law of informed consent contains a great deal of uncertainty. There are many gray areas and different states have different views, either in their statutory laws (legislation) or in their common law (judge-made law or precedent).

In caring for the trauma victim, emergency physicians (EPs) and surgeons rarely have the luxury to seek legal consultations, let alone wait for a court to render a decision concerning the legal nuances of consent. In these situations it is helpful for physicians to follow the "When in Doubt Rule" to guide their immediate actions. In any consent case, the "When in Doubt Rule" should be "Do what you believe in the patient's best interest and worry about the legal consequences later." It is true that physicians risk criminal and civil charges of false imprisonment, battery, and even negligence suits for failure to obtain appropriate informed consent. But it is always more defensible to help the patient than let them die for lack of informed consent. The courts consistently rule in favor of physicians who act in good faith on behalf of their patients. Successful civil litigation on a consent theory against an EP or surgeon acting reasonably and consistent with the appropriate standard of care, in the setting of acute trauma, is extremely rare. In fact, an EP is far more likely to be sued for failure to treat than for providing reasonable treatment without consent. When in doubt, act.

GENERAL RULES

Both federal and state laws govern consent. Federal law, The Emergency Medicine Treatment and Active Labor Act (EMTALA),[2,3] comes into play primarily in the evaluation of minors and when patients refuse an examination, stabilizing treatment, or transfer. State consent laws vary widely and may be set by statutes, case law, or both. The concepts discussed in the following section are generally applicable to emergency trauma care, but physicians should be keenly aware of the consent laws particular to their own state.

Doctrine of Informed Consent

The law presumes that barring certain circumstances, an adult is mentally competent to make medical decisions. The competent adult is entitled to sufficient information to make an informed decision concerning the physician's proposed course of examination and treatment.[4]

Elements of Informed Consent

Physicians have the duty to disclose the following information to patients:[4-6]

1. The patient's condition and/or diagnosis.
2. The nature and purpose of the proposed treatment, including the likelihood of success in the physician's practice.
3. Reasonable alternative measures related to the diagnosis and treatment and the probable outcome of these or the absence of any treatment.
4. The particular known inherent risks that are material to make an informed decision about whether to accept or reject the proposed treatment, and the consequences of refusing that treatment.

Standards of Disclosure

The states are split on the standard to determine what should be disclosed for patients to make informed decisions, but the modern trend is toward the "reasonable patient standard" of disclosure. Under the "reasonable patient standard," a physician must disclose all the information that a reasonable person would require to make a decision under the facts and circumstances of the case. Under the second standard, "the professional disclosure standard"[7,8] a physician must provide the same information that other physicians in the community would provide to patients in the same or similar circumstances. This standard is generally less stringent than "the reasonable person standard."[6,9]

What Needs to Be Disclosed?

Physicians do not need to disclose every remote risk associated with a surgical procedure. Nor do physicians have a duty to disclose risks that are common knowledge or obvious to the patient, such as the risk of infection following an operation.[10] The law only requires disclosure of risks that are *material,* judged by their seriousness or chance of occurrence. One court defined material information as "information . . . which the physician knows or should know would be regarded as significant by a reasonable person in the patient's position when deciding to accept or reject the recommended medical procedure."[11]

Some states legally require physicians to disclose specific risks, such as death.[12] Some states statutorily require that a physician meet both the reasonable person standard and the professional disclosure standard.[13,14]

Who Obtains a Patient's Informed Consent?

The physician who proposes to undertake a surgical procedure must be the one to obtain the patient's informed consent. The duty to obtain consent is nondelegable; physicians cannot ask nurses or other healthcare providers to obtain the patient's consent on their behalf. Obviously, the physician who's going to be taking care of the patient is the one best qualified to discuss that treatment and its risks and benefits with the patient.

A common practice in some hospitals is for a physician about to perform a procedure or an operation to write an order for the nurse to "obtain a signed consent form for the patient's chart." Consent forms obtained by nurses are worthless. Nurses, or for that matter a physician who is not skilled in performing the actual procedure, cannot obtain valid informed consent. If such practices only evidence that the physician explained to the patient the consent, that the patient had no further questions, and that the patient is signing the form to acknowledge that the physician obtained consent, then the form has some validity.

Documentation of Informed Consent

The physician should dictate into the patient's medical record a summary of the discussion held with the patient and the family concerning the enumerated elements of informed consent. Particular attention should be made to documenting those material risks discussed with the patient before obtaining the patient's consent.

Consent is a *process,* not a signature. A written, signed, separate consent form is not legally required under the doctrine of informed consent; however, hospitals and/or medical staffs may require its completion and the patient's signature on a standardized consent form. It is important to recognize that the signed form is not a substitute for the consent process. The signed piece of paper cannot replace the dialogue and exchange of information that occurs between the physician and the patient and the family, the answering of questions, and the ultimate agreement of the patient to undergo the medical or surgical intervention.[4]

However, a signed, written consent form does constitute some evidence of a valid consent. In some states, a written, signed consent form is presumed to be valid consent unless that presumption is rebutted by proof that the consent was obtained by fraud, deceit, or misrepresentation of a material fact.[15] Standard "blanket" authorization consent forms a patient signs when registering into the emergency department (ED) do not constitute "informed consent." No dialogue or consent process has yet taken place.

SPECIFIC SITUATIONS

Emergency Exception to Informed Consent

If a patient is unconscious or incapacitated such that he or she is unable to express consent, the law assumes the patient consented to treatment for the emergency situation. This implied legal consent is premised on first, the duties of informed consent are excused if irreparable harm and even death may result if the physician delays providing treatment, and second, the law assumes that a reasonable, competent, lucid adult would consent to life-saving treatment.[16,17]

Physicians need to recognize that the emergency treatment allowed is limited to the circumstances of the emergency; without consent, the physician should provide only that treatment required to resolve the emergency. Similarly, the emergency condition must require immediate medical attention, meaning there is not sufficient time to inform the patient or seek consent from another person.[18]

The courts disagree on the definition of a "true emergency." Whether the emergency exception applies depends on the definition accepted by the court and the particular set of facts. Fortunately, the courts generally stretch the doctrine to protect the physicians who act in good faith during a perceived emergency.[19,20] In these situations, documentation of the physician's concerns weigh greatly in the court's determination. Although physicians can further protect themselves by obtaining a second opinion that a true emergency exists, this scenario is not always practical.

In a major trauma case, the trauma team generally does not have time to agonize over these issues. At least one (and if possible, two) physicians should document that an emergency is present, and treat without obtaining consent. Documentation of a life or limb threat and the need for prompt action should protect the physicians from any liability. The physicians should attempt to secure and involve family members and obtain consent by other means as discussed earlier in the "General Rules" and in the following under the "Incompetent Patient" section.

Minors

MINOR ACCOMPANIED BY PARENT(S) OR LEGAL GUARDIAN

Parents or a child's legal guardian have the right to consent on behalf of their minor children. However, parents must act reasonably and in the best interest of their children. If they do not, their right to consent may be abrogated by the state or the courts. Parents are not allowed to refuse treatment for life-threatening injuries to a child. The management of injured children whose parents refuse to give their consent to treatment is discussed in the "Refusal of Care" section.

The general rules of consent apply equally to informing parents. Parents need the same understanding, material information, and risks and benefits one would give a competent adult to make an informed decision.

Either natural parent of the minor child may provide legally binding consent. If one parent agrees with your proposed treatment and the other does not, accept consent from the agreeing parent. Even if separated or divorced, either parent may give consent unless one parent has been judicially granted sole legal custody of the child. In this case, only the custodial parent may consent. The child's biological father, even if never married to the mother, may also consent for his child.

UNACCOMPANIED MINOR

Federal Law, the Emergency Medicine Treatment and Active Labor Act (EMTALA)[2] mandates that *all* persons presenting to an ED requesting care be examined to determine if an emergency condition is present. This federal law vitiates all state consent laws regarding the initial evaluation of a minor child. In essence, the child's request for an examination or treatment (or a request made by anyone on behalf of the minor) constitutes legal consent to determine if an emergency condition is present. For example, if a 14-year-old babysitter brings in a 2-year-old child because the child fell down the stairs, the hospital must, by law, evaluate the child to decide if an emergency condition is present. Furthermore, the hospital should never delay this initial screening evaluation to wait for consent. Examine the child; if no emergency is identified, then one can wait to obtain consent from the parents or guardian. If an emergency condition is present, proceed with treatment, since both EMTALA and legal exceptions to parental consent will protect the EP.

EMERGENCY MEDICAL CONDITION IDENTIFIED

If an emergency condition is discovered through the initial screening examination,[2,3] then the physician may treat the emergency under either state or federal legal theories. First, under state laws, the standard emergency exception doctrine applies. State laws allow physicians to proceed with treatment of an unaccompanied minor anytime an emergency exists. No uniform legal definition of emergency exists amongst the states, but state laws tend to liberally define an emergency. For example, an emergency may be defined as "any threat to the minor's life or health"[17] and the courts almost always affirm a physician's judgment regarding an emergency condition. States rarely question the treatment given to a minor without parental consent.[21] Preserving life, preventing permanent disability, alleviating pain and suffering, and avoiding eventual harm are used as guidelines for emergency treatment without consent.[21] The physician should perform a medical screening examination on any minor presenting to the ED to determine if an emergency exists.

If a physician *treats* (as opposed to simply examining) a minor without consent, the mere presence of an emergency is insufficient grounds to act. Not only must an emergency be present, but also the need for emergency treatment (before parental consent) must be clear. Two example cases illustrate this point. In *Jackovach v. Yocum*, a 7-year-old boy was injured in a train accident and required immediate surgery to amputate an arm and prevent exsanguination. The court very bluntly said "that when the surgeon was confronted with an emergency, endangering the life or health of the patient, he had a duty to do what the occasion demanded within the usual and customary surgical practice without the consent of the patient.[22] In the second case, *Rogers v. Sells*, a 14-year-old boy suffered a crush injury to one leg. The surgeon amputated the boy's foot without the permission of the parents. After expert testimony, the court held that the extremity was viable and the situation was not such an emergency that the physician couldn't wait to obtain consent from the parents before proceeding with the amputation.[23]

Under federal law, if an emergency medical condition is present, the hospital and physicians must provide "stabilizing treatment," since that term is defined by law.[3] Federal law also gives the physician broad discretion to decide what stabilization treatment should be done and in what time frame it should be accomplished. However, to date there are no federal cases on this point. Additionally, this stabilization requirement includes transfer to an institution capable of handling the minor's injuries if the initial hospital and physicians are unable to stabilize the patient.[1] Thus, under federal law, a minor could be examined, stabilized, and transferred to another institution for his or her traumatic injuries before consent from the family. Not only would the care be in the patient's best interest, but it would be legally correct.[2,3]

Nowhere does the "When in Doubt Rule" come into play more forcefully than in the treatment of unaccompanied minors. Physicians are much more likely to be held negligent for delaying care (and also potentially held in violation of federal law) if they wait to obtain parental consent, than if they acted in the child's best interest.[24] Simply asking oneself, "What would you want done if it was your child?" would generally lead the physician to the correct action on behalf of the minor.

NONEMERGENCY MEDICAL CONDITION IDENTIFIED

Generally, if the initial screening examination of the minor does not reveal an emergency condition, physicians need to obtain proper consent from the minor's parents or legal guardian. However, there are a number of exceptions that either state law or the courts have applied to allow minors to seek treatment on their own without parental consent. These exceptions vary widely from state to state, and most are applied on a case-by-case basis by the courts.

Under the *mature minor exception*, minors who possess the understanding of the nature and consequences of the treatment and appear competent to make their own decisions will be allowed to consent.[25] This exception is despite not having reached the age of the majority. Generally, a mature minor will be in the age range of 15 to 17 years.

The *emancipated minor* is also an exception to the need for parental consent. If the minor is living on his or her own, self-supporting, or in the Armed Forces, the courts may recognize the minor as emancipated and able to consent on his or her own. Again, this decision is determined by the courts on a case-by-case basis.[7] Additionally, most states have statutory reasons a minor may seek care without the consent of his or her parents. These reasons are generally non–trauma-related such as in the case of sexually transmitted diseases and pregnancy, but may also include domestic violence injuries.[26-28]

Incompetent or Incapacitated Adults

If an individual has been declared "legally incompetent" by a court, obtain routine consent from the person's court-appointed legal guardian. Even if not declared "legally incompetent" by a court, an individual may have appointed a surrogate to make legal decisions in case of incompetence. State sanctioned living wills, advanced directives, or durable medical powers of attorney all transfer consent powers from an individual who becomes incompetent to his or her legally appointed surrogate.[29]

If an incompetent adult has neither a legal guardian nor an appointed surrogate, physicians typically look to the patient's family for consent to treat. However, consent to treatment by the family, even the patient's spouse, is generally not acceptable under American law (unless the spouse or family member has been appointed legal guardian by a court of proper jurisdiction).[30] Marriage does not confer one spouse the legal capacity consent to medical treatment for the other spouse, even when that spouse is incompetent. However, never forget that it is *always* the family that sues for wrongful death. Flippant disregard for a family's wishes or a callous neglect for their input in medical decisions inevitably results in legal action.

Some states recognized this problem and enacted "family consent statutes," which provide a hierarchy of family members who can provide consent when a family member becomes incapacitated.[31] However, even when families have no legal standing to consent for the incompetent relative, it is always wise to involve family in the medical decision-making process. Communication and concern for the family avoids misunderstandings, surprise, and anger–the primary reasons for litigation. Fortunately, if a trauma emergency exists, no authorization from family is necessary to provide such reasonable care necessary to correct the life-threatening situation.

Once the emergency is resolved, or in nonemergency circumstances, consent will need to be obtained from someone authorized to act on behalf of the incompetent patient. If there is no legal guardian or surrogate appointed, and no state family consent statute, then the physicians need to seek consent authorization from the courts. The courts may appoint a guardian at that time, generally, but not always, a family member or the court itself. Under state statute and after judicial review, the family or the court may grant consent on behalf of the incapacitated person.[32]

Prisoners

COMPETENT PRISONERS

Competent prisoners generally do not surrender the right to consent by virtue of being incarcerated. However, a state or court may compel treatment based on interests perceived as paramount to the prisoner's interests.[33] For example, in North Carolina, if a prisoner refuses to consent to treatment for an intentionally self-inflicted injury, the chief medical officer of the prison may grant or withhold consent on behalf of the prisoner—over the objections of the prisoner.[34]

The elements usually necessary to treat self-inflicted injuries over the objection of the competent prisoner include the following:

1. The injury to the prisoner was willful and intentionally self-inflicted
2. The proposed operation or treatment is necessary to preserve or restore the health of the prisoner
3. The prisoner refused consent
4. The prison medical officer documents his or her findings in the prisoner's record[35]

INCOMPETENT PRISONER

If the prisoner is a trauma victim and needs immediate surgery or other treatment and is unconscious, incompetent, or otherwise incapacitated and incapable of giving consent, then the chief medical officer of the prison may consent on behalf of the prisoner. However, the consent of the prison medical office would be superfluous, since the "emergency doctrine" would be sufficient to allow the trauma surgeon to proceed with the emergency operation in the best interest of the patient.

Alchohol-Intoxicated Patients

Alcohol is the primary risk factor for motor vehicle crashes (MVCs) and all other types of trauma such as fractures, burns, drowning, assaults, and cases of domestic violence.[36] In one study, over 50% of patients presenting with major trauma were intoxicated with alcohol.[37] These patients frustrate the EP, both regarding consent and through their propensity to disrupt the ED.

Alcohol intoxication itself may not render a patient incompetent to give informed consent.[38] The EP must evaluate each situation individually to determine if the patient is incapacitated by alcohol to the extent that he or she is no longer able to understand the proposed treatment, risks and benefits, and rational alternatives. In essence, just because the patient is intoxicated with alcohol the EP can't disregard the general rules for determining whether the individual is competent to make informed decisions.

The "When in Doubt Rule" is particularly applicable in these cases, since alcohol intoxication causes a high incidence of occult serious injuries in trauma patients. If the EP feels that the intoxication has rendered the patient incompetent to refuse necessary emergency treatment, the EP should document this finding and proceed with his or her best judgment.

CONTROLLING THE AGITATED, COMBATIVE INTOXICATED TRAUMA PATIENT

Alcohol-intoxicated patients with altered mental status or who are combative become the responsibility of the emergency staff. These patients need to be protected from harming themselves, but also from harming other staff members, other patients, and potentially the public at large. Physicians should give verbal interventions only seconds to effect proper constraint. If words are not adequate, and the behavior potentially dangerous, then promptly initiate physical and/or chemical restraints. Physical restraints require an appropriate number of people to prevent harm to all concerned. State laws provide both criminal and civil immunity to physicians who in good faith restrain and treat patients after determining that the patients are a threat to themselves or others.[39]

Chemical restraints in the trauma patient are probably best done with the butyrophenones, haloperidol or droperidol (see Chapter 10). These drugs work within 5 to 10 minutes when given intravenously, and they have a very safe hemodynamic profile, particularly applicable in the trauma patient. Additionally, their half-life of 10 to 20 hours allows prolonged periods of control, which are necessary for the surgical and/or observational management of the traumatized patient. Benzodiazepines may be a better choice to chemically restrain patients intoxicated with cocaine or those who have recently seized.[40,41] In general however, butyrophenones are probably safer than benzodiazepines in the trauma victim.

Always consider organic causes of altered mental status such as closed head injury, hypoxia, hypoglycemia, hypotension, or ingestion of other intoxicating substances in the combative intoxicated trauma patient.

USE OF BLOOD ALCOHOL LEVELS

Any traumatized patient with significant altered mental status should have a serum alcohol done to determine if alcohol intoxication is a cause of the altered mental status. Alcohol intoxication, particularly if documented by a measured blood alcohol level, is strongly suggestive to courts and juries of impaired mental status, even though healthcare workers know many alcoholics who are entirely rational and competent at fairly high blood concentrations.[42] An example of how physicians can be protected by the courts by use of a serum level is the case of *Miller vs. Rhode Island Hospital.*[38] In this case, the court determined as a matter of law that a person's intoxication rendered him incapable of giving informed consent in an emergency situation. The patient, brought to the ED after a MVC, had a measured blood alcohol level of 0.233 mg%. The trauma team was concerned about potential internal injuries and informed the patient that a diagnostic peritoneal lavage was indicated, but the patient refused. The trauma team determined the patient lacked the capacity to fully understand and comprehend the extent of his injuries and judged him to be medically incompetent to refuse treatment. The patient tried to leave the ED but was physically restrained and the procedure carried out after intravenous anesthesia was administered. The patient sued the hospital for battery. The Supreme Court of Rhode Island ultimately determined that the patient's intoxication had the propensity to impair the patient's ability to give informed consent. It stated that the determination of whether a patient's intoxication rendered the patient incapable of giving informed consent depended on the specific circumstances, not solely the intoxication itself. The court stressed that medical competency depends on whether the patient could reasonably understand the medical condition and the nature of the proposed medical procedure, including the risks, benefits, and the available alternatives.[38]

Thus the patient's clinical capacity is more important than the specific level of alcohol in determining if the patient is competent. Conversely, low alcohol levels do not guarantee competence. Other processes such as hypoglycemia, blood loss, or other illicit substances may cause the patient to be incompetent.[43]

Another advantage of obtaining a serum alcohol level is that the level may be used in a criminal charge against the individual who may have been driving and caused a MVC. Approximately 14 states allow physicians discretion to report an intoxicated driver to authorities on the basis of a medical serum alcohol.[44] States may also allow blood alcohols drawn only for medical purposes to later be subpoenaed by the prosecutor for use against the driver in a driving while intoxicated (DWI) prosecution or other criminal charges.[45]

It is important to recognize that the state "legal limit" of intoxication is not a measure of a patient's competence. The legal level for driving has little, if anything, to do with capacity to make informed decisions. However, this situation is sometimes difficult for judges and juries to understand, and the EP can actually use the level to support his or her judgment that the patient was not competent to make informed decisions in a particular instance.

Drawing a blood alcohol can also make the care of an intoxicated patient more difficult. Some physicians believe that if they draw an alcohol level that returns above the legal limit to drive, they are mandated to draw a second level that is below the limit before discharge. They fear that if the patient is injured after discharge they will be liable. Indeed this situation may be a concern if the EP allows the patient to drive home while intoxicated. Apart from the DWI issue, there is no legal basis for the expensive practice of serial alcohol levels; however, it is a common medical-legal myth. Sometimes it is better to not have a "number" so the only relevant criterion for determining the patient's competence is the physician's judgment.

Patients Treated with Pain Medications

Obtaining informed consent from patients treated with pain medications before an operation is a common issue in trauma care. Similar to alcohol intoxication, *the mere fact that the patient's been administered narcotic analgesia does not render the patient incapable of consenting to surgical procedures.* Plaintiff attorneys can always argue "the patient was too snowed with drugs to give consent," but on the other hand, they can equally argue that the patient was "in too much pain to consent; they would've consented to anything to resolve the pain." The jury may consider it coercion if pain medication was withheld until the patient gave consent for a procedure. In regards to medical analgesics or anxiolytics and informed consent, the physician must judge (and document!) the patient's ability to understand the issues pertaining to the procedure. It is a good idea to involve the family in the process if possible. If narcotics are given before consent was obtained, the physician should document that the premedicated state was considered when judging the patient's competence to make an informed decision.

INFORMED REFUSAL OF MEDICAL CARE (AGAINST MEDICAL ADVICE)

The corollary to a patient's right to informed consent is the patient's right to refuse medical care, *even if such refusal results in death.* In *Cruzan v. The Director of Missouri Department of Health,* the United States Supreme Court determined that a *competent* adult has a constitutionally protected liberty interest to refuse medical care.[46] However, that right is not absolute. Under particular circumstances courts will consider countervailing compelling state interests such as preventing suicide, preserving life, and protecting innocent third parties.

General Rules

If a competent adult wants to refuse indicated medical intervention, it often is the result of fear, anger, misunderstanding, or some other failure in communications of the doctor-patient relationship. Before allowing a patient to refuse care, the physician should try to determine and resolve the underlying reasons behind the patient's refusal. Nurses and residents should always involve the attending physician when a patient expresses intent to leave against medical advice (AMA).[47]

As with consent, *refusal of medical care is a process,* not a signature. It must be an 'informed' refusal; merely having the patient sign an "Informed Consent to Refuse Examination, Treatment, or Transfer" form (or an "Against Medical Advice" form) is not enough. The four essential components of that process are:

1. **Competence.** The physician must determine that the patient is competent to make decisions. A normal mental status examination without evidence of diminished mental capacity from closed head injury, severe pain, hypoxia, hypotension, alcohol intoxication, mental retardation, or mind-altering substances is good evidence of competency. If a patient is permitted to leave AMA, document that he or she is alert, oriented times three, and appears to understand the issues involved.
2. **Informed Decision.** To be legally binding, a refusal/AMA decision must be an informed decision. The physician must explain the severity of the patient's condition, the potential complications, and the alternative treatments available. The physician should use terms that the patient can understand and provide the patient an opportunity to ask questions. The patient must understand that the risks of leaving include the possibility of permanent disability and death. Ideally a witness is present when the physician informs the patient and any family members.
3. **Family.** Involve the patient's family, friends, and personal physician whenever possible. These persons should hear the same message as the patient; they may be able to persuade the patient to accept the recommended therapy. If the patient expressly forbids you to speak with others, as is his or her legal right, explain this decision to the family and document it in the medical record.
4. **Documentation.** Appropriate documentation of the refusal process is necessary to protect the physician and hospital from litigation. Ask the patient to sign the refusal form; if he or she refuses to sign the form, document that fact, and have the form signed by a hospital representative who witnessed the patient's refusal. The medical record should reflect the patient's mental status examination and competency to make informed decisions, the risks and benefits of recommended treatments, the available alternatives, and identify the participating family or friends.

    Documenting the patient's rationale for refusing treatment, that the patient was treated to the extent allowed by the patient, and that the patient was welcome back at any time offers added protection.

Informed consent to refuse:

Examination Treatment Transfer

I understand that the hospital has offered: (Check all that apply).

A. To examine me (the patient) to determine whether I have an emergency medical condition, or

B. To provide medical treatment or to provide stabilizing treatment for my emergency condition (AMA), or

C. To provide a medically appropriate transfer to another medical facility.

The hospital and physician have informed me that the *benefits* that might reasonably be expected from the offered services are:

____

and the ***risks*** of the offered services are:

____

Physician Documentation

The patient appears competent and capable of understanding risks.

Alternative treatments discussed with the patient.

Patient's family involved. Family not available. Patient does not want family involved.

Signature of Physician ______________________________

I understand that if I refuse offered services, I am doing so against medical advice. I understand that my refusal may result in a worsening of my condition and could pose a threat to my life, health, and medical safety. I understand I am welcome to return at any time. I choose to refuse the offered services.

Signature/Patient or Legally Responsible Person ______________________________

Print Name ______________ Address ______________

City ______________ State/Zip ________ Date ________ Time ________

Witness/Signature ______________ Print Name ______________

Patient or person legally responsible for patient was offered but refused to sign form after explanation of their rights and the risk/benefits of the services offered:

Hospital representative who witnessed refusal to sign: ______________________________

Date ______________ Time ______________

Fig. 48-1 Example of an informed consent to refuse.

Physicians who honor a competent patient's decision to refuse treatment will not be subject to liability for any resulting bad outcome.[48,49] To avoid legal peril, have the patient sign a document that addresses the above four concerns (Fig. 48-1). Today, the physician is more likely to be successfully sued for treating competent patients over their objections even when the treatment is life saving.[50]

Parent(s) or Guardian Refuses Care of Blood Transfusion for Minor

Generally, state laws support parental control of health issues affecting their children. However, the state will not allow parents to deny children needed emergency medical care under the doctrine "parens patriae"—the state's paternalistic interest in children.[51] All states empower EPs to intercede under their child abuse and child neglect laws.[52]

Any time a child's injuries are potentially life threatening, the EP or surgeon can take custody of the child under the child abuse laws and provide indicated treatment, including blood transfusions. When treating against the parents' wishes, always document the life threats and the need for immediate action. When deciding whether to act, the "when-in-doubt-rule" definitely applies. All jurisdictions statutorily protect physicians from criminal and civil liability for acting in good faith to protect children.[52]

The courts have specifically addressed the issue of

Jehovah's Witness parents who refuse emergency blood transfusions for their minor children. All jurisdictions hold that a parent's right to freedom of religion does not include the right to deny life-sustaining medical intervention for their minor children.[53,54] One judge best summarized the feelings of the courts: "Not even a parent has unbridled discretion to exercise his or her religious beliefs when the state's interest in preserving the health of the children within its borders weighs in the balance."[55]

Some states specifically address the issue of overriding parental refusal of indicated medical intervention. For example, in North Carolina, if the parents refuse to consent to treatment, a physician can render treatment without parental consent if the following conditions are met: (1) the delay to obtain a court order would seriously worsen the child's physical condition or endanger life; and (2) a second physician agrees that the procedure is necessary to prevent immediate harm. If it is not possible to contact a second physician before initiating treatment, then the physician may still perform the indicated procedure without parental consent.[56]

Conversely, courts refuse to rule against the wishes of the parents when the child's medical condition is not serious or life threatening.[57] If there is no life threat or potential for serious impairment, the parent's refusal should be respected. Parental refusal of indicated nonemergency medical treatment is usually statutorily defined as child neglect, which is not legally sufficient to take custody of the child. Child neglect should still be reported to the appropriate authorities; treatment for the child may then be obtained under a court order.[52]

Adult Jehovah's Witnesses and Blood Transfusions

> *"Nothing in Life Is More Wonderful than Faith–The One Great Moving Force Which You Can Neither Weigh in the Balance nor Test in the Crucible"*
>
> **Sir William Osler 1910**

There are approximately 1 million Jehovah's Witnesses in the United States. They steadfastly believe blood transfusion destroys their relationship with God and forfeits their chance for eternal life; accepting transfusion is not a minor infraction of their faith.[58] They do not accept whole blood, packed cells, platelets, white cells, plasma, or autotransfusion of stored blood. Most will allow the use of crystalloids, albumin, hemophiliac preparations, immunoglobulins, dialysis, and heart-lung machines.[58,59] However, autotransfusion of blood salvaged from the chest or peritoneum is often acceptable. Jehovah's Witnesses and the issue of blood transfusion presents very difficult medical-legal issues in the emergency care of the trauma patient.[60] State courts may have widely divergent views or may not have yet addressed the difficult situations faced by trauma specialists. There are no clear-cut answers, but the trend is definitely toward greater autonomy to refuse blood, even when the state asserts compelling interests to override a person's refusal.

General principles and the 'when-in-doubt-rule' apply, but hospitals and medical staff should additionally undertake the following:

1. Develop Policies and Procedures in an advance to resolve potential conflicts and deal with Jehovah's Witness patients.
2. Coordinate each case with hospital legal counsel, in contact with a judge who can issue court orders when appropriate, if time allows.
3. Have other physician consultants write notes of agreement regarding the need to give blood.
4. Communicate effectively with patients and family, in advance when possible.

COMPETENT ADULT JEHOVAH'S WITNESS

"The competent adult has the right to refuse a transfusion regardless of whether his refusal to do so arises from fear of adverse reaction, religious belief, recalcitrance, or cost,"[61] and "even though we may consider a patient's beliefs unwise, foolish, or ridiculous."[62] However, even this right is not absolute. If the individual's refusal conflicts with compelling state interests such as the preservation of life, the prevention of suicide, or the protection of innocent third parties, the courts may order transfusions despite the individuals objections.[60,63,64]

Typical scenarios where the courts override a competent person's refusal include pregnant women to protect the life of the fetus, mothers of young children to promote the general welfare of the children, or a sole supporting father or mother to avoid offspring from becoming wards of the state.[64-66]

However, recent court decisions significantly restrict hospitals' or the state's ability to assert compelling interests challenging a competent individual's right of self-determination. In the case of *In re Fetus Brown*, the Illinois Appellate Court recently held that the state could not force a 34-week pregnant woman to accept a blood transfusion to save the life of her fetus.[67] The state asserted its interest in preserving the life of the fetus and the welfare of the woman's other children at home. The husband and grandparents testified they were willing and able to take care of the other children. The court balanced the mother's constitutional right to refuse treatment against the state's interest in the fetus, and concluded the state could not override a competent pregnant woman's decision.[67]

Three other state courts recently refused to allow transfusion of a pregnant female over her religious objections when a hospital (often asserting the state's interest in preventing the "abandonment" of the infant) went to court to obtain a court order to initiate transfusions. The courts ruled the hospitals did not have legal standing to assert the state's interests to override a competent patient's choice.[68-71] The implication of these cases is that hospitals must request the State's attorney general to intervene, who then decides whether to seek a court order authorizing the transfusion. The courts may or may not decide the issue differently when the state itself petitions the court.

UNCONSCIOUS OR MEDICALLY INCOMPETENT ADULT JEHOVAH'S WITNESSES

Religious Beliefs and Transfusion Preferences *Unknown* to the Physician. In an emergency, if the Jehovah's Witness' beliefs are unknown, physicians may transfuse the patient because consent is implied under the emergency doctrine.[72,73] It is irrelevant if the spouse, mother, or other family members adamantly refuse to allow the transfusion for religious reasons. The state's compelling interest in preserving life outweighs the family's expression of the patient's religious preferences.[72]

Religious Beliefs and Transfusion Preferences *Known* to the Provider. In the past, when a Jehovah's Witness's beliefs and transfusion preferences were known in advance but the patient was incompetent at the time of the emergency, the courts tended to support transfusion until the patient became competent and could refuse transfusion contemporaneously.[53,74] However, the law in this area is in a state of flux, and the immediate care of the trauma patient is best addressed by answering the enigmatic question:

Should cards carried by patients identifying them as members of the Jehovah's Witness Faith, setting out their religious objection to blood transfusion, be considered adequate evidence for physicians to rely on to not administer blood transfusions in an emergency?

Presently in the United States, the trend is toward accepting the card as a form of advanced directive binding on hospitals and physicians. In at least six states, if the card is dated and signed before two witnesses, it is statutorily valid.[70,75] Michigan's state's Patient Advocate Designation Statute requires patient advocates to follow the instructions given by the patient, including clear and convincing instructions to refuse life-sustaining treatment the patient would find objectionable on religious grounds.[76]

Even if the blood refusal card does not conform to a state's advanced directive statute, it should be considered strong evidence, but not necessarily determinative, of the Jehovah's Witness's wishes. Advanced directives are merely a means to express an individual's rights, they are not the exclusive means to legally express those rights.[29,70] Jehovah's Witnesses are learning to use state statutorily defined advanced directive methods to legally express their intentions.[8]

The Canadian case of *Malette v. Shulman*[77] awarded the patient $20,000 for the physician administering a transfusion despite knowledge of the refusal card. The court stated "Only if there is evidence to cast doubt on whether the card was a true expression of the patient's opinion is a physician justified in transfusing a patient."

Failure to honor Jehovah's Witnesses' expressed refusal of blood exposes hospitals and physicians to monetary damages under battery or negligence theories.[8,78,79] Increasingly, plaintiffs are winning suits for six-figure damages against physicians who treat patients against their expressed wishes.[8,50]

Interestingly, no Jehovah's witness has successfully sued a healthcare provider to recover damages in cases where blood was *withheld* on the basis of an apparently valid blood refusal card.[80] In addition, according to one author "Criminal, civil, or professional misconduct liability has never been imposed on healthcare providers for forgoing treatment the patient did not want."[81]

If the EP finds a card in the wallet of an unconscious trauma patient stating that the carrier will not accept a blood transfusion, most current legal thinking suggests that the physician should honor the document. However, some EPs may decide to give blood despite this card, because the patient *might* accept blood in the *current* life-threatening circumstances (if they were conscious). This line of reasoning has some historic support in U.S. courts. Some courts have stated that the mere carrying of the card is not conclusive evidence of the patient's understanding and wishes.[53,74,82,83] The courts inquire further into how recently the card had been executed, circumstances surrounding its execution, or whether the individual had signed the card as an affirmation of faith and unity with members of his or her congregation, or whether he or she had actually contemplated it to be binding in life-threatening situations. Courts also want to examine intervening circumstances to determine if the card currently expresses a patient's true, firm convictions regarding blood transfusions. In other words, how strong is the person's present religious conviction?[53,74]

These courts believe that, "Where there is an emergency, calling for an immediate decision, nothing else than a fully conscious *contemporaneous* decision by the patient himself would be sufficient to override evidence of medical necessity."[53]

The Michigan case of *Werth v. Taylor*[74] provides an excellent example of just how contemporaneous the event must be. A woman was admitted to the hospital to deliver twins. Two months previously she had completed a form expressing her refusal to accept blood transfusion on religious grounds. At the time of admission to the hospital, she and her husband signed another form reaffirming their opposition to blood transfusion. A few days after delivery she had uterine bleeding necessitating a D&C. Physicians again discussed the issue of possible blood transfusions with the patient and husband, who again reiterated their refusal to accept transfused blood. Hours later, when the patient was placed under general anesthesia and the procedure performed, hemorrhage ensued and the anesthesiologist determined blood transfusion was necessary to save the plaintiff's life.

The court pointed out that the patient was unconscious when the transfusion was needed and that the urgency of the transfusion was not anticipated since it was thought the surgery would relieve the bleeding. In the court's view, these circumstances prevented the woman's previously expressed views from being a truly informed and contemporaneous refusal of treatment, and thus did not override the implied consent recognized by the law for treatment of a life-threatening emergency, which is necessary to preserve a patient's life.[74]

Refusal of Care Summary

1. A competent, nonsuicidal adult who is fully informed of the risk of his or her decision may refuse treatment, including life-saving treatment or emergency transfusions.
2. A noncompetent adult, a suicidal patient, or a minor child with a life-threatening illness cannot refuse emergency medical treatment, and EPs have an affirmative duty to treat these individuals and protect them from harm. In the case of the noncompetent adult, document the reasons why the physician believes the patient to be incompetent.
3. If a minor child is not suicidal or suffering from a life-threatening condition, then competent parents may refuse care on behalf of their child in the ED. However, the courts may intervene on behalf of the child under the state's child neglect laws.
4. When in doubt about any competency or consent issue, err on the side of patient safety. The courts usually protect physicians from legal consequences.

CONCLUSIONS

Consent issues in the emergency management of the trauma patient can be difficult, frustrating, and of significant consequence to both the patient and the physician. Respect for an individual's right of self-determination, a truly informed consent process, and appropriate communication with patients and families can resolve the vast majority of consent situations. In immediate life-threatening emergencies, the "emergency doctrine" exception and the "when-in-doubt" rule should guide the physician. However, all physicians need to have a working knowledge of the general consent statutes and the common law of the state in which they practice. Physicians also need to work with the hospital administrators and legal counsel to educate the clinical staff and to develop policies and procedures to resolve problems with informed consent issues when they arise.

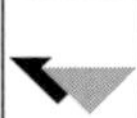

PEARLS & PITFALLS

- Documentation—juries may believe the "not documented, not done" rule. They may suspect trial testimony as self-serving. The medical record made at the time of the patient encounter is usually accepted as the best account of actual events.
- Sources of malpractice litigation. Although a bad outcome certainly prompts lawsuits, misunderstandings, surprise, and anger are primary motivations for litigation.
- Delaying treatment in an emergency to obtain informed consent is a much more serious and a much more common medicolegal problem than failure to obtain proper informed consent.
- In any consent case, use the "When in Doubt Rule." This rule is "Do what you believe in the patient's best interest and worry about the legal consequences later."

- During a trauma resuscitation, a physician might not obtain consent to treat an incompetent patient, or may treat despite a patient's refusal. This intervention is legal if the physician can document why they believed the patient was incompetent, *and* attest to the fact that the emergency condition was life or limb threatening.
- A written, signed, separate consent form is not legally required under the doctrine of informed consent; however, hospitals and/or medical staffs may require its completion.
- Emergency exception: If a patient is unconscious or incapacitated such that they are unable to express consent, the law will assume the patient consented to treatment for the emergency.
- The physician should perform a medical screening examination on any minor presenting to the ED to determine if an emergency exists.
- Simply asking oneself, "What would you want done if it was your child?" would generally lead the physician to the correct action on behalf of the minor.
- Alcohol and Drugs. The EP must evaluate each situation individually to determine if the patient is incapacitated by alcohol to the extent that they no longer understand the proposed treatment, risks and benefits, and rational alternatives.
- Alcohol levels. The patient's clinical capacity is more important than the specific level of alcohol in determining if the patient is competent. Drawing a blood alcohol level for medico-legal reasons (as opposed to medical reasons in a trauma patient with an altered sensorium) is a sword that cuts both ways.
- Pain medication and consent. The law does not require pain medications to be withheld before obtaining informed consent. If such medication is given before the consent process, document the patient's clinical capacity to understand the procedure.
- Restraints. State laws provide both criminal and civil immunity to physicians who in good faith restrain and treat patients after determining that the patients are a threat to themselves or others. Document the need for restraints and the fact that the patient does not appear competent.
- Leaving Against Medical Advice. As with consent, refusal of medical care is a process, not a signature. It must be an "informed" refusal.
- Jehovah's Witnesses. Most legal theory holds that a physician should honor a "Do Not Transfuse" card under most circumstances. If a competent patient refuses a life-saving transfusion, they are within their rights.

REFERENCES

1. Schloendoff v. The Society of New York Hospital, 211 N.Y. 125 (NY 1914).
2. 42 USC 1395dd(a).
3. 42 USC 1395dd(b).
4. Katz J: *The silent world of doctor and patient,* 1984, Free Press.
5. Cobbs v. Grant, 502 P2d 1 (Calif.1972).
6. Furrow B, et al: The liability of health care professionals, *Health Law* 409-447, 1995.
7. Cal Civ Code Section 62 (West 1979) Wyo. Stat. Section 14-1-101 (1981).
8. Ridley DT: Honoring Jehovah's Witnesses' advanced directives in emergencies: a response to Drs. Migden and Braen, *Acad Emerg Med* 5:824-835, 1998.
9. Wells v. Van Nort, 125 NE 910 (Ohio 1919).
10. Percle v. St Paul Fire and Marine Insurance Co., 349 So2d 1289(1977).
11. Truman v. Thomas, 611 P.2d 902 (1980).
12. Iowa Code Ann Section 147.137(West 1989).
13. ALA Code Section 6-5-484 (1990).
14. N.C. Gen. Stat. Section 90-21.13.
15. N.C. Gen. Stat. Section 90-21.13(b).
16. Canterberry v. Spence, 464 F2d 772(D.C. Cir) *cert denied,* 409 US 1064 (1972).
17. Dunham v. Wright, 423 F 2d 940 (3rd Cir. 1970) – Emergency Exception.
18. Wheeler v. Barker, 208 P2d 6068 (1949).
19. Sullivan v. Montgomery 279NYS 575(1935) definition of EMC for minors stretched.
20. Thomson v. Sun City Community Hospital, 668 P 2d 605 (1984).
21. Tsai AK, et al: Evaluation treatment of minors: reference on consent, *Ann Emerg Med* 22:1211-1217, 1993.
22. Jackovach v. Yocum 237 NW 444 (1931).
23. Rogers V. Sells, 178 Okla 103 (1936).
24. Holder A: Minors' right to consent to medical care, *JAMA* 257: 3400-3402, 1987.
25. Cardwell v. Bechtol, 1724 S.W.2d 739(TN 1987).
26. Colo. Rev. Stat. Section 13-22-103 (1979).
27. Mass. Gen. Laws Ann. Chapter 112, Section 12F (West 1975).
28. N.C. Gen. Stat. Section 130A-135; Section 90-21.5(a).
29. Collin F, Lombard J, Moses A, Spitler H: *Durable powers of attorney and health care directives*, ed 3, Colorado Springs, 1997, Shepard's.
30. In Re Quinlan, 335 A2d 647 (1976).
31. Ark. Stat. Ann. Section 41-41-3 (1984); Idaho Code Section 39-4305 (1975); Wells v. Van Nort, 125 NE 910 (Ohio 1919).
32. Cal. Probate Code Section 3,200-3,211(West 1981); Va. Code Section 371.1-134.2 (1982).
33. Commissioner of Corrections v. Myers, 399 NE2d 452 (1979).
34. N.C. Gen. Stat. Section 148-46.2.

35. N.C. Gen. Stat. Section 148-22.2; La. Rev. Stat. Ann. Section 15.860.
36. 7th Special Report to Congress on Alcohol and Health: National Institute on Alcohol Abuse and Alcoholism. Rockville, MD, Department of Health and Human Services, 1990.
37. Fantus RJ, et al: Driving under the influence: a level one trauma center's experience, *J Trauma* 31:1517-1520, 1991.
38. Miller v. Rhode Island Hospital, 625 A2d 778 (R.I. 1993).
39. Henry GL: Risk Management and high-risk issues in emergency medicine, *Emerg Med Clin North Am* 11:905-922, 1993.
40. Thomas H Jr, Schwartz E, Petrilli R: Droperidol versus haloperidol for chemical restraint of agitated and combative patients, *Ann Emerg Med* 21:407-13, 1992.
41. Richards JR, et al: Chemical restraints for the agitated patient in the emergency department: lorazepam vs. droperidol, *J Emerg Med* 16:567-573, 1998.
42. Siegel DM: Consent and refusal of treatment, *Emerg Med Clin North Am* 11:833-840, 1993.
43. Etherington JM: Emergency management of acute alcohol problems, *Can Fam Physician* 42:2423-2431, 1996.
44. Emerg Med News Vol 18, No 7, July 1996, page 1.
45. Mich. Comp. Laws Ann. Section 257.625a(9).
46. Cruzan v. Director, Missouri Department of Health, 497 U.S. 261,279 (1990).
47. Dubow D, Propp D, Narasimhan K: Emergency department discharges against medical advice, *J Emerg Med* 10:513-516, 1992.
48. Rodriguez v. Pinol, 634 So2d 681 (Fla. Ct. App.1994).
49. Wons v. Public Health Trust, 500 So. 2d 679, 686 (Fla. Dist. Ct. App. 1987).
50. Rodriguez KF: Suing health care providers for saving lives: Liability for providing unwanted life-sustaining treatment, *J Leg Med* 20:1-66, 1999.
51. Goldstein J: Medical care for the child at risk: state supervision of parental autonomy, *Yale Law J* 86:645-670, 1977.
52. Sullivan DJ. Patient discharge against medical advice, *Emerg Depart Legal Letter* 7:91-100, 1996.
53. In Re Estate of Dorone, 534 A. 2d 1271 (PA. 1985).
54. Jehovah's Witness of Washington v. Kings County Hospital, 278 F Supp 488 (D.C. 1967) affirmed *per curiam* 390 US 598 (1968).
55. Nowak v. Cobb County-Kennestone Hosp. Authority, 74 F2d 1173, (1996).
56. N.C. Gen. Stat. Sections 90-21.1-3.
57. In Re Green, 292 A2D 387, (Pa. 1972).
58. Cox M, Lumley J: No blood or blood products, *Anaesthesia* 50: 583-585, 1995.
59. Migden DR, Braen GR: The Jehovah's Witness blood refusal card: ethical and medicolegal considerations for emergency physicians, *Acad Emerg Med* 5:815-824, 1998.
60. Spence RK: The Jehovah's Witness patient and medicolegal aspects of transfusion medicine, *Semin Vasc Surg* 7:121-126, 1994.
61. St. Mary's Hospital v. Ramsey, 465 So2d 666 (1985).
62. In re Brooks Estate, 205 NE2d 435 (1965).
63. Hartman KM, Liang BA: Exceptions to informed consent in emergency medicine, *Hosp Physician* 35:53-60, 1999.
64. In re Osborne, 294 A2d 372 (DC Ct. App. 1972).
65. Hamilton v. McAuliffe, 352 A2d 634 (MD 1976).
66. In re Winthrop Univ. Hosp. 490 NYS2d 996 (Sup.Ct. 1985); In re Melideo, 390 NYS2d 523 (1976).
67. In re Fetus Brown, No. 1-96-2316, Dec. 31, 1997, Ill. App. Ct.
68. Fosimire V. Nicholeau, 551 NE2d 77 (NY 1990).
69. In re Dubreuil, 629 So2d 819 (Fla. 1993).
70. Md. Ann. Code 43 Section 135C (1980).
71. Stamford Hosp. v. Vega, 236 Conn. 646 (1996).
72. John F. Kennedy Mem. Hosp. v. Heston, 279 A2d 670 (NJ 1971).
73. University of Cincinnati Hospital v. Edmond, 506 NE2d 299 (1986).
74. Werth v. Taylor, 475 N.W.2d 426 Mich. App. (1991).
75. Colo. Rev. Stat. Ann §§ 15-14-504(b), -504(b)(3), -505(2), -506(1); Fla. Stat. Ann. § 765.101(1); Ky. Rev. Stat. Ann. §§ 311.621(2), .637(6); Me. Rev. Stat. Ann. Tit. 18A, §§ 5-801(a), -801(I), -802(a), -804; Md. Code Ann., Health-Gen. §§ 5-601(b), -602(c), -603, -611(e)(2); 79 Op. Att'y Gen. No. 94-028 n.13 (Md. 1994); N.M. Stat. Ann. §§ 24-7A-1(A), -2, -4, -16(A).
76. Mich. Comp. Laws Ann. Section 700.496(9).
77. Malette v. Shulman, 72 O.R.2d 417 (Ont. Ct. App. 1990).
78. Jones v. Wrona, No. 94 L 2935 (Cir. Ct. Will County (Ill.) Nov. 12, 1997).
79. Sargeant v. New York Infirmary-Beekman Downtown Hospital, No. 16068-91 (Sup. Ct. NY County July 25, 1994).
80. Zeitz E: Legal reasoning and medical decision making, *Acad Emerg Med* 5:755-757, 1998.
81. Cohen: Refusing and foregoing treatment, *Treatise on Health Care Law* 18.07[2], 1997.
82. Corlett V. Caserta, 562 N.E.2d 257 (1990).
83. In re Hughes, 611 A2d 1148, 1152 (NJ Super App Div 1992).

Trauma Team Response: Management and Leadership

49

THOM A. MAYER

"A team is a small number of people with complementary skills who are committed to a common purpose, performance goals, and approach for which they hold themselves mutually accountable."

Jon R. Katzenbach and Douglas K. Smith
The Wisdom of Teams[1]

The care of the trauma patient is a team activity. The trauma team comprises multiple providers from diverse backgrounds practicing in a unique and challenging setting. Its central goal is to produce the best outcome for injured patients. At its best, the care of the trauma patient is like a symphony in which the team members anticipate each other's needs before they are even articulated. Leadership may vary between the surgeon and emergency physician (EP), but the focus is constant. This emphasis is on the needs of the patient, not on issues of turf, ego, or prestige. Indeed it is instructive to note that Katzenbach and Smith do not mention the leader or team captain in their definition.[1]

At its worst, the trauma "team" exists in name only—a crowd working at different purposes, with no common goals. A dysfunctional team produces a cacophony of shouts and commands, often contradictory and competitive—inarticulate, and unfocused. Further, during quality improvement review, interaction degenerates into recriminations, focusing on "Whose fault was it?" These interactions are the "other" ABCs of trauma care: accuse, blame, and criticize. All measures should be taken to avoid this paradigm, to ensure that the care of all injured patients is exemplary—not dysfunctional.

NATURE OF A TEAM

Although Katzenbach and Smith did not focus on trauma teams specifically in their seminal work, they accurately described the most important elements of the trauma team, which include the following:

1. Diverse people
2. Complementary skills
3. Clearly defined goals
4. Defined approach to the problem
5. Mutual accountability

DIVERSE PEOPLE

The composition of the trauma team varies, depending on institutional resources and the acuity of the patient. Academic institutions typically have more available manpower and, consequently, larger trauma teams than community hospitals. It should be pointed out that numbers do not always equal strength. In fact, too many people in the room may be as great a handicap as too few. A small, well-organized team can provide excellent care to even the most severely injured patient. When designing a trauma team, many institutions follow the guidelines developed by the American College of Surgeons Committee on Trauma[2-3] and the American College of Emergency Physicians Trauma Committee.[4] Special teams may be needed for pediatric or obstetrical resuscitations.

To an increasing degree, trauma activation systems have used a tiered response to match the needs of each individual patient. This tiered classification of trauma victims occurs through a blend of anatomic, physiologic, and mechanism of injury criteria (Box 49-1). Patients are categorized from the most severely injured to least severely injured, and designated with easily recognizable terminology, such as Code Blue, Code Yellow, Code White, and Trauma Consult.[5] The more severely injured the patient, the more intensive the response. Based on accumulated data, the criteria for identification of these patients are continuously updated and revised. This concept ensures that the

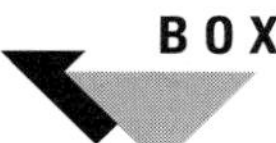

BOX 49-1

Code Blue, Yellow, White Trauma Response Criteria

1. *Code Blue Trauma Triage Parameters*
   The purpose of a Code Blue with full trauma team response is to ensure the rapid and orderly arrival of the patient to the operating suite and the immediate management of traumatic life-threatening airway, breathing, and circulatory problems identified in the prehospital setting.
   A. Airway and breathing emergencies
   B. Systolic blood pressure of <90 with signs and symptoms of shock
   C. Glasgow Coma Scale (GCS) score of <8
   D. Paralysis
   E. Penetrating injury to the head/neck/torso
   F. Crush to torso/upper thighs
   G. Major amputations
2. *Code Yellow Trauma Triage Parameters*
   The purpose of a Code Yellow with a modified trauma team response is to rapidly assess patients who have no significant physiologic impairments but have a high index of suspicion for occult injury because of the mechanism of injury or anatomic alterations and need a rapid evaluation. If necessary, these patients will be upgraded to CODE BLUE should the patient's condition warrant. Code Yellow requires a physiologic or anatomic alteration, or a significant mechanism of injury.
   A. Physiological alterations
      - Loss of consciousness >5 minutes
      - Pregnancy of >3 months
   B. Anatomic alterations
      - Maxillofacial trauma
      - Significant subcutaneous air
      - Evidence of pelvic instability
      - Two or more long bone deformities
      - Major lacerations involving fascia
   C. Mechanism of injury
      - *Stab wound* to the head/neck/torso *AND* stable vital signs
      - Ejection from vehicle
      - Pedestrian struck >15 miles per hour (mph)
      - Motorcycle accident >25 mph
      - Motor vehicle crash >35 mph
      - Documented falls >20 feet
      - Burns (meeting ABA Referral Criteria)
        * Second and third degree burns of >10% body surface area (BSA) in patients <10 years or >50 years of age
        * Second and third degree burns of >20% BSA in other age groups
        * Second and third degree burns with serious threat of functional or cosmetic impairment that involve face, hands, feet, genitalia, perineum, or major joints
        * Third degree burns >5% BSA in any age group
        * Significant electrical burn injuries including lightning injury
        * Chemical injuries with serious threat of functional or cosmetic impairment
        * Inhalation injury with burn injury
        * Circumferential burns of an extremity or chest
        * Burn injury in patients with preexisting medical disorders that could complicate management, prolong recovery, or affect mortality
        * Any burn patient with concomitant trauma (e.g. fractures) in which the burn injury poses the greatest risk of morbidity/mortality. However, if the trauma poses the greater immediate risk, the patient may be treated in a trauma center initially until stable, before being transferred to a burn center. Physician judgment will be necessary in such situations, and should be in concert with the regional medical control plan and triage protocols.
        * Burned children should be transferred to a hospital with qualified personnel and equipment
3. *Code White Trauma Triage Parameters*
   A. Trauma victims for whom cardiopulmonary resuscitation (CPR) has been initiated before arrival, with no evidence of patient response, *AND* trauma is due to:
      1. Blunt trauma
      2. Gunshot wound to the head
      3. Traumatic asphyxiation
      4. Burn
      5. Lightning strike/electrical shock
   B. Code White status patients should be upgraded to a Code Blue or Code Yellow patient should the patient become viable.

specific needs of patients are met in a cost-effective manner.

The trauma team members are listed in Box 49-2. This list typifies an academic level 1 trauma center team and is comprehensive. Trauma teams at regional community hospitals are typically smaller. One of the primary differences between Code Blue and Code Yellow patients is the necessity of immediate bedside consultation by the trauma surgeon, since a small percentage of such patients require an immediate operation.[6-8]

BOX 49-2
Trauma Team Members*

CODE BLUE RESPONSE TEAM
Emergency Medicine Physician
Trauma Surgeon
Emergency Medicine Resident†
Senior Surgical Resident†
Trauma Surgical Resident†
Trauma Critical Care Fellow†
Trauma Nurse Responder
Emergency Medicine Trauma Nurse
Recorder Nurse
Respiratory Therapist
X-ray Technician (2)
ED Technician
Social Worker
Total: 12-14 Team Members

CODE YELLOW RESPONSE TEAM
Emergency Medicine Physician
Emergency Medicine Resident†
Senior Surgical Resident
Trauma Critical Care Fellow†
ED Trauma Nurse (2)
Respiratory Therapist
X-ray Technician
Total: 8 Team Members

CODE WHITE RESPONSE TEAM
Emergency Medicine Attending
Emergency Medicine/Senior Surgical Resident†
Trauma RN Team Leader
Respiratory Therapist
Trauma Nurse Team Leader (Recorder)
Social Worker
ED Registrar
Total: 7 Team Members

*Additional personnel may also be involved in any trauma case at the discretion of the team captain. These might include: Operating Suite Nurse(s), Administrative Director, trauma Research Assistant, ED Technician, Consultants, Pediatric Intensivist (Pediatric Code Blue), OB/GYN Physician, Flight RN or paramedic.
†Additional Emergency Medicine Physicians and trauma surgeons may substitute for Residents and Fellows at community hospitals without training programs.

COMPLEMENTARY SKILLS

Nurses and Physicians

Physicians and nurses are educated with a different emphasis and focus. Physicians are educated in an "ends driven" manner, and are likely to modify their management approach depending on the clinical circumstances. Physicians reason through the potential diagnoses and consider various treatments, to develop a course of action.[9] Nursing education is more "process-driven."[10] Nurses tend to adhere to protocols and may resist deviations from historical precedent. The degree to which protocols are followed may be a source of tension between physicians and nurses. Residents unfamiliar with the trauma algorithms may create further friction or unease. Physician and nursing leaders must remain sensitive to these important philosophic and operational differences.

Nurses coordinate many vital activities within the trauma bay, including bedside care, trauma circulation, recording of the trauma flow sheet (see the following discussion), transition to in-patient care, participation in trauma quality improvement, and the ongoing design of trauma protocols.

In some trauma facilities, a specified and limited group of emergency department (ED) and/or intensive care unit (ICU) nurses function as trauma responders. However, it is advantageous to cross-train all ED nurses in trauma resuscitation. In situations where only an isolated group of the nurses are trained in trauma response, vacations, illness, and multiple-trauma incidents can strain the system.

Surgeons and Emergency Physicians

Although the vast majority of trauma surgeons and EPs work in a close, cooperative, and collegial fashion, others do not. In some centers, battles rage regarding who is the "captain of the ship" or the "admiral of the fleet."[11] Each camp believes the patient is "theirs." In the playground vernacular, the trauma surgeon might feel the EP should "move out of the way," whereas the EP resents the surgeon coming into his or her yard and "stealing the ball." These attitudes are team destroying and impede patient care. To maintain a cohesive team, EPs and trauma surgeons must work cooperatively.[3-5] Both parties should possess considerable expertise in the early assessment and stabilization of the injured patient. In many centers the team captain role is alternated between emergency medicine and trauma. This set-up provides an equitable and shared approach to leadership, and allows individuals to maintain their skills.

Controversy of Airway Management

One of the most contentious areas of early trauma care relates to management of the airway. Emergency physicians, surgeons, and anesthesiologists each have a sense of ownership, a different approach, and strong opinions on this matter. However, few would argue that airway management is the most important intervention in the acute stabilization of the injured patient. Success requires the highest level of cooperation and mutual understanding.

Although opinions and local practice may vary, the EP is the team member best suited for airway management for several reasons: (1) he or she is immediately available to respond to the trauma room, (2) he or she is skilled in the assessment of the injured patient, (3) he or she should possess substantial experience with airway management techniques, including rapid sequence intubation (RSI), and (4) he or she should be familiar and proficient with alternative airway management techniques. To fill this role in a credible and effective manner, the EP must strive to develop and maintain the skills required to provide nothing short of expert airway management. Interdepartment cooperation during the development of protocols and quality assurance facilitates the process.

CLEARLY DEFINED GOALS

The common purpose of the trauma team is clear: to offer the best possible clinical care for each patient evaluated and treated and to set the stage for healing for the patient and his or her family at the earliest possible time. In academic institutions, a related but secondary goal is the education of medical students, residents, fellows, and allied health personnel who constitute the future of trauma care. A commitment to research is essential to the future of our specialty. The attainment of these goals requires constant effort (Box 49-3).

Mission Statement

First, the team needs to be guided by clearly stated goals or mission statement, mutually agreed to by the respective members of the team. Leaders must communicate the central goals and mission to new team members during the course of orientation.

Second, it is important that leaders constantly promote these goals. They can be accentuated during quality improvement review, trauma morbidity and mortality conference, educational conferences, the trauma committee, and through daily interaction in the trauma room.

Third, the leaders must empower members of the team to use talent and creativity to improve trauma care. In the spirit of quality improvement, each team member should participate in quality review and morbidity and mortality conferences, with the purpose of improving both individual skills and the protocols. These discussions should be data-driven, with an understanding of trends within the existing trauma center, as well as data available from regional and national resources.

Fourth, there should be careful integration of patient care with education. At times these goals may not be shared by all. The creative tension between clinical care and education must always be at the forefront of the attending physicians, whether from the trauma service or the emergency medicine service.

Finally, the trauma center must be integrated within the trauma system locally, regionally, and nationally. Affiliations may include regional EMS councils, trauma planning groups, state and national committees, and professional organizations such as the American College of Surgeons, the American College of Emergency Physicians, the American Trauma Society, and the Emergency Nurses Association. Team members must understand the trauma system concept, delineated by the American College of Emergency Physicians on trauma care systems.[4]

Team Building

Although the importance of a cooperative approach to trauma resuscitation and evaluation is unquestioned, it is less clear how to attain it. Turf battles, academic skirmishes, and ego confrontations destroy teams. These problems can be circumvented by an unswerving commitment to the needs of our patients

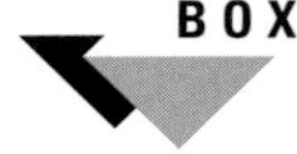

BOX 49-3
Maintaining Clearly Defined Goals

1. Mutually defined goals and a mission statement must be established
2. The goals and mission must be constantly reinforced and visible
3. Team members must be empowered to meet the goals
4. Clinical and educational goals must be balanced, with the primary focus on patient care

and their families and by the following team building strategies.

Set an Example

First, the leaders of the trauma and emergency medicine services set the tone for the rest of the team (Box 49-4). The physician and nursing leaders of the trauma service and the ED must reach agreement on the central goals, processes, and operative details. When areas of disagreement on policies or procedures occur, as they unquestionably will, these differences should be resolved collegially and not by executive fiat unless necessary. The best approach is through negotiation and consensus. The leaders of the respective services should always give the other a "heads up" on any difficult, controversial, or potentially divisive issues that need to be raised. On rare occasions, differences may need to be resolved by medical staff or administrative hierarchies. However, it is preferable for the ED and trauma service to resolve issues themselves.

Mutual Support

The leadership of the ED and trauma service must support each other, especially when dealing with the medical staff, and academic and administrative structures. As the healthcare dollar tightens and reimbursement for inpatient and outpatient services declines, it is imperative that the ED and trauma service leadership work jointly. They must often join forces to lobby for space, capital equipment purchases, marketing and public relations, and other related issues.

ONGOING COLLABORATION

Ongoing collaboration includes routine meetings, defined quality improvement processes, research, morbidity and mortality review, educational conferences, and the trauma committee. The monthly meeting should be an absolute priority. Joint research projects between nursing, emergency medicine, and surgery also promote esprit de corps.

BOX 49-4
Establishing Cooperative Trauma Approach

1. The leaders set the tone for the department
2. The leaders must be visible clinically and administratively
3. The leaders must demonstrate mutual support
4. The leaders should have a defined structure for ongoing collaboration and communication
5. The leaders should be prospective in managing problems
6. The leaders should always focus on the best interests of the patient

DEFINED APPROACH
Development of Protocols

Evidence from the United States and abroad indicates that a defined approach to critically ill and injured patients improves outcome.[12,13] Clinical pathways are certainly not new and have been utilized effectively in trauma since the genesis of the Advanced Trauma Life Support (ACLS) guidelines in the early 1970s.[14-15] In many respects, trauma was among the first diseases addressed by guidelines and a protocol-oriented approach, aspects that have since formed the basis of what has come to be recognized as evidence-based medicine.[16-17]

There are several advantages to a defined approach to trauma care (Box 49-5). Protocols extend beyond initial clinical evaluation and management to laboratory, intensive care unit, operating suite, social work, rehabilitation, and quality improvement review. (See Trauma Essential Services covered later in the chapter.)

Development of protocols requires time and planning. First, consider the experience of trauma centers across the region, state, and nation. Their protocols may provide innovative approaches that can refine local practice. The *process* of developing the protocols, roles and responsibilities, goals, and mission are as important as the result. Protocols simply dictated from the top are less likely to be followed than those developed by the team. A multidisciplinary team should generate these trauma protocols. This "buy in" promotes adherence to established guidelines. Similarly, trauma protocols should be updated and revised on a regular basis and these revisions should be guided by a multidisciplinary approach.

BOX 49-5
Advantages of a Protocol Approach to Trauma Care

1. Widely known and disseminated knowledge of how team members approach the patient
2. Maximizes speed and efficiency in the care of the patient
3. Decreases variability and improves predictability
4. Assists the evidence-based medicine approach
5. Improves patient care and outcome

Although flexibility is necessary in providing optimal care, capricious deviations from protocols can lead to poor patient care, destroy team morale, and call leadership into question. Trauma centers must continually study the impact of these clinical pathways on outcome. The relationship between practice and outcome is a fundamental principle of the evidence-based medicine approach.[14,15,18] In addition to their impact on patient care, clinical pathways also foster team learning essential to healthy, growing organizations.[19-21]

MUTUAL ACCOUNTABILITY

In the most productive teams, all successes are team successes, failures are team failures, and problems are "our problems."[1,22] This spirit of mutual accountability should be readily visible in the trauma resuscitation process. Further, the spirit of mutual accountability requires an open and candid dialogue in the quality improvement review process. This process does not concentrate on assigning blame, but rather finds ways to improve care.[23,24] Problems and deviations from protocols should be kept in perspective, so that small issues are kept small. "Don't let the incident report become bigger than the incident."

TRAUMA ESSENTIAL SERVICES

There are a number of people who represent services that contribute immeasurably to the care of the trauma patient, some of whom never see the patient, including imaging, laboratory services, registration, social services, and managed care planning. In the past, these services were often referred to as "ancillary." The origins of the term *ancillary* are particularly instructive. Ancillary derives from the Latin "ankilla," meaning female slave or maid servant. Given this meaning, there is no room on a trauma team for "ancillary services." Instead, these services are truly *essential* services.

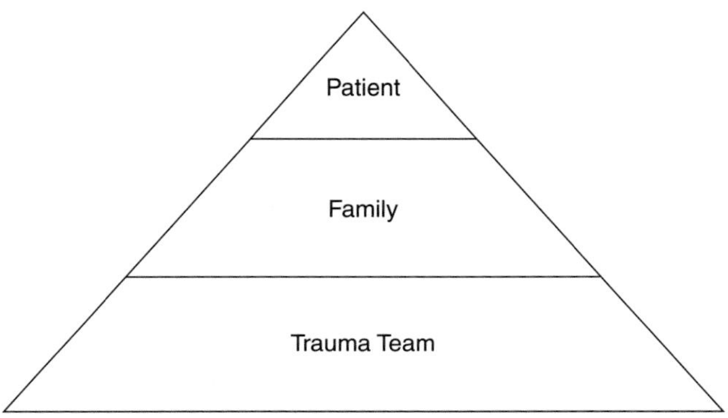

Fig. 49-1 The trauma pyramid.

The focus in trauma care should always begin with the patient, closely followed by the family members of the injured victim (Fig 49-1). Unfortunately, the trauma team is often slow in communicating with the family of the victim.[25] For that reason, in the best of trauma systems, the social worker, or patient representative, is involved early and consistently through the course of care.

Essential service team members also must be familiar with the protocol approach to the patient. For example, most trauma centers have a defined approach to clearing the cervical spine in trauma victims. The radiology technician assigned to the trauma team must be familiar with this protocol. Such team members should sit on the quality improvement review and the trauma committee.

TRAUMA RESUSCITATION AREA

Trauma resuscitations require sufficient space and supplies to allow for adequate care of the patient. However, no definitive guidelines define the space necessary to accomplish this goal. Some centers use an area as small as 12 feet by 12 feet, whereas others utilize a space greater than 22 feet by 22 feet. The 1993 guidelines of the American College of Surgeons Committee on trauma states, "The space should be large enough to allow an assembly of the full trauma team plus necessary equipment . . . ".[3] The area should also prevent unauthorized access and maintain patient privacy. OSHA and CDC Guidelines mandate a physical or visual barrier to ensure that blood and infectious risks are followed within the proscribed area. An alternate way of setting up the trauma bay is shown in Fig. 49-2, which provides an elevated trauma recording and viewing area.

In most cases, it is wise to dedicate a specific room for the majority of trauma resuscitations. This room serves a number of purposes, not the least of which is ensuring the necessary equipment. This equipment includes surgical packs, chest tube trays, blood-warming equipment, a wide array of airway equipment, and peritoneal lavage trays. In many cases, specific equipment may be delineated by state, regional, or national organizations.[3-4]

Many trauma centers designate areas for members of the trauma team, particularly at the bedside of the patient. This plan ensures that each trauma team member knows his or her responsibilities and roles, and is aware of the specific space that he or she is to occupy during the resuscitation. A suggested template for the roles of each team member, and their position at the bedside is provided in Appendix A.

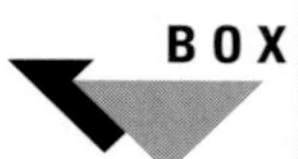

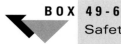

BOX 49-6
Safety and Security

RESPONSIBILITIES OF LAW ENFORCEMENT OFFICERS IN THE EMERGENCY DEPARTMENT

Purpose

To maintain the peace and function in a safe environment a security officer is stationed in the triage area of the emergency department from 19:00 through 03:00 weekdays and 20:00 through 04:00 weekends. Also, because of the nature of the ED, law enforcement officers are frequently in the department to interview or assist with patients and their families. Following are guidelines for law enforcement officers in the ED.

Policy

1. Officer will identify himself or herself to charge nurse on entering the department.
2. Charge nurse and primary nurse for the injured patient will inform officer when he or she may talk with the patient and enter the patient's room.
3. Number of officers with an arrested patient will be determined by law enforcement protocols.
4. Numerous law enforcement officers in the ED will be directed by the charge nurse to an area for their use and will be informed of a "point person" for contact in the ED.
5. Any officer present in the ED to conduct interviews of witnesses must do so away from the ED waiting room or patient care area.
6. Security for ED staff and patients during an "unusual incident" (e.g., patient with multiple gun shot wounds, stabbing, or related violent crimes) will be enforced by hospital security officers and police, if needed, as deemed necessary in collaboration with the ED charge nurse and ED charge physician, per "Lock Down of the Emergency Department" policy.
7. Only officers primarily responsible for a situation in the Emergency Department may park in the upper deck/ambulance bay. All other police vehicles (motorcycles, cars, vans) must park in another designated area. The charge nurse may request that police vehicles be removed from the ambulance bay at any time to facilitate ambulance parking and patient care.

The trauma room should facilitate "crowd control" and exclude nonessential personnel. In addition to ensuring patient confidentiality and privacy, this design also diminishes noise during resuscitation so that communication can occur. Fixed overhead radiographic and videotaping equipment (for quality improvement purposes) is available at some centers. A specific nurse is assigned to recording and occupies a dedicated space close to the telephones. Effective prehospital and in-hospital communications should be available nearby, as well as the capability of interfacility communication for regional trauma centers.

There should be a defined path from the trauma resuscitation area to key areas of the hospital, including imaging, the operating suite, the intensive care units, and prehospital/helicopter access. Develop a process by which the trauma room is restocked, cleaned, and "reloaded" for the next trauma resuscitation. This procedure should coordinate nursing, physician, housekeeping, registration, and other personnel.

Trauma protocols and equipment in the trauma room should follow OSHA and CDC Guidelines for control of infectious and blood-borne diseases. Each trauma center should address these requirements in hospital-wide policies. Bedside providers need to be appropriately protected by barrier gowns, masks, shoe covers, and lead x-ray gowns. The area in which all providers with direct patient contact are required to wear such equipment should be clearly marked.

Airway control:
Anesthesia
Emergency physician
Head of Bedside
Team leader:
Senior surgical
or
ED Resident
Evaluator:
ED Resident
or
Surgical resident
Primary nurse
Registered nurse
Consultative:
ED Attending
Trauma attending
Trauma recorder

Fig. 49-2 In the majority of institutions it is helpful to ensure that there are designated areas for specific members of the trauma team, particularly at the bedside of the patient.

TRAUMA FLOW SHEET

A standardized trauma flow sheet allows for improved patient care, quality improvement, trauma registry, trauma research, and risk management. The essential data elements vary by institution. Appendix B is a representative trauma flow sheet. Usually an ED or critical care unit nurse is designated as the trauma recorder. However, if multiple providers will be using the flow sheet, clearly delineate who is responsible for filling out specific sections of the form. A single trauma recorder is preferred and key providers review and sign the flow sheet by way of verification. The physician performing the physical examination calls out appropriate clinical information to be recorded on the trauma flow sheet.

MANAGEMENT OF MULTIPLE VICTIMS

The ability to handle multiple victims is essential for *all* trauma centers, regardless of the level of designation. All trauma centers should plan for multiple casualties including designated areas for resuscitation, back-up personnel, and appropriate equipment. Multiple casualty incidents should be a part of the hospital disaster plan, including both internal, external, and "mini-disaster" capabilities

Clearly delineated mechanisms are necessary to ensure that the various patients and data do not become mixed during resuscitation. Because registration of patients into the hospital computer system can be problematic, many hospitals have developed alphabetic or numeric systems to designate patients until definitive identification of victims can be made. One commonly used scheme is the "Alpha, Baker, . . . Zulu Doe" system. Medical record numbers are established in advance and matched to the "Doe" names, with packets including the chart, trauma flow sheet, and requisitions. When definitive identification is made, the previously selected medical record numbers of the "Doe" system are married to the patient's demographic information. This system ensures coordination of imaging results, laboratory studies, blood typing, and medical records. In many cases, color coordination of initial radiographic films and laboratory studies are necessary to match the correct films to the patient. Multiple casualties provide opportunities for quality improvement, and a review following each incident can improve future response.

COMMUNITY VERSUS ACADEMIC TRAUMA CENTERS

A primary difference between academic and community centers is the focus on research. In fact, the American College of Surgeons' Guidelines do not specifically distinguish community from academic medical centers, but instead focus on research as a primary distinction between level I and level II centers.[3] From a practical standpoint, academic centers integrate residents and medical students within these trauma teams.

Residents should function as fully empowered members of the team. They must be familiar with policies and procedures, roles and responsibilities, and the overall mission of the trauma team. It should be made clear during orientation that a collegial relationship is *expected* and not simply anticipated.

In institutions where they exist, upper level emergency medicine residents must be given the opportunity to lead trauma resuscitations. This role should be coordinated with the senior surgical resident and may be shared by alternating days. For example, on even days, emergency medicine runs trauma resuscitations and on odd days surgery is in charge. Emergency medicine residents should rotate on the trauma service to learn more about intensive care unit management, surgical experience, inpatient care, rehabilitation, and trauma service management.

TRAUMA AND MANAGED CARE

Dealing with managed care plans is a necessity for all trauma programs. Managed care is a generic term that generally describes healthcare insurance plans. Common features include the following:

- Risk is transferred to the provider.
- Contracts are awarded selectively.
- The plan preferentially refers their patients to less costly providers.

Many managed care plans have failed to contract with trauma centers for the care of injured patients. Prehospital personnel usually take trauma patients to the nearest appropriate trauma center for care. This approach limits managed care's ability to contract selectively with less costly providers. Managed care plans have attempted to transfer some financial risk to the provider by simply negotiating reduced fees based on contractual agreements. In some regions, capitation based on a fixed number of enrollees pays for trauma services, but this situation is rare. In dealing with managed care plans, it is usually best to try to align strategic incentives with clinical pathways. These pathways may incorporate cost-effective strategies that both appeal to managed care and are safe for the patient. Data regarding cost-of-care should be available to the physicians and hospital representatives before negotiations.

It is important to remember the dictum that "Form follows finance." For example, in discounted fee-for-service systems, higher volumes of trauma result in higher payments. In such a case, the incentive to the provider is "Treat, Treat, Treat." In discounted fee-for-service systems, profligate testing is in the hospital's financial interest.

In fully capitated systems (in which trauma centers are paid a fixed amount per member per month for the care of trauma victims) there is a strong incentive to utilize only clearly necessary imaging studies and laboratory services in the care of the patient. In the capitated environment, the incentive is "Prevent, Prevent, Prevent."

In addition to aligning strategic incentives, it is best to offer managed care payors high-quality, cost-effective care that returns the patient to preinjury function at the earliest possible time. In many environments, trauma centers offer to promptly transfer patients, after appropriate intervention, to participating hospitals and physicians. It is imperative that trauma providers do not compromise the best interests of their patients and families as they seek cost-efficient solutions.

TRAUMA: THE DISINTEGRATIVE EMERGENCY DEPARTMENT DISEASE

Trauma patients are essentially disintegrative to ED care. They consume resources, personnel, and time, and disrupt overall patient flow. The child with a cough must wait for his or her chest radiograph, the patient awaiting transport to the floor lingers while trauma resuscitations divert doctors, nurses, and technicians to the trauma room. Trauma patients by nature are labor-intensive and take priority over virtually any other patient in the ED. This reality presents issues regarding resources and waiting times for all patients in the ED. Some medical staff members feel trauma victims pull resources away from their patients, including operating suite time, intensive care unit beds, and capital investments. The leadership and management of the ED and trauma service must jointly address these issues with the administration and medical staff. As trauma volumes and acuity rise, their effect on the ED and the hospital grows. The best way to ensure that trauma is *not* disintegrative is to match resources to volume and acuity.

EMERGENCY DEPARTMENT SECURITY AND VIOLENCE

The rise in violence in EDs across the country has presented substantial problems for patients, their families, and for the staff. Because trauma centers care for victims of violent crime, they are at higher risk for violence. Gang warfare may erupt when rivals meet in the ED waiting room following a street fight. Domestic violence victims and their care providers may be assaulted in the treatment room by an enraged spouse. In the case of gunshot victims, some would-be killers may even come to the trauma room to "finish the job" they started. All trauma centers should have a "lock down" security policy that describes in detail how to coordinate trauma center operations, hospital security, and local law enforcement in appropriate circumstances (Box 49-6). Specific protocols should address gang-related issues and protection of patient confidentiality. Like all issues facing the trauma center, careful prospective cooperation among ED, trauma services, security, and law enforcement personnel is essential. Each activation of lock down in the ED should be subject to rigorous quality improvement review.

In some urban EDs, up to 25% of gunshot victims transported by paramedics are found to be armed.[26] Emergency departments must develop protocols regarding patient searches to secure weapons. These protocols should be applied in a manner that will not appear discriminatory or capricious. Indications for a weapons search may include victims of penetrating trauma, patients who are intoxicated, or those with altered mental status, and especially those with homicidal ideation.

CONCLUSION

The trauma team is composed of a relatively small number of people with complementary skills who are committed to a common purpose. The objective is excellent clinical care of injured patients, with clearly defined performance goals, and a specified approach for which they hold themselves mutually accountable. The members, goals, and approach should be arrived at in a collaborative fashion, guided by national, regional, and local guidelines. The best teams are fiercely loyal to each other, as well as to the patients and their families. Leaders must work hard to build this team loyalty. Without careful nurturing and team building, chaos and acrimony reign.

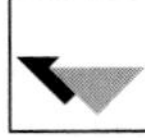

PEARLS & PITFALLS

- Team building must be an important goal of both emergency medicine and trauma services.
- The interaction between the emergency department and trauma services is influenced by the attitude of the leaders.

- Recognize that too many people in the trauma room may be as great a handicap as too few.
- A tiered response to trauma is both safe and cost effective.
- Clinical pathways can standardize trauma management and prevent diagnostic or therapeutic oversights.

REFERENCES

1. Katzenbach JR, Smith DK: *The wisdom of teams: creating the high-performance organization,* Boston, 1993, Harvard Business School Press.
2. Committee on Trauma, American College of Surgeons: *Resources for optimal care of the injured patient,* Chicago, 1990, American College of Surgeons.
3. Committee on Trauma, American College of Surgeons: *Resources for optimal care of injured patient: 1993,* Chicago, 1993, American Colleges of Surgeons.
4. Sacra J, et al: Trauma care systems quality improvement guidelines: ensuring quality care in the trauma care setting, *Ann Emerg Med* 21:740-741, 1992.
5. Dekeyser FG, et al: Decreasing the cost of trauma care: a system of secondary in-hospital triage, *Ann Emerg Med* 23:841-844, 1994.
6. Keller MS, Stafford PW, Vane DW: Conservative management of pancreatic trauma in children, *J Trauma* 42:1097-1100, 1997.
7. Sacco WJ, et al: Status of trauma patient management as measured by survival/death outcomes: looking toward the 21st century, *J Trauma* 36: 297-298, 1994.
8. Shackford SR, Molin M: Management of splenic injuries, *Surg Clin North Am* 70: 595-620, 1990.
9. Mayer TA: Leadership, management, stewardship and motivation. In Salluzzo R, et al (editors): *Emergency department management: principles and applications,* St Louis, 1997, Mosby.
10. Mayer TA: The role of the emergency department medical director. In Salluzzo R, et al (editors): *Emergency department management: principles and applications,* St Louis, 1997, Mosby.
11. Eichelberger MR: Be prepared. In Harris BH (editor): Progress in pediatric trauma. Proceedings of the First National Conference on Pediatric Trauma. The Kiwanis Pediatric Trauma Institute, Boston, September, 1985.
12. West JG, Trunkey DD, Limb RC: Systems of trauma care: a study of two counties, *Arch Surg* 114:455-460, 1979.
13. Centers for Disease Control Panel on Trauma Care Systems: Trauma care systems. In *The Third National Injury Conference: setting the national agenda for injury control in the 1990's,* Atlanta, 1991, U.S. Department of Health and Human Services, Centers for Disease Control.
14. Committee on Trauma, American College of Surgeons: *Advanced trauma life support course,* Chicago, 1973, American College of Surgeons.
15. Committee on Trauma, American College of Surgeons: *Advanced trauma life support course,* Chicago, 1994, American College of Surgeons.
16. Evidence-based Medicine Working Group: Evidence-based medicine: a new approach to teaching the practice of medicine, *JAMA* 268: 2420-2425, 1992.
17. Waeckerle JF, et al: Evidence-based emergency medicine: integrating research into practice, *Ann Emerg Med* 30:626-628, 1997.
18. Ellrodt G, et al: Evidence-based disease management, *JAMA* 278:1687-1692, 1997.
19. Senge PM: The leader's new work: building learning organizations, *Sloan Manag Rev* 10:7-23, 1990.
20. Garvin DA: Building a learning organization, *Harv Business Rev* 71: 78-91, 1993.
21. Kotter JP: What leaders really do, *Harv Business Rev* 68: 103-111, 1990.
22. Eisenhardt KM, Kahwajy JL, Bourgeois LJ: How management teams can have a good fight, *Harv Business Rev* 75:77-86, 1997.
23. Pellegrino ED, Thomasma DC: *For the patient's good: the restoration of beneficence in healthcare,* New York, 1989, Oxford University Press.
24. Pellegrino ED, Thomasma DC: *The virtues in medical practice,* New York, 1993, Oxford University Press.
25. Cross ML, et al: Interaction between trauma team and families: lack of timely communication, *Am J Emerg Med* 14:548-550, 1996.
26. Wasserberger J, et al. Violence in the community emergency room, *Arch Emerg Med* 6:266-269, 1989.

Appendix A: Roles and Responsibilities of the Trauma Team

STATEMENT

The Emergency Medicine Physician and trauma surgeons work collaboratively in the initial resuscitation and stabilization of the trauma patient. This resuscitation and stabilization should blend smoothly with the overall trauma management plan for the patient and should never occur in isolation. The following information is intended to maximize the ability to deliver optimal patient care, provide for a framework in which the emergency medicine and surgical members of the team can cooperate best, and allow a smooth transfer of the patient from the emergency service to the trauma service.

It is the responsibility of all authorized code team members to ensure that they work as a coordinated team and that each member performs assigned duties in a priority that is most beneficial to the patient.

POLICY

I. Team Captain
   A. Definition
      1. Emergency Physician (EP): Team captain until the trauma surgeon arrives. Shares responsibility after trauma surgeon arrives. Alternate day schedule most effective in academic institutions. Will report immediately to the trauma receiving area for CODE BLUES and CODE YELLOWS. Following arrival of the trauma surgeon, the EP will give a clinical update, complete tasks started, and when appropriate from a clinical standpoint, transfer the management of the patient to the trauma surgeon or admitting attending surgeon if the patient is not admitted to the trauma service. Refer to Trauma Service Administrative Protocol Code Yellow Trauma Case Policy.
      2. Trauma Surgeon: Will report immediately to trauma receiving area on all CODE BLUE patients. Will respond either in person or by phone for CODE YELLOW patients.
   B. Responsibilities
      1. Obtain prehospital history (A.M.P.L.E.) and integrate this information into the assessment and treatment plan.
      2. Perform primary survey as defined and prioritized in the Advanced Trauma Life Support Curriculum. The team captain may designate a physician to assess the patient and call out his or her findings.
         Airway
         Breathing
         Circulation
         Disability
         Expose
      3. To designate an individual to perform procedures. If sufficient personnel are available the team captain should not perform procedures, but remain at the foot of the bed and designate a "procedure" physician to provide:
         a. Airway management
         b. Ventilation management
         c. Secure venous access and laboratory studies
         d. Management of circulation to include appropriate external hemorrhage control.
         e. Emergency procedures such as, but not limited to:
            i. Tube thoracostomy
            ii. Thoracotomy
            iii. Pericardiocentesis
            iv. Diagnostic peritoneal lavage
            v. Endotracheal intubation
            vi. Cricothyrotomy
      4. Communicate patient care needs to the trauma RN team leader.
      5. Ensure that the trauma RN team leader has accurately recorded information regarding primary survey and resuscitation management.
      6. Perform secondary survey as defined in Advanced Trauma Life Support.
      7. Ensure timely completion of priority radiographs, trauma lab profile, ABGs.
      8. Repeat appropriate examination as necessary to address changes in the patient's condition.
      9. Communicate to trauma RN team leader all findings of above examinations.
      10. Request necessary consultants through trauma RN team leader.

11. Collaborate with residents and consultants regarding patient's problems.
12. Coordinate multidisciplinary approach to comprehensive patient management and serve as patient advocate.
13. Manage crowd control.
14. Communicate with patient's family members (as soon as possible) the patient's condition, extent of injuries and the comprehensive plan.

II. Emergency Department Resident
  A. Responsibilities
    1. Assume duties of team captain as delegated.
    2. Assume duties delegated to him or her by the team captain.
    3. Manage the airway.

III. Senior Surgical Resident
  A. Responsibilities
    1. Assume duties of team captain as delegated.
    2. Assume duties delegated to him or her by the team captain.

IV. Junior Emergency Medicine and Surgical Residents
  A. Responsibilities
    1. Will be included in trauma assessment and resuscitation when and if the team captain feels it is compatible with quality patient care.

V. Anesthesia
  A. Determined in each institution. May be called by the emergency physician if there are difficulties securing the airway.

VI. Trauma RN
  A. Definition: Primary Nurse, physically located at patient's left.
  B. Responsibilities
    1. In the case of a nonintubated Code Yellow, assume duties of intensive care unit (ICU) trauma RN.
    2. Coordinate immediate equipment set-up in trauma room.
    3. Confirm field report and identify potential needs based on mechanism of injury.
    4. Identify physician team captain and identify self as primary nurse.
    5. Coordinate nursing care.
    6. Receive and acknowledge physician orders.
    7. Assist with set-up/initiation/maintenance of:
      a. Peripheral IV (L)
      b. Peritoneal lavage
      c. Chest tube placement (L)
      d. Central line placement (L)
    8. Utilize the nursing process in the continual care of the trauma patient.
    9. Communicate information for documentation and equipment requirements to the trauma RN team leader.
    10. Assumes total care of patient and role of trauma nurse team leader when initial resuscitation and stabilization of patient allows for reassignment of staff.
    11. Review documentation for completeness prior to patient's final disposition.
    12. Accompany patient based on final disposition as follows:
      a. Direct to operating suite
         ICU trauma RN
      b. Floor/IMC admit
         Trauma RN team leader
      c. Computed tomography (CT), special procedures (angio)
         Code Blue or Intubated Yellow
         ICU trauma RN
         Code Yellow
         Trauma RN team leader
      d. ICU 2
         ICU trauma RN
      e. ED Discharge
         Trauma RN team leader
    13. Notify Blood Bank when uncrossmatched blood has been utilized and ensure that complete slips are sent to Blood Bank via pneumatic tube system.

VII. Trauma Nurse Team Leader
  A. Definition: Facilitates flow of care and information within the trauma bay and ensures accurate and complete documentation.
  B. Responsibilities
    1. Jointly determine with the team captain who may remain in the trauma bay as observers (should be done before the arrival of the patient, when possible).
    2. Monitor team response times/names.
    3. Provide accurate, on-going documentation and ensure completion of:
      a. Trauma flow sheet
      b. ED chart
      c. Trauma bay standing orders
      d. ED charge sheet
      e. Uncrossmatched blood slips
    4. On arrival of the patient, start lapse timer in admitting area.
    5. Begin video tape recorder for all Code Blue patients.
    6. Ensure primary and secondary survey are completed and results recorded.

7. Advise resuscitation team members of time lapse every 10 minutes for the first 30 minutes.
8. Act as a liaison for ED charge nurse.
9. Ensure that blood specimen is obtained within 5 minutes of patient arrival and that all specimens are sent for processing as they are obtained.
10. Notify via the ED core:
    a. CT, special procedures.
    b. Bed assignment request.
    c. Need for specialist consultation
11. Provide medicines as needed.
12. Inform team of lab results.
13. Call the operating suite with update when decision is made to go to the operating suite or as the patient leaves the trauma bay for further diagnostics.
14. Passes role of nurse team leader to trauma RN team leader when initial resuscitation and stabilization of patient allows for reassignment of staff.
15. Review documentation with team captain and trauma RN team leader before leaving the trauma bay.

VIII. ICU trauma RN
  A. Definition: Physically located on the patient's right side.
  B. Responsibilities
    1. Assume responsibilities delegated by team captain and trauma nurse team leader.
    2. Assist with equipment set-up.
    3. Prepares patient:
       a. Cut away clothes if deemed appropriate.
       b. Apply restraints (when necessary) with physician order.
    4. Obtain initial and serial vital signs (including temperature) and communicate these to the trauma RN team leader.
    5. After initial manual BP, utilize equipment to monitor:
       a. ECG
       b. Noninvasive BP
       c. O_2 saturation
    6. Assist with set-up/initiation/maintenance of:
       a. Peripheral IV (R)
       b. Chest tube placement (R)
       c. Central line placement (R)
    7. Obtain ABGs from arterial line set-up with physician order.
    8. Insert nasogastric or orogastric tube and connect to low continuous suction on direction of team captain.
    9. Insert Foley catheter to straight drainage on direction of team captain.
    10. Obtain urine specimen for:
       a. Complete urinalysis
       b. Toxicology screen
       c. Urine dipstick for blood
       d. Urine pregnancy
    11. Utilize nursing process in the continual care of trauma patient.
    12. Accompany patient based on final disposition as follows:
       a. Direct to operating suite
          ICU trauma RN
       b. Floor/IMC admit
          Trauma RN team leader
       c. CT, special procedures (angio)
          Code Blue or Intubated Yellow–ICU trauma RN;
          Code Yellow–Trauma RN team leader
       d. ICU
          ICU trauma RN
       e. ED discharge
          Trauma RN team leader

IX. Radiology Technician
  A. Responsibilities
    1. Respond to trauma room and report to trauma RN team leader to identify radiographic needs and need for additional resources.
    2. Respond with sufficient number of cassettes to perform standard trauma radiograph series, as directed by team captain. (Runner to get film developed and return with radiograph.)

X. Computed Tomography Technician
  A. Responsibilities
    1. Called at discretion of ED charge physician/trauma surgeon before the patient's arrival in the trauma room based on mechanism of injury and patient report from scene.
    2. Make CT scanner available in a timely manner based on trauma patient needs.

XI. Respiratory Therapist
  A. Responsibilities
    1. Assist emergency medicine resident in securing airway.
    2. Monitor airway and ventilation.
    3. Provide mechanical ventilators in CT scanner/ICU and monitors continual function of ventilators while in CT scan.
    4. Suction PRN.
    5. Set up and maintain functioning of A-Line monitoring equipment.

XII. ED Charge RN
   A. Responsibilities
      1. Assume duties of the communication nurse in the implementation of codes when communication nurse is absent. (See Responsibilities for Implementation of a Code.)
      2. Liaison with family members and social worker.
      3. Assign ED nurses to trauma team.
      4. Oversee relocation of those patients in the trauma room.
      5. Offer assistance as needed for CODE YELLOWS.
      6. In the event of multiple codes, coordinates the assignment of the nursing trauma teams.

XIII. Social Services
   A. Definition: Provide family support and crisis counseling for the trauma patient and their family members.
   B. Responsibilities
      1. Respond to all CODE BLUES and to CODE YELLOWS when available.
      2. Secure patient valuables.
      3. Make initial contact with family or significant others.
      4. Assess need for crisis intervention with patient and family members—see on-call criteria for ED.
      5. All trauma cases are opened for disposition/discharge planning and shall remain open until the patient is out of the system or when a request has been made to close it by the attending physician.
      6. Facilitate demographic data collection between ED registrar and the patient, family or friends, in a crisis situation.

XIV. ED Registrar
   A. Definition: Obtain vital demographic and financial information for the trauma patient. Registrar will focus on obtaining all data within 30 minutes of patient arrival.
   B. Responsibilities
      1. Respond to all CODES BLUES, CODE YELLOWS, and CODE WHITES.
      2. Secure vital information to include: Name, DOB, SSN, Address, Home and Work Phone, Employer, Guarantor (G) Name, G Home and Work Phone, Emergency Contact (EC) Name, EC Home and Work Phone, Health Insurance, and automobile insurance if applicable.
      3. Obtain essential information from the patient, police, EMS, transferring facility, helicopter crew, EMS Run Sheet, CAD sheet, family members, and friends.
      4. Collaborate with social worker to obtain vital information in a crisis situation.

XV. ED Core Secretary
   A. Definition: Provide on-going support for the trauma team.
   B. Responsibilities
      1. Order tests as needed.
      2. Page consultants as needed.
      3. Calls operating suite with initial patient information.

Trauma Response Team Members

To provide guidelines for crowd control in the trauma bay and to provide the best environment for optimal patient care, the following are authorized members of the trauma response team.

CODE BLUE TRAUMA TEAM (TOTAL 14)

Hands-On Zone

Team leader
Trauma RN team leader
ICU trauma RN
ED resident
Respiratory therapy
Junior surgical resident

Periphery

Trauma surgeon/Fellow
Radiology technicians (2)

Observers

Surgical acting intern
Social work
Trauma nurse team leader (recorder)
ED registar

CODE YELLOW TRAUMA TEAM (TOTAL 12)

Hands-On

Team leader
Primary RN
Respiratory therapy
ED resident
Junior surgical resident

Periphery

Radiology technicians (2)
ED attending

Observer

Surgical acting intern
Trauma nurse team leader (recorder)
Social worker
ED registrar

CODE WHITE TRAUMA TEAM (TOTAL 7)

Emergency medicine attending
Trauma nurse team leader (recorder)
Emergency medicine/senior surgical resident
Social worker
Trauma RN team leader
ED registrar
Respiratory therapy

Additional personnel may also be involved in any trauma case on an as-needed basis:

Operating room nurse(s)
Administrative director
Trauma research assistant
ED technician
Consultants
Pediatric intensivist
OB/GYN physician
Flight RN or paramedic–assigned at the discretion of the trauma RN team leader

In addition to the defined team members, two to three additional observers may be present provided they are approved by the nurse team leader and the team captain. They may be medical, nursing, or other allied health students, EMS personnel, or other designated visitors.

Approved observers must remain on the recording platform behind the shield unless otherwise permitted. Sufficient lead aprons must be available for all designated code team members. If unauthorized personnel arrive in the trauma bay, it is the responsibility of the trauma RN team leader and the team leader to ask excess observers to leave. Additional assistance may be requested from the emergency medicine attending or the trauma surgeon.

Appendix B: Inova Fairfax Hospital Trauma Flow Sheet

Date: ________ Time called: ________ CODE: ❑ Blue ❑ Yellow ❑ Changed to: ________ Time: ________

Arrival time: ________ Arrival by: ❑ Walk-in ❑ Ground ❑ Air – Unit number/ name ________

From ❑ Scene ❑ Hospital ________ Mechanism: ________

Sex ____ Age ____ Allergies ________ PMH ________

Arrived with: ❑ Cervical Collar ❑ Long Back Board ❑ Intubated ❑ MAST Inflated ❑ 0_2@ via ________

PRIMARY SURVEY

AIRWAY: ❑ patient maintained ❑ mechanically maintained by: ________

BREATHING: ❑ spontaneous ❑ assisted by: ________

CIRCULATION:

pulse: ❑ present ❑ absent CPR started at: ________

color: ❑ normal ❑ abnormal: ________

cap refill: ❑ normal ❑ delayed: ________

vitals: b/p ____ / ____ pulse rate ____ resp. rate ____ pulse ox ____ temp ____ route ____

SECONDARY SURVEY

HEAD: ❑ pupils equal ❑ pupils unequal: ________

❑ TM's normal ❑ TM's abnormal: ________

❑ Nose normal ❑ Nose abnormal: ________

❑ Mouth normal ❑ Mouth abnormal: ________

NECK: ❑ trachea normal ❑ trachea abnormal: ________

❑ c-spine normal ❑ c-spine abnormal: ________

Cleared ❑ Yes ❑ No By: ________

CHEST: ❑ BS equal ❑ BS unequal: ________

❑ wall normal ❑ wall abnormal: ________

ARMS: ❑ color normal ❑ color abnormal: ________

❑ movement normal ❑ movement abnormal: ________

❑ sensation normal ❑ sensation abnormal: ________

ABD: ❑ normal ❑ abnormal: ________

PELVIS: ❑ stable ❑ unstable: ________

❑ rectal normal ❑ rectal abnormal: ________

❑ meatus normal ❑ meatus abnormal: ________

LEGS: ❑ color normal ❑ color abnormal: ________

❑ movement normal ❑ movement abnormal: ________

❑ sensation normal ❑ sensation abnormal: ________

BACK ❑ normal ❑ abnormal: ________

INJURY SUMMARY

1 - Abrasion
2 - Amputation
3 - Avulsion
4 - Crepitus
5 - Ecchymosis
6 - Fx/Dislocation
7 - Gunshot
8 - Hematoma
9 - Laceration
10 - Puncture
11 - Stab wound
12 - Swelling
13 - Burn

Comments: ________

____

____

____

PATIENT IDENTIFICATION

79

FAIRFAX HOSPITAL

TRAUMA RESUSCITATION FLOWSHEET

PAGE 1 OF 3

Original White: Chart
Canary: ED Physician
Pink: Trauma Services
White: Emergency Department

NUR-4858.A/R11-95 • PKGS OF 100 SETS

VITAL SIGNS

Time	B/P	Pulse	Resp	Pulse Ox	
	/				
	/				
	/				
	/				
	/				
	/				
	/				
	/				
	/				
	/				
	/				
	/				
	/				
	/				
	/				
	/				
	/				

INTAKE

Route	IV #	Site	Solution	Time Up	By	Time Down	Total

OUTPUT

	Time/Amount	Time/Amount	Time/Amount	Total
Urine	/	/	/	
Gastric	/	/	/	
L. Chest	/	/	/	
R. Chest	/	/	/	
	/	/	/	
TOTAL				

MEDICATIONS

Time	Drug	Dose	Route	Site	Initials

X-RAYS

Film	Time Taken	Time Back	Result
Cervical Spine			
Thoracic Spine			
Lumbar Spine			
AP Chest			
AP Pelvis			

PROCEDURES

	Time	Size/Site	By Whom
Foley catheter			
NG/OG			

LABS

Bloods Sent at: ______________ **Drawn by:** __________

Prep used: ❑ Betadine ❑ Alcohol ❑ Other: __________

Urine Sent at: ________ ❑ Voided ❑ Foley ❑ Other: ____

Gross Blood: ❑ yes ❑ no **Dip:** ❑ positive ❑ negative

PATIENT IDENTIFICATION

FAIRFAX HOSPITAL

TRAUMA RESUSCITATION FLOWSHEET
PAGE 2 OF 3

NUR-4858.B/R11-95 • PKGS OF 100 SETS

G.C.S.
● 2
● 3
● 4
● 5
● 6
● 7
● 8
● 9

Glasgow Coma Scale		Initial		Peds GCS & WT	
EYES OPEN	Spontaneously	4	4		4
	To Speech	3	3		3
	To Pain	2	2		2
	None	1	1		1
BEST VERBAL RESPONSE	Oriented	5	5	Social smile, orients to sound follows objects	5
	Confused	4	4	Cries, anes., consolable	4
	Inappropriate Sounds	3	3	Inappropriate, consistent crying	3
	Incomprehensible Sounds	2	2	Agitated, resteless	2
	None	1	1	None	1
BEST MOTOR RESPONSE	Obeys Commands	6	6	Spontaneous	6
	Localizes Pain	5	5		5
	Withdraws to Pain	4	4		4
	Flexes to Pain	3	3		3
	Extends to Pain	2	2		2
	None	1	1		1
	Glasgow Coma Total			Glasgow Coma Total	
	Paralytic Agents On Board?	YN	YN	Paralytic Agents On Board?	YN

Revised Trauma Score		Initial	
GLASCOW COMA TOTAL	13-15	4	4
	9-12	3	3
	6-8	2	2
	4-5	1	1
	3	0	0
SYSTOLIC BLOOD PRESSURE	>89 mm Hg	4	4
	76-89 mm Hg	3	3
	50-75 mm Hg	2	2
	01-49 mm Hg	1	1
	No pulse	0	0
RESPIRATORY RATE	10-29/min	4	4
	>29/min	3	3
	6-9/min	2	2
	1-5/min	1	1
	None	0	0
	TOTAL REVISED TRAUMA SCORE		

TRAUMA RESPONSE	Name	Arrival Time
Trauma Surgeon		
ED Physician		
Surgical Resident		
Recorder		
ED Trauma RN		
Anesthesia		
ICU Nurse		
	CONSULTANTS	
Time Called	Name	Arrival

NOTES: ____________________

DISPOSITION INFORMATION

Patient to: ____________________ Time: ____________

CT Ordered: ____________________

Accompanied by: ❑ Tech ❑ ED Nurse ❑ ICU Nurse ❑ Physician

LOC: ❑ aware ❑ lethargic ❑ comatose ❑ sedated

Family notified by: ____________________

C-spine: ❑ clear ❑ not clear ❑ stabilized by: ____________

Valuables: ❑ to safe ❑ with patient ❑ to family ❑ to police

Documenting RN: ____________________

Bedside RN: ____________________

PATIENT IDENTIFICATION

FAIRFAX HOSPITAL

TRAUMA RESUSCITATION FLOWSHEET
PAGE 3 OF 3

NUR-4858.C/R11-95 • PKGS OF 100 SETS

Myths in Trauma

50

D. MATTHEW SULLIVAN

From the dogma that is ingrained during a trauma rotation as a medical student, to the Advanced Trauma Life Support (ATLS) recertification process, many precepts in trauma care often go unchallenged. We often cling to practices that remain unsupported by scientific research. In this chapter, we examine some of these myths of trauma. Although we do not advocate a complete moratorium on these practices, our readers should understand that tradition and unfounded tenets drive much of trauma care.

MYTH 1: PREHOSPITAL NEEDLE DECOMPRESSION OF THE CHEST SAVES LIVES

Most prehospital protocols call for needle decompression of suspected tension pneumothorax (PTX). This apparently reasonable policy relates to the life-threatening nature of tension PTX, and the fact that needle decompression seems a facile solution.[1]

The sensitivity of clinical examination alone for PTX varies. The absence of breath sounds is specific for PTX, but insensitive.[2-4] In practice, however, needle decompression is often erroneously[5] attempted simply because of a penetrating mechanism, and not in response to lung findings. Paramedics may attempt to decompress both sides of the chest when treating shock unresponsive to standard ATLS therapy.

The procedure has potential for complications. A needle may lacerate the intercostal vessels if inserted below, rather than above, the rib,[6] and if driven deeply, can lacerate the lung or damage the mammary artery.[1,7] If patients who receive needle decompression do not initially have a PTX, they may develop one from needle injury to the lung.

A needle in the chest may not decompress a tension PTX. Catheter malfunctions occur from failure to penetrate the chest wall cavity,[8,9] kinking or clogging of the catheter,[10] or dislodgment.[11] One case report noted that a needle failed to release a tension PTX despite proper technique.[12] The single prospective series demonstrated that only 5% of patients had improved vital signs and 7% had a decrease in subjective dyspnea after needle decompression in the field.[9] This modest impact suggests that either most patients had no indications for needle decompression, or that needle decompression alone is inadequate.[13]

Some design advancements may improve chest decompression. A spring-loaded needle with a blunt tip and side hole may decrease the potential for lung damage.[14] However, this device remains untested in the prehospital setting, and the potential for vascular injury still exists. In one small series, researchers showed the advantages of a 15-cm 16-gauge mini-trocar device, but complications were relatively high.[15]

The one comparative trial between needle decompression and tube thoracostomy in the field by air-medical prehospital personnel illustrates the following critical points:

- Thirty-eight percent of the patients who underwent initial needle decompression underwent tube thoracostomy before transport.
- On-scene time is significantly greater with tube thoracostomy compared to needle decompression (approximately 5 minutes).
- Significantly fewer patients were dead on arrival with tube thoracostomy than with needle decompression.[11]

Given the poor performance of needle aspiration, the next logical step appears to be prehospital tube thoracostomy. Although tube thoracostomy is the definitive therapy for tension hemopneumothorax, the extended scene time required for placement is disadvantageous.[16,17] For years physicians and prehospital providers have argued over the safety and efficacy of this procedure in the hands of prehospital personnel.[10,18] Some argue that only hospital-based physicians should perform this procedure,[19] but other studies show that prehospital tube thoracostomy is safe, effective, and can have fewer nontherapeutic placements compared to a trauma service.[10,20] These findings hold with non-physician responders.[21]

Most data demonstrate a clear link between morbidity and the use of a trocar chest tube both in[18,22,23] and out[24] of the hospital setting. Complications comprise tube malposition,[18] lung perforation,[25] diaphragmatic injury,[24] pulmonary edema,[26] and subsequent empyema.[27] However, immediate complications relating to the initial insertion are only 1% to 1.8%.[24,27]

How do we achieve the necessary clinical success for life-threatening tension PTX without extending scene times, and maintain a high safety profile? One English trial demonstrated that after the prehospital identification of hemopneumothorax, which compromised ventilation, some patients benefited from thoracostomy without the placement of a chest drainage tube.[28] An incision in the chest wall alone allowed air and/or blood to vent.[29] The wound was then covered with a sterile gauze dressing. This technique was as effective, took less time, and required less training than tube thoracostomy, "Tubeless" field thoracostomy avoids the common complications of a chest drain. Territorial issues of who should perform an invasive maneuver to the chest will always be debated, and training prehospital personnel to perform this task requires extra effort.

In summary, simple needle decompression of chest injuries is frequently ineffective or performed without good indications. Prehospital personnel should perform needle decompression only in patients with markedly decreased or absent unilateral breath sounds in combination with severe respiratory distress or hypotension. Additional research may determine the usefulness of field thoracostomy with or without tube placement.

MYTH 2: HELICOPTER RESPONSE TO TRAUMA SCENE CALLS IS BENEFICIAL

Civilian prehospital use of helicopter rescue began in 1972.[30] Since then proponents and skeptics have battled over the value of helicopter scene response for the transport of the trauma patient. The benefit seen by the military during combat is not as easily observed in civilian systems.

Early studies were descriptive,[31,32] but argued for round-the-clock helicopter scene response.[33] One study indicated improved mortality in blunt trauma within an individual air-medical system compared with ground transport.[34] They evaluated patients using Glasgow Coma Scale (GCS) score,[35] the Injury Severity Score (ISS),[36] the Trauma Score (TS),[37] and the TRISS methodology.[38] This methodology was then applied across multiple flight programs,[39] which revealed that 5 out of 7 air-medical response programs had statistically significant decreases in mortality compared to that predicted by the Major Trauma Outcome Study data.[40] However, detailed analysis of this data indicated that the subset of patients with minor injuries did *worse* than predicted despite air transport. Experience in other air-medical programs showed no justification for urban helicopter transport of a patient with a low to moderate trauma score.[41]

There is little or no advantage to the helicopter transfer of blunt trauma patients within an advanced metropolitan emergency medical system (EMS).[41,42] In the study by Schiller et al,[42] those patients transferred by helicopter had a *higher* mortality despite similar TS and GCS. Multiple studies confirm that in the urban setting, helicopter transport takes longer than ground transportation.[16,43-46]

One land versus air comparison study for severely head-injured patients showed a 9% reduction in mortality with air transport.[45] Aggressive advanced life support (ALS) interventions in the helicopter cohort may be responsible for some of this benefit.

Medical interventions requiring physician skills are necessary in less than 1% of air-medical flights.[47] Although aggressive prehospital resuscitation and airway management decreases mortality,[48] non-physician providers can perform many of these procedures.

In a large prospective trial of helicopter versus ambulances, air transport resulted in 16% more deaths than predicted.[49] In this study, care providers in both cohorts performed intubation. These conclusions sharply contradicted earlier urban air-medical studies.

In a study of over 1300 patients Cunningham et al[50] was able to show that while overall patients transported by helicopter were more severely injured, after stratification of injury severity score there was no significant improvement in survival for those transported by helicopter. Although this study did describe a trend towards improvement of those patients with a trauma score of 5 to 12 and an ISS of 21 to 30, there was no significant difference in mortality when stratified by calculated probability of survival.

The most recent analysis of the Pennsylvania trauma system compared scene calls transported by ALS ground units to helicopter scene transports. They found that after adjusting for risk factors, helicopter transportation does not affect overall survival compared to ALS ground unit transport.[51] Although helicopter transport may benefit some patients with an ISS 16 to 45, those at the extremes of the injury spectrum are not helped by air transport.

The criteria for "appropriate" transport are often loosely defined and have no uniformity across various programs. In a recent panel review of a Canadian helicopter system, only 25% of the transported patients had a condition that merited the speed and skill provided by the air-medical crew. They defined this group by the need for critical intervention, clinical instability, major respiratory problems with cyanosis, and amputations requiring reimplantation.[52] When helicopter programs audit the appropriateness of urban transports, the numbers of inappropriate flights declines.[53] Refining the criteria for initiating scene response is important. Several groups have tried to define criteria for emergency air-medical trauma response.[54,55] One report suggests that unresponsiveness to verbal stimulus is the best marker for activating a helicopter scene response.[56] However, no consensus currently exists.

Two other subgroups of trauma helicopter scene response require attention: the rural scene response and the patient suffering traumatic arrest. A criterion-based review of trauma transports in a rural setting show that anywhere from 14% to 27% of patients derive some benefit from helicopter transport. However, only 18% were scene responses, nor were conclusions based on outcome data.[57] Other studies demonstrate a benefit in rural settings where significant time delays exist for ground personnel.[41,58]

In more certain terms, the literature supports no role in helicopter transport of the trauma victim in cardiac arrest.[59-62] Patients with a traumatic arrest in the field or at an outlying hospital are not revived by a helicopter flight. The expense and danger of helicopter activation is unjustified for trauma cardiopulmonary resuscitation.

In summary, helicopter service at the scene of trauma may help if it provides a substantial increase in the level of care available at the scene, or if it will significantly decrease time to arrival at a trauma center. Clearly there is no benefit in the setting of traumatic arrest. In a rural setting, characterized by long scene response times and limited training of responders, helicopters may be useful. The majority of studies note that within an urban area, air transport is of limited value.

One advantage of helicopters is the advanced training of the medical staff. However, in the modern urban EMS system, it may be more cost effective to train existing ground paramedics in advanced interventions,[63] than to routinely "call for the chopper."

MYTH 3: PREHOSPITAL USE OF LIGHTS AND SIRENS IS BENEFICIAL IN TRAUMA

Some people revel at the site of the local ambulance speeding by with lights and sirens ablaze. For the uninitiated, this scenario represents the standard of care for any emergency. Although many EMS systems have condemned the use of lights and sirens in most emergency calls,[64,65] the literature is sparse. Concerning trauma, the data barely exists. However, several studies suggest a very limited role for their use.

A convenience sample of 50 transports in the small city of Greenville, NC, demonstrated a 40.5 *second* mean time savings using lights and sirens in transporting patients from the scene to the emergency department.[66] Other studies show that lights and sirens are inappropriately used in nearly 40% of patient transports.[67] The most recent prospective trial demonstrated a timesaving of only 3 minutes using lights and sirens in a heavily populated urban environment.[68] Previous abstracts have demonstrated a timesaving of anywhere from 1 second[69] to 3 minutes.[70] In most cases, lights and sirens save 3 minutes or less. Does this difference matter for the trauma patient?

Most authorities recommend a "scoop and run"[44] philosophy of trauma transport. The question is, "How fast to run?" No controlled study has answered this question.

We are left with a public expectation for the "need for speed." However, high-velocity ambulances careening through cities endanger many lives.[71-75] A less than 3-minute difference in time of arrival probably matters to only a select few.

MYTH 4: SEPTAL HEMATOMA

Reviews of nasal trauma routinely state that septal hematoma requires emergent drainage to prevent cosmetic deformity. Authors state that septal damage arises from separation of the mucoperichondrium from the cartilage, disrupting capillary flow, and causing pressure-mediated, septal cartilage necrosis.[76-79] There are even isolated case reports that claim that septal hematoma is potentially life threatening and requires immediate action.[80] For this reason, emergency physicians (EPs) search earnestly in all patients with facial trauma for the dreaded septal hematoma. However, the literature surrounding this issue is scarce, based on case reports filled with selection bias. Furthermore, the number of patients studied is surprisingly low.

Most septal hematomas are identified more than 5 days after acute injury[81,82] and are often bilateral. The majority occur after minor trauma such as a fall, punch, or sports injury and are not always associated with nasal bone fracture.[82-85] Nasal obstruction is the most common presentation, but swelling, headache, nasal pain, and rhinorrhea also occur.

How common is septal hematoma? The few studies that address this issue note a very low incidence: 13 out of 162,109 admissions in an 8-year period at The Hospital for Sick Children,[86] 3 abscesses in 10 years at the Children's Hospital of Los Angeles,[87] 46 septal hematoma referrals to an ENT clinic in Nigeria over a 5-year period,[83] and in a 10-year review from the Massachusetts Eye and Ear Infirmary only 16 patients presented with septal abscess and no sterile hematomas were seen.[85] Judging from these reports, the average EP may never see this entity during their career.

What are the consequences of missed septal hematoma? Most complications appear to involve nasal abscess. In a retrospective evaluation over an 18-year period, physicians at the Royal Children's Hospital in Melbourne found only 20 cases of patients admitted for hematoma and abscess of the nasal septum.[82] Eight of these cases (40%) were identified as isolated hematoma at surgery. Of those eight, only two had any identifiable cartilaginous destruction and one was secondarily infected with *Staphylococcus aureus*. Chukuezi[83] presented 46 consecutive patients who presented more than 1 week after the injury was identified and only 4 had nasal deformity. Clearly cartilaginous destruction is not instantaneous. Although cartilaginous deterioration may result in cosmetic complications, septal abscess is a more likely sequelae of a septal hematoma.

Septal abscess may be serious. In one study,[83] eight patients had staphylococcal abscesses on presentation and four later developed brain abscess—three of whom died. A septal abscess may progress to meningitis[87] or cavernous sinus thrombosis after delay of 3 weeks or more.

How should an EP manage a septal hematoma? Some texts suggest incision and drainage. However, early authorities realized that the incidence of abscess after hematoma formation was low and advocated that in simple cases "firm nasal packing and external dressing for a few days may be the only treatment necessary."[88] Others feel that the management of septal hematoma is to prevent abscess formation usually through a drainage procedure.[88,89] Whether or not the nose is drained, most recommend some form of packing ranging from simple gauze[83] to internal packing with external splinting.[90] Technologic advance allows the use of a Miracil sponge for nasal packing. There is no clear evidence that one form of packing is superior, and there are no controlled studies to demonstrate the efficacy of packing.

Bottom Line

If a patient after acute minor trauma complains of difficulty breathing through the nose or pain in the nose, it is not unreasonable to examine the septum. However, septal hematoma is exceedingly rare. The number that progress to abscess is even lower. The literature is silent in regards to the number of patients with unrecognized hematomas who go on to good outcome.

Hematomas may present in delayed fashion, in which case ruling out infection becomes a primary goal. Needle aspiration and culture is a reasonable approach.[85] Cosmetic complications are linked to infected hematoma, not pressure necrosis, and all serious complications appear to be associated with septal abscess formation. It seems that drainage may only be necessary for patients with a definable septal abscess.

Although large-scale studies regarding initial treatment of septal hematoma would be valuable, this endeavor would take decades as a result of the scarcity of the condition. Numerous options appear acceptable for this "once in a career" diagnosis. Alternatives include drainage and/or nasal packing in the emergency department, or simple referral for follow-up.

MYTH 5: THE RECTAL EXAMINATION IS VALUABLE IN TRAUMA ASSESSMENT

How many trauma victims have shuddered at the phrase "there will be a little pressure in your bottom"? Performance of a rectal examination is a dictum handed down by generations of EPs and surgeons and the phrase "a finger or tube in every orifice" is routinely taught in ATLS. There is little evidence behind this universal dictum. The purported need for the rectal examination includes detection of the following:

- Decreased rectal tone
- Absent bulbocavernosus reflex
- Blood per rectum
- A high-riding prostate

Although decreased rectal tone may be important in the evaluation of the head-injured or spinal-injured patient, in others the indication is less clear. Does the initial assessment warrant this rigid alphabetic approach; A, B, C . . . R? What does decreased rectal tone mean in the obtunded? Has the interrater reliability among assessors ever been evaluated? How many times has the finding of decreased rectal tone been the sole neurologic finding?

These questions remain unanswered. In the patient with paraplegia, there is little value in acutely determining rectal tone. In the rare circumstance that sacral fracture yields a sensory loss to the posteromedial thigh and buttocks, then assessment of the S2-4 motor function may be valuable.

The physician will assess the bulbocavernosus reflex after Foley catheter insertion (implying that one rectal examination has already been completed). Someone alludes to the bulbocavernosus reflex and the trauma intern dutifully inserts a finger in the anus and tugs on the catheter. In the late summer months, this examination is followed by a puzzled look and a repeat examination by a more experienced EP. Having confirmed its absence, the medical students on service are then summoned. While they are digitizing, the students might ponder the following:

- The presence of a normal bulbocavernosus reflex does not rule out a significant lesion[91]
- Sixteen percent of patients with documented conus medullaris and cauda equina injury have a normal bulbocavernosus reflex[92]
- The bulbocavernosus reflex may be delayed or absent in those with baseline impotence, particularly diabetics[93]
- The sensitivity for residual bladder dysfunction in patients with spinal injury is only 39%[94]

Has the absence of a bulbocavernosus reflex ever been documented as the isolated finding in a patient with a spinal cord injury? An investigation reveals the answer to be no.

Rectal Bleeding

Despite being a "mandatory" aspect of the examination,[95] there is no study that evaluates the significance of rectal bleeding in the trauma patient. Even reviews of penetrating abdominal trauma[96] and trauma assessment and resuscitation[97] make no mention of this finding. Patients with a diagnosis of gastrointestinal hemorrhage based on rectal examination alone include those with insertional injuries.[98] However, this population typically does not present as trauma. Trauma-related rectal bleeding includes those with hemobilia, but the bleeding rarely occurs in the first week after blunt abdominal trauma.[99] In the era of ultrasound, spiral computed tomography scanning, and interventional angiography, one must question whether rectal examination should determine the need to further study the pelvis or abdomen.

The rectal examination is also used to search for a high-riding prostate. Few may recognize this finding; fewer check for prostatic mobility. A recent experience involved an elderly gentleman after a minor motor vehicle collision. After a period of moaning, he was asked if he had ever had a rectal examination performed before. His response was "yes, but my doctor doesn't do all that rolling around in there." His prostate was not high riding.

Evaluation of the literature reveals no reports of a traumatic urethral disruption without coexisting external soft tissue or bony injury. Isolated prostatic injury probably does not exist. Indeed, rectal examination findings are not pertinent in most cases of urogenital trauma. Penetrating urogenital injuries are associated with injury to other organs,[100,101] and clearly require operative exploration.[102] Anterior urethral injuries are not identified during rectal examination and typically present with signs of external trauma.[103-105] Posterior urethral injuries cause the high-riding or mobile prostate.

Using the posterior urethral injury classification system based on urethrography (Fig. 50-1), classifications I to III may result in an upwardly mobile prostate.[106] The type I urethral stretch injury is secondary to rupture of the puboprostatic ligaments, presumably from pelvic hematoma. In this injury, the intact urethra is treated with catheterization. The supposed rationale for a rectal examination is that blood may not be evident at the urethral meatus in these injuries. Without assessment of the prostate, passage of a catheter may theoretically result in further injury to types II and III or result in a missed type I injury. However, one may miss the injury in young men with small prostates or inadvertently palpate the hematoma itself. Prostatic mobility is all but impossible to ascertain.[107] If the physician suspects posterior urethral injury regardless or rectal findings, imaging is mandatory.

The most telling argument against routine evaluation for urethral disruption lies in a simple fact. All traumatic urethral injuries are associated with pelvic fractures. Barring a pelvic fracture, the search for the high-riding prostate is for naught. The literature supports the following indications for rectal examination in the trauma patient:

- Pelvic fracture without blood at the male urethral meatus
- High suspicion for sacral nerve injury with posteromedial thigh and buttock sensory loss.
- Re-presentation 3 to 4 weeks after blunt trauma with the suspicion for hemobilia.

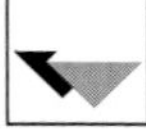

PEARLS & PITFALLS

- Most needle decompressions of the chest are either not indicated or ineffective.
- Helicopter transport is usually not indicated in an advanced urban EMS system.

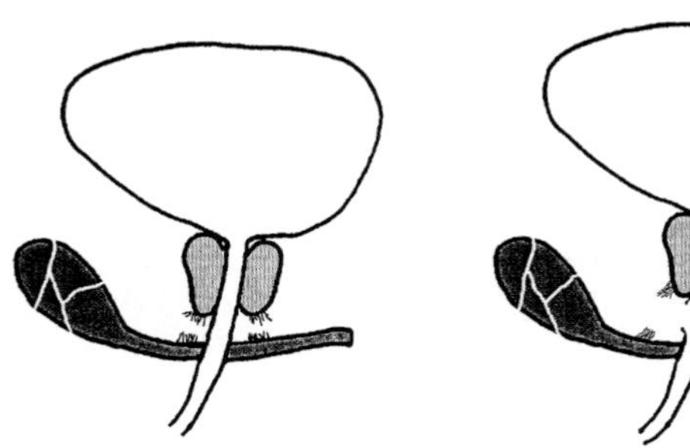

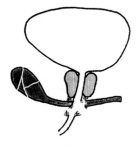

Type 1 Injury pattern

Type 2 Injury pattern

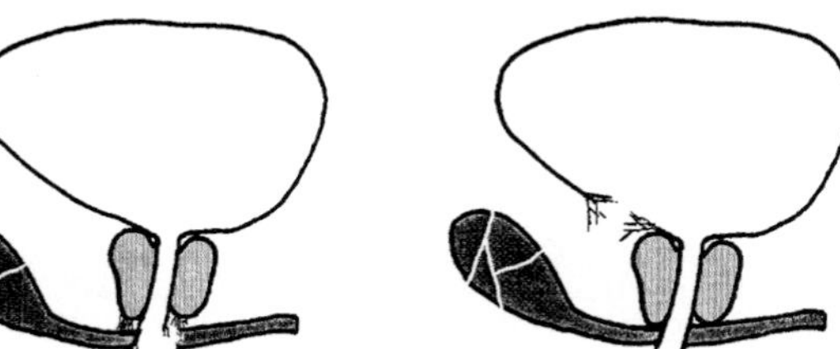

Type 3 Injury pattern

Type 4 Injury pattern

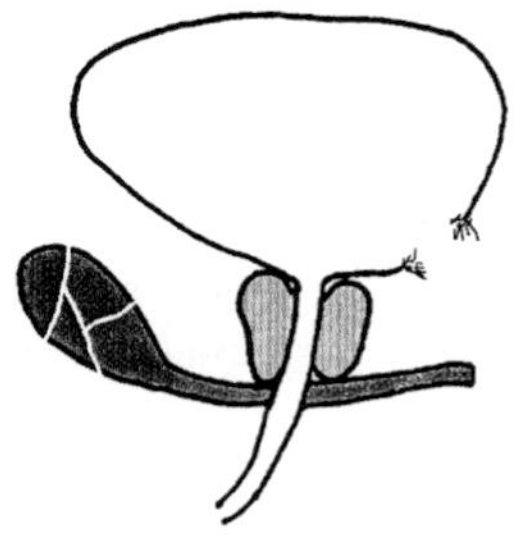

Type 4 A Injury pattern

Fig. 50-1 Classification of blunt urethral trauma. (Adapted from Goldman SM, et al: *J Urol* 157:85-89, 1997 and Colapinto V, McCallum RW: *J Urol* 118:575-580, 1977.)

- Patients in traumatic arrest should not be transported by helicopter.
- Lights and sirens are probably not indicated in most trauma patients.
- Septal hematomas are extremely rare. There is little evidence that they produce pressure necrosis.
- The rectal examination rarely changes patient management. It provides useful information in a small, defined subset of patients.

REFERENCES

1. Kaye W: Invasive therapeutic techniques: emergency cardiac pacing, pericardiocentesis, intracardiac injections, and emergency treatment of tension pneumothorax, *Heart Lung* 12:300-319, 1983.
2. Brown LH, et al: Assessment of breath sounds during ambulance transport, *Ann Emerg Med* 29:228-231, 1997.
3. Hunt RC, et al: Inability to assess breath sounds during air medical transport by helicopter, *JAMA* 265:1982-1984, 1991.
4. Chen SC, et al: Hemopneumothorax missed by auscultation in penetrating chest injury, *J Trauma* 42:86-89, 1997.
5. Graham JM, Mattox KL, Beall AC Jr: Penetrating trauma of the lung, *J Trauma* 19:665-669, 1979.
6. Carney M, Ravin CE: Intercostal artery laceration during thoracentesis: increased risk in elderly patients, *Chest* 75:520-522, 1979.
7. Hansbrough JF, Chandler JE: Lung laceration following catheter insertion in the chest for pneumothorax, *Emerg Med Serv* 8:48, 1979.
8. Britten S, Palmer SH, Snow TM: Needle thoracentesis in tension pneumothorax: insufficient cannula length and potential failure, *Injury* 27:321-322, 1996.
9. Eckstein M, Suyehara D: Needle thoracostomy in the prehospital setting, *Prehosp Emerg Care* 2:132-135, 1998.
10. Coats TJ, Wilson AW, Xeropotamous N: Pre-hospital management of patients with severe thoracic injury, *Injury* 26:581-585, 1995.
11. Barton ED, et al: Prehospital needle aspiration and tube thoracostomy in trauma victims: a six-year experience with aeromedical crews, *J Emerg Med* 13:155-163, 1995.
12. Mines D, Abbuhl S: Needle thoracostomy fails to detect a fatal tension pneumothorax, *Ann Emerg Med* 22:863-866, 1993.
13. Mattox KL, Allen MA: Systematic approach to pneumothorax, hemothorax, pneumomediastinum and subcutaneous emphysema, *Injury* 17:309-312, 1986.
14. Wung JT, et al., A spring-loaded needle for emergency evacuation of pneumothorax, *Crit Care Med* 6:378-379, 1978.
15. Wayne MA, McSwain NE Jr: Clinical evaluation of a new device for the treatment of tension pneumothorax, *Ann Surg* 191:760-762, 1980.
16. Sampalis JS, et al: Impact of on-site care, prehospital time, and level of in-hospital care on survival of severely injured patients, *J Trauma* 34:252-261, 1993.
17. Clevenger FW, Yarbrough DR, Reines HD: Resuscitative thoracostomy: the effect of field time on outcome, *J Trauma* 28:441-445, 1988.
18. Baldt, MM, et al: Complications after tube thoracostomy: assessment with CT, *Radiology* 195:539-543, 1995.
19. McSwain NE Jr: Chest tube decompression of blunt chest injuries by physicians in the field: effectiveness and complications (editorial comment), *J Trauma* 44:101, 1998.
20. Schmidt U, et al: Chest tube decompression of blunt chest injuries by physicians in the field: effectiveness and complications, *J Trauma* 44:98-101, 1998.
21. York D, et al: A comparison study of tube thoracostomy: aeromedical crews vs in hospital trauma service, *J Air Med Transport* October:69, 1991.
22. Mattox KL: Prehospital care of the patient with an injured chest, *Surg Clin North Am* 69:21-29, 1989.
23. Lechleuthner A, et al: Prehospital chest tubes: incidence and analysis of iatrogenic injuries in the emergency medical service Cologne, *Theor Surg* 9:220, 1994.
24. Millikan JS, et al: Complications of tube thoracostomy for acute trauma, *Am J Surg* 140:738-741, 1980.

25. Moessinger AC, Driscoll JM, Wigger HJ: High incidence of lung perforation by chest tube in neonatal pneumothorax, *J Pediatr* 92:635-637, 1978.
26. Childress ME, Moy G, Mottram M: Unilateral pulmonary edema resulting from treatment of spontaneous pneumothorax, *Am Rev Respir Dis* 104:119-121, 1971.
27. Daly RC, et al: The risk of percutaneous chest tube thoracostomy for blunt thoracic trauma, *Ann Emerg Med* 14:865-870, 1985.
28. Deakin CD, Davies G, Wilson A: Simple thoracostomy avoids chest drain insertion in prehospital trauma, *J Trauma* 39:373-374, 1995.
29. Beall AC Jr, et al: Considerations in the management of penetrating thoracic trauma, *J Trauma* 8:408-417, 1968.
30. Cleveland H, et al: A civilian air emergency service: a report of its development: technical aspects and experience, *J Trauma* 16:452-463, 1976.
31. Mackenzie CF, et al: Two-year mortality in 760 patients transported by helicopter direct from the road accident scene, *Am Surg* 45:101-108, 1979.
32. Duke JH Jr, Clarke WP: A university-staffed, private hospital-based air transport service. The initial two-year experience, *Arch Surg* 116:703-708, 1981.
33. Schwab CW, et al: The impact of an air ambulance system on an established trauma center, *J Trauma* 25:580-586, 1985.
34. Baxt WG, Moody P: The impact of a rotorcraft aeromedical emergency care service on trauma mortality, *JAMA* 249:3047-3051, 1983.
35. Teasdale G, Jennett B: Assessment of coma and impaired consciousness: a practical scale, *Lancet* 2:81-84, 1974.
36. Baker SP, et al: The injury severity score: a method for describing patients with multiple injuries and evaluating emergency care, *J Trauma* 14:187-196, 1974.
37. Champion HR, et al: An anatomic index of injury severity, *J Trauma* 20:197-202, 1980.
38. Champion HR, et al: Trauma score, *Crit Care Med* 9:672-676, 1981.
39. Baxt WG, Moody P: Hospital-based rotorcraft aeromedical emergency care services and trauma mortality: a multicenter study, *Ann Emerg Med* 14:859-864, 1985.
40. Champion HR, Frey CF, Sacco WJ: Determination of national normative outcomes of trauma *J Trauma* 24(abstract):651, 1984.
41. Fischer RP, et al: Urban helicopter response to the scene of injury, *J Trauma* 24:946-951, 1984.
42. Schiller WR, et al: Effect of helicopter transport of trauma victims on survival in an urban trauma center, *J Trauma* 28:1127-1134, 1988.
43. Feero S, et al: Does out-of-hospital EMS time affect trauma survival? *Am J Emerg Med* 13:133-135, 1995.
44. Gervin AS, Fischer RP: The importance of prompt transport in salvage of patients with penetrating heart wounds, *J Trauma* 22:443-448, 1982.
45. Baxt WG, Moody P: The impact of advanced prehospital emergency care on the mortality of severely brain-injured patients, *J Trauma* 27:365-369, 1987.
46. Cocanour CS, Fischer RP, Ursic CM: Are scene flights for penetrating trauma justified? *J Trauma* 43:83-86, 1997.
47. Rhee KJ, et al: Is the flight physician needed in helicopter emergency medical services? *J Trauma* 24(abstract):680, 1984.
48. Schmidt U, Fraet al., On-scene helicopter transport of patients with multiple injuries: comparison of a German and an American system, *J Trauma* 33:548-553, 1992.
49. Nicholl JP, Brazier JE, Snooks HA: Effects of London helicopter emergency medical service on survival after trauma, *Br Med J* 311:217-222, 1995.
50. Cunningham P, et al: A comparison of the association of helicopter and ground ambulance transport with the outcome of injury in trauma patients transported from the scene, *J Trauma* 43:940-946, 1997.
51. Brathwaite CE, et al: A critical analysis of on-scene helicopter transport on survival in a statewide trauma system, *J Trauma* 45:140-144, 1998.
52. Powell DG, et al: The impact of a helicopter emergency medical services program on potential morbidity and mortality, *Air Med J* 16:48, 1997.
53. Norton R, et al: Appropriate helicopter transport of urban trauma patients, *J Trauma 41:886-891, 1996.*
54. Burney RE, Fischer RP: Ground versus air transport of trauma victims: medical and logistical considerations, *Ann Emerg Med* 15:1491-1495, 1986.
55. National Association of EMS Physicians, Position paper: Air medical dispatch: guidelines for scene response, *Air Med J* 13: 315, 1994.
56. Rhodes M, et al: Field triage for on-scene helicopter transport, *J Trauma* 26:963-969, 1986.
57. Urdaneta LF, et al: Role of an emergency helicopter transport service in rural trauma, *Arch Surg* 122:992-996, 1987.
58. Anderson TE, Rose WD, Leicht MJ: Physician-staffed helicopter scene response from a rural trauma center, *Ann Emerg Med* 16:58-61, 1987.
59. Wright SW, et al: Aeromedical transport of patients with post-traumatic cardiac arrest, *Ann Emerg Med* 18:721-726, 1989.
60. Heller MB: Aeromedicine and trauma arrest: a question of perspective (editorial), *Ann Emerg Med* 18:791-792, 1989.
61. Law DK, et al: Trauma operating room in conjunction with an air ambulance system: Indications, interventions, and outcomes, *J Trauma* 22:759-765, 1982.
62. Shimazu S, Shatney CH: Outcomes of trauma patients with no vital signs on hospital admission, *J Trauma* 23:213-216, 1983.
63. Jacobs LM, et al: Prehospital advanced life support: benefits in trauma, *J Trauma 24:8-13, 1984.*
64. Elling R: Dispelling myths on ambulance accidents, *JEMS* July:60, 1989.
65. Quinlavin J: Case in point, *Emergency* March:30, 1993.
66. Hunt RC, et al: Is ambulance transport time with lights and siren faster than that without? *Ann Emerg Med* 25:507-511, 1995.
67. Lacher ME, Bausher JC: Lights and siren in pediatric 911 ambulance transports: are they being misused? *Ann Emerg Med* 29:223-227, 1997.
68. Ho J, Casey B: Time saved with use of emergency warning lights and sirens during response to requests for emergency medical aid in an urban environment, *Ann Emerg Med* 32:585-588, 1998.
69. Grillo A, et al: Does the routine use of lights and sirens shorten transport times from the scene to the hospital? *Acad Emerg Med* 1(abstract):A56, 1994.
70. Dhindsa HS, et al: Impact of the use of lights and sirens by ambulances on elapsed travel times in an urban emergency medical services setting *Acad Emerg Med* 3(abstract):454, 1996.
71. Biggers W, Zachariah B, Pepe P: Emergency medical services collisions in an urban system, *Prehosp Disast Med* 9(suppl 3): S54, 1994.
72. Auerbach PS, et al: An analysis of ambulance accidents in Tennessee, *JAMA* 258:1487-1490, 1987.
73. US Department of Transportation, National Highway Safety Administration: Ambulance involvement in fatal crashes by person type of fatalities and crash type, In Fatal Accident Reporting System 1996: A review of information on fatal traffic

crashes in the United States, Washington DC, National Traffic Safety Administration, 1997.
74. Burrailo RG, Swor RA: Characteristics of fatal ambulance crashes during emergency and non-emergency operation, *Prehosp Disast Med* 9:125, 1994.
75. Saunders CE, Heye CJ: Ambulance collisions in an urban environment, *Prehosp Disast Med* 9:118, 1994.
76. Surkov VK: The veins of the nasal septum with regard to the formation of hematomas and abscesses, *Vestn Otorhinolaringol* 25:14, 1963.
77. Colton JJ, Beehkuis GJ: Management of nasal fractures, *Otolaryngol Clin North Am* 19:73-85, 1986.
78. East CA, O'Donaghue G: Acute nasal trauma in children, *J Pediatr Surg* 22:308-310, 1987.
79. 79. Fry HJ: The pathology and treatment of haematoma of the nasal septum, *Br J Plast Surg* 22:331-335, 1969.
80. Ginsburg CM, Leach JL: Infected nasal septal hematoma, *Pediatr Infect Dis J* 14:1012-1013, 1995.
81. Feinberg AN, et al: Picture of the month: bilateral nasal septal hematomas, *Arch Pediatr Adolesc Med* 152:601-602, 1998.
82. Canty PA, Berkowitz RG: Hematoma and abscess of the nasal septum in children, *Arch Otolaryngol Head Neck Surg* 122:1373-1376, 1996.
83. Chukuezi AB: Nasal septal hematoma in Nigeria, *J Laryngol Otol* 106:396-398, 1992.
84. Grymer LF, Gutierrez C, Stoksted P: Nasal fractures in children: influence on the development of the nose, *J Laryngol Otol* 99:735-739, 1985.
85. Ambrus PS, et al: Management of nasal septal abscess, *Laryngoscope* 91:575-582, 1981.
86. Fearon B, McKendry JB, Parker J: Abscess of the nasal septum in children: a case history of meningitis secondary to a septal abscess, *Arch Otolaryngol* 74:408, 1961.
87. Eavey RD, Malekzakeh M, Wright HT Jr: Bacterial meningitis secondary to abscess of the nasal septum, *Pediatrics* 60:102-104, 1977.
88. Salinger S, Traumatic diseases of the nasal septum, *Ann Otol Rhinol Otolaryngol* 53:274, 1944.
89. Facer GW: Management of nasal injury, *Postgrad Med* 57:123-126, 1975.
90. Olsen KD, Carpenter RJ III, Kern EB: Nasal septal injury in children: diagnosis and management, *Arch Otolaryngol* 106: 317-320, 1980.
91. Blaivas JG, Zayed AA, Labib KB: The bulbocavernosus reflex in urology: a prospective study of 299 patients, *J Urol* 126:197-199, 1981.
92. Pavlakis AJ, et al: Neurourologic findings in conus medullaris and cauda equina injury, *Arch Neurol* 40:570-573, 1983.
93. Sarica Y, Karacan I: Bulbocavernosus reflex to somatic and visceral nerve stimulation in normal subjects and in diabetics with erectile impotence, *J Urol* 138:55-58, 1987.
94. Watanabe T, et al: High incidence of occult neurogenic bladder dysfunction in neurologically intact patients with thoracolumbar spinal injuries, *J Urol* 159:965-968, 1998.
95. Colucciello SA: Blunt abdominal trauma, *Emerg Med Clin North Am* 11:107-123, 1993.
96. Marx JA: Penetrating abdominal trauma, *Emerg Med Clin North Am* 11:125-135, 1993.
97. Levison M, Trunkey DD: Initial assessment and resuscitation, *Surg Clin North Am* 62:9-16, 1982.
98. Wanebo HJ, Hunt TK, Mathewson C Jr: Rectal injuries, *J Trauma* 9:712-722, 1969.
99. Sedgwick CE, Coburn RJ: Evaluation of the patient with hemobilia, Surg Clin North Am 50:683-690, 1970.
100. Tucak A, et al: Urogenital wounds during the war in Croatia in 1991/1992, *J Urol* 153:121-122, 1995.
101. Diggs CA: Suicidal transurethral perforation of bladder, *Am J Foren Med Pathol* 7:169-171, 1986.
102. Herwig KR, Blumberg N, Hubbard H: Injuries of the penile and bulbous urethra, *Mil Med* 135:289-292, 1970.
103. Palaniswamy R, et al: Urethro-cavernous fistula from blunt penile trauma, *J Trauma* 21:242-243, 1981.
104. Pode D, Shapiro A: Traumatic avulsion of the female urethra: case report, *J Trauma* 30:235-237, 1990.
105. Witherington R, McKinney JE: An unusual case of anterior urethral injury, *J Urol* 130:564-565, 1983.
106. Goldman SM, et al: Blunt urethral trauma: a unified, anatomical mechanical classification, *J Urol* 157:85-89, 1997.
107. Colapinto V, McCallum RW: Injury to the male posterior urethra in fractured pelvis: a new classification, *J Urol* 118:575-580, 1977.

PART SIX

PROCEDURES

51 Procedures in the Trauma Patient

SUSAN M. DUNMIRE

Teaching Case

A 20-year-old man is ejected from his car at high speed. He has massive midface trauma and his prehospital blood pressure is persistently less than 80 mmHg. On arrival to the emergency department (ED), he is obtunded and still hypotensive. He is unable to be intubated orally because of distortion of his airway anatomy. His neck is rapidly prepared with iodine solution, lidocaine is injected into the skin overlying the cricothyroid membrane, and a cricothyrotomy is successfully performed. Breath sounds are clear on the left, but diminished on the right, and there is right-sided chest subcutaneous air. After preparation of the fifth intercostal space in the midaxillary line with iodine solution and lidocaine, a 32 French tube thoracostomy is performed immediately, with a rush of air and 200 cc of blood. The chest tube is placed to water suction and secured to the chest wall. A chest radiograph confirms proper placement of the chest tube. His blood pressure remains at 85/40 mmHg. A urinary catheter and orogastric tube are placed in preparation for a diagnostic peritoneal lavage (DPL), since the ultrasound machine is currently out of service. A pelvic radiograph done before the DPL shows bilateral pubic rami fractures. After preparing the abdomen with iodine and lidocaine, an open DPL is performed supraumbilically to avoid entering a pelvic hematoma. After aspirating 10 cc of gross blood, the procedure is halted and the patient is rushed to the operating suite, where his fragmented spleen is removed and a tracheostomy performed. ■

AIRWAY MANAGEMENT

Obtaining and maintaining an adequate and reliable airway is an essential step in trauma resuscitation. Indications for active airway management include airway protection in the obtunded patient, airway protection in patients with significant facial or neck trauma, profound shock, and provision of adequate ventilation. **Rapid sequence induction (RSI)** followed by endotracheal intubation is the procedure of choice for definitive airway management in the trauma patient. This procedure can be challenging as a result of facial trauma, blood and secretions in the airway, or distortion of the anatomy. Should endotracheal intubation be unsuccessful, alternative methods of establishing a definitive airway include **cricothyrotomy** or **needle cricothyrotomy with transtracheal jet ventilation**.

Cricothyrotomy

Cricothyrotomy is a valuable airway procedure in trauma patients when endotracheal intubation is unsuccessful or impossible (Box 51-1).[1-3] Although cricothyrotomy is considered to be an easier procedure than tracheostomy, it has the potential for significant complications, including bleeding and great vessel injury. The instruments needed for cricothyrotomy are few and should be available at all times.

PROCEDURE (Fig. 51-1)

In patients with potentially unstable cervical spines, the anterior aspect of the cervical collar should be removed from the patient and in-line stabilization provided at all times during the procedure. The right-handed operator should stand at the right side of the patient. Using the nondominant hand, stabilize the trachea between the thumb and third fingers and identify the cricothyroid membrane with the index finger. The cricothyroid membrane is bordered by the thyroid cartilage superiorly and the cricoid cartilage inferiorly. If the patient remains conscious and if time permits, 1% lidocaine should be injected subcutaneously for local anesthesia. The neck should be prepared with povidone-iodine solution. Using a scalpel,

BOX 51-1
Cricothyrotomy

EQUIPMENT REQUIRED

Scalpel blade
Curved hemostat or Trousseau dilator
Tracheal hook
#4 Shiley tube or a 6.0 endotracheal tube

INDICATIONS

Inability to perform orotracheal intubation
Partial or complete airway obstruction
Maxillofacial injuries making oral or nasal endotracheal intubation difficult or hazardous

CONTRAINDICATIONS

There are no absolute contraindications other than complete transection of the trachea with loss of the distal end
Cricothyrotomy in children less than 8 years of age is extremely difficult, leads to multiple serious sequelae such as tracheal stenosis, and should be avoided when possible
Coagulopathies, distorted external anatomy, and profound obesity may all be relative contraindications

COMPLICATIONS

Bleeding
Incorrect tube placement
Injury to the great vessels
Injury to the recurrent laryngeal nerve with vocal cord paralysis
Laryngeal stenosis

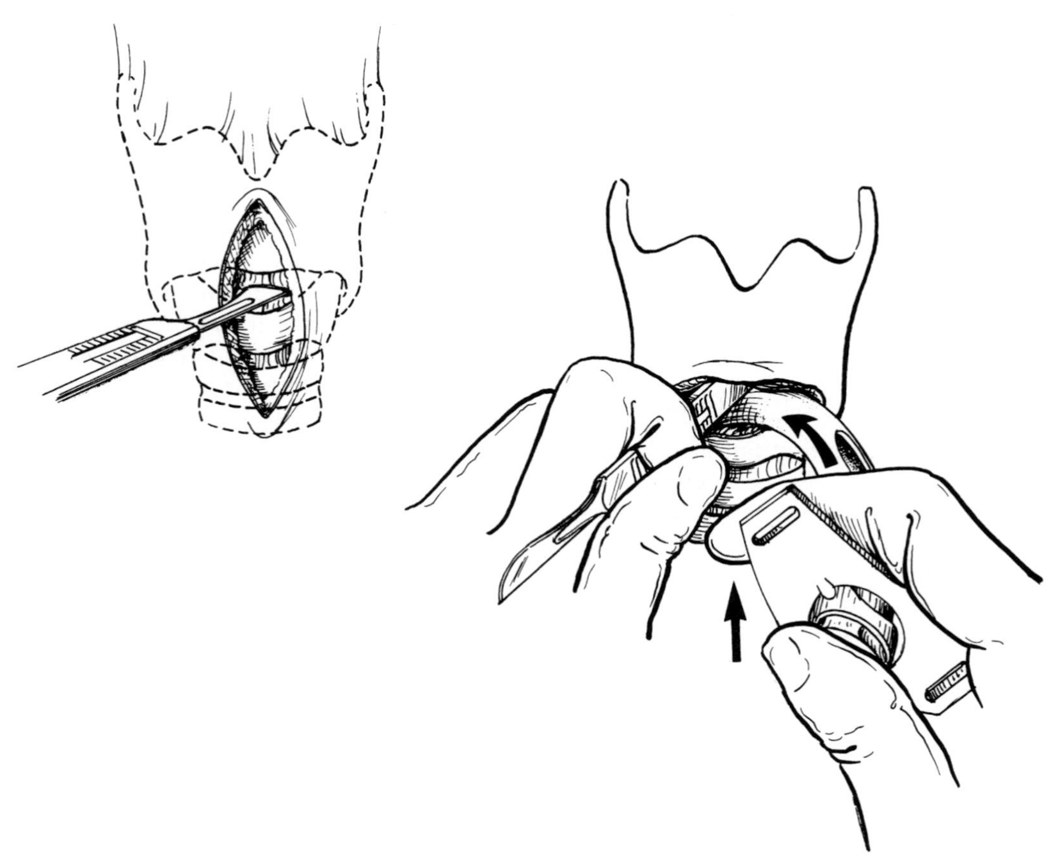

Fig. 51-1 Cricothyrotomy. (From Dunmire SM, Paris PM: *Atlas of emergency procedures,* Philadelphia, 1994, Saunders.)

make a 3 to 4 cm skin incision over the cricothyroid membrane. There is a great deal of controversy regarding the choice of a vertical or horizontal incision. The advantage to a vertical incision is better exposure of the anatomy. The disadvantage is that should the isthmus of the thyroid be incised, there is increased bleeding from the wound. Immediately after the skin has been incised, insert your index finger into the incision to once again locate the cricothyroid membrane. Stabilizing the trachea, make a 2 cm horizontal stab incision with the scalpel through the cricothyroid membrane and into the trachea. Insert either the handle of the scalpel or a Trousseau dilator into the incision. Some authors recommend placing a tracheal hook into the incision immediately after making the stab wound and before removing the scalpel blade. The hook grasps the thyroid cartilage above the cricothyroid membrane and can be given to an assistant, who will maintain traction. If the handle of the scalpel is used, rotate it 90 degrees to spread the incision. While spreading the incision, insert either a #4 or #5 Shiley tracheostomy tube or a 6.0 endotracheal tube into the opening and secure it after inflating the balloon. Auscultate for breath sounds to confirm placement of the tube and secure the tube to the neck with either tape or ties.

One important consideration regarding cricothyrotomy is the possible loss of visualization of the membrane, which may be obscured by blood or tissue. Once the membrane is identified, always keep *something* in the membrane (e.g., finger, tracheal hook, or dilator). A new, more rapid technique involving fewer steps and using the tracheal hook to grasp the cricoid cartilage has recently been described, but clinical data on its effectiveness are lacking.[4]

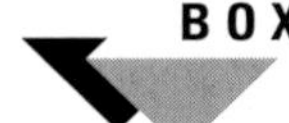

BOX 51-2
Needle Cricothyrotomy With Transtracheal Jet Ventilation

EQUIPMENT
10- or 12-gauge needle
10 cc syringe
High-pressure ventilation tubing attached to a standard wall oxygen outlet at 55 psi
Manual valve for intermittent delivery of oxygen

INDICATIONS FOR TRANSTRACHEAL JET VENTILATION
Inability to perform orotracheal intubation in cases where cricothyrotomy relatively contraindicated (e.g., children <8 years of age, altered neck anatomy, coagulopathy)
Partial or complete airway obstruction

CONTRAINDICATION FOR TRANSTRACHEAL JET VENTILATION
Lack of proper equipment (Using a standard bag-valve-mask to attempt ventilation through a 10-gauge transtracheal catheter does not allow for adequate ventilation. There must be availability of oxygen at 55 psi through high-pressure tubing.)
Total obstruction of proximal airway
Suspected tracheal or bronchial injury

COMPLICATIONS
Subcutaneous emphysema
Bleeding
Pneumothorax
Pneumomediastinum

Needle Cricothyrotomy with Transtracheal Jet Ventilation

Needle cricothyrotomy with transtracheal jet ventilation (TTJV) offers the physician an alternative to surgical cricothyrotomy when endotracheal intubation is either unsuccessful or contraindicated (Box 51-2). Although TTJV was originally thought to offer only a temporary airway, studies show that it will adequately oxygenate a patient for more than 24 hours.[5] TTJV is an excellent alternative in patients under the age of 8 years, in whom cricothyrotomy is relatively contraindicated. *It is essential that the TTJV equipment be prepared ahead of time and be available for immediate use, and that the faculty and nursing staff understand how to use it.* A patient with a difficult airway should not stimulate a frantic assembly. The TTJV equipment requires high-pressure ventilation tubing attached directly to a standard wall oxygen outlet providing 55 psi of oxygen pressure.[6] To achieve this goal, remove both the standard "Christmas tree" adaptor and oxygen flow meter that is usually present in the wall outlet. A manual valve located along this tubing controls oxygen flow. This tubing is directly connected to a 10- or 12-gauge catheter inserted into the cricothyroid membrane.

There are several needle cricothyrotomy kits available. These kits are easy to assemble, and the airway catheter includes a flange, which secures the catheter to the neck. If these kits are unavailable, a 10- or 12-gauge intravenous (IV) angiocatheter is an alternative.

PROCEDURE (Fig. 51-2)

Prepare the patient's neck by scrubbing with a povidone-iodine solution and then draping in a sterile fashion. Inject local anesthetic. Attach a 10 cc syringe to the 10- or 12-gauge catheter hub. Using the nondominant hand, stabilize the trachea between the

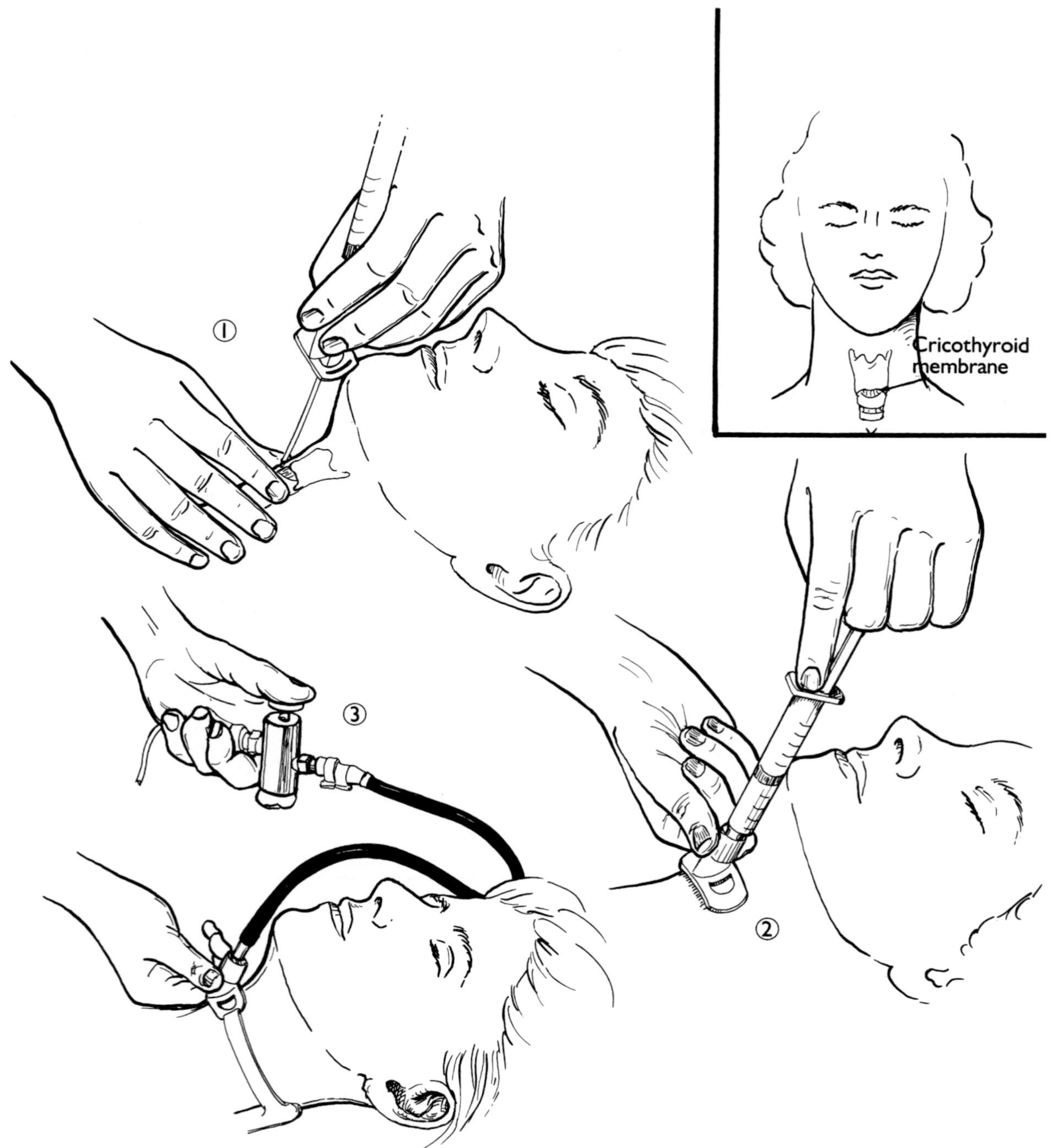

Fig. 51-2 Needle cricothyrotomy with transtracheal jet ventilation. (From Dunmire SM, Paris PM: *Atlas of emergency procedures,* Philadelphia, 1994, Saunders.)

middle finger and thumb, and identify the cricothyroid membrane with the index finger. Insert the needle into the cricothyroid membrane, directing the needle at a 60° angle caudad (toward the sternal notch). Aspirate continuously until a free flow of air fills the syringe. Then advance the plastic catheter into the trachea and remove the needle. Attach the high-pressure oxygen tubing to the hub of the catheter. Secure the catheter so that it does not pull back and allow air entry into the subcutaneous space. Intermittently inflate the lungs pressing on the delivery valve for 1 second and then releasing for 2 to 3 seconds. Check

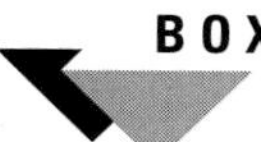

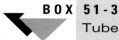

BOX 51-3
Tube Thoracostomy

EQUIPMENT REQUIRED
Scalpel blade
Large Kelly clamp
Thoracostomy tube
Size: Adult 28-40 French
Pediatric Pneumothorax 14-16 French
Hemothorax 20-24 French

INDICATIONS
Pneumothorax
Hemothorax
Hemopneumothorax
Any size pneumothorax in patients on positive pressure ventilation

CONTRAINDICATIONS
Requirement for immediate open thoracotomy (traumatic arrest)

COMPLICATIONS
Bleeding (damage to the intercostal vein or artery)
Laceration of the lung
Damage to the great vessels or heart
Intraabdominal placement of the thoracostomy tube
Malfunctioning of the thoracostomy tube
Infection

for breath sounds. An efflux of air through the mouth is not uncommon.

If there is significant subcutaneous emphysema, the catheter has become dislodged and should be removed and reinserted.

Tube Thoracostomy

Blunt and penetrating injuries to the chest can result in a simple, tension, or open pneumothorax (PTX), and hemothorax. The initial treatment of a tension PTX is either immediate **tube thoracostomy** (Box 51-3) or initial **needle decompression** followed by a tube thoracostomy. A PTX is usually graded as being small (≤15%), moderate (15% to 60%), or large (≥60%).[7] A small PTX from blunt trauma can simply be observed if the patient is awake, alert, and oriented and hemodynamically stable. Should a patient with any size PTX require ventilator support with positive pressure ventilation, a tube thoracostomy will be required.[8,9] Most penetrating injuries resulting in a PTX require tube thoracostomy.

It is often difficult to diagnose a small-to-moderate PTX in a blunt trauma patient because most initial chest radiographs are supine. It is helpful to get an upright chest radiograph as soon as the cervical spine can be radiographically and clinically cleared. Often a small PTX is identified during abdominal computed tomographic (CT) scanning when the scan includes the lower thorax.[10]

In placing a tube thoracostomy there are several precautions that will minimize complications. This procedure is extremely painful and if clinical circumstances allow, requires both local anesthesia and parenteral sedation. The physician must be careful to insert the Kelly clamp just over the top of the rib to avoid traumatic injury to the intercostal vessels. We recommend not using the trocar, which is packaged with the chest tube, during this procedure. A Kelly clamp will guide the tube into the chest wall. To ensure proper passage of the tube into the pleural cavity, a finger should be inserted into the pleural cavity first to ensure that there is a proper tract above the diaphragm. In penetrating trauma, the physician can use his or her finger to "sweep" the diaphragm and search for a tear.

PROCEDURE (Fig. 51-3)

Perform a povidone-iodine scrub of the lateral and anterior chest wall and drape in a sterile fashion. Locate the fourth or fifth intercostal space at the midaxillary line. Inject a subcutaneous weal of 1% lidocaine with or without epinephrine using a 25-gauge needle. Replace the 25-gauge needle with a 1½ inch 20- or 22-gauge needle. Inject approximately 5 to 10 cc of 1% lidocaine while advancing this needle over the rib to the pleura. Once local anesthesia is achieved, use a scalpel blade to make a 5 cm incision through the skin and subcutaneous tissue *over* the chosen rib between the anterior axillary and midaxillary line. The incision should be made parallel to the rib. Some authorities suggest starting the incision an interspace lower, and tunnel upwards to the next rib. This subcutaneous tract is thought to prevent air entry into the chest on tube removal. Once a skin incision has been made, place the Kelly clamp through your incision. Push the Kelly clamp *over* the rib until it pops into the pleural space. Once the clamp has entered the pleural space, spread the prongs of the clamp in order to widen the tract. Remove the Kelly clamp and insert a finger into the hole, ensuring that there is a viable tract into the pleural space and that there is no lung adherent to the chest wall. The lung tissue should be palpable at the top of your finger.

The tube is marked in centimeter increments from the tip. Holding the chest tube over the patient's chest before insertion allows the physician to estimate to

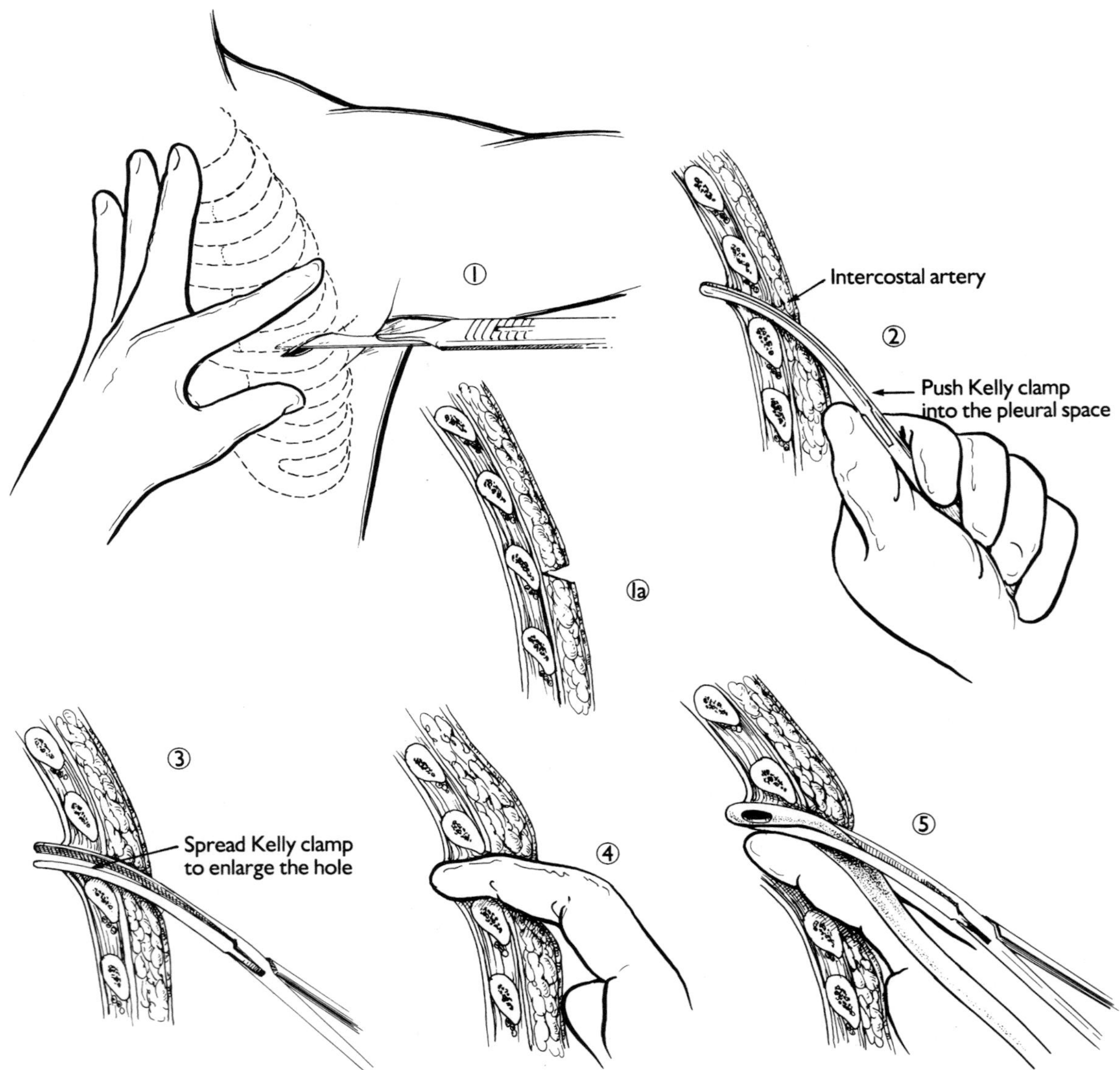

Fig. 51-3 Tube thoracostomy. (From Dunmire SM, Paris PM: *Atlas of emergency procedures,* Philadelphia, 1994, Saunders.)

which centimeter mark the tube must be inserted. All holes in the chest tube must be within the pleural space. Clamp the end of the chest tube with the Kelly clamp and, using your finger as a guide, insert the chest tube into the pleural space. Continue to insert the tube, aiming superiorly and posteriorly until very mild resistance is met. Pull back 2 to 3 cm. Attach the end of the chest tube to a Pleur-evac suction device. Close the incision with a 3-0 or 4-0 nylon suture. Place a horizontal mattress suture and tie once and wrap the suture ends around the chest tube. Place an occlusive dressing over the insertion site. Tape the lateral chest and abdominal walls first, then place the exposed portion of the chest tube over this tape. Place more tape over the chest tube to firmly secure it to the lateral thoracoabdominal wall. Some data suggests that antibiotics, such as cefazolin, decreases the incidence of subsequent empyema, if given around the time of chest tube insertion.[11,12]

Thoracotomy

A **thoracotomy** should be performed in patients in actual or impending cardiac arrest who have sustained penetrating thoracic trauma (Box 51-4). It is extremely controversial as to whether thoracotomy

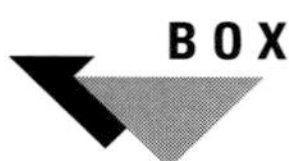

BOX 51-4
Thoracotomy

INDICATIONS
Impending (e.g., worsening hypotension) or full cardiac arrest in patients with penetrating thoracic trauma
Cardiac tamponade in the trauma patient
Witnessed cardiac arrest in the emergency department in victims of blunt trauma (controversial)

CONTRAINDICATIONS
Cardiac arrest with obvious massive head trauma
Patients with no vital signs at the scene
Patients with no ECG evidence of cardiac activity (flatline)

EQUIPMENT
Povidone-iodine solution
Scalpel
Mayo scissors
Rib spreaders
Tissue Forceps
10-inch needle holder
2-0 or larger suture on a curved needle
Suture scissors
15 French Foley catheter with a 30 cc balloon

COMPLICATIONS
Laceration of the intercostal vessels
Lung laceration
Phrenic nerve transection
Myocardial rupture
Infection
Coronary artery laceration
Air embolism
Laceration of internal mammary artery

benefits victims of blunt trauma.[13,14] Although some trauma textbooks recommend the procedure in victims of blunt trauma who arrive in the ED with a pulse and blood pressure and subsequently arrest, survival is dismal in this circumstance. Thoracotomy is also indicated in the trauma patient with cardiac tamponade.

PROCEDURE (Fig. 51-4)

Rapidly prepare the entire left chest wall with a povidone-iodine solution. With a scalpel blade, make a single incision through skin and subcutaneous tissue at the level of the fifth intercostal space extending from the left sternal border to the posterior axillary line. (Note: If the patient sustained a penetrating injury on right side, open the right side of the chest first.) The incision should follow the course above the fifth rib. Using the blade, then make a 5 to 10 cm incision through intercostal muscle above the rib to the pleural space. The Mayo scissors can then extend this incision from the posterior axillary line to the left sternal border. Cutting through the sternum may increase exposure of the heart. Heavy shears will rapidly open the sternum in a horizontal direction. Insert a rib spreader and spread the ribs; if this maneuver is impossible, use the Mayo scissors and extend the incision posteriorly. Once the ribs have been spread, use the nondominant hand to move the lung medially so that the heart can be visualized.

Inspect the heart for any sign of blood within the pericardial sac. Grasp the pericardium with forceps and, using the Mayo scissors, incise the pericardial sac in a vertical direction anterior to the phrenic nerve. The phrenic nerve runs in a vertical course along the left lateral aspect of the pericardial sac and has the appearance of a white fibrous line. Once the pericardial incision extends the entire length of the heart, "deliver" the heart through the pericardial sac.

Inspect the heart thoroughly for penetrating wounds. There are several techniques described for controlling hemorrhage from a penetrating cardiac wound. The most effective is to place the thumb over the hole while the remainder of that hand performs cardiac compression. If the patient must be transported to the operating suite before repair of the cardiac wound, a Foley catheter can be inserted through the hole and 10 to 20 cc of saline should be used to inflate the balloon of the catheter. Very gentle traction applied to the catheter will slow the bleeding.

Ideally, the cardiac wound should be sutured before transporting the patient to the operating suite. However, if the operating suite and surgeon are ready, the EP can run beside the stretcher, keeping his or her finger in the wound. Since sutures may tear the heart muscle, some authors recommend using cotton pledgets; the needle is driven through the pledget then through the myocardium and out through another pledget. A dog study showed that a skin stapler is faster and as effective as sutures plus pledgets.[15]

CARDIAC MASSAGE

If **cardiac massage** is necessary, use the two-handed technique with one hand over the posterior aspect of the heart and one on the anterior aspect. Compress the heart from the base to the apex at approximately 60 compressions per minute. Once patients are resuscitated by thoracotomy and their penetrating cardiac wounds controlled with either sutures, Foley catheter, or digital pressure, transport the patient to

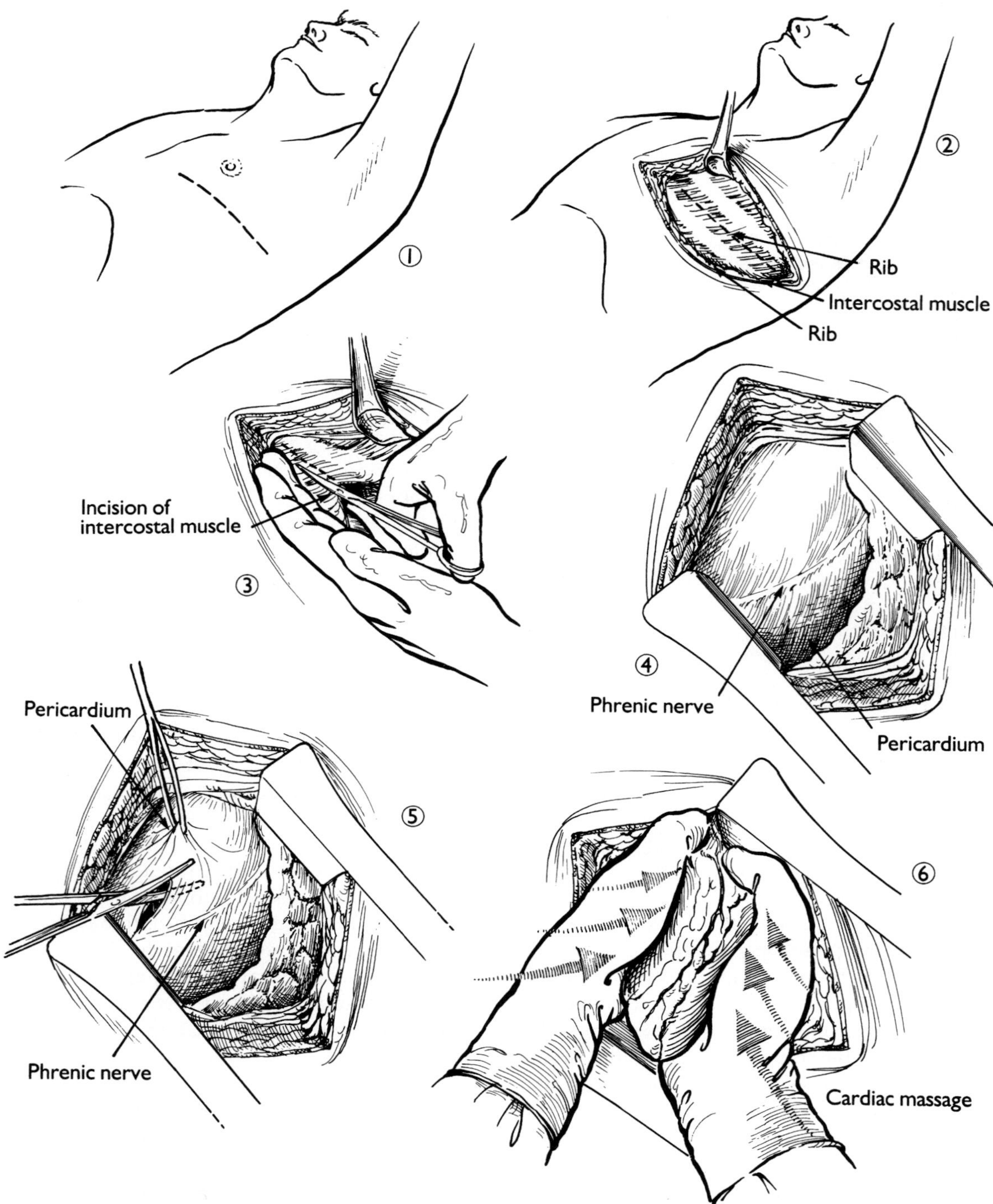

Fig. 51-4 Thoracotomy. (From Dunmire SM, Paris PM: *Atlas of emergency procedures,* Philadelphia, 1994, Saunders.)

the operating suite for definitive repair of all other intrathoracic wounds, as well as closure of the thoracotomy.

The first priority in ED thoracotomy is to release a pericardial tamponade. However, compression of the aorta remains an important secondary goal. Aortic occlusion diverts blood to the cerebral and coronary arteries. Once the chest is opened, have an assistant place his or her hand in the chest, and press on the aorta over the lumbar spine. A variety of specially designed vascular clamps will also serve this purpose.

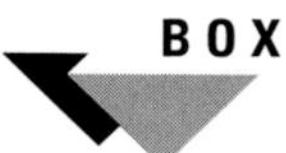

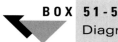

BOX 51-5
Diagnostic Peritoneal Lavage

INDICATIONS

Evaluation of blunt abdominal trauma in patients with associated
- Transient hypotension
- Altered level of consciousness
- Inability to evaluate the abdomen as a result of the following:
    - Spinal cord injury
    - Drugs and/or alcohol

A trauma patient who is hemodynamically unstable and requires emergent surgical interventions for other injuries

Penetrating stab wounds to the lower thorax (controversial)

CONTRAINDICATIONS

Absolute
- Hemodynamic instability with clear signs of significant abdominal trauma (peritoneal signs) requiring immediate operative intervention
- Evisceration

Relative
- Pregnancy (greater than 12 weeks); consider ultrasound in the stable patient
- History of prior abdominal operations; recent studies suggest this situation is not a contraindication

EQUIPMENT—OPEN DIAGNOSTIC PERITONEAL LAVAGE

1% lidocaine with epinephrine
5 cc syringe with 25-gauge needle
Scalpel blade
Curved hemostats
Self-retaining retractor
Army-Navy retractors
Peritoneal catheter
1 liter of 0.9% saline solution
Intravenous tubing
0 polypropylene suture
Skin stapler
10 cc syringe
Povidone-iodine
Sterile towels

COMPLICATIONS

Perforation of intraabdominal organs
Iatrogenic hemoperitoneum
Peritonitis

Diagnostic Peritoneal Lavage

Diagnostic peritoneal lavage (DPL) remains a valuable tool in diagnosing hemoperitoneum in patients who have undergone blunt trauma to the abdomen (Box 51-5).[16,17] Indications for DPL include the following: (1) hemodynamic instability; (2) patients who have a significant mechanism of injury but an unreliable examination as a result of altered mental status, effects of drugs or alcohol, or spinal cord injury; or (3) patients who need immediate surgical intervention for other injuries. Although CT scanning and ultrasound are alternative diagnostic modalities for hemoperitoneum, DPL can rapidly rule out hemoperitoneum. It is the most sensitive diagnostic test for intraperitoneal blood. DPL is particularly useful in patients who are hemodynamically unstable or those who need immediate operation for another injury (e.g., subdural hematoma). DPL is useful to evaluate penetrating abdominal stab wounds, but is not indicated for gunshot wounds to the abdomen (see Chapter 20). There are three techniques for performing DPL: the closed percutaneous technique, semiclosed technique, and open technique. In this chapter, we discuss both the closed percutaneous technique and the open technique. Before initiating DPL, place a urinary catheter to decompress the bladder and insert a nasogastric tube (or orogastric tube in patients with midface trauma) under suction for gastric decompression.

CLOSED PERCUTANEOUS TECHNIQUE

The closed percutaneous technique for peritoneal lavage is simple and rapid to perform. It is associated with a low complication rate. Numerous studies show it as accurate and much faster than the open technique. Previous authors suggested that it should not be used in patients who have had a history of abdominal surgery or intraabdominal adhesions. However, a recent review showed that "the complication rate and accuracy of closed DPL in patients with previous abdominal surgery were similar to those for DPL performed in patients without previous abdominal surgery."[18]

The Seldinger ("wire through a needle") approach

is the basis for the closed technique. There are many DPL catheter kits available, which simplify equipment assembly. Place the patient in a supine position. The abdominal wall is prepared with a povidone-iodine solution and draped in a sterile fashion. Inject 1% lidocaine with epinephrine in the subcutaneous tissue inferior to the umbilicus, then insert an 18-gauge needle directly through the skin or through a stab incision, aiming at a 45° angle toward the pelvis. Two "pops" are felt as the needle penetrates the linea alba and then the peritoneum. After the second pop, pass a J-tipped guide wire through the needle and into the peritoneal cavity, again directing the wire at a 45° angle toward the pelvis. After the wire is in place, remove the 18-gauge needle and guide the peritoneal catheter over the wire into the peritoneal cavity. A stab incision at the base of the wire will ease passage of the catheter. Remove the guide wire and attach a 10 cc syringe to the catheter. Aspirate into the 10 cc syringe; if 10 cc of free blood or intestinal contents return from the peritoneal catheter, the procedure is complete and the patient should be transported quickly to the operating suite. If there is no return of gross blood, infuse 1 liter of normal saline solution through IV tubing into the peritoneal cavity in adults (15 cc/kg in children). After 1 liter of normal saline solution is instilled, drop the bag to the floor, which will drain the peritoneal cavity by gravity. Some authors suggest temporarily placing the patient in Trendelenburg or gently rocking them to allow the lavage fluid to reach all of the peritoneal spaces. A minimum of 300 cc of lavage fluid must return to give a representative sample. Once the lavage fluid has been collected, the catheter is removed, any skin incision stapled, and the fluid sent to the laboratory.

OPEN TECHNIQUE (Fig. 51-5)

The open technique may be better for patients who are obese, have pelvic fractures, are pregnant, or who have had prior abdominal operations and the possibility of adhesed bowel. The abdomen is prepared with povidone-iodine and draped in a sterile fashion. Sterile techniques should be used throughout this procedure. A 5 cm vertical midline incision is made just inferior to the umbilicus. (*Note:* In patients with intrauterine pregnancies, or suspected pelvic fractures, a supraumbilical incision is preferred.) The incision is carried down through subcutaneous tissue to the linea alba. Use Army-Navy retractors for good visualization of each layer as it is incised. Once the linea alba is visualized, grasp it on two sides by hemostats, lift and incise. Just beneath the linea alba, identify the peritoneum. Lift the peritoneum by two hemostats in a tent-like fashion and make a 1 cm incision in the peritoneum. Then insert a peritoneal catheter into the peritoneal cavity under direct visualization and advance it inferiorly toward the pelvis. Never force the catheter, since this action may perforate the bowel. Once the catheter has been positioned, attach a 10 cc syringe to the catheter and aspirate for gross blood. If there is a return of 10 cc of gross blood or if intestinal contents are obtained, the procedure is terminated and the patient is taken immediately to the operating suite. If there is no return of gross blood, 1 liter of normal saline solution (15 cc/kg in children) should be infused through the peritoneal catheter and drained by gravity. The fascia should be closed with interrupted or running 0-polypropylene sutures. The skin incision can then be closed with skin staples or running 3-0 nylon suture.

INTERPRETATION OF RESULTS OF DIAGNOSTIC PERITONEAL LAVAGE

Positive results of DPL include the following:

1. Immediate return of 10 cc of gross blood or intestinal contents with initial aspiration
2. RBC count >100,000 cells per ml in blunt trauma
3. RBC count >10,000 cells per ml in abdominal stab wounds
4. RBC count >5,000 cells per ml in penetrating chest trauma
5. WBC count >500 cells per ml
6. If lavage fluid exits urinary, nasogastric, or tube thoracostomy tubes

Pericardiocentesis

Pericardiocentesis is a useful tool in the diagnosis and treatment of nontraumatic cardiac tamponade in the unstable patient (Box 51-6). It is not as useful in the setting of traumatic cardiac tamponade. With traumatic hemopericardium, there is a high incidence of clotted blood present in the pericardium, resulting in a false-negative pericardiocentesis. A thoracotomy with pericardiectomy or a pericardial window is a far superior diagnostic and therapeutic procedure. On occasion emergency pericardiocentesis temporarily stabilizes a patient until the arrival of a surgeon.

PROCEDURE (Fig. 51-6)

Place all patients undergoing pericardiocentesis on a cardiac monitor, oxygen, and pulse oximetry. Cardiac resuscitation equipment should be readily available. Prepare the skin over the xiphoid process with a povidone-iodine (Betadine) solution, and sterilely drape the area. In the awake patient, inject 1% lidocaine solution subcutaneously at the site of insertion prior to initiation of the procedure. Attach a 50 cc

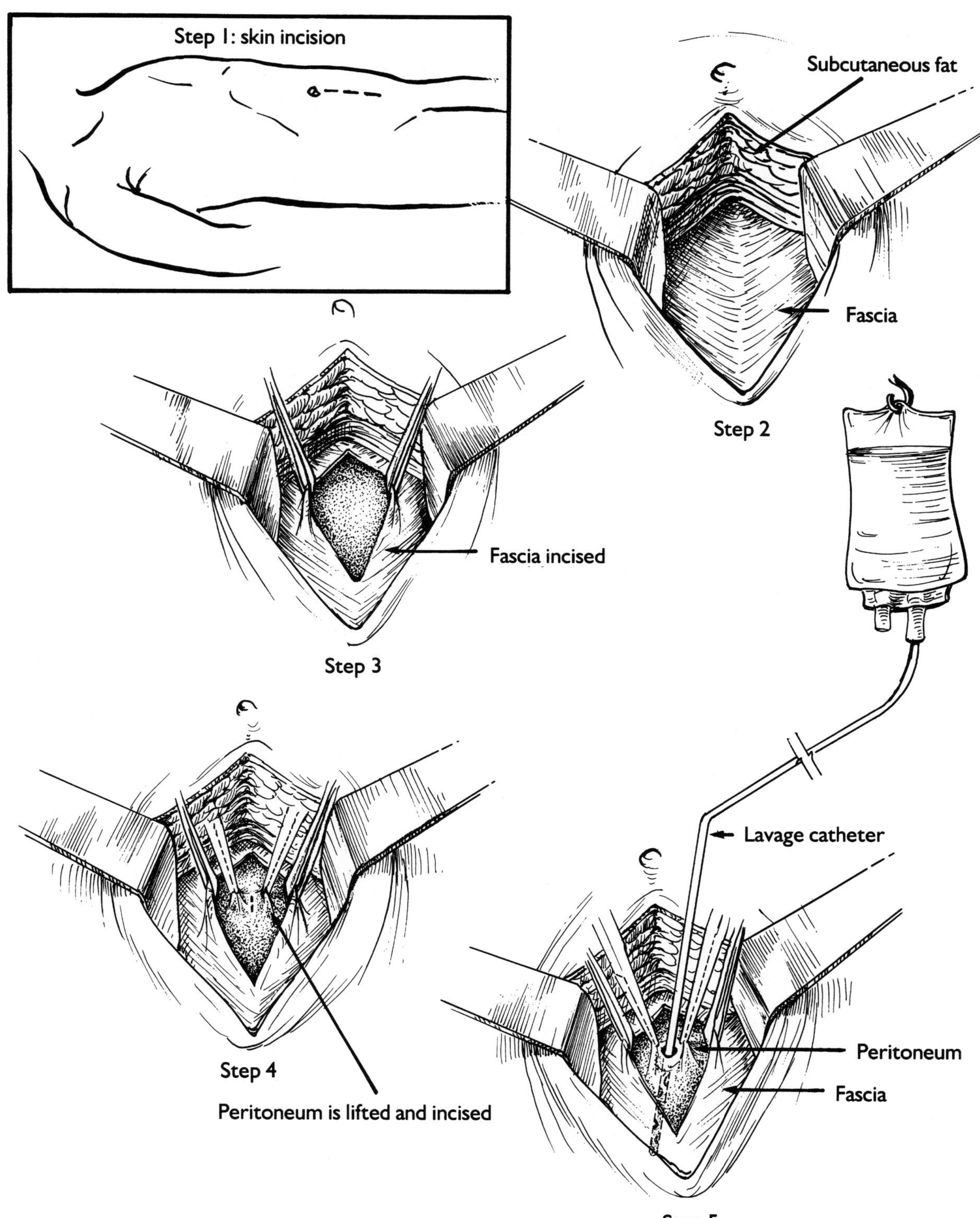

Fig. 51-5 Diagnostic peritoneal lavage (open technique). (From Dunmire SM, Paris PM: *Atlas of emergency procedures,* Philadelphia, 1994, Saunders.)

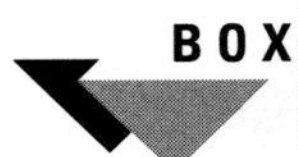

BOX 51-6 Pericardiocentesis

INDICATION

Diagnosis of pericardial tamponade in a hemodynamically unstable patient (in the stable patient, make the diagnosis of hemopericardium by echocardiography)

EQUIPMENT

Local anesthetic (1% lidocaine)
25-gauge needle and a 10 cc syringe for anesthetic injection
Povidone-iodine solution
Sterile towels and clips
50 cc syringe
Two 3/4-inch 18-gauge spinal needle
Immediate availability of resuscitation cart with a defibrillator

COMPLICATIONS

Pneumothorax
Pneumopericardium
Dysrhythmia
Laceration of myocardium
Laceration of coronary artery
Laceration of thoracic great vessels

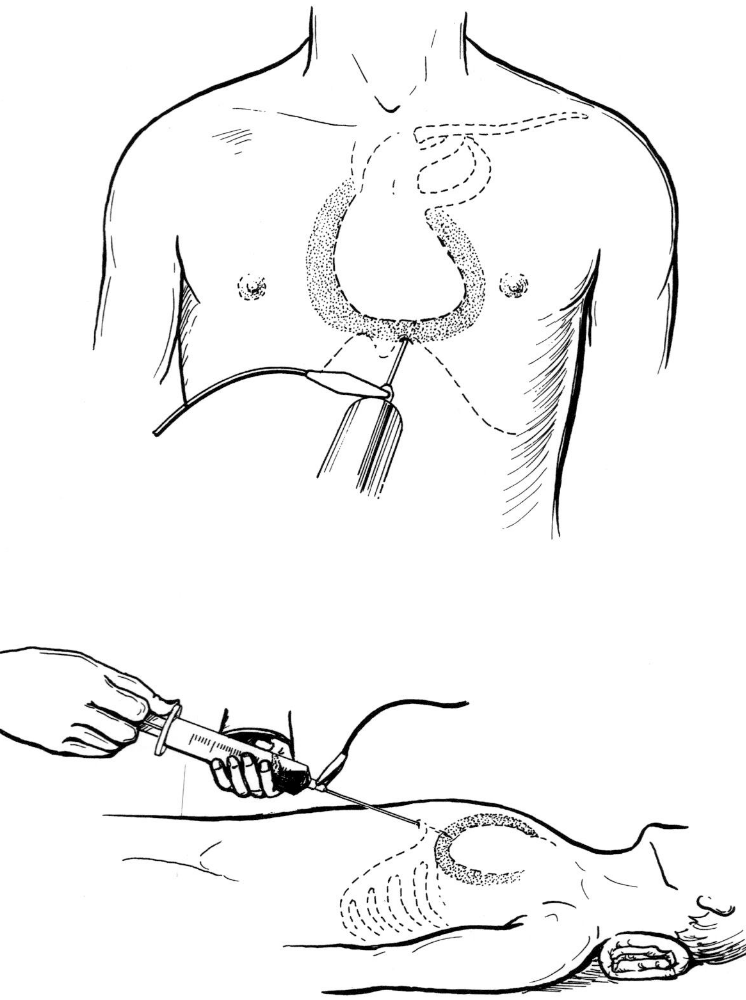

Fig. 51-6 Pericardiocentesis. (From Dunmire SM, Paris PM: *Atlas of emergency procedures,* Philadelphia, 1994, Saunders.)

syringe to an 18-gauge spinal needle. Insert the needle just below the xiphoid process at a 30° angle to the skin, aiming at the left midclavicular line. Aspirate as the needle is advanced until fluid or blood is obtained. Aspirate up to 50 cc of fluid and then withdraw the syringe and needle. If hemorrhagic fluid is obtained, it can be difficult to determine whether this fluid was obtained from the pericardial sac or the heart chamber itself. Clotting or nonclotting of the blood obtained is a nonspecific finding and is not helpful in delineating the source of the fluid. If the blood is suspected to come from the pericardium, a catheter can be left in place for repeat aspirations. All trauma patients in whom the diagnosis of hemorrhagic pericardial tamponade is entertained should undergo a pericardial window or thoracotomy.

Venous Access

SAPHENOUS VEIN CUT-DOWN

All clinicians who treat trauma patients should be familiar with the procedure of the **saphenous vein cut-down** (Box 51-7). It is an extremely valuable technique for vascular access when attempts at central venous or peripheral cannulation have failed, and particularly useful in children.

Procedure (Fig. 51-7). Cleanse the entire ankle area with Betadine solution and drape with sterile towels. The saphenous vein is located two fingers' breadth superior and anterior to the medial malleolus. The vein is usually palpable. Anesthetize the area with 1% lidocaine. Using a scalpel, make a 2.5 cm transverse incision through the dermal layer over the area of the vein. This incision should be made perpendicular to the vein (i.e., horizontally across the leg). Use a curved hemostat to bluntly dissect in the direction of the vein and isolate the saphenous. Once the vein is isolated, pass the curved hemostat under the vein and grasp the end of one of the silk ties, pulling it beneath the vein. Repeat this maneuver with the second silk tie. Position the two silk ties such that they are separated by approximately 2 cm along the vein. Tie off the distal suture, to prevent bleeding during venotomy. Select the appropriate catheter size, depending on the diameter of the vein. In the adult, a cordis kit using the Seldinger technique allows passage of an 8 French catheter.[19]

Maintain steady gentle traction on the two silk ties while a 0.5 cm incision is made through the vein wall parallel to the vein. Approach the vein from the side with the tip of a scalpel blade with the sharp edge up. By stabbing the middle of the vein in this manner, a compete transection is unlikely. Insert the end of the catheter into the incision and advance it proximally while relaxing the silk tie on the proximal end of the vessel. Aspirate to confirm that the catheter is within the lumen. Knot the proximal suture line over the cannula. The wound can then be closed with either sutures or skin staples.

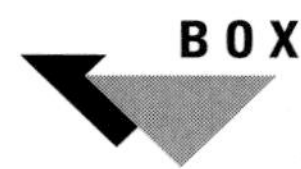

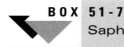

BOX 51-7
Saphenous Vein Cut Down

INDICATIONS
Inability to obtain peripheral or central venous access in adults
Inability to obtain peripheral or central intravenous access in infants or small children who are hemodynamically unstable

CONTRAINDICATIONS
Blunt or penetrating trauma to the ipsilateral leg or pelvis
Potential vascular injury on the ipsilateral leg or pelvis
Cellulitis over the site of insertion

EQUIPMENT
Scalpel blade with handle
Two curved hemostats
Straight hemostat
Self-retaining retractor
1% lidocaine
5 cc syringe with 25-gauge needle for injection of lidocaine
Sterile towels
Povidone-iodine solution
Two 3.0 silk ties
Needle holder
Intravenous tubing
Sterile dressing

COMPLICATIONS
Transection of the saphenous vein
Venous thrombosis
Infection
Air embolism

INTRAOSSEOUS ACCESS

The **intraosseous (IO)** space is an easily accessible site (Box 51-8). The EP should imagine a horizontal line between the tibial tuberosity and the medial edge of the tibia. The site of insertion should be halfway along this line and 2 cm distal to the line. The lateral distal femur is another acceptable site, although the needle

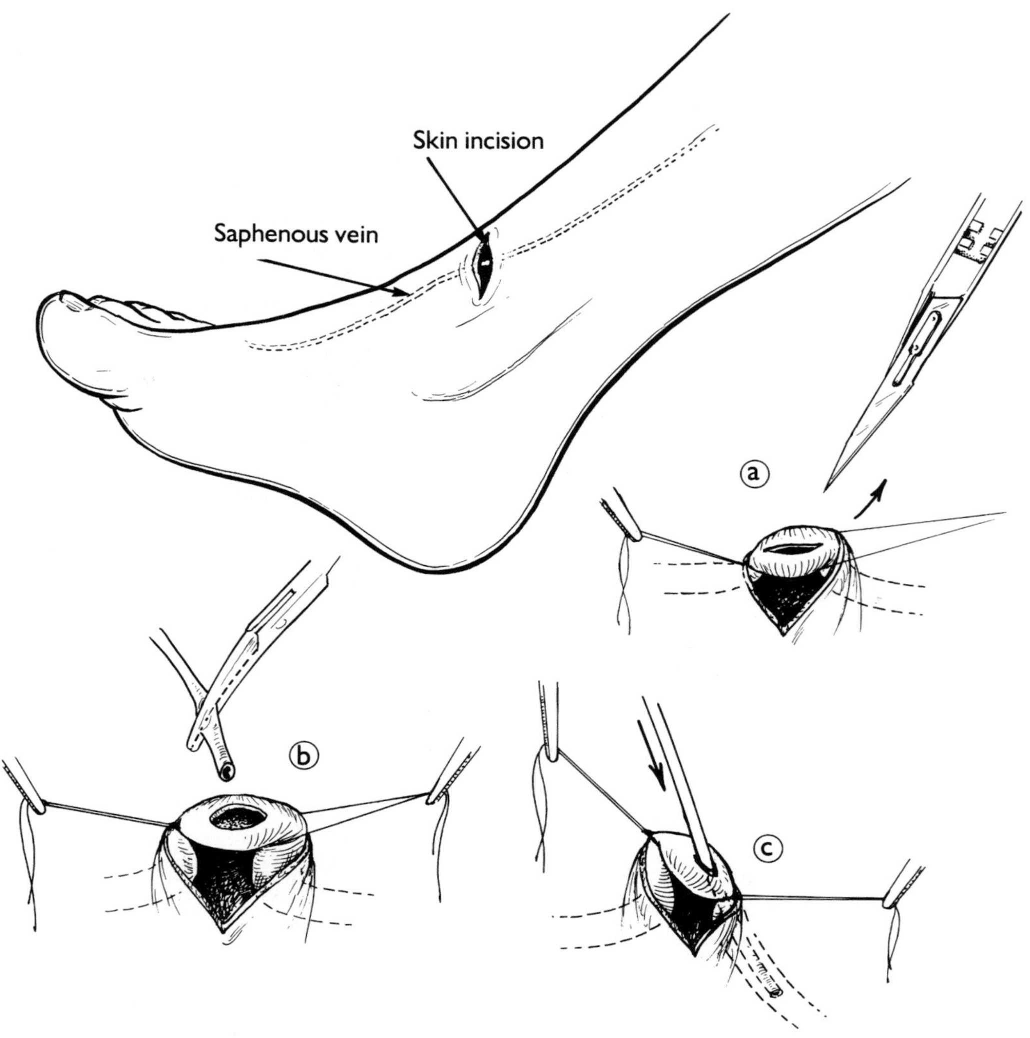

Fig. 51-7 Saphenous vein cutdown. (From Dunmire SM, Paris PM: *Atlas of emergency procedures,* Philadelphia, 1994, Saunders.)

is more likely to slip off the bone during insertion because of the greater curvature.

Procedure (Fig. 51-8). Cleanse the area with povidone-iodine solution. Using a rotary motion, insert the intraosseous needle at approximately a 60° angle to the skin, aiming away from the knee joint and growth plate. Do not place your hand under the leg near the insertion site; it is easy to drive the needle entirely through the child's leg and into your hand. Once a decrease in resistance is felt, remove the stylet and slowly aspirate with a 5 cc syringe. If there is a free flow of blood and marrow content, infuse 3 to 5 cc of sterile saline solution, palpating over the tibial plateau for extravasation. If no extravasation occurs, attach IV tubing to the intraosseous needle and infuse blood or crystalloid under pressure into the marrow cavity. If a line infiltrates, use the opposite tibia or the ipsilateral femur to start a new line.

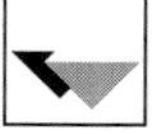

PEARLS & PITFALLS

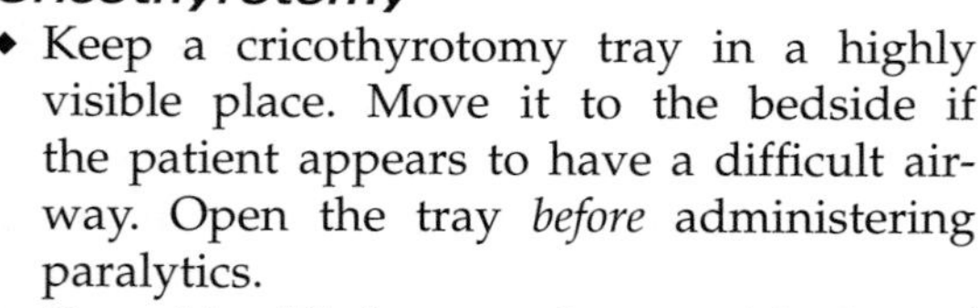

Cricothyrotomy

- Keep a cricothyrotomy tray in a highly visible place. Move it to the bedside if the patient appears to have a difficult airway. Open the tray *before* administering paralytics.
- Once identified, never lose positioning of the cricothyroid membrane.

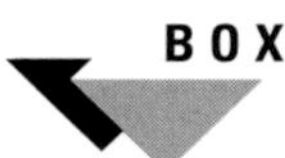

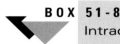

BOX 51-8
Intraosseous Access

INDICATIONS
Intraosseous infusion is indicated in the hemodynamically unstable infant or young child, 6 years of age or younger, in whom peripheral or central venous access is unsuccessful. Crystalloid fluid and blood are readily absorbed from the marrow space.

CONTRAINDICATIONS
Fracture to the bone of entry
Infection at the puncture site
History of severe bone disorders (osteogenesis imperfecta, leukodystrophies, rickets)

EQUIPMENT
14- to 20-gauge intraosseous infusion needle with an attached 5 cc syringe
Intravenous tubing
Resuscitative crystalloid or packed red blood cell solution
Pressure bag for infusion
Povidone-iodine solution

COMPLICATIONS
Extravasation of the fluid (resulting from either incomplete penetration of the bone or leakage from the marrow space)
Clot formation within the intraosseous needle
Infection
Fracture
Growth plate injuries

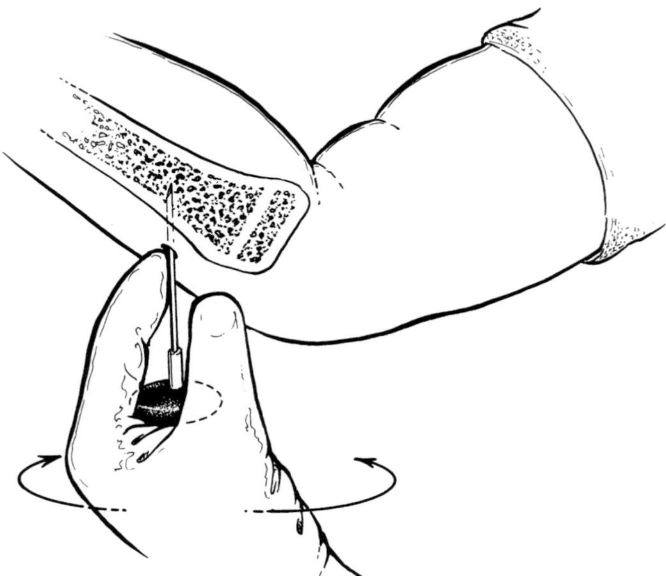

Fig. 51-8 Intraosseous access. (From Dunmire SM, Paris PM: *Atlas of emergency procedures,* Philadelphia, 1994, Saunders.)

- The procedure is based on touch (digital identification of the membrane) *not* on sight. Surgical lamps and retractors are unnecessary for the emergency physician.

Needle Cricothyrotomy with Transtracheal Jet Ventilation

- Prepare the TTJV equipment ahead of time and make it available for immediate use.
- Allow sufficient time for expiration during TTJV. The small size of the catheter allows breaths to "stack," increasing the risk of barotrauma.
- Become familiar with the set-up, since TTJV is rarely needed and physicians are unlikely to be comfortable during emergency situations.

Tube Thoracostomy

- Use a large tube in patients with hemothorax (36 to 40 French in adults); smaller tubes may clot off.
- Set up an autotransfuser device for patients with significant hemothorax, before connecting the drainage system to the tube.
- Before inserting the chest tube, place a finger in the thoracostomy site to avoid placement into adherent lung tissue or into organs such as the liver or spleen.
- Place the chest tube in the third or fourth interspace in pregnant women in the second half of pregnancy. Their diaphragms rise during pregnancy and a lower tube may enter the abdomen.
- Make sure the tube is in the pleural cavity and not obstructed. All side ports must be inside the chest cavity. Water in the water seal chamber of the drainage system should rise and fall slightly with the respiratory cycle, and a cough will usually cause bubbling. A kink or obstruction in the system or an extrapleural location of the tube will prevent the respiratory variation in the water seal compartment.
- A trocar can spear important structures in the chest or abdomen. Do not use it.[20-22]

- Search for persistent air leaks. Continuous bubbling of the chest tube apparatus off suction may indicate an air leak within the lung or within the drainage system.

Thoracotomy

- Quickly call for help. If a patient is to survive an ED thoracotomy, a surgeon will need to take the patient to the operating suite.
- Make a large incision. To "deliver" the heart, open the chest from the sternum to the left posterior axillary line; opening the sternum provides greater access.
- Relieve tamponade. Release of a pericardial tamponade is the goal of ED thoracotomy. If a tense hemopericardium is present, it may be difficult to pick up the pericardium with toothed forceps–make a small incision first and then pick up the pericardium.
- Despite the need for speed, be deliberate. Thoracotomy is associated with lacerations to the physician and assistants. In some cities, nearly one quarter of patients with penetrating trauma are HIV positive.

Diagnostic Peritoneal Lavage

- Before initiating DPL, place a urinary catheter to decompress the bladder. A nasogastric tube should also be inserted and placed on continuous suction for gastric decompression.
- If transferring a patient to a trauma center, consider leaving the DPL catheter in place to allow resampling of the abdomen.
- If a CT is performed after a DPL, inform the radiologists of the DPL. Otherwise they will interpret remaining lavage fluid as blood and free air as intestinal perforation.
- A positive RBC criteria for DPL does not mandate an operation in a hemodynamically stable patient, especially in children. DPL is indicated in children only if they remain hemodynamically unstable despite resuscitation.

Pericardiocentesis

- Pericardiocentesis in trauma is only a temporizing measure.
- ED echocardiography may quickly demonstrate a pericardial tamponade.

Saphenous Vein Cut-Down

- A simple laceration tray supplies nearly all of the equipment necessary for a venous cut-down.
- Avoid a deep initial skin incision that might transect the saphenous vein.
- Blunt dissection in the same direction as the vein will avoid tearing this structure.

Intraosseous Access

- The most common mistakes regarding IO lines is either failure to consider them or reluctance to use them.
- IO lines are frequently dislodged during resuscitation. Once the line is established, stabilize it using a Styrofoam cup or other device.
- Many physicians do not realize the high pressures needed to infuse adequate fluid volumes through an IO line. Use a large syringe to pump blood or fluids in by hand. A gravity drip is inadequate for volume resuscitation.
- Avoid multiple punctures in the same bone, which allow IO fluids to extravasate.

REFERENCES

1. DeLaurier GA, et al: Acute airway management: role of cricothyroidotomy, *Am Surg* 56:12-15, 1990.
2. McGill J, Clinton JE, Ruiz E: Cricothyrotomy in the emergency department, *Ann Emerg Med* 11:361-364, 1982.
3. Salvino CK, et al: Emergency cricothyroidotomy in trauma victims, *J Trauma* 34:503-505, 1993.
4. Holmes JF, et al: Comparison of 2 cricothyrotomy techniques: standard method versus rapid 4-step technique, *Ann Emerg Med* 32:442-446, 1998.
5. Yealy DM, Stewart RD, Kaplan RM: Myths and pitfalls in emergency translaryngeal ventilation: correcting misimpressions, *Ann Emerg Med* 17:690-692, 1988.
6. Carl ML, et al: Pulmonary mechanics of dogs during transtracheal jet ventilation, *Ann Emerg Med* 24:1126-1136, 1994.
7. Kirsh MM and Sloan H (editors): *Blunt chest trauma: general principles of management*, Boston, 1977, Little, Brown.
8. Collins JC, Levine G, Waxman K: Occult traumatic pneumothorax: immediate tube thoracostomy versus expectant management, *Am Surg* 58:743-746, 1992.
9. Enderson BL, et al: Tube thoracostomy for occult pneumothorax: a prospective randomized study of its use, *J Trauma* 35:726-730, 1993.
10. Bridges KG, et al: CT detection of occult pneumothorax in multiple trauma patients, *J Emerg Med* 11:179-186, 1993.
11. Gonzalez RP, Holevar MR: Role of prophylactic antibiotics for tube thoracostomy in chest trauma, *Am Surg* 64:617-620, 1998.
12. Evans JT, et al: Meta-analysis of antibiotics in tube thoracostomy, *Am Surg* 61:215-219, 1995.
13. Cogbill TH, et al: Rationale for selective application of emergency department thoracotomy in trauma, *J Trauma* 23:453-460, 1983.
14. Esposito TJ, et al: Reappraisal of emergency room thoracotomy in a changing environment, *J Trauma* 31:881-885, 1991.
15. Bowman MR, King RM: Comparison of staples and sutures for cardiorrhaphy in traumatic puncture wounds of the heart, *J Emerg Med* 14:615-618, 1996.

16. Bilge A, Sahin M: Diagnostic peritoneal lavage in blunt abdominal trauma, *Eur J Surg* 157:449-451, 1991.
17. Henneman PL, et al: Diagnostic peritoneal lavage: accuracy in predicting necessary laparotomy following blunt and penetrating trauma, *J Trauma* 30:1345-1355, 1990.
18. Moore GP, Alden AW, Rodman GH: Is closed diagnostic peritoneal lavage contraindicated in patients with previous abdominal surgery? *Acad Emerg Med* 4:287-290, 1997.
19. Klofas E: A quicker saphenous vein cutdown and a better way to teach it, *J Trauma* 43:985-987, 1997.
20. Meisel S, et al: Another complication of thoracostomy: perforation of the right atrium, *Chest* 98:772-773, 1990.
21. Fraser RS: Lung perforation complicating tube thoracostomy: pathologic description of three cases, *Human Pathol* 19:518-523, 1988.
22. Millikan JS, et al: Complications of tube thoracostomy for acute trauma, *Am J Surg* 140:738-741, 1980.

Appendix

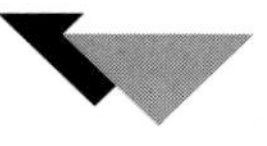

Prehospital Triage Criteria—Variables Associated with a Higher Risk of Significant Injury

PATIENT ASSESSMENT

1. Pulse <60 or >100
2. Respiratory rate <10 or >29
3. Systolic blood pressure <90
4. Glasgow Coma Scale score <13
5. Anatomic location of injuries may predict the need for emergent surgical or specialty care
   a. Penetration injuries to chest, abdomen, head, neck, or groin
   b. Flail chest
   c. Multiple proximal long bone fractures
   d. Burns with >50% body surface area, face, or airway burns
   e. Pelvic fractures
   f. Paralysis
   g. Extremity amputation

MECHANISM OF INJURY

1. Ejection from automobile
2. Death of victim in the same passenger compartment
3. Extrication time >20 minutes
4. Fall >20 feet
5. Rollover accident
6. High-speed vehicle crash
7. Auto versus pedestrian >5 mph
8. Motorcycle crash >20 mph or separation of rider from bike

PREMORBID CONDITION

1. Age <5 or >55 years
2. Cardiac or respiratory disease
3. Psychosis
4. Diabetic taking insulin
5. Cirrhosis
6. Malignancy
7. Obesity
8. Coagulopathy

OTHER ISSUES

1. Potential for decline in patient condition
2. Availability of resources
3. Personnel and level of training
4. Equipment and supplies
5. Transport vehicles (ground versus air)
6. Turnaround time for vehicles
7. Local facilities and bed availability
8. Adult and pediatric trauma centers
   Burn centers
   Other specialized care centers
9. Presence of on-going hazards or environmental dangers

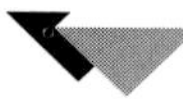

Tetanus Immunizations

NUMBER OF TETANUS TOXOID DOSES RECEIVED	CLEAN, MINOR WOUNDS		ALL OTHER WOUNDS*	
	Td†	TIG	Td†	TIG
Unknown or < three	Yes‡	No	Yes	No
≥three§	No‖	No	No¶	No

*Such as highly contaminated wounds (e.g., feces, soil, saliva); puncture wounds, avulsions; missile, crushing, burn, and frostbite wounds.
†DPT for children <7 years of age (Td if pertussis vaccine contraindicated).
‡Complete the primary immunization series (second dose at 4 weeks, third dose at 6 months).
§If only three doses of fluid toxoid have been received, a fourth dose of adsorbed toxoid should be given.
‖Yes, if >10 years since last dose.
¶Yes, if >5 years since last dose.

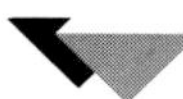

Revised Trauma Score

SCORE	GLASGOW COMA SCALE SCORE	SYSTOLIC BLOOD PRESSURE	RESPIRATORY RATE
4	13-15	>89	10-29
3	9-12	76-89	>29
2	6-8	50-75	6-9
1	4-5	1-49	1-5
0	3	0	0

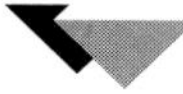

Glasgow Coma Scale Score

EYE OPENING (E)		VERBAL RESPONSE (V)		MOTOR RESPONSE (M)	
Spontaneous	4	Alert and oriented	5	Follows commands	6
To voice	3	Confused speech	4	Localizes pain	5
To pain	2	Inappropriate words	3	Withdraws to pain	4
No response	1	Unintelligible sounds	2	Decorticate flexion	3
		No response	1	Decerebrate extension	2
				No response	1

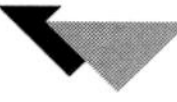

Pediatric Trauma Score

	−1	+1	+2
SIZE (kg)	<10	10-20	>20
Airway	Unmaintained	Maintained	Normal
Systolic blood pressure (mmHg)	<50	50-90	>90
Level of consciousness	Comatose	Altered	Awake
Wounds	Major open	Minor open	None
Skeletal trauma	Open/multiple	Closed	None

Index

B

D

F

M

X

Z